Introductory Nutrition and Nutrition Therapy

Introductory Nutrition and Nutrition Therapy

THIRD EDITION

Marian Maltese Eschleman, MS, RD, CDE
Nutrition Consultant
Ewing, New Jersey

Formerly Director of Nutrition
Princeton Diabetes Treatment and Education Center
Princeton, New Jersey

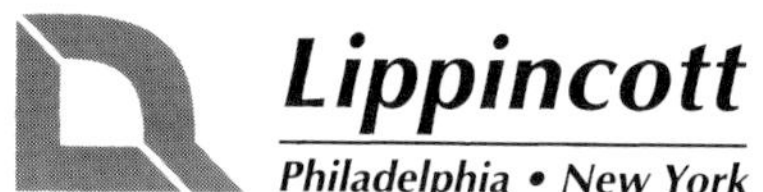

Acquisitions Editor: Donna L. Hilton, RN, BSN
Editorial Assistant: Susan M. Keneally
Project Editor: Barbara Ryalls
Indexer: Michael Ferreira
Senior Design Coordinator: Kathy Kelley-Luedtke
Designer: OX & Company, Inc.
Cover Designer: Lou Fuiano
Production Manager: Helen Ewan
Production Coordinator: Nannette Winski
Compositor: Tapsco, Incorporated
Printer/Binder: R. R. Donnelley & Sons Company/Crawfordsville

3rd Edition

1 3 5 6 4 2

Eschleman, Marian Maltese.
Introductory nutrition and nutrition therapy / Marian Maltese Eschleman.—3rd ed.
p. cm.
Rev. ed. of: Introductory nutrition and diet therapy. 2nd ed. c1991.
Includes bibliographical references and index.
ISBN 0-397-55108-8
1. Nutrition. 2. Diet therapy. I. Eschleman, Marian Maltese. Introductory nutrition and diet therapy. II. Title.
[DNLM: 1. Nutrition. 2. Diet Therapy. QU 145 E738ia 1996]
QP141.E77 1996
613.2—dc20
DNLM/DLC
for Library of Congress 95-19854
CIP

To Ned, my husband—the ghostwriter of Introductory Nutrition and Nutrition Therapy. *Without his unfailing support, devotion, and willing sacrifices, this book, all three editions, would not have been written.*

Contributors

Monica W. Luby, MS, RD
Director of the Dietetic Internship Program
Department of Foods and Nutrition
College of Saint Elizabeth
Morristown, New Jersey
Chapter 29, Nutrition Therapy Related to Surgery and Following Burns: Alternative Feeding Methods
Chapter 30, Nutrition Therapy in Cancer, AIDS, and Other Special Problems

Nena Loney, RD, CDE
Renal Nutritionist
Burlington County Dialysis Center
Lumberton, New Jersey
Nutrition Consultant, Private Practice
Lumberton, New Jersey
Chapter 27, Nutrition Therapy in Renal Disease

Reviewers

Virginia R. LaFond, RN, MSN
Nurse Educator
Helene Fuld School of Nursing
Trenton, New Jersey

Mary A. Johnson, MS, RD, CDE
Director of Nutrition
Joslin Center for Diabetes
Saint Barnabas Medical Center
Princeton Division
Princeton, New Jersey

Susan A. Jones, RD, CNSD
Nutrition Support Dietitian
The Graduate Hospital
Philadelphia, Pennsylvania

PREFACE

The third edition of *Introductory Nutrition and Nutrition Therapy* enters an age of health information explosion, an era of heightened public interest in health and nutrition. Numerous scientific reports support the view that good nutrition is key to health promotion and disease prevention. The science of nutrition is growing rapidly and with this growth comes new knowledge that challenges traditional concepts. The latest (1994) nutrition recommendations of the American Diabetes Association are one of many such developments discussed in this edition.

This book provides a foundation in the science of normal nutrition and nutrition therapy for students of nursing, dietetic technology, and other health technologies that include a nutrition component such as dental hygiene, dental assisting, physical therapy, and respiratory therapy. It is also useful in refresher courses.

Central Focus

Practical application of the science of nutrition continues to be the central focus of this book. Ways in which the student can apply the information and concepts presented are integrated into each chapter and are emphasized in "Keys to Practical Application," a feature that accompanies each chapter.

The subject matter focuses on major health concerns that are relevant to student goals. All are presented in a comprehensive yet straightforward and easily understood style.

Organization

Introductory Nutrition and Nutrition Therapy is divided into four parts. Part 1, "Introduction to Nutrition Care in Health and Illness," begins with improved nutrition as a national health priority and a discussion of current social and economic influences on American food habits. The components of nutrition care and the responsibilities of the various health care team members are delineated. In Part 1, two basic questions are answered—"Why is it important to be well nourished," and "How do we know if a person is well nourished?" Chapter 2, devoted to nutrition assessment, examines not only the physical needs for food but also its social, cultural, and psychological meanings to better prepare the student to work with clients toward enhancing nutritional status.

The phenomenal rise in recent years of the number of pathogens recognized as causing foodborne illness and the devastating effects on the health of persons with weakened immune systems has prompted increased emphasis on food safety. In this edition an entire chapter, placed prominently in the first section of this book, is devoted to this issue.

This text makes a departure from traditional sequence in that hospital food service and client feeding are covered in the first part of the book. This change was made to provide background information for the student's early clinical experience, when client feeding is frequently a first assignment. If desired, the topic can easily be discussed at a later point in the course.

The essential nutrients are considered in Part 2, "The Role of Nutrients in the Maintenance of Normal Health," which opens with an overview of nutrient functions serving to unify the concepts of cellular nutrition. Here, recognized standards such as the *Recommended Dietary Allowances* and guidelines such as the *Dietary Guidelines for Americans* and the *Food Guide Pyramid* are introduced. Recommendations of the Advisory Committee for the 1995 revision of the Dietary Guidelines for Americans are discussed. As each nutrient is described, emphasis is placed on food sources of nutrients, knowledge of which is basic to practical application. An abstract understanding of the properties and functions of nutrients is of little value unless the student can readily identify food sources and assist clients to incorporate them in the diet.

Relevant concerns of the public also come into the discussion. For example, the material on carbohydrates is followed by such topics as overconsumption of sugars, dental caries, dietary fiber, low-carbohydrate reducing diets, and diseases that require carbohydrate modification. The purpose of these brief discussions is to help the student connect the study of nutrients to dietary goals.

Part 3, "Nutrition in the Life Cycle," translates the information of the preceding two parts into practical terms. This section discusses such topics as choosing foods that meet nutritional requirements in various stages of life; fast foods; culture, lifestyle, and nutrition; vegetarianism; teenage pregnancies; eating disorders; fraudulent health claims; and food management.

Nutrition therapy is addressed in Part 4, "Nutrition Therapy in Illness." The opening chapter of this section relates the scientific method of problem solving to client-centered nutrition care. Nutrition education is stressed as an essential part of that care. Techniques that promote learning and empower the client and the student's role in nutrition education are covered. An entire chapter (22) is devoted to teaching aids in nutrition therapy, including the exchange lists. The preparation of low literacy materials is also covered in this chapter. The practical aspects of nutrition therapy, such as the purchase and the preparation of food, are discussed. Included also is the most recently available information on the nutritional aspects of weight control, diabetes, cholesterol-lowering, end-stage renal disease, gastrointestinal disease, and AIDS. The latest information on alternative feeding methods, including tube feeding is presented.

New Content

The dynamic nature of the nutrition field is evident in the many new developments included in this third edition. One of the most notable is the 1995 revision of the Exchange Lists for Meal Planning (Chapter 22). The new Exchange Lists are more user friendly than in previous editions and include vegetarian choices and commercial lowfat foods. The 1995 Exchange Lists have been designed so they can be used in carbohydrate counting, an alternative to the traditional exchange-list approach to meal planning in diabetes.

Labeling regulations that became effective in 1994 have been integrated into all sections of this book. The basic provisions of this comprehensive labeling reform are given in Chapter 5 and the use of food labeling as a teaching tool is presented in Chapter 22. Labeling regulations relative to specific nutrients are discussed in those chapters in which the nutrients are presented. Regulations relative to the prevention and treatment of chronic diseases are discussed in appropriate chapters, such as those dealing with diabetes mellitus, cardiovascular disease, and weight control.

In addition to the new exchange lists and food labeling regulations, other exciting new developments covered in this edition include:

- Report of the Dietary Guidelines Advisory Committee on the revision of the Dietary Guidelines for Americans, 1995 edition
- Results and implications of the Diabetes Control and Complications Trial
- The 1994 Nutrition Recommendations of the American Diabetes Association
- Definition of women's health issues and nutrition-related concerns
- The new approach to treating nausea (morning sickness) in pregnancy

- Recognition of binge eating (without purging) as an eating disorder
- The Hazard Analysis Critical Control Point (HACCP) concept for controlling foodborne illness
- Empowerment, a holistic, patient-centered approach to the management of chronic illness
- Carbohydrate counting, one of several meal planning strategies in diabetes
- Update of recommendations for the management of high blood cholesterol in adults (Adult Treatment Panel II)
- Recommendations for the management of high blood cholesterol in children and adolescents
- A new philosophy in the treatment of obesity
- Peptic ulcer as a disease caused largely by bacterial infection
- Gastroparesis, a disease of gastrointestinal motility
- Update of nutrition guidelines in end-stage renal disease.

These new developments have necessitated substantial revision of the previous edition. Much effort and interest have gone into making this book as up-to-date as possible.

Expanded Content

The content related to nutrition in the life cycle has been expanded substantially. In this edition, separate chapters are devoted to each of the following categories: pregnancy and lactation; infancy; childhood and adolescence; and adulthood, with emphasis on the older adult. Additionally, nutrition therapy in diseases of infancy and childhood has been integrated into the appropriate chapters. For example, the discussion of phenylketonuria appears in the chapter that covers nutritional needs during infancy; eating disorders are discussed in the chapter devoted to childhood and adolescent nutrition. Diabetes, hypercholesterolemia and obesity in childhood and adolescence are covered in chapters that deal with nutrition therapy in these disorders.

Energy Metabolism (Chapter 7) has been expanded to include more information on physical fitness. Food habits of the American Indian and Alaska Native have been added to Chapter 14, "Meeting Nutrition Needs in Various Cultures and Lifestyles." Also added to this chapter are discussions of cultural diversity and nutrition-related health problems, plus more demographic information about the various cultural groups. A chapter (Chapter 4) devoted entirely to food safety has been added. Nutrition Therapy in Gastrointestinal Diseases (Chapter 28) has been expanded to include discussions of gastroparesis and irritable bowel syndrome.

Content related to nutrition guidelines for Canadians has been added. *Nutrition Recommendations for Canadians* and *Canada's Guidelines for Healthy Eating* are included in this edition (See Appendix D). Recommended Nutrient Intakes for Canadians have been updated. (Appendix C).

Learning Aids and Key Features

Numerous learning aids help students understand and retain information. Each chapter is preceded by Objectives, new in this edition. As in previous editions, *Key* features in each chapter highlight significant concepts, skills, and behaviors. *Key Terms,* found at the start of each chapter, provide a glossary of terms the student should know. *Keys to Practical Application* translate theory into practice, identifying desirable attitudes, insights, approaches, and actions. *Key Ideas* summarize the essential points of the chapter. *Keys to Learning* present thought-provoking questions and case studies.

Key Issues, highlighting contemporary topics and controversies, are relevant to the students' personal interests and make the subject matter more enjoyable. Topics covered in *Key Issues* include:

- Nutrition and Athletic Performance
- Fiber: Fact and Fiction
- Fish Oils: Protective or Destructive?
- Osteoporosis: Common and Complex
- Vitamin and Mineral Supplements: Use or Abuse?
- Premenstrual Syndrome: Does Diet Help?

- Fast Foods: Are They Junk Food?
- How Reliable Are Health Claims?
- Anorexia Nervosa and Bulimia Nervosa.

Included is the latest revision (1991) of the Nutritive Value of the Edible Part of Food (Home and Garden Bulletin Number 72). This handy Appendix (E) lists the nutritive value for household measures of 908 common foods. Also included are the saturated fat, monounsaturated fat, polyunsaturated fat, cholesterol, and sodium contents of these foods. In addition, the Appendix also provides the Metropolitan Height and Weight Tables, the Recommended Dietary Allowances, and the Canadian information discussed above.

In *Introductory Nutrition and Nutrition Therapy,* persons receiving nutritional care services are referred to as *clients.* This is because they are viewed as consumers of health services with the rights and responsibilities this term implies. Moreover, because these consumers could be either well persons or sick persons, the term *clients* is more appropriate than patients.

My aim has been to provide a practical, current, comprehensive, and easily understandable basic clinical nutrition text for students of nursing, dietetic technology, and the other health technologies. The "Key" theme has been employed to facilitate learning and to spark interest in normal nutrition and nutrition therapy.

At every opportunity, I have stressed the importance of food and eating situations in nourishing the human spirit—their role in enhancing the quality of life. Hopefully, the student will have a greater awareness of the emotional and social aspects of food—the uplifting effect of being fed by a caring, patient caregiver; the feelings of security and unity conveyed to a young child by family mealtimes; and the comforting nature of a shared meal for the elderly adult. I sincerely hope this text will meet these goals and the needs of the reader. I welcome suggestions and critical comments from readers.

Marian Maltese Eschleman, MS, RD, CDE

ACKNOWLEDGMENTS

I wish to express my sincere appreciation to those who provided assistance and encouragement during the preparation of this third edition.

I am deeply indebted to the two contributors to this revision. Monica W. Luby MS, RD, Director of the Dietetic Internship Program, College of Saint Elizabeth, Morristown, New Jersey has updated and expanded Chapter 29, Nutrition Therapy Related To Surgery and Following Burns: Alternative Feeding Methods and Chapter 30, Nutrition Therapy in Cancer, AIDS, and Other Special Problems. Nena Loney, RD, CDE, Renal Nutritionist, Burlington County Dialysis Center has included the most current developments in the treatment of chronic renal disease in her revision of Chapter 27, Nutrition Therapy in Renal Disease.

Several reviewers have made valuable suggestions that have greatly enhanced this third edition. Virginia R. Lafond, RN, MSN, Nurse Educator, Helene Fuld School of Nursing, Trenton, New Jersey, reviewed the entire book. Mary A. Johnson, MS, RD, CDE, Director of Nutrition, Joslin Center for Diabetes, Saint Barnabas Medical Center, Princeton, New Jersey, Division, and Susan A. Jones, RD, CNSD, Nutrition Support Dietitian, The Graduate Hospital, Philadelphia, PA, reviewed selected chapters.

At Lippincott, I have been privileged to have the expert guidance of Donna L. Hilton, Vice President and Publisher. I am especially grateful for the support and reliable assistance of Susan M. Keneally, Editorial Assistant, who so efficiently and meticulously managed the many details associated with manuscript preparation. Barbara Ryalls, Project Editor, skillfully and patiently guided the production of this third edition. The fresh, new, modern design of this edition is due to the diligence and competence of Kathy Kelley-Luedtke, design coordinator.

I wish to express my gratitude to my husband, Ned Eschleman, to whom this book is dedicated. His trust, encouragement, and willing sacrifices, are largely responsible for this book. I also am most grateful to my sister, Rosemary Maltese, for her unfailing support and to my daughter, Annemarie, and son, Tom, for their patience and encouragement. Finally, I wish to acknowledge the example of diligence and perseverance provided by my dear and loving parents, Mary and the late Thomas Maltese.

CONTENTS

CHAPTER 6
Digestion and Absorption 95

CHAPTER 7
Energy Metabolism 112

CHAPTER 8
Carbohydrates 133

CHAPTER 9
Fats 154

CHAPTER 10
Proteins 174

CHAPTER 11
Minerals 192

CHAPTER 28
Nutrition Therapy in Gastrointestinal Disease 567

CHAPTER 29
Nutrition Therapy Related to Surgery and Following Burns; Alternative Feeding Methods 592

CHAPTER 30
Nutrition Therapy in Cancer, AIDS, and Other Special Problems 613

Appendixes

Index 685

Introductory Nutrition
and
Nutrition Therapy

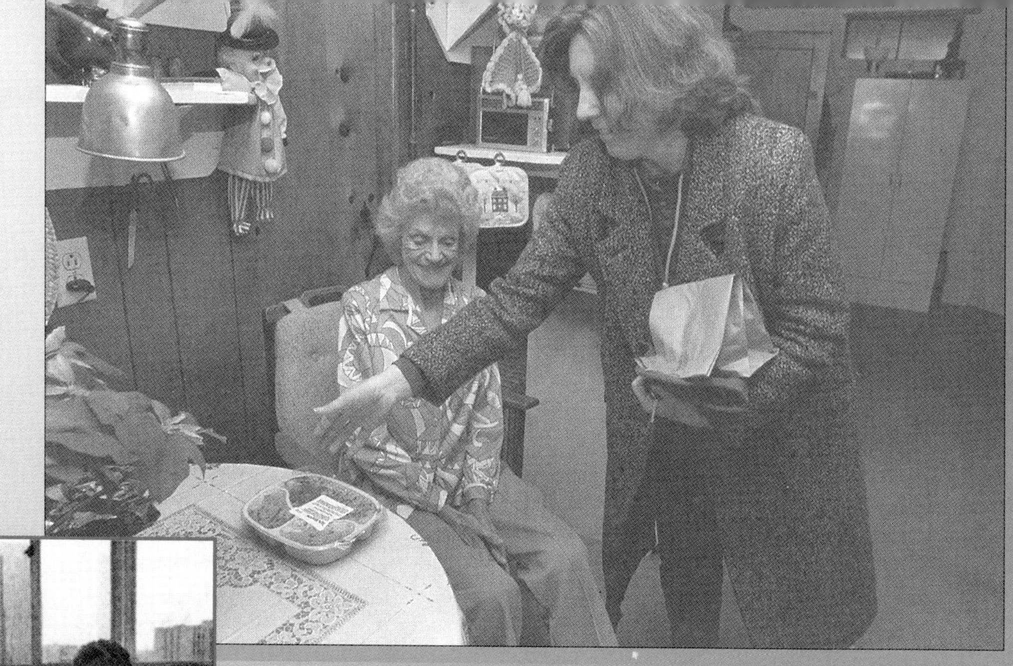

PART ONE

Introduction to Nutrition Care in Health and Illness

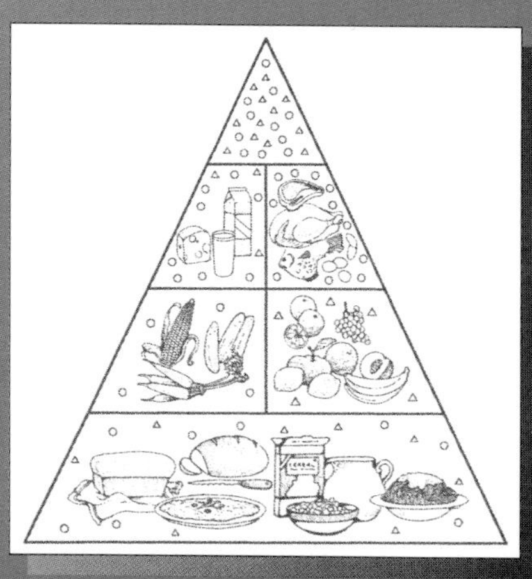

CHAPTER

1

Nutritional Concerns: Opening the Door to the 21st Century

KEY TERMS

chronic/long-term diseases diseases that have symptoms of long duration and that frequently are incurable

client the receiver of health care; replaces the word *patient,* which usually implies illness

fragmented broken up and scattered

health care care aimed at the prevention of illness and achievement of good health, as well as care provided during illness

incidence the extent to which a disease occurs in a given population

morbidity disease rate

mortality death rate

nutrition the science of food and its relation to health and disease; the processes by which the body ingests, absorbs, transports, uses, and excretes food substances

nutrition care the application of the science of nutrition to the care of people

nutrition therapy nutrition intervention used to treat a condition or disease

obesity excessive deposit and storage of fat in the body

sedentary involving mostly sitting; little physical activity

OBJECTIVES

After completing this chapter, the student will be able to:

1. Identify the factors that place nutrition care in the forefront of present and future health concerns in the United States.
2. Assess commitment to a healthy lifestyle.
3. Identify the various factors in society that influence American eating habits and the nutrition concerns associated with them.
4. Identify the components of nutrition care and the responsibilities of the various members of the health care team in the delivery of this care.

As the health care system evolves into the 21st century, nutrition and nutrition therapy are on the cutting edge. Increasing emphasis on cost control, health promotion, disease prevention, medical technology, and home care are among the factors that contribute to the growth of nutrition science and nutrition therapy. Other factors, such as an increasing elderly population, greater public health consciousness, and cultural diversity also contribute to the focus on nutrition.

Nutrition intervention is among the most cost-effective means of promoting health and helping to prevent disease. Shorter hospital stays and more home care (including the use of medical technology in the home) require health care providers to have a thorough understanding of nutrition and be able to teach and monitor clients and families. Health promotion through nutrition and nutrition therapy will continue to grow in importance as the focus of health care continues to shift from treatment to prevention.

IMPROVED NUTRITION: A NATIONAL PRIORITY

HEALTH PROMOTION/ DISEASE PREVENTION

In 1990, the US Department of Health and Human Services issued national objectives that emphasize prevention of major health problems. This report, entitled *Healthy People 2000: National Health Promotion and Disease Prevention Objectives,* aims to improve the health of all Americans during the 1990s. It comprises 298 objectives in 22 areas of high public health priority (Display 1-1). Each of the 22 priority areas has subobjectives for special high-risk populations. Nutrition is one of 22 priority areas in the report. Within the nutrition priority area, there are 21 objectives, some of which are shared with other priority areas such as physical activity and fitness and heart disease and stroke.

Nutrition is key to health promotion and disease prevention. According to *The Surgeon General's Report on Nutrition and Health,* two thirds of Americans die of diseases linked to diet. Eating habits in the United States are associated with five of the 15 leading causes of death: heart disease, some cancers, stroke, diabetes, and *atherosclerosis,* or hardening of the arteries (Table 1-1). Excessive intake of fat is considered a major contributing factor.

Obesity, the most common nutrition-related problem, affects 34 million Americans. People who are obese have an increased risk of high blood pressure, high cholesterol levels, diabetes, gallbladder disease, and some cancers. Diet, according to the surgeon general's report, also contributes to the incidence of osteoporosis, dental caries, and anemia.

Among the nutrition-related problems affecting children are hunger, growth retardation, iron-deficiency anemia, dental disease, and obesity. Poor maternal nutrition during pregnancy is one of the main causes of infant mortality and morbidity.

For elderly people, adequate nutrition is an essential factor in the quality of life contributing to physical, social, and mental well-being and the maintenance of independent living. At all ages, people who are well-nourished are more resistant to disease and recover more quickly from acute illness, injury, and surgery.

DISPLAY 1-1 HEALTHY PEOPLE 2000: PRIORITY AREAS

HEALTH PROMOTION

1. Physical activity and fitness
2. Nutrition
3. Tobacco
4. Alcohol and other drugs
5. Family planning
6. Mental health and mental disorders
7. Violent and abusive behavior
8. Educational and community-based programs

HEALTH PROTECTION

9. Unintentional injuries
10. Occupational safety and health
11. Environmental health
12. Food and drug safety
13. Oral health

PREVENTIVE SERVICES

14. Maternal and infant health
15. Heart disease and stroke
16. Cancer
17. Diabetes and chronic disabling conditions
18. Human immunodeficiency virus (HIV) infection
19. Sexually transmitted diseases
20. Immunization and infectious diseases
21. Clinical preventive services

SURVEILLANCE AND DATA SYSTEMS

22. Surveillance and data systems

TABLE 1-1 DEATH RATES AND PERCENTAGE OF TOTAL DEATHS FOR THE 15 LEADING CAUSES OF DEATH: UNITED STATES, 1991 (RATES PER 100,000 POPULATION)

RANK ORDER*	CAUSE OF DEATH†	RATE	TOTAL DEATHS (%)
...	All causes	860.3	100.0
1	Diseases of heart‡	285.9	33.2
2	Malignant neoplasms, including neoplasms of lymphatic and hematopoietic tissues‡	204.1	23.7
3	Cerebrovascular diseases‡	56.9	6.6
4	Chronic obstructive pulmonary diseases and allied conditions	35.9	4.2
5	Accidents and adverse effects§	35.4	4.1
...	Motor vehicle accidents	17.3	2.0
...	All other accidents and adverse effects	18.2	2.1
6	Pneumonia and influenza	30.9	3.6
7	Diabetes mellitus‡	19.4	2.3
8	Suicide§	12.2	1.4
9	HIV Infection	11.7	1.4
10	Homicide and legal intervention	10.5	1.2
11	Chronic liver disease and cirrhosis§	10.1	1.2
12	Nephritis, nephrotic syndrome, and nephrosis	8.5	1.0
13	Septicemia	7.8	0.9
14	Atherosclerosis‡	6.9	0.8
15	Certain conditions originating in the perinatal period	6.7	0.8
...	All other causes	117.4	13.7

* Rank based on number of deaths.
† From Ninth Revision International Classification of Diseases, 1975.
‡ Causes of death in which diet plays a part.
§ Causes of death in which excessive alcohol consumption is instrumental.
(National Center for Health Statistics. *Monthly Vital Statistics Report* Aug 31 1993;42:2(S).)

Wellness is more than the absence of disease. Both the quality and quantity of life are enhanced by a healthier lifestyle. Some experts believe that, although the life span has increased, the quality of life has not increased proportionately. How would you rate your lifestyle? (See Display 1-2.)

CHALLENGES FOR THE HEALTH WORKER

As a health worker, you face clear challenges in this new approach to health care that is not limited to sick care but also encompasses and supports health promotion and disease prevention. In the present health care setting, you must be able to offer sound nutrition information, apply this information to everyday eating, and help the public distinguish between unreliable, reliable, and controversial information. The informed health worker also recognizes when to refer clients to physicians, dietitians, or other resources for assistance with problems related to nutrition and nutrition therapy.

INFLUENCES ON EATING HABITS

Knowing the principles of good nutrition is of little value unless the health worker can apply this knowledge to people's everyday needs and circumstances. These considerations challenge health workers to apply the science of nutrition to the ever-changing environment.

(text continues on page 9)

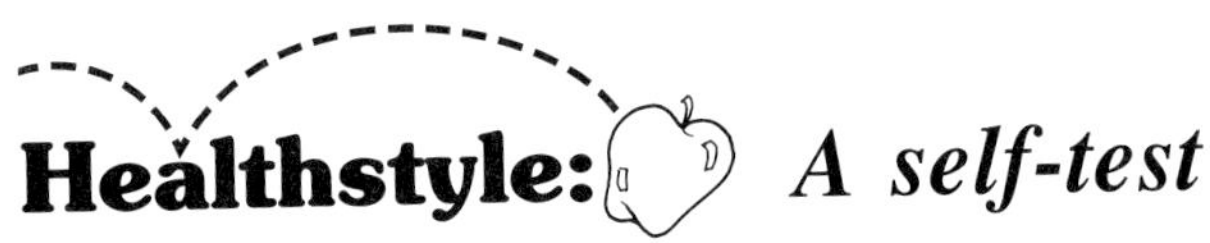

Healthstyle: A self-test

All of us want good health. But many of us do not know how to be as healthy as possible. Health experts now describe *lifestyle* as one of the most important factors affecting health. It is estimated that as many as seven of the ten leading causes of death could be reduced through commonsense changes in lifestyle. That is what this brief test, developed by the Public Health Service, is all about. Its purpose is simply to tell you how well you are doing to stay healthy. The behaviors covered in the test are recommended for most Americans. Some of them may not apply to people with certain chronic diseases or disabilities or to pregnant women. Such people may require special instructions from their physicians.

If you *never smoke*, enter a score of 10 for this section and go to the next section on *Alcohol and Drugs*.

	Almost Always	Sometimes	Almost Never
1. I avoid smoking cigarettes.	2	1	0
2. I smoke only low-tar and nicotine cigarettes *or* I smoke a pipe or cigars.	2	1	0

Smoking Score: ____________

	Almost Always	Sometimes	Almost Never
1. I avoid drinking alcoholic beverages *or* I drink no more than one or two drinks a day.	4	1	0
2. I avoid using alcohol or other drugs (especially illegal drugs) as a way of handling situations or the problems in my life.	2	1	0
3. I am careful not to drink alcohol when taking certain medicines (for example, medicine for sleeping, pain, colds, and allergies), or when pregnant.	2	1	0
4. I read and follow the label directions when using prescribed and over-the-counter drugs.	2	1	0

Alcohol and Drugs Score: ____________

	Almost Always	Sometimes	Almost Never
1. I eat a variety of foods each day, such as fruits and vegetables, whole-grain breads and cereals, lean meats, dairy products, dry peas and beans, and nuts and seeds.	4	1	0
2. I limit the amount of fat, saturated fat, and cholesterol I eat (including fat on meats, eggs, butter, cream, shortenings, and organ meats such as liver).	2	1	0
3. I limit the amount of salt I eat by cooking with only small amounts, not adding salt at the table, and avoiding salty snacks.	2	1	0
4. I avoid eating too much sugar (especially frequent snacks of sticky candy or soft drinks).	2	1	0

Eating Habits Score: ____________

	Almost Always	Sometimes	Almost Never
1. I maintain a desired weight, avoiding overweight and underweight.	3	1	0
2. I do vigorous exercises for 15–30 minutes at least three times a week (examples include running, swimming, brisk walking).	3	1	0
3. I do exercises that enhance my muscle tone for 15–30 minutes at least three times a week (examples include yoga and calisthenics).	2	1	0
4. I use part of my leisure time participating in individual, family, or team activities that increase my level of fitness (such as gardening, bowling, golf, and baseball).	2	1	0

Exercise/Fitness Score: ____________

(Continued)

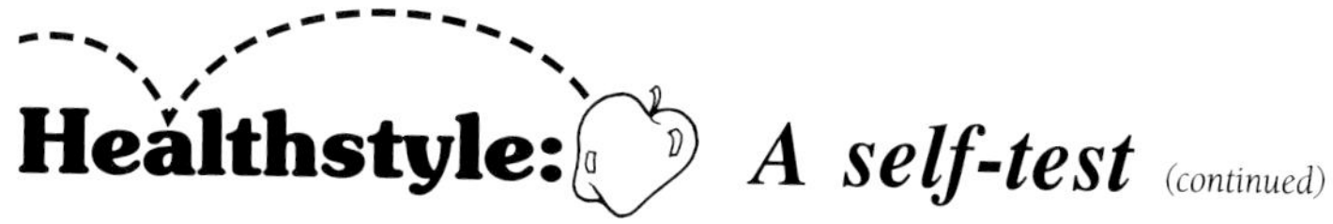

	Almost Always	Sometimes	Almost Never
1. I have a job or do other work that I enjoy.	2	1	0
2. I find it easy to relax and express my feelings freely.	2	1	0
3. I recognize early, and prepare for, events or situations likely to be stressful for me.	2	1	0
4. I have close friends, relatives, or others to whom I can talk about personal matters and call on for help when needed.	2	1	0
5. I participate in group activities (such as church and community organizations) or hobbies that I enjoy.	2	1	0

Stress Control Score: ____________

	Almost Always	Sometimes	Almost Never
1. I wear a seat belt while riding in a car.	2	1	0
2. I avoid driving while under the influence of alcohol and other drugs.	2	1	0
3. I obey traffic rules and the speed limit when driving.	2	1	0
4. I am careful when using potentially harmful products or substances (such as household cleaners, poisons, and electrical devices).	2	1	0
5. I avoid smoking in bed.	2	1	0

Safety Score: ____________

SCORES OF 9 AND 10

Excellent! Your answers show that you are aware of the importance of this area to your health. More important, you are putting your knowledge to work for you by practicing good health habits. As long as you continue to do so, this area should not pose a serious health risk. It is likely that you are setting an example for your family and friends to follow. Because you got a high test score on this part of the test, you may want to consider other areas where your scores indicate room for improvement.

SCORES OF 6 TO 8

Your health practices in this area are good, but there is room for improvement. Look again at the items you answered with a "Sometimes" or "Almost Never". What changes can you make to improve your score? Even a small change can often help you achieve better health.

SCORES OF 3 TO 5

Your health risks are showing! Would you like more information about the risks you are facing and about why it is important for you to change these behaviors? Perhaps you need help in deciding how to successfully make the changes you desire. In either case, help is available.

SCORES OF 0 TO 2

Obviously, you were concerned enough about your health to take the test, but your answers show that you may be taking serious and unnecessary risks with your health. Perhaps you are unaware of the risks and what to do about them. You can easily get the information and help you need to improve, if you wish. The next step is up to you.

(Continued)

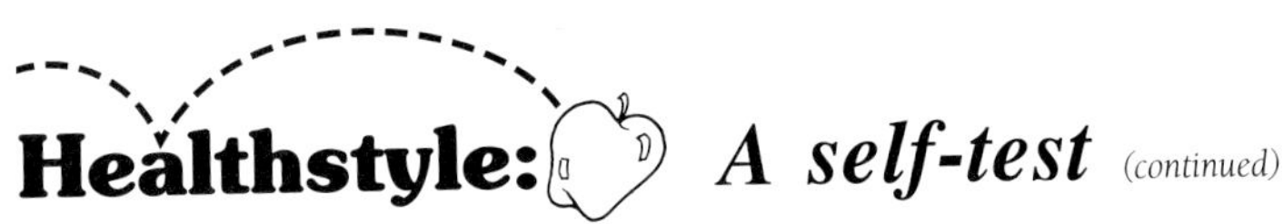

Healthstyle: A self-test (continued)

In the test you just completed were numerous suggestions to help you reduce your risk of disease and premature death. The following are some of the most significant.

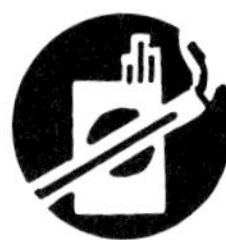

AVOID CIGARETTES. Cigarette smoking is the single most important preventable cause of illness and early death. It is especially risky for pregnant women and their unborn babies. People who stop smoking reduce their risk of getting heart disease and cancer. So if you are a cigarette smoker, think twice about lighting that next cigarette. If you choose to continue smoking, try decreasing the number of cigarettes you smoke and switching to a low-tar and nicotine brand.

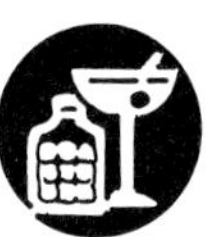

FOLLOW SENSIBLE DRINKING HABITS. Alcohol produces changes in mood and behavior. Most people who drink are able to control their intake of alcohol and to avoid undesired, and often harmful, effects. Heavy, regular use of alcohol can lead to cirrhosis of the liver, a leading cause of death. Also, statistics clearly show that mixing drinking and driving is often the cause of fatal or crippling accidents. So if you drink, do it wisely and in moderation. *Use care in taking drugs.* Today's greater use of drugs—both legal and illegal—is one of our most serious health risks. Even some drugs prescribed by your doctor can be dangerous if taken when drinking alcohol or before driving. Excessive or continued use of tranquilizers (or "pep pills") can cause physical and mental problems. Using or experimenting with illicit drugs such as marijuana, heroin, cocaine, and PCP (phencyclidine) may lead to a number of damaging effects or even death.

EAT SENSIBLY. Overweight individuals are at greater risk for diabetes, gall bladder disease, and high blood pressure. So it makes good sense to maintain proper weight. But good eating habits also mean holding down the amount of fat (especially saturated fat), cholesterol, sugar, and salt in your diet. If you must snack, try nibbling on fresh fruits and vegetables. You will feel better—and look better, too.

EXERCISE REGULARLY. Almost everyone can benefit from exercise—and there is some form of exercise almost everyone can do. (If you have any doubt, check first with your doctor.) Usually, as little as 15–30 minutes of vigorous exercise three times a week will help you have a healthier heart, eliminate excess weight, tone up sagging muscles, and sleep better. Think how much difference all these improvements could make in the way you feel!

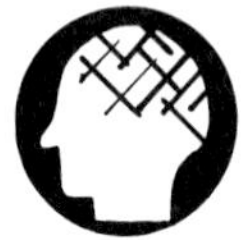

LEARN TO HANDLE STRESS. Stress is a normal part of living; everyone faces it to some degree. The causes of stress can be good or bad, desirable or undesirable (such as a promotion on the job or the loss of a spouse). Properly handled, stress need not be a problem. But unhealthy responses to stress—such as driving too fast or erratically, drinking too much, or prolonged anger or grief—can cause a variety of physical and mental problems. Even on a busy day, find a few minutes to slow down and relax. Talking over a problem with someone you trust can often help you find a satisfactory solution. Learn to distinguish between things that are "worth fighting about" and things that are less important.

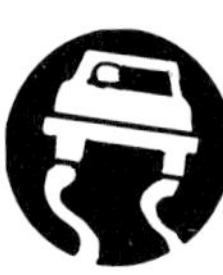

BE SAFETY CONSCIOUS. Think "safety first" at home, at work, at school, at play, and on the highway. Buckle seat belts and obey traffic rules. Keep poisons and weapons out of the reach of children, and keep emergency numbers by your telephone. When the unexpected happens, you will be prepared.

(Continued)

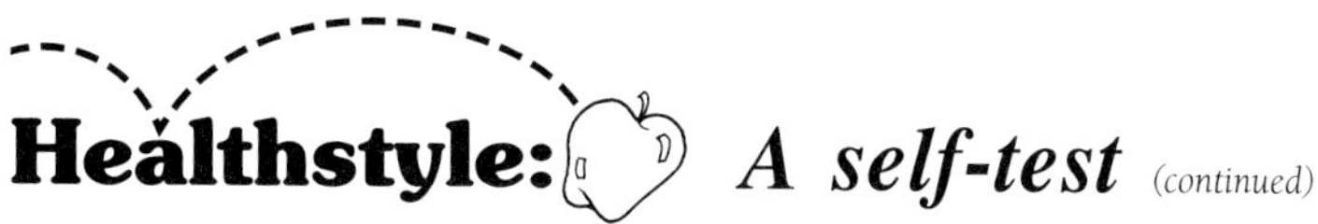

Start by asking yourself a few frank questions: *Am I really doing all I can to be as healthy as possible? What steps can I take to feel better? Am I willing to begin now?* If you scored low in one or more *sections* of the test, decide what changes you want to make for improvement. You might pick that aspect of your lifestyle which you feel you have the best chance for success and tackle that one first. Once you have improved your score there, go on to other areas.

If you already have tried to change your health habits (to stop smoking or exercise regularly, for example), do not be discouraged if you have not yet succeeded. The difficulty you have encountered may be due to influences you have never really thought about—such as advertising—or to a lack of support and encouragement. Understanding these influences is an important step toward changing the way they affect you.

THERE'S HELP AVAILABLE. In addition to personal actions you can take on your own, there are community programs and groups (such as the YMCA or the local chapter of the American Heart Association) that can assist you and your family to make the changes you want to make. If you want to know more about these groups or about health risks, contact your local health department or the National Health Information Center. There is a lot you can do to stay healthy or to improve your health—and there are organizations that can help you. Start a new HEALTHSTYLE today!

For assistance in locating specific information on these and other health topics, write to National Health Information Center, P.O. Box 1133, Washington, DC 20013-1133.

THE CHANGING AMERICAN DIET

Eating habits have undergone many changes as a result of the family's changing lifestyle. For example, family members may arise at different times and prepare their own breakfasts. Some may skip breakfast. They may purchase lunch at the factory or office cafeteria, the school cafeteria, a restaurant, or a fast-food establishment. They may hurriedly prepare, serve, and eat dinner to accommodate family members' many activities. Or, each family member may heat prepared foods or a frozen meal in the microwave oven when convenient. Snacking may begin with the midmorning coffee break and continue through to bedtime. Children may get into the habit of snacking from the time they return from school until dinnertime. Even the elements in a single meal may be fragmented, as in a new trend call *grazing*, in which people eat fewer meals, eating instead snacks, soups, vegetables, and desserts throughout the day. Are all the essential foods being provided by this fragmented style of eating? Or are foods with little nutritional value making up too large a part of the American diet?

Changes in family structure and child care have important nutrition implications. Many children live in poverty. In these circumstances, money for food and nutrition knowledge are frequently lacking. Families are relying more on takeout and costly convenience foods. Are these meals balanced in nutrients? Are they contributing excessive amounts of energy, fat, salt, and sugar?

More than half of mothers with children younger than age 6 years work outside the home, and approximately 14.6 million preschool children require day care. Some are cared for in in-home day care, whereas others are in community-based child care centers. How well informed about nutrition are the care-givers? What is the nutritional quality of food served in day care programs? Are nutrition standards established and monitored?

In addition, approximately 34.4 million school-age children attend day care. Many children participate in after-school child care programs held in the school setting. Some schools provide all-day food services offering breakfasts, snacks, lunches, and, in many cases, after-school snacks. For many children, school and day care food services provide the bulk of their food intake. Are parents aware of what foods the child has actually consumed throughout the day?

Because so many meals are eaten away from home and because family members may eat at different times, many children seldom, if ever, enjoy the sharing of a family mealtime. Are parents aware of the role of food and feeding in building a secure and supportive family environment?

SMALLER HOUSEHOLDS

Another change is the composition of the American household. Estimates indicate that, by the year 2000, more than 60% of households will consist of only one or two people. Household size affects nutrition. Meal patterns frequently change with the shift from family to nonfamily households. Are people who live alone preparing well-balanced meals for themselves? Are they as motivated as those who must provide for a family?

THE INCREASING OLDER POPULATION

Of those people living alone, at least half are age 65 years or older. The elderly population aged 85 years and older is growing six times faster than the rest of the population. How well are elderly people adapting their eating habits to their declining strength, immobility, isolation, and chronic illnesses? Some rely on home delivery services for the bulk of their meals. Are the needs for high-quality, home-delivered meals being met?

Our aging population will have a significant impact on the types of foods available in the future. Some manufacturers are considering fortifying foods with antioxidants such as vitamin E and beta carotene, which are believed to slow the aging process. Flavors with greater intensity may be added to foods to compensate for the loss of taste and smell that frequently accompany aging. Packaging design is also likely to become more user friendly. Will elderly consumers be able to achieve a moderate, balanced, and varied diet when confronted with a maze of new technologies and products?

CULTURAL DIVERSITY

The US population is becoming increasingly diverse. Food habits are closely related to ethnic and religious identity. Most traditional food habits yield a nutritionally adequate diet. More often, nutrition problems arise when immigrants adapt to contemporary US food habits—giving up more desirable food habits and preparation methods for less desirable ones.

Easily prepared ethnic foods are expected to become more available. The growing Hispanic, African American, and Asian populations are now looked on as major markets by food manufacturers and supermarkets.

EATING OUT

The number of meals eaten away from home has increased to approximately one third. The rise in the number of women employed outside the home, smaller households, greater mobility, improved financial status, lack of time for food preparation, and easy access to inexpensive fast food are factors that promote restaurant eating. In the mid-1960s, people spent 30% of the food budget on eating out; by 1980, they spent 39%, and by 1992, 43%. Fast-food meals lack variety, may be high in calories relative to the amount of nutrients they provide, and tend to be excessively high in fat. Because the trend of eating out is not likely to decline, how can we encourage better consumer choices and more variety in the foods offered?

CONVENIENCE FOODS

The fast pace of life has made the use of convenience foods increasingly attractive. As many as 20,000 food products confront consumers at the supermarket. In addition, supermarkets are attempting to capture some of the large amount of money spent on take-out meals. An increasing variety of ready-to-eat supermarket foods are being marketed. Attractive packaging and displays and ease of preparation may entice people to buy foods that are nutritionally inadequate—overrefined and excessive in fats, salt, and calories.

HEALTH AND FITNESS TRENDS

Within the realm of convenience and restaurant foods, the trend, however, is toward lighter foods, health consciousness, and wellness. Increased public awareness of the relationship between diet and health and the aging of the "baby boomers" are believed to be the primary forces behind this trend. The well-educated baby boom generation is interested in convenience but wants quality, safety, and good taste as well. They are willing to pay more for foods with less fat and less salt. But how can consumers be sure that they are getting less fat, less salt, and fewer calories? Do they know how to evaluate food advertisements and use the comprehensive nutrition labeling on commercial food products?

The emergence of biotechnology in the agricultural field provides another avenue through which the demand for leaner, lowfat foods is being met. In animal production, biotechnology makes it possible to genetically engineer desirable traits into animals. As a result, biotechnology techniques have been used to produce pork with 75% less fat.

STRESS

It is widely believed that we live in a more stressful time than did our grandparents. The stress factors may be related to employment, frequency of moving from one place to another, the general pace of life, or other factors. Whatever the cause, many people find that what they eat, when they eat, and how they eat are all influenced by these stress factors.

SUBSTANCE ABUSE

A substance dependency, whether on alcohol, drugs, tobacco, or another substance, may strongly influence a person's eating habits. The cost of the substance and its relationship to the foods that are eaten may be significant factors.

SEDENTARY LIFESTYLES

Although studies have shown that Americans consume fewer calories than in the past, obesity is increasing. The implication is that Americans are becoming increasingly sedentary. In many cases, lack of physical activity is so extreme that weight reduction or even maintenance can occur only at low caloric levels. When calories are so severely restricted, are all the essential nutrients being provided? Is reducing food intake, alone, the answer to maintaining an appropriate body weight?

THE CHANGING CONSUMER

Consumer groups have heightened public concern about the nutritional quality of food, safety of food additives, freshness of shelf foods, methods of pricing foods, and the role of government in food safety. The consumer movement has prompted increasing concern for consumer rights and demand for greater control over one's own health. In the health field, clients have become prominent members of the health team, making choices and decisions and assuming a greater role than before in managing their health problems.

The eating habits of today's consumers are greatly influenced by the mass media, especially television. Children and adults alike are the targets of commercial messages aimed at persuading them to purchase various food items and so-called health foods and supplements.

THE CHANGING ECONOMY

Changes in economic conditions have strongly influenced eating habits. The US homeless population is estimated to be as high as 3 million. Hunger appears to be more widespread than at any time in the past 20 years. The economic recession of the late 1980s through the early 1990s—the worst since the 1930s—coupled with cuts in national welfare programs are believed to be largely responsible for this situation.

In times of inflation and unemployment, many people may have to cut their food budgets to meet the rising costs of such necessities as heating fuel, housing, and transportation. The amount spent for food becomes the only flexible item in their budget. When the food budget is low, people can meet nutrition needs only if they carefully plan purchases and limit purchases to those foods that provide the most food value at the lowest cost. At the same time, developing industries may help create a group of newly wealthy people with money available to spend on food but who may not know how to spend it wisely. These people may increase their intake of rich foods that are low in nutritional value. Good and poor diets are found at all income levels.

PROVIDING NUTRITION CARE

COMPONENTS OF NUTRITION CARE

Nutrition care involves applying the art and science of nutrition to promote the health and well-being of people. It includes

- evaluating nutritional status and assessing nutrition needs and nutrition-related psychosocial and economic issues
- planning food consumption patterns and guidelines that meet the physical, psychological, and lifestyle needs at all stages of the life cycle
- providing education and counseling so that individuals may apply the science of nutrition to their needs both in health and disease
- providing meals and other forms of nutrition support to individuals in community facilities such as hospitals and nursing homes and in programs such as congregate meals for elderly people and home-delivered meals
- evaluating the client's progress toward nutrition goals; revising plans as needed.

TEAM APPROACH

The health care delivery system has changed from an exclusive relationship between the physician and client to one that includes an increasing number of allied health personnel (Fig. 1-1).

The client is the central player in the health care team. Clients should control key decisions about their care. The need for client control is especially evident in cases of chronic disease that require the client or the family to manage the disease on a day-to-day basis. Clients who have a role in determining the goals and objectives of their care are more likely to take an active part in achieving them. People do not respond well to personal goals others have set for them.

RESPONSIBILITIES OF THE HEALTH TEAM

Successful maintenance or improvement of nutritional well-being or treatment of disease by means of nutrition intervention requires teamwork. However, the clinical dietitian and the public health nutritionist (registered dietitians, or RDs) are the nutrition authorities and carry the major responsibilities for nutrition care (Display 1-3).

In the hospital or nursing home, the dietitian assesses the client's nutritional status, develops a plan for meeting the nutrition needs identified, manages nutrition therapy, and evaluates results. The dietetic technician or DT assists the dietitian

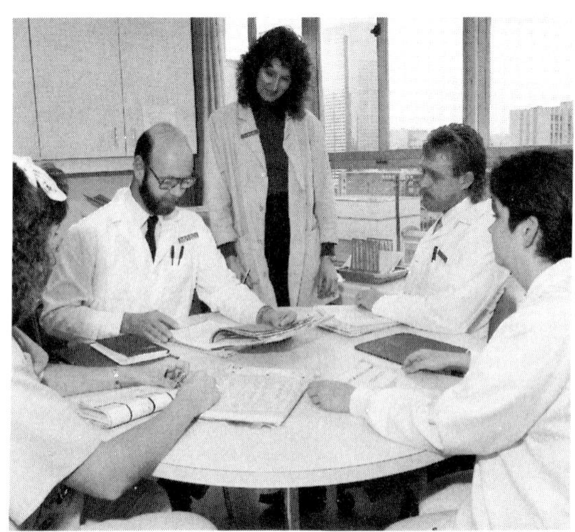

FIGURE 1-1

Health care delivery has changed to include an increasing number of allied health personnel, shown here in an interdisciplinary team conference.

DISPLAY 1-3 RESPONSIBILITIES OF VARIOUS MEMBERS OF THE HEALTH CARE TEAM

CLIENT

The focus is on the client, who should participate in his or her care to the extent possible. The client and his or her family are kept informed and take part in making decisions about care. The client and the family members involved ultimately make the decisions regarding the management of the client's health care.

PHYSICIAN

Responsible for the diagnosis and treatment of the client's medical problems. Orders laboratory tests and treatment procedures and prescribes medication. May assess nutritional status and prescribe the care plan. Explains to the client the role of nutrition care in the treatment plan.

REGISTERED DIETITIAN (RD)

Carries the major responsibility for the client's nutrition care. Assesses the nutritional status of the client. In consultation with the physician, determines the client's nutrition needs and care plan. Develops nutrition care plans and meal plans that meet the client's nutritional and personal needs. Responsible for nutrition education and counseling. Together with the physician, has primary responsibility for the client's nutrition care.

DIETETIC TECHNICIAN (DT)

Assists the RD in providing nutrition care. May assist in taking nutrition histories and body measurements, screening records, checking on client's acceptance of food, and providing nutrition education.

REGISTERED NURSE (RN)

Responsible for client's daily care as ordered by the physician. Identifies nutrition problems. Maintains communication with the physician and dietitian about the client's nutrition needs. Plans nursing functions needed such as assisting the client at meal times; observing, recording, and reporting the client's responses to food; reinforcing nutrition education; and providing diet instruction in the absence of a dietitian.

LICENSED PRACTICAL NURSE (LPN)

Under the supervision of an RN, provides nutrition care such as feeding clients, checking food consumption, and maintaining intake and output records.

CLINICAL PHARMACIST

A specialist in drug actions and interactions and in the uses and side effects of drugs. Provides consultation and assistance in the selection of intravenous nutrition products.

LICENSED SOCIAL WORKER

Helps client solve social, emotional, and financial problems. Makes referrals to community agencies that can assist the client after discharge from the hospital.

MEDICAL TECHNOLOGIST

Performs laboratory procedures that aid in diagnosing disease states and monitoring the effects of treatment.

(Continued)

DISPLAY 1-3 *(Continued)*

RESPIRATORY THERAPIST

Assists client with breathing difficulties by using therapeutic techniques or equipment.

PHYSICAL THERAPIST

Evaluates and assists client with physical disabilities to restore function and alleviate pain by using treatments that involve exercise, massage, heat, cold, and other techniques.

OCCUPATIONAL THERAPIST

Evaluates and assists the disabled client to learn ways of performing the activities of daily living and to live a productive life. Assists with the mechanical aspects of feeding the disabled by recommending appropriate adaptive equipment.

SPEECH PATHOLOGIST

Evaluates and provides services for the client with communication disorders involving speech, language, or hearing. Diagnoses and recommends diet modification and other aspects of treatment for swallowing disorders.

by taking diet histories and participating in nutrition education. The nurse may assist in the nutrition assessment and help to develop, support, and carry out the care plan. The nursing staff makes the mealtime atmosphere as encouraging to the client's appetite as possible. The nursing staff observes and records the quantity of food consumed and alerts the physician and dietitian when food intake appears inadequate. The nurse assists in providing nutrition education, taking advantage of daily opportunities to reinforce the dietitian's nutrition education and counseling efforts.

In the ambulatory care setting, such as the clinic, health center, physician's office, or home, nurses have an excellent opportunity to provide nutrition education. Because they see the client periodically over an extended time and because a change in eating habits is usually slow, the nurse is able to help the client make a gradual adjustment to recommended dietary changes. A dietitian is frequently available to assist. Sometimes, the dietitian is a member of the staff and provides diet counseling for clients with complex nutrition problems.

In the home, community, or public health settings, nurses have a unique opportunity to observe eating habits and the circumstances that influence them. They provide health education and bedside nursing care in the home and may supervise home health aides. The public health nurse is more aware than other members of the health team of the effects of circumstance such as income, cultural factors, family organization, and housing on eating habits. With a knowledge of these factors and repeated contacts with clients over extended periods, the public health nurse can provide practical and meaningful assistance. A public health nutritionist or a community nutrition counselor is frequently available to assist the nurse with nutrition care in the home.

In the school or day care center, nurses may be more successful than the child's parent in influencing eating habits. They may be able to help parents with children's eating problems and may be involved in nutrition education programs for both children and parents.

In business and industry, nurses provide nutrition education as part of preventive health programs offered to employees. They may also provide guidance to personnel who require nutrition therapy.

KEYS TO PRACTICAL APPLICATION

Keep informed of and be sensitive to the changes and trends in the health care system. Seek to understand how these changes influence your role as a health worker.

Change those lifestyle habits that are damaging your health.

Remember that example is the best teacher.

Keep in mind the everyday circumstances of your clients as you study nutrition and apply what you learn.

Seek to understand how social issues affect your client's eating habits and nutritional status.

Always keep your focus on the needs of your clients—they are the reason for all our efforts.

KEY IDEAS

Trends and forces shaping the health care industry today are expected to bring profound changes in the health care field. These trends involve cost control, emphasis on health promotion and prevention, proactive health consumers, an aging population, increased home care, decreased hospitalization, medical technology, cultural diversity, and increased focus on maternal and child health issues.

Promoting health and preventing disease is the focus of health care in the 1990s. This is the emphasis in the government report *Healthy People 2000: National Health Promotion and Disease Prevention Objectives.*

Emphasis on prevention and self-care places more responsibility on clients than in the past. Many consumers are taking a more aggressive role in their health care.

Improved nutrition plays a prominent role in health promotion and disease prevention. Two thirds of Americans die of diseases linked to diet. Present nutrition problems are related mostly to excess, especially excessive calories and fat.

Good nutrition has a profound effect on the health and well-being of infants and children and on the quality of life of elderly people.

Well-nourished people of all ages are more resistant to disease and recover more quickly from acute illness, injury, and surgery.

The new emphasis on wellness and disease prevention requires that health care personnel be more involved and more knowledgeable than before in providing nutrition education.

Changes in family structure and child care affect the way people eat and bring about changes in patterns of eating.

To be effective, knowledge of nutrition must be applied to the everyday needs and circumstances of people.

Influences on eating habits include

- fewer family meals and a fragmented style of eating for family members
- more children consuming food outside the home with no family supervision or family togetherness and many children living in poverty
- an increasing older population, with the greatest growth in the age group 85 years and older
- merging of ethnic food habits with contemporary US food habits
- an increase in eating out spurred by easy access to inexpensive fast-food restaurants
- increased use of convenience foods, with the trend toward lighter, lowfat, low-sodium foods
- a more stressful environment
- substance abuse
- sedentary lifestyles, resulting in obesity despite the consumption of fewer calories
- increased public concern about nutritional quality and safety and the freshness and cost of food
- increased concern for consumer and client rights

- inflation and unemployment, resulting in lowered expenditures for food.

Nutrition care involves applying the art and science of nutrition to promote the health and well-being of people. It involves evaluation of nutritional status, planning meal patterns and guidelines, providing education and counseling, providing meals and other forms of nutritional support, and evaluating progress.

The complex nature of health care requires a team approach. The client is the central team player; people do not respond well to personal goals that others set for them.

Health personnel most directly involved in providing nutrition care include the physician, registered dietitian, nurse, dietetic technician, and home health aide.

The clinical dietitian and the public health nutritionist (RD) are the nutrition authorities who carry the major responsibility for nutrition care.

The need exists for nutrition care in many areas of health care; the services of dietitians, public health nutritionists, and diet counselors are available to assist health workers with nutrition-related problems.

KEYS TO LEARNING

STUDY–DISCUSSION QUESTIONS

1. Discuss one of the trends or forces shaping health care in the 1990s. How do you think it impacts on your health career? On nutrition care?
2. Use the lifestyle profile in Display 1-2 to find out how your lifestyle may be affecting your health. How does your lifestyle score? What changes would you like to make? Take one unhealthy behavior and develop a plan for change.
3. Increasing responsibility for health care is being placed on the shoulders of consumers. Why?
4. Based on your knowledge of the subject, discuss the ways in which nutrition is involved in achieving and maintaining good health, preventing disease, and treating illness.
5. Explain why the preventive self-care movement requires that health care personnel become more involved in nutrition education.
6. What facilities for preventive health care are available in your community? What kinds of nutrition services, if any, are provided?
7. Bring to class an example from a newspaper or magazine of one of the current influences on eating habits. Explain to the class how the example you have chosen may affect eating habits.
8. What does nutrition care involve? Why is the team approach important in delivering this care? Explain the client's role as a member of the health care team.
9. What do you hope to achieve from this study of nutrition?

BIBLIOGRAPHY

BOOKS

Bureau of Labor Statistics. Consumer expenditure survey 1992. Washington, DC: US Dept of Labor, 1994.

US Dept of Health and Human Services, Public Health Service. Health, United States, 1991, and prevention profile. Washington, DC: US Government Printing Office, 1992. US Dept of Health and Human Services publication PHS 92-1232.

US Dept of Health and Human Services, Public Health Service.

Healthy people 2000: national health promotion and disease prevention objectives. Washington, DC: US Government Printing Office, 1990.

US Dept of Health and Human Services, Public Health Service. The surgeon general's report on nutrition and health (summary and recommendations). Washington, DC: US Government Printing Office, 1988. US Dept of Health and Human Services publication PHS 88-50211.

PERIODICALS

American Dietetic Association. Position of the American Dietetic Association: affordable and accessible health care services. J Am Diet Assoc 1992;92:746.

American Dietetic Association. Position of the American Dietetic Association; nutrition in comprehensive program planning for persons with developmental disabilities. J Am Diet Assoc 1992;92:613.

American Dietetic Association. White paper on health care reform. J Am Diet Assoc 1992;92:749.

Bronner, Y. Healthy people 2000: A call to action for ADA members. J Am Diet Assoc 1991;91:1520.

Clarke DL. Moving into a biotech world. Food News 1991;7:4:12.

Danford DE, Stephenson MG. Healthy people 2000: development of nutrition objectives. J Am Diet Assoc 1991;91:1517.

Fast foods: the current state of affairs. Dietetic Currents 1991;18:4:1.

Ferguson T. Patient, heal thyself. The Futurist 1992;Jan–Feb:9.

National Center for Health Statistics. Monthly Vital Statistics Report Aug 31 1993;42:2(s):5.

Selker LG, Broski DC. Forces and trends shaping allied health practice and education. J Allied Health 1991;20:5:13.

Sousa AM. Benefits of dietitian home visits. J Am Diet Assoc 1994;94:1149.

Splett PL, Story M. Child nutrition: objectives for the decade. J Am Diet Assoc 1991;91:665.

Sucher KP, Kittler PG. Nutrition isn't color blind. J Am Diet Assoc 1991;91:297.

Warshaw HS. America eats out: Nutrition in the chain and family restaurant industry. J Am Diet Assoc 1993;93:17.

CHAPTER

2

Assessing Nutrition Needs: Physical and Psychological

KEY TERMS

anthropometrics measurement of body size (height and weight) and body composition (fat, muscle, and water)
antigen foreign substance such as a germ or virus that causes the body to produce antibodies
assessment evaluation of a person's nutritional well-being through the collection of data such as nutrition history, physical examination, laboratory values, and radiographic studies
composite made up of various parts
creatinine a substance normally found in blood and urine; it is a waste product of creatine, which is found mostly in muscle tissue
criteria standards on which judgments may be based
culture beliefs, art, and customs that make up a way of life for a group of people
energy capacity to do work; body fuel provided by certain nutrients (carbohydrate, fat, and protein)
hunger an unpleasant sensation caused by inadequate intake of food
kyphosis curvature of the spine causing hunching or stooping of the body
linear of length
lymphocyte a white blood cell formed in lymph tissue that is involved in the immune system
malnutrition a state of impaired health due to undernutrition, overnutrition, an imbalance of nutrients, or by the body's inability to use the nutrients ingested
monitor to watch over or observe for an extended period
nutrients chemical substances supplied by food that the body needs for growth, repair, and general functioning
overnutrition excessive intake of one or more nutrients; frequently refers to excessive intake of nutrients that provide energy
recumbent reclining position
serum a clear liquid that separates from clotted blood
serum albumin the chief protein of blood plasma
serum transferrin iron-carrying protein in the blood serum
standard an approved model used as a basis for comparison
stature height while standing
undernutrition deficiency of one or more nutrients; also may refer to a deficiency of nutrients providing energy

OBJECTIVES

After completing this chapter, the student will be able to:

1. Define the science of nutrition, nutrients, nutritional status, malnutrition, marginal nutritional status, nutritional imbalance, nutrition assessment, and nutrition screening.
2. Identify at least four ways in which nutrition affects physical health.

3. Discuss the incidence of malnutrition worldwide and in the United States.
4. Identify at least four components of nutrition assessment and briefly describe each.
5. Discuss the psychological importance of food and its specific importance to clients in health care facilities.
6. Identify some of the factors that have shaped the student's food habits.
7. Discuss the impact of the psychological aspects of food on health education efforts.
8. Develop a greater awareness of the feelings that clients communicate by their attitudes toward food.

PHYSIOLOGIC IMPORTANCE OF FOOD

As long as we are not hungry, does it really matter what we eat? Most of us have been warned of the dire consequences of missing breakfast or eating lunches consisting of soda and potato chips. Nevertheless, we may have skipped breakfast and satisfied our hunger with snack foods or sweets at mealtime and felt no ill effects. A person who eats poorly today most likely will live to tell the tale tomorrow. What, however, will be the long-range effects of the many days of poor eating? Will it be anemia, with its symptoms of weakness and fatigue that sap the body of strength to enjoy life to the fullest? Will it be overweight, which is frequently damaging to emotional health and increases the risk of serious chronic diseases? Will it be premature hardening of the arteries, a condition responsible for heart attacks and strokes? Or, will it be decreased resistance to disease, resulting in frequent colds and infections, which take their toll on an individual's productive days?

Nutrition is the science that deals with the chemical substances in food—called *nutrients*—that the body needs for life and growth. Nutrition provides information about how much of each nutrient is needed and under what circumstances, and about the types and quantities of food that provide the necessary nutrients. Nutrition also identifies foods that may need to be limited and the reasons why. Included in the science of nutrition are the functions of nutrients; how they interact; what happens when there is a lack, an excess, or an imbalance of nutrients; and the processes by which the body digests, absorbs, uses, and excretes the end products of food eaten. The psychological, social, and cultural factors that influence food selection also are considered. Nutrition draws on many other sciences, including biology, chemistry, physiology, medicine, psychology, anthropology, and sociology.

The terms *nutritional status* and *malnutrition* are used frequently in this book. Nutritional status refers to the state of the body as a result of the body's intake and use of nutrients. Malnutrition is a state of impaired health resulting from *undernutrition*—a lack of nutrients—or from *overnutrition*—an excessive intake of nutrients. The person who is obese, for example, is malnourished. Malnutrition also may result if the body cannot properly use the food it receives. For example, a child who has frequent bouts of diarrhea may be poorly nourished because the nutrients in the food he or she eats cannot be absorbed adequately from the intestinal tract.

Marginal nutritional status refers to a condition in which the store of a nutrient may be low and in which food consumption, laboratory data, and other indicators may be abnormal but there are no outward signs of impaired health. People in this nutritional state are considered to be at risk of nutritional deficiency, especially when subjected to stress such as surgery or infection. *Nutritional imbalance* refers to health problems arising from insufficient or excessive intakes of one nutrient or food component relative to another. For example, a high intake of phosphorous in a diet that is low in calcium may result in gradual loss of calcium from bone tissue because the body maintains a balance of these two nutrients in the bloodstream. Calcium that is not supplied in food is gradually leached from the bones.

ROLE OF NUTRITION IN GROWTH AND DEVELOPMENT

SKELETAL GROWTH AND SEXUAL DEVELOPMENT

Nutrients in food are required by the cells for growth, repair, rebuilding, and regulation of function. Retarded growth and delayed sexual development result from deficiencies of certain nutrients. Although heredity limits a person's ultimate build, the state of nutrition determines whether the person will achieve hereditary limits. The growth pattern of a child is a useful means for judging nutritional well-being. When a child is poorly nourished, the growth rate diminishes partly because of a delay in bone development. Both the quality of the bone (the amount of calcium and phosphorus it contains) and its capability for growth are influenced by nutrition.

Sexual maturity appears to occur later in populations that are malnourished than in developed countries. Furthermore, in developed countries, sexual maturity occurs at an earlier age in each succeeding generation.

MENTAL DEVELOPMENT

The most rapid growth of the brain occurs from 5 months before birth to 10 months after birth. At the end of the first year of life, the brain, the first organ to attain full development, has achieved 70% of its adult weight. Poorly nourished babies have fewer and smaller brain cells than babies who are adequately nourished. Whether inadequate nutrition in infants damages later intellectual development is unknown because it is difficult to separate the effects of nutrition on mental development from the effects of other factors, such as heredity, presence of disease, emotional state, and the home environment. Most studies, however, have indicated that early and severe malnutrition is an important factor in deficiencies in later mental development apart from social and hereditary influences. The effects of mild or moderate undernutrition on intellectual development are less clear.

Severe deficiencies of specific nutrients can cause adverse structural changes and impaired functioning of the central nervous system. Symptoms such as anxiety, irritability, depression, mental confusion, and physical and mental apathy are associated with certain deficiency diseases. Such symptoms most certainly influence learning ability. Infants with iron deficiency score lower on the Bayley Scale of Mental Development. Iron deficiency anemia among schoolchildren may interfere with motivation and the ability to concentrate for extended periods. A study conducted by the National Heart, Lung, and Blood Institute suggested that iron deficiency states may cause a reduction in iron-containing enzymes in brain tissue, which in turn causes alterations in brain function.

Hunger, the unpleasant sensation of stomach pangs caused by insufficient food intake, can affect learning. Hungry children are distracted by their hunger pangs and are unable to pay attention and respond to educational stimulation. Although many factors influence behavior, it is safe to assume that poorly nourished people who tire easily, have little energy, and are unable to concentrate will have difficulty achieving their intellectual potential.

MALNUTRITION, ILLNESS, AND CHRONIC DISEASE

The severe undernutrition that health workers are most likely to see is the result of illness. Many illnesses interfere with appetite or with the body's ability to use food. Surveys have indicated that malnutrition is widespread among clients hospitalized more than 2 weeks. Undernourished people do not tolerate illness well. They show delayed wound healing, are particularly susceptible to infection and complications of illness, and may be unable to withstand demanding medical treatments. In a study of 200 patients admitted to a health care facility, 73% developed pressure sores despite good nursing care. Those who developed pressure sores had lower nutrient intakes than those who did not. More attention is being focused on maintaining or improving the nutritional status of clients in hospitals and other health agencies.

Other cases of severe undernutrition are the result of ignorance, extreme poverty, neglect, mental illness, or unusual environmental conditions. Although severe malnutrition is not widespread in the United States, it does exist. Malnutrition is considered a contributing factor in the high death tolls among children of migrant farmers, among American Indians, and among elderly people.

Babies born to poorly nourished women and teenagers are likely to have a low birth weight, the cause of about half of all infant deaths. Those babies who survive are about twice as likely to have physical, mental, and developmental disabilities.

Most problems of nutritional deficiency in the United States are moderate in severity. Although this undernutrition is not severe enough to threaten their lives, malnourished children grow at a slower rate and are more susceptible to infection than well-nourished children.

Overnutrition, not deficiency, is responsible for the major nutrition problems in the United States today. A number of chronic diseases have been linked to diet. Many scientists believe that diets high in fat and cholesterol promote *atherosclerosis* (a form of hardening of the arteries), which is the underlying cause of most heart attacks and strokes. *Hypertension* (high blood pressure) has been associated with a high intake of salt, obesity, and the use of alcohol. Hypertension also increases the risk of stroke and heart disease. Obesity makes some people more susceptible to a type of diabetes mellitus that does not require treatment with insulin. A high percentage (10% to 20%) of people who consume large quantities of alcohol for extended periods develop *cirrhosis of the liver,* a serious, frequently fatal disease characterized by fatty deposits in the liver and damaged liver cells. Lack of fiber in the diet has been associated with the incidence of colon cancer and also blamed for the high occurrence of *diverticulosis,* a condition in which abnormal sacs form at points of weakness in the intestinal wall. Furthermore, diet is a basic factor in tooth decay, one of the most widespread of all chronic diseases.

MALNUTRITION WORLDWIDE

Undernutrition is widespread in the developing countries of the world. It is estimated that 400 million people suffer from serious nutritional deficiencies. In Asia, Africa, and Latin America, 25% to 30% of the population suffers from semistarvation. Millions more suffer from a serious deficiency of a specific nutrient such as iron, iodine, or vitamin A (Fig. 2-1).

Children are hardest hit. Working together, nutritional deficiency and infection create a vicious cycle. The poorly nourished child is highly susceptible to infection, and infections are more severe and last longer in a malnourished than in a well-nourished child. The child is then more vulnerable to the next infectious disease to which he or she is exposed. The annual death toll due to common childhood diseases is extremely high in developing countries—15 million children younger than age 5 years. This number represents one fourth of all the deaths throughout the world.

NUTRITION ASSESSMENT: MEASURING NUTRITIONAL STATUS

Well-nourished people have a general appearance of vitality and well-being. They are alert, have sufficient energy to perform physical activities, and recover rapidly from periods of stress. A lack of these attributes, however, is not necessarily due to inadequate nutrition; it could be caused by nonnutritional factors such as a lack of rest or emotional stress.

Because the symptoms of malnutrition tend to be vague and difficult to detect in the United States, the well-nourished appearance of some clients may be misleading with regard to their ability to withstand physical stress. Evaluation of an individual's nutritional status should be done as part of a routine health checkup. In particular, the nutritional needs of high-risk clients such as elderly people, people scheduled for surgery, clients with cancer, people with chronic disease, or those people living in deprived environments should be monitored. Nutritional assessment also is conducted on groups of people to determine which problems are likely to exist in a given population or age group.

How do we determine whether an individual is well nourished? The physician, registered dietitian, or other health professional trained in the diagnosis of nutrition problems uses a number of tools to measure an individual's nutritional status, including the medical and social history, clinical examination, biochemical measurements (laboratory data), food intake records and diet

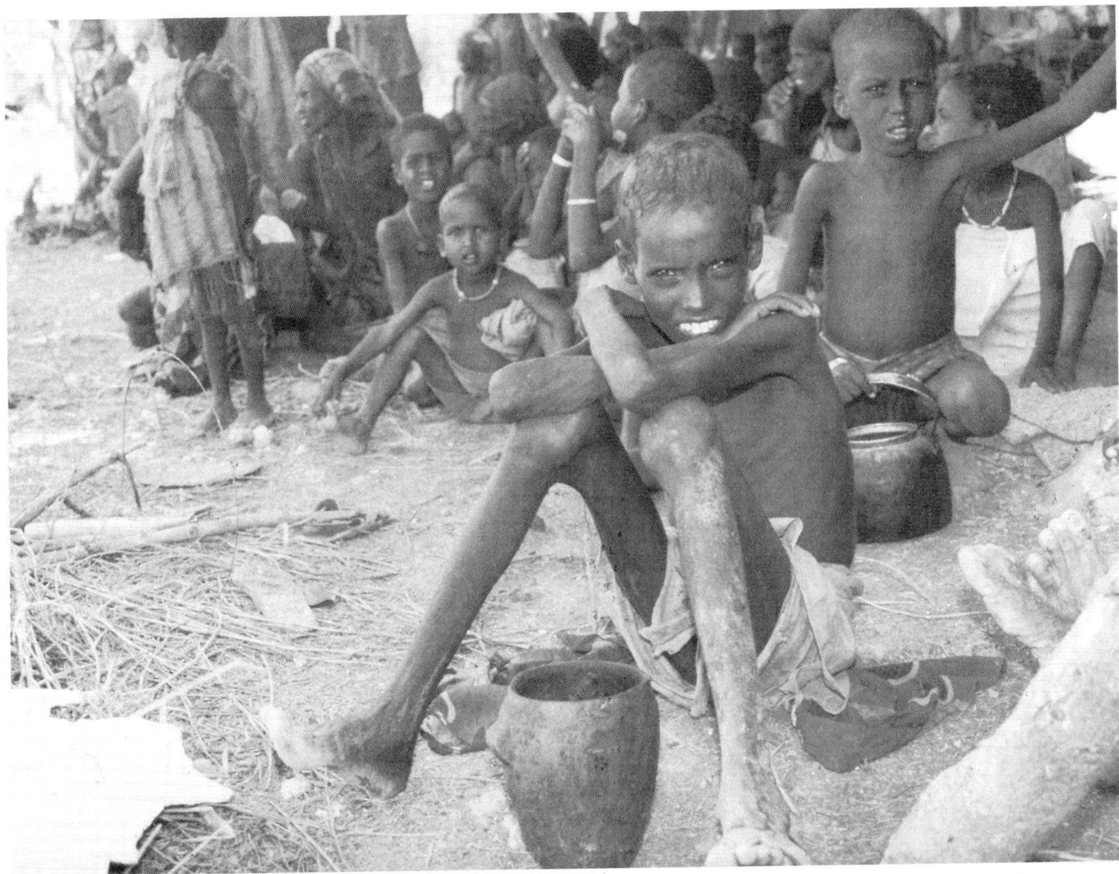

FIGURE 2-1

Severe undernutrition is widespread in the developing countries. Children are hardest hit, frequently caught in a vicious cycle of nutritional deficiency and infection. *(Courtesy US Dept of Agriculture.)*

history, and, if appropriate, radiographic (x-ray) studies.

The measurement of these indicators of nutritional status is called *nutrition assessment.* The health professional uses the data obtained from these measurements to evaluate the client's nutritional status and to determine the possible causes of any existing nutrition problems. These data form the basis from which goals and objectives of nutrition care are developed and to which progress is compared (see Chapter 20).

Assessment may be a brief screening when time and resources are limited or a comprehensive gathering of information. *Nutrition screening* is a process of identifying individuals who have characteristics that are known to be associated with nutrition problems—clients who are potentially at high risk. Those clients identified at high risk are given a more in-depth assessment, which includes most or all of the components discussed previously.

Criteria used in screening must be simple, relatively straightforward, and easy to administer. The idea is to take a few critical measurements that are strongly associated with malnutrition as a means of identifying those clients at nutritional risk. These critical measurements might include height, weight, unintentional weight loss, change in appetite, and serum albumin level. Each of the components of a nutrition assessment is discussed as follows.

CLINICAL EXAMINATION

MEDICAL HISTORY AND PHYSICAL SIGNS

A person's medical history can provide many clues about nutritional status. Does the person have a history of hypertension, alcoholism, recent weight loss or gain, recent surgery, or physical disabilities? What drugs is he or she taking that might interact with nutrients? Social data such as educational background, occupation, and family environment usually are included. Many circumstances of a person's life can affect nutritional status.

During the physical examination, the examiner looks for physical signs and symptoms associated with malnutrition (Table 2-1). Examination of skin, mouth, and eyes is particularly important. The cells in these tissues are replaced at a high rate, so signs of malnutrition appear more quickly in these tissues. Easily plucked hair, scaling skin, and sores at the corners of the mouth or eyelids are examples of signs that may be associated with nutritional deficiencies. The examiner also asks the client questions about how he or she functions and feels. Most symptoms of malnutrition indicate two or more nutrient deficiencies.

Because signs associated with malnutrition also can be attributed to other causes, the examiner must interpret physical findings in light of other data, such as laboratory findings and diet history. For example, easily plucked hair might be caused by malnutrition, a hormone imbalance, or chemotherapy. Vital signs such as pulse rate, respiration, temperature, and blood pressure provide additional physical data.

ANTHROPOMETRIC MEASUREMENTS

Anthropometrics are body measurements such as height, weight, skinfold thickness, and midarm circumference (MAC) that reflect growth and development or an increase or decrease in body fat and muscle tissue. The measurements taken on an individual are compared with standard measurements for people of the same sex and age. Standards are based on measurements taken on large numbers of people. They are most reliable when they are taken on people of the same race and geographic location as those being measured.

Anthropometric measurements are especially useful when compared with the individual's own measurements taken previously. Repeated measurements on an individual can be used to evaluate the degree of change in nutritional status over time. Most changes take 3 to 4 weeks to become evident.

Anthropometric measurements are relatively easy to perform and require little equipment. Their accuracy and usefulness, however, are limited by poor techniques, inaccurate measuring equipment, incorrect readings, or inaccurate recording. Obtaining accurate measurements requires skill, which is developed through practice.

HEIGHT AND WEIGHT

Children

Growth rate is largely the result of nutritional status and certain hormonal functions. Because nutritional deficiency can result in retarded growth, nutrition problems may be detected when a child's height and weight are compared with those of other children of the same sex, age, and body build. Growth charts have been devised by the National Center for Health Statistics (NCHS) for this purpose (see Fig. 17-3). If a child's measurements differ substantially from standard measurements, nutrition problems should be suspected. The chance of a problem increases substantially if a single measurement falls above the 95th percentile or below the 5th percentile on the NCHS charts. Although heredity influences the linear growth of children, the height of parents is rarely the cause of height below the 5th percentile.

A child's own height and weight measurements taken periodically give the greatest insight into health status. The trends in growth revealed by these periodic measurements can detect abnormal growth, monitor nutritional status, and give evidence of the effects of medical treatment. A child

TABLE 2-1 Signs Associated With Malnutrition

Criterion	Normal	Possible Malnutrition
Growth, body size	Normal rate of growth in children Normal weight for height, frame size, age in adults	Failure to increase in stature or to gain weight Excessive fatness or thinness, sudden gain or loss of weight
Muscular and skeletal systems	Good muscle tone; can walk or run without pain	Wasted muscles; infant's skull bones are thin and soft; delayed closing of soft spots (fontanelles) on infant's head; beading of ribs; knock-knees or bowlegs; bleeding into muscle; inability to get up or walk properly; calf tenderness
Hair	Shiny, firm, not easily plucked	Lusterless, dry, thin, sparse; easily plucked; changes in pigmentation occurring in distinct bands
Skin	Clear, slightly moist; pink mucous membranes	Dry and flaky; sandpaper feel; red swollen pigmentation of exposed areas; excessive bruising; pinpoint hemorrhages
Lips	Smooth, not chapped or swollen	Puffy, swollen; grooves at corners of the mouth
Nails	Firm, pink, smooth	Spoon shaped, brittle, ridged, pale nail beds
Face	Skin color uniform; smooth, not swollen	Pale; skin dark over cheeks and under eyes; skin flaky around nose and mouth; scaling around nostrils
Mouth	Pink tongue with surface papillae (small projections from the mucous membrane that covers the tongue); not swollen Pink, firm, nonbleeding, nonswollen gums Bright teeth, no pain, no cavities	Tongue pale or raw, scarlet red or purplish red; smooth in appearance (papillae not evident); sores on tongue Spongy, swollen; bleed easily; receding from tooth line Mottled (gray or black spots); cavities; reduced sense of taste and smell
Eyes	Bright, clear, shiny; no sores at corners of eyelids; no prominent blood vessels	Pale or red eye membranes; redness and fissuring of eyelid corners; dryness of eye membranes; dull appearance of cornea; ring of fine blood vessels around cornea
Glands	Face, neck not swollen	Enlarged thyroid (front of neck); enlarged parotid (cheeks appear swollen)
Behavior	Alert, energetic, good attention span, cheerful, productive	Listlessness; tendency to tire easily; inability to concentrate; irritability, nervousness; poor work capacity
Cardiovascular system	Normal heart rate and rhythm, normal blood pressure	Rapid heart rate; abnormal rhythm; elevated blood pressure; labored breathing
Gastrointestinal system	No palpable organs or masses (in children liver edge may be felt); normal digestion and elimination; good appetite	Liver enlargement; indigestion; diarrhea or constipation; poor appetite
Nervous system	Normal reflexes and vibratory sense; good coordination; psychological stability	Reduced knee and ankle reflexes; loss of position and vibratory sense; burning and tingling of hands and feet; weakness and tenderness of muscles; poor coordination; paralysis of eye muscles; mental irritability and confusion
Immune system	Resistant to infection	Frequent infections such as colds; poor wound healing; slow convalescence

who shows steady growth along the 5th percentile may be in a normal growth pattern. However, the weight shift of an infant from the 50th to 95th percentile in a few months may signal the danger of becoming obese.

Up to age 2 years, length is measured while the child is *recumbent* (in a reclining position), preferably on a measuring board. For children older than 2 years, *stature* (height while standing) is measured using a measuring device or a nonstretchable tape attached to a vertical flat surface. A right-angle headboard also is needed. Extension rods to measure height found on most clinical scales are unreliable.

Accurate weight measurements require the use of a beam scale with nondetachable weights. Infants and young children are weighed while lying down on a pan-type pediatric scale. Older children are weighed on a platform beam scale. The scale should be checked and adjusted frequently, if necessary, at zero weight on the beam. Figure 2-2 shows measuring methods.

Adults

Once adult height has been reached, changes in body weight are useful in evaluating nutritional status. Platform beam scales should be used to measure weight.

The height of an adult should also be measured. Asking adults to recall their height is not a good practice because previous measurements may have been inaccurate. Also, men tend to overestimate and women tend to underestimate their height. Equipment for measuring standing height is the same as that used for children. When the person being measured is taller than the measurer, the measurer should stand on a stool so that an accurate measurement can be made. Measuring rods on platform scales are not as accurate as a measuring device attached to a vertical surface.

The height of people who are bedridden or in a wheelchair can be estimated from arm span measurement. For people with spinal deformity such as the elderly person with *kyphosis* (curvature of the spine causing hunching or stooping), knee height may be a more reliable guide for estimating stature. Mathematical formulas are used to estimate height from these measurements.[1] (See Display 19-1 on page 384.)

Height–Weight Tables

Height and weight tables, such as the Metropolitan Life Insurance tables (see Appendix A), may be used to evaluate an individual's weight as it corresponds to his or her height. Which tables best represent ideal body weight is a controversial subject. The policies of the individual health care facility determines which set of tables is used. Because ideal weight for height differs depending on a person's frame size, it is useful to estimate frame size using wrist circumference or elbow breadth. These methods are detailed in Displays 2-1 and 2-2.

Body Mass Index

Body mass index (BMI) has been recommended by experts as the preferred means of evaluating the health of individuals. The BMI is the body weight in kilograms divided by height in meters squared. Display 23-1 gives formulas for determining the BMI using either kilograms and meters or pounds and inches. The index relates well to body fat content. The BMI ranges associated with the lowest risk to health are 22 to 25. The BMIs at various heights and weights are given in Table 23-1.

Percent Usual Body Weight

Comparing current weight with usual body weight frequently is a more useful guide than ideal body weight. This is especially true when evaluating the effects of illness, such as rapid unintentional weight loss or a weight increase due to water retention. The percentage of usual body weight can be determined by dividing the actual weight by the usual weight as follows:

$$\%\text{ usual body weight} = \frac{\text{actual weight}}{\text{usual weight}} \times 100$$

[1] Chumlea WC, Roche AF, Mukherjee D. Nutritional assessment of the elderly through anthropometry. Columbus, OH: Ross Laboratories, 1988.

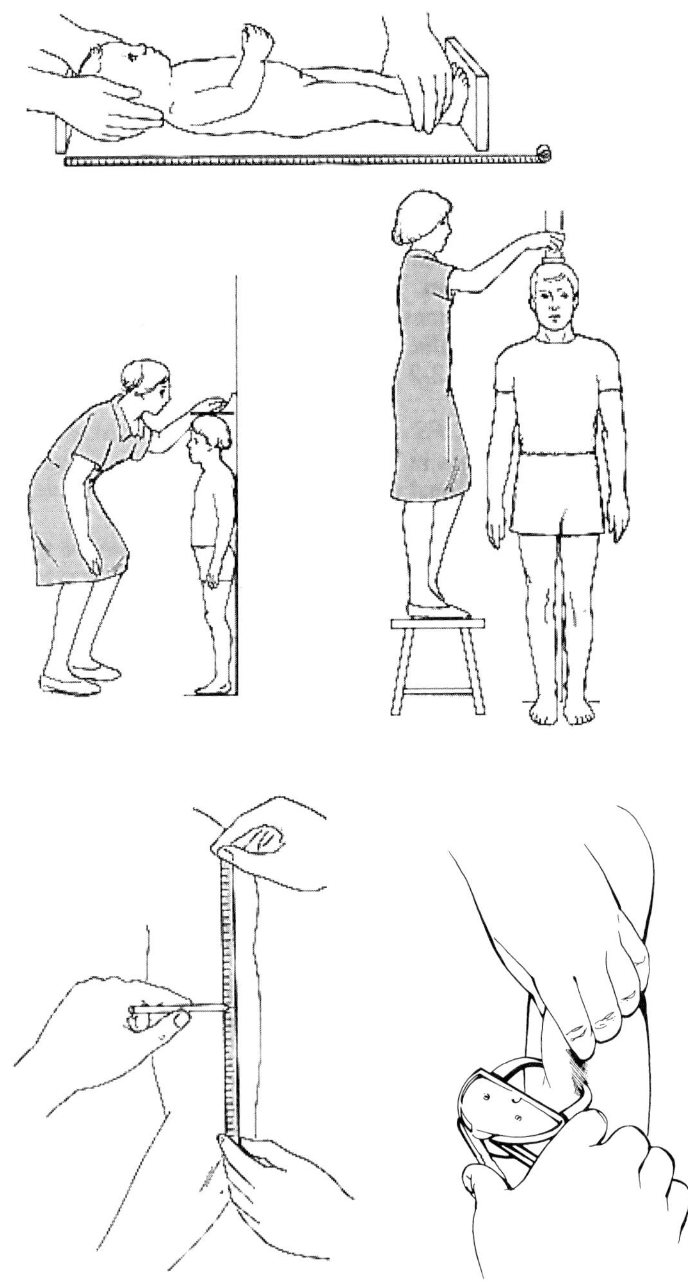

FIGURE 2-2

Techniques of anthropometric measurements.

DISPLAY 2-1 ESTIMATING BODY FRAME SIZE USING THE HEIGHT/WRIST CIRCUMFERENCE RATIO (R)

Divide the height in centimeters by the wrist circumference in centimeters. The wrist of the nondominant arm is measured where it bends. (To convert height in inches to centimeters, multiply by 2.54.)

$$r = \frac{\text{height (cm)}}{\text{wrist circumference (cm)}}$$

Compare the results to the following table:

FRAME	MALE *R*	FEMALE *R*
Small	>10.4	>11.0
Medium	9.6–10.4	10.1–11.0
Large	<9.6	<10.0

An unplanned and recent weight loss or gain of 10% or more requires further evaluation.

HEAD CIRCUMFERENCE

Head circumference is an important measurement when assessing infants and children younger than age 3 years. Although head circumference measurements can reflect the effect of nutrition on brain growth, abnormal head growth usually is due to nonnutritional factors.

When measuring head circumference, the tape is positioned just above the eyebrows, above the ears, and around the prominent bony structure at the back of the head, the largest occipitofrontal circumference. Several measurements should be made to determine the largest.

DISPLAY 2-2 ESTIMATING BODY FRAME SIZE USING ELBOW BREADTH

Extend the arm and bend the forearm upward at a 90° angle. Keep the fingers straight and turn the inside of the wrist toward the body. Place the thumb and index finger of the other hand on the two prominent bones on either side of the elbow. Measure the space between the fingers against a ruler or a tape measure.* Compare this measurement with the measurements shown below.

This table lists the elbow measurements for men and women of medium frame at various heights. Measurements lower than those listed indicate that you have a small frame, whereas higher measurements indicate a large frame.

HEIGHT IN 1-IN HEELS (IN)	ELBOW BREADTH (IN)	HEIGHT IN 2.5-CM HEELS (CM)	ELBOW BREADTH (CM)
MEN			
62–63	$2\frac{1}{2}$–$2\frac{7}{8}$	158–161	6.4–7.2
64–67	$2\frac{5}{8}$–$2\frac{7}{8}$	162–171	6.7–7.4
68–71	$2\frac{3}{4}$–3	172–181	6.9–7.6
72–75	$2\frac{3}{4}$–$3\frac{1}{8}$	182–191	7.1–7.8
76	$2\frac{7}{8}$–$3\frac{1}{4}$	192–193	7.4–8.1
WOMEN			
58–59	$2\frac{1}{4}$–$2\frac{1}{2}$	148–151	5.6–6.4
60–63	$2\frac{1}{4}$–$2\frac{1}{2}$	152–161	5.8–6.5
64–67	$2\frac{3}{8}$–$2\frac{5}{8}$	162–171	5.9–6.6
68–71	$2\frac{3}{8}$–$2\frac{5}{8}$	172–181	6.1–6.8
72	$2\frac{1}{2}$–$2\frac{3}{4}$	182–183	6.2–6.9

* For the most accurate measurement, measure the elbow breadth with a caliper.

(Source of basic data: 1979 Build Study, Society of Actuaries and Association of Life Insurance Medical Directors of America, 1980. Reprinted from Metropolitan Life Insurance Company, Medical Department, Health and Safety Education Division. Copyright 1993, 1900 Metropolitan Life Insurance Company).

SKINFOLD THICKNESSES

Skinfold thickness is a measurement of a double layer of skin and subcutaneous fat that accounts for about half the fat in the body. Skinfold thickness measurements are a more accurate estimate of fatness than body weight, because weight includes not only fat but also muscle mass, water, and bone components, which can change unpredictably. These measurements are most reliable when taken from several body sites. Triceps, biceps, and subscapular and suprailiac skinfold measurements are most commonly used.

The width of the fat layer is measured with a device called a *skinfold caliper* (see Fig. 2–2). Skinfold thickness measurements are compared with averages for people of the same age and sex or with the client's previous measurements. The amount and rate of change over time can help determine whether the client is malnourished or how well the client is recovering after treatment. Periodic measurements are most useful in the management of infants, children, and adults with undernutrition or overnutrition and in the follow-up of disease status.

The *triceps skinfold thickness (TSF)* is the most frequently used fatfold measurement. The TSF is measured on the back of the nondominant (usually the left) arm, midway between the shoulder and elbow. Using a flexible, nonstretchable tape, the midpoint between the shoulder and elbow at the back of the arm is located and marked. Slightly above this midpoint, the health worker gently pulls the skinfold away from underlying muscle tissue and holds it in a vertical fold of skin and subcutaneous fat with the thumb and index finger. The jaws of the caliper are placed over the fold at the midpoint mark. The jaws are closed and the TSF is read from the dial.

MIDARM AND MIDARM MUSCLE CIRCUMFERENCES

The midarm circumference (*MAC*) measures muscle mass and subcutaneous fat. At the midpoint of the upper arm, the arm circumference is measured with a flexible, nonstretchable tape. The tape is drawn snugly but not so tight as to make an indentation. The MAC is not a reliable indicator of nutritional status when used alone. This measurement is usually taken because it is needed to calculate the *midarm muscle circumference (MAMC)*. The MAMC is a means of indirectly estimating the midarm muscle mass. This measurement provides an estimate of the amount of skeletal muscle that decreases in protein malnutrition.

MAMC is calculated from the TSF and the MAC using the following formula: Divide the TSF in millimeters by 10 to convert to centimeters. Then,

$$\text{MAMC (cm)} = \text{MAC (cm)} - [3.14 \times \text{TSF (cm)}]$$

The measurement obtained is compared with standards for the MAMC and to previous measurements to determine change. Measurements below the 10th percentile indicate a lack of protein.

LABORATORY DATA

Blood, urine, and stool tests reveal much about what foods have been eaten, the quantity of certain nutrients in body stores, and how the nutrients are being used. A low blood level of a particular nutrient may suggest that the body is poorly nourished in regard to that nutrient. Certain blood tests, for example, indicate the adequacy of iron intake. Laboratory tests frequently signal a nutrition problem before outward symptoms appear.

The following are tests used most commonly to determine nutritional status in hospitalized patients:

Serum albumin levels—Measurement of the amount of this main protein in the blood is used to determine protein status.

Serum transferrin levels—The amount of this iron-carrying protein in the blood increases above normal if iron stores are low; it decreases when the body is lacking protein.

Total lymphocyte count—The count of white blood cells, which defend the body against infection, is a measure of the body's immune function, and may or may not reflect nutritional status. When protein intake is inadequate, the lymphocyte count decreases.

Creatinine excretion levels—Creatinine is a substance that comes from the breakdown of creatine, which is found mainly in muscle tissue. The level of creatinine excretion in the urine reflects the amount of skeletal muscle mass. If muscle mass is depleted as a result of malnutrition, creatinine excretion is less than normal.

IMMUNOLOGIC MEASUREMENTS

Antigen skin testing is a test of the body's immune system. Organisms to which most people are immune are injected under the skin. A reaction that develops on the skin surface indicates that the immune system is working. Deficiencies of calories, protein, and individual nutrients have been associated with a depressed immune system. Other factors, however, such as age, allergies, and chemotherapy, can interfere with the body's immune response. The total lymphocyte count (discussed previously) is also an indicator of the body's immune response.

RADIOGRAPHIC STUDIES

Radiographic studies are a useful tool in determining whether bones have developed as would be expected for age. Nutrition influences the size and quality of bone as well as its rate of development. Radiographs of the wrist bones of children are particularly useful. These bones appear earlier and develop earlier in well-nourished children than in poorly nourished children. Films are also useful in detecting bone deformities caused by nutritional deficiency diseases such as rickets and scurvy. These abnormalities are the result of deficient intake that has existed for a long time.

DIET HISTORY AND FOOD INTAKE RECORDS

Information about the client's eating habits signals the possibility of malnutrition, serves as a check on the findings of the physical examination and laboratory tests, and provides a basis for making changes in eating habits, if necessary. Information about a client's food intake can be obtained through diet recall, the food diary, and the food frequency record.

A *diet recall* is a record based on the client's remembrance of food items eaten during the previous 24 hours (Display 2-3). A *food diary* is a record of specific foods and the quantities consumed over a certain period, usually 3 to 7 days. The information is recorded in the diary as soon as possible after the food has been eaten. A *food frequency record* is a list of food items on which the client indicates how frequently he or she consumes each item. It may be used together with a diet recall or food diary as a means of cross-checking to provide as complete and accurate a picture as possible. After an estimate of food intake is obtained, it is compared with a recognized standard to determine the likelihood of deficiency or excess.

In a health care facility, a dietitian or physician may request that a detailed 24-hour food intake record be kept for a client for a period of days. This record should indicate all foods and liquids consumed at meals and between meals and any foods obtained from other sources, such as visiting family and friends. The amount of food and fluid left on the tray is subtracted from the amount initially served. Nutrients obtained in intravenous feedings and nutrient supplements are also included.

While obtaining a diet history, a skillful interviewer tries to elicit information about environmental, cultural, economic, and behavioral factors that may affect nutritional status. Poverty, food fads, lack of family support, and mental disturbance are examples of factors that can significantly influence nutritional status.

Through questioning and the analysis of the food intake records, the dietitian determines the usual pattern of eating, its nutritional quality, the number of meals eaten away from home—what are these foods and where are they obtained—and how heavily the individual relies on convenience foods. Other important determinations involve level of physical activity, the setting of meals and with

DISPLAY 2-3 FORMS USED TO ASSESS FOOD INTAKE

DIET RECALL

What foods do you choose for your usual meals and snacks?

Morning ______________________
Noon ______________________
Night ______________________
Snacks ______________________

What specific foods have you eaten in the past 24 hours?

Morning ______________________
Noon ______________________
Night ______________________
Snacks ______________________

FOOD FREQUENCY CHECKLIST

HOW OFTEN HAVE YOU EATEN THE FOLLOWING FOODS?	NEVER LESS THAN 1 TIME PER WEEK	1–2 TIMES PER WEEK	MORE THAN 3–7 TIMES PER WEEK	ONCE A DAY
MILK (8 OZ)				
Whole				
2% fat				
1% fat				
Skim				
Chocolate				
JUICES (4 OZ)				
Citrus (orange, grapefruit)				

FOOD DIARY

TIME B—BEGIN F—FINISH	FOOD	AMOUNT	KCAL	PLACE	ACTIVITY (TV, READING, ETC.)	POSITION S—SITTING ST—STANDING R—RECLINING	MOOD*	DEGREE OF HUNGER, 0–5

* A, angry; B, bored; D, depressed; H, happy; N, neutral; Ner, nervous; T, tired.

whom, and, if obesity is present, is it due to poor choices, small excesses or compulsive eating. Also determined is the impact of psychosocial factors such as family support, stress level, educational level, previous nutrition education, financial status, and attitudes toward health and eating behavior.

The dietitian adds the dietary data to the nutrition-related factors in the client's medical record. From this composite of information, he or she together with the client and other health team members develops the goals and objectives of nutrition care (see Chapter 20).

PSYCHOLOGICAL IMPORTANCE OF FOOD

Assessing an individual's need for food does not stop with an understanding of the role of food and eating in fulfilling the person's physical needs.

This assessment also includes an understanding of the role of food and eating in fulfilling the person's psychological and emotional needs. Sociologists have expressed concern about the lack in many homes of family-centered meals. At all socioeconomic levels, fewer meals are being eaten at home or in a family setting. It is believed that this practice could seriously weaken the stability of the family, the most basic and important institution in our society. As one sociologist put it, "The family that eats together stays together." Although this concern focuses on children, the psychological aspects of eating are equally important for elderly people. Food intake has a tremendous impact on the quality of life of elderly people—over and above its impact on health. "Eating is one of the greatest pleasures in old age and one of the most important ties to life."[2]

You may wonder how these concerns relate to your study of nutrition and ultimately to your health career. Perhaps you already know, because it does not take a long association with hospitalized people to appreciate the significance of meals to them. Hospitalized clients spend considerable time choosing menus, anticipating meals, and evaluating the food served them. In the anxiety that accompanies illness and hospitalization, food and food service assume great importance. To the client and family, who may not understand the intricate tests and treatments that have been prescribed, the client's appetite and food acceptance may be one of the best indicators of progress.

People attach particular meanings to food. These meanings reflect a person's values and beliefs and are strongly influenced by social factors. In nonindustrialized societies, custom is an important influence. In Western countries, fashion and accepted modes of behavior, strengthened by advertising and other commercial techniques, are powerful forces in food selection.

The health worker soon learns that teaching clients the concepts of nutrition does not guarantee that they will put them into practice. Health workers need an acute awareness of the meaning of food if they are to be successful in helping others meet their nutritional needs. If changes in eating habits are necessary, they must be in harmony with the meanings that food holds for individuals.

PSYCHOSOCIAL FACTORS

From the beginning of life, food and the act of eating play a vital role in growth and development. A newborn's entire world centers around the eating–feeding situation. It is the basic experience through which newborns perceive the world around them and through which they establish their most important relationship—with their mother or other care-giver. Ideally, this early eating–feeding experience conveys feelings of warmth, tenderness, and love.

As children grow, attitudes and feelings continue to be communicated to them through food. The family mealtime is an important means of affording all members a sense of togetherness and unity. Mealtime establishes family relationships, and through it some cultural patterns are passed from one generation to the next. Mealtime also provides an occasion for parents and children to interact and share and develop understanding.

In adulthood, warm human relationships also are fostered when food is offered. Food—even just a cup of tea or coffee—is a symbol of hospitality. We honor our friends by inviting them to eat with us. In most cultures, for a family to share a meal with someone is a strong expression of social acceptance and commitment. When a person fell from favor in ancient China, his rice bowl was broken and he was no longer permitted to eat with the family or group.

Problems arise when mealtime is no longer shared. Aloneness is said to be the great tragedy of aging. Eating alone, as many elderly people must,

[2] Schlettwein-Gsell D. Nutrition and the quality of life: a measure for the outcome of nutritional intervention. Am J Clin Nutr 1992;55:1265S.

dampens the appetite and the motivation to prepare meals. To meet the problem of aloneness faced by the hospitalized person, many hospitals and other health care facilities encourage clients to eat in the company of others by making available dining rooms where clients can eat together. Many communities offer group mealtimes for elderly people, providing social contacts for people who otherwise would be isolated.

Reward and punishment and anxiety and depression also find expression in ways that center around food. A child's behavior may be rewarded or punished by the giving or withholding of a prized dessert or sweet. Adults may reward themselves after a particularly trying day by eating a special food or eating out. Some people react to anxiety by overeating, whereas others lose their appetite. During intensive study for an examination, for example, a student may take frequent snack breaks not because of hunger but to seek relief from tension.

CULTURAL FACTORS

Acquiring food is a basic need. How people meet this need, however, varies greatly among cultural groups. According to Niehoff, *culture* "is a system of customs transmitted from one generation to the other, mainly by means of language. And among these customs none is more significant than the ways of procuring and consuming food" (p. 54). Culture is learned, beginning with the earliest childhood experiences.

It is as important to consider cultural differences in this country as it is when dealing with a person from a foreign country. In days past, people in the United States tended to resist the idea that there are important differences separating people. The revival of interest in American Indians, African Americans, Italian Americans, and the increased cultural diversity has helped to overcome this tendency and to make us more aware of cultural differences.

What is considered acceptable food by one society may be deemed inedible by another. Undoubtedly, the kinds and quantities of food available in a particular locality and the economic capacity to obtain foods are important influences. Certain plants, animals, and insects may be commonly eaten in some cultures but considered taboo in others. Most Americans react negatively to the idea of eating insects, which are widely consumed by other peoples. Indians who were starving because of a lack of rice found the wheat offered by the United States an unacceptable substitute. In World War II, Japanese prisoners became ill when they first tried to eat the food prepared by their American captors. Only in extreme circumstances will people eat something that they consider inedible.

Every food in a given culture is endowed with meaning. Sometimes the meanings associated with a particular food are dramatic—for example, Americans attach vivid symbolism to such words and phrases as *Thanksgiving turkey, champagne, birthday cake,* and *Fourth of July picnic.* Differences in sex, age, and level of sophistication also may be expressed through food likes and dislikes. A jellied fruit salad may be considered feminine fare, whereas a steak-and-potatoes meal may provoke thoughts of strength and manliness. Peanut butter sandwiches and hot dogs are thought to be the delight of children, whereas artichokes and lobster are more likely the choice of the sophisticated adult. Even the relation between food intake and body weight is interpreted culturally. In some societies, overweight is considered natural and a sign of well-being, whereas the slim, almost skeletonlike figure is held as desirable in others.

Religious beliefs frequently find expression in food customs. Fasting is common to many religions. Certain foods may be forbidden, such as pork to the Orthodox Jew and Muslim and beef to the Hindu. Closely akin to eating habits related to religious beliefs are those associated with a life philosophy, such as the yoga diet or macrobiotics. Some people do not eat meat for philosophical reasons. Strong emotional factors are involved in the choice of these patterns.

FOOD BELIEFS AND HEALTH PRACTICES

Many cultures around the world use food and herbs as therapy for illness. Display 2-4 lists foods used as home remedies by people from the Dominican

DISPLAY 2-4 FOODS FREQUENTLY USED AS HOME REMEDIES BY PEOPLE FROM THE DOMINICAN REPUBLIC

FOOD	TO CURE
Honey with onions, garlic, castor oil, snake oil, or cod fish oil (mixture)	Asthma and chest colds
Honey with lemon	Colds, sore throat
Garlic tea	High blood pressure
Sweet and sour water	To calm nerves
Hot milk with cinnamon	For low blood pressure
Anise tea	Gas, bloating, infant colic
Grass ground up with salt	Skin warts

Republic. In a study of 200 Korean American women attending a prenatal clinic of a large New York City hospital, 20% avoided eating blemished fruit and 3% avoided chicken. These practices were based on the beliefs that blemished fruit might produce an infant with skin disease or an unpleasant face and that the child might have prickly skin if chicken were eaten.[3]

Another example of the effect of cultural beliefs on eating habits is a type of folk medicine practiced among Latin American people known as the *hot–cold theory of disease.* Many Puerto Ricans living in the United States, especially elderly people and recent immigrants, believe in this system of disease. Diseases, as well as medications and foods, are grouped into hot and cold classes. Illnesses such as arthritis and colds, which are classified as *frio* (cold), are treated with hot medications and foods, whereas *caliente* (hot) illnesses, such as rashes and ulcers, are treated with cool substances. The temperature of the food or medications is not necessarily related to its classification. For example, hot linden tea is considered a cool food, whereas cold beer, because of its alcoholic content, is considered hot.

It is not difficult to imagine how these beliefs can conflict with medical advice. Puerto Rican mothers have been known to discontinue feeding formula, a hot food, in favor of cool foods such as whole milk or barley water when their infants develop rashes.

[3] Ludman EK, Kang KJ, Lynn LL. Food beliefs and diets of pregnant Korean-American women. J Am Diet Assoc 1992;92:12:1519.

YOUR PERSONAL FOOD PREFERENCES

Everyone accepts certain foods and rejects others for different reasons. What are your feelings about food? Do peanut butter and jelly sandwiches give you a comfortable feeling when you are worried or anxious? Maybe they remind you of an earlier time when you felt more secure and life was less complicated. Is chocolate cake a favorite dessert, perhaps because you associate it with special family celebrations? Are peas on your hate list because you were forced to eat them when you were a child? Or, perhaps, you dislike lamb because your father would not eat it, so your mother never served it.

If you have insight into your own food likes and dislikes, you will be less likely to impose your feelings on others. Moreover, you will have greater understanding and respect for preferences that differ from your own. If you are aware that you dislike lamb because it is unfamiliar to you, you are unlikely to make an unpleasant remark about the lamb being served on a client's tray. Similarly, you will be understanding of the client who uses olive oil to flavor his vegetables and the one who refuses her tray because it includes bacon. Every individual has had particular life experiences that have contributed to the formation of eating habits. This is as true for health workers as it is for the people they serve.

WHAT THE CLIENT'S EATING BEHAVIOR TELLS YOU

By their responses to food, clients may be telling you that they are worried and afraid or that they feel insecure. Clients may express their feelings by being fussy about food, by lack of appetite, or by demands for extra attention. Hospitalized clients may feel a greater need to have favorite foods that give them a feeling of comfort or security. They may make requests for custards and puddings or extra servings of milk, foods associated with infancy or childhood—periods of dependency and security. Some adults may refuse these same foods, despite their nutritional value, because, to them, the foods symbolize their dependency on others during illness, and they fear the loss of their independence. When under stress and in need of psychological reward, some people eat too many sweets and desserts, foods that are frequently associated with rewards for good behavior in childhood. Others may express their discouragement through anorexia. Providing for groups of clients to eat together in a dining room or solarium can help stimulate the appetite. When anxieties are shared, problems may seem less threatening.

By their eating behaviors, clients may indicate that they are dissatisfied because the hospital foods and meal patterns are so different from those to which they are accustomed. This is especially true for clients with strong cultural preferences. Or, clients may be telling us that their modified diets are depressing reminders of the incurable nature of their chronic diseases. To be denied the pleasures of eating food with seasonings they like and to keep reminding themselves that they cannot have them is not easy to accept.

Health workers need to be aware of what food means to clients under different circumstances. Nurses who are aware of how their clients communicate through food will be better able to help them. If changes in eating habits are necessary for the client's health, these changes must respect his or her psychological as well as physical needs. Food is more than nourishment for the body; it feeds the spirit as well.

KEYS TO PRACTICAL APPLICATION

What we eat does matter; let your clients know that you think good eating habits are important and why.

When taking weights, heights, and other body measurements, take them carefully because inaccurate measurements can lead to false conclusions.

Measure the height of your adult clients; do not rely on their memory.

Develop an understanding of your own eating habits. Why do you like some foods and dislike others?

Respect the eating habits of your clients. Never display an aversion to their food preferences. Remember that these eating habits hold meanings that are important to them.

When clients are fussy, complain about food, reject food, or overeat, try to understand what they are communicating by this behavior.

Remember that nutrition education efforts will most likely be unsuccessful if the psychosocial aspects of food are ignored.

KEY IDEAS

Nutrition is the sum total of all the processes involved in using food to meet bodily needs; it also includes consideration of the factors that influence a person's food choices.

The nutrients in food are necessary for life—for the growth, repair, rebuilding, and regulation of the body.

The adverse effects of poor eating habits are not immediate but develop gradually.

In developing countries, the vicious cycle of malnutrition and infectious disease is responsible for the high death toll due to common childhood diseases.

Although malnutrition in the form of the classic vitamin deficiency diseases such as scurvy or beriberi rarely is seen in the United States, other less dramatic effects are widespread: growth retardation, weight loss, decreased resistance to infection, increased risk of chronic illness, depression, weakness, delayed recovery from disease, complications in newborns, impaired learning, and possibly, impaired mental development.

Accurate diagnosis of nutritional problems requires that the health professional use a variety of assessment techniques, including medical history and physical signs, anthropometric measurements, immunologic measurements, radiographic studies, laboratory data, and a diet history.

When time and resources are limited, nutrition screening (taking a few critical measurements that are strongly associated with malnutrition) may be used to identify those clients at nutritional risk.

Anthropometric measurements are useful only if they are accurate and reliable. This form of measurement requires good technique and accurate equipment.

Height and weight measurements in children are used to help evaluate the pattern of growth. In adults, weight as it corresponds to height is used to indicate body fatness and to help determine an appropriate body weight.

Authorities consider the BMI to be the preferred means of evaluating height–weight status.

Skinfold thickness is used to estimate body fatness. The MAC measures muscle mass and body fatness. The MAMC estimates muscle mass.

Laboratory tests can uncover a nutritional problem before outward physical signs become apparent. Serum albumin and serum transferrin levels and the total lymphocyte count reflect the adequacy of protein. The total lymphocyte count and antigen skin testing measure the body's immune response. Deficiencies in protein, energy, and individual nutrients (vitamins and minerals) are associated with a depressed immune system.

Tools used in gaining information about a person's eating habits include a 24-hour diet recall, food diary, and food frequency record.

Through questioning and the analysis of food intake records, the dietitian determines the usual pattern of eating, its nutritional quality, and the impact of psychosocial factors on food habits.

A composite of information including the diet history and nutrition-related factors in the client's medical record is used to develop goals and objectives of nutrition care.

The meanings people attach to food reflect their values, beliefs, culture, and emotional state.

Health workers who understand the cultural influences that have helped shape their own eating habits will be more respectful of the eating habits of clients and more sensitive to the ways in which they and clients communicate to each other through food behaviors.

KEYS TO LEARNING

STUDY–DISCUSSION QUESTIONS

1. Discuss in class some of the nutrition problems you have observed within the community. To what causes do you attribute these problems?
2. Why are the effects of malnutrition, especially mild and moderate degrees of malnutrition, difficult to determine? Why is obesity considered a form of malnutrition?
3. What tools are involved in making an accurate evaluation of an individual's nutritional status? Why would it be unwise to draw conclusions based on one method of evaluation?
4. Consider in class discussion the effects of the following factors on eating habits: ethnic background, religious background, anxiety, size of family, family income, hospitalization, and living alone.
5. Record all the food you eat or drink for 3 days. Classify the major items (meat and meat substitutes, breadstuffs, vegetables, fruits, desserts, snack foods, and beverages) into the following

categories: favorite foods, foods you like, foods you tolerate, and foods you do not eat (foods that do not appear on your record). Try to determine why you feel as you do about each item listed. Take one item in each category and explain your feelings about that food.

CASE STUDY

Rosita, age 57 years, born in El Salvador, has been in the United States for 5 years. She speaks little English. She has recently learned that her daughter in El Salvador is pregnant and has been confined to bed because of complications. Rosita is worried about her.

Rosita was admitted to the hospital 8 days ago for treatment of pneumonia. Her weight before her illness of 3 weeks' duration was 135 pounds. She now weighs 126 pounds. Rosita, previously a hearty eater, has no appetite. Her family is worried about her and she is worried about herself and the hospital bill.

Because Rosita has high blood pressure, her physician has ordered a sodium-controlled diet for her. She eats her breakfast well but sends her lunch and dinner trays back untouched. Her son has asked the nurse if he can bring food that she likes from home but has been told that this is not permitted because Rosita is on a sodium-controlled diet.

This evening, Rosita is tempted by the aroma of the soup on the tray of the other patient in the room. The patient offers Rosita the soup and she accepts. As she is eating the soup, the nurse enters the room and scolds both patients for swapping food because Rosita is on a special diet.

Rosita's son comes to visit and finds his mother in tears. After hearing what happened, he threatens to sign his mother out of the hospital.

1. What are some possible reasons for Rosita's poor appetite?
2. Her current weight is what percentage of her usual body weight? Is this cause for concern?
3. What could have been done to increase Rosita's food consumption? List at least three alternatives.
4. How would you have handled the situation involving the soup?

BIBLIOGRAPHY

BOOKS AND PAMPHLETS

Chicago Dietetic Association and South Suburban Dietetic Association. Manual of clinical dietetics. 4th ed. Chicago: The American Dietetic Association, 1992:3–30.

Chumlea WC, Roche AF, Mukherjee D. Nutritional assessment of the elderly through anthropometry. Columbus, OH: Ross Laboratories, 1988.

Committee on Nutrition, American Academy of Pediatrics. Pediatric nutrition handbook. Elk Grove Village, IL: American Academy of Pediatrics, 1993:193–201.

Dwyer JT. Dietary assessment. In: Shils ME, Olson JA, Shike M. Eds. Modern nutrition in health and disease. 8th ed. Philadelphia: Lea and Febiger, 1994:842–860.

Dwyer JT. Screening older Americans' nutritional health: current practices and future possibilities. Washington, DC: Nutrition Screening Initiative, 1991.

Grivetti LE. Nutritional anthropology: an integrated approach to pregnancy and delivery. In: Shils ME, Olson JA, Shike M. Eds. Modern nutrition in health and disease. 8th ed. Philadelphia: Lea and Febiger, 1994:1517–1525.

Heymsfield SB, Tighe A, Wang Z. Nutritional assessment by anthropometric and biochemical methods. In: Shils ME, Olson JA, Shike M. Eds. Modern nutrition in health and disease. 8th ed. Philadelphia: Lea and Febiger, 1994:812–841.

Niehoff A. Food, science, and society. New York: The Nutrition Foundation, 1969.

Nutrition Screening Initiative. Nutrition screening manual for professionals caring for the older Americans. Washington, DC: The Nutrition Screening Initiative, 1991.

Seventh report of the director. Washington, DC: National Heart, Lung, and Blood Institute; 1979. Publication NIH 80-1672.

Watson RC, Grossman H., Meyers MA. Radiologic findings in nutritional disturbances. In: Shils ME, Olson JA, Shike M. Eds. Modern nutrition in health and disease. 8th ed. Philadelphia: Lea and Febiger, 1994:861–882.

PERIODICALS

Elmore MF, Wagner DR, Knoll DM, et al. Developing an effective adult nutrition screening tool for a community hospital. J Am Diet Assoc 1994;94–113.

Lieberman LS. Cultural sensitivity and problems of interethnic communication. Dir Appl Nutr 1987;1:1.

Ludman EK, Kang KJ, Lynn LL. Food beliefs and diets of pregnant Korean-American women. J Am Diet Assoc 1992;92:1519.

Pachter LM. Culture and clinical care: folk illness beliefs and behaviors and their implications for health care delivery. JAMA 1994;271:690.

Schlettwein-Gsell D. Nutrition and the quality of life: a measure for the outcome of nutritional intervention. Am J Clin Nutr 1992;55:1263S.

Terry RD. Needed: a new appreciation of culture and food behavior. J Am Diet Assoc 1994;94:501.

CHAPTER

3

Nutrition Care in the Health Care Facility

KEY TERMS

acute illness illness that has a rapid onset with severe and pronounced symptoms of short duration

adaptive equipment eating utensils and other commonly used items of daily living changed or adjusted to accommodate a physical disability

anorexia absence of appetite

dysphagia difficulty swallowing

empathy the act of mentally putting oneself in the place of another person; sensitivity to the plight of another person

modified changed from the normal to suit special needs, for example, a modified diet

primary care care provided in a coordinated way at the client's entry point into the health care system; the health care professional who provides the primary care is responsible for coordinating the care for the client's health problems

pulmonary aspiration the process of sucking in or out that causes food or other substances to be inspired into the lungs

stomatitis inflammation of the mouth

OBJECTIVES

After completing this chapter, the student will be able to:

1. Explain the need for giving high priority to overseeing the client's meal acceptance and describe the activities involved in fulfilling this responsibility.
2. Discuss the ways in which both verbal and nonverbal communication can influence the client's food intake.
3. Describe the kinds of assistance—the little things—that can make a significant difference in the client's food acceptance.
4. Give five techniques that are useful when feeding clients.
5. Discuss opportunities for informal teaching.
6. Explain the basic food service procedures and routines that serve to simplify and clarify communication in clinical settings.
7. Describe the indications for use and the composition of the standard or routine diets provided in hospitals and other health care facilities.

In many educational programs for nurses and other health workers, clinical experience is provided early in the curriculum. Within a few weeks, students are assigned to providing care, which frequently includes feeding hospitalized clients. By learning some basics about the food service system in your clinical setting, you can be more helpful to clients and you may save yourself needless stress and frustration.

Hospitals, nursing homes, and other health care facilities have specific, basic food service procedures. These routines simplify and clarify communication and make service more uniform and convenient. This chapter discusses these basic components of client food service and the communication related to it. See Chapter 20 for a more in-depth discussion on planning and providing nutrition care in the health-care setting.

YOUR ROLE IN NUTRITION CARE

Without an adequate supply of food, tissues break down—no body cell is immune to the effects of poor nutrition. Add to this the damaging effects of illness: the increased losses of energy and nutrients in the client with fever, the poor absorption of nutrients in the client who has severe diarrhea, and the massive losses of fluids and nutrients in the extensively burned client. Malnutrition prolongs illness and may even cause death. Unfortunately, more attention usually is given to medication than to food. *At mealtime, few other tasks should take priority over seeing that clients are eating the food served them.*

You who are nursing staff members hold a key position in maintaining and improving nutrition because you frequently interact with clients. Although you do not plan the diet and may not serve the tray, you are responsible for knowing what clients eat and how they react to food served. You are responsible for seeing that clients are fed or assisted, if necessary.

You may be the first person to become aware of circumstances that discourage clients from eating or of problems related to clients' understanding of their nutrition therapy. Poorly fitted dentures or a sore tongue or mouth may hinder a client's efforts to eat. You may observe that food portions are too small for an adolescent boy or that a Mexican American adult is eating little of the food served her. Conversely, you may notice that a particular food is well taken by someone who generally eats poorly.

COMMUNICATION

Words are only one means of communication. We also communicate nonverbally, by the way we listen, by facial expressions, and by our hurriedness or leisurely attitude. You can learn a good deal about your clients' attitudes and concerns by observing responses to the food served and by listening to what is said about it.

Any change in food service that may make clients feel better or improve food intake is worth trying. Sometimes you can accomplish these changes yourself; more frequently, you must report your observations to the nursing supervisor, dietitian, or physician, depending on the circumstances. Your observations, when communicated to appropriate members of the health care team, are the link to improving nutrition care.

The importance of your own personal commitment to the routine task of feeding and assisting clients at mealtime cannot be overestimated. What you say to clients and what you do to make them comfortable, to make eating easier, and to accommodate their needs and preferences can make the difference between eating and not eating—a speedy recovery or a delayed one. You—not the menus, diet manuals, or diet orders—are the most important aspect of nutrition care.

CREATING A PLEASANT ENVIRONMENT

Showing enthusiasm is an important factor. The person who understands his or her own feelings about food makes only positive remarks about the client's meal. Conversation should be cheerful and encouraging. The person who "wouldn't eat" or "wasn't hungry" may have needed the encouragement of a concerned, unhurried person. Some elderly clients may have to be made aware that it is mealtime. They may fall asleep while eating and have to be awakened and reminded to eat.

Mouth care before meals can improve the appetite of anorexic clients. Good mouth care can help prevent *stomatitis* (ulcerative lesions in the mouth), which can seriously affects one's ability or desire to eat. This condition may develop in people who receive chemotherapy. When feeding a client who complains of a dry mouth, offer sips of water before offering food.

When the tray arrives, the client should be ready to receive it: hands and face washed, positioned at a comfortable angle, and screened from offensive sights. The extension table should be positioned over the bed or chair and cleared. The meal then can be served and eaten as soon as it arrives.

INTERPRETING THE NUTRITION PRESCRIPTION

You may often be the first person to become aware that the client is confused or worried about the diet prescribed for him or her. The situation may provide the opportunity for some informal teaching. In response to questions, or as a means of encouraging the client to eat, you might explain that the specific meal plan has been ordered by the physician and explain the benefits.

Similarly, if the client has been given a selective menu, helping the client choose items that are balanced in nutritional content and appropriate for his or her particular diet provides opportunity for education. You are not expected to know all the answers about nutrition; when asked a question you cannot answer, you should consult with the nurse in charge or the dietitian.

MAKING FOOD APPEALING

When a person is being cared for in the home or in a small residential or health care facility, the nurse or other health worker may have some responsibilities for supervising the food service. Making the food attractive and appetizing is of utmost importance. To the extent that the individual's diet permits, variety in the color, texture, flavor, and temperature of food adds interest and attractiveness to a meal. The use of colorful garnishes, favors for special occasions and holidays, and an occasional flower or item of interest to the client add that special touch that says someone cares.

Whether the client is served at a table or by tray, all items should be spotlessly clean, including the table or tray cover, silverware, dishware, glassware, and tray card and holder. All dishware and glassware should be free of chips and cracks. Hot foods should be served hot and cold foods cold. Portions of food should be appropriate to the client's appetite. Nothing is more discouraging to a person with little appetite than to be confronted with a plate piled high with food.

If tray service is used, the tray should be large enough that the items on it are not crowded. The items should be placed conveniently so that the client can reach them easily.

ASSISTING THE CLIENT

How much help clients need depends on their ability to feed themselves. Clients should be encouraged to feed themselves to the extent possible, and most prefer to do so. Clients such as those in traction or those who have lost hand or arm strength may need assistance opening an eggshell, cutting meat, buttering bread, opening milk and juice containers and single-service items such as salad dressings, creamers, and jelly packets, and placing food within reach. Others may need to be fed.

Anorexia, gastrointestinal discomfort, inactivity, and some drugs may reduce the desire for food. Some clients may be so anxious or depressed that, although they are physically capable of feeding themselves, they are unable to eat. Helping clients to talk about concerns, encouraging them to eat some of the food on the tray, and determining what kinds of food might tempt their appetite are ways in which you can assist. Your show of concern may be all that is needed to get a client to eat.

FEEDING THE CLIENT

Some clients require total assistance. To feed someone successfully requires sensitivity to each individual's feelings and an awareness of the importance of providing nourishment for people who cannot do so for themselves. It also requires patience. Imagine that you are weak, are depressed about your condition, and have little appetite, and that you are being fed by someone who is hurried, distracted, and clearly bothered by the task. How much food do you think you would consume? If you have empathy (i.e., identify with the experiences of your clients), you will be better able to provide understanding and support (Fig. 3-1).

Before beginning to feed the client, position and support him or her so that the client is comfortable and the head is elevated to promote easy swallowing. If it is permitted, place the client in as nearly upright a position as possible. A client whose head cannot be elevated should be fed lying on his or her side with head turned toward the side. Eating while lying flat on the back increases the possibility that liquid or food will enter the trachea.

A pleasant, unhurried manner does much to stimulate the client's appetite. Assume a relaxed, comfortable position; sit, if possible, so that the client does not feel rushed. Ask about eating preferences: whether the preference is for tea with the meal, the meat and potatoes together, and so on. Offer small amounts of food at a time. A drinking tube, preferably a disposable one for sanitary reasons, is useful for people who have difficulty drinking from a cup. Caution the client to take only small sips of warm liquids. If the client is permitted and able, suggest that he or she hold a slice of toast or roll or hold the drinking tube in the beverage while sipping so that he or she may become involved in the feeding process to the extent possible.

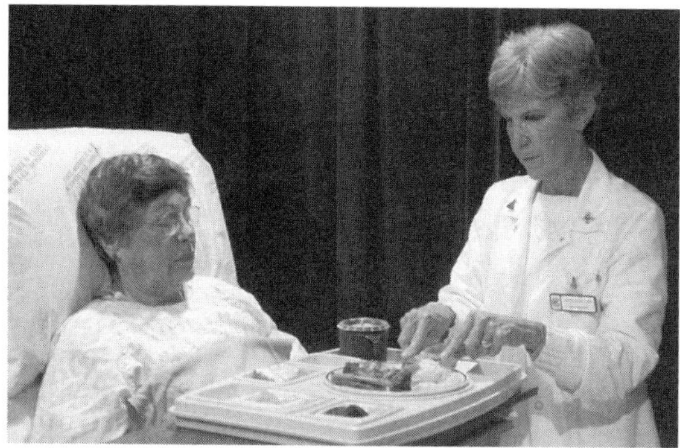

FIGURE 3-1

Feeding a client successfully requires sensitivity, patience, and a commitment to the importance of providing nourishment.

DISABLED CLIENTS

You will encounter clients among all age groups who have physical disabilities that hamper their ability to obtain an adequate diet. Clients with conditions such as severe arthritis, Parkinson's disease, stroke, or neuromuscular diseases such as cerebral palsy may have difficulty feeding themselves or may be unable to suck, chew, bite, or swallow normally. Special training is needed to learn how to position and feed people who, because of brain dysfunction, cannot control movements of the jaw, lips, tongue, and swallowing.

If the client cannot see, describe the food on the tray and indicate the position of each item. If the sightless client can feed himself or herself, describe the face of a clock to indicate the position of food on the plate: for example, potatoes are at 12 o'clock, peas at 3 o'clock, and meat between 6 o'clock and 9 o'clock. If the client needs to be fed, establish a method of signaling, such as moving the hand to indicate when he or she is ready for more food.

Disabled clients who must be fed should be evaluated on a regular basis to determine nutritional needs and physical abilities. As soon as possible, a self-feeding training program is begun to help clients do all they can for themselves. Consultation with physical, occupational and/or speech therapists can provide useful information about techniques and equipment that are appropriate for each individual's needs. Helping a disabled person to eat independently promotes self-esteem and helps prevent mental and physical deterioration.

The person who is being trained to feed himself or herself needs support and understanding from health care personnel who are sensitive to the client's feelings. The client may feel frustrated because of difficulty cutting food and opening cartons, may feel embarrassed because his or her table manners are unacceptable to others, may be too proud to ask for help, may be angry because of disabilities, and may feel isolated, especially if blind or deaf.

Techniques and Aids Useful in Self-Feeding

Certain techniques and equipment are beneficial in self-feeding programs. A disabled client who cannot maintain head balance could inhale fluid or food into the lungs (*pulmonary aspiration*). To prevent pulmonary aspiration, position the client so that he or she is comfortable and stable. The use of a binder or strap at the pelvis may be helpful. Pillows and a headrest, as well as a footstool, may afford additional support. A high chair for a small child or a cutout table for an older child may provide the needed stability. The parent of an infant who has difficulty sucking is taught how to stimulate the mouth to encourage the sucking reflex. The infant may need to be tube-fed until able to obtain sufficient amounts of food on his or her own.

The client who cannot swallow is fed by tube. The client is continually evaluated to assess the ability to swallow before feeding by mouth can be started. The ability to swallow saliva is one indication of this ability. An ice cube can be rubbed on the skin over the throat to induce swallowing.

Physical Characteristics of Food

If the client has eating problems that involve the mouth or throat, the physical characteristics of the food—its consistency and texture—may assume great importance. Liquids are frequently difficult to handle; soft or semisolid foods may be more easily managed. Liquids may be provided in the form of fruit ices or slush prepared by blending concentrated fruit juice with ice. The gelling of food has become a useful technique for those who have difficulty handling liquids (see Chapter 21). Some disabled children can handle only a single texture or consistency at a time. The consistency, texture, shape, and size of the food should be suited to the individual's needs.

Offering semisolid food in the form of finger food is useful in self-feeding programs for elderly clients. Semisolids appear to be more acceptable than pureed food. It has been suggested, too, that children receiving pureed or ground food also be given the opportunity to see the foods in their customary form.

Hard or brittle foods that do not soften quickly in the mouth should be avoided. Nuts, dry raisins, whole-kernel corn, and coconut are examples of such foods, which could be inhaled and cause choking.

Care must be taken to see that the client receives an adequate diet regardless of the consistency of the food. In an effort to provide foods of a suitable consistency, it is easy to overlook the nutritional balance of the diet.

Equipment

Adaptations in utensils can help the handicapped person eat independently. This special equipment, called *adaptive equipment,* can be purchased or can be made in the health facility or at home. A long straw, a universal cuff holder, and a rocker knife are examples of equipment that require less strength than normal for self-feeding. Built-up handles make grasping easier. A plate guard and covered plastic cup help the client with poor coordination (Fig. 3-2). A placemat, frame, or wet facecloth on which the plate can rest can turn a slick tabletop into a nonskid surface.

Bibs, which are sometimes used to protect the clothing, can cause embarrassment and damage to a client's self-image as well as the image the client presents to the staff and other clients. It is suggested that the less obvious vest-type bib be used.

Keep in mind the usefulness of these special techniques and adaptive equipment as you work with clients. The elderly person with osteoarthritis, the person in traction, and others not necessarily classified as disabled may find eating easier when a special technique or aid is used.

FOOD SERVICE IN THE CLINICAL SETTING

The dietary or food service departments of hospitals, nursing homes, and other extended care facilities are responsible for providing the re-

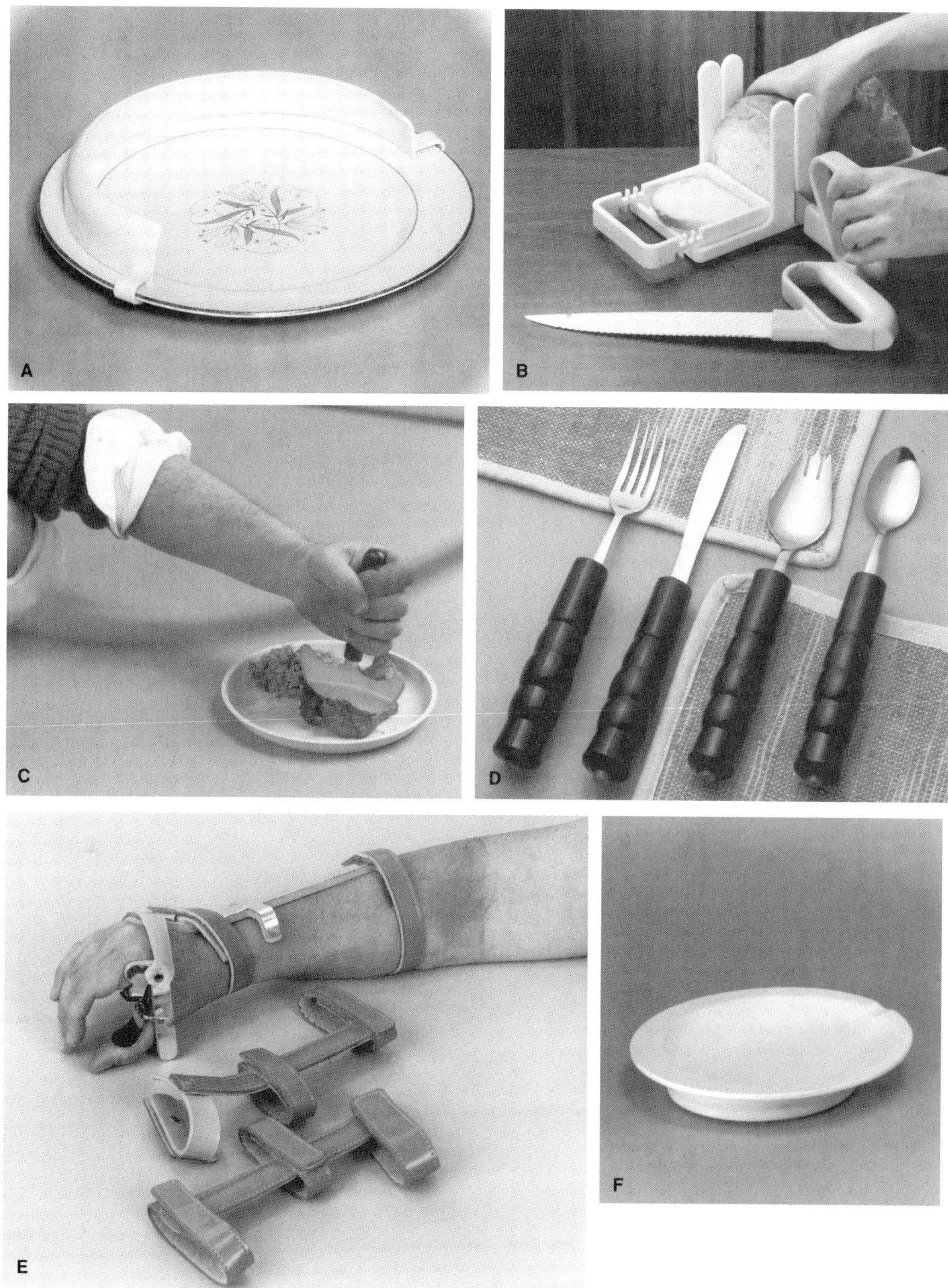

FIGURE 3-2

Adaptive equipment used in self-feeding of the disabled: (*A*) plate guard, (*B*) even slicer and right-angle knife, (*C*) rocker knife, (*D*) built-up handled utensils, (*E*) wrist support with Palmar Clip, (*F*) scoop dish. *(Courtesy of Fred Sammons, Inc., a Bissel Healthcare Co.)*

quired diet for each client. The chief administrative dietitian or food service manager directs the overall operation of the food service department. Duties include supervising menu planning and food purchasing, preparation, and service. Clinical dietitians are responsible for the nutrition care of clients. They work with the medical and nursing staffs to see that the nutritional needs of individual clients are met and that nutrition education is provided when necessary. Dietetic technicians and diet aides or clerks assist the administrative and clinical dietitians. The dietary staff also includes cooks, maids, porters, and receiving clerks.

In larger hospitals, the primary care nurse coordinates communication among the client, physician, and dietitian, assists the client at mealtime, observes the client's response to the food served, charts nutrition-related information, and reinforces the nutrition instruction provided by the dietitian. In small hospitals, nursing homes, and community nursing services, the nurse may have some responsibility for planning and supervising nutrition care and may need to interpret the diet to the client, client's family, and food service personnel. Once you know how the nursing and nutrition-related services interact, you will know where to turn if your client receives the wrong tray, requires a delayed meal, has a diet change, asks for a special food, or has some other nutrition- or food-related problem.

Nursing homes are required, as a result of the Omnibus Budget Reconciliation Act of 1987, to employ a qualified dietitian on a full-time, part-time, or consultant basis. This legislation also requires that residents have nutrition assessments on admission and periodically thereafter, and that palatable, adequate meals that include some choice of foods and service in a dining-room setting be provided.

Case management is an approach used in some health care settings—hospital, extended care facility, or home—to coordinate the care provided by numerous professionals and health care workers. Case managers oversee, manage, and are responsible for the complete health care, including nutrition-related care, of a group of clients over time. Case managers may be nurses, social workers, or other members of the health care team.

DIET ORDER

When the client is admitted to the hospital or other health care facility, a diet is prescribed to meet individual needs. In many cases, the physician prescribes the diet and writes the order in the client's medical chart, but a nutrition specialist or a dietitian also may do so. In either case, the physician, dietitian, and nurse work together to prescribe the most appropriate diet and make changes when necessary.

The order may vary from "nothing by mouth" to "normal diet." The diet may be changed during the course of the client's stay because of a change in condition or because the diagnosis necessitates a modified diet. Modified diets (also called *therapeutic diets*) are meal plans that have a specific purpose in the treatment of symptoms or disease conditions. Clients who cannot consume sufficient food by mouth may be fed by tube or intravenously.

Diet orders should be specific; otherwise, the client may not receive the diet that the physician intended. For example, a 1200- or 1500-kcal diet rather than a "low-calorie" or "reducing" diet should be ordered. A "low-sodium" diet order should specify the amount of sodium, such as 1000 mg or 2000 mg. When the diet order is unclear, ask the physician for clarification. If the physician is unavailable, the dietitian usually determines the specific diet and records the diet modification in the medical chart.

Sometimes the diet order is inappropriate for the client because the physician may be unaware of nutrition-related problems when ordering a diet. The physician may not know that the client has difficulty chewing or an intolerance to spices, or that the client has been following a sodium-controlled diet at home. When anyone on the health team realizes that the diet order is inappropriate, the dietitian or physician should be notified.

Open communication between the dietary and nursing departments is absolutely essential to successful food service. Neither can provide for the client's nutritional needs without the help of the other. The nurse communicates to the dietitian the client's special needs.

DIET MANUAL

The *diet manual* is an important communication tool. All the diets provided in the health care facility are compiled in the diet manual, which describes what foods are allowed and not allowed on each diet, the purpose of the diet, the conditions under which the diet is ordered, and the nutritional adequacy of the diet. Diets should be ordered using the terminology given in the manual to avoid misunderstandings among medical team members.

A copy of the diet manual is usually available at each nurses' station. The diets are described in technical terms and are intended for health care team use. They usually are inappropriate for distribution to clients. Materials used in diet counseling are adapted from diets in the manual and are adjusted to the needs and preferences of clients. Diet manuals often differ in minor ways from one facility to another. You should become familiar with the diets served in the facility in which you work.

The diet manual frequently lists policies regarding food service in the facility, including meal hours and procedures to use in requesting a new diet, changing diets, reporting problems, or requesting nutrition counseling. The student should become familiar with these policies.

CHECKING ACCURACY

When many people are involved in the communication chain, mistakes can occur easily. Regardless of who is responsible for delivering the tray to the client, there can never be enough checking to see that the client is receiving the correct tray. Check to see that the tray is delivered to the person designated on the tray. Sometimes the room number is incorrectly recorded in the food service department or the client has been moved and another person admitted to the room. Check also to see that the correct diet has been delivered.

SELECTIVE MENUS

Most hospitals offer a daily menu from which a client can make selections (Fig. 3-3). Two or more items are offered for each course. For example, for dinner, the choices may be roast chicken or salisbury steak, rice or baked potatoes, and tossed green salad or Waldorf salad. Sometimes the client on a modified diet also is offered a selective menu. The client indicates selections on the printed menu the day before the meal. Some clients need assistance in making choices, and some may need help marking their menus.

Selective menus have considerably improved the acceptance of foods in hospitals and other health care institutions. The choices offered accommodate most food preferences. When selective menus are not used, allowance should be made for food preferences. Even minor choices such as whether to have tea, coffee, or cocoa with a meal or jelly, butter or margarine with toast can do much to make a meal more enjoyable.

Selective menus are effective in client teaching. For example, if the client repeatedly selects less than adequate meals, assistance in making more balanced selections from the menu is needed. If the selective menu is the basis of a modified diet, the client needs instruction to make appropriate choices. Client selections can serve as a test of understanding of the diet and as an aid in follow-up instruction.

MEDICAL RECORD

All elements of the client's care including nutrition care are included in the medical record. It is a communications tool by which the health care team shares information and coordinates activities. The medical record usually includes a database, problem list, and progress notes.

Breakfast SUNDAY

FULL DIET

Mark X as large as possible in the box ☒

Portion Size: ☐ Small ☐ Regular ☐ Large

- ☐ ORANGE JUICE
- ☐ PEAR NECTAR
- ☐ FRESH BANANA

- ☐ HOMINY GRITS
- ☐ SPECIAL K
- ☐ CORN FLAKES

- ☐ SCRAMBLED EGG
- ☐ EGG OMELET w/Mushroom sauce
- ☐ SAUSAGE LINK

☐ SUGAR ☐ SUGAR SUB. ☐ SALT ☐ PEPPER
☐ MILK ☐ SKIM MILK ☐ CREAM

☐ HARD ROLL ☐ WHITE BREAD ☐ WHOLE WHEAT ☐ RYE BREAD
☐ MARGARINE ☐ JELLY

☐ COFFEE BLACK ☐ DECAF COFFEE ☐ HOT CHOC. ☐ TEA ☐ ICE TEA ☐ LEMON

NAME________________ ROOM________

DIET________________________________

Luncheon SUNDAY

FULL DIET

Please No Substitutions

Portion Size: ☐ Small ☐ Regular ☐ Large

- ☐ CREAM OF MUSHROOM SOUP

- ☐ ROAST BEEF w/Gravy
- ☐ MANICOTTI

- ☐ BAKED POTATO
  - ☐ SOUR CREAM
- ☐ BROCCOLI SPEARS
- ☐ CORN SOUFFLE

- ☐ TOSSED SALAD
  Italian or Blue Cheese Dressing

- ☐ GRAPEFRUIT SECTIONS
- ☐ CHEESE CAKE
- ☐ JELLO

☐ SUGAR ☐ SUGAR SUB. ☐ SALT ☐ PEPPER
☐ MILK ☐ SKIM MILK ☐ CREAM

☐ HARD ROLL ☐ WHITE BREAD ☐ WHOLE WHEAT ☐ RYE BREAD
☐ MARGARINE ☐ JELLY

☐ COFFEE BLACK ☐ DECAF COFFEE ☐ HOT CHOC. ☐ TEA ☐ ICE TEA ☐ LEMON

NAME________________ ROOM________

DIET________________________________

Dinner SUNDAY

FULL DIET

Please Do Not Leave Menu on Tray

Portion Size: ☐ Small ☐ Regular ☐ Large

- ☐ CRANBERRY JUICE

- ☐ SHAKE 'N BAKE CHICKEN
- ☐ HAMBURGER ON ROLL
  Mustard-Catsup-Relish

- ☐ RICE FIESTA
- ☐ PEAS & CARROTS
- ☐ CAULIFLOWER

- ☐ LETTUCE & TOMATO SALAD
  Italian Dressing or Mayonnaise

- ☐ APRICOT HALVES
- ☐ GERMAN CHOCOLATE CAKE
- ☐ VANILLA PUDDING

☐ SUGAR ☐ SUGAR SUB. ☐ SALT ☐ PEPPER
☐ MILK ☐ SKIM MILK ☐ CREAM

☐ HARD ROLL ☐ WHITE BREAD ☐ WHOLE WHEAT ☐ RYE BREAD
☐ MARGARINE ☐ JELLY

☐ COFFEE BLACK ☐ DECAF COFFEE ☐ HOT CHOC. ☐ TEA ☐ ICE TEA ☐ LEMON

NAME________________ ROOM________

DIET________________________________

FIGURE 3-3

Selective hospital menu for 1 day. *(Courtesy Mercer Medical Center, Trenton, NJ.)*

The dietitian and dietetic technician record nutrition-related information in the medical record. These notations might include a summary of the diet history and weight history, nutrition care goals and objectives, progress made in achieving goals, acceptance of meals and supplements, and the nutrition education provided. The physician and nurse also make notations regarding nutrition care as it relates to their roles.

Each health facility has its own policies regarding the format and organization of the client's medical chart. The medical record is covered in more detail in Chapter 20.

FOOD SERVED VERSUS FOOD CONSUMED

Although almost all the diets served are nutritionally adequate, meeting or exceeding the Recommended Dietary Allowances (RDAs), it is important to remember that the food served does not necessarily represent the food consumed by the client. Observation and accurate recording of the client's food intake are important to prevent the development of malnutrition. When a considerable quantity of the food served is left on the tray, the appropriate health team member should be notified immediately.

OTHER CLINICAL SETTINGS

HOME CARE

Complicated medical and nutrition services can be provided in the client's home. Greater emphasis is being placed on home care, and this trend is expected to continue and to expand. All levels of nutrition care can be provided in the home including tube feedings and intravenous nutrition therapy. The majority of people referred to home care are on modified diets. When nutrition services are applied early, health outcomes improve and health care costs are reduced.

Some home health agencies provide a wide spectrum of services including nursing; home health aides; physical, occupational, and speech therapies; nutrition; and social work. Dietitians who work for these agencies provide direct services to clients in the home, act as consultants to other health team members, and provide education for clients and staff.

HOSPICE

Hospice is not a facility. It is a philosophy of care for terminally ill people that focuses on comfort and quality of life. Pain alleviation, respect for client preferences, and consideration of care-givers' needs are components of hospice care. This type of care can be provided in the home or in a health care facility. Nutrition care involves accommodating client preferences and using techniques that help control symptoms and pain.

STANDARD OR ROUTINE DIETS

The diets served in most hospitals, nursing homes, and larger residential care facilities are classified into two categories: routine or standard diets and modified (or therapeutic) diets. The standard diets provided consist of some or all of the following: normal or general, soft, full liquid, and clear liquid diets (Tables 3-1 and 3-2). Some institutions may offer a light diet—a step between the soft and general diets.

The calorie-controlled and sodium-controlled diets are examples of diets classified as modified or therapeutic. This classification is somewhat misleading for two reasons. First, all diets, whether normal or modified, are important in therapy from the standpoint of healing and recovery. Second, the routine soft and liquid diets also qualify as modified diets, differing mainly in texture and consistency from the normal diet.

Because the majority of clients in health care facilities are placed on routine diets, a knowledge of these diets is useful to you at this point. To understand nutritional needs during illness, however, you first need to understand normal nutrition. After you have studied normal nutrition, reference again is made to this chapter. The following is a descrip-

(text continues on page 51)

TABLE 3-1 Routine Hospital Diets

Regular Diet	Light or Soft Diet	Pureed Soft Diet	Full Liquid Diet	Clear Liquid Diet
Beverages				
All	All except alcoholic beverages	Milk and milk drinks, carbonated beverages, coffee, tea, decaffeinated coffee, cereal beverages, fruit drinks	Same as pureed soft diet; coffee, tea, as allowed and tolerated; high-protein, high-calorie oral supplements (see Chapter 29)	Carbonated beverages; tea, coffee as allowed and tolerated, decaffeinated coffee, cereal beverages; fruit-flavored drinks (some strained fruit juices may be permitted); no milk or milk products
Breads				
All	Enriched white, refined wheat, and light rye breads; soft rolls and refined crackers; melba toast, rusk, zwieback	Soft, crustless bread may be pureed with milk, if tolerated; breadcrumbs added to soups, casseroles, vegetables	None	None
Cereals				
All	Cooked cereals and refined ready-to-eat cereals made from corn, rice, oats	Cooked cereals without added fruits or nuts	Cooked refined cereals or strained cooked cereals	None
Desserts				
All	Cakes, cookies, puddings; custard, ice cream; fruit ices, sherbets, gelatin desserts; fruit whips; frozen pops—all without nuts, coconut, seeds, dried fruit, or tough skins	Plain custards, puddings; ice cream; sherbet, fruit-flavored ices and frozen pops; fruit whips; flavored yogurt; flavored gelatin; cakes and pies pureed with milk or other liquids—all without seeds, nuts, coconut	Custard, puddings; gelatin desserts; rennet desserts; smooth ice cream; sherbet, fruit ice, frozen pops—all without seeds, nuts, coconut, or fruit	Clear flavored gelatin; fruit ice made from clear fruit juice; frozen pops

Eggs				
All	All	Scrambled eggs and egg substitutes may be pureed and used as tolerated; eggnog made from commercial mix*	Soft custard; eggnog made from commercial mix*	None
Fats				
All	Butter, margarine; cream; vegetable shortening and oils; mild salad dressings; white sauce; whipped cream and whipped toppings	Same as soft diet	Butter, margarine, cream, vegetable oils	None
Fruit, Fruit Juices				
All	All fruit juices; cooked or canned fruits (without seeds, skins, coarse fibers); ripe banana, orange and grapefruit sections, peeled ripe peach or pear	All fruit juices and nectars; peeled, pureed cooked or canned fruits	All fruit juices	Clear and strained fruit juices (apple, grape, orange, pineapple, cranberry, cranapple); (Fruit juices sometimes omitted)
Meat, Fish, Poultry, Cheese				
All	Tender beef, lamb, veal, liver, lean pork; chicken, turkey; fish, seafood (prepared any way except highly seasoned, fried, or pickled); cottage cheese; mild natural or processed cheese; creamy peanut butter; plain or flavored yogurt	Pureed or finely ground beef, lamb, veal, lean pork, chicken, turkey, fish thinned with broth or cream sauce; cottage cheese; yogurt without seeds, nuts, or whole fruit pieces	Plain or flavored yogurt without seeds, nuts, or fruit pieces; pureed meat added to broth or cream soup, if allowed	None (commercially prepared low residue nutritional supplements may be used if diet is required for more than 3 days; see Chapter 29)

(Continued)

TABLE 3-1 *(continued)*

Regular Diet	Light or Soft Diet	Pureed Soft Diet	Full Liquid Diet	Clear Liquid Diet
Potato or Substitutes				
All	White and sweet potatoes; hominy; barley; enriched rice; spaghetti, macaroni, other pasta	Mashed or creamed potatoes; pureed rice or pasta thinned with sauce or gravy	Mashed white potato in cream soup	None
Soups				
All	Broth-based and cream soups made from foods allowed	Broth, bouillon, consommé; broth soups and cream soups made with pureed foods	Consommé, broth, bouillon, strained soup	Clear broth, consommé
Sugar, Sweets				
All	Sugar; sugar substitute; syrup; honey; molasses; seedless jam, clear jelly, fruit butters; plain candy, marshmallows—all used in moderation	Sugar; sugar substitute; honey; syrup; clear jelly, seedless jam, fruit butters	Sugar; honey; syrups; clear sugar candy; sugar substitute	Same as full liquid diet
Vegetables, Vegetable Juices				
All	All vegetable juices; cooked or canned tender vegetables, including asparagus tips, beets, carrots, green and wax beans, eggplant, mushrooms, peas, pumpkin, spinach, squash, tomatoes; pureed lima beans and corn; lettuce, if tolerated	All vegetable juices, purees of the following cooked vegetables: asparagus, beets, green and wax beans, carrots, corn, lima beans, peas; pumpkin, spinach, squash; tomatoes if tolerated	All vegetable juices	None

* A pasteurized commercial eggnog preparation or pasteurized dried egg powder should be used rather than fresh raw eggs. The danger of *Salmonella* infection, a type of food poisoning, exists when raw egg is used.

TABLE 3-2 TYPICAL MENUS FOR ROUTINE HOSPITAL DIETS

REGULAR DIET	LIGHT OR SOFT DIET	PUREED SOFT DIET	FULL LIQUID DIET
Breakfast			
Orange juice	Orange juice	Orange juice	Orange juice
Bran flakes	Rice Krispies	Farina	Farina
Banana	Banana	Margarine	Margarine
Whole wheat toast	White toast	Ripe banana or pureed pears	Instant breakfast drink
Margarine	margarine	Instant breakfast drink	Coffee/tea
Jelly or jam	Jelly	Coffee/tea	
2% milk	2% milk	Midmorning snack: eggnog (from mix)	Midmorning snack: eggnog (from mix)
Coffee/tea	Coffee/tea		
Lunch			
Chicken with rice soup	Chicken with rice soup	Strained cream soup	Strained cream soup
Sliced turkey sandwich on seeded rye bread	Sliced turkey sandwich on light rye bread (no seeds)	Pureed chicken	Grape juice
Lettuce and sliced tomato	Lettuce, if tolerated	Mashed potatoes with gravy	Chocolate pudding
Mayonnaise (light)	Mayonnaise (light)	Pureed green beans	2% milk
Fresh fruit salad	Canned peach salad	Pureed peaches	Afternoon snack: milk shake
Chocolate pudding	Chocolate pudding	Chocolate pudding thinned with milk	
Sugar cookie	Sugar cookie	2% milk	
2% milk	2% milk		
Dinner			
Roast beef sirloin	Roast beef sirloin	Pureed beef	Strained cream soup
Mashed potatoes	Mashed potatoes	Mashed potatoes with gravy	Tomato juice
Broccoli	Sliced cooked carrots	Pureed carrots	2% milk
Tossed salad with French dressing	Tomato juice	Tomato juice	Ice cream
Whole wheat roll	Snowflake rolls	Applesauce	Evening snack: malted milk or allowed supplement
Margarine	Margarine	Ice cream	
Apple	Applesauce	Tea/coffee	
Angelfood cake	Angelfood cake	Evening snack: malted milk	
Tea/coffee	Tea/coffee		

tion of the routine diets you are likely to find in your health care facility.

GENERAL OR REGULAR DIET

The general or regular diet (also called a full diet) is based on the principles of an adequate diet pattern discussed in Chapters 5 and 14. It is planned to meet or exceed the RDAs. All foods are permitted, but fried foods, spicy foods, and pastries may be offered in moderation. Many hospitals and nursing homes have a selective menu that permits clients to avoid foods they dislike or cannot tolerate.

Some hospitals and other health care facilities have tailored their general diets to meet the recommendations for the general population outlined in the Dietary Guidelines for Americans (see Chapter 5). These diets are reduced in fat, cholesterol, sugar, and salt.

SOFT DIET

The soft diet (may also be called a light diet) differs from the normal diet in texture, seasonings, and methods of preparation. It usually is ordered for people who are recovering from surgery or acute illness such as infections and gastrointestinal disturbances and who are unable, physically or psychologically, to tolerate a general diet. Fried, highly seasoned, and high-fiber foods, including most raw fruits and vegetables, are omitted. The soft diet, as planned, is nutritionally adequate, meeting or exceeding the RDAs.

MECHANICAL SOFT DIET

The mechanical soft diet (also called dental soft) includes all easily chewed foods: small cubed, ground, or minced meat, fish, and poultry and tender cooked vegetables and canned fruits. Raw fruits and vegetables and foods containing seeds, nuts, and dried fruits are usually excluded. All seasonings and methods of preparation are permitted. This diet is suited for clients who have undergone head, neck, or mouth surgery, have dental problems that cause chewing difficulties, or when facial muscles should not be used, such as after eye surgery. This diet, as planned, is nutritionally adequate.

If dysphagia (swallowing difficulty) is suspected, a swallowing evaluation is performed and the diet is individualized. The nutrition management of dysphagia is discussed in Chapter 21.

PUREED DIET

The pureed diet consists of foods that require little or no chewing and can be swallowed easily. It includes soft or ground and pureed meats, pureed fruits and vegetables, and soft desserts. Fried, spicy, and gas-forming foods are omitted. This diet is provided for clients who have gastrointestinal problems, extreme weakness, or chewing or swallowing difficulties due to inflammation, ulceration, or neurologic or structural changes in the mouth or esophagus.

Liquids that complement the food being served, such as broth, milk, gravies, or sauces can be added to achieve a consistency that makes swallowing easier. To increase the caloric content of the pureed foods, fats such as butter, margarine, or gravy may be added to vegetables, soups, and meats, and sweeteners such as sugar or honey may be added to beverages, cereals, fruits, and desserts.

The pureed diet is nutritionally adequate if sufficient quantities of food are eaten. If the client cannot eat enough food, a liquid nutritional supplement (e.g., Ensure, Meritene, or Sustacal) can be added.

FULL LIQUID DIET

The full liquid diet consists of foods that pour or are liquid at body temperature such as milk, ice cream, gelatin, custards, puddings, refined cooked cereals, cereal gruels (strained and liquefied cooked cereals), pureed or strained soup, and egg in custard or eggnog (made with pasteurized powdered egg rather than raw egg to avoid the possibility of *Salmonella* infection, a type of food poisoning). This diet is ordered for people who are acutely ill with infection or gastrointestinal disturbances, who are weak and too ill to chew, who have dental wiring, or who, for other reasons, are unable to chew, swallow, or digest foods normally. It may be used after surgery as an intermediate step between the clear liquid diet and solid foods.

Because milk-based foods form a large part of this diet, people who have difficulty digesting milk (i.e., are lactose intolerant; see Chapter 28) may require the use of lactose-free products or lactose-reduced milk.

The full liquid diet is likely to be inadequate in nutrients except calcium, vitamin C, and protein. The nutritional value can be improved with the use of high-protein, high-calorie, and fiber-containing liquid supplements.

CLEAR LIQUID DIET

The clear liquid diet supplies fluid and energy in a form that requires little digestion and work by the gastrointestinal tract. It includes clear fruit juices (e.g., apple, cranberry, or grape), strained fruit juices (e.g., orange, grapefruit, or lemonade), clear broths or bouillon, clear fruit-flavored or unflavored gelatin, fruit ices, frozen pops, plain hard candy, sugar, honey, and sugar substitutes. Clear coffee, clear tea, and carbonated beverages are used as allowed and tolerated. No milk or milk products are permitted.

The clear liquid diet is frequently ordered after surgery to provide fluids and energy after the return of gastrointestinal function. It is also used in acute gastrointestinal disturbances (such as acute vomiting or diarrhea), in preparation for bowel surgery or before colonoscopic examination, and as a first step in refeeding of a nutritionally debilitated person.

This diet is totally deficient in nutrients and caloric content. The average clear liquid diet contains 400–500 calories derived from the sugar content of fruit juice and the sugar as an ingredient in gelatin dessert, fruit ices, carbonated beverages, and the sugar added to coffee and tea. Severe malnutrition can result if this diet is used for an extended period. Appropriate health care team members should be reminded if the client remains on the diet beyond 48 hours. If the diet is required for a longer period or the client's condition is nutritionally poor, commercially prepared low-residue or clear liquid oral supplements (see Chapter 29) are included if the client's medical condition permits.

See Table 3-1 for a summary of foods included in routine hospital diets and Table 3-2 for typical menus. See Table 3-3 for a sample menu for a clear liquid diet.

TABLE 3-3 CLEAR LIQUID DIET MENU

Breakfast	4 oz strained orange juice 1/2–1 cup flavored gelatin (plain or fortified) 1 cup coffee/tea Sugar, if desired
Midmorning	1/2 cup flavored gelatin (plain or fortified)
Lunch	1 cup broth or consommé 4 oz apple juice 1/2 cup flavored gelatin (plain or fortified) 1 cup coffee/tea Sugar, if desired
Midafternoon	1/2 cup fruit juice
Evening meal	1 cup broth or consommé 4 oz grape juice 1/2 cup flavored gelatin (plain or fortified) 1 cup coffee/tea Sugar, if desired
Evening	4 oz cranberry–apple juice 1/2 cup flavored gelatin (plain or fortified)

This sample meal does not meet the National Research Council RDAs. Nutritional adequacy cannot be met with clear liquids unless highly specialized commercial supplements are used.

KEYS TO PRACTICAL APPLICATION

At mealtime, give priority to seeing that your clients are eating.

Be aware of how each client reacts to the food served.

When a client eats poorly, try to find out why and communicate your findings to the nurse in charge.

Be positive. Show enthusiasm for the food served; be cheerful and encouraging at mealtime.

Have the client ready for his or her meal when the tray arrives: hands and face washed, mouth care provided, if necessary, client positioned properly, and room environment made conducive to a good appetite.

Remember that your attentiveness, facial expressions, and hurriedness or unhurried manner convey, as much as words do, how much you care.

Circulate among your clients at mealtime; they frequently need help cutting meat and opening milk and juice cartons and condiment containers.

When you feed a client, let him or her know that you consider this an important assignment worthy of your time.

Be sensitive to the feelings of frustration, embarrassment, anger, dependence, and isolation that a disabled client with feeding problems is likely to feel.

Acquire or make adaptive equipment to help disabled clients feed themselves.

If a diet order does not appear to be appropriate for the client, discuss this issue with the head nurse or dietitian.

Find out where the diet manual is kept; become familiar with its contents.

Learn to scan the tray quickly: verify that the client has received the correct tray and correct diet and all the foods that were ordered.

Be aware that clients' nutritional needs can be met only when good communication exists between the nursing and dietary departments.

KEY IDEAS

Attending to the client's nutritional needs deserves high priority.

The nurse holds a key position in meeting clients' nutritional needs. The nurse's responsibilities include creating an environment conducive to a good appetite, seeing that the client is fed or assisted if necessary, observing and recording food consumption, communicating the client's nutritional needs to the dietitian and other appropriate members of the health care team, and assisting in nutrition education.

Providing for clients' nutrition care requires teamwork; good communication among the various members of the health team is essential.

Feeding situations that involve helplessness or disabling conditions require a special sensitivity and empathy for the feelings the client is likely to experience and an awareness of the importance of providing adequate nourishment.

Positioning techniques, changes in texture and consistency of food, and adaptive equipment are useful in feeding disabled clients.

Health care facilities have some basic food service procedures or routines that simplify and clarify communication. The student should know the food service policies related to meal hours, delayed meals, procedures for requesting diets, changing diets, or making special requests, and where to find the composition of diets served in the facility (diet manual).

Diet orders should be given in specific terms using the terminology given in the facility's diet manual. Diet orders that appear inappropriate should be discussed with the physician or dietitian.

The medical record includes all elements of the client's care, including the nutrition component; it assists in communication and in coordinating activities of the health care team.

Trays should be checked at all points to see that the client receives the correct tray and correct diet.

Selective menus accommodate the client's food preferences and are also an effective teaching tool.

Hospital diets fall into two general categories: routine hospital diets and modified diets. The routine hospital diets include the regular, soft, full liquid, and clear liquid diets; the modified diets include such diets as the calorie-controlled and sodium-controlled diets.

All levels of nutrition care including tube feedings and intravenous therapy can be provided in home care, a rapidly growing clinical setting.

Nutrition care provided in hospice focuses on comfort and quality of life.

KEYS TO LEARNING

CASE STUDY

Mary is a 78-year-old frail woman who suffers from severe arthritis and osteoporosis. She was admitted to the hospital 2 days ago for a cough accompanied by expectoration of blood. Although weak, Mary is mentally alert. Mary is worried about her health and about giving consent to having a bronchoscopy, a procedure that seems painful and frightening. Although she has always been a good eater, she has lost her appetite totally since the bronchial condition developed.

The dietary aide delivers Mary's tray and places it on the overbed table. The table is near the foot of the bed. Mary tries to pull the table toward her, but it is too painful for her to reach that far. A nurse's aide enters the room to help the client in the next bed. Mary asks the aide to move the table. The aide tells her she will come back in a minute. Mary puts her head back on the pillow and falls asleep.

Twenty minutes later, Mary's daughter, Joan, enters the room to find her mother asleep and an untouched tray of cold food at the foot of the bed. Joan notices that the tray card reads "Diabetic Diet" and that the name on the card is not her mother's. Joan storms to the nurses' station and complains bitterly that her mother has not eaten and that she has received the wrong tray.

1. What went wrong? What steps should have been taken to avoid this situation?
2. Do you think Joan's feelings are justified? How would you answer Joan's complaints?
3. The physician ordered a soft diet for Mary. Check the diet manual in your hospital. What foods permitted on a regular diet would not be offered on a soft diet?
4. According to the policies in your hospital, how would you report the mistake and obtain another tray for Mary?
5. Mary's hands are severely deformed because of arthritis. She has difficulty cutting meat and poultry. What type of adaptive equipment would help her?
6. What adaptive equipment useful in self-feeding of disabled clients is available in your hospital? Make a display of this equipment and explain the usefulness of each item.
7. Select two clients in your clinical setting who, like Mary, have been eating poorly. Try to determine possible causes by questioning the clients and examining information in their medical records. With your classmates, compile a list of reasons for poor food consumption and, for each cause, list possible ways of resolving these difficulties.

BIBLIOGRAPHY

BOOKS

Chicago Dietetic Association and the South Suburban Dietetic Association. Manual of clinical dietetics. 4th ed. Chicago: The American Dietetic Association, 1992.

Mahan LK, Arlin MT. Krause's food, nutrition and diet therapy. Philadelphia: WB Saunders, 1992:415–429.

PERIODICALS

Anderson EG. Getting through to elderly patients. Geriatrics 1994;46:5:74.

Dubé L, Trudeau E, Belanger M. Determining the complexity of patient satisfaction with food services. J Am Diet Assoc 1994;94:394.

Lane SJ, Cloud HH. Feeding problems and intervention: an inter-disciplinary approach. Topics Clin Nutr 1988; 3:23.

Sanders HN, Hoffman SB, Lund CA. Feeding strategy for dependent eaters. J Am Diet Assoc 1992;92:1389.

CHAPTER 4 Food Safety

KEY TERMS

interstate commerce the buying and selling of goods or services between states; business that crosses state boundaries

mycotoxin a poisonous product produced by a mold

pathogens any living agent capable of causing disease

septicemia serious infection in the blood produced by microorganisms and their poisonous products

spore a reproductive cell produced by microorganisms; spores are resistant to heat

OBJECTIVES

After completing this chapter, the student will be able to:

1. Appreciate that people with weakened immune systems are at greatly increased risk of serious, possibly fatal, illness from foodborne disease.
2. Explain the responsibilities of health care workers regarding the prevention of foodborne illness.
3. List three pathways by which pathogens enter food.
4. Give the symptoms, source of infection, and preventive methods for foodborne illness caused by each of the following:
   - *Salmonella*
   - *Staphylococcus aureus*
   - *Clostridium perfringens*
   - *Campylobacter jejuni*
   - *Clostridium botulinum*
   - *Escherichia coli* 0157:H7
   - *Listeria monocytogenes*
5. Explain the danger posed by molds on food.
6. Explain the dangers posed by eating raw or undercooked meat, fish, and poultry.
7. State the three basic food safety concepts for preventing foodborne illness.
8. List four rules of food safety.
9. Identify five ways by which foods can become chemically toxic.
10. Explain how the federal government controls the use of pesticides and the use of food additives.
11. Explain the relationship of a varied diet to chemical toxicity.
12. List the three US government agencies most involved in promoting food safety.

The safety of food can be adversely affected by bacterial infections, bacterial toxins, viruses, parasites, molds, and chemicals. The chemicals may be naturally present, added intentionally during food production and processing, or added unintentionally due to pollution, carelessness, accident, or ignorance.

FOODBORNE ILLNESS DUE TO PATHOGENS

The most common cause of illness related to food consumption is the contamination by *pathogens* (disease-causing organisms) or harmful toxins produced by them. The appearance, taste, and odor of the contaminated food may be unaffected, and the consumer often is completely unaware that the food is unsafe.

The organisms that cause foodborne illness are all around us. Safe food practices prevent the harmful organisms from multiplying and causing foodborne illness. Although foodborne illnesses can be traced to foods of every food group, foods of animal origin are the most common carriers.

Pathogens enter food by several pathways. An animal that later is eaten as food may be infected with salmonellae or trichinae. A food handler may introduce disease organisms into food by hands soiled with feces or urine, or by coughing or sneezing over the food during preparation. Equipment, such as cutting boards or meat slicers, and working surfaces, such as countertops, can become contaminated from infected food. Cross contamination can occur if these surfaces are not cleaned properly and other foods prepared on them become infected. Household pets, dust, and the feces and bodies of insects are other sources of contamination.

Since 1970, there has been a phenomenal rise in the number of pathogens recognized as capable of causing foodborne illness. Foodborne illness affects as many as 80 million Americans each year. Many cases go unrecognized because the symptoms—chills, fever, diarrhea, cramps, and vomiting—resemble flu symptoms. For many people,the symptoms are mild, but in some rare cases, the results are devastating, leading to the death of 9000 Americans annually.

The US Public Health Service Centers for Disease Control and Prevention reported that 97% of foodborne illnesses reported between 1983 and 1987 could have been prevented by safe food handling practices, including proper selection, cooking, holding, and storage of food and appropriate hygienic practices of food handlers.

WEAKENED IMMUNITY AND FOODBORNE ILLNESS

The health of people with weakened immune systems and gastrointestinal disorders can be seriously threatened by foodborne illness. High-risk clients include pregnant women, infants and young children, elderly people, and people who have diseases or disorders that weaken the immune system or involve the gastrointestinal tract. These people are not only more susceptible to foodborne disease, but also are more likely to develop serious complications.

The immune systems of the fetus, infant, and young child are immature and vulnerable. In elderly people, a number of factors—inadequate nutrition, poor blood circulation, and chronic debilitating disease—are likely involved in a poor immune response.

Foodborne illness is a serious problem for people with liver disease, diabetes mellitus, and immune disorders, including acquired immunodeficiency syndrome, cancer, and reduced immunity due to steroid or immunosuppressant therapy (as in organ transplantation). People who have a diminished amount of hydrochloric acid in the stomach due to previous gastric surgery or a gastrointestinal disorder or antacid therapy are also more prone to foodborne illness because gastric acid protects the body from harmful bacteria.

Health care workers have an especially important role to play in the prevention of foodborne illness because they interact daily with people who have weakened immunity. This responsibility involves using safe food practices themselves, seeing that the people whom they supervise use safe food practices, and educating their clients to use them.

BACTERIAL CONTAMINATION

Some of the bacteria responsible for foodborne illness in the United States include *Salmonella, Staphylococcus aureus, Clostridium perfringens, Clostridium botulinum, Shigella, Campylobacter jejunum, Listeria monocytogenes, Escherichia coli* (*E. coli*), *Yersinia enterocolitica,* and *Vibrio vulnificus.* In addition, to these organisms, 20 or so others can cause foodborne illness. The sources, symptoms, and preventive measures for each of these pathogens are given in Table 4-1. Safe food handling measures, such as those given in Display 4-1, are the only way to effectively prevent illness caused by harmful bacteria.

SALMONELLA

Salmonellosis is the most commonly reported foodborne illness in the United States. It can be extremely serious in infants, the elderly, and people weakened by illness. *Salmonella* bacteria are found in raw or undercooked animal foods such as eggs, poultry, meats, unpasteurized milk, and other dairy products. Fruits, vegetables, chocolate, and yeast have also been implicated. *Salmonella* on the outer rind of melons can contaminate interior melon tissues when cut.

Heat destroys *Salmonella* bacteria. Thoroughly cook meat and poultry according to the guidelines in Table 4-2. Purchase eggs only from refrigerated cases and keep refrigerated until used. Thoroughly cook eggs, especially for people with weakened immune systems. Do not use cracked eggs unless they can be hard cooked or used in baking. Use pasteurized dried egg powder or eggnog mix instead of raw eggs in eggnogs. Wash vegetables and fruits well, including the outer rind of melons before cutting. Thoroughly wash utensils and surfaces used in preparing raw foods to prevent contamination of other foods.

Typhoid fever caused by a species of *Salmonella* usually is transmitted to food by a food handler who is a carrier. The disease affects the gastrointestinal tract, liver, gallbladder, spleen, and kidneys.

STAPHYLOCOCCUS AUREUS

Staphylococci produce a toxin that can cause food poisoning if enough of the organisms are present in the food. The organisms are found in the respiratory passages and on the skin. They enter food from boils or infected cuts or when the food handler coughs or sneezes. If the contaminated food is kept unrefrigerated for a long period or is not reheated thoroughly, the toxin can accumulate and cause illness. Environments in which these bacteria produce toxin include meats, poultry, and egg products; tuna, potato, and macaroni salads; and cream-filled pastries.

CLOSTRIDIUM PERFRINGENS

C. perfringens is a spore-forming bacterium. Its spores are resistant to heat, ordinary cooking, and methods of food preservation such as freezing and drying. Food poisoning from *C. perfringens* most often occurs when large amounts of prepared foods have been held for long periods on steam tables or at room temperature. For this reason, it is referred to as the "cafeteria or buffet germ." It can also occur when foods are not cooled properly after serving. Large leftover portions of food such as roasts, turkey, stuffing, gravy, soups, and refried beans are common carriers. Because the organism lives in the soil, contamination from unwashed vegetables is also possible.

When serving foods in cafeteria or buffet style, keep them above 140°F or below 40°F. Store large portions of leftover cooked foods in small batches in shallow pans and heat leftovers to at least 165°F or until steaming hot before serving. Wash vegetables thoroughly to remove all soil.

CLOSTRIDIUM BOTULINUM

C. botulinum produces a toxin that even in small amounts causes serious illness and is fatal in about two thirds of all cases. The spores grow only in *anaerobic* (without oxygen) conditions and are destroyed by high temperatures. Botulism most frequently occurs from the use of home-canned low-acid foods that have been inadequately processed. Foods packed too densely can cause a problem for commercial canners as well. Recently,

DISPLAY 4-1 FOOD SAFETY RULES

- Do not work with food if you have an infectious disease or infected cuts or other skin infections.
- Always work with clean hands, clean fingernails, and clean hair, and wear clean clothing.
- Wash hands thoroughly after handling raw meat, poultry, or eggs and before working with other food.
- Keep hands away from the mouth, nose, and hair.
- Avoid using the same spoon more than once for tasting food while preparing, cooking, or serving.
- Do not serve baby foods directly from the jar or can to avoid contaminating any remaining food.
- Never store cleaning supplies, pesticides, and drugs with food or in food containers such as soda bottles and food jars.
- Refrigerate perishable foods at 40°F or below. Store perishable and frozen foods in the refrigerator and freezer as soon after shopping as possible.
- Keep hot foods hot—above 140°F—and cold foods cold—below 40°F. Foods that are held for more than 2 hours at a temperature between 60°F and 125°F may not be safe to eat.
- Keep food that contains milk or egg products and little vinegar or other acids refrigerated. This includes cream, custard, and meringue pies; foods that contain custard fillings, such as cakes, cream puffs, and eclairs; and salads and sandwich fillings. On summer outings, keep these foods in a cooler with ice or reusable cold packs.
- Cook commercially frozen stuffed poultry from the frozen state and keep it in the refrigerator until time to start cooking. If stuffing is made in advance at home, store it separately in the refrigerator. Stuff the bird just before putting it into the hot oven.
- Remove the stuffing from all leftover cooked meat, poultry, or fish before storing, and store it in the refrigerator in separate container.
- Refrigerate leftover meat, fish, poultry, broth, and gravy immediately after a meal. Freeze them if they are to be kept longer than a few days.
- Clean all dishes, utensils, and work surfaces thoroughly with soap and water after each use. It is especially important to clean equipment and work surfaces that have been used for raw food, such as raw poultry or meat before they are used for cooked food or foods such as salads that are eaten without cooking. A solution prepared with 1 tbsp chlorine laundry bleach in 1 qt of cold water destroys bacteria. This solution can be used for rinsing utensils and work surfaces. Equipment such as cutting boards, meat grinders, blenders, and can openers particularly need to be sanitized in this way.
- Cook meat, poultry and fish thoroughly. See guidelines in Table 4-2.
- Serve foods immediately after cooking or refrigerate promptly. Hot foods can be placed in the refrigerator as long as they do not raise the temperature of the refrigerator above 45°F. Large quantities of food can be cooled more quickly if refrigerated in shallow containers.
- Thaw frozen meat, fish, and poultry in the refrigerator. These meats may be cooked from the frozen state if cooked for at least $1^1/_2$ times as long as required for the unfrozen product. Undercooked foods may be unsafe. Cook stuffing to a temperature of at least 165°F, even if you are cooking it separately. Use a meat thermometer.
- Heat leftovers thoroughly; boil broths and gravies for several minutes before reusing.
- Handle foods to be put in your home freezer as little as possible to keep bacteria at a minimum before freezing. Freezing does not kill bacteria but merely stops their growth; the bacteria then continue to multiply when the food is thawed.
- Avoid home canning of meat and poultry. It is too risky.
- Can low-acid vegetables in a pressure canner at the proper temperature and for the time specified in the directions. The boiling water–bath method is safe only for fruits, high-acid red tomatoes, and jellies and jams.
- Simmer all home-canned vegetables, meat, and poultry for 10 to 20 minutes before tasting.
- Heating makes the odor of spoilage more noticeable. If a food looks spoiled, foams, or has an off-odor, destroy it without tasting.
- Do not eat moldy foods. Discard the entire food, including those portions on which the mold is not apparent. Hard cheese with small mold spots can be saved. Cut off at least 1 inch around and below the mold. Keep knife out of the mold itself.
- Do not use fresh raw eggs in eggnog or soft custard, especially when serving the food to small children or people in a weakened condition. Use pasteurized dried egg powder instead.
- Use cracked eggs only if thoroughly cooked, as in hard-cooked eggs or baked dishes.
- Use a microwave oven safely (see Display 4-2).

TABLE 4-1 Bacteria Causing Foodborne Illness

Foodborne illness, caused by harmful bacteria, normally produces intestinal flulike symptoms lasting a few hours to several days. But in cases of botulism, *E. coli* 0157:H7, or listeriosis, or when food poisoning strikes infants or ill or elderly people, the situation can be serious. Harmful bacteria, microscopic in size, surround us—in the air, soil, water, and in our own digestive tracts and in those of many animals. The only way they can be stopped effectively is by careful attention to food handling rules such as those outlined in this table and in Displays 4-1, 4-2, 4-3 and Table 4-2.

Bacteria	How it Attacks	Symptoms	Prevention*
Staphylococcus aureus	Staph spreads from someone handling food; it is found on the skin and in boils, pimples, and throat infections; at warm temperatures, staph produces a poison Susceptible foods are meat; poultry; meat and poultry salads; cheese; egg products; starchy salads (potato, macaroni, pasta, and tuna); custards; cream-filled desserts	2–8 h after eating, vomiting and diarrhea develop and last 1 or 2 days	Cooking does not destroy the staph poison, so Wash hands and utensils before preparing food Do not leave food out for more than 2 h
Salmonella	You can get *Salmonella* infection when infected food—meat, poultry, eggs, fish—is eaten raw or undercooked; other cases include cooked and uncooked food that comes in contact with infected raw food and food contaminated by an infected person	6–48 h after infection, diarrhea, fever, and vomiting develop and last 2–7 days	Keep raw food away from cooked food Thoroughly cook meat, poultry, fish, eggs Be especially careful with poultry, pork, roast beef, hamburger Do not drink unpasteurized milk Avoid raw eggs, eggnogs made with raw eggs
C. perfringens	This "buffet germ" grows rapidly in large portions of food that are cooling slowly; it also can grow in chafing dishes that do not keep food sufficiently hot and even in the refrigerator if food is stored in large portions that do not cool quickly	8–24 h after infection, diarrhea and gas pains begin, ending usually in less than 1 day; older people and patients with ulcers can be badly affected	Keep food hot (>140°F) Divide bulk cooked foods into smaller portions for serving and cooling Be careful with poultry, gravy, stews, casseroles
Campylobacter jejuni	You can become infected by drinking untreated water on an outing; by eating raw or undercooked meat, poultry, or shellfish; or by coming into contact with an infected pet	2–5 days, after infection, severe (possibly bloody) diarrhea, cramping, fever, and headache develop and last 2–7 days	Do not drink untreated water or unpasteurized milk Thoroughly clean hands, utensils, and surfaces that touch raw meats Thoroughly cook meat, poultry, fish
C. botulinum	Bacteria often occur in home-canned or any canned goods that show warning signs—clear liquids turned milky, cracked jars, loose lids, swollen or dented cans or lids; beware of any jar or can that spurts liquid or has an off-odor when opened Also found in warm, airtight conditions such as tightly foil-wrapped baked potato and garlic in oil held at room temperature	12–48 h after infection, the nervous system is affected; symptoms include double vision, droopy eyelids, trouble speaking and swallowing, difficult breathing Untreated botulism can be fatal	Carefully examine home-canned goods before use Do not use any canned goods showing danger signs If you or a family member has botulism symptoms, get medical help immediately; then call health authorities Store foods in the refrigerator

TABLE 4-1 *(continued)*

BACTERIA	HOW IT ATTACKS	SYMPTOMS	PREVENTION*
E. coli 0157:H7	Recent outbreaks traced to undercooked hamburgers; can also become infected from other undercooked meats and poultry, raw milk, improperly processed fruit and vegetable juice such as "roadstand cider"	3–9 days after infection, severe abdominal pain and watery diarrhea, that often becomes bloody, develop; possible complications include severe anemia and renal failure in children (called HUS-hemolytic uremic syndrome) and a similar condition in adults accompanied by strokes	Thoroughly cook meat, fish and poultry; avoid raw milk; buy pasteurized cider; avoid unprocessed juices; wash fruits and vegetables thoroughly
Shigella	Food becomes contaminated when *Shigella*-infected food handler contaminates food that is not cooked thoroughly afterward; carried by milk and dairy products and cold tuna, chicken, and potato salads	1–7 days after infection, person develops abdominal cramps; diarrhea, sometimes bloody; nausea, headaches, chills, and dehydration	Practice good personal hygiene and follow sanitary food preparation measures; care-givers of children should wash hands with warm soapy water after every diaper check and change; teach children to wash hands after going to the bathroom
Yersinia enterocolitica	Organism can grow at normal refrigeration temperatures; can be found in meats, poultry, unpasteurized milk and dairy products, seafood from sewage-contaminated water, produce fertilized with raw manure	1–7 days after infection, abdominal pain, diarrhea (sometimes bloody), and sometimes vomiting develop; immuno-compromised individuals may be at risk of reactive arthritis, heart problems, and, in rare cases, meningitis	Thoroughly cook and reheat foods; thoroughly wash fruits and vegetables; avoid unpasteurized milk and dairy products; practice good personal hygiene
Listeria monocytogenes	Commonly found in intestines of animals and humans; frequent carriers are unpasteurized dairy products, soft cheeses, meat patés, and processed meats; can grow slowly at refrigerator temperature	Symptoms appear 24 h to several weeks following infection Symptoms of Listeria infection: Sudden onset fever, chills, headache, backache and occasional abdominal pain and diarrhea. In newborns respiratory distress, refusal to drink, vomiting Complications include spontaneous abortions, stillbirths, septicemia, meningitis, meningoencephalitis	Avoid unpasteurized milk and dairy products; cook meats and poultry thoroughly; wash produce thoroughly; avoid cross-contamination
V. vulnificus	Lives in coastal waters; infects humans through open wounds or consumption of raw or undercooked seafood	Appear abruptly; chills, fever, or prostration	Avoid eating raw shellfish; cook shellfish thoroughly

* Although the table highlights the preventive measures most important in avoiding each type of bacteria, you should follow all the rules of prevention with all food. (Adapted from Young MK. Safe food backgrounder. Chicago, IL: National Live Stock and Meat Board, 1994, and various publications of the Food and Drug Administration and the Food Safety and Inspection Service cited in the Bibliography.)

TABLE 4-2 COOKING FOODS SAFELY

For safe cooking, never use an oven temperature below 325°F. When testing for doneness, insert meat thermometer or microwave temperature probe into the thickest part of meat or poultry away from bone or fat. Temperature-check microwaved foods after the standing time that completes their cooking.

PRODUCT	COOK TO THIS INTERNAL TEMPERATURE (°F)	VISUAL CHECKS
Fresh Beef, Veal, Lamb		
Ground products like hamburger (prepared as patties, meat loaf, meatballs, etc.)	160	No longer pink
Roasts, Steaks, and Chops		
Medium rare	145	Pink center
Medium	160	Pale pink center
Well done	170	Grey or brown throughout
Fresh Pork		
All cuts including ground product		
Medium	160	Pale pink center
Well done	170	Not pink
Poultry		
Ground chicken, turkey	165	Cook until juices run clear
Whole chicken, turkey		
Medium, unstuffed	170	
Well done	180	
Whole bird with stuffing (stuffing must reach 165°)	180	
Poultry breasts, roasts	170	
Thighs, wings		
Fully Cooked Meat and Poultry Leftovers		
To reheat	165	Steaming hot
Ham		
Fresh (raw)	160	Pale pink center
Fully cooked, to reheat	140	Hot
Fish and Shellfish		
Fish, filleted and whole	160	Flesh is opaque, flakes easily
Shellfish	160	Opaque, steaming hot
Eggs		
Fresh		Both yolk and white firm
Egg-based sauces and custards	160	Sauces coat spoon, custards are firm
Pasteurized egg substitutes	Safe uncooked	Cook as desired

(Adapted from Wiliamson C. Why experts say "cook it." Food News for Consumers 1991;8:1:10; and US Dept of Agriculture, Food Safety and Inspection Service. A quick consumer guide to safe food handling. Washington, DC: US Government Printing Office, 1994. Home and Garden bulletin 254.

the Food and Drug Administration (FDA) expressed concern that commercial low-acid canned foods that are reduced in sugar or salt may pose a higher risk of botulism. These ingredient changes may make processing ineffective for controlling this bacterium.

Botulism also can form in bacon or smoked meats that have been prepared without the use of nitrites as preservatives. Home canning of meat and poultry is not recommended. Can low-acid vegetables in a pressure canner at the proper temperature and for the time specified in the directions. The boiling water–bath method is unsafe for low-acid foods.

Destroy, without tasting the contents, any can that bulges, looks spoiled, foams, or has an off-odor. However, canned foods are not the only foods that can cause a problem. The botulism toxins thrive in warm, oxygen-free environments. An unrefrigerated, tightly wrapped baked potato and unrefrigerated garlic in oil have been reported to be sources of botulism. Other uncanned foods responsible for botulism include peppers, asparagus, eggs, tomatoes, salmon, beets, pickles, and onions. It is important to refrigerate these foods.

Babies are especially susceptible to *C. botulinum,* which often is found in honey. Never use honey in foods or on pacifiers of infants younger than age 1 year.

SHIGELLA

Shigella bacteria are found in the fecal matter of infected humans. The disease shigellosis usually is caused by the contamination of food by a food handler who is infected with *Shigella.* Because the *Shigella* bacteria are destroyed by cooking, contaminated cold foods such as tuna, chicken, or potato salads are the primary food carriers. Plant foods that have been fertilized with raw manure, irrigated with contaminated water, or contaminated by humans may also carry the bacteria.

Good personal hygiene and sanitary food handling practices are important in the prevention of shigellosis. This disease is most common in children aged 1 to 4 years. Care-givers of children in diapers must wash hands with warm, soapy water after every diaper check and change and teach children to wash their hands after going to the bathroom. Care-givers of infants and children in diapers should wash the infant's or child's hands after each diaper change.

CAMPYLOBACTER JEJUNI

Campylobacteriosis has recently been recognized as one of the leading causes of diarrhea in the United States. Foodborne illness caused by *C. jejuni* is now believed to cause as much or more illness than *Salmonella* and *Shigella* combined.

C. jejuni is present in the intestinal tracts of healthy cattle, chickens, turkeys, and household pets. It can contaminate meat and poultry during the slaughtering process. *C. jejuni* grows slowly, taking 3 to 5 days after ingestion to produce the symptoms of cramps, diarrhea (possibly bloody), and fever. Convulsions may occur in some young children who experience high fever due to the disease. Most cases have been attributed to undercooked meat and poultry, unpasteurized milk, and untreated water. This bacterium is destroyed by heat.

Cook and heat meats and poultry thoroughly according to guidelines in Table 4-2 and avoid cross-contamination of foods. Do not permit dogs and other pets in food preparation areas.

LISTERIA MONOCYTOGENES

L. monocytogenes is a bacteria commonly found in intestines of humans and animals, milk, soil, leafy vegetables, and food processing plants. Frequent food carriers of the disease are unpasteurized dairy products (especially soft cheese), meat patés, and processed meats. The bacteria can grow slowly at refrigerator temperatures.

The symptoms vary in adults and newborns and are especially serious in people with depressed immune systems. Symptoms range from influenza-like symptoms to, in severe cases, potentially fatal complications such as septicemia, meningitis, and meningoencephalitis. Newborns can contract listeriosis from an infected mother during birth. It can cause spontaneous abortions and stillbirths.

Because *L. monocytogenes* is commonly found in the environment, controlling the growth and preventing the survival of this bacterium are the basic means of avoiding illness. Avoid unpasteurized milk and milk products and undercooked meats and poultry. Wash produce before preparation, thoroughly clean equipment and food surfaces, and practice good personal hygiene.

ESCHERICHIA COLI/E. COLI 0157:H7

E. coli are a group of bacteria found in the intestines of some animals used for food and in humans. *E. coli* can be transmitted through contamination of food during processing and improper food handling or through a contaminated water supply.

E. coli 0157:H7 is a highly infectious, potentially fatal, strain of *E. coli* that has received much media attention in recent years due to a serious outbreak traced to undercooked hamburgers in a fast-food chain. Several people died as a result of this disease.

Hemorrhagic colitis (inflammation of the colon) can occur as a result of *E. coli* 0157:H7 infection. This condition may lead to *hemolytic uremic syndrome*, which is characterized by severe anemia and kidney failure. These kidney complications occur in 2% to 7% of cases. It is a leading cause of acute kidney failure in children and also can pose a serious kidney risk for elderly people. Adults may develop kidney symptoms similar to those of children but with involvement of the central nervous system, including strokes and seizures.

E. coli 0157:H7 can be effectively controlled by thorough cooking of meats and poultry and thorough reheating of leftovers. Avoid unprocessed fruit and vegetable juices (including "roadstand ciders") and unpasteurized milk and milk products. Wash fruits and vegetables thoroughly.

YERSINIA ENTEROCOLITICA

Y. enterocolitica are bacteria found in the fecal matter of animals. Only certain strains produce disease. *Y. enterocolitica* can be found in meats, poultry, unpasteurized milk and dairy products, seafood from sewage-contaminated waters, and produce fertilized with raw manure. *Y. enterocolitica* bacteria are of increasing concern because they can grow at normal refrigeration temperatures and can reach infectious levels in 4 days in milk and meat products.

Yersiniosis usually affects young children. Although it is not a commonly reported disease, serious complications may occur in elderly people and people with compromised immune systems. These complications include septicemia, reactive arthritis, anemic conditions, heart problems, and in rare cases, meningitis.

Important preventive measures include thoroughly cooking and reheating foods. In addition, maintain good sanitation and personal hygiene.

VIBRIO VULNIFICUS

V. vulnificus lives in coastal waters and can infect humans either through open wounds or through the consumption of contaminated seafood. Symptoms include sudden chills, fever, nausea, vomiting, and stomach pain. It can sometimes cause septicemia. People with weakened immune systems are especially vulnerable.

The disease is usually caused by eating raw molluscan shellfish—oysters, mussels, clams, and whole scallops. The bacteria can multiply even when refrigerated. However, the bacteria are completely killed when the shellfish are thoroughly cooked.

VIRUSES

Hepatitis A virus is carried by mollusks from beds polluted by untreated sewage. Symptoms include malaise, appetite loss, and fever; after 3 to 10 days, the client develops jaundice with darkened urine. Severe cases can result in liver damage and death. Certain other viruses known as Norwalk viruses can contaminate mollusks and cause severe diarrhea. Thorough cooking kills the Norwalk virus but may not always kill hepatitis A virus. Eating raw shellfish is hazardous. Mollusks in the shell should always be alive when purchased. Buy seafood only from reputable dealers. Ask to see the shipper's tag for molluscan shellfish.

MOLDS

Mold is a result of spoilage. It is a type of fungus consisting of "root" threads that permeate the food, a stalk that rises above the foods, and spores that form at the ends of the stalks. The spores can spread the mold from place to place. Some molds cause allergic reactions and respiratory problems. A few molds produce poisonous substances called *mycotoxins*.

Aflatoxin, a mycotoxin produced by certain molds, is a cancer-causing substance that develops in spoiled peanuts, peanut butter, nuts, soybeans, grains, spices, and animal products. Apparently, aflatoxin cannot be completely eliminated from the food supply, but the FDA strictly limits the amount permitted to 15 parts per billion in food for sale in interstate commerce.

Because the long-term effects of mold toxins (mycotoxins) are unknown, it is advisable to avoid eating moldy foods and to avoid sniffing mold, which can enter the body through the respiratory tract. The mold that is seen is only the spore-bearing part; the rest of the mold is buried deep inside the food substance. Cooking does not destroy mold toxins. Molds can continue to grow also at refrigerator temperatures.

Mold-ripened cheese such as bleu cheese or Roquefort apparently is safe to use. However, cut off mold on other hard cheeses to a depth of 1 inch surrounding the mold spot and eat the remainder. Discard all other foods with mold on them.

There is continual federal monitoring of crops at high risk for toxic mold growth. These crops include grains, nuts, celery, apples, and tomatoes. Examine foods carefully before purchasing. Check the stem areas on fresh produce. Keep foods covered to prevent exposure to mold spores in the air. Mold spores from moldy foods can build up in the refrigerator and affect other food. Clean the refrigerator frequently, using a disinfectant solution to remove visible mold on rubber casings.

PARASITES

CRYPTOSPORIDIUM

Cryptosporidium is a parasite found in the intestinal tracts of many species of birds and animals. It was first discovered as a cause of human disease in 1976. It is now considered to be one of the foremost causes of diarrhea in the world, especially among children. Recent problems with contaminated water in Milwaukee were traced to this microscopic parasite. Foods of animal origin, vegetables, and improperly treated water are potential carriers. *Cryptosporidium* is resistant to chlorine, so it is controlled only through proper water filtration methods.

The parasite attaches to intestinal cells and causes profuse watery diarrhea, abdominal cramps, and fever. Healthy people rid their bodies of the parasite in 1 or 2 weeks. In contrast, the infection may take hold in immune-compromised individuals, progressing into a debilitating and wasting disease. Safe food handling practices and good personal hygiene can control the spread of cryptosporidiosis.

Giardia lamblia and *Entamoeba histolytica* are two parasites carried by polluted water and foods grown in polluted soil. Both are characterized by severe gastrointestinal symptoms similar to those of other foodborne illnesses. The diseases are caused by the consumption of uncooked contaminated foods or cooked foods contaminated by infected food handlers.

TRICHINELLA SPIRALIS

Trichinosis occurs when a person consumes raw or undercooked pork that is infected with the parasite *T. spiralis. Trichinella* levels in pork products have been reduced considerably in recent years due to efforts by the US Department of Agriculture (USDA) and the pork industry. However, cook pork to a temperature high enough to kill bacteria that may be in the raw food. For optimum safety, cook all meat and poultry to an internal temperature of 160°F, which is medium for pork. For well-done pork, cook to an internal temperature of 170°F.

ANISAKIS MARINA

Although raw fish (sushi) is popular, it may be unsafe to eat. Occasionally, sushi is contaminated with a tightly coiled, clear worm $\frac{1}{2}$ to $\frac{3}{4}$ inches long called *A. marina,* which imbeds itself in salmon, herring, and other fish. Symptoms of this disease include diarrhea and abdominal pain.

Parasites in fresh, raw fish can be killed by commercially freezing (at temperatures lower than home freezers) the fish and then thawing the fish before eating. However, freezing **does not** kill the bacteria in raw fish. Both parasites and bacteria are killed by thorough cooking.

PREVENTING FOODBORNE ILLNESS: RULES OF FOOD SAFETY

Preventing foodborne illness caused by harmful organisms involves three basic concepts: handling food in a careful, sanitary manner, cooking food to a temperature that will destroy harmful pathogens, and controlling the temperature at which perishable foods are held and stored—keeping hot foods hot and cold foods cold (Figure 4-1).

Most harmful bacteria enter food through careless handling and a contaminated environment (such as countertops, utensils, can openers, and cutting boards). Temperature control keeps the harmful bacteria that are in food from multiplying. Cooking foods to an internal temperature of 160°F or more kills most harmful bacteria.

Recently, serious outbreaks of foodborne illness traced to undercooked hamburgers have focused attention on the importance of cooking meat to a temperature that will destroy harmful bacteria. In late 1993, it became mandatory that all packages of raw or partially cooked meat and poultry contain "Safe Handling Instructions." Ground meat and ground poultry are more risky than steaks and roasts because of the kind of handling and preparation they receive. Bacteria on the surface of the meat or poultry may spread throughout the food during grinding. Cook ground meats to an internal temperature of at least 160°F or until the center is no longer pink. Cook ground poultry to at least 165°F or until juices run clear. Properly cooked fish should flake easily with a fork and should be opaque and firm, not translucent.

Holding and storing food properly is also important. Keep cooked food that is not served immediately hot at a temperature of 140°F to 165°F. Even at this temperature, do not keep hot food out

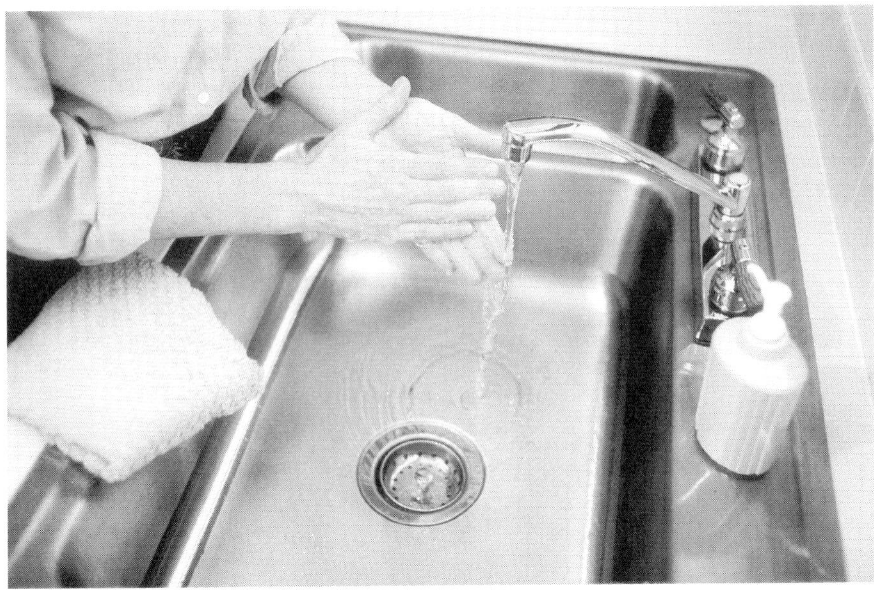

FIGURE 4-1

Handling food in a careful, sanitary manner is basic to safe food preparation. Personal cleanliness is the first critical step.

more than 2 hours. A cold environment also slows the growth of bacteria. The colder the environment, the less chance the bacteria have to grow. Store food at below 40°F in the refrigerator or at 0°F or below in the freezer. These three basic concepts are translated into the food safety rules given in Display 4-1 and illustrated in Figure 4-2.

Microwave cooking does not always cook food evenly. Some spots are not thoroughly cooked. The friction caused by the microwaves inside the food actually does the cooking. Cooking begins just below the surface of the food. Full cooking is achieved as the heat starts to spread throughout the rest of the food. To complete cooking the food throughout without overcooking the high-heat spots, many microwave recipes call for a 10- to 15-minute standing time following the power cooking. It is important to observe these instructions to allow cooking to continue after removing the food from the microwave while the heat spreads evenly through the food. Display 4-2 gives safety rules for cooking meat in the microwave.

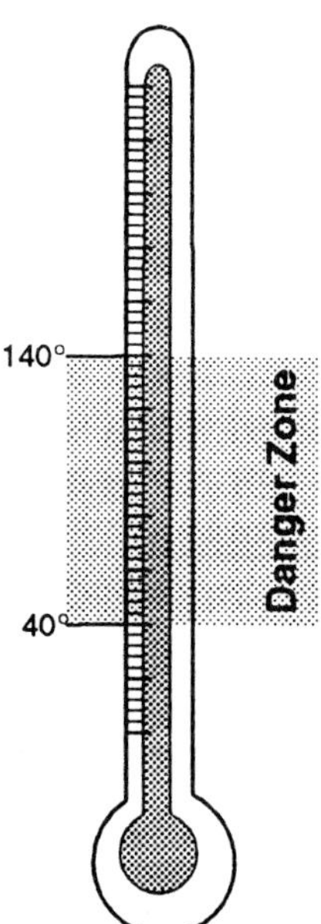
Danger Zone
140°
40°
Danger Zone
Keep Hot Foods Hot: above 140° F
Keep Cold Foods Cold: below 40° F
Avoid The Danger Zone

FIGURE 4-2

When holding or storing food, temperature control keeps the harmful bacteria that are in food from multiplying. Even at temperatures of 140°F or more, hot foods should not be kept out more than 2 hours.

HAZARD ANALYSIS CRITICAL CONTROL POINT (HACCP) SYSTEM

HACCP is a preventive system used widely in the commercial food industry to ensure food safety. This approach has resulted from the heightened concern about food safety in recent years and appears to offer the greatest promise for resolving safety concerns before the food reaches the consumer. The Food and Drug Administration of the US Department of Health and Human Services and the Food Safety and Inspection Service of the US Department of Agriculture are working to make HACCP the basis for their food safety regulations.

The Hazard Analysis Critical Control Point System is developed and implemented by the food processor or retail food outlet (restaurant, hospital, nursing home, food market) and includes:

- a breakdown of the production of a product or of food preparation into a series of identifiable steps
- identification of those steps where hazards (pathogens, metals, chemicals, pollutants) could develop and cause the food to be unsafe for consumers
- identification of "critical control points" in the process where failure could cause the hazard to occur
- identification of operating procedure for each critical control point (e.g. proper refrigerator temperature)
- establishment of monitoring procedures for tracking performance of critical control points (e.g. checking temperature of refrigerators twice daily)
- establishment of corrective action to be taken if monitoring shows a problem
- establishment of record-keeping procedures to record results of monitoring
- verification that control system is working by

DISPLAY 4-2 SAFETY GUIDELINES FOR MICROWAVE COOKING

DEFROSTING

- *When using a microwave to defrost, finish cooking the food immediately.* Some areas begin to cook during defrost cycle, raising food to temperatures that promote bacterial growth.
- *Remove food from store wrap before thawing in a microwave.* Foam trays and plastic wraps are not heat stable; they may cause chemicals in the wraps to migrate into the food.
- *Do not defrost or hold food at room temperature for more than 2 hours.* It is easy to forget a food item thawing in the microwave.

COOKING

- *Debone meat and cook it slowly at a lower temperature.* Bone may shield some of the meat from heating through.
- *Arrange food items uniformly in a covered dish and add a little liquid.* When covered, steam helps kill bacteria and ensures uniform heating. Vent plastic wraps to allow steam to escape. If plastic wrap is used as a cover, it should not touch food.
- *Cook large pieces of meat at 50% power for longer period.* This allows the heat to reach deeper portions without overcooking outer areas.
- *Move the food inside the dish several times during cooking.* Stir soups and stews. If the microwave does not have a turntable, turn entire dish several times during cooking. This is especially important for casseroles.
- *Do not cook whole, stuffed poultry in microwave.* Both poultry and stuffing may not cook adequately.
- *Never partially cook food.* If planning to combine microwave cooking with conventional cooking such as broiling, transfer microwaved food to conventional heat immediately.
- *Use oven temperature probe or meat thermometer to check that food is done.* Insert it at several places, avoiding bone and fat. Red meat should reach 160°F; poultry should reach 180°F.
- *Make allowances for differences in oven wattage.* Make sure food is well cooked.
- *Observe standing time specified in recipe.* It is necessary to complete cooking process.

WARMING PRECOOKED FOODS

- *Cover precooked foods with a microwave-safe plastic, waxed paper, or a glass lid.* This keeps moisture in and provides even cooking.
- *Heat leftovers and precooked food to at least 165°F.* Food should be very hot and steaming.
- *Do not heat infant formula in a microwave* because of the risk of burning the infant's mouth. *Commercial infant foods containing a substantial amount of protein such as meat, poultry, meat dinners, or egg yolks should not be heated in a microwave;* these foods heat unevenly, resulting in the possibility of explosion. Other baby foods should be thoroughly mixed and taste-tested before given to an infant.

UTENSILS, WRAPS, AND COOKWARE

- *Use of glass and ceramic cookware is safe.*
- *Use only those containers and products approved for microwave use.* These products are designed to withstand high temperatures when cooking foods that have a high fat or sugar content.
- *Avoid using cold storage containers,* such as margarine, cottage cheese, or whipped topping tubs. High heat could cause chemicals to transfer into food.
- *Use of waxed paper is safe.* Other paper products such as towels, plates, and napkins have not been tested for microwave use. If used, use only plain white paper goods.
- *Avoid letting plastic wrap touch foods during microwaving.* If not a heavy duty type, it could melt in contact with hot food.
- *Do not reuse trays and containers provided with microwave convenience foods.* They have been designed for one-time use with that specific food only.
- *Use of oven cooking bags is safe in microwaves.* They are made from tough nylon material and promote even cooking of food.
- *Never use brown grocery bags and newspapers.* These contain recycled materials and metals that could start a fire.
- *Follow package directions when heating microwavable foods with special browning or crisping devices in the package.* Do not reuse these browning devices and do not eat from a package that becomes charred.

Adapted from Conley S, Williamson C, Johnston M. A microwave handbook. Food News for Consumers 1993;9:4:4–5.)

both the company or the food establishment and regulators (city, state, federal).

The system is gaining in popularity in hospital dietary departments as a means of ensuring food safety and quality. The system can be applied to clinical nutrition services, e.g. as a means of preventing foodborne illness among clients who are tube fed.

FOOD TOXICITY DUE TO CHEMICALS

We rarely think of foods in their natural state as a group of chemicals. Nevertheless, a food seemingly as simple as a potato consists of far more than 100 chemicals. Harmful chemicals can enter the food supply as a result of nature, accident, carelessness, or environmental pollution, or during production and processing.

NATURAL TOXICITY

Some foods contain toxic substances as part of their chemical makeup. Potatoes contain *solanine,* a compound that can interfere with the transmission of nerve impulses. Spinach and rhubarb contain *oxalates,* which combine with calcium, making it unavailable for its functions. Cabbage and turnips contain *goitrogens,* substances that may interfere with the proper functioning of the thyroid gland and cause it to enlarge. A cancer-causing substance in pollen has been found in honey. These are a few examples of potentially harmful substances that occur naturally in foods. The quantity of toxic substances found in commonly eaten foods is low, however, and extremely large amounts would have to be ingested over a long period to do harm. Interactions between chemicals may block the toxic substances, and the heat of cooking can destroy certain toxic substances, as in legumes. When there is a wide variety of foods in the diet, there is little chance that the toxic properties of any one food will be harmful.

TOXIC METALS

Toxic metals such as mercury, lead, and cadmium contaminate the environment and may enter the food supply. The high levels of mercury occurring in fish are, in some cases, due to pollution and, in other cases, due simply to a high mercury concentration occurring naturally in some unpolluted waters. Industrial pollution is the main cause of freshwater fish contamination. In contrast, fish such as swordfish, which have a long life span, tend to accumulate the mercury that is naturally present in the ocean. The federal government has set a limit of 5 parts per million as an acceptable level of mercury in fish.

Foods can become contaminated when placed in containers made with toxic materials. Lead poisoning can occur when an earthenware pitcher is used to store orange juice. Copper poisoning can be caused when soft drinks are dispensed through tubing that has eroded to its copper base.

Acceptable levels of lead and cadmium in earthenware products also have been established. The FDA recently proposed the ban of all lead-soldered cans used for food either from US or foreign markets. The purpose of the ban is to reduce harmful effects of lead in fetuses, infants, and children who are especially sensitive to lead exposure. Because most US manufacturers and food processors no longer make or use lead-soldered cans, imported canned foods are the target of the proposal.

ENVIRONMENTAL POLLUTION AND FISH

Reports of contamination with polychlorinated biphenyls (PCBs) from industrial wastes and harmful bacteria have raised questions about the safety of eating fish. Fish tend to concentrate pollutants in their bodies as big fish consume smaller fish and plants. Also, they filter gallons upon gallons of water through their systems, leaving pollutants and contaminants behind. Unfortunately, rivers, streams, and oceans are full of sewage, dangerous heavy metals such as mercury and lead, and industrial wastes.

Fish caught offshore or deep at sea, where the water is significantly cleaner, are less likely to be affected. Industrial pollution is most likely to be a problem in sheltered ocean bays, harbors, and recreational freshwater lakes and streams that are near industrial plants. Bacterial contamination primarily affects mollusks and shellfish. Bacterial contamination can be overcome by adequately cooking mollusks and shellfish rather than eating them raw or undercooked.

Polychlorinated biphenyls (PCBs) are most likely to concentrate in large fatty fish. Bluefish is one of the species of saltwater fish most susceptible to contamination. Some experts believe that PCBs pose a problem only for recreational fishers and their families who eat bluefish regularly.

Fish is an excellent food with many health benefits. These benefits can be enjoyed with a little caution and common sense. Guidelines for using fish safely are given in Display 4-3.

ACCIDENTS

Accidents in which poisonous substances are mistaken for food are another cause of illness and death. Rat poison has been mistaken for flour and boric acid, for sugar. Death has resulted from mistakenly drinking cleaning fluid stored in a soda bottle. **Never** store household chemicals in empty food containers.

DISPLAY 4-3 SAFETY PRECAUTIONS FOR FISH

- Never eat fish or shellfish raw. People who insist on eating raw fish and shellfish should ensure that it has been frozen at least 3 days before preparation.
- Cook fish thoroughly until it flakes easily with fork and is opaque and firm. It should not be translucent.
- Boil molluscan shellfish (oysters, clams, mussels, and whole scallops), until shells open. Continue cooking 3–5 minutes more after shells open; steamed shellfish should be cooked at least 5 minutes (not just until they open). Discard any clams, mussels, or oysters that do not open during cooking.
- Boil or simmer shucked oysters for at least 3 minutes; fry in oil at least 10 minutes at 375°F; or bake at least 10 minutes at 450°F.
- Check that mollusks in the shell are alive when purchased. Discard any that do not close tightly. Store live mollusks in refrigerator covered loosely with a clean, damp cloth so they can breath. Do not store in airtight containers or water.
- Remove the skin and dark-colored flesh of fatty fish because chemicals tend to concentrate in fish fat. Also grill or broil fatty fish to allow drippings to run off.
- Buy fish from reputable fish stores. Ask to see the shipper's tag for molluscan shellfish.
- Vary the species of the fish you eat.
- Be sure the fish is displayed on thick layers of ice; fish should have a pleasant ocean smell. The flesh of the fish should be shiny, moist, and firm—not soft or spongy. Avoid fish with drying or browning around the edges.
- Keep cooked and raw seafood separate. Be sure your deli does not display raw fish next to cooked fish.
- Cook fish no later than 2 days after purchase. Cook shrimp and pawns as soon as possible because they have probably been frozen and then thawed.
- Store fresh fish in coldest part of your refrigerator in the same wrapper it had in the store. Thaw frozen fish in the refrigerator. Marinate fish in the refrigerator.
- Treat raw fish like raw chicken. Be sure to wash hands and all utensils and surfaces in hot soapy water before touching anything else to avoid cross contamination.
- Heed advisory warnings put out by the state and fishing associations to stay away from certain species. Call state wildlife associations or the health department for advisories. Do not fish downstream from industrial complexes.

Adapted from US Food and Drug Administration. Get hooked on seafood safety: important information for people with gastrointestinal disorders. U.S. Food and Drug Administration. Washington, DC, 1992. DHHS publication FDA 92-2259.)

ADDITIVES

A *food additive* is any substance that becomes part of a food when added either intentionally or accidentally. Food additives are not new. Salt, herbs, and spices have been used for years as preservatives. In the 20th century, the increase in food additives has been a result of mass production of food, long-distance transportation, long storage periods, and increased demand for convenience foods. The effect of additives on health, especially in the long term, is frequently questioned.

Intentional food additives all have some useful purpose in the food product; they include food supplements (vitamins and minerals), preservatives, antioxidants, stabilizers, emulsifiers, and coloring and flavoring agents. Some 2800 of these substances are used presently. Another 10,000 are incidental additives that find their way into food, although their presence is not desired. These additives include pesticides, fertilizers, hormones and tranquilizers given to animals used for meat, and chemicals used in packaging to preserve freshness.

LEGISLATIVE CONTROL OF FOOD ADDITIVES

Intentional food additives added to food by manufacturers serve many useful purposes: they retard spoilage, improve nutrition, add leavening, enhance flavor and color, and maintain texture. The FDA is authorized by amendments to the Food, Drug, and Cosmetic Act of 1938 to regulate the safety of food additives. This legislation requires that manufacturers prove that each proposed additive is safe for human consumption. The steps required for approval of an additive may take several years, during which time a manufacturer must prove by various tests and procedures that the additive is not a cause of cancer or birth defects and has no other known harmful effects. The Delaney Clause in the Food Additives Amendment of 1958 specifies that no additive can be permitted that produces cancer in test animals, even if the risk for humans is remote. The FDA also monitors the food packaging materials to ensure they are not hazardous.

Because sulfites can cause serious allergic reactions in persons who are sulfite-sensitive, FDA issued the following regulations in 1986: sulfites used as preservatives must be listed on the label regardless of amount; sulfites used in food processing must be listed if present at levels of 10 ppm or higher; use of sulfites on fruits and vegetables intended to be eaten raw, such as in salad bars and grocery store produce sections, is banned.

GRAS LIST

In the 1958 Food Additives Amendment, two categories of additives were exempted from the testing and approval process. One group consists of substances that were approved for use in food before 1958; the second consists of some 700 additives known as the GRAS list. A *GRAS additive* is one that experts have judged to be *g*enerally *r*ecognized *a*s *s*afe. GRAS additives did not undergo extensive testing to determine their safety and were not strictly regulated. The reasoning behind the GRAS list is that it is unnecessary to prove the safety of substances that have been in use for long periods with no known harmful effects.

In 1968, prompted by the uncertainty that had developed about the safety of cyclamates, the FDA decided to review the GRAS list. Most of the additives have been approved; others have been reclassified and further testing recommended.

PESTICIDES

Pesticides are an example of an incidental or indirect additive. Farmers use pesticides to control pests that cause their crops to become diseased and damaged. Pesticides control such pests as harmful insects, molds, fungi, and weeds. Many molds and fungi are a danger to humans as well as to crops. Although exposure to minute pesticide residues in foods do not immediately or in the short term cause ill effects, the possibility of harmful cumulative effects over a lifetime is cause for concern.

The federal government determines what pesticides may be used and what residue levels are permissible. Farmers are legally obligated to use pesticides according to established standards—to use no more than is necessary and to wait an established period from the last application of a pesticide until they harvest the food.

The US Environmental Protection Agency (EPA) evaluates scientific information to determine if a pesticide is safe to use. The pesticides are subjected to more than 120 separate tests. These tests assess the possible effects of the pesticide on humans, fish, wildlife, and the environment. If the pesticide meets EPA standards, the manufacturer is granted a "product registration" or license to sell, which stipulates how the product can be used.

The EPA establishes an *Acceptable Daily Intake (ADI)*, also called "reference dose," for each pesticide. The ADI is the maximum level of residue recommended in our diet and considers the cumulative contribution of all food residues to our diets. The ADI is 100 to 1000 times lower than the level at which no health effects are observed in laboratory animals. *Tolerances* are then established both for fresh and processed food. A tolerance is a maximum residue level of a specific pesticide legally permitted on or in a food, feed, or food constituent.

Tolerances are used in monitoring to ensure the safety of the food supply. The FDA monitors the incidence and levels of pesticide residues in food products other than meat and poultry. The Food Safety and Inspection Service (FSIS) of the USDA monitors chemical residues in meat, poultry, and dairy products. According to the FDA's Residue Monitoring Program, little or any residue remains on the food we buy.

PREVENTING CHEMICAL TOXICITY: IMPORTANCE OF A VARIED DIET

A diet consisting of a wide variety of foods provides the best protection against potentially harmful chemicals in food. The body tolerates small quantities of many toxic substances but has only a limited ability to cope with large quantities of any single one.

Almost any chemical can have a harmful effect if it is taken in a large enough quantity—even sodium or vitamin D. It is important to understand the difference between toxicity and hazard. Many foods contain toxic chemicals, but these chemicals do not present a hazard in the usual amount consumed.

GOVERNMENT'S ROLE IN REGULATING THE FOOD SUPPLY

The consumer has an important role in safeguarding the food supply once the food is purchased. The consumer, however, must rely on federal, state, and local government agencies to protect the food supply before it reaches the point of purchase.

The federal government regulates the shipment of foods over state lines, foods manufactured in US territories and the District of Columbia, and the import and export of foods. State governments control most foods manufactured and sold within state boundaries.

FOOD AND DRUG ADMINISTRATION (FDA)

The FDA of the US Department of Health and Human Services is responsible for protecting the consumer against unsafe, unsanitary, and improperly labeled products. The FDA enforces food safety standards for all processed foods other than meat, poultry, or eggs that are in interstate commerce. Adulterated and misbranded foods are prohibited for sale by the FDA. A food is considered adulterated if it contains spoiled or filthy products, meat from diseased animals, or noncertified colors; if it is diluted or a substitute ingredient is used; if an essential ingredient is omitted; if the packaging material is made from hazardous substances; if it contains additives that conceal nutritional deficiencies or additives that have not been approved by the FDA; or if it is produced or stored under unsanitary conditions.

The agency sets sanitary standards and inspects establishments that produce, process, store, or transport food other than meat or poultry to see that standards are met. The FDA provides educational materials and programs for industry, professional, and consumer groups on food safety and health issues under its jurisdiction. The FDA also monitors the incidence and levels of pesticide residues in food products other than meat and poultry.

FOOD SAFETY AND INSPECTION SERVICE (FSIS)

The Food Safety and Inspection Service (FSIS) of the USDA develops safety standards and labeling regulations for meat and poultry products. The FSIS inspects sanitation and operating procedures of meat and poultry processing plants. The FSIS provides educational materials and programs on food sanitation and safety for industry, professional, and consumer groups. The FSIS also monitors the incidence and levels of pesticide residues in meat, poultry, and dairy products.

ENVIRONMENTAL PROTECTION AGENCY (EPA)

The EPA regulates the manufacturing, labeling, and use of pesticides. The Safe Drinking Water Act of 1974, administered by the EPA, established minimum standards for drinking water, including limitation of potentially harmful substances. States are responsible for enforcing the regulations. The FDA, however, is responsible for regulating the purity of bottled water and water used in food and food processing.

FEDERAL TRADE COMMISSION (FTC)

The Federal Trade Commission regulates the advertising of foods, drugs, and cosmetics through media such as television and radio. Its responsibility is to protect the public against false and misleading advertising.

STATE AND LOCAL AGENCIES

State departments of health and agriculture work with federal agencies such as the FDA, FSIS, and the EPA to assure food safety. Most states play a role in monitoring residues and reviewing safety test results within their state territories.

The pasteurization of milk and the inspection of cattle and goats that produce milk are under state control. State agencies are also responsible for regulating the production and processing of food products that are sold within state boundaries and are not in interstate commerce. Local governments also may have sanitary codes that regulate food production and processing and provide for the inspection of public eating establishments.

SOURCES OF RELIABLE FOOD SAFETY INFORMATION

Local field offices of the FDA and local or county offices of the Cooperative Extension Service are excellent sources of information and educational materials on food safety. Also, state and local health and agriculture agencies sponsorcational programs and provide information and educational materials. They also process complaints regarding food sanitation and safety.

KEYS TO PRACTICAL APPLICATION

Be aware of the devastating effect of foodborne illness on immunocompromised people.

Accept the responsibility for upholding the highest standards of food sanitation that working in the health care system requires.

Follow the rules of food safety given in Displays 4-1, 4-2, and 4-3 and Table 4-2.

Know where to go for information regarding food sanitation and safety in your local area.

KEY IDEAS

Contamination of food by disease-causing organisms or harmful toxins produced by organisms is the most common cause of illness due to food consumption. People with weakened immune systems are more likely to develop serious complications from foodborne illness.

Campylobacter jejuni, Listeria monocytogenes, and *E. coli* 0157:H7 are more recently identified disease-causing bacteria.

Salmonella bacteria are carried by raw meats, poultry, eggs, milk, fish, and household pets. They are destroyed by heat.

Infection with *C. perfringens* usually occurs when food is left at room temperature for long periods.

Staphylococcal poisoning is caused by toxins from staph bacteria, which enter food from boils, infected cuts, and coughing and sneezing; the toxins accumulate when food is held at an improper temperature.

Botulism, a rare but deadly form of food poisoning, most frequently is caused by homecanned, low-acid foods. Botulism also can form in bacon or smoked meats that have been prepared without the use of nitrites as preservatives and in food stored in warm, oxygen-free environments.

Campylobacter jejuni, present in the intestinal tract of healthy cattle and poultry, contaminates the meat and poultry during slaughter. The bacteria is destroyed by heat.

Listeria monocytogenes, although destroyed by cooking, may contaminate foods such as cheese and ice cream that do not require cooking. Avoid unpasteurized milk and products made from unpasteurized milk.

Shigellosis is usually caused by the contamination of food by a food handler who is infected with the *Shigella* bacteria; careful hand-washing is important.

E. coli 0157:H7 is a highly infectious, potentially fatal strain of bacteria recently associated with outbreaks due to undercooked hamburger; thorough cooking of ground meat, ground poultry, and all other cuts of meat and poultry is necessary.

Yersinia enterocolitica is of increasing concern because it can grow at normal refrigeration temperatures; thorough cooking and reheating of food and good sanitation and personal hygiene are important preventive measures.

V. vulnificus infects humans through the consumption of raw molluscan shellfish; thorough cooking completely destroys the bacteria.

Hepatitis A and the Norwalk virus are carried by mollusks; buy shellfish from reputable dealers and avoid eating raw shellfish.

Poisons produced by molds may have long-term harmful effects; it is advisable to discard moldy food.

Aflatoxin is a cancer-causing mold that develops in spoiled peanuts, peanut butter, nuts, soybeans, grains, spices, and animal products.

Trichinosis is caused by eating raw or undercooked pork. Raw fish (sushi) may be contaminated with a worm called *Anisakis marina.*

Cryptosporidium is now considered to be one of the foremost causes of diarrhea in the world; in the United States, it was recently associated with contaminated water.

Foodborne illness is prevented by protecting food from contamination and by temperature control. Thoroughly cook and reheat food and keep hot foods hot (above 140°F) and cold foods cold (below 40°F).

The consumer's role in food safety involves good food handling practices, such as good personal hygiene, proper food storage, temperature control, and sanitary practices in preparing and cooking food (see Display 4-1, 4-2, and 4-3 and Table 4-2).

Chemical contamination of food can result from food containers made with toxic materials, environmental pollution, the accumulation of toxic metals in animals and fish, and radioactive fallout. Poisoning also can occur through ingestion of toxic substances mistaken for food.

Fish are subject to contamination from water polluted with industrial wastes and from harmful bacteria. See Display 4-3 for suggestions for ensuring a safe fish supply.

The EPA controls pesticides and the FDA and the FSIS monitor pesticide residues in food.

The FDA controls the use of food additives. Manufacturers must prove by extensive tests that an additive is safe.

The GRAS list is a list of food additives that experts have recognized as generally safe and, by law, are exempt from testing. As a result of a review of these substances, some additives have been reclassified and recommended for further testing.

Eating a varied diet and consuming no single food in excessive amounts provide the best protection against harmful chemicals in food.

Various government agencies protect the food supply in aspects of food safety that are beyond the control of the individual. These agencies receive their authority from federal laws designed to protect the public.

The three major agencies most involved in promoting food safety are the Food and Drug Administration, the Food Safety and Inspection Service (of USDA), and the Environmental Protection Agency.

KEYS TO LEARNING

STUDY–DISCUSSION QUESTIONS

1. The consumer can prevent foodborne disease by controlling the number of bacteria in food eaten at home. In what three basic ways can the consumer accomplish this control? Discuss the sanitary food handling practices that promote the control of harmful bacteria.
2. Discuss the effects of foodborne illness on people with weakened immune systems. What sanitary food handling practices can be used in client areas of hospitals and nursing homes to prevent foodborne illness?
3. Give the recommended temperatures and visual checks for

    cooked hamburger
    cooked ground turkey
    cooked meat (not ground)
    cooked poultry (not ground)
    holding hot foods
    holding cold foods

4. What is the proper method for home-canning low-acid foods? Why is the use of this method so important? What precautions should a person take before eating home-canned, low-acid foods? What conditions promote botulism? Are canned foods the only source of this disease? Explain.
5. Why is it important to observe the standing time specified in recipes when microwave cooking meat and poultry?
6. Discuss the importance of a varied diet from the standpoint of food safety.
7. Contact the consumer information officer of the FDA field office in your area. Become informed of the services this office provides for consumers. Obtain the most recent FDA publications relating to food additives, nutrition labeling, or related subjects of interest to the class. Discuss with the class the information you have obtained.
8. Visit your local Cooperative Extension Service. Discuss with the Extension home economist or agricultural agent the food safety services provided by this agency.
9. Visit your local health department or have a representative from the department speak to the class about the department's role in protecting the safety of the food supply.

BIBLIOGRAPHY

BOOKS AND PAMPHLETS

Hathcock JH, Rader JI. Food additives, contaminants and natural toxins. In: Shils ME, Olson JA, Shike M. Eds. Modern nutrition in health and disease. 8th ed. Philadelphia: Lea and Febiger, 1994:1593–1611.

Hecht A. The unwelcome dinner guest: preventing foodborne illness. Rockville, MD: Food and Drug Administration, 1991. DHHS publication FDA 91-2244.

Pariza MW. Diet, cancer, and food safety. In: Shils ME, Olson JA, Shike M. Eds. Modern nutrition in health and disease. 8th ed. Philadelphia: Lea and Febiger, 1994:1545–1558.

US Dept of Health and Human Services, Public Health Service/Food and Drug Administration. Eating defensively: food safety advice for person with AIDS. Bethesda, MD: US Dept of Health and Human Services, 1990. DHHS publication FDA 90-2232.

US Dept of Health and Human Services, Public Health Service/ Food and Drug Administration. Get hooked on seafood safety: important health information for people with gastrointestinal disorders. Bethesda, MD: US Dept of Health and Human Services, 1992. DHHS publication FDA 92-2259.

US Dept of Health and Human Services, Public Health Service/ Food and Drug Administration. News release, January 21, 1994.

PERIODICALS

Cabelof DC. Preventing infection from foodborne pathogens in liver transplant patients. J Am Diet Assoc 1994;94:1140.

Conley S, Williamson C, Johnston M. A microwave handbook. Food News for Consumers 1993;9:4:4.

Gantz H. Answering your questions on *E. coli*. Food News for Consumers 1993;10:3(summer suppl):4.

Golden DA, Rhodehamel EJ, Kautter DA. Growth of *Salmonella* spp in cantaloupe. J of Food Protection 1993;56:194.

Institute of Food Technologists' Expert Panel on Food Safety and Nutrition. Government regulation of food safety: interaction of scientific and societal forces. Food Technology 1992;46:73.

Moriarty P. *Campylobacter* control. Food News for Consumers 1991;8:1:14.

O'Brien B. FSIS moves to adopt HACCP. The new "gold standard" in modern food inspection. Food News for Consumers 1991;8:2:14.

O'Brien B. USDA researcher develops new *Yersinia* tests. Food News for Consumers 1991;8:2:14.

Parmley MA. What to do about mold—a consumer handbook. Food News for Consumers 1993;9:4:8.

Ross EE, Guyer L, Varnes J, et al. *Vibrio vulnificus* and molluscan shellfish: the necessity of education for high-risk individuals. J Am Diet Assoc 1994;94:132.

Schiller MR, Catakis, A. Hazard analysis critical control points: Implications for clinical nutrition service delivery. Topics in Clinical Nutrition 1992;7:4:52.

Williamson C. *Cryptosporidium* update. Food News for Consumers 1993;10:3(summer suppl):11.

Winter CK. Pesticide residues and the Delaney Clause. Food Technology 1993;47:7:81.

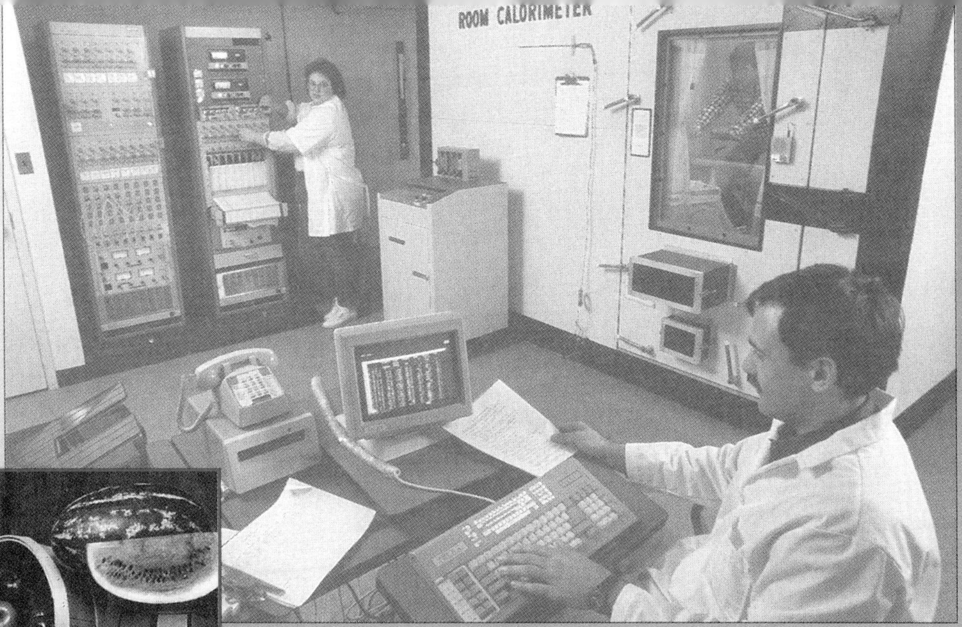

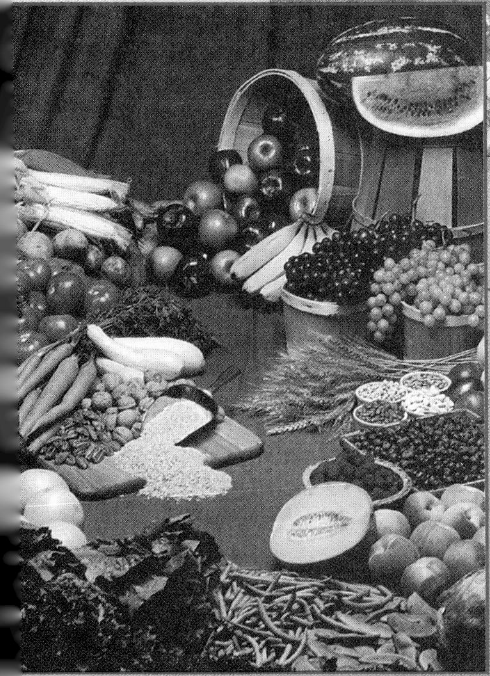

PART TWO

The Role of Nutrients in the Maintenance of Normal Health

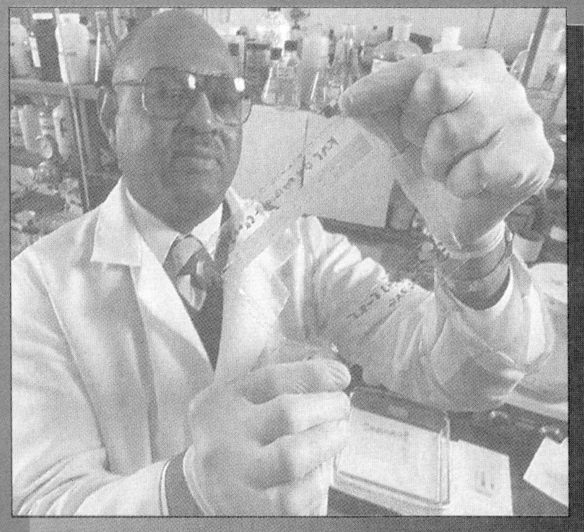

CHAPTER

5

Food and Its Functions; Food Guidelines, Guides, and Labeling

KEY TERMS

bioavailability the amount of a nutrient absorbed from the intestinal tract

catalyst a substance that causes or speeds up a chemical change without being changed itself

contemporary belonging to the same period

Daily Reference Values (DRVs) a set of dietary references used in food labeling that apply to fat, saturated fat, cholesterol, carbohydrate, fiber, protein, sodium, and potassium

Daily Value (DV) a dietary reference term used on food labels indicating what percentage a serving of a food contributes to recommended daily amounts; Daily Reference Values and Reference Daily Intakes serve as the basis for calculating the percentage of the Daily Value

Dietary Guidelines for Americans a US government publication presenting seven guidelines designed to promote good eating and reduce risk of chronic disease

enzyme a substance, usually a protein, that is formed in living cells and brings about chemical changes; the enzyme itself remains unchanged

extracellular outside the cell

graphic a diagram or pictorial presentation of an idea

intracellular inside the cell

kilocalorie (kcal) the unit of heat that measures the energy values of food or the energy needs of the body; it represents the amount of heat required to raise the temperature of 1 kg of water 1°C

median in the middle; the middle number of a series of numbers (as in lists of weights or heights)

Recommended Dietary Allowances (RDAs) a national standard that lists all the nutrients known to be essential for health and the recommended daily intake; it provides for variation among most healthy people in the United States

Reference Daily Intakes (RDIs) a set of dietary references used in food labeling that are based on the Recommended Dietary Allowances for essential vitamins and minerals and, in selected groups, protein

standard an approved model or pattern that serves as a basis for comparison

OBJECTIVES

After completing this chapter, the student will be able to:

1. Cite the six categories of nutrients and the three basic functions of the nutrients.
2. Explain what is meant by the interaction of the nutrients, the storage of nutrients, and the stages in the development of deficiency diseases.
3. Identify the standard in the United States to which food consumption is compared to determine adequacy.

4. Cite at least one important publication that identifies excessive food consumption as a health problem in the United States.
5. Explain the significance of the Dietary Guidelines for Americans.
6. Cite the seven Dietary Guidelines for Americans.
7. Explain the role of a food guide.
8. Describe the Food Guide Pyramid; cite its food groups and recommended servings from each group; and explain how it conveys proportion, moderation, and variety.
9. Evaluate the student's own food intake in comparison with the Pyramid and identify shortcomings, if any.
10. Use food labeling—both nutrition and ingredient labeling—in a more informed and comprehensive manner. Explain how food labeling regulations help consumers follow the Dietary Guidelines for Americans.

This chapter is a brief overview preparatory to our study of the individual nutrients. It offers an opportunity to see the whole as a means of better understanding the individual parts, and to see how what we know about the science of nutrition is interpreted in terms of the food we eat daily.

NUTRIENTS

There are more than 50 known nutrients, yet all can be classified into six categories: (1) carbohydrates, (2) proteins, (3) fats, (4) vitamins, (5) minerals, and (6) water. Fiber, which also plays a role in the diet, is not considered a nutrient because it is not absorbed by the bloodstream.

Most foods contain more than one nutrient group. Milk, for example, contains water, protein, carbohydrate, fat, the minerals calcium, phosphorus, and sodium and the vitamins A, riboflavin, thiamin, and niacin. Foods usually are identified by the amount of protein, carbohydrate, or fat they contain. A *protein food* is one that contains more protein than fat or carbohydrate (e.g., fish). In contrast, bacon is considered a fat food, although it contains some protein. This classification is useful, yet many exceptions exist. Peanut butter usually is classified as a protein food; however, it contains significant amounts of fat and carbohydrate as well as protein. Beef usually is considered a protein food; however, some fatty cuts of beef, such as the steak or rib portion, may contain more fat than protein.

For the cells to be nourished, food eaten must be changed to a form cells can use. This is done by the digestive system. Once food has been reduced to its simplest form, it passes through the intestinal tract into the blood and lymph and eventually is carried to the liver. In the liver, additional changes in the nutrients occur before distribution to other body cells. By means of the circulatory system, the nutrients finally reach the extracellular fluid from which the cells select the nutrients they need. The waste products that result from cellular activity are released into the extracellular fluid and enter the bloodstream to be excreted from the body, primarily through the lungs and kidney.

Each cell, such as a blood cell or a nerve cell, has its own work or specific activity. Each cell also has specific nutritional needs; the nutrient needs of one type of cell differ from those of another. Adequate nutrition of all the cells is the goal—the health of the cells determines the health of the tissues, which in turn determines the health of the organs and bodily systems.

FUNCTIONS OF NUTRIENTS

Nutrients perform three basic functions: (1) building and maintaining body tissue, (2) furnishing energy, and (3) regulating body processes. All of the nutrient classes are involved in the building and maintenance of body tissue. Some nutrients, such as protein and minerals, are major structural components of the body, whereas others, such as vitamins, play supporting roles in tissue growth and maintenance. All of the nutrient classes also are involved in regulating body processes. Although only protein, fat, and carbohydrate furnish energy, all the other nutrient classes play crucial roles in this bodily process.

BUILDING AND MAINTAINING TISSUES

Water makes up one half to two thirds of an adult's weight. It is an essential part of every cell and is the basic substance of blood, lymph, and body secretions. All body cells require protein. Fat rounds the body contours and provides protective padding and support for vital organs. Calcium and phosphorus are deposited in bones and teeth. Various minerals are found in body tissues. Carbohydrates used mainly for energy occurs only in small amounts in body tissues. Even when the body has reached its final growth, material that composes the cells is continually exchanged. The body is constantly renewing itself.

FURNISHING ENERGY

The body uses carbohydrates, fats, and proteins as fuel. Providing energy is a main function of carbohydrates and fats. Proteins provide energy when carbohydrates and fats do not meet the body's energy needs.

The energy value of food or the energy needs of the body are measured in units called *calories*. Calories represent the amount of heat produced by ingested food. The large calorie, or kilocalorie (kcal), is the amount of heat required to raise 1 kg (1000 g) of water 1°C. The calorie used in nutrition is always the larger calorie or kilocalorie.

The body requires energy for its ongoing activities. These activities include not only such obvious ones as breathing and walking but also the infinite number of hidden tasks carried out by the trillions of body cells.

REGULATING BODY PROCESSES

The cell has been aptly described as a chemical factory. The chemicals the cells produce are called *enzymes*. An enzyme is a protein that directs the activities of the cell. Enzymes are catalysts, that is, they cause chemical reactions to occur but do not themselves change. Vitamins and minerals combine with specific proteins to form enzymes.

In addition to enzymes, the body produces other substances that act as regulators. For example, hemoglobin is an iron-containing substance in the blood that transports oxygen to the cells. The hormone insulin is needed to convert blood glucose to energy.

Water is an important regulator because all chemical reactions in the body occur in its presence. As the basic ingredient of body fluids, water permits nutrients to be digested, absorbed, and circulated to the cells. Water provides for the elimination of waste products and also regulates body temperature.

NUTRIENTS WORKING TOGETHER

Like the cells, the nutrients each have a part to play. They cannot function independently, however. The functions of the nutrients are related in a complex fashion. Any changes in the consumption of one nutrient may lead to changes in the activity of others. For example, the absorption of calcium depends on the supply of vitamin D. Calcium, in turn, is needed for the absorption of vitamin B_{12}.

NUTRIENT STORAGE

Some nutrients can be stored in the body as a reserve that is called on when food intake is low, as in illness, or when need is increased, as in pregnancy. Excess nutrients that cannot be stored are excreted, principally in the urine.

The ability to store certain nutrients is not always an advantage. Obesity can result from excessive caloric intake; an excess of certain vitamins and minerals also may cause harmful effects. Toxic effects have resulted from excessive intake of vitamins A, D, and others in the form of vitamin supplements. Excessive intake of minerals usually is due not to food itself but to minerals that contaminate the food supply. For example, copper poisoning has been know to develop from deteriorating copper tubing through which sodas and other fountain drinks are served.

DEVELOPMENT OF DEFICIENCY DISEASES

Inadequate intake of a nutrient does not produce immediate, dramatic effects. At first, the body goes through a period of exhausting its reserves. This time varies from a few hours in the case of protein to as long as 7 years for calcium. During this period of depletion, the body attempts to cope with the deficiency. Eventually, the individual cells become depleted of the nutrient, and the symptoms of deficiency disease become evident. Scurvy, beriberi, pellagra, and simple goiter are examples of deficiency diseases.

PROVIDING FOR ADEQUACY: NUTRIENT STANDARDS

What nutrients do we need and in what amounts to keep physically fit? What foods supply these nutrients? Do we only need to be concerned about getting enough of the nutrients? Or is it possible to consume too much? To answer these questions, reference guides, standards to which we can compare the nutrient content of the food we eat, have been developed.

RECOMMENDED DIETARY ALLOWANCES

How much of each nutrient is required by the body is the subject of intensive and continual study. In the United States, standards of nutrition are set by the Committee on Dietary Allowances, appointed by the Food and Nutrition Board of the Institute of Medicine of the National Academy of Sciences. The committee recommends the amounts of nutrients required at all age levels to keep the normal population well nourished. The committee recommendations are summarized in Appendix B, Recommended Dietary Allowances (RDAs), revised, 1989. The RDAs are revised periodically to reflect new information.

The RDAs shown in Appendix B and the recommended energy intakes (see Table 7-1) are expressed in terms of reference individuals—individuals of a specific height and weight. In the 10th edition of the RDAs, heights and weights of references adults in each of the age–sex categories are the actual median heights and weights for the US population of a given age, as reported in the second National Health and Nutrition Examination Survey (NHANES II). They are actual heights and weights and should not be considered ideal.

The RDAs are guides, not requirements. Individuals differ in their precise nutritional requirements. To consider these differences among healthy people, the RDAs provides a margin of safety. That is, allowances are set high enough to cover the needs of most healthy people. It provides not only for individual differences but also for storage of nutrients as a means of protection during periods of stress.

Energy requirements are an exception in that they are based on average requirements. They are listed separately from the RDA table (see Table 7-1). The RDAs do not apply to people who are ill or who have increased or decreased requirements because of disease or use of medications.

USE OF THE RDAS

The dietary allowances are intended for professional use. They are used most appropriately when applied to broad areas such as evaluating the adequacy of the national food supply, setting standards for publicly funded programs and community agencies that serve clients in the area of nutrition, and developing nutrition education materials.

In practice, however, the RDAs frequently are used to evaluate the adequacy of an individual's food intake. If a healthy individual consumes food that meets or exceeds the RDAs, it is likely that the person is meeting his or her nutritional needs to the fullest. Failure to meet the RDAs, however, does not necessarily indicate that the person is malnourished, because the RDAs are higher than the requirements of most people. If a person consumes considerably less than the RDA for a nutrient over

a prolonged period, the risk of deficiency increases. To determine the nutritional status of an individual requires a thorough assessment, as described in Chapter 2.

STANDARDS IN OTHER COUNTRIES

Other countries, including Canada, have established dietary allowances for their populations. The World Health Organization also has adopted dietary recommendations. Dietary recommendations may differ from country to country because of factors such as differing climate, occupations, and availability of food and also because of the way the committee that develops the standards interprets the research. The Canadian equivalent of the RDAs is called the Recommended Nutrient Intakes for Canadians (see Appendix C).

AVOIDING EXCESS: RECOMMENDATIONS AND GUIDELINES

The victory over infectious diseases (such as diphtheria, small pox, and polio) and the prevention of nutritional deficiency diseases (such as scurvy, pellagra, and beriberi) that occurred in the early 1900s have led to an increased life expectancy in the United States and other developed nations. Americans today face early death and/or disability from chronic health problems such as obesity, hypertension, coronary heart disease, stroke, cancer, diabetes mellitus, diseases of the liver, and osteoporosis.

In the mid-1900s, health professionals began to realize that there was more to nutritional health than providing all the essential nutrients in adequate amounts. They expressed concern that food habits involving *excess* consumption of calories, saturated fat, cholesterol and salt were promoting the potential for chronic disease. Although the RDAs provided guidance in achieving an adequate diet, they did not address these other aspects of American eating habits.

SURGEON GENERAL'S REPORT

In 1988, the Public Health Service of the US Department of Health and Human Services (DHHS) published *The Surgeon General's Report on Nutrition and Health*, the first devoted exclusively to nutrition. The publication reviewed the large body of scientific evidence that linked diet to chronic disease. Based on this evidence, the report recommended dietary changes that could improve health prospects for many Americans. The chief recommendation was to reduce the intake of fat, especially saturated fat, and to increase intake of foods high in complex carbohydrates and fiber, such as fruits, vegetables, and whole grains. Although the report did not present any new information, it underscored the fact that these recommendations were well supported by scientific evidence. The recommendations received overwhelming acceptance from authorities and from the leading US health organizations.

The report was prepared primarily for use by institutions, agencies, and the food industry in developing nutrition policies. The recommendations also were used in the development of national health goals including *Healthy People 2000* (see Chapter 1).

DIET AND HEALTH REPORT OF THE FOOD AND NUTRITION BOARD

Another expert group of nutrition scientists, the Food and Nutrition Board of the National Academy of Sciences, also decided to study diet and its relationship to chronic disease. The Food and Nutrition Board is the recognized authority for setting standards of nutrition in the United States, notably the RDAs.

In 1984, the board established the Committee on Diet and Health to evaluate the scientific evidence relating dietary factors to chronic disease risk and to propose appropriate dietary guidelines. In 1989, the committee issued its first report in the publication *Diet and Health: Implications for Reducing Chronic Disease Risk*. The committee plans to provide periodic updates, much like the RDAs revisions, as new information becomes available. The eight dietary recommendations in this report are as follows:

1. Reduce total fat intake to 30% or less of calories. Reduce saturated fat intake to less than 10% of calories and cholesterol intake to less than 300 mg daily. The intake of fat and cholesterol can be reduced by substituting fish, poultry without skin, lean meats, and lowfat or nonfat dairy products for fatty meats and whole milk dairy products; by choosing more vegetables, fruits, cereals, and legumes; and by limiting oils, fats, egg yolks, and fried and other fatty foods.
2. Eat five or more servings of a combination of vegetables and fruits daily, especially green and yellow vegetables and citrus fruits. Increase intake of starches and other complex carbohydrates by eating six or more daily servings of a combination of breads, cereals, and legumes.
3. Maintain protein intake at moderate levels.
4. Balance food intake and physical activity to maintain appropriate body weight.
5. Limit consumption of alcohol to less than 1 oz of pure alcohol in a single day. This is the equivalent of two cans of beer, two small glasses of wine, or two average cocktails. However, the committee does not recommend that people drink alcoholic beverages. Pregnant women should avoid alcoholic beverages.
6. Limit total daily intake of salt (sodium chloride) to 6 g (2.4 g of sodium) or less. Limit use of salt in cooking and avoid adding it to food at the table. Consume salty, highly processed salty, salt-preserved, and salt-pickled foods sparingly.
7. Maintain adequate calcium intake.
8. Avoid taking dietary supplements in excess of the RDAs in any one day.
9. Maintain an optimal intake of fluoride, particularly during the years of primary and secondary tooth formation growth.

(These recommendations are referred to in the discussions of various nutrients in chapters that follow.)

DIETARY GUIDELINES FOR AMERICANS

In 1980, to address the issue of dietary excess with the general population, a publication entitled *Nutrition and Your Health: Dietary Guidelines for Americans* was issued jointly by the US Department of Agriculture (USDA) and the US Department of Health and Human Services (DHHS) (Consumer Information Center, Pueblo, CO 81009). This publication presents seven guidelines designed to promote health through moderation. The dietary guidelines serve as the main dietary message from the federal government for healthy Americans. The basic messages remained the same in the 1985 and 1990 revisions of the dietary guidelines. According to the 1995 Report of the Dietary Guidelines Advisory Committee, the changes to the latest revision are not substantial.

The new guidelines are as follows:

1. Eat a variety of food.
2. Balance the food you eat with physical activity. Maintain or improve your weight.
3. Choose a diet with plenty of grain products, vegetables and fruits.
4. Choose a diet low in fat, saturated fat, and cholesterol.
5. Choose a diet moderate in sugars.
6. Choose a diet moderate in salt and sodium.
7. If you drink alcoholic beverages, do so in moderation.

In the most recent revision, there is increased emphasis on foods with key nutrients such as calcium and folate. More emphasis has been given to the importance of physical activity in maintaining or improving weight status, as well as increased emphasis on the use of grains, fruits, and vegetables. The Food Guide Pyramid, discussed below, and the new nutrition label will be incorporated into the dietary guidelines pamphlet.

Nutrition Recommendations for Canadians and *Canada's Guidelines for Healthy Eating* are given in Appendix D.

FOOD GUIDES

Nutritional standards are of little value unless they can be translated into practical everyday food choices. Consumers need to know the kinds and amounts of food needed to obtain the recommended intake of nutrients.

Since the early 1900s, contemporary nutrition knowledge has been translated into *food guides* such as the basic four, also called the four food groups. Food guides are patterns or outlines for daily food choices based on food groups. The guides indicate the kinds and amounts of food that should be eaten daily to meet nutrition recommendations. In the past, food guides, including the basic four, focused on nutrient needs that would support growth and development and prevent deficiency diseases. Food guides emphasized a *foundation diet* to which other foods could be added to satisfy caloric needs. In the 1980s, with the increasing focus on the prevention of chronic degenerative diseases, the emphasis of food guides began to shift from a basic foundation diet to a *total diet.*

Food guides are based on choices from various food groups comprising foods of similar composition and nutritive value. Each food group is noted for its specific nutrient contributions to the diet. For example, the milk group is noted as a source of calcium; the fruits and vegetables groups are noted for their contributions of vitamins A and C and fiber.

In 1992, two new food guides were introduced: (1) the Food Guide Pyramid from the USDA and (2) the revised *Guide to Good Eating* from the National Dairy Council. Both are discussed as follows.

FOOD GUIDE PYRAMID

The Food Guide Pyramid, released in April 1992 by the USDA and the DHHS, is the official graphic of federal dietary guidelines and outlines what foods to eat daily. It is an exciting and sound educational tool for members of the health care team. The Food Guide Pyramid replaces the Four Food Group Wheel as the visual symbol representing the foods that compose the daily diet (Fig. 5-1). The Pyramid is intended to help Americans choose a diet that is higher in grains, fruits, and vegetables, and lower in fat and sugar.

The pieces of the Pyramid represent the five food groups (breads, cereals, rice, pasta; fruits; vegetables; meats, poultry, fish, dry beans and peas, eggs, and nuts; milk, yogurt, and cheese) and the fats, oils, and sweets commonly found in the diet. The size of the food-group piece corresponds to the number of daily servings recommended from that food group. For example, the largest number of servings recommended are in the bread–cereal group, which is the largest piece in the Pyramid. The Pyramid Food Guide to Daily Food Choices (see Table 14-1) provides information on portion sizes.

The need for moderation in the consumption of fats, oils, and sweets is conveyed by placing this group in the small tip of the Pyramid and by using a fat symbol (circle) and a sugar symbol (triangle) scattered throughout the Pyramid pieces to represent the naturally occurring and added fats and oils as well as added sugars in certain foods (see Fig. 5-1). The Pyramid conveys the following three essential elements of a healthy diet:

1. *Proportion,* that is, the relative amount of food to choose from each major group.
2. *Moderation* in eating fats, oils, and sugar sparingly.
3. *Variety,* by emphasizing the importance of eating a selection of different foods from each of the major food groups daily.

Unlike the Four Food Groups Wheel, the Pyramid suggests *total* amounts from each group rather than *minimum* recommendations. Also, the Pyramid emphasizes not only variety as in the four food groups, but also proportion and moderation. See Displays 14-5 and 14-6 for examples of how a daily food guide can be used in planning

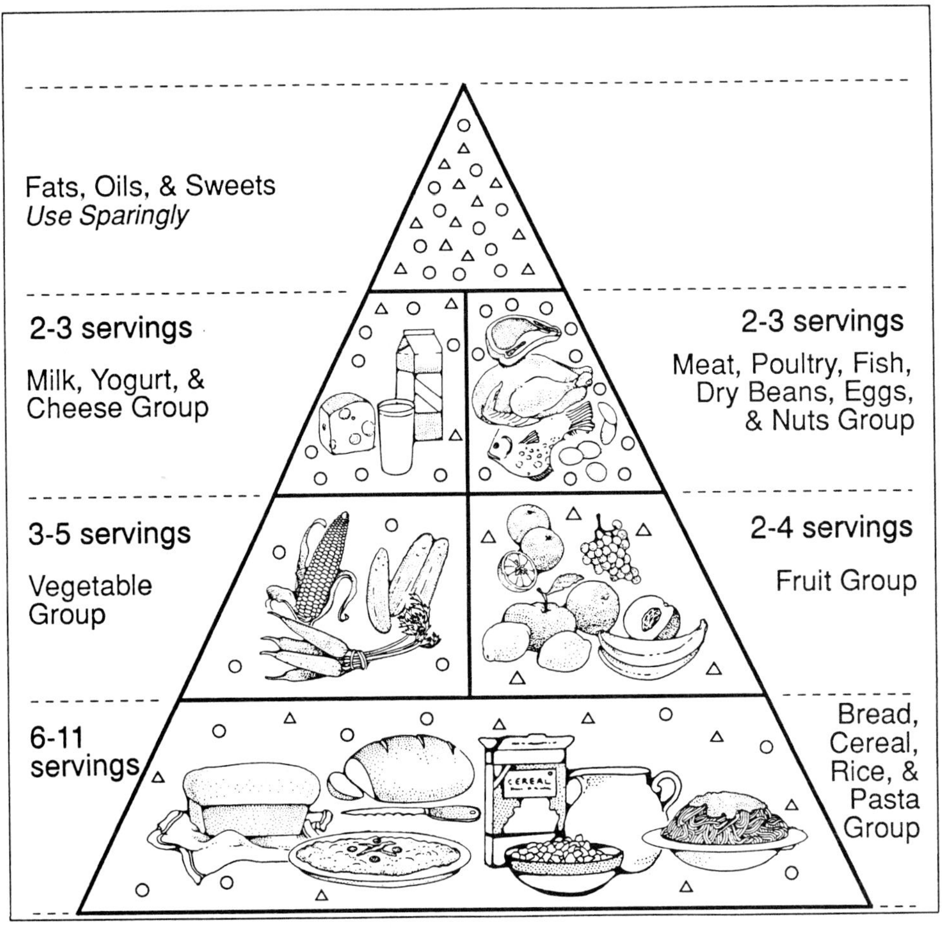

FIGURE 5-1

The Food Guide Pyramid: A Guide to Daily Food Choices. (*Circle*) Fat (naturally occurring and added). (*Triangle*) Sugars (added). These symbols show fats, oils, and added sugars in food. *(Adapted from US Dept of Agriculture, Human Nutrition Information Service. The food guide pyramid. Washington, DC: US Government Printing Office, 1992. Home and Garden Bulletin No. 252, p. 3.)*

daily meals. See Display 14-3 for lists of foods in the six groups represented in the Food Guide Pyramid.

A number of government publications targeting various audiences (such as teenagers, low-level readers, and so forth) and incorporating the *Dietary Guidelines for Americans* and the Food Guide Pyramid have been published. These publications are available from the USDA–Human Nutrition Information Service (USDA–HNIS) and the US Government Printing Office.

GUIDE TO GOOD EATING

The National Dairy Council released its revised *Guide to Good Eating* in 1992 as a tool to complement the Pyramid. It identifies the same five food groups as the Pyramid—(1) milk, (2) meat, (3) vegetables, (4) fruits, and (5) grains—and recommends the same number of servings for each food group except for the milk group. The *Guide to Good Eating* recommends three servings instead of two for adults aged 25 years and older and four servings instead of three for teenagers, young adults to age 25 years, and pregnant or breastfeeding women.

TABLES OF FOOD COMPOSITION

How do we know the nutrient composition of the foods we eat? The nutritive values of foods have been chemically analyzed in laboratories of universities, USDA, and the food industry. The results of these analyses are published in tables of food composition. Most of the food composition tables in print and those in computerized nutrient data programs are derived largely from the USDA nutrient data bank.

The value given in a table of food composition represents the average value of a number of samples of the food analyzed in a laboratory. Many factors, such as the climate in which the foodstuff was grown, the method of processing, and the method of preparation, affect nutritional value. For this reason, the nutritive values given for a particular food may differ in various tables. Such differences, however, are usually slight. (See Appendix E for a table of food composition.)

It is also important to understand that the amount of a nutrient chemically present in food, does not necessarily represent the amount of that nutrient that is biologically available for use by the body. The bioavailability of a nutrient may depend on factors such as body need and interaction with drugs or other nutrients and with antinutrients (substances that block the absorption of nutrients such as fiber and starch blockers). Also, the condition of the body may affect the way in which the body processes each nutrient. For example, if severe diarrhea is present, the nutrients in food may be poorly absorbed.

In the field of nutrition, we depend on nutrient data banks and food composition tables to determine

- the nutritional value of a particular diet for comparison with a standard such as the RDA
- the nutritional value of one food as compared with another in regard to a specific nutrient or in total caloric value
- what foods must be included in, limited in, or omitted from a diet to meet specific needs such as high protein, controlled fat, or high iron
- the foods required to meet specific nutrient and caloric needs (as in diabetes).

In the study of nutrition, as in other sciences, the metric system of weights and measures is used instead of the customary pounds and quarts. In using tables of food composition, it is important to understand the relationship between the metric units and the way to convert household measure to and from metric measures. See Table 5-1 for useful equivalents.

FOOD LABELING

NUTRITION LABELING

Thanks to food labeling regulations enacted in 1994, consumers now have available on a daily basis the nutritional composition of most of the com-

TABLE 5-1 USEFUL CONVERSIONS TO AND FROM METRIC MEASURES

Weight

1 kg = 1000 g
1 g = 1000 mg
1 mg = 1000 mcg (or μg)
1 kg = 2.2 lb
1 lb = 454 g
1 oz = 28.35 g (usually rounded off to 30 g)

Volume

1 tsp = 5 mL
1 tbsp = 15 mL
1 fl oz = 30 mL
1 cup (8 oz) = 240 mL
1 qt = 1060 mL or 1.06 liters

Length

1 in = 2.54 cm
1 ft = 30 cm

kg = kilogram
g = gram
mg= milligram
mcg = microgram
mL = milliliter
cm = centimeter

mercially processed foods. It had become apparent that without this information, consumers would be unable to follow the nutritional guidelines being recommended.

In the early 1990s, the most comprehensive and consumer-oriented food labeling reform occurred in the United States. The new food labeling regulations of the Food and Drug Administration (FDA) of the DHHS and the Food Safety and Inspection Service (FSIS) of the USDA were designed to help consumers choose a healthier diet and to encourage food manufacturers to improve the nutritional quality of their products.

The FSIS is responsible for the safety and nutrition labeling of meat and poultry and the FDA controls the labeling of all other products. The Federal Trade Commission, which regulates food advertising, also plays a role in ensuring that nutrition information in the marketplace is accurate.

Under the previous nutrition labeling regulations established in 1973, nutrition labeling was voluntary unless a nutrient was added to a food or a nutritional claim was made about the product. In 1990, the Nutritional Labeling and Education Act was enacted by Congress, giving the FDA the authority to require nutrition labeling on practically all foods that are meaningful sources of nutrition. Although the act does not mandate labeling of processed meat and poultry products, the FSIS followed suit by issuing regulations for these foods. Nutrition labeling regulations became fully effective in mid-1994.

In addition to providing nutrition labeling for almost all foods, nutrition labeling regulations

- provide information on how a food fits into the overall daily diet
- emphasize nutrients that are of greatest health concern to consumers: total fat, saturated fat, cholesterol, dietary fiber, and sodium
- designate specific definitions for terms that describe the nutrient content of a food such as *free, low, light,* and *lean;* these terms will always mean the same thing regardless of the product on which they appear
- allow, for the first time, health claims on labels—but only those claims that have been supported by scientific evidence
- specify serving sizes that are more like the amount people eat and that are standardized for various foods so that comparison shopping will be easier (previously, portion sizes were up to the discretion of each food manufacturer); portion sizes are to be given in both common household and metric measures
- provide a consistent format for most processed foods that makes it easier to compare the nutritional content of foods (Fig. 5-2).

Voluntary and Exempt Products

A voluntary nutrition labeling program has been developed for the 20 most popular varieties of raw fruits, vegetables, and fish and for raw, single-ingredient meat and poultry products such as beef roasts and raw chicken. The nutrition information for these products are provided on cards or signs at the point of purchase. If voluntary compliance is poor, nutrition labeling may be made mandatory for these products.

Food products exempt from nutrition labeling are plain coffee and tea; some spices; medical foods; and foods produced by small businesses or packaged in small containers. Foods sold in restaurants, hospital cafeterias, and airplanes are also exempt. Nutrition labeling may voluntarily be provided for these foods. If a nutrient or health claim is made about an exempt food, nutrition labeling must be provided.

"NUTRITION FACTS" PANEL

The nutrition information panel, entitled "Nutrition Facts," must include the following dietary components on the label: total calories; calories from fat; and amounts of total fat, saturated fat, cholesterol, sodium, total carbohydrate, dietary fiber, sugars, protein, vitamin A, vitamin C, calcium, and iron. Dietary components that may be listed voluntarily include calories from saturated fat; stearic acid (on meat and poultry products); amounts of polyunsaturated fat, monounsaturated fat, potassium, soluble fiber, insoluble fiber, sugar alcohol (i.e., the sugar substitutes xylitol, mannitol, and sorbitol), and other carbohydrate; the percentage of vitamin A present as beta carotene; and other essential vitamins and minerals.

Only these mandatory and voluntary components are permitted on the label. If a food is fortified or enriched with one of the optional in-

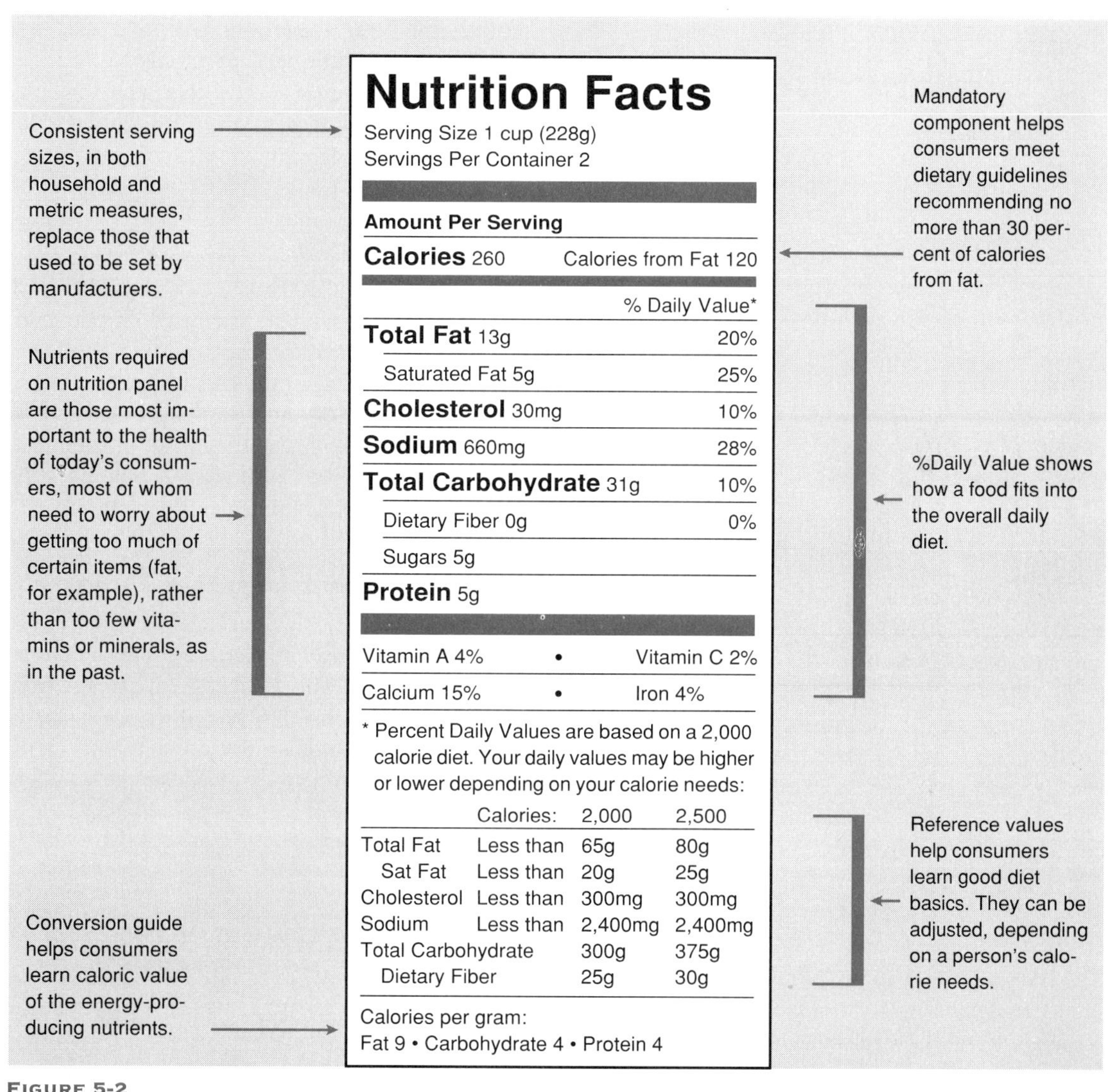

Nutrition Facts
Serving Size 1 cup (228g)
Servings Per Container 2
Amount Per Serving
Calories 260 Calories from Fat 120
% Daily Value*
Total Fat 13g 20%
Saturated Fat 5g 25%
Cholesterol 30mg 10%
Sodium 660mg 28%
Total Carbohydrate 31g 10%
Dietary Fiber 0g 0%
Sugars 5g
Protein 5g
Vitamin A 4% • Vitamin C 2%
Calcium 15% • Iron 4%
* Percent Daily Values are based on a 2,000 calorie diet. Your daily values may be higher or lower depending on your calorie needs:
Calories: 2,000 2,500
Total Fat Less than 65g 80g
Sat Fat Less than 20g 25g
Cholesterol Less than 300mg 300mg
Sodium Less than 2,400mg 2,400mg
Total Carbohydrate 300g 375g
Dietary Fiber 25g 30g
Calories per gram:
Fat 9 • Carbohydrate 4 • Protein 4
Consistent serving sizes, in both household and metric measures, replace those that used to be set by manufacturers.
Nutrients required on nutrition panel are those most important to the health of today's consumers, most of whom need to worry about getting too much of certain items (fat, for example), rather than too few vitamins or minerals, as in the past.
Conversion guide helps consumers learn caloric value of the energy-producing nutrients.
Mandatory component helps consumers meet dietary guidelines recommending no more than 30 percent of calories from fat.
%Daily Value shows how a food fits into the overall daily diet.
Reference values help consumers learn good diet basics. They can be adjusted, depending on a person's calorie needs.

FIGURE 5-2

Nutrition label format.

gredients or if a claim is made about any one of them, the nutrition information about this nutrient becomes mandatory.

Nutrient Content

The amount of fat, cholesterol, carbohydrate, sodium, fiber, and protein are given in grams or milligrams per serving. The amount of these nutrients are also expressed in terms of a percentage of a dietary reference value called the *Daily Value (DV)*. The content of vitamins and minerals are given only as a percentage of the DV. The "% Daily Value" is based on a 2000-kcal diet. The purpose of declaring nutrients as a percentage of the DV is to help consumers understand the nu-

TABLE 5-2 REFERENCE DAILY INTAKES (RDIs)*

NUTRIENT	AMOUNT
Vitamin A	5,000 IU
Vitamin C	60 mg
Thiamin	1.5 mg
Riboflavin	1.7 mg
Niacin	20 mg
Calcium	1.0 g
Iron	18 mg
Vitamin D	400 IU
Vitamin E	30 IU
Vitamin B_6	2.0 mg
Folic acid	0.4 mg
Vitamin B_{12}	6 mcg
Phosphorus	1.0 g
Iodine	150 mcg
Magnesium	400 mg
Zinc	15 mg
Copper	2 mg
Biotin	0.3 mg
Pantothenic acid	10 mg

* Based on the National Academy of Sciences 1968 Recommended Dietary Allowances. (Taken from Kurtzweil P. "Daily values" encourage healthy diet. FDA Consumer [Special Report: Focus on food labeling], May 1993. DHHS Publication No. [FDA] 93-2262. p. 43.)

tritional impact of the food in the context of the total daily diet.

Daily Value

The DV comprises two sets of references—the Reference Daily Intakes (RDIs) and the Daily Reference Values (DRVs). These reference points help give the consumer a perspective on nutritional recommendations. The RDIs are based on the RDAs and are established estimated values for vitamins, minerals, and, in selected groups, protein. The nutrient values temporarily being used for the RDIs are the former U.S. RDAs used by the FDA in previous nutrition labeling (Table 5-2).

The DRVs are a set of dietary references that have been established for total fat, saturated fat, cholesterol, total carbohydrate, dietary fiber, sodium, potassium, and protein based on current recommendations (Table 5-3). The DRVs for fat, carbohydrate, protein, and fiber are based on the number of calories consumed each day as follows:

fat based on 30% of calories
saturated fat based on 10% of calories
carbohydrate based on 60% of calories
protein based on 10% of calories (for adults and for children aged 4 years and older)
fiber based on 11.5 g of fiber per every 1000 calories.

The "% Daily Value" of these nutrients are based on a total intake of 2000 kcal. The DVs for cholesterol, sodium, and potassium are not based on caloric intake and are the same regardless of caloric level.

On larger packages, the DVs for selected nutrients for both a 2000- and 2500-kcal diet may be given. Manufacturers have the option of listing additional calorie levels. Labeling regulations affecting vitamin and mineral supplements are discussed in Chapter 12.

Foods for Children Younger Than 2 Years

Labels on foods for children under 2 years of age cannot carry information related to calories from fat and saturated fat. This is to prevent parents from wrongly assuming that they should restrict the fat intake of infants and toddlers. Dietary fat is needed during these years to ensure adequate growth and development.

TABLE 5-3 DAILY REFERENCE VALUES (DRVs)*

FOOD COMPONENT	DRV
Fat	65 g
Saturated fatty acids	20 g
Cholesterol	300 mg
Total carbohydrate	300 g
Fiber	25 g
Sodium	2400 mg
Potassium	3500 mg
Protein†	50 g

* Based on 2000 calories a day for adults and for children ages 4 years and older.

† DRV for protein does not apply to certain populations; RDI for protein has been established for these groups: children ages 1 to 4 years: 16 g; infants younger than 1 year: 14 g; pregnant women: 60 g; breastfeeding mothers: 65 g.

Taken from Kurtzweil P. "Daily values" encourage healthy diet. FDA Consumer [Special Report: Focus on food labeling], May 1993. DHHS Publication No. [FDA] 93-2262, p. 42.

HEALTH CLAIMS

Although previously forbidden by the FDA, manufacturers may now make health claims for food–disease relationships approved by the FDA. They may make these claims through statements, symbols, or descriptions. Strict rules apply to the use of health claims, and manufacturers must use caution so that they do not overstate the case. Health claims may be made for the following relationships:

calcium and reduced risk of osteoporosis
sodium and increased risk of hypertension
dietary saturated fat and cholesterol and an increased risk of coronary heart disease
dietary fat and an increased risk of several types of cancer
fiber-rich grain products, fruits and vegetables, and reduced risk of cancer and coronary heart disease
fruits and vegetables and a reduced risk of cancer.

Regulations regarding the use of health claims on labels of vitamin and mineral supplements differ from those permitted on foods (see Chapter 12).

NUTRIENT CONTENT DESCRIPTORS

Labeling regulations provide specific definitions and specific conditions under which descriptive terms such as *low, light, lean,* and so forth can be used. See Display 22-3 for definitions of these terms.

INGREDIENT LABELING

Labeling regulations that became effective in 1993 and 1994 also have affected ingredient labeling. People who use the ingredient label to avoid substances to which they are allergic or sensitive or who avoid certain substances for religious or cultural reasons will be helped by present labeling regulations.

All ingredients in a food must appear on all processed, packaged foods, including standardized foods that previously were exempt from ingredient labeling. Standardized foods are those made by prescribed recipes in which the ingredients are fixed by law. Some standardized foods are dairy products, mayonnaise, ketchup, jelly, and orange juice. The ingredients must be listed in decreasing order according to weight.

Food manufacturers are also required to list FDA-certified color additives by name such as Red No. 3. Colors in butter, cheese, and ice cream are exempt. Colors that do not have to be identified and may be listed simply as "artificial colors" are caramel, paprika, and beet juice.

Another ruling is important to people with milk allergy. The milk derivative caseinate, which may be used in foods that claim to be nondairy, must now be identified on the ingredient label as a milk derivative.

Protein hydrolysates (proteins broken down by acids or enzymes) used in foods as leavening agents, thickeners, flavor enhancers, or other purposes that previously were listed as "flavorings" must be listed by their common name. Also, their source must be identified, such as "hydrolyzed corn protein" or "hydrolyzed casein."

Consumers are now informed of how much fruit juice is actually in their juice-containing beverages. Beverages must state the exact percentage of juice that is present. Also, if a product contains several juices and the "featured" juice is only present in small amounts, the label must state that the beverage is "flavored" with the juice or declare the amount of that juice within 5%, for example, "raspberry flavored juice blend" or "juice blend, 2 to 7 percent raspberry juice."

KEYS TO PRACTICAL APPLICATION

Do not expect the effects of poor eating habits to be felt immediately, but be assured that prolonged poor eating habits will take their toll.

Be suspicious when foods are promoted as miracle foods.

Be cautious about the use of vitamin and mineral supplements; changes in the intake of one nutrient may affect the functioning of other nutrients, and excessive amounts of some nutrients can be toxic.

Be aware that too much food is as harmful as too little. Study the recommendations made in the *Dietary Guidelines for Americans*. This publication has a lot of useful information for both the health worker and the client.

Use the Food Guide Pyramid or other reliable food guide in choosing your own food and in helping others choose a healthy diet. Take time to explain how the principles of proportion or balance, moderation, and variety are symbolized in the graphic.

Learn the details of food labeling regulations. Show your clients how the nutrition label can help them eat a healthful diet and how ingredient labeling can help them avoid foods to which they are allergic or sensitive.

KEY IDEAS

Nutrients—chemical substances in food needed by the body—are classified into the following categories: carbohydrates, proteins, fats, vitamins, minerals, and water.

Nutrients provide for growth and maintenance of the body, furnish energy, and regulate body processes.

Adequate nourishment of the body as a whole depends on adequate nutrition of the cell, the basic unit of life.

The functions of nutrients are interrelated; changes in the consumption of one nutrient may lead to changes in the activities of others.

Some nutrients can be stored, providing a reserve supply for use in periods of stress; when taken, and thus stored, in excess, however, these nutrients can have adverse effects.

Deficiency diseases develop slowly. The body first attempts to adjust to a reduced supply of the involved nutrients, and eventually symptoms of disease appear.

The RDAs represent the opinion of an expert committee concerning the amounts of energy and nutrients required to keep the population of the United States well nourished.

Two major reviews of the scientific literature, *The Surgeon General's Report on Nutrition and Health* and the National Academy of Sciences *Diet and Health: Implications for Reducing Chronic Disease Risk*, underscored the need to address eating habits involving excess consumption of calories, saturated fat, cholesterol, salt, and alcohol.

Dietary Guidelines for Americans, a publication of the USDA and the DHHS, is aimed at helping Americans avoid or delay chronic illness. It recommends that Americans avoid excessive calories, fat, cholesterol, sodium, and alcohol and consume more vegetables, fruits, and grains.

The Food Guide Pyramid visually represents the Dietary Guidelines for Americans. The pieces of the Pyramid represent five food groups: (1) bread, cereal, rice, and pasta; (2) fruits; (3) vegetables; (4) milk, yogurt, and cheese; and (5) meat, poultry, fish, dry beans, eggs, and nuts.

The Pyramid conveys the need for consuming fats, oils, and sweets sparingly by putting these foods in the smallest piece of the Pyramid. Symbols for fat and added sugar scattered throughout the Pyramid alert consumers to the potential for fat and sugar in the five food groups.

The size of the food group piece in the Pyramid corresponds to the number of daily servings recommended from that group. The bread, cereal, rice, and pasta group form the base of the Pyramid.

The *Guide to Good Eating* (revised in 1992) is the food guide of the National Dairy Council. It differs from the Pyramid only in its recommendation for an additional serving from the milk group.

Tables of food composition are indispensable tools in the field of nutrition.

Food labeling regulations, which became effective in mid-1994, are designed to help consumers choose a healthier diet and encourage manufacturers to improve the nutritional quality of their products.

The FSIS (of the USDA) is responsible for the labeling of meat and poultry; the FDA (of the DHHS) controls the labeling of all other products.

Nutrition labeling is mandatory for most processed foods; a voluntary nutrition labeling program has been developed for raw foods.

The "Nutrition Facts" panel emphasizes those nutrients of greatest health concern to consumers: total fat, saturated fat, cholesterol, dietary fiber, and sodium.

The energy nutrients as well as cholesterol, sodium, and fiber are given in grams and milligrams per serving and also are expressed as a "% Daily Value." Vitamins and minerals are expressed only as a percentage of the DV.

The DV is a dietary reference term comprising two sets of references—(1) Reference Daily Intakes (RDIs) and (2) Daily Reference Values (DRVs).

RDIs are established estimated values for vitamins, minerals, and, in selected groups, protein known formerly as the USRDAs and based on the RDAs.

DRVs are a set of dietary references that have been established for total fat, saturated fat, cholesterol, total carbohydrate, dietary fiber, sodium, potassium, and protein based on current dietary recommendations.

The "% Daily Value" is based on a caloric intake of 2000 kcal.

The "% Daily Value" for cholesterol, sodium, and potassium are the same regardless of caloric level.

Health claims for food–disease relationships approved by the FDA may appear on the label and are subject to strict conditions.

Descriptive terms such as *low, light, free,* and *reduced* have been clearly defined (see Display 22-3).

KEYS TO LEARNING

STUDY-DISCUSSION QUESTIONS

1. Discuss in class the meaning of *interrelationships of nutrients* and *storage of nutrients.* In light of these explanations, what is your opinion of the practice of taking vitamin, mineral, or other nutrient supplements without a physician's advice?
2. Explain each of the following:
   RDAs
   The Surgeon General's Report on Nutrition and Health
   Dietary Guidelines for Americans
   The Food Guide Pyramid
3. What are the advantages of recommending the consumption of nutrients in quantities that provide a margin of safety?
4. Deficiency diseases develop slowly. What effect might this fact have on nutrition education efforts?
5. List all the foods and beverages you consume for 1 day. Include all items, even gum, candy, diet drinks, tea, and coffee. State the amount you have eaten: for example, $^1/_2$ cup of peas; two slices of baked ham; one glass (8 oz) of whole milk; and $^1/_8$ of a 9-inch apple pie. Estimate the amount of fat and sugar used in cooking and added at the table and add the information to your record. (Save this record for use in subsequent chapters.) Compare your record to the Food Guide Pyramid. What aspects of your diet, if any, fall short of the recommendations?
6. Discuss the ways in which you use nutrition labeling. Does it affect your food choices? Explain. Identify specific ways in which nutrition labeling can help consumers follow recommendations in the *Dietary Guidelines for Americans.*
7. Using the "Nutrition Facts" panel, compare the nutritional value and cost of 8 oz of each of the following products: homogenized whole milk; 2% fat milk; 1% fat milk; nonfat milk; commercial buttermilk; nonfat dry milk powder reconstituted to 8 oz fluid milk; plain yogurt; and lowfat plain yogurt.

BIBLIOGRAPHY

BOOKS AND PAMPHLETS

Bureau of Nutritional Sciences. Recommended nutrient intakes for Canadians. Dept of National Health and Welfare, Canada, 1989.

Committee on Diet and Health, Food and Nutrition Board, National Research Council. Diet and health: implications for reducing chronic disease risk (executive summary). Washington, DC: National Academy Press, 1989.

National Academy of Sciences, National Research Council, Food and Nutrition Board, Recommended dietary allowances. 10th ed. Washington, DC: National Academy Press, 1989.

National Dairy Council. Guide to good eating: leader's guide. Rosemont, IL: National Dairy Council, 1992.

US Dept of Agriculture and US Dept of Health and Human Services. Nutrition and your health: dietary guidelines for Americans. 3rd ed. Washington, DC: US Government Printing Office, 1990. Home and Garden bulletin 232.

US Dept of Agriculture. Dietary Guidelines Advisory Committee. Report of the Dietary Guidelines Advisory Committee on the dietary guidelines for Americans, 1990. Hyattsville, MD: US Dept of Agriculture, Human Nutrition Information Service, 1990.

US Dept of Agriculture, Human Nutrition Information Service. The food guide pyramid. Washington, DC: US Government Printing Office, 1992. Home and Garden bulletin 252.

US Dept of Health and Human Services, Public Health Service. The surgeon general's report on nutrition and health (summary and recommendations). Washington, DC: US Government Printing Office, 1988. US Dept of Health and Human Services publication PHS 88-50211.

Woteki CE, Thomas PR. Eds. Eat for life. Washington, DC: National Academy Press, 1992.

PERIODICALS

Anderson J. US Government dietary guidelines: past review and present opportunity. Nutrition Update 1993;3:1.

Farley D. Look for "legit" health claims on foods. FDA Consumer (Special Report: Focus of Food Labeling), May 1993. DHHS Publication No. (FDA) 93-2262.

Kurtzweil P. "Daily values" encourage healthy diet. FDA Consumer (Special Report: Focus on Food Labeling), May 1993. DHHS Publication No. (FDA) 93-2262.

Kurtzweil P. Good reading for good eating. FDA Consumer (Special Report: Focus of Food Labeling), May 1993. DHHS Publication No. (FDA) 93-2262.

Kurtzweil P. "Nutrition facts" to help consumers eat smart. FDA Consumer (Special Report: Focus on Food Labeling), May 1993. DHHS Publication No. (FDA) 93-2262.

McBean LD. The food group approach to eating in the 1990's. Dairy Council Digest 1993;64:3:1.

Peterkin BB. What's new about the 1990 Dietary Guidelines for Americans. J Nutr Educ 1991;23:183.

Segal M. What's in a food. FDA Consumer (Special Report: Focus on Food Labeling), May 1993. DHHS Publication No. (FDA) 93-2262.

Soergel D, Pennington JA, McCan A, et al. A network model for improving access to food and nutrition data J Am Diet Assoc 1992;92:78.

CHAPTER

6

Digestion and Absorption

KEY TERMS

absorption the transfer of nutrients from the intestinal tract to the bloodstream

active transport movement of molecules that requires energy expenditure

amylase an enzyme that digests carbohydrates

bacterial flora bacteria in the gastrointestinal (GI) tract

bolus food mass

chyme the semifluid mass formed by the mixing and partial digestion of food in the stomach

diffusion movement of molecules from regions of higher to regions of lower concentration

digestion the chemical breakdown of complex nutrient molecules to a form that the cells can use; digestion is accomplished mainly through the action of enzymes found in digestive fluids

emulsification the production of a liquid substance in which small globules of one liquid, such as a fat, are dispersed evenly throughout a second liquid

epithelium the tissue that forms the outer part of the skin and lines the blood vessels and the passages that lead to the outside of the body

flatus intestinal gas expelled through anus

herbivores animals that eat only plant foods

hydrolysis a chemical reaction in which a large molecule is split into simpler compounds by the addition of water

lamina propria the connective tissue in the villus that is supplied with blood and lymph vessels

lipase an enzyme that digests fat

metabolism the total of all the chemical and biologic processes that occur in the body

mucus a fluid with a slippery consistency that is secreted by mucous membranes and glands; it lubricates and protects the GI mucosa

parietal cells cells that form the wall of a structure

peristalsis rhythmic muscular contractions of the GI tract that break up food into smaller particles, mix these particles with digestive fluids, and move the food along the intestinal tract

pH symbol used to express hydrogen ion concentration in a solution; a pH of 7.0 is neutral; a lower pH is acid; a higher pH is basic

proteinase an enzyme that digests protein

pyloric sphincter a ringlike muscular valve located between the stomach and the small intestine; it determines the length of time food stays in the stomach

pylorus the opening of the stomach into the duodenum

residue contents remaining in the large intestine after the digestion of food

rugae ridges or folds

simultaneous occurring at the same time

synthesize to form or build complex substances from simpler ones

vagus nerve a nerve that controls muscular contractions of the stomach and the secretion of digestive chemicals

villus a fingerlike projection of the mucosa that lines the small intestine; it is supplied with blood and lymph vessels; the epithelial cells of each villus have tiny rodlike projections, called *microvilli;* these microscopic hairlike projections form the *brush border*

OBJECTIVES

After completing this chapter, the student will be able to:

1. Discuss the role of each part of the digestive system in the digestion and absorption of nutrients.
2. Discuss the roles of the accessory organs in the digestive process.
3. Have a greater awareness of the possible effects of pathology of the digestive tract on nutritional status.
4. Explain the relationship between common digestive disturbances and conditions that hinder or affect the digestive process.

Humans and other animals must obtain the nutrients they need from foods. Most of the major nutrients in food are present in the form of large molecules or in an insoluble form that prevents absorption from the intestinal tract. The role of the digestive system is to reduce these large molecules to their simplest units and to convert insoluble molecules into soluble forms. Once the nutrients have been digested—reduced to their basic units—they are transported across the wall of the intestine into the blood and lymph; this process is called *absorption.* The absorbed nutrients are transported by the blood, lymph, and tissue fluids to the cells of the liver, where they may be modified to suit the body's needs. They are then transported to all body cells to be used for energy or for the production of body tissue and regulatory compounds, such as enzymes, hormones, and body fluids.

Understanding the body's digestive and absorptive functions is essential to the study of nutrition. Any problem or abnormality that affects the body's ability to digest or absorb foods may profoundly affect a person's nutritional status. The body cannot use foods that it cannot digest or absorb; consequently, malnutrition can occur even though the individual is consuming a nutritionally adequate diet.

DIGESTION

Digestion involves all the activities in the digestive tract that prepare food for absorption into the bloodstream and that reject unabsorbed substances. Some nutrients such as simple sugars (monosaccharides), water, vitamins, minerals, and alcohol require little or no digestion. Most nutrients need considerable change to enable them to pass through the lining of the intestine into the blood or lymph. These nutrients include complex carbohydrates (starches) and disaccharides (double sugars), lipids (fats and fatlike substances), and protein.

DIGESTIVE PROCESS

Digestion is accomplished by simultaneous mechanical and chemical means. When the digestive process is completed, the nutrients are reduced to their basic units as follows:

Carbohydrate is reduced to simple sugars: glucose, fructose, and galactose.
Protein is reduced to amino acids.
Fat is reduced to fatty acids and glycerol.

Some vitamins also must be broken down before they can be absorbed.

Mechanical digestion involves the chewing of food and the muscular movement of the gastrointestinal (GI) tract. Mechanical digestion prepares the food for chemical digestion by breaking it into small particles, which increases the surface area, and by mixing the particles with digestive fluids. *Emulsification,* the suspension of one substance in another, also prepares fats and fatlike materials for chemical breakdown. Emulsification occurs in the small intestine through the action of bile salts. The bile coats the tiny fat particles and prevents them from coming together and forming larger particles. The surface area of the fat is thus increased, allowing digestive fluids greater access to the fat molecules. Bile salts are produced by the liver and released in the bile.

Chemical digestion of carbohydrates, proteins, and fats to their basic forms involves the process of *hydrolysis*. Hydrolysis is the addition of water to each molecule, resulting in the splitting of the molecule into simpler compounds. In the case of especially large molecules, hundreds of smaller molecules are formed. In contrast, simple sugars such as fructose require no digestion.

Enzymes in digestive fluids are largely responsible for the chemical reactions that bring about the hydrolysis of nutrients. The enzymes are specific in their activity; for example, pepsin acts only on protein, and ptyalin acts only on starch. The enzymes involved in the digestive process are named for the substances on which they act. For example, lipase is an enzyme that digests lipids (fats) and proteinase is an enzyme that digests protein. The ending *-ase* signifies *enzyme*.

Hormones also are involved in GI activity. The mucous membranes of the tract produce these chemical substances, which travel through the bloodstream and stimulate target glands and organs to release their secretions. The hormones are produced in the presence of specific substances; for example, the entrance of fats into the duodenum stimulates the secretion of *cholecystokinin*, a hormone that causes the gallbladder to contract and release *bile*, a yellow–green liquid.

In addition to its role in hydrolysis, water dilutes the foods in the intestinal tract and holds them in suspension, which in turn, promotes the activity of the digestive enzymes. Water also promotes *peristalsis*, the muscular activity of the digestive tract. Digestive secretions supply an abundant amount of water along the digestive tract.

Because body tissue comprises proteins, fats, and other nutrients similar to the composition of food, enzymes that digest foods could also digest the tissues that line the intestinal tract. This does not normally occur because of various protective mechanisms. Digestive enzymes are secreted in their inactive form and are not activated until they are free within the lumen (cavity) of the GI tract. The secretion of *mucus*, a thick slippery substance, is another mechanism that protects the GI wall. It also aids in mixing the food mass and lubricating the tract so that food moves more readily along it. The lining of the stomach (gastric mucosa) is subjected to especially harsh conditions, not only due to the presence of digestive enzymes but also because of the highly acidic nature of the gastric juice. In addition to a protective alkaline mucus covering, the epithelial cells of the gastric mucosa are tightly joined, which prevents acid from leaking into the submucosa. Also, the cells that are damaged are shed. The entire epithelial lining is replaced every 3 days.

DIGESTIVE TRACT

The *digestive tract* is a long, unbroken muscular tube passing through the body; it begins at the mouth and ends at the anus. The organs of the GI tract include the oral cavity, pharynx, esophagus, stomach, small intestine, and large intestine (Fig. 6-1). The GI tract consists of two holding or receiving areas connected by a tube (the small intestine) designed to provide close contact between the food in the tract and the circulatory system. The first of the holding areas (the stomach) receives the ingested food, and the other (the large intestine) collects the indigestible waste. Strong rings of muscle, called *sphincters*, separate segments of the tube. A sphincter is an opening or valve surrounded by a circular set of muscles. The passageway closes when muscles contract and opens when they relax. Sphincters prevent food from passing too rapidly through the digestive tract. They also prevent regurgitation. The functions of each part of the GI tract are interdependent.

Peristalsis is responsible for the movement of food through the entire length of the GI tract. Peristalsis functions independently of gravity, enabling astronauts, for example, to digest food in space. Two sets of muscles control peristalsis. One set is circular and squeezes inward; the second set consists of muscle fibers that run the length of the GI tract. These two sets alternately contract and relax, creating a wavelike movement. In the stomach, a third set of muscles churns the food, reducing it to small particles and mixing it thoroughly with digestive secretions.

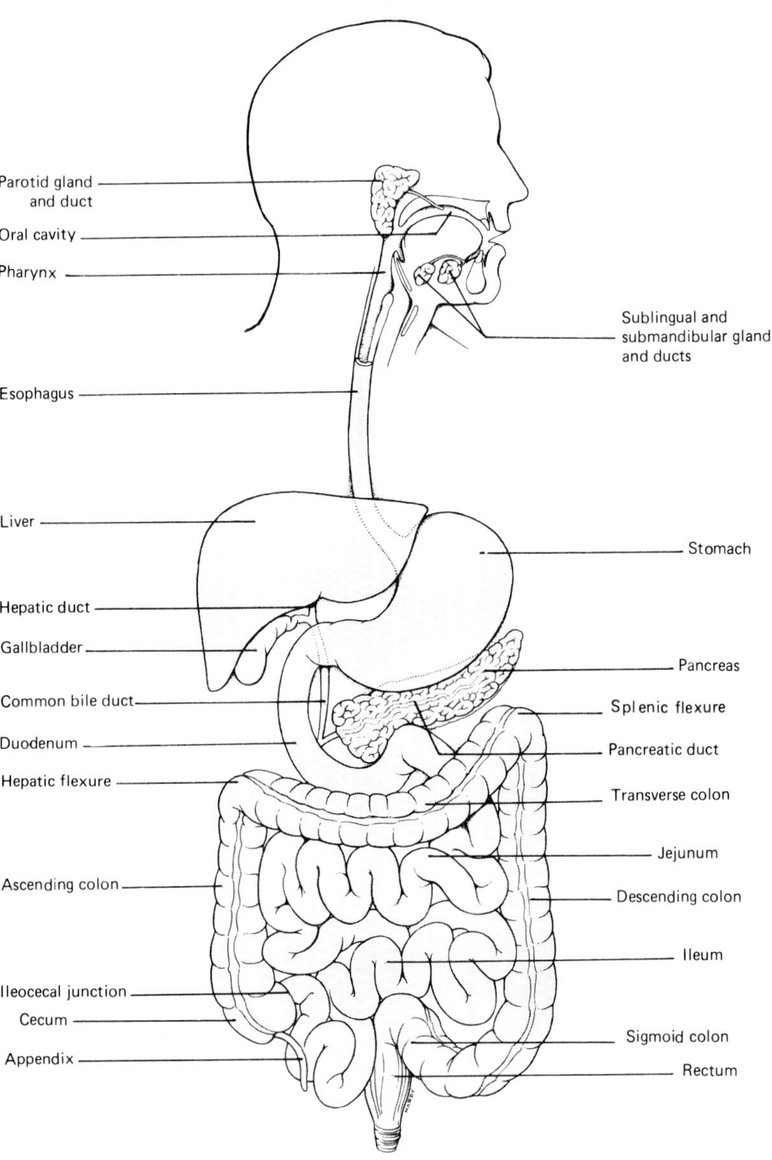

FIGURE 6-1

Digestive tract.

These muscular actions as well as the secretory activities of the GI tract are controlled by a network of nerves within the GI wall extending from the esophagus to the anus.

The GI tract is lined with a mucous membrane that produces secretions. The characteristics of the mucous membrane and its secretions vary; the mucous lining of the stomach differs from that of the small intestine, which differs from that of the esophagus and of the large intestine. Other organs essential to digestion, called *accessory organs,* include the liver, pancreas, and gallbladder. The secretions of these organs are important in the digestive process (Fig. 6-2). The teeth, tongue, and salivary glands are also considered to be accessory organs.

The digestive tract protects the body from harmful substances that may be ingested along with food, such as parasites, bacteria, viruses, and chemical poisons. Many of these potentially harmful sub-

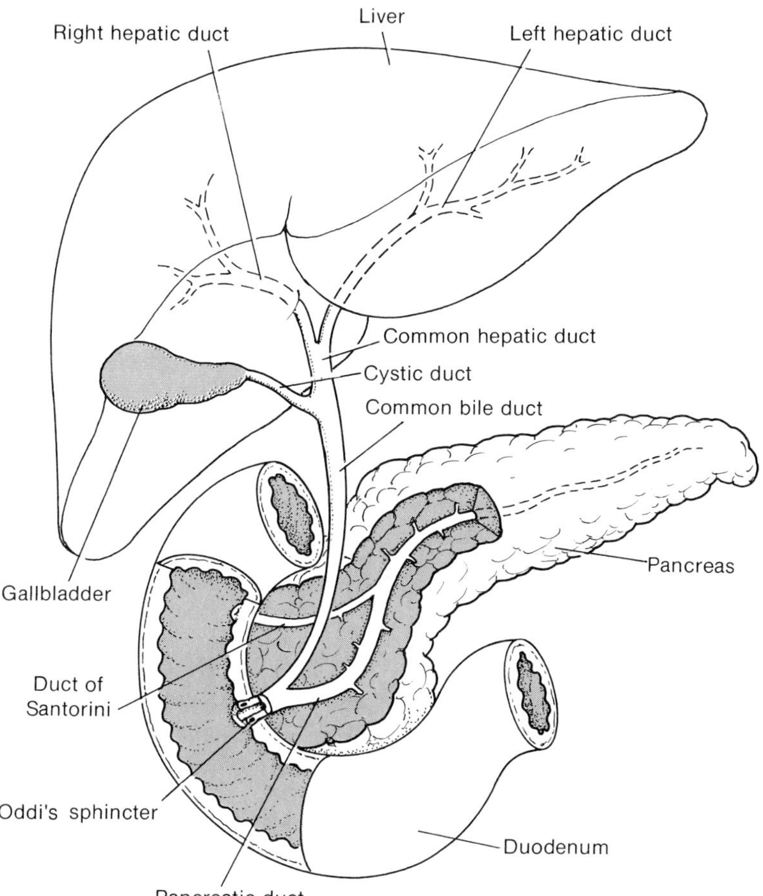

FIGURE 6-2

Accessory organs. The digestive secretions produced by the liver and pancreas play a vital role in digestion. The gallbladder acts as a storage organ.

stances pass through the GI tract without entering the bloodstream. They are then excreted in the feces. Table 6-1 summarizes the functions of the digestive system.

STAGES OF DIGESTION

Digestion normally occurs in stages. Large molecules are broken down to medium-sized molecules by a specific enzyme, and the medium-sized molecules are in turn reduced to smaller molecules through the action of another enzyme. Any unabsorbed food materials are moved onward by peristalsis to the end of the tube and are excreted. Fiber is one of these indigestible materials. Humans lack enzymes capable of breaking down fiber.

DIGESTION IN THE MOUTH

Chewing aids digestion by breaking up food into smaller particles and by mixing these food particles with *saliva.* Saliva, which is secreted by salivary glands in the mouth, lubricates food so that it may readily pass down the esophagus. Ptyalin, also called *salivary amylase,* is an enzyme occurring in saliva. It begins the digestion of starch, breaking down some of the starches to sugars.

The reflex action of swallowing pushes the bolus of food down the *pharynx,* a muscular passage from the mouth to the esophagus, into the esophagus. The esophageal sphincter opens as food is passed from the pharynx. It then closes, and peristalsis pushes the food down the esophagus. At the

(text continues on page 102)

TABLE 6-1 SUMMARY OF FUNCTIONS OF THE DIGESTIVE SYSTEM

STRUCTURE	DESCRIPTION	ACTIVITY	TIME TAKEN
Mouth	Contains the cheeks, lips, tongue, taste buds, opening of the salivary glands, teeth	The cheeks and lips keep the food between the teeth, which grind and break down the food to increase the area exposed to chemicals in the saliva; the tongue maneuvers the food and rolls it into a bolus to be swallowed; nerve impulses from the taste buds to the brain stimulate salivation, moistening and softening the food and cleansing the mouth 0.5 to 2 liters (3.5 to 4.5 pt) produced daily	Minutes
Pharynx	Muscular passage between the back of the mouth and the esophagus	The tongue forces the bolus of food into the pharynx, which continues the swallowing process by reflex action; the air passageways are closed and the opening to the esophagus is widened	Seconds
Esophagus	A muscular tube about 25 cm (10 in) long that connects the pharynx and the stomach	Forces the bolus into the stomach by peristaltic waves of muscular contraction; secretion of mucus aids the process	5–10 sec for solids, 1 sec for liquids
Cardiac sphincter	A muscular band that closes the entrance to the stomach	The sphincter opens to receive food pushed along by peristaltic waves in the esophagus; normally, it is shut to prevent reflux of contents	Seconds
Stomach	A *J*-shaped muscular sac, folded into rugae to increase the surface area; has a capacity of about 1 liter; gastric and mucous glands secrete about 2 liters/day (3.6 pt) of gastric juice	The rugae allow the stomach to distend; the muscular walls churn and macerate the food, mixing it with gastric juices and reducing it to chyme; peristaltic waves force the chyme through the stomach to the pyloric sphincter; the storage of food in the stomach prevents the need for many small meals	2–6 h
Pancreas	A soft, oblong organ lying behind and below the stomach; it is made up of islets of Langerhans which secrete glucagon and insulin, and other masses of cells that secrete about 800 mL of pancreatic juice daily; connected to the duodenum by the pancreatic duct and duct of Santorini	Pancreatic juice consists of three protein-digesting enzymes, one carbohydrate-digesting enzyme, and one fat-digesting enzyme; hormones from the duodenum stimulate the activity of the gland; glucagon and insulin control the fate of digested and absorbed carbohydrates	

(Continued)

TABLE 6-1 *(continued)*

STRUCTURE	DESCRIPTION	ACTIVITY	TIME TAKEN
Liver	The largest organ in the body, located below the diaphragm on the right of the abdomen, and divided into two lobes; connected to the duodenum by the common bile duct	A complex organ that has a variety of vital functions; as far as digestion is concerned, it manufactures and secretes watery green bile used in the small intestine to emulsify fats	
Gallbladder	A small sac attached to the underside of the liver, folded into rugae to enable it to expand; connected to the duodenum by the common bile duct	Stores bile, which it concentrates until stimulated to contract by the presence of acid and fat in the duodenum, when it ejects bile into the duodenum	
Small intestine	A tube about 3 m (10 ft) long that begins at the pyloric valve of the stomach and coils through the central and lower abdomen to merge with the large intestine; divided into three segments: duodenum, jejunum, ileum; intestinal and mucous glands secrete about 2 or 3 liters of intestinal juice daily; the inner wall has villi, increasing the surface area	Most digestion and absorption of food occurs here; hormones secreted here stimulate the pancreas, liver, and gallbladder to pour their digestive juices into the duodenum; the muscular walls mix the chyme with digestive juices and bring all the food particles into contact with the villi for absorption; peristalsis moves the chyme forward	5–6 h
Appendix and cecum	Closed sacs at the junction of the small and large intestine	Have no function in humans; in herbivores, they contain bacteria that digest cellulose	
Large intestine	A tube about 1.5 m (5 ft) long that extends from the ileum to the anus; divided into four regions: cecum, colon, rectum, anal canal; the ileocecal valve ensures one-way movement of materials; mucous glands secrete mucus into the large intestine	Bacteria digest any remaining foods; water is absorbed, creating solid or semisolid feces that are excreted from the anus by muscular action; mucus lubricates the feces and protects the tissue from the small intestine's digestive juices	12–24 h

(Bisacre M, Carlisle R, Robertson D, Ruck J. Eds. The illustrated encyclopedia of the human body. New York: Exeter Books, 1984.)

lower end of the esophagus, the cardiac sphincter controls entry of food to the stomach.

DIGESTION IN THE STOMACH

The stomach is a *J*-shaped bag that has three distinct functional parts: the cardiac, fundus, and pyloric areas. These sections differ in structure and in the secretions they produce. Gastric secretions contain primarily hydrochloric acid, pepsin, and mucus. Parietal cells in the fundus of stomach (the middle region) produce large amounts of hydrochloric acid. The pH of gastric juice is less than 2. This is more acidic than lemon juice or vinegar. This strong acid has several important functions: it activates the enzyme pepsin, it prepares the protein molecule for partial digestion by pepsin, it destroys harmful bacteria, and it makes certain minerals such as iron and calcium more soluble.

Food entering the stomach is temporarily stored. The digestion of carbohydrate begun in the mouth continues until the food mass mixes with hydrochloric acid.

The partial digestion of protein is the principal chemical function of the stomach. In adults, this purpose is achieved by the enzyme *pepsin,* which partially digests protein, reducing large protein molecules to smaller ones. Pepsin is first secreted in the inactive form pepsinogen. *Pepsinogen* prevents the enzyme from digesting the cells that produce it. Once pepsinogen is free within the stomach, it is converted to active pepsin through the action of hydrochloric acid.

Another gastric enzyme, *rennin,* is important in digestion for infants. Rennin breaks up the molecules of the milk protein casein. Curds are formed when the breakdown products of casein react with calcium. Rennin works best in the less acidic environment of the infant's stomach; hydrochloric acid accomplishes milk curdling in the adult's stomach.

Gastric lipase, another enzyme, also functions best in the more alkaline environment of the infant's stomach. This enzyme breaks the butterfat molecules of milk into smaller molecules. Hydrochloric acid accomplishes this function in the adult.

Secretions in the stomach are under the control of hormones and nerves. The thought, sight, taste, and smell of food cause nerve stimulation, which causes the flow of stomach secretions. The vagus nerve is of particular importance in both the control of peristalsis and the production of gastric secretions in the stomach. Even before food is consumed, the stomach prepares to receive it. The presence of food further stimulates gastric secretions. This secretory action begins through the action of *gastrin,* a hormone secreted by the pyloric region of the stomach.

When the food is thoroughly mixed and in a milky liquid state, called *chyme,* strong peristaltic waves beginning in the middle of the stomach push the food toward the *pyloric sphincter,* the valve separating the stomach from the duodenum. When the pressure in the stomach is greater than that in the small intestine, chyme is forced through the pylorus at a rate of about $\frac{1}{2}$ to 1 tsp per peristaltic wave. The stomach empties in about 2 to 6 hours. Carbohydrate foods leave first, followed by protein, and, last, fats.

Little absorption of food occurs in the stomach. Some water and minerals, certain drugs, and alcohol pass through the stomach wall. Consequently, the effects of alcohol are felt so soon after drinking it.

DIGESTION IN THE SMALL INTESTINE

The small intestine, so named because of its diameter, is the longest part of the digestive tract—about 6.1 m (20 ft) long. It consists of three parts: the duodenum, jejunum, and ileum. About 90% of the digestion of food occurs in the small intestine. For this reason, people who have had all or part of their stomach surgically removed are able to survive well.

The chyme enters the duodenum. The acid and fat contents of the chyme stimulate the cells lining the walls of the duodenum to produce hormones. Some of these hormones travel to their target organs—the pancreas, liver, and gallbladder—causing these organs to fulfill their roles in the digestive process. The peristaltic action of the small intestine mixes the chyme with the intestinal fluids. These fluids consist of bile manufactured by the liver, pancreatic juice secreted by the pancreas, and intestinal juice produced by the walls of the intestine. The secretions contain *bicarbonate,* an alkaline substance that neutralizes the acidity of the chyme as it comes from the stomach. Large quantities of mucus also are secreted into the intestine to protect the intestinal lining and to lubricate the moving food mass.

The pancreas secretes a number of the most important digestive enzymes in the body. These enzymes are necessary for the breakdown of carbohydrates, proteins, and fats. The pancreas produces about 800 mL (1.6 pt) of pancreatic juice daily. This digestive fluid pours down the pancreatic duct, joins with the common bile duct from the liver and gallbladder, and is secreted into the duodenum. The pancreas is stimulated to produce pancreatic juice by the hormones secretin and pancreozymin, which are produced by the cells of the duodenum.

Carbohydrate digestion, which begins in the mouth, is completed in the small intestine through the action of the enzymes secreted by the pancreas and the intestinal mucosa. Pancreatic amylase splits the remaining starch into sugar. Three enzymes in the intestinal juice (sucrase, lactase, and maltase) act on the sugars, reducing them to monosaccharides.

Protein digestion, begun in the stomach, is completed in the small intestine through the action of three enzymes in pancreatic juice and by a group of enzymes known as *peptidases* in the intestinal juice. Trypsin is a powerful enzyme. To prevent its digesting the cells of the pancreas, trypsin is secreted in an inactive form and is not activated until it contacts one of the intestinal enzymes. The pancreatic proteinases break down proteins to smaller molecules. The peptidases reduce these molecules to amino acids, the form in which proteins enter the bloodstream.

Fat digestion occurs primarily in the small intestine. Bile and a pancreatic enzyme are responsible for the digestion of fats.

When fat and acid contact the cells of the intestine, the hormone cholecystokinin is released into the blood. This hormone causes the gallbladder to contract and secrete bile into the common bile duct, which opens into the duodenum just below the stomach. The liver produces bile; the gallbladder merely stores and concentrates it. The liver synthesizes about 950 mL/day (2 pt) of bile. The bile consists of water, bile salts, bile acids, cholesterol, and two pigments. The breakdown products of one of these pigments, bilirubin, give feces its characteristic brown color. The bile salts mix with the chyme and split the fat into tiny droplets so that they can be more easily acted on by enzymes.

When the gallbladder is surgically removed, there is no longer a storage place for bile. Instead, bile is continually secreted in small amounts directly into the small intestine, regardless of whether fatty foods are present. When large amounts of fat are eaten, there may not be enough bile in the intestinal tract to emulsify the fat. The fat globules tend to cluster together, and consequently the digestive enzymes take longer than normal to do their job. For this reason, some people who have had their gallbladder removed experience discomfort after eating a high-fat meal.

The lipase called *steapsin,* which is secreted in pancreatic juice, completes the digestion of fats. Through the action of this pancreatic enzyme, fats are reduced to fatty acids and glycerol, and then absorbed.

Through the process of digestion, proteins, fats, and carbohydrates are reduced to their simplest forms—amino acids, fatty acids, and monosaccharides (Table 6-2). In these forms, the nutrients can be absorbed and used.

The time required for food material to pass through the intestine varies with the rate of peristaltic movements. Toxic materials, irritating substances (including some laxatives), and emotional stress can cause *hypermotility,* or abnormally rapid peristalsis. Hypermotility results in diarrhea and causes the digestion and absorption of nutrients to be greatly reduced.

ABSORPTION

Absorption is the transfer of nutrients from the GI tract into the blood and lymph vessels. Most absorption occurs in the small intestine, principally in the lower part of the duodenum and the first part of the jejunum. Diseases such as celiac disease and disorders such as lactose intolerance and cystic fibrosis may seriously hinder the absorption of nutrients. Problems may result from the lack of certain

TABLE 6-2 SUMMARY OF CHEMICAL CHANGES IN DIGESTION

PLACE OF ACTION	JUICES AND GLANDS	ENZYMES	RESULTS OF ENZYME ACTIVITY
Mouth	Saliva from salivary glands	Ptyalin (salivary amylase)	Begins starch digestion
Stomach*	Gastric juice from stomach wall	Pepsin (proteinase)	Begins protein digestion
		Rennin (proteinase)	Curdles milk protein
		Lipase	Breaks down emulsified fats to fatty acid and glycerol
Small intestine†	Pancreatic juice from the pancreas	Proteinase: Trypsin, Chymotrypsin, Carboxypeptidases	Reduce protein to smaller molecules
		Steapsin (lipase)	Breaks down fats to fatty acids and glycerol
		α-mylase (amylase), Isomaltase	Reduces starch to sugar
	Intestinal juice from the small intestine	Peptidases (proteinases)	Completely break down protein to amino acids
		Sucrase, Maltase, Lactase	Reduce sugars to simplest form

* Hydrochloric acid in the gastric juice softens the connective tissue of meat and activates the enzyme pepsin.
† Bile, produced by the liver, reduces fat to tiny globules so that the pancreatic lipase can more readily act on it.

digestive enzymes or from defects in the intestinal mucosa.

The anatomy of the small intestine is uniquely suited to promoting absorption. The mucosa of the small intestine is gathered into folds. Millions of fingerlike projections, called *villi*, cover the mucosa. Each epithelial cell of the villi has a brush border that consists of 500 to 600 *microvilli*, tiny, hairlike rodlets that can be seen only through an electron microscope. The surface area provided by these combined structures is estimated to be more than 61 m^2 (200 ft^2) in the average adult.

The villi are extremely small (0.04 in long) but have a complex structure (Fig. 6-3). Beneath the epithelium of each villus is a layer of connective tissue, the *lamina propria*, that is supplied with small arteries and veins connected by capillaries. The villus also is supplied with lymphatic capillaries called *lacteals*.

Absorption is a complex process involving two basic mechanisms of transport across the cell membranes lining the intestinal tract: *diffusion* and *active transport*. Diffusion is the movement of particles in solution from regions of higher to regions of lower concentration. This process does not require energy. Some nutrients require a carrier to transport them across a membrane containing fatlike substances, a process called *carrier facilitated diffusion*.

Other nutrients require active transport—movement that involves the input of energy. These nutrients are "pumped" from a region of lower concentration to one of higher concentration. Energy is required because the nutrients are moving across cell membranes against pressure. Usually some sort of carrier is needed to help in the transport process.

Sometimes larger particles such as proteins and fats are engulfed by the absorbing cells in a process called *pinocytosis*. Foreign proteins that get into the bloodstream in this way may cause allergic reactions.

Once the nutrients are transported across the epithelium into the lamina propria, they enter the blood or lymph vessels. Monosaccharides, amino

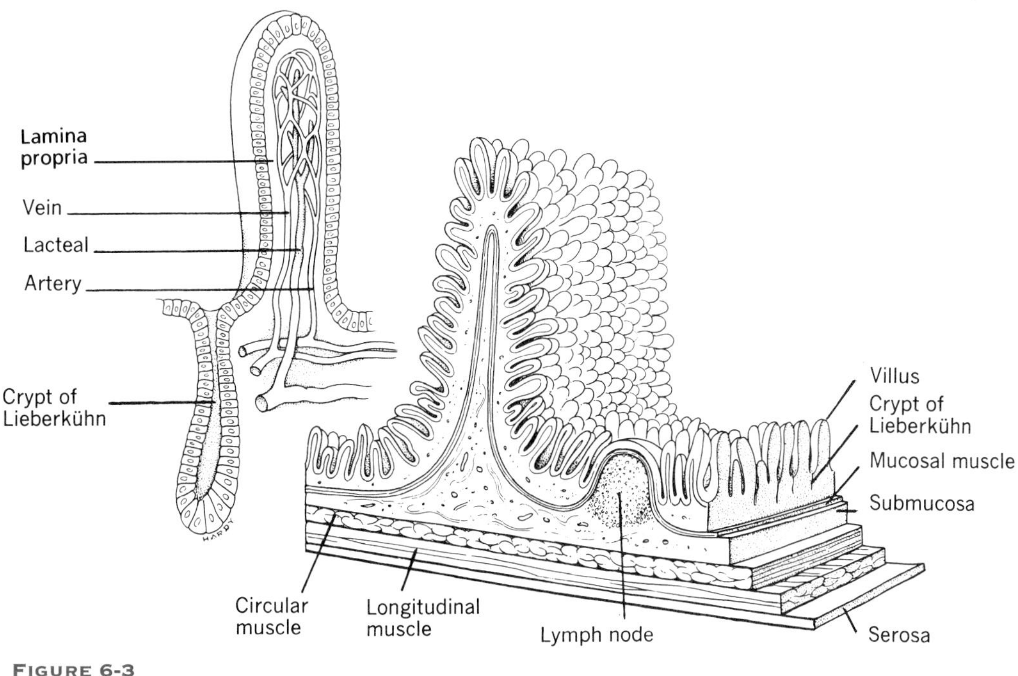

FIGURE 6-3

Diagram of the mucous membrane of the small intestine showing numerous villi on one circular fold. At left is an enlarged drawing of a single villus.

acids, glycerol, mineral salts, and water-soluble vitamins enter the blood capillaries, which run into small blood vessels draining each villus. Eventually, they enter the hepatic portal vein, which leads to the liver. In the liver, additional changes in the nutrients occur before they are delivered to other cells. Fatty acids and other fat-soluble substances, such as cholesterol and fat-soluble vitamins, are absorbed into the lacteals and then transported by the lymph vessels to the thoracic duct, which empties into the vena cava in the neck region. They are then carried by the blood to the liver for further changes before distribution to body cells.

EXTENT OF ABSORPTION

In healthy people, practically all digested carbohydrate, protein, and fat are absorbed. Some minerals, such as sodium, potassium, and iodine, also are absorbed to a high degree.

Absorption of other minerals is less complete. A well-nourished adult absorbs only 10% of the iron, 20% to 30% of the zinc, and about 40% of the calcium ingested. Higher amounts of iron and calcium are absorbed if body stores are low or if there is greater need than normal, as in pregnancy. The mechanisms in the small intestine that regulate absorption protect the body because excessive amounts of these minerals can be toxic. The amount of minerals absorbed is influenced by the form in which the minerals occur and by the presence of other substances. Iron found in flesh foods is absorbed more readily than iron from plant foods. The presence of vitamin C improves the absorption of iron, and the presence of vitamin D increases the absorption of calcium.

Some nutrients form insoluble compounds with other substances in food. Minerals bound in these insoluble compounds are not absorbed even when body stores are low. The calcium in spinach, for example, is not absorbed because it forms an insoluble compound with oxalate, a substance also present in spinach.

EXCRETION OF WASTE

Whatever remains of food after digestion and absorption have occurred is excreted by way of the large intestine, so named because of its diameter, which is three times the diameter of the small intestine. The mucous lining contains no villi, and no enzymes are secreted. The large intestine, which is 1.2 m to 1.5 m (4 ft to 5 ft) long, consists of four parts: the *cecum,* which receives undigested material from the small intestine; the *colon,* which removes most of the water content from the undigested material; the *rectum,* which temporarily stores the solid waste material, called *fecal matter;* and the *anal canal,* through which the feces are excreted. The colon forms the largest part of the large intestine. The muscular walls of the colon form pouchy segments, which give the tube a puckered appearance and a great capacity to expand. The anus is controlled by a muscular valve called the *anal sphincter.* The lower part of the rectum and the anal sphincter are continuations of the skin. These structures contain sensory nerves, which are responsible for the pain a person feels when the anal veins become enlarged and inflamed (hemorrhoids).

A narrow sac about 7.6 cm (3 in) long, the *appendix,* is connected to the cecum. This structure is no longer useful. When humans were herbivores, living only on plant foods, the appendix played a part in digesting the large amount of fiber found in plant material.

Chyme, still in a liquid state, passes slowly from the ileum into the cecum. Most of the water is extracted in the cecum and the first part of the colon. The chyme becomes solid or semisolid; in this state, it is called *feces.* Mucus secreted by the walls of the large intestine provides lubrication and protects the walls of the intestine from the digestive enzymes that may remain in the food residue as it comes from the small intestine. By the time the feces reach the rectum they consist of water, bacteria, food residues (mainly fiber), intestinal secretions, and dead cells.

The bacteria found in the large intestine have important functions. They synthesize some B vitamins and vitamin K, which is essential in the blood-clotting process. Bacteria found in the intestinal tract are referred to as *bacterial flora.*

DIGESTIVE DISTURBANCES

Disturbances of the GI tract are extremely common. These disturbances may indicate a serious underlying disease. In many cases, however, digestive disturbances are due to conditions that hinder the digestive process. These conditions include a poor mental or emotional state, overeating, eating of high-fat meals, insufficient chewing of food, and eating when overly tired. Promoting the best conditions for digestive function can do much to relieve digestive problems. The health worker's knowledge of the digestive process can be a vital tool in conveying scientifically sound information. Circumstances that may help or hinder digestion are described as follows.

PSYCHOLOGICAL FACTORS

Emotional stress is the primary cause of disturbances in digestive function. Fear, worry, anger, nervous fatigue, and emotional excitement can adversely affect the digestive process. These stresses cause changes in the flow of digestive juices and in the muscular activity of the GI tract. Some emotions may cause hypermotility, abnormally increased movement of the tract with increased secretion of digestive juices. Others may cause *hypomotility,* depressed or abnormally slow movement of the digestive tract. Irritable bowel syndrome is a disorder influenced by emotional stress. Contrary to previous opinion, however, peptic ulcer is not influenced by emotional factors but by bacteria, smoking, and other factors that weaken the body's mucosal defense system. These disorders are discussed in Chapter 28.

A lack of appetite frequently accompanies a depressed emotional state. People who are certain that particular foods will disagree with them may find that their apprehension actually causes them to feel discomfort after eating these foods.

A peaceful environment, cheerful companionship, and attractively served food all promote good digestion. The dinner table is not the place for controversy or scolding. In the hospital setting, mealtimes are inappropriate for unpleasant procedures, sights, smells, or sounds.

INDIGESTION

Pain or discomfort in the abdominal region or chest is often referred to as *indigestion* or *poor digestion.* This discomfort usually is not caused by foods that are hard to digest but by emotional factors, poor eating habits such as a high-fat diet, and hurried and irregular meals or other conditions that adversely affect digestion.

The typical American diet is almost completely digested: 98% of the carbohydrates, 95% of the fats, and 92% of the proteins. The digestion of carbohydrates is reduced to about 85% in diets that contain large amounts of the indigestible fiber found in fruits, vegetables, and whole-grain cereals, such as vegetarian diets. Some foods are digested more slowly than others, and thus remain in the stomach longer. Foods that are considered hard to digest are merely foods that are digested more slowly. Slowing of the digestive process may be caused by the nature of the food itself, the size of the meal, the way the food is cooked, or the manner in which the food is eaten. Foods that are not chewed properly can slow the digestive process and cause distress. Large lumps of food require more churning action by the stomach and more time for the hydrochloric acid and enzymes to do their work.

Foods that by nature are more slowly digested than others are more satisfying because they delay the emptying of the stomach and have greater staying power. Such foods are said to have a high satiety value. Carbohydrates leave the stomach first, followed by protein, and then fat. Fats and foods rich in fat, especially mixtures of protein and fat, such as meat, milk, and eggs, have a high satiety value. It is no wonder that a person who eats a breakfast of juice, toast, and coffee is hungry by midmorning. The addition of an egg or a glass of milk improves the satiety value of this breakfast. Foods containing excessive amounts of fat, especially fried foods, may cause digestive discomfort because of the long time required to digest them.

Under normal conditions, the body can digest almost any food or combinations of food without any trouble. True allergic reactions to foods do exist but are relatively rare. Foods that can be eaten separately should not cause discomfort when eaten together. This applies to eating seafood and milk products in the same meal and to other widely held taboos. People who always avoid certain foods to prevent discomfort may be masking the symptoms of a serious disorder. Because symptoms of indigestion can be signs of organic disease, a person who frequently experiences "indigestion" should seek the advice of a physician.

GASEOUSNESS

Gas formation is a normal result of the digestive process. Most of the gas that is formed is absorbed into the blood. The remainder (1 pt to 2 qt daily) is eliminated by belching through the mouth or passing through the rectum. Much of the gas is expelled insensibly (without being felt). If the gas does not readily move out of the digestive tract, it may accumulate in some part of the digestive tract and cause bloating and pain. If gas collects in the left side of the colon, it can be mistaken for heart disease; on the right side, it can be confused with gallbladder disease or appendicitis. Eating fatty foods delays the stomach emptying and allows gas to build up and cause bloating and discomfort. In some cases, complaints of excessive gas are due to increased intestinal movement, which does not permit time for normal absorption of gas through the intestinal wall. Although gaseousness is usually nothing to be concerned about, it can be the sign of an intestinal obstruction, gastritis, or lactose intolerance. People with persistent and extreme flatulence should discuss this issue with a physician.

Belching results from the swallowing of air and not from excessive gas production in the stomach. The swallowing of air can be excessive when a person is under stress, has a postnasal drip, chews gum, smokes, eats rapidly, or has poorly fitting dentures. Drinking through straws or drinking carbonated beverages may also produce excessive gas in the intestinal tract. Frequent belching may also be the result of gastroesophageal reflux or gastritis (see Chapter 28).

Intestinal gas in the large intestine (flatus) is mostly the result of bacterial action on undigested food residues. The bacteria causes the undigested material to ferment (decompose) and produce gas. High-fiber foods and certain vegetables and fruits seem to promote excessive gaseousness for many people. These foods include dried peas, beans, lentils, broccoli, brussels sprouts, cabbage, onions, peppers, and melons. The gas-producing property of dried beans has been traced to the presence of specific indigestible carbohydrates—stachyose and raffinose.

A carefully kept diary of foods eaten and symptoms of gaseousness can help clients identify problem foods. People with GI disorders in which carbohydrates are poorly absorbed often experience excessive gas production; lactose intolerance is such a disorder (see Chapter 28).

Some people may find relief in medications such as over-the-counter drugs to relieve gassiness, lactase enzymes (in lactose intolerance), or prescribed GI stimulants that help move gas through the intestine more quickly.

Suggestions for reducing gas in the intestinal tract are as follows:

- Have a dentist check the fit of dentures.
- Eliminate carbonated beverages and avoid drinking through straws.
- Avoid chewing gum or sucking on hard candies (especially avoid products containing sorbitol, which is absorbed very slowly and can lead to gas build-up).
- Avoid excessive use of high-fat foods (delay stomach emptying).
- Limit or avoid milk products if you are lactose intolerant.
- Limit intake of gas-producing foods such as cabbage, cauliflower, dried beans, and brussels sprouts.
- Increase walking, jogging, and calisthenics to help stimulate movement of gas through intestinal tract.

People who have made a conscious effort to increase fiber in their diets may experience increased gassiness. They should add high-fiber foods gradually and in small quantities to the diet. Most people adapt to these foods within 3 to 4 weeks; others may continue to experience symptoms.

GASTRIC ACIDITY

The stomach is normally acidic. This strongly acidic environment has important functions in the digestive process. Psychological factors can stimulate the flow of gastric juice. The presence of food in the stomach, however, stimulates acidic gastric secretion more than anything else. Meat, alcohol, caffeine, and substances other than caffeine in both regular and decaffeinated coffee have an especially stimulating effect on acid secretion.

Heartburn, a common digestive disorder, is caused by a backup of the acid contents from the stomach into the esophagus and not from excessive acid production. It occurs when the lower esophageal sphincter relaxes or is very weak and fails to hold down the stomach's contents (see Chapter 28). Sometimes digestive disturbances are caused by abnormally low amounts of stomach acid, which may indicate serious illness. A person suffering from such a digestive disturbance may mistake the condition for excess acidity and take antacid medications. The regular use of nonprescription antacids is a dangerous practice. These self-prescribed medications can mask the symptoms of serious illness and delay a person from seeking treatment. The excessive use of antacids also can upset the acid–base balance in the body.

CONSTIPATION

Constipation may be caused by dehydration or intestinal disease. Uncomplicated constipation (not due to disease) frequently is a result of eating and health habits. One of the most common causes of constipation is failure to respond to the defecation reflex. Another major cause is a lack of muscle tone, characterized by inadequate muscular movements along the digestive tract. Lack of exercise and a low intake of fibrous foods contribute to this lack of tone. Frequently, the affected person resorts to the use of self-prescribed laxatives. The intestine then becomes dependent on this artificial stimulation, and a vicious cycle results (see Chapter 21).

MEDICATION

Some medications irritate the lining of the stomach and can cause discomfort if not taken with food. Among them are iron preparations, potassium, chloride, levodopa, and analgesics.

KEYS TO PRACTICAL APPLICATION

To prevent digestive disturbances, encourage your client to do the following:

- Create as pleasant an atmosphere as possible at mealtime.
- Chew food well; eat slowly.
- Avoid excessive amounts of fat, especially fried foods.
- Eat small to moderate amounts of food at one time because large meals take longer to digest,
- Add high-fiber foods gradually to the diet to avoid excessive gas formation.

Advise client to see a physician if he or she repeatedly experiences digestive discomfort.

Discourage the regular use of self-prescribed antacids because these medications can mask the symptoms of serious illness and delay the client from seeking treatment.

Be aware that persistent problems of digestion or absorption can have profound effects on nutritional status.

KEY IDEAS

The functioning of the GI tract greatly influences nutritional status.

The digestive tract reduces the size of nutrient particles to a form that can be absorbed, protects the body from harmful substances ingested with food, and eliminates the undigested wastes.

Digestion is accomplished by both mechanical and chemical means.

The digestive tract is a long muscular tube consisting of two hold areas (stomach and large intestine) connected by the small intestine, where most of the digestive process occurs (see Table 6-1).

The functions of the accessory organs—the liver, pancreas, and gallbladder—are important in digestion.

Secretions in the stomach are under the control of hormones and nerves.

The rhythmic muscular movements of the GI tract and the emulsification of fats through the action of bile salts prepare food for chemical digestion, which occurs mainly by the action of enzymes.

The stomach is normally acidic; hydrochloric acid secreted in gastric juice activates pepsin, prepares protein for partial digestion by pepsin, increases the solubility of certain minerals, and destroys harmful bacteria.

Several protective mechanisms including the secretion of mucus protect the GI lining from being digested.

Digestion occurs in stages; the chemical breakdown of nutrients and absorption occur mostly in the small intestine.

Hydrolysis results in the splitting of the nutrient molecule into simpler compounds; hydrolysis is accomplished mainly by the action of enzymes.

The process of digestion reduces proteins to amino acids, carbohydrates to simple sugars, and fats to fatty acids and glycerol (Table 6-2).

The anatomy of the small intestine including the folds of the small intestine and the villi and microvilli lining the small intestine provides enormous absorptive area.

Nutrients are absorbed mainly by two mechanisms: diffusion and active transport.

Almost all digested protein, fat, and carbohydrate are absorbed. The degree of absorption of some minerals is less complete. Mineral absorption depends on body stores, need, the form in which the nutrient occurs, and the presence of other substances.

Whatever remains of food after digestion and absorption have occurred is excreted from the body by way of the large intestine; the main function of the large intestine is to remove water from waste material.

Bacteria in the intestinal tract synthesize some B vitamins and vitamin K.

Poor mental and emotional states, overeating, high-fat meals, improperly chewed food, swallowing of air, and eating when overly tired hinder the digestive process and may cause digestive disturbances.

The frequent use of antacids to relieve GI discomfort is dangerous because it may delay a person from getting medical treatment for serious illness.

Fats and proteins are more slowly digested in the stomach than carbohydrates, and thus tend to delay hunger.

Frequent belching can be due to excessive swallowing of air, gastroesophageal reflux, or gastritis.

Gas in the large intestine is produced mostly by bacterial activity on nonabsorbable carbohydrates.

KEYS TO LEARNING

STUDY–DISCUSSION QUESTIONS

1. Describe the mechanical and chemical aspects of digestion.
2. Describe the differences in appearance and function of the stomach, small intestine, and large intestine.
3. Discuss the effects of psychological factors on the functioning of the digestive tract. What evidence do you see of these effects among your clients?
4. What are some of the common causes of gastric distress or indigestion? Why is the repeated use of nonprescription remedies a dangerous practice?
5. What is meant by the *satiety value* of food? What foods have a high satiety value? Name some of the factors that influence the speed with which foods are digested.
6. Give five suggestions for reducing excessive gaseousness.

BIBLIOGRAPHY

BOOKS

Greene HL, Moran JR. The gastrointestinal tract: regulator of nutrient absorption. In: Shils ME, Olson JA, Shike M. Eds. Modern nutrition in health and disease. 8th ed. Philadelphia: Lea and Febiger, 1994:549–568.

Mahan KL, Arlin M. Krause's food, nutrition and diet therapy. Philadelphia: WB Saunders, 1992:Chapters 26, 27.

Memmler RL, Cohen BJ, Wood DL. Structure and function of the human body. Philadelphia: JB Lippincott, 1992.

Meyer JH. The stomach and nutrition. In: Shils ME, Olson JA, Shike M. Eds. Modern nutrition in health and disease. 8th ed. Philadelphia: Lea and Febiger 1994:1029–1035.

PERIODICALS

Montes RG, Perman JA. Lactose intolerance: pinpointing the source of nonspecific gastrointestinal symptoms. Postgraduate Medicine 1991;89:8:175.

CHAPTER

7

Energy Metabolism

KEY TERMS

adenosine triphosphate (ATP) a high energy compound involved in the transfer of energy within the cell

aerobic requiring oxygen

anabolism the phase of metabolism in which new molecules are synthesized and more complex substances are made from simpler ones

anemia a decrease in the number of red blood cells or hemoglobin

basal metabolic rate (BMR) the expression of the number of calories used hourly in relation to the surface area of the body

basal metabolism the amount of energy required to carry on the vital processes when the body is at rest

caloric density the number of calories in a unit of weight of a specific food

catabolism the chemical breakdown of more complex substances in living cells to simpler compounds with the release of energy

coenzyme a substance, such as a vitamin, required for the activation of some enzymes

energy metabolism all the chemical changes that result in the release of energy in the body

ergogenic work producing

hemoglobin the oxygen-carrying red pigment in blood cells

hyperthyroidism excessive secretion of the thyroid gland resulting in an increased basal metabolic rate

hypothyroidism deficiency of thyroid secretion resulting in a lowered basal metabolic rate

intensity (of exercise) how hard a person works during exercise as determined by heart rate

joule an international unit of energy; 1 kcal = 4.184 kJ

Krebs cycle (also called ***tricarboxylic acid cycle***) a set of complex chemical reactions within the cell that produces energy through the oxidation of carbohydrate, protein, and fat

nutrient density the nutritional content of a food in relation to its caloric value; usually determined in terms of specific nutrients

oxidation the chemical process by which a substance combines with oxygen

ratio a numeric or quantitative comparison of two things

synthesis the process of building up; the formation of complex substances from simpler ones

thermic effect of food the increase in metabolism caused by the digestion of food and the absorption, and transport of nutrients to the cells

OBJECTIVES

After completing this chapter, the student will be able to:

1. Identify the nutrient sources of energy.
2. Identify the important role of respiration in energy metabolism.
3. Discuss the distinct role of each of the three energy nutrients in supplying energy to the body.
4. Estimate the energy value of a food given the amounts of the energy nutrients it contains.

5. Identify and explain the factors that affect basal energy requirements.
6. Identify and explain the three factors that compose the total energy requirements for an individual.
7. Estimate his or her own energy requirements.
8. Explain the concept of energy balance and its relationship to weight maintenance, weight gain, and weight loss.
9. Discuss the recommendations of authorities regarding the contributions that each of the energy nutrients should make to total energy needs.
10. Identify the characteristics that determine the energy values of specific foods and give examples of foods that illustrate these characteristics.
11. Define *caloric density* and *nutrient density;* identify foods that are examples of each.
12. Discuss the benefits of exercise as a consistent lifestyle component and discuss precautions.
13. Identify and define the three essential components of aerobic exercise needed to improve cardiorespiratory functioning.
14. Discuss the benefits of resistance exercises and of low to moderate intensity exercises.
15. Explain the nutritional requirements of athletes for each of the following: carbohydrate, protein, fat, vitamins, minerals, and fluids.
16. Identify the different energy sources needed for different physical activities.
17. Discuss the proneness of athletes to "magic" claims about foods and dietary supplements and its possible effects.

Metabolism refers to all the processes by which the body cells use nutrients to support life. These processes involve chemical changes that occur in nutrients after they have been absorbed from the digestive tract. Metabolism has two parts: synthesis and breakdown of nutrients. Synthesis involves the conversion of simple compounds into more complex molecules. This process, by which the body forms new tissue, is called *anabolism.* The breakdown of nutrients involves the reconversion of complex molecules into simpler ones. This process is called *catabolism.* The production of energy is a catabolic process. Because the formation of new compounds requires energy, both catabolic and anabolic processes occur simultaneously.

Anabolism and catabolism occur continuously and are normally in balance. During periods of rapid tissue growth, such as in childhood, pregnancy, and convalescence, anabolism exceeds catabolism. Some catabolic processes occur as a result of disease, injury, immobility, or aging and are not beneficial. Under these conditions, catabolism exceeds anabolism.

Within each cell, hundreds of enzymes direct the use of nutrients so that the bodily needs for energy, building and maintenance of tissue, and regulation of body processes are satisfied. Carbohydrates and fats combine with oxygen to supply energy or are converted to stored energy in the form of adipose tissue. Amino acids are used to build new cells, to form hormones and enzymes, or as a form of energy. Vitamins and minerals become a part of the cell structure or combine with other nutrients to form substances that regulate body processes.

CONVERTING FOOD TO ENERGY

Energy metabolism refers to chemical changes that result in the release of energy. The light energy of the sun is converted to chemical energy in food. The body has the ability to transform food energy from one form to another. The chemical energy of food can be converted to mechanical, electrical, and heat energy and other forms of chemical energy in the body.

The carbohydrates, proteins, and fats in food are the nutrients that provide energy. Alcohol (ethanol), which is derived from glucose, also yields energy. Vitamins, minerals, and water do not supply energy.

After food is digested and the nutrients are absorbed into the bloodstream, the nutrients are carried by the blood to every cell in the body. It is within the cell that metabolism occurs. To follow the metabolism of proteins, fats, and carbohydrates, we must think of them in terms of their basic units—amino acids, fatty acids and glycerol, and glucose. If not needed by the cell for energy, these basic units can be stored: glucose units are used to form a body starch called *glycogen;* fatty acids and glycerol are recombined into *triglycerides* (fats); and amino acids are used to make a variety of body protein. These are examples of anabolic reactions.

If the cell needs energy, any or all of these basic units—glucose, amino acids, and fatty acids and glycerol—can be split further. During the process of energy metabolism, the carbon atoms in these nutrient molecules are separated and the energy that held them together is released. This release of energy by splitting compounds into smaller units is a catabolic reaction.

The energy that results from the breakdown of nutrients in the body is either converted to heat, which maintains body temperature, or temporarily held by a phosphorus-containing compound called *adenosine triphosphate (ATP)*. The chemical bonds that hold this compound together are strong, high energy bonds. The energy stored in ATP has been described as a loaded spring that releases its energy when it is triggered. ATP provides energy for all the work performed by the cell. Some is converted to mechanical energy needed by muscle tissue, some to electrical energy involved in the transmission of nerve impulses, and some to chemical energy needed for the synthesis of new compounds.

The process by which energy is released within the cell involves many steps, each requiring the assistance of a specific enzyme. Many enzymes require other substances called *coenzymes*. The coenzymes involved in energy metabolism comprise, in part, the B vitamins. The vitamin thiamin, for example, is needed for the formation of a coenzyme involved in one of the steps in carbohydrate metabolism. Other nutrients such as minerals also act as coenzymes. Various hormones play important roles in energy metabolism. Insulin, a hormone secreted by the islets of Langerhans in the pancreas, must be present for glucose to enter the cell.

RESPIRATION

Oxygen is required for the complete release of the energy available in the fuel-producing nutrients, just as it is required for the complete burning of substances outside the body. The chemical process in which a substance combines with oxygen is called *oxidation*. Oxidation is called an *aerobic* process. By-products of oxidation are water and carbon dioxide, a gas that is toxic to the body.

Ventilation (breathing) makes possible the exchange of gases—oxygen and carbon dioxide—between the air and the blood. This gas exchange occurs entirely by diffusion through lung tissue. Both the respiratory and circulatory systems must be working normally and in coordination to supply sufficient oxygen for the metabolism of food and to eliminate carbon dioxide and water.

Most of the oxygen in the blood is chemically bonded to hemoglobin. Normal hemoglobin levels are necessary if adequate amounts of oxygen are to be available for the efficient use of body fuel. Hence, people suffering from low hemoglobin levels (anemia) become tired with physical effort.

ENERGY CYCLE

The series of steps or chemical reactions that results in the complete oxidation of carbohydrate, protein, and fat is known as the *Krebs cycle* or *tricarboxylic acid cycle*. Within this cycle of reactions, energy is removed bit by bit from the energy-producing nutrients and stored as ATP. Before entering the cycle, the nutrients are broken down to the compound acetyl coenzyme A (CoA; Fig. 7-1).

GLUCOSE

Glucose is the body's major source of energy. When needed for energy, glucose is split in half, releasing energy and forming two molecules of a substance called *pyruvate*. At this point, the reaction can be reversed and glucose can be reformed. If the cell still needs energy, pyruvate is broken down to a smaller compound, acetyl CoA. Once acetyl CoA is formed, the reaction cannot be reversed to form glucose. If energy is needed, acetyl CoA enters the Krebs cycle, further releasing energy by a complex series of steps. If energy is not needed, acetyl CoA is converted to fatty acids, which are stored as body fat. In this way, excessive amounts of carbohydrate contribute to body fat.

The extent to which energy nutrients can be converted to pyruvate determines how much glu-

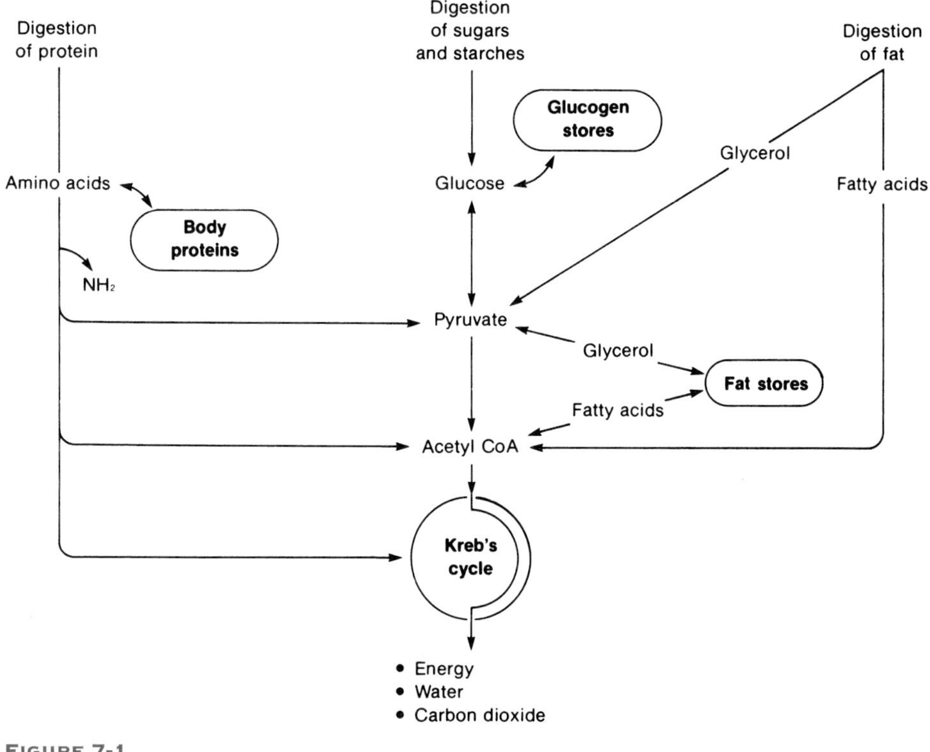

FIGURE 7-1

Simplified diagram of the aerobic pathway for energy production.

cose they can provide. This is important because brain and nervous tissue *require* glucose for energy. Those parts of protein and fat that can be converted to pyruvate can provide glucose for the body. Those parts that are converted directly to acetyl CoA cannot be converted to glucose.

FATTY ACIDS AND GLYCEROL

Fats comprise one molecule of a glycerol and three molecules of fatty acids. The glycerol part can be readily converted to pyruvate and then converted to glucose or further broken down to acetyl CoA. Glycerol represents only a small amount by weight of the fat molecule; only about 5% of the fat molecule can be converted to glucose.

The fatty acids part of the fat molecule can be broken down to acetyl CoA and then further broken down in the Krebs cycle to yield energy. Alternatively, the fatty acids part is used to make other fatty acids, cholesterol, or ketones. Fat is not a good source of glucose and cannot provide energy for the brain and nervous tissue.

AMINO ACIDS

Proteins are absorbed as amino acids. Ideally, they are used to build or maintain body proteins. If the body's energy needs are not being met by carbohydrates and fats, however, amino acids can be used to provide energy. In this case, nitrogen is removed from the amino acid and the remaining atoms are treated in a variety of ways. About half can be converted to pyruvate and therefore can provide glucose. Protein is a fairly good source of glucose when carbohydrate is unavailable.

The other half of the amino acids are converted to acetyl CoA or enter the Krebs cycle directly. Amino acids also break down when both excessive calories and excessive proteins are consumed because protein cannot be stored in the body. The excessive amino acids are stripped of their nitrogen and most are converted to acetyl CoA. Because energy is not needed, the acetyl CoA is not broken down further. Instead, it is converted to fatty acids and stored as body fat.

ENERGY PRODUCTION WITHOUT OXYGEN

The Krebs cycle requires high levels of oxygen. At times, however, the oxygen supply to the cells is inadequate. For example, during strenuous exercise, the muscles become depleted of oxygen and the respiratory and circulatory systems cannot keep up with the demand. In this situation, glucose takes another pathway. Instead of being broken down to pyruvate, it is reduced to lactic acid. Some energy is released in this reaction. The lactic acid, however, cannot be broken down further to yield more ATP or energy. The lactic acid causes the muscle environment to become more acidic. Fatigue sets in and cramps may result. The most limiting factor to exercise is the ability of a person's respiratory and cardiovascular systems to deliver oxygen to the tissues.

DISPOSAL OF END PRODUCTS OF ENERGY PRODUCTION

Oxidation of the fuel-producing nutrients results in heat and other forms of energy, water, and carbon dioxide. The carbon dioxide is carried to the lungs, where it is exhaled. The water, called *metabolic water,* can be used by the body just like the water obtained from food and beverages. The portion of water that is not needed is excreted by the kidneys in the urine. Some water also may be lost in expired air or through the skin. Nitrogen, which results from the breakdown of amino acids, is synthesized into urea in the liver and is excreted by the kidneys in the urine.

MEASURING ENERGY

Heat is a measure of energy produced. Food energy is measured in kilocalories. The kilocalorie represents the amount of heat required to raise 1 kg (1000 g) of water 1°C. In popular usage, the kilocalorie is referred to as a *calorie*. The international unit for measuring energy is the joule. One kilocalorie is equal to 4.184 kJ.

ENERGY FROM FOOD

The caloric value of the three fuel-producing nutrients differs because the relationship of carbon to hydrogen to oxygen in each of the nutrients differs. The less oxygen the nutrient contains, the more calories it supplies. Approximate energy values have been established for the three fuel-producing nutrients as follows: carbohydrate, 4 kcal/g; protein, 4 kcal/g; and fat, 9 kcal/g. Alcohol, which is produced from the fermentation of glucose, provides 7 kcal/g. Fat has more than twice the caloric value of protein or carbohydrate. Foods that contain a high percentage of fat, therefore, provide a substantial amount of calories.

The energy value of an individual food is determined by burning a weighed portion of the food in a bomb calorimeter. The amount of heat (or calories) produced by the burning is determined by the change in temperature of a measured amount of water that surrounds the insulated chamber in which the food is burned.

Because the energy value of a particular food depends on the amount of protein, fat, and carbohydrate it contains, energy value can be estimated if the composition of the food is known. For example, a ½-cup portion of baked macaroni and cheese contains 8 g of protein, 11 g of fat, and 20 g of carbohydrate. From this information, with the fuel values given earlier, its approximate energy value is determined as follows:

Protein	8 g × 4 =	32
Fat	11 g × 9 =	99
Carbohydrate	20 g × 4 =	80
		211 kcal

ENERGY PRODUCED BY THE BODY

The amount of energy produced by the body can be measured directly or indirectly. In the direct method, a person is placed in an insulated heat-sensitive chamber and the heat given off by his or her body is measured. This method is expensive, and is used only in scientific research.

In the indirect method, a respiration apparatus is used. It records the amount of oxygen consumed or carbon dioxide exhaled by the person in a given number of minutes. From this information, one can calculate the number of calories produced by the body. This method, now used in research, was once used in clinical practice. It has been replaced by thyroid function tests, which are discussed in the section Basal Metabolism. Various other indirect methods, including heart rate, are being used to assess energy expenditure.

FACTORS INFLUENCING ENERGY NEEDS

Total energy needs are based on three factors: basal metabolism or resting energy expenditure (REE), voluntary physical activity, and the thermic effect of food (Figure 7-2).

BASAL METABOLISM

Basal metabolism is the energy required to carry on vital body processes at rest. These processes include all cellular and glandular activities, skeletal muscle tone, body temperature, circulation, and respiration. In people who are generally inactive physically, basal metabolic needs make up the largest part—about two thirds—of the total energy requirements.

The *basal metabolic rate (BMR)* is the rate at which a person requires energy for these vital body processes. It is measured in the morning after awakening from sleep, at least 12 hours after the last meal. More recently, the REE has been used as a measure of the body's energy needs at rest. The REE is not measured under the same conditions and may include the influence on metabolism of a previous meal. There is less than 10% difference between the REE and the BMR; thus the terms are used interchangeably.

Various equations can be used to estimate the REE. One is the Harris-Benedict equation. This equation normally is not used for people younger than age 18 years:

$$\text{Female: REE} = 655 + (9.6 \times W) + (1.8 \times H) - (4.7 \times A)$$

$$\text{Male: REE} = 66 + (13.7 \times W) + (5 \times H) - (6.8 \times A)$$

where A = age in years, H = height in centimeters, and W = weight in kilograms. Although frequently used to determine BMR, Harris and Benedict's data collection methods more closely measure REE.

The BMR for the average woman is about 0.9 kcal/kg of body weight per hour and for the average man is 1 kcal/kg of body weight per hour. Thus, a man weighing 150 lb would require 1632 calories for basal metabolic needs: 150 lb = 68 kg (1 kg = 2.2 lb); 68 kg × 1 kcal/kg/h × 24 h = 1632 kcal.

FACTORS INFLUENCING BMR

The BMR or REE differs among people because of differences in body size and shape, gender, physical condition, age, state of nutrition, presence of disease, glandular activity, body temperature, and environmental temperature. Body composition affects heat lost by the body. The greater the skin area, the greater the amount of heat lost and the higher the BMR. A tall slender person has more surface area and therefore a higher BMR than a shorter stout person of the same weight.

Muscle and glandular tissue are active and have a higher BMR than fatty tissue. An athlete tends to have a higher BMR than a sedentary person of the same age and size. The BMR for women is about 10% lower than for men because of the difference in muscle mass.

The BMR or REE differs with age because the amount and composition of metabolically active tissue (lean body mass) differs with age. The BMR is high in infancy because the infant has a higher proportion of metabolically active organ tissue than the adult. In the adult, lean body mass in the form of skeletal muscle has the greatest effect on resting metabolism. Muscle tissue declines at the rate of about 2% to 3% per decade after early adulthood, and the BMR or REE declines proportionately. The activity component of total energy needs is affected more by age than by the BMR or REE. Adults who continue to consume the same number of calories as they did earlier in life experience a gradual weight gain. This is frequently the case among middle-aged people.

Growth increases the BMR because of the additional energy needed to synthesize protein and fat and deposit it in the tissues. Except for the first year of life, however, the effect of growth on total energy requirements is only about 1%. The BMR of a woman increases during pregnancy and lactation.

The state of nutrition, especially in the case of severe starvation or prolonged periods of inadequate caloric intake, can affect the BMR because the body attempts to adapt to a decrease in intake by decreasing its BMR. Disease conditions that produce fever raise the BMR in proportion to the increase in body temperature. The BMR increases about 7% for each increase of 1°F.

Environmental temperatures below 68°F and hot temperatures increase BMR. If a hot climate reduces the amount of work done, then the total energy expenditure may actually decrease.

Secretions of certain endocrine glands, especially those of the thyroid and adrenal glands, affect basal metabolism. They have more influence on basal energy needs than any other single factor. Thyroxine, produced by the thyroid, regulates the speed of energy metabolism, and epinephrine, from the adrenal glands, provides for the rapid conversion of glycogen (carbohydrate stored in the liver) to glucose when a source of quick energy is needed.

Blood tests that measure the activity of the thyroid gland are used in clinical practice to measure basal metabolism. Two thyroid hormone compounds, T_3 (the prethyroxine hormone) and T_4 (thyroxine), are measured, and from these measurements the level of energy production is calculated. Also, because iodine is found only in the secretions of the thyroid gland, two other blood tests may be performed to evaluate thyroid function: serum levels of protein-bound iodine and radioactive iodine uptake tests. Excessive production of thyroxine, called *hyperthyroidism*, causes the rate of metabolism to be abnormally high. A reduced secretion of thyroxine, *hypothyroidism*, results in a lower than normal rate of metabolism. Pituitary hormones, which stimulate thyroid and adrenal secretions, also may affect the BMR.

PHYSICAL ACTIVITY

The influence of physical activity on total caloric needs depends on the type of activity, intensity, length of time it is performed, and size (or build) of the person (Figure 7-2). Most Americans are expending fewer calories for physical activity than in the past. The activity pattern of Americans is generally sedentary to light. The RDAs committee's recommended energy intakes (Table 7-1) for adults, however, are based on a light to moderate activity level. The committee encourages adults, even those older than age 50 years, to maintain this level of activity.

It may be surprising to discover how few calories are required to perform various activities (Table 7-2). People tend to be busy with a myriad of tasks, yet, because of the type of work being done, they are mostly inactive physically. For example, a student may be wholly occupied but sedentary at the same time. Mental activity requires practically no increase in energy expenditure over the BMR. Brain cell activity is part of the BMR and does not vary whether one is sleeping or studying. Any increase in energy expenditure that results from mental work usually is due to muscle tension rather than brain cell activity. People who engage in strenuous physical activity for prolonged periods, however, may require as many as 4000 kcal to 5000 kcal/day.

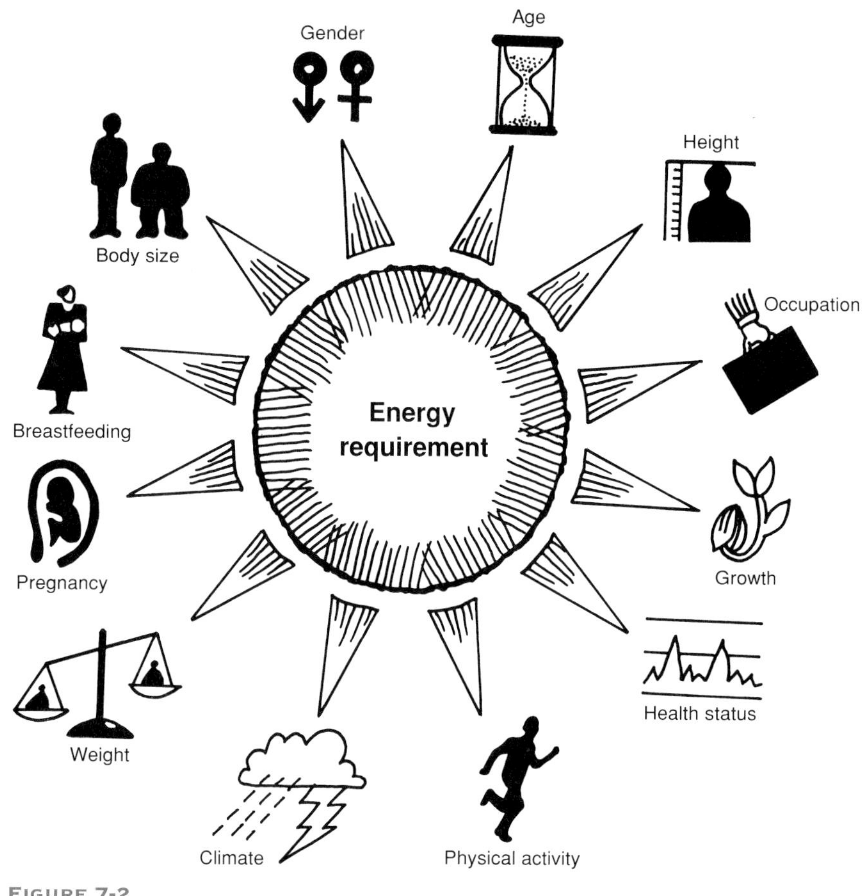

FIGURE 7-2

Factors affecting energy requirements. *(US Dept of Agriculture. Eating for good health. Washington, DC: US Government Printing Office, 1994. Agricultural Information Bulletin 685:68.)*

The larger the body, the more energy is needed for activities that require body movement, such as walking. The energy expenditures needed for the activities listed in Table 7-2 increase as the weight of the person increases. Overweight people frequently make up for the greater effort required of them for activity by becoming less active.

As a general rule, sedentary activity increases a person's total energy needs to 130% of the BMR, light activity to 150% to 160%, moderate activity to 160% to 170%, and strenuous activity to 190% to 210%. Display 7-1 provides examples of activities at each level.

THERMIC EFFECT OF FOOD

The BMR increases for about 4 hours after a meal. It reaches a peak about 1 hour after the meal. Digestion, absorption, transport of nutrients to the cells, and the changes the nutrients undergo all require energy. The production of heat following a meal is known as the *thermic effect* of food or the *specific dynamic action* of food. The effect varies according to the kinds and amounts of food eaten and the person's metabolic needs. The use of nutrients to build new tissue requires more energy than the breakdown of nutrients to provide energy. The thermic effect of food varies from about 5% to 10% of total energy needs.

TABLE 7-1 MEDIAN HEIGHTS AND WEIGHTS AND RECOMMENDED ENERGY INTAKE

Category	Age (yr) or Condition	Weight kg	Weight lb	Height cm	Height in	REE* (kcal/day)	Average Energy Allowance (kcal)† Multiples of REE	Per kg	Per Day‡
Infants	0.0–0.5	6	13	60	24	320		108	650
	0.5–1.0	9	20	71	28	500		98	850
Children	1–3	13	29	90	35	740		102	1300
	4–6	20	44	112	44	950		90	1800
	7–10	28	62	132	52	1130		70	2000
Males	11–14	45	99	157	62	1440	1.70	55	2500
	15–18	66	145	176	69	1760	1.67	45	3000
	19–24	72	160	177	70	1780	1.67	40	2900
	25–50	79	174	176	70	1800	1.60	37	2900
	51+	77	170	173	68	1530	1.50	30	2300
Females	11–14	46	101	157	62	1310	1.67	47	2200
	15–18	55	120	163	64	1370	1.60	40	2200
	19–24	58	128	164	65	1350	1.60	38	2200
	25–50	63	138	163	64	1380	1.55	36	2200
	51+	65	143	160	63	1280	1.50	30	1900
Pregnant	1st trimester								+0
	2nd trimester								+300
	3rd trimester								+300
Lactating	1st 6 months								+500
	2nd 6 months								+500

* Calculation based on Food and Agriculture Organization equations, then rounded.
† In the range of light to moderate activity, the coefficient of variation is ±20%.
‡ Figure is rounded.
(National Academy of Sciences, Food and Nutrition Board, National Research Council. Recommended dietary allowances. 10th ed. Washington, DC: National Academy Press, 1989:33.)

ESTIMATING ENERGY NEEDS

Total energy needs are the sum total of basal metabolism (or REE) plus energy expenditure for physical activity plus energy expenditure due to the thermic effect of food (after meals). To estimate the caloric needs of an individual, each of these factors is determined as follows:

1. Determine the BMR or REE by one of the following methods:
   a. Multiply body weight in kilograms by 0.9 for women and 1 for men, then multiply by 24 (0.9 × weight in kilograms × 24 [hours in a day]).
   b. Use the Harris-Benedict equation.
2. Select an activity level appropriate for the individual based on the nutrition history (occupation, lifestyle, and age). Multiply the BMR or REE by the figure associated with that activity level (see activity levels and activity factors in Display 7–1).
3. Add calories for the thermic effect of food. Multiply the calories determined in step 2 by 0.1 (10%). Add this amount to the calories in step 2.

ENERGY BALANCE

An infallible guide exists for determining whether food intake is meeting energy needs. This guide is body weight. If the number of calories you consume is equal to the number you use for energy, your

TABLE 7-2 CALORIE VALUES FOR 10 MINUTES OF ACTIVITY

ACTIVITY	BODY WEIGHT		
	125 lb	175 lb	250 lb
Sleeping	10	14	20
Sitting, writing	15	21	30
Walking downstairs	56	78	110
Walking			
At 2 mph	29	40	58
At 4 mph	52	72	102
Running			
At 5.5 mph	90	125	178
At 7 mph	118	164	232
Cycling at 5.5 mph	42	58	83
Light gardening	30	42	59
Mowing grass (power)	34	47	67
Golfing	33	48	68
Swimming, crawl	40	56	80
Racquetball	75	104	144
Tennis	56	80	115
Dancing (vigorous)	48	66	94

(Adapted from Brownell KD. The LEARN Program for weight control. Copyright © KD Brownell, Philadelphia: University of Pennsylvania, 1989:55.)

body weight will be constant. If you consistently consume more calories than you use for energy, you will gain weight. Excess calories are stored in the form of fat. If you usually eat fewer calories than you use, you lose weight. Energy must come from somewhere, so needed calories not provided by food are drawn from body stores.

One pound of body fat represents 3500 kcal. For every 3500 kcal lacking in the diet, 1 lb of body weight is lost, and for every 3500 kcal excess, 1 lb is gained. It does not matter whether the excess or shortage occurs over a period of 1 week or 1 year.

EXCESS ENERGY

Balancing energy needs with energy intake is difficult for many people, as is clearly demonstrated by the fact that obesity is a major nutritional problem in the United States. Although it may be seen in people of any age, obesity is especially prevalent among adults, mostly because of a gradual reduction in BMR together with a decrease in physical activity. Whereas energy needs decrease, the intake of calories often remains the same as it was earlier in life, when energy expenditure was greater.

Regardless of what weight reduction ads frequently imply, weight loss can occur only when caloric intake is lower than energy needs. Even when attempting to lose weight, the diet should include all the basic foods necessary to provide the essential nutrients. An appropriate strategy is to reduce portion sizes and replace rich desserts with fruits.

For many of us, everyday living demands little physical activity. Advances in technology often reduce the physical activity required to do a task. Exercise is a valuable aid in achieving a balance between energy intake and energy output. Over months or years, even small increases in daily exercise can make a difference in weight. For example, a 150-lb person who spends 5 minutes a day walking up and down stairs will experience a weight loss of 12 lb a year if food consumption remains the same.

The National Academy of Sciences Food and Nutrition Board has suggested it is healthier to achieve weight control by increasing physical activity than by reducing calories. It is difficult to obtain essential nutrients and proper use of protein on diets that are low in calories. Exercise has many other advantages, which are discussed more fully later in this chapter.

ENERGY DEFICIT

When energy intake fails to meet the body's needs, weight loss occurs. Excessive weight loss can cause serious problems. It is frequently seen as a result of diseases that dampen the appetite, interfere with the intake, digestion, or absorption of food, or greatly increase the body's BMR. Excessive weight loss also may result from severe dieting.

Providing energy is the body's first priority. Not only physical activity, but all the body's chemical reactions and other metabolic activities require fuel. When fuel from food is lacking, the body must supply the fuel from within itself. Fat stores are called

DISPLAY 7-1 ESTIMATING TOTAL CALORIC NEEDS

STEP 1

Determine calories required for basal metabolic expenditure (or resting energy expenditure):

Body weight ÷ 2.2 × 0.9 (woman) × 24 =
in pounds × 1.0 (men) × 24 =

(May also use Harris-Benedict equation in text.)

STEP 2

Multiply calories needed for BMR or REE times appropriate activity factor

× 1.3 Very light activity

× 1.6 (men) / × 1.5 (women) — Light activity

× 1.7 (men) / × 1.6 (women) — Moderate activity

× 2.1 (men) / × 1.9 (women) — Heavy activity

STEP 3

Add calories for the thermic effect of food. Estimate this by multiplying kilocalories determined in step 2 by 0.10 (10%). Add this amount to the calories determined in step 2.

Total caloric needs = Calories required for BMR or REE × activity factor + calories for thermic effect of food

EXAMPLE

The estimated caloric requirement for a 125-lb woman, light activity:

Step 1. 125 ÷ 2.2 = 57 kg; 57 × 0.9 × 24 = 1231
Step 2. 1231 × 1.5 = 1846.5
Step 3. 1846.5 × 0.10 = 184.65
1846.5 + 184.65 = 2031.15

Estimated caloric need = 2031 kcal

ACTIVITY LEVELS

Very light: Seated and standing activities; writing, typing, laboratory work, driving, cooking, sewing.
Light: Teaching, light gardening, housecleaning, garage work, golf, electrical trades.
Moderate: Yard work such as pulling weeds, mowing lawn (not motorized), walking up and down small hills, skiing, tennis, cycling.
Strenuous: Chopping wood, felling trees, heavy manual digging, basketball, football, climbing.

on to provide energy. Fat, however, can provide little glucose. Therefore, body protein breaks down to provide the glucose required as fuel for brain tissue. Whenever fat is used almost exclusively as the source of energy, body protein also is used. The gradual loss of body protein causes muscle loss and decreases resistance to disease.

RECOMMENDED ENERGY INTAKES

Recommended energy intakes are given in Table 7-1. The adult allowances are based on light to moderate activity. In each age category, a reference person—a person of a given height and weight—

has been used as a standard. For example, the reference man is 25 to 50 years old, weighs 174 lb, and is 70 inches tall. Changes are required for differences due to body size or physical activity; for example, a man whose ideal weight or activity is higher than that of the reference man requires more calories.

Energy needs increase during pregnancy and in infancy and childhood. These needs are discussed in Chapters 16, 17, and 18.

FOOD SOURCES OF ENERGY

CONSUMPTION PATTERNS

In the typical American diet, the energy value of food is derived 48% from carbohydrate, 35% from fat, and 14% to 18% from protein. Alcohol contributes up to 1800 kcal/day for some people. Many authorities believe that the entire population would benefit from dietary changes. The National Academy of Sciences Committee on Diet and Health has recommended an increase in carbohydrates (mostly from starches and naturally occurring sugars) to more than 55% of energy intake and a reduction in fat to 30% or less of energy intake. Carbohydrate foods are the least expensive source of energy.

ENERGY CONTENT OF FOOD

Foods vary greatly in energy value, depending on the proportion of energy-producing nutrients (protein, fat, and carbohydrate), water, and fiber they contain. For example, energy-producing nutrients make up less than 3% of lettuce and 100% of cooking oil.

Because fats provide more than twice as many calories per gram as either carbohydrates or proteins, foods that contain even a moderate amount of fat have a high energy value. Cream, cream cheese, butter, margarine, oils, cheese, and fatty meats have a high caloric content. In contrast, because water and fiber do not yield calories, foods that contain high proportions of water and fiber have a low caloric content. Fruits and vegetables, especially green leafy vegetables, fall into this category. Between these two extremes are foods that are intermediate in fuel value, such as lean meats, cereal foods, and starchy vegetables.

Some foods that do not contain fat and are low in water are high in fuel value. These foods include sugar, dried legumes, and dried fruits. For example, a $^{2}/_{3}$-cup portion of fresh grapes has 67 kcal, whereas a $^{2}/_{3}$-cup portion of raisins (dried grapes) has 290 kcal. The caloric content of hard cheese is high, not only because the food has a high-fat content, but also because it is a highly concentrated food with a low moisture content. Table 7-3 demonstrates the influence of fat, alcohol, water, and fiber content on the energy value of selected foods.

Method of food preparation is another factor that greatly influences the energy value of food. For example, poultry and fish, which tend to be low in calories, become high energy dishes when fried or served with cream sauces.

To call foods *fattening* or *nonfattening* is scientifically incorrect. Whether a person gains weight depends on whether total caloric intake exceeds energy needs. Unfortunately, some nutritious foods such as potatoes, bread, and milk have been labeled *fattening*. Potatoes are an excellent food, providing essential vitamins and minerals. A medium-sized baked potato, which yields about 140 kcal, is well worth its calories in nutrient content. It is the addition of gravy, butter, sour cream, or crumbled bacon that greatly increases its energy content.

CHOOSING CALORIES WISELY

People who are concerned about energy balance should aim to obtain all the essential nutrients while staying within the caloric level required to maintain their ideal weight. For this goal to be accomplished, the diet should be built around the most nutritious foods: milk; small portions of lean meat, fish, poultry; eggs; lowfat cheese; fruits; vegetables; whole-grain breads, and cereals. As long as these foods provide the essential nutrients, additional calories may be added or subtracted as individual needs change.

TABLE 7-3 Effects of Fat, Alcohol, Water, and Fiber Content on the Energy Values of Selected Foods*

Food	Portion	Kcal
Fat Content		
High fat content → high energy value		
Ground beef, broiled (lean)	3 oz	230
Ground beef, broiled (regular)	3 oz	245
Whole milk (3.3% fat)	1 cup	150
Skim milk (0.1% fat)	1 cup	85
Cottage cheese, creamed (4% fat)	½ cup	118
Cottage cheese, lowfat (2% fat)	½ cup	103
Peanut butter (2 tbsp)	1 oz	190
Turkey, light meat	1 oz	45
Cheddar cheese	1 oz	115
Alcohol Content		
High alcohol content → high energy value		
Beer	12 oz	150
Beer, "light"†	12 oz	96–100
Manhattan	3½ oz	164
Tom Collins	10 oz	180
Water Content		
High water content → low energy value		
Peaches, fresh, sliced	½ cup	38
Dates	½ cup	245
Grapes, fresh	2 oz	39
Raisins	2 oz	160
Fresh peas, cooked	½ cup	63
Split peas, dried, cooked	½ cup	115
Fiber Content		
High fiber content → low energy value		
Lettuce, raw	½ cup	5
Celery, raw	½ cup	10
Endive, raw	½ cup	5
Method of Preparation		
High-energy ingredients → high energy value		
Potato, medium, boiled (1)	4½ oz	115
Potato with 1 tsp margarine	4½ oz	150
Potato, french fried	4½ oz	400
Hash brown	4½ oz	278

* Sources of nutritive values: Nutritive value of foods. USDA Home and Garden Bulletin, no. 72, And Pennington JAT. Bowes & Church's Food values of portions commonly used. 16th ed. Philadelphia: JB Lippincott, 1994.)

† Label information

For many people with a low level of physical activity, there is little room for foods that furnish calories but few or no nutrients. Many Americans obtain 30% or more of their calories from foods such as pure sugars, fats, and alcohol, which provide limited amounts of vitamins and minerals. In the United States, sugar is consumed—mostly in hidden forms—at an average of 138 lb per person per year. The more calories people derive from such foods, the more likely they are to be poorly nourished.

CALORIC DENSITY AND NUTRIENT DENSITY

Two terms describe the energy value and the nutritional value of individual foods: caloric density and nutrient density. *Caloric density* refers to the number of calories per unit of weight of a specific food. One cup of lettuce (about 2 oz) yields 5 kcal and is said to have low caloric density; 2 oz of cheddar cheese yields 230 kcal; thus this food has a high caloric density.

Nutrient density refers to the nutritional quality of a food in relation to the calories it supplies. Knowledge of the general characteristics of different foods enables us to choose those foods that have a good nutrients/calories ratio. Greens are foods of low caloric density but high nutrient density with respect to a number of important nutrients. Carbonated beverages have a poor nutrient density for all nutrients. Peanut butter is high in caloric density but also high in nutrient density for a number of nutrients.

PHYSICAL FITNESS

BENEFITS OF EXERCISE

The study of energy metabolism would be incomplete without a discussion of the benefits of physical activity. It is difficult to overstate the importance of making exercise a consistent part of life at all age levels. People who are least fit appear to reap the greatest benefits when they become more active, even if the activities are of low intensity.

Exercise enhances flexibility, increases muscle strength and endurance, and improves heart and lung efficiency. It reduces body fat and increases muscle mass. Exercise increases the resting metabolic rate, which is the greatest single influence on our total energy expenditure.

Strong research evidence has linked regular physical activity with lower rates of illness and longer life expectancy. Exercise helps reduce the risk of cardiovascular disease and osteoporosis and it plays a significant role in the treatment of certain medical conditions such as hypertension, abnormal blood fat levels, and non–insulin-dependent diabetes (type II). Improvements in health can be achieved with even modest levels of activity. Furthermore, physical activity has important psychological benefits: it decreases mild anxiety, stress, and depression and enhances self-esteem and self-confidence.

TYPES OF EXERCISE

Aerobic exercises require large amounts of oxygen and involve movements of large muscle groups (arms and legs). When done for long periods, aerobic exercises use a lot of energy, and when performed under certain conditions, can strengthen the heart and lungs. Walking, swimming, jogging, cycling, and dancing are examples of aerobic exercises.

Anaerobic (without oxygen) exercises are performed at intense levels for short periods. These activities are called anaerobic because they exceed the ability of the heart and lungs to deliver oxygen to the tissues; exhaustion sets in quickly. Examples of anaerobic activities are football, tennis, and housecleaning.

Resistance or strength training involves muscle strengthening exercises such as curl-ups and push-ups and the use of weight lifting or strength-training equipment such as Nautilus or Universal. It is important to learn the proper technique for using this equipment in a supervised setting with qualified instructors. The American College of Sports Medicine now suggests that both aerobic and strength training should be included in a well-rounded exercise program.

EXERCISING SAFELY

Low to moderate exercise such as walking is safe for most people. However, people with certain physical problems should not begin an exercise program without first being carefully checked by a physician. These problems include a history or evidence of heart disease, stroke, hypertension, diabetes, kidney disease, liver disease, arthritis, orthopedic problems, and osteoporosis. Many people with these disorders may be able to exercise but will need expert guidance regarding the kind and amount of exercise that is appropriate.

A person should stop exercise and consult a physician if the person develops any of the following symptoms: chest pain, dizziness, nausea, unusual fatigue, and visual disturbances. It is recommended that people older than age 40 years get their physician's approval before beginning an exercise program.

STARTING AN EXERCISE PROGRAM

The following are general considerations before starting an exercise program:

- Follow exercise precautions. (See the section Exercising Safely.)
- Choose exercises that you enjoy. Choosing to do more than one type of exercise may add interest and prevent injury.
- Wear a good pair of well-fitted exercise shoes.
- Drink plenty of water before, during, and after exercise.
- Start slowly, and build strength and endurance gradually.

EXERCISING TO IMPROVE CARDIORESPIRATORY FITNESS

Exercise that improves cardiorespiratory functioning is aerobic exercise that consists of three essential components: intensity, duration, and frequency. Each exercise session should consist of warm-up, aerobic activity, and cool down.

Warm-up is a period of 5 minutes to 15 minutes that allows the heart rate and body temperature to rise in preparation for more intense activity. Warm-up might include walking or other movements at a slow to moderate pace and stretching exercises.

Aerobic activity is the portion of the exercise session that builds endurance and overall fitness. The three essential components are as follows:

1. *Intensity* is how hard the body should work while doing the exercise. Pulse rate must be kept within 60% to 85% of the maximum heart rate. The maximum heart rate varies from person to person. It can be roughly estimated by subtracting the person's age from 220. Multiply this number by .60 and .85 to determine a range of 60% to 85%. Divide this number by 6 to determine the heart rate for 10 seconds. The heart rate is monitored by the pulse rate, which tells how many times the heart is beating. The beginner should start at an intensity of 50% to 60% of the maximum heart rate. A higher percentage of calories are burned from fat when exercise is at the lower end of the heart rate zone.
2. *Duration* of exercise must be at least 20 minutes to 30 minutes at the target pulse rate. The beginner should start with 3-minute to 5-minute segments of exercise separated by 1 minute of rest or more relaxed exercise. As the individual's endurance increases, he or she should reduce the number of rest periods.
3. *Frequency* refers to how many times per week a person performs exercise. To strengthen heart and lungs, exercise must be done three to four times per week.

Cool down is a period of 10 minutes to 15 minutes following the "training period," during which activity decreases gradually until heart rate and body temperature return to normal resting levels. Muscle strengthening and stretching exercises are beneficial at this time.

EXERCISING AT LOW TO MODERATE INTENSITY

Even low levels of activity can provide health benefits. Long-term participation in exercise at low to moderate intensity levels (below 60% of maximum heart rate) may be better advice for some people than a prescription of vigorous exercise. Consistent low intensity activity is associated with greater weight loss over time. Kelly D. Brownell, an internationally known expert in weight control, and his associates believe that the preceding cardiorespiratory exercise formula regarding intensity may be inappropriate for overweight people—it may deter such people from exercising. It is important to help individuals become more active. The best exercise is the one people will practice.

KEY ISSUES

Nutrition and Athletic Performance

NUTRITIONAL REQUIREMENTS

Athletes are always looking for ways to improve their physical performance or appearance; consequently, they are prone to following fad diets. Fad diets include increasing or decreasing one or more nutrients in the diet and taking vitamins and mineral supplements and special dietary aids, which athletes may believe will give them extraordinary power.

Active people can meet their nutritional requirements by eating a well-balanced, varied diet with sufficient calories to meet their increased energy needs. Although increasing physical activity increases the need for energy, water, and some nutrients, athletes can meet most of these needs by increasing caloric intake, frequently ranging from 3000 kcal to 6000 kcal/day. This assumes, however, that they will choose wholesome foods such as whole-grain cereals, vegetables, and fruits to increase caloric intake. Studies have shown that the food choices of female athletes, in particular, tend to be poor. Their nutrient intakes frequently are inadequate to maintain health, let alone promote good athletic performance. The desire to maintain a slim appearance seems to underlie this situation.

Energy

Caloric needs depend on many factors including body size, age, gender, metabolic rate, fitness level, and type of physical activity as well as the intensity, duration, and frequency of the activity. The energy demands of the specific sport or activity need to be understood. Display 7-1 can be used to estimate energy needs.

Ideal Body Weight

For athletes, use of percentage body fat measurements may be a more accurate means of evaluating body composition than usual methods such as height–weight tables. Body fat measurements for athletes range from 4% to 12% in men and 10% to 20% in women.

Carbohydrates

Carbohydrate (starches and sugars) is the most important source of fuel for the physically active person. It maintains glycogen (stored carbohydrate) reserves in the muscles, which is of critical importance during prolonged exercise. Training diets that supply 55% to 65% of total calories from carbohydrate are recommended. People who compete in endurance events of long duration should consume 60% to 70% of calories from carbohydrates.

Protein

A popular belief is that large amounts of protein and protein supplements are needed for muscle strength and endurance. Recent research has suggested that athletes may have an increased need for protein, slightly above the RDA of 0.8 g/kg of body weight. Approximately 10% to 15% of total calories from protein is recommended. During the initial stages of training, an increased protein intake of about 1.2 g protein per kg of body weight is recommended to support the increased muscle development. During intensive training or competition, the protein requirement increases to 1.5 g per kg of body weight. Weight lifters, bodybuilders, and people involved in intensive strength training may need up to 2.0 g per kg body weight. It is important that athletes consume sufficient calories to meet their energy needs; otherwise, their bodies will use protein to supply energy rather than tissue maintenance and growth.

Many athletes consume at least twice the recommended allowance of protein in eating enough food to meet their energy needs. The use of prepackaged protein and amino acid drinks, powders, and pills, sometimes at a cost of $50/lb, is totally unnecessary. Some athletes consume high-protein diets containing large quantities of eggs and meats, which tend to elevate blood cholesterol and thus promote hardening of the arteries. Because the end products of protein metabolism are excreted by the kidneys, excessive protein increases urination, possibly causing dehydration (in people restricting fluids) and calcium loss. It is important to remember, also, that protein consumed in amounts that exceed the body's caloric needs is stored as fat and not muscle.

Fat

A fat intake of less than 30% of total calories is recommended. During aerobic activity of low to moderate duration, fat is the main source of energy. However, during intense exercise and during anaerobic activity, carbohydrates (glucose and glycogen) are the body's main source of energy. When diets are high in fat, the amount of sugar that is stored in the muscle as glycogen is reduced, thus limiting the athlete's endurance.

Fluids

Athletes can lose up to 5% of their body weight in perspiration during an event. Dehydration hinders performance and, if severe, can cause death. Athletes cannot depend on the sensation of thirst to remind them to replace lost water; they are encouraged to drink liberal amounts of water before an event and small cups (3 oz to 6 oz) of water at 15-minute intervals during the event. Checking body weight (nude) before and after events is the best way to monitor the athlete's fluid status. For each pound of weight lost during the event, 16 oz of fluid should be consumed before the next event.

Plain water is the best fluid because it is rapidly absorbed. Sweet beverages with more than 10% sugar slow the emptying time of the stomach. Consequently, water is drawn from the circulating blood into the intestinal tract, further increasing the danger of dehydration. If athletes consume soft drinks, they should dilute then with three parts water. Endurance athletes who expend energy for more than 60 minutes may benefit from drinking sports beverages, which contain small amounts of glucose, during exercise, thus replacing both fluids and energy.

Vitamins, Electrolytes, and Other Minerals

Certain minerals (sodium, chloride, potassium, and magnesium) called *electrolytes* are lost in sweat. For moderate exercise in moderate environmental conditions lasting fewer than 60 minutes, electrolytes lost can be replaced within 24 hours by consuming a well-balanced diet. Athletes who participate in heavy exercise lasting more than 60 minutes or under poor environmental conditions (high heat and humidity) may benefit from sports drinks that replace electrolytes as well as fluid. Salt tablets are not recommended because they draw fluids from the plasma into the intestinal tract, causing cramps and dehydration.

Iron supplements may be needed if anemia exists. *Sports anemia* occurs in some athletes, reducing the oxygen supply to the cells, and thus reducing exercise capacity. Some possible causes of sports anemia are inadequate diet, decreased absorption, increased losses in sweat, the rupture of red blood cells resulting from exercise stress, and the increase in plasma volume that occurs during training, which may dilute the hemoglobin.

Athletes do not have increased calcium needs. However, female athletes who experience an absence of menstrual periods due to decreased estrogen (female sex hormone) levels may have reduced bone density and increased risk of early onset osteoporosis. Treatment may involve calcium supplements and estrogen replacement.

Caffeine and Other Performance-Enhancing (Ergogenic) Aids

In an effort to improve physical performance or appearance, athletes are prone to accept magic claims about foods and dietary supplements. Among the products promoted are amino acids, bee pollen, alcohol, coenzyme Q10, inosine, and vitamin supplements. Some of these substances are safe at appropriate doses, whereas others may pose safety risks. Caffeine and alcohol, for example, may actually impair performance. The performance-enhancing properties of most of the ergogenic aids are questionable. A well-balanced diet is the surest way to maximize athletic performance.

There appears to be evidence that caffeine has a glycogen-sparing effect because it increases the level of free fatty acids in the blood. Some athletes find that caffeine enhances their performance. However, adverse effects such as anxiety, nervousness, headaches, and irritability impair performance for others. Both caffeine and alcohol increase urination and may hinder the regulation of body temperature during exercise. In some competitions, the use of caffeine is banned. In certain sports such as marksmanship, the use of alcohol is also illegal.

The use of anabolic steroids (synthetic derivatives of the male sex hormone testosterone) to promote muscle mass has serious side effects such as liver and heart damage, psychological changes, and growth stunting. The use of steroids in sports competitions is illegal and banned.

Carbohydrate Loading

Carbohydrate loading is a technique used to increase endurance in long-distance events. The goal is to store as much glycogen in the muscle as possible. Carbohydrate loading involves two steps. One week before the event, the athlete consumes high-protein, high-fat, low-carbohydrate meals and also exercises heavily, depleting the glycogen in the muscle. Then, after 2 or 3 days, the athlete switches to a high-carbohydrate diet and reduces exercise. This increases muscle glycogen two to three times normal levels. Water content in the muscle increases, causing heaviness and stiffness. Cardiac pain and abnormal electrocardiograms also have been reported.

Because of possible harm to heart function, carbohydrate loading is not recommended, especially for high school athletes. Experienced athletes who use carbohydrate loading, though, should be supervised by a physician. The technique should not be used more than two or three times a year. A less drastic carbohydrate loading technique involves eating a mixed diet in which carbohydrate is not restricted 3 to 6 days before competition while training is reduced. This diet is followed by a high-carbohydrate diet in the days before competition.

Pregame Meal

A light small meal that is low in fat and protein and rich in complex carbohydrates should be eaten 3 or 4 hours before the event to provide time for the food to be digested and absorbed. High-protein and high-fat meals delay the emptying time of the stomach and do not contribute to glycogen stores.

KEYS TO PRACTICAL APPLICATION

Choose foods that provide the most nutrients for the fewest calories.

Watch out for fatty foods, sweets, and alcohol. They provide calories and little else.

Avoid calling foods *fattening* or *nonfattening*. Whether a person gains weight depends on total caloric intake, not on the consumption of any specific foods.

Maintain a high level of physical activity. It can help you control your weight and has many other benefits.

Through exercise, develop and maintain good muscle tone. Muscle tissue uses more calories than fat tissue.

Encourage your clients to become more active at whatever level is comfortable.

KEY IDEAS

Metabolism includes all the processes by which body cells use nutrients to support life. Anabolism is the use of nutrients to build more complex substances, as in the formation of new tissue; catabolism is the breakdown of nutrients or body tissue, as in the production of energy.

Enzymes direct the use of the nutrients within each cell.

Proteins, fats, and carbohydrates provide energy; carbohydrates are the preferred source.

Energy metabolism involves splitting of the carbon atoms in glucose, fatty acids, glycerol, and amino acids; splitting causes the energy that held the carbon atoms together to be released. This energy is converted to body heat or temporarily stored as ATP, a substance that provides energy for all the work performed by the cell.

Release of energy in the cells is a complex process requiring the activity of enzymes, coenzymes, and hormones.

Oxygen is required for the efficient release of energy in the cells; water and carbon dioxide also are produced by the oxidation of the fuel-producing nutrients.

Respiration provides the oxygen needed for energy metabolism and removes carbon dioxide and water, the end products of energy metabolism.

Energy is removed bit by bit from the energy nutrients in a series of chemical reactions known as the Krebs cycle or tricarboxylic acid cycle; all nutrients enter this common pathway after being broken down to acetyl CoA. If energy is not needed, excess proteins, fats, and carbohydrates are converted to fatty acids and stored as fat in the body.

The energy value of a food depends on its protein, fat, and carbohydrate content; protein provides 4 kcal/g; fat, 9 kcal/g; and carbohydrate, 4 kcal/g.

A person's total energy needs are based on basal metabolism, voluntary physical activity, and the thermic effect of food.

The BMR is the speed at which fuel is needed to maintain the vital body processes at rest. It is influenced by body composition, age, gender, physical condition, state of nutrition, disease conditions, secretions of endocrine glands, body temperature, and environmental temperature.

The effect of physical activity on total caloric needs depends on the type of activity, intensity, length of time it is performed, and size of the person doing it.

Energy balance results when the number of calories consumed equals the number used for energy; body weight indicates the relationship of energy intake to energy output. Exercise is a valuable aid in achieving energy balance.

When the body uses mostly body fat for energy because of a lack of carbohydrate, it also uses protein.

Foods vary in energy value according to the proportion of energy-producing nutrients they contain: foods that contain fat or alcohol or have a low water content tend to have a high energy value; lean meats, cereals, and starchy vegetables are intermediate in energy value; and fruits and vegetables are low in energy value.

All the essential nutrients should be provided within the caloric level required to maintain ideal weight; the more calories people obtain from pure sugars, fats, and alcohol, the more likely they are to be poorly nourished.

People at all age levels should make exercise a consistent part of life; the benefits in overall fitness, disease prevention, and disease treatment are many.

Aerobic exercise that strengthens the heart and lungs must have three essential components: intensity, duration, and frequency. Resistance exercises also should be a part of the exercise prescription.

Low to moderate exercise may be more appropriate for overweight individuals.

Athletes have increased needs for some nutrients, most of which can be easily met by the athlete's increased caloric intake. The following distribution of total calories is recommended for the athlete: 10% to 15% protein, 55% to 60% carbohydrate (mainly complex carbohydrates), and less than 30% fat.

Replacement of fluids lost in perspiration during athletic events is essential; the athlete cannot depend on sensation of thirst for adequate fluid replacement.

In addition to replacement of electrolytes lost in sweat, iron and calcium are other minerals that may require attention. Carbohydrate loading is a risky technique that may impair heart function.

A pregame meal 3 to 4 hours before the event should be low in fat, protein, and fiber and consist mainly of complex carbohydrates.

A well-balanced diet is the best way to maximize performance; the value of most ergogenic aids is questionable and some are unsafe.

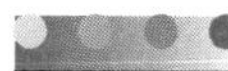

KEYS TO LEARNING

STUDY–DISCUSSION QUESTIONS

1. What nutrients provide energy? When a person's energy needs are being met, what happens to excessive intake of any or all of these nutrients?
2. What is the most efficient source of energy? If this nutrient is lacking, how are the body's energy needs met?
3. A ½-cup serving of New England clam chowder contains 5 g of protein, 5 g of fat, and 7 g of carbohydrate. Using this information, calculate the approximate energy value of this food serving.
4. What are the three factors that determine a person's total energy needs? Describe each of these factors.
5. Using Display 7-1, estimate your total caloric needs for the day using your present weight.
6. Using the 1-day food diary you kept in Chapter 5, calculate your energy intake. How does your energy intake compare with your estimate in question 5? What is the infallible guide for determining whether your caloric intake is in balance with your energy needs? Explain. What happens to excess calories?
7. Discuss the value of exercise in maintaining energy balance and in other aspects of health.
8. More than 30% of the total energy intake of many Americans consists of pure sugars, fats, and alcohol. Why are these people apt to be malnourished?
9. Explain the fallacy in the statement, "Potatoes are fattening."
10. Mr. K is a 45-year-old accountant who is unhappy with his steady weight gain. He has gained another 4 lb in the past 28 days. Mr. K thinks that he eats moderately, no more than he ate when he was 25 years old and 50 lb lighter. What are some possible reasons for his weight gain? About how many excess calories is he eating daily to have gained 4 lb in 28 days?
11. Develop what you would consider to be an ideal exercise program for yourself. What safety factors should you consider? How would you schedule this exercise program within the week?
12. Interview several athletes and obtain information about their nutrition-related philosophies and practices. In class, discuss this information in the light of the material in this chapter.

BIBLIOGRAPHY

BOOKS

Benardot D. Ed. Sports nutrition: a guide for the professional working with active people. 2nd ed. Chicago: The American Dietetic Association, 1993.

Chicago Dietetic Association and the South Suburban Dietetic Association. Manual of clinical dietetics. Chicago: The American Dietetic Association, 1992:87–97.

Hultman E, Harris RC, Spriet LL. Work and exercise. In: Shils ME, Olson JA, Shike M. Eds. Modern nutrition in health and disease. 8th ed. Philadelphia: Lea and Febiger, 1994:663–681.

National Academy of Sciences, National Research Council, Committee on Diet and Health, Food and Nutrition Board. Diet and health: implications for reducing chronic disease risk (executive summary). Washington, DC: National Academy Press, 1989.

National Academy of Sciences, National Research Council, Food and Nutrition Board. Recommended dietary allowances. 10th ed. Washington, DC: National Academy Press, 1989.

Schutz Y, Jequier E. Energy needs: assessment and requirements. In: Shils ME, Olson JA, Shike M. Eds. Modern nutrition in health and disease. 9th ed. Philadelphia: Lea and Febiger, 1994:101–111.

PERIODICALS

Anderson RE. Making exercise fun. Weight Control Digest. 1992;2:164.

Dietz WH, Bandini LG, Morelli JA, et al. Effect of sedentary activities on resting metabolic rate. Am J Clin Nutr 1994;59:556.

Grilo CM, Wilfley DE. Weight control: exercise adherence and abuse. Weight Control Digest 1992;2:161.

Grilo CM, Wilfley DE, Brownell KD. Physical activity and weight control: why is the link so strong? Weight Control Digest 1992;2:153.

Horton TJ, Geissler CA. Effect of habitual exercise on daily energy expenditure and metabolic rate during standardized activity. Am J Clin Nutr 1994;59:13.

International Olympic Academy. Declaration of Olympia on nutrition and fitness. J Am Diet Assoc 1992;92:1282.

Klesges RC, Shelton ML, Klesges LM. Effects of television on metabolic rate: potential implications for childhood obesity. Pediatrics 1993;91:281.

Rosenbloom C, Millard-Stafford M, Lathrop J. Contemporary ergogenic acids used by strength/power athletes. J Am Diet Assoc 1992;92:1264.

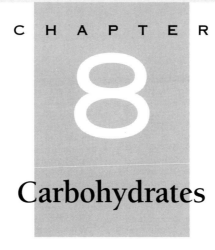

CHAPTER 8

Carbohydrates

KEY TERMS

caries dental cavities
cellulose plant fiber; a fibrous form of carbohydrate that makes up the framework of plants
complex carbohydrates a class of carbohydrates called *polysaccharides;* foods composed of starch and cellulose
empty calories foods that provide calories but few, if any, other nutrients such as vitamins and minerals
fiber a group of compounds that make up the framework of plants; fiber includes the carbohydrates cellulose, hemicellulose, gums, mucilages, and pectin and a noncarbohydrate called *lignin;* fiber cannot be digested by the human digestive tract
glucagon a hormone produced in the pancreas that raises blood sugar by increasing the conversion of glycogen in the liver to glucose
glycogen animal starch; the form in which carbohydrate is stored in animals
insulin a hormone that is secreted by the beta cells of islets of Langerhans in the pancreas; insulin is necessary for the proper metabolism of blood sugar
ketosis the accumulation in the body of ketones, substances that result from the incomplete metabolism of fatty acids
naturally occurring sugars sugars found in foods in their natural state; for example, glucose occurs naturally in grapes and other fruits
nonnutritive sweetener sweetener that produces no calories or only negligible amounts
nutritive sweetener sweetener that produces calories
periodontal disease gum disease
plaque transparent sticky film on teeth and gums that harbors acid-producing bacteria
refined food food that has undergone many commercial processes, which results in the loss of nutrients
simple carbohydrates a class of carbohydrates composed of monosaccharides and disaccharides; also known as *sugars*
somatostatin a hormone produced in the pancreas and hypothalamus; somatostatin helps maintain blood sugar levels by inhibiting the production of insulin and glucagon as needed

OBJECTIVES

After completing this chapter, the student will be able to:

1. Appreciate the role of carbohydrate as the primary energy source for the body and its sparing effect on protein.
2. Identify the two general types of carbohydrates and the food sources of each.
3. Describe the digestion and absorption of carbohydrate and describe the metabolism of carbohydrate and how it is affected by various hormones.

4. Explain why carbohydrates are needed for the normal metabolism of fats.
5. Explain the effects of milling on the nutritive value of grains and describe the practices used to counteract these effects.
6. Discuss the reasons that underlie recommendations that carbohydrates be increased to more than 55% of total calories in the diet.
7. Identify and discuss the characteristics of the non-nutritive sugar substitutes.
8. Discuss the association of carbohydrates with dental disease; identify factors that can minimize their adverse impact on dental health.
9. Define fiber and the two general types; identify its beneficial effects and possible adverse effects on health; identify its food sources.

What do intravenous glucose, tooth decay, fiber, and diabetes mellitus have in common? In one way or another, all are associated with a class of food called *carbohydrates.* Carbohydrates, which are composed of carbon, hydrogen, and oxygen, are the basic fuel source for the body. Through the process of photosynthesis, plants use the carbon dioxide in the air and water from the soil to manufacture carbohydrate (sugars and starches). Chlorophyll, the pigment in green leaves, acts as a chemical catalyst in this process, which transforms the sun's energy to food energy.

Sugars, starches, and celluloses are the main forms in which carbohydrate occurs in food. Starches and sugars are the major energy sources and the cheapest and most easily used form of fuel for the body. Celluloses are fibrous materials that provide bulk, aiding digestion. Although most carbohydrates occur in plant life, two are of animal origin: lactose, the sugar in milk, and glycogen, the form in which animals store sugar.

Worldwide, carbohydrates are the major source of food energy. The proportion of energy supplied by carbohydrates depends on agricultural and economic conditions. Peoples of Asia, the Middle East, Africa, and Latin America obtain as much as 80% of their total energy from carbohydrates such as cereal grains and starchy vegetables. In contrast, Americans obtain about 46% of their caloric intake from carbohydrate.

Generally speaking, the proportion of carbohydrate in the diet is greater when income is low. Carbohydrates such as rice, pasta, bread, legumes, potatoes, and other starchy vegetables are considerably less expensive than meat, poultry, eggs, and dairy products. Also, compared with other types of foods, carbohydrate foods are easily stored and do not spoil readily.

The kind of carbohydrate foods eaten determines the nutritional contribution to the diet. Highly refined and overprocessed carbohydrate foods such as sugars and products made from unenriched white flour contribute little to the diet other than calories. Refined and processed foods undergo changes in processing that cause a loss of nutrients. In contrast, whole-grain and enriched carbohydrate products, fruits, and vegetables provide vitamins, minerals, and fiber as well as energy.

CLASSIFICATION OF CARBOHYDRATES

Carbohydrates are classified into three major types: monosaccharides, disaccharides, and polysaccharides. The monosaccharides are the simplest form of carbohydrate and are referred to as *simple sugars.* They are composed of one (mono-) carbohydrate unit (saccharide). The disaccharides, called *double sugars,* are composed of two (di-) carbohydrate units. The polysaccharides contain many (poly-) carbohydrate units. The monosaccharides and disaccharides are referred to as *sugars* or *simple carbohydrates;* polysaccharides are called *complex carbohydrates* because they have a more intricate chemical structure.

SIMPLE CARBOHYDRATES

MONOSACCHARIDES

Monosaccharides require no digestion and are readily absorbed from the intestinal wall directly into the bloodstream. The nutritionally important monosaccharides are glucose, fructose, and galactose.

Glucose, also called *dextrose,* is found in sweet fruits, such as grapes and berries, and in corn and some vegetables, such as carrots. It is found in corn syrup, which is made commercially by treating the starch from corn with enzymes. The main source of glucose results from the digestion of disaccharides and starches in the body. Glucose is blood sugar, the form of carbohydrate that circulates in the bloodstream and the form that body cells use for energy. All carbohydrates either are absorbed as glucose or are converted to glucose in the liver.

Fructose, also called *fruit sugar* or *levulose,* is found in ripe fruits, some vegetables, and honey. Fructose also is formed from sucrose (table sugar) during digestion. It is the sweetest of all sugars.

Galactose in combination with glucose forms lactose, the sugar in milk. Galactose is formed by the digestion or hydrolysis of lactose. During lactation, glucose is converted to galactose in the body so that breast milk can be produced. A few plant foods contain significant amounts (more than 10 mg galactose/100 g fresh weight). These include dates, papayas, bell peppers, persimmons, tomatoes, and watermelon.

DISACCHARIDES

Disaccharides are sugars composed of two monosaccharides joined together. Three disaccharides that are important in nutrition are sucrose (one glucose plus one fructose), lactose (one glucose plus one galactose), and maltose (two glucose). In the process of digestion, the disaccharides are reduced to the monosaccharides that compose them.

Sucrose is table sugar. It comes from sugarcane and sugar beets. It is purified and processed into various forms, such as white, brown, and powdered sugars. *Lactose,* or milk sugar, is found in the milk of mammals. *Maltose* is found in beer, some infant formulas, and malted breakfast cereals and other malt products. Maltose is an intermediate product in the breakdown of starch. It is produced commercially by the malting and fermentation of grains and in the body during the process of starch digestion.

SWEETNESS

Sugars vary in sweetness and in solubility (the ability to dissolve in water). The sweetness of a sugar is an important consideration in efforts to reduce the use of sugar (as in diabetes and obesity) or to increase the use of sugar (when extra calories are needed and appetite is poor). Because fructose is very sweet, a small amount of it yields the same sweetness as larger amounts of table sugar for fewer calories. Although lactose is about one sixth as sweet as table sugar, it is seldom used to increase the caloric value of beverages. It is poorly soluble and tends to cause gastrointestinal discomfort when consumed in large quantities. Regardless of how sweet they taste, all sugars have the same energy value. One teaspoon of fructose has the same energy value as 1 tsp of sucrose.

SUGAR ALCOHOLS

Sugar alcohols are obtained from chemical reactions involving sugar. Sorbitol, mannitol, and xylitol are sugar alcohols used as alternatives to sucrose for sweetening food products. All provide 4 kcal/g, as do sucrose and glucose. Because they are more slowly absorbed from the gastrointestinal tract, they do not raise blood sugar or stimulate insulin secretion as much as sucrose. Also, they do not promote tooth decay because they are not useful to mouth bacteria.

Xylitol is as sweet as sucrose but is not commonly used because its safety is questioned. Sorbitol and mannitol are less sweet than sucrose. They are commonly used in sucrose-free candies and desserts. Eating excessive amounts may cause diarrhea.

COMPLEX CARBOHYDRATES

Polysaccharides are composed of many single sugar units. They must be reduced to monosaccharides by the process of digestion before they can be absorbed into the bloodstream. The polysaccharides that are important in nutrition are starch, cellulose, dextrins, and glycogen.

Starch is the chief form of carbohydrate in the diet. Cereal grains, some vegetables, and other plants provide starch. Plant starches are the main food source for humans.

Cellulose is one of the polysaccharides that compose the framework of plants. It occurs in the stalks and leaves of all plants, in the skins of fruit and vegetables, and in the outer covering of seeds and cereals. Cellulose cannot be broken down in the human digestive tract and therefore is not absorbed. Cellulose together with other indigestible substances found in the skeletal walls of plants are commonly called *fiber* or *roughage.* Although fiber is not a true nutrient, it plays an important role in the functioning of the intestinal tract.

Other nondigestible polysaccharides in plants, including pectin, agar, carrageenan, and vegetable gums, have the ability to dissolve in water and form a gel. This property is useful in food processing and in the production of cosmetics and drugs.

Soluble fiber also appears to be useful in controlling blood sugar and blood cholesterol levels. See Key Issues section at the end of this chapter.

Dextrins occur primarily as products in the partial breakdown of starch due to enzymes or in cooking, such as in toasting bread.

Glycogen, or animal starch, is the form in which carbohydrate is stored in the body. Glycogen is found in liver and muscle tissue.

DIGESTION AND METABOLISM OF CARBOHYDRATES

Before carbohydrates can be absorbed into the bloodstream, they must be reduced to monosaccharides by the process of digestion. Table 8-1 summarizes carbohydrate digestion, which was discussed in Chapter 6.

The monosaccharides are absorbed and carried by the portal circulation to the liver. In the liver, fructose and galactose are converted to glucose. Ultimately, all carbohydrates become glucose. Glucose is then released by the liver into the bloodstream and distributed to the cells. Any excess glucose is converted in the liver to glycogen (*glycogenesis*) for storage. When energy is needed, the liver converts the glycogen back to glucose (*glycogenolysis*) and releases it into the bloodstream in sufficient amounts to maintain a normal blood sugar level. Muscle tissue also is able to store glucose as glycogen. Glycogen is present in most body organs. The ability to form glycogen is limited, however. When more carbohydrate is eaten than is needed for energy or storage as glycogen, it is converted to fat and stored as fat tissue.

When insufficient carbohydrate is consumed, some amino acids and the glycerol portion of fats can be converted to glucose. This process is called *gluconeogenesis.*

While glucose is being absorbed from the digestive tract, the blood sugar level rises to no higher than 130 mg/dL to 140 mg/dL, even after the heavy consumption of sweets. As the tissues take the needed glucose from the bloodstream and the liver converts glucose to glycogen, the blood sugar gradually returns to its normal level of less than 100 mg/dL of venous whole blood (less than 115 mg/dL of venous plasma).

The hormone *insulin,* produced by the beta cells of islets of Langerhans of the pancreas, greatly influences the way the body uses carbohydrates and regulates the blood sugar level. When blood sugar rises, the pancreas is stimulated to produce insulin. Insulin regulates the use of glucose for energy by the cells, the storage of carbohydrate as glycogen in the liver, and the conversion of excess glucose to fat.

Other hormones cause a rise in blood sugar. *Glucagon,* a hormone secreted by the alpha cells of islets of Langerhans, raises the blood sugar level by promoting the conversion of glycogen in the liver to glucose. *Somatostatin,* secreted by delta cells in the pancreas and in other regions of the body, including the hypothalamus, is a hormone that suppresses the production of insulin, glucagon, and growth hormone as needed to maintain a normal blood glucose level. Other hormones, released in response to stress, raise the blood sugar level by blocking the effects of insulin and are therefore called *insulin antagonists.* These include *epinephrine* (from the adrenal medulla), *glucocorticoids* (from the adrenal cortex), and *growth hormone* (from the pituitary), as well as glucagon. People who take glucocorticoid medications such as cortisone acetate, prednisone, and dexamethasone may have elevated blood sugar levels. In healthy people, a balance exists between hormones that lower blood sugar and those that raise it.

TABLE 8-1 SUMMARY OF CARBOHYDRATE DIGESTION

Site of Action	Carbohydrate	Enzyme	End Products	
Mouth	Starch	Amylase in saliva (ptyalin) →	Dextrins, maltose, glucose	
Small intestine	Starch	Amylase in pancreatic juice →	Dextrins, maltose, glucose	
	Dextrins	→	Maltose, glucose	
		Enzymes in brush border of small intestine		
	Dextrins	Isomaltase	Maltose, glucose	
	Maltose	Maltase →	Glucose	Absorbed into the bloodstream
	Sucrose	Sucrase →	Glucose and fructose	Absorbed into the bloodstream
	Lactose	Lactase →	Glucose and galactose	Absorbed into the bloodstream

FUNCTIONS OF CARBOHYDRATES

Carbohydrates provide the most efficient form of energy, compose parts of certain body substances, promote the growth of beneficial bacteria, and provide fiber for the proper functioning of the gastrointestinal tract.

PROVIDE ENERGY

Carbohydrates are the most economical and efficient energy source. Each gram of carbohydrate supplies an average of 4 kcal. One tablespoon of sugar contains 12 g of carbohydrate and yields 48 kcal ($12 \times 4 = 48$ kcal).

Protein and fat also can be used to produce energy; however, the body uses carbohydrate first. When not enough carbohydrate is provided, the body uses protein and fat for its energy needs. This occurs at the expense of the other functions of protein and fat. Under normal conditions, the tissue of the central nervous system can use only glucose as its form of energy, whereas skeletal muscles can use either glucose or fatty acids (fats) as fuel.

When more carbohydrate is consumed than is needed immediately for energy, the excess is stored in two ways: in limited amounts as glycogen and the remainder as body fat. The amount of carbohydrate that is stored as glycogen in the liver and muscle tissue represents about half of an adult's daily energy needs. Glycogen stored in the liver is converted to glucose to maintain a normal blood glucose level. Glycogen stored in the muscle can supply energy only for the muscle cells. Athletes sometimes use a practice called *carbohydrate loading,* which causes the body to increase glycogen stores in the muscle. This practice is potentially dangerous (see Key Issues: Nutrition and Athletic Performance in Chapter 7). Although the amount of carbohydrate that is stored in the body is limited, the amount of excess carbohydrate that can be stored as fat is unlimited.

SPARE PROTEIN

Meeting energy needs takes priority over other bodily functions. Carbohydrates are needed to provide energy quickly so that the available protein can be used for building and repairing tissue. If a person does not eat enough food to meet energy needs, the body burns its own tissues to supply energy. In starvation, death eventually results from the breakdown of vital body tissue (protein). The protein-sparing effect of carbohydrate is extremely important in diseases of the kidneys (see Chapter 27) and liver (see Chapter 28) and after surgery (see Chapter 29).

HELP THE BODY USE FAT EFFICIENTLY

Carbohydrates are necessary for the proper use of fats. If carbohydrate intake is low, larger than normal amounts of fat are called on to supply energy. The body is unable to handle the excessive breakdown of fat, however. As a result, the fat does not burn completely, and abnormal amounts of certain breakdown products (ketones) accumulate in the blood, causing a condition known as *ketosis*.

ARE COMPONENTS OF BODY SUBSTANCES

Carbohydrates are components of body substances needed for the regulation of body processes. Heparin, which prevents blood from clotting, contains carbohydrate. Nervous tissue, connective tissue, various hormones, and enzymes also contain carbohydrates. Ribose, another carbohydrate, is a part of deoxyribonucleic acid (DNA) and ribonucleic acid (RNA), the substances that carry the hereditary factors in the cell. Carbohydrate also is a component of a compound in the liver that destroys toxic substances.

ENCOURAGE GROWTH OF USEFUL BACTERIA

Carbohydrates encourage the growth of beneficial intestinal bacteria that are involved in the production of certain vitamins and the absorption of calcium and phosphorus.

PROMOTE NORMAL FUNCTIONING OF THE LOWER INTESTINAL TRACT

Cellulose and other indigestible carbohydrates are the components of dietary fiber. Fiber absorbs and holds water, resulting in a softer, bulkier stool and faster movement through the lower intestinal tract. Other benefits of fiber are discussed in the Key Issues section at the end of this chapter.

CARBOHYDRATE SOURCES

Cereal grains, vegetables, fruits, nuts, milk, and concentrated sweets provide significant amounts of carbohydrates. Milk is the only important animal source of carbohydrate. Table 8-2 compares the carbohydrate content of various foods.

CEREAL GRAINS

Cereal grains have been the staple food of humans since prehistoric times. Worldwide, rice is the most widely used cereal. It is the basic food for more than half of the world population, including the peoples of Asia, the Far East, and some Latin American and African countries. Wheat, the next most common cereal, is most widely used in Europe and the Americas. Corn is widely used in Mexico, Latin America, and the southern United States. Rice and products made from cereal grains, such as breads and other baked goods, breakfast cereals, and macaroni products, contribute substantial amounts of carbohydrate to the American diet.

Whole grains are products that contain all of the grain that is edible. They include the bran and germ portions as well as the starchy portion (endosperm). The bran and germ portions contain most of the vitamins, minerals, and fiber. Examples of whole grains are whole wheat, cracked wheat, bulgur, oatmeal, whole cornmeal, popcorn, brown rice, whole rye, and scotch barley.

TABLE 8-2 COMPARISON OF THE CARBOHYDRATE CONTENT OF SELECTED FOODS*

FOOD	SERVING SIZE	CARBOHYDRATE CONTENT (G)
Milk	1 cup	12
Cheddar cheese	1 oz	Trace
Creamed cottage cheese	1/2 cup	3
Grapefruit	1/2 cup	12
Banana	1	27
Dried prunes	5 large	31
Bread	1 slice	13
Oatmeal, cooked	1/2 cup	12
Cornflakes	1 1/4 cup	24
Macaroni	1/2 cup	16
Rice	1/2 cup	25
Asparagus	1/2 cup	4
Mashed potato	1/2 cup	19
Split peas	1/2 cup	21
Peanut butter	2 tbsp	6
Walnuts	1/4 cup	5
Sunflower seeds	1/4 cup	5
Sugar	1 tbsp	12
Yellow cake with icing	1/16th 8-in cake	39
Apple pie	1/6th 9-in pie	60

* Source of food values: US Dept of Agriculture, Human Nutrition Information Service. Nutritive value of foods. Washington, DC: US Government Printing Office, 1991. Home and Garden Bulletin 72.

MILLED GRAINS

The milling of wheat to produce a pure white flour results in the removal of bran and the germ layers of the grain, those parts that contain most of the vitamins and minerals (Fig. 8-1). Similarly, much of the vitamin and mineral content of rice is lost in milling to produce white rice. Oat products retain more of the original grain kernel than do other processed cereals and thus lose fewer nutrients. Cereals that have the outer layers of the kernel removed by milling are called *refined cereals.*

Because breads and cereals are basic foods, the federal government took measures some years ago to improve the nutritional quality of refined wheat products through enrichment—the addition of nutrients. The label *enriched* on flour or bread means that iron and the vitamins thiamin, niacin, and riboflavin have been added, within amounts specified by law. Most white flour, white bread, pasta products such as macaroni, noodles, and spaghetti, and ready-to-eat cereals are enriched.

The practice of enriching refined grain products has been expanded to include corn and rice products. In the southern United States, state laws requiring enrichment of corn products have been enacted. Enriched rice, which is fortified with thiamin, niacin, and iron, is widely available in the United States. Converted rice also has a higher nutritional value than unenriched rice. Converted rice is commercially parboiled before milling, which forces some of the vitamins and minerals into the center of the kernel. Although enriched regular rice and enriched converted rice have the same iron, thiamin, and niacin content, converted rice has more calcium, potassium, and phosphorus. It is a wise practice to read the labels on refined grain products and purchase only enriched products.

WHOLE-GRAIN VERSUS ENRICHED WHITE BREAD

The milling of wheat eliminates at least 20 nutrients. Enrichment restores only four of these. Some of the nutrients that are not replaced, including vitamin B_6, folacin, and zinc, are lacking in many Americans' diets. Enriched white bread also lacks fiber, which whole-grain bread contains. Enriched

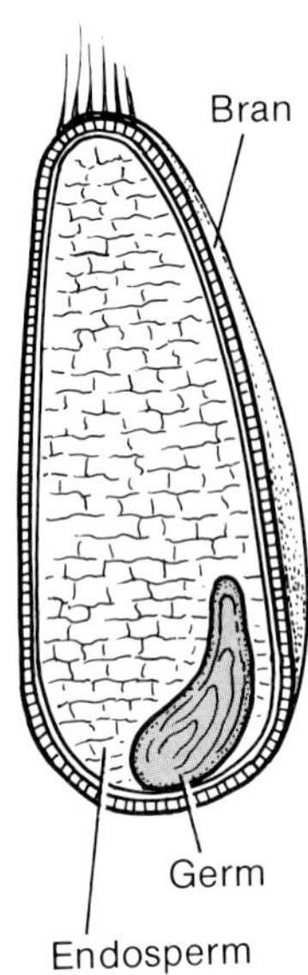

FIGURE 8-1

Edible parts of grain. *Whole grain:* May be eaten as is (e.g., brown rice) or may be flaked into whole-grain cereal (e.g., oatmeal) or ground into whole-grain cereal or flour. *Endosperm:* Mainly starch and protein (refined white grains contain little else). *Germ:* High in vitamin E, many B vitamins, minerals, and protein; a source of polyunsaturated fat. *Bran:* High in fiber, many B vitamins, and minerals.

white bread is not a totally worthless food, as some have claimed, but whole-grain products are preferred over enriched products because they contain fiber trace minerals, and additional vitamins.

By law, bread that is labeled *whole wheat* must be made from 100% whole wheat flour. Consumers are sometimes misled by the label *wheat bread,* which may be made from varying amounts of white flour and whole wheat flour. The type of flour listed first on the label is present in the largest amount. Sometimes a dark color is produced by caramel coloring.

FRUITS

Fruits are a less concentrated source of carbohydrate than cereals because of their high water content. Cantaloupe and watermelon are the lowest in carbohydrate content; bananas are among the highest. Dried fruits, such as prunes, dried apricots, raisins, dates, and figs, have a much higher concentration of sugar than fresh fruit because of their low moisture content. Many canned fruits and some frozen fruits are packed in a sugar syrup, which increases their carbohydrate content. The plantain, a fruit related to the banana, must be cooked before being eaten. In tropical countries in which they are an important carbohydrate source, plantains are part of the main course of the meal. Avocados and olives, classified as fruits, are high in fat and low in carbohydrate.

VEGETABLES

Vegetables contain carbohydrate in the forms of starch, sugar, and cellulose. Because of their high water and fiber content, vegetables that represent the leaf, flower, or stem of the plant are low in carbohydrate. These include the green leafy vegetables, celery, asparagus, cauliflower, broccoli, and brussels sprouts. The roots, tubers, and seeds of plants have a higher starch and sugar content and less water. These include potatoes, beets, carrots, turnips, parsnips, peas, lima beans, dried beans, and lentils.

NUTS

Although nuts are noted for their fat and protein content, they also contain 10% to 27% carbohydrate. Peanut butter is about 15% digestible carbohydrate. Peanuts are actually legumes, although we usually think of them as nuts.

SUGARS AND SWEETS

Most people think of sugar as sucrose or white table sugar. There are many forms of caloric sweeteners that are considered sugars, however. The following is a list of the names of sugars used in foods:

- Sugar
- Sucrose
- Glucose
- Dextrose
- Sorbitol
- Fructose
- Maltose
- Lactose
- Mannitol
- Honey
- Corn syrup
- High-fructose corn syrup
- Molasses
- Maple syrup
- Fruit juice concentrate

Sugar is 100% carbohydrate and yields 4 kcal/g but contains no other nutrients. For this reason, sugar and foods high in sugar content—jellies, jams, candy, cake, cookies, and sugar-sweetened soft drinks—are considered empty calories.

Sucrose is the most commonly used sugar. It is processed from either sugarcane or beet sugar. Corn-based sweeteners are used in large amounts in food processing. Honey, maple syrup, and brown sugar add variety in flavor to the diet. They are slightly more nutritious than table sugar, but the quantities of vitamins and minerals they contain are too small to make an important contribution to the diet. Molasses contains a significant amount of iron: 1.2 mg/tbsp. Blackstrap molasses supplies iron in the amount of 3.2 mg/tbsp, but its strong flavor limits its use. Molasses also provides B vitamins and calcium.

Consumption of table sugar, syrups, and jelly has decreased since 1974, but consumption of sugar in processed food and soft drinks has increased. In addition to its presence in obviously sugary foods such as cake, cookies, and pies, sugar is found in an endless number of other products, such as cereals, soups, canned vegetables, tomato sauce, and luncheon meats.

The "Nutrition Facts" panel of the food label takes the guesswork out of determining the sugar content of food. The total sugar content (both naturally occurring and added sugar) of the food in grams per serving must be listed on the label. The quantity of sugar alcohols such as mannitol and sorbitol also must be included in the amount of sugar listed. See a sample label in Figure 8-2.

MILK AND MILK PRODUCTS

Fresh cow's milk contains carbohydrate in the form of lactose. Cottage cheese contains about half the lactose of an equal quantity of milk. Hard cheeses contain only traces.

DIETARY FIBER

The best sources of dietary fiber are whole-grain breads and cereals, especially those containing bran, leafy vegetables, legumes, vegetables and

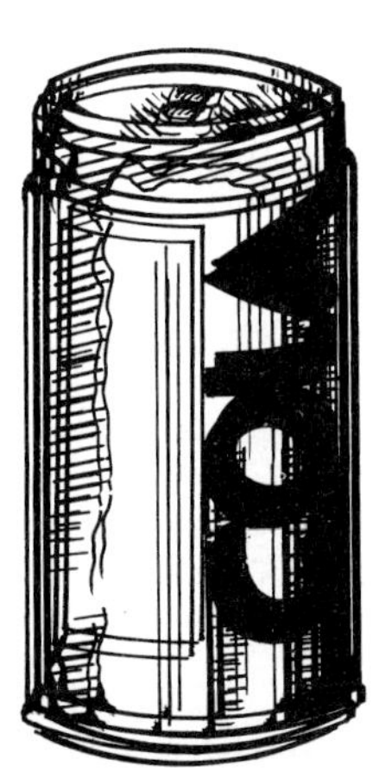

Nutrition Facts

Serving Size 1 can (360 mL)

Amount Per Serving	
Calories 140	
	% Daily Value*
Total Fat 0g	0%
Sodium 20mg	1%
Total Carbohydrate 36g	12%
Sugars 36g	
Protein 0g	0%

* Percent Daily Values are based on a 2,000 calorie diet.

FIGURE 8-2

Nutrition labeling requires that the sugar content in grams per serving be listed. *(From Kurtzweil P. "Nutrition facts" to help consumers eat smart. FDA Consumer [Special Report: Focus on Food Labeling], May 1993, 36.)*

fruits with skins and seeds, and nuts and seeds. See the Key Issues section on Fiber: Fact and Fiction at the end of this chapter.

RECOMMENDED CARBOHYDRATE INTAKE

About 100 g/day of digestible carbohydrate are needed to prevent ketosis and the excess breakdown of tissue protein and to supply glucose to the central nervous system. The total carbohydrate in the following foods equals this amount: two slices of bread, one small potato, two glasses of milk, and two servings of fruit. Because carbohydrate is the most efficient energy source and because its storage in the body is limited, carbohydrate foods should be eaten regularly and spaced throughout the day.

Desirable amounts of carbohydrate are considerably higher than these minimal levels, however. In the 10th edition of *Recommended Dietary Allowances,* the National Academy of Sciences Food and Nutrition Board recommended that carbohydrates provide more than half of an individual's energy requirement after infancy. If RDA recommendations to reduce fat and possibly protein in the diet (see Chapters 9 and 10) are implemented, carbohydrates must make up the caloric shortages these reductions would cause. In its 1989 report, the National Academy of Sciences Committee on Diet and Health recommended that carbohydrates be increased to more than 55% of total calories, primarily by increasing complex carbohydrates. A 2100-kcal energy intake would require a minimum of 290 g of carbohydrate.

Suggestions that carbohydrate intake be increased have met with considerable resistance from the general public. Carbohydrates frequently are thought to be fattening; however, this is a misconception. Carbohydrates provide 4 kcal/g—the same as protein. Fats yield 9 kcal/g, more than twice as much as either carbohydrate or protein. Protein foods usually are higher in calories than carbohydrate foods because protein is combined with fat in most foods (as in meat, cheese, eggs, and peanut butter). Complex carbohydrates and naturally occurring sugars, as are found in fruits, vegetables, whole-grain breads and cereals, dried peas and beans, and seeds and nuts, provide many essential vitamins and minerals plus fiber, in addition to calories.

Refined sugars and sugars in processed foods perhaps deserve the label *fattening.* People tend to overeat these foods, which frequently take the place of more nutritious foods in the diet. Display 8-1 gives the sugar content of some commonly used foods.

CONSUMER-RELATED ISSUES

FOOD LABELING

The food label reform that became law in May 1994 helps to clear up confusion regarding several carbohydrate-related issues. Consumers now have available the total carbohydrate, fiber, and sugar content of almost all the products they buy. Manufacturers must list these three components. Manufacturers may voluntarily list the following components: soluble fiber, insoluble fiber, sugar alcohols (such as sorbitol and mannitol), and "other carbohydrate" (the difference between total carbohydrate and the sum of dietary fiber, sugars, and sugar alcohols, if declared). See the sample label in Figure 5-2. Uniform definitions have been established for descriptive words used on labels, such as sugar-free, reduced sugar, and high fiber. See Display 8-2 for the definitions of carbohydrate-related descriptive terms.

It is important to note, however, that the total sugar content listed on the label represents both naturally occurring and added sugar. For example, 8 oz of milk contain 12 g sugar in the form of lactose, which is naturally present in the milk. Eight ounces of chocolate milk contain 26 g sugar, 12 g of which are naturally present in the milk and 14 g of added sugar. The ingredient label can help you determine if some or all of the sugar in a product is naturally occurring or added.

DISPLAY 8-1 SUGAR CONTENT OF COMMON FOODS

WHERE ARE THE ADDED SUGARS?

FOOD GROUPS	ADDED SUGARS (TSP)*
BREAD, CEREAL, RICE, AND PASTA	
Bread, 1 slice	0
Muffin, 1 medium	*1
Cookies, 2 medium	*1
Danish pastry, 1 medium	*1
Doughnut, 1 medium	**2
Ready-to-eat cereal, sweetened, 1 oz	†
Pound cake, no-fat, 1 oz	**2
Angel food cake, 1/12 tube cake	*****5
Cake, frosted, 1/16 average	******6
Pie, fruit, 2 crust, 1/6 8-in pie	******6
FRUIT	
Fruit, canned in juice, 1/2 cup	0
Fruit, canned in light syrup, 1/2 cup	**2
Fruit, canned in heavy syrup, 1/2 cup	****4
MILK, YOGURT, AND CHEESE	
Milk, plain, 1 cup	0
Chocolate milk, 2%, 1 cup	***3
Lowfat yogurt, plain, 8 oz	0
Lowfat yogurt, flavored, 8 oz	*****5
Lowfat yogurt, fruit, 8 oz	*******7
Ice cream, ice milk, or frozen yogurt, 1/2 cup	***3
Chocolate shake, 10 fl oz	*********9
OTHER	
Sugar, jam, or jelly, 1 tsp	*1
Syrup or honey, 1 tbsp	***3
Chocolate bar, 1 oz	***3
Fruit sorbet, 1/2 cup	***3
Gelatin dessert, 1/2 cup	****4
Sherbet, 1/2 cup	*****5
Cola, 12 fl oz	*********9
Fruit drink, ade, 12 fl oz	************12

* 4 g sugar = 1 tsp.
† Check product label.
(US Dept of Agriculture, Human Nutrition Information Service. The food guide pyramid. (Washington, DC: US Government Printing Office, 1992. Home and Garden bulletin 252:16.)

NONNUTRITIVE SUGAR SUBSTITUTES

Consumer interest in health issues and weight loss has led to a tremendous increase in the use of sugar substitutes, a $1 billion industry. Sweeteners are classified as nutritive or nonnutritive. *Nutritive sweeteners* are those that provide calories such as sucrose, fructose, honey, and sorbitol. *Nonnutritive sweeteners* supply no calories or only negligible amounts. Three nonnutritive sweeteners, saccharin, aspartame, and acesulfame-potassium (ACE-K or acesulfame-K), are available in the United States. The nonnutritive sweetener cyclamate is banned in the United States but is permitted in Canada. The Food and Drug Administration (FDA) is presently evaluating several nonnutritive sweeteners, including alitame, sucralose, and cyclamate.

In approving both aspartame and ACE-K, the FDA established an *Acceptable Daily Intake* (ADI). The ADI is the amount that is determined to be safe to consume daily over a person's lifetime without any adverse effects. It includes a 100-fold safety factor so that there would be no adverse effects, even if a person reached the ADI consumption levels.

SACCHARIN

Saccharin, 300 times sweeter than sucrose and derived from petroleum, is the oldest sugar substitute. It is not metabolized by the body and is excreted unchanged by the kidneys. Sweet'n Low and Sugar-Twin are two popular saccharin sweeteners.

Because of its link to bladder cancer at high doses in laboratory animals, there is some question about its safety. There is no evidence of increased risk in humans. Some health authorities advise "prudent" use of saccharin in pregnancy. The American Academy of Pediatrics Nutrition Committee on Insulin Dependent Diabetes Mellitus (IDDM) has advised that the use of saccharin and cyclamate be limited by children with IDDM and that the use of aspartame is a better choice.

No ADI has been established for saccharin. Recommendations have been made to limit consumption to 500 mg/day for children and 1000 mg/day for adults weighing 70 kg. A tabletop packet of saccharin contains 40 mg saccharin. A 12-oz serving

DISPLAY 8-2 CARBOHYDRATE-RELATED FOOD LABELING TERMS: WHAT THEY MEAN

SUGAR

Sugar free: Less than 0.5 g per serving

No added sugar, Without added sugar, No sugar added:

- No sugars added during processing or packing, including ingredients that contain sugars (e.g., fruit juices, applesauce, or dried fruit).
- Processing does not increase the sugar content above the amount naturally present in the ingredients. (A functionally insignificant increase in sugars is acceptable from processes used for purposes other than increasing sugar content.)
- The food that it resembles and for which it substitutes normally contains added sugars.
- If the food does not meet the requirements for a low- or reduced-calorie food, the product bears a statement that the food is not low calorie or calorie reduced and directs consumers' attention to the nutrition panel for further information on sugars and calorie content.

Reduced sugar: At least 25% less sugar per serving than reference food

FIBER

High fiber: 5 g or more per serving (foods making high-fiber claims must meet the definition for lowfat, or the level of total fat must appear next to the high-fiber claim)

Good source of fiber: 2.5 g to 4.9 g per serving

More or Added fiber: at least 2.5 g more per serving than reference food

(Stehlin D. A little "Lite" reading. FDA Consumer. [Special Report: Focus on Food Labeling]. May 1993. DHHS publication FDA93-2262:32.)

of a saccharin–aspartame blend carbonated beverage contains 96 mg of saccharin.

CYCLAMATE

Cyclamate has been banned in the United States since 1969 but is permitted in Canada. It is 30 times sweeter than sucrose, heat stable, and most useful when used together with other high-intensity sweeteners. Although the FDA concluded that cyclamate is not cancer causing, there are concerns about its safety for some people who metabolize cyclamate to the potentially harmful substance cyclohexylamine.

ASPARTAME

Aspartame, derived from protein, is 180 to 200 times sweeter than sucrose. Such small amounts are required for sweetness that negligible calories are produced. Because it loses sweetness when exposed to high heat, its usefulness in cooked foods is limited.

Extensive research has failed to show any relationship of aspartame to reported side effects. A product of the metabolism of aspartame is a toxic alcohol methanol. However, the amount produced from aspartame is no greater than the methanol produced by the foods normally in the diet (fruits and vegetables). It is approved for use by all people, including pregnant women. The only exception is for people with phenylketonuria, a genetic condition diagnosed at birth by a test performed on all infants. The label on products containing aspartame must read, "Phenylketonurics: contains phenylalanine." An ADI of 50 mg/kg of body weight has been established by the FDA. A 12-oz can of soda sweetened 100% with aspartame contains 180 mg; one tabletop sweetener packet contains 35 mg aspartame.

Aspartame is found on the market as NutraSweet and Equal. It is also available under other brand names, one of which is NatraTaste, because the patent held by the Nutrasweet Co. expired in December 1992.

ACESULFAME-K

ACE-K is the most recently approved nonnutritive sugar substitute. It is not metabolized by the body and is excreted unchanged by the kidneys. It has been in use in foreign countries since 1983. It is approximately 200 times sweeter than sucrose and can be subjected to heat in cooking. Some bitterness may be detected when used in high concentrations.

An ADI of 15 mg/kg body weight has been established by the FDA. One tabletop sweetener packet contains 50 mg of ACE-K. It is marketed as Sunette and Sweet One.

CARBOHYDRATES AND HEALTH

Knowledge of the carbohydrate sources, their characteristics, and their nutritional value helps both in the prevention of disease (as in dental caries) and in the treatment of disease involving the use of carbohydrate (as in diabetes mellitus). It also helps correct widespread misunderstandings about this group of foods.

OVERCONSUMPTION OF SUGARS

Foods with a high sugar content provide energy but few nutrients. This is the basis for calling sugary foods *empty calories*. In the United States, daily sugar intake ranges from 18% to 32% of total calories. Diets that contain a high percentage of sugar are likely to lack vital nutrients such as vitamins and minerals. Everyone should limit the consumption of sugar, especially people whose total caloric needs are low.

Although there is no direct link between obesity and excessive sugar consumption, sugar consumption certainly contributes to obesity. A good way to cut back on caloric intake without reducing nutrients is to reduce consumption of foods containing a high percentage of sugar.

DENTAL DISEASE

The major health problem associated with eating sugar is tooth decay. Dental caries are symptoms of a complex disease to which individuals are subject in varying degrees. Both kinds of carbohydrate—sugars and starches—are linked to the development of tooth decay. Foods containing refined cooked starch are transformed into sugars in the mouth through the action of enzymes in saliva and those produced by bacteria. Foods previously thought to have a low potential for promoting dental caries—such as breads, muffins, crackers, and chips—are no longer considered safe for teeth especially when eaten between meals. Mixtures of starches and sugars may be retained longer in the plaque than high-sugar foods. *Dental plaque* is a transparent, sticky substance comprising microorganisms, proteins from the saliva, and polysaccharides. The plaque adheres to the teeth and gums and harbors the acid-forming bacteria.

The more frequently the carbohydrate is eaten and the longer the food stays in the mouth, the greater the risk. Every time bacteria on the tooth surface are exposed to carbohydrates, they produce acid for 20 to 30 minutes. This acid causes loss of mineral from the teeth. Because most foods contain starch or sugar, excessive between-meal snacking should be avoided. When carbohydrate foods are eaten as part of a meal, they mix with other foods, such as protein, which may protect against tooth decay. Proteins stimulate the production of saliva, which protects the teeth from decay, and keep the saliva from becoming acidic. Fats also may affect the pH of the saliva in a beneficial way. Foods that have an abrasive texture, such as apples, have a detergentlike action that may help clean the teeth. Other factors, such as dental hygiene and fluoridation of water, also are important in the prevention of dental decay.

LACK OF FIBER

The increased use of convenience foods, which are made from highly refined ingredients, has resulted in diets that are low in fiber. A high-fiber diet has proved useful in reducing the symptoms of chronic constipation and diverticulosis. Research has suggested that a high-fiber diet also may be useful in preventing some types of cancer, reducing serum cholesterol, and reducing blood sugar levels in diabetes (see Chapter 24).

FAD DIETS

Low carbohydrate–reducing diets that promote the use of fats and protein and severely restrict or eliminate the use of carbohydrates can cause serious harm. When there is too little carbohydrate, fat is not burned completely, and a condition known as *acidosis* (also called *ketosis*) results. Excessive quantities of water and sodium are excreted, body tissue breaks down, and there is a general deterioration in physical condition. Also, the replacement of carbohydrate with fat predisposes the individual to high serum cholesterol levels and some types of cancer.

ABNORMAL USE OF CARBOHYDRATES

In several disease conditions, the body is unable to use carbohydrates normally. The most common of these diseases is *diabetes mellitus,* in which the cells are unable to burn glucose for energy at a normal rate. This causes the quantity of glucose entering the cell to decrease and therefore the quantity of sugar circulating in the blood to increase. Diabetes may be due to a lack of insulin or to factors that inhibit the functioning of insulin (see Chapter 24).

Lactose intolerance is due to a deficiency of the enzyme lactase, which is necessary for the digestion of lactose (milk sugar). The condition is uncommon in infancy. Many people, however, lose their ability to digest milk sugar in adulthood. These people suffer from cramps, diarrhea, and flatulence after drinking milk (see Chapter 28).

In *galactosemia,* the liver is unable to convert the sugar galactose to glucose. This disorder, which occurs in infancy, is caused by the lack of a certain enzyme. Digestive disturbances, physical and mental retardation, and cataracts are some of the consequences of the disease (see Chapter 17).

ALCOHOL ABUSE

Alcohol is produced by the fermentation of glucose. It is considered a foodstuff because it yields 7 kcal/g. One-half fluid ounce of 80-proof alcohol contains 12 g of alcohol and 84 kcal. Alcohol does not require digestion and is absorbed intact from the gastrointestinal tract. It is water soluble and immediately disperses throughout the body fluids.

Chronic alcohol abuse creates serious physiologic, psychological, and social problems for an estimated 9 million Americans. Chronic alcoholics may eat poorly because of a lack of money to support an adequate diet or because alcohol depresses their appetite. Excessive alcohol intake can seriously impair liver function and cause disorders of the nervous and cardiovascular systems. It also contributes to the development of certain cancers.

Heavy drinking during pregnancy can result in the birth of a baby with fetal alcohol syndrome, which is characterized by physical defects and behavioral disturbances. Even light to moderate drinking can result in adverse effects. A woman who is pregnant or planning a pregnancy should not drink alcohol.

KEY ISSUES

Fiber: Fact and Fiction

Fiber in the diet has been the focus of much attention in recent years. The value of fiber in promoting normal bowel function has long been recognized. In the 1970s, new interest was sparked by the observations of a British physician that there might be a connection between the high-fiber diet of rural Africans and the low incidence of *diverticular disease* (outpouching of the walls of the colon) in that population. This led to many other investigations into the possibility of a link between fiber intake and diseases that plague the Western world.

WHAT IS FIBER?

Fiber, commonly called bulk or roughage, is a group of compounds found in plant foods. These compounds cannot be broken down by acids and enzymes in the digestive tract. For the most part, fiber passes through the digestive tract and is eliminated in bowel movements. Some fiber is partially broken down by bacteria in the colon, producing gas, water, and short-chain fatty acids. The compounds that compose fiber include cellulose, hemicellulose, pectin, gums, mucilages, and lignin. All are polysaccharides except lignin, a substance that forms the woody parts of plants.

The compounds that make up fiber are of two general types: water soluble and water insoluble. Soluble fiber dissolves in water and forms a gel-like consistency in the digestive tract. It delays the emptying time of the stomach and slows the movement of food along the digestive tract. Insoluble fiber holds water in the gastrointestinal tract, thus increasing bulk. It speeds gastric emptying time and speeds movement through the tract (Display 8-3). Insoluble fiber includes the woody or structural parts of plants such as skins and the outer coating of wheat and corn kernels.

Foods contain both soluble and insoluble fiber, but differ in the amounts of each type they contain. Some foods are better sources of soluble fiber, whereas others contain predominantly insoluble fiber. It is important to eat a variety of plant foods to benefit from the effects of the different kinds of fiber (Display 8-4).

DISPLAY 8-3 TYPES AND FUNCTIONS OF FIBER

SOLUBLE FIBER (PECTINS, GUMS, GUAR, HEMICELLULOSE)

Sources: Oats, barley, some vegetables and fruits, legumes)

Delays gastric emptying time
Prolongs intestinal transit time
Flattens blood sugar rise after meals
Reduces serum cholesterol

INSOLUBLE FIBER (CELLULOSE, LIGNIN)

Sources: Whole-grain wheat, vegetables, fruit, corn bran, nuts)

Speeds gastric emptying time
Speeds intestinal transit
Little effect on after-meal rise in blood sugar
Minimal effect on serum cholesterol

HOW DOES FIBER PROMOTE GOOD HEALTH?

Much hype in the press and in advertising has been given to the benefits of fiber. Fiber has been said to prevent or cure such a variety of diseases that one would think most diseases would disappear if people ate more fiber. Although many claims are exaggerations, fiber appears to be play some role in the prevention or treatment of several diseases. Not all authorities agree on the benefits attributed to fiber, however, because of conflicting research results.

Gastrointestinal Disorders

Fiber clearly plays a role in preventing and alleviating constipation. Insoluble fiber, especially wheat and corn bran, holds water in the gastrointestinal tract. The water softens and increases the stool volume and causes faster movement along the tract, thus aiding elimination.

Because fiber reduces pressure in the intestinal tract, it appears to be useful in such diseases as diverticulosis, appendicitis, and hemorrhoids. In these diseases, excessive pressure causes the intestinal tract to weaken and give out in certain places.

Colon Cancer

Some scientists believe that insoluble fiber protects us from colon cancer. Fiber may dilute the concentration of cancer-causing substances in the intestinal tract. Because it speeds movement, it also reduces the time the tract is exposed to these harmful substances.

Scientists have differed, however, concerning the value of soluble fiber in cancer prevention.

DISPLAY 8-4 AVERAGE FIBER CONTENT OF FOODS

FOOD	FIBER (G)
Milk, meat	0
Fruits (1 serving)	2
Vegetables, nonstarchy	
Cooked (1/2–3/4 cup)	2
Raw (1–2 cups)	2
Vegetables, starchy (1/2 cup)	3
Brown rice, barley (1/3 cup)	3
Dried beans, lentils (1/2 cup)	4–5
Whole-grain breads, crackers (1 serving)	2
Shredded wheat, bran flakes (1/2–3/4 cup)	3–4
Other whole-grain cereals (1/2–3/4 cup)	2
Concentrated bran cereals (1/3–1/2 cup)	8–9
Nuts, seeds (1 oz)	3

Some have suggested that protective substances are formed when soluble fiber is broken down by the bacteria in the intestinal tract. Others have claimed that soluble fiber has been shown to increase tumor production in laboratory animals by increasing the concentration of bile acids in the intestines. Studies of vegetarians, who typically consume large quantities of fiber, have shown a lower incidence of colon cancer but a higher incidence of stomach cancer.

Elevated Blood Cholesterol

Soluble fiber appears to lower blood cholesterol levels by binding bile salts and bile acids that are in the intestinal tract. These substances are made from cholesterol. Fiber increases their excretion and in this way reduces the amount of cholesterol that is reabsorbed into the bloodstream.

Elevated Blood Glucose

Starches and sugars appear to be more slowly absorbed when they are part of a diet high in soluble fiber. This slow absorption keeps the blood sugar from rising rapidly after a meal. Some people with diabetes are able to reduce insulin dosage when consuming a diet high in soluble fiber. The American Diabetes Association has recently acknowledged, however, that the quantity of fiber needed to achieve these results is difficult to attain without the use of fiber supplements. People with diabetes are encouraged to increase dietary fiber consumption to the level recommended for the general public (20 g to 35 g/day).

Weight Control

Soluble fiber may aid in weight loss because it slows gastric emptying time and increases the feeling of fullness after a meal. Bulky high-fiber foods also take longer to eat and cause lower caloric intake when used in place of fatty and sugary foods.

DOES FIBER HAVE ANY HARMFUL EFFECTS?

High-fiber foods may interfere with the absorption of some minerals, including zinc, calcium, iron, and magnesium. Fiber binds these nutrients and interferes with their absorption. The various types of fiber affect absorption differently. When the diet contains a variety of high-fiber foods, the absorption of nutrients is not a problem. Fiber-containing commercial laxatives may interfere with the absorption of nutrients if taken with meals.

Intestinal discomfort may occur, at first, when fiber is increased. Some people may experience gaseousness, cramping, and even diarrhea. This usually is a temporary problem that subsides as the body adjusts to a diet higher in fiber. Increasing fiber gradually helps reduce digestive problems. However, excessive fiber intake occasionally leads to intestinal obstruction.

Increased fluid is required when fiber intake is increased. If fluid is inadequate, the fiber is constipating rather than stimulating to the digestive tract.

WHAT FOODS CONTAIN FIBER?

Fiber is found in whole-grain products; vegetables, especially those with edible skins, stems, and seeds; whole fruits with edible skins and seeds; dry peas, beans, and lentils; and nuts and seeds (see Display 8-4). Some contain primarily soluble fiber, whereas others contain more insoluble fiber (Display 8-3).

All vegetables contribute some insoluble fiber; fruits eaten with the skins on also are excellent insoluble fiber sources. Whole-grain breads, cereals, and crackers and brown and wild rice add insoluble fiber to the diet. Wheat bran is a rich insoluble fiber source.

Oats, barley, some fruits and vegetables, and legumes (dried peas, beans, and lentils) are good soluble fiber sources. Kidney, navy, pinto, and lima beans are excellent sources of both soluble and insoluble fiber. Apples, peaches, plums, bananas, citrus fruits, broccoli, carrots, and cabbage are good soluble fiber sources.

Oat bran is an excellent soluble fiber source and has been shown to be helpful in lowering blood cholesterol levels. It should not be considered a cure-all, however, and should be a part of a diet low in saturated fat and cholesterol. The effectiveness of oat bran appears to be based on its soluble fiber content. Other foods such as barley and dried peas and beans may be equally effective.

Measuring fiber in food is difficult. Many tables of food composition give what is called the *crude fiber* content of food. The crude fiber represents the fiber that remains in food after treatment in the laboratory with hot acid and hot alkali. More than half of the fiber in food is destroyed in this process, which is much harsher than the treatment food receives in the body. The term *dietary fiber* represents all the fiber in food and more accurately conveys what we need to know about the fiber content of food. In recent years, better methods have been developed for determining the amount of total fiber in foods. Total dietary fiber is a required component of nutrition labeling. The manufacturer may voluntarily provide, in addition, the soluble and insoluble fiber contents.

HOW MUCH FIBER DO WE NEED?

In light of the uncertainties, exactly how much fiber we should eat is unclear. The average fiber intake of Americans is quite low: only about 11 g. A daily dietary fiber intake of 20 g to 35 g from a wide variety of plant sources is recommended. This means selecting fiber-rich whole-grain breads and cereals, all types of fruits and vegetables, legumes, and, in moderation, nuts. All are excellent sources of essential vitamins and minerals, as well.

The following are suggestions for increasing fiber in the diet:

- Increase fiber intake *gradually* to minimize digestive problems that may result. Slowly replace refined, processed foods with unrefined high-fiber foods (Display 8-5).
- Use raw whole fruits in place of juice. The skins, seeds, and membranes are rich in fiber.
- Increase the use of whole-grain and unrefined foods. Whole-grain or bran cereals, breads, and crackers; brown rice; scotch barley; bulgur; popcorn; and whole cornmeal are good choices.
- Increase the use of raw and cooked vegetables. Avoid mashing or grinding vegetables.
- Start with small servings of legumes, which may cause gaseousness and discomfort. Len-

DISPLAY 8-5 AN EXAMPLE OF A GRADUAL INCREASE IN FIBER INTAKE

STEP 1	FIBER (G)
3 servings fruit	6
1 cup cooked vegetables	4
1 serving starchy vegetables	3
4 servings whole-grain bread, crackers, cereal	8
Subtotal	21
STEP 2	
Add: 1 cup raw vegetables	2
1/3 cup concentrated bran cereal	8
Subtotal	31
STEP 3	
Add: 1/2 cup cooked dried beans or lentils	4–5
Total	35–36

tils, split peas, and lima beans are the most easily digested.

- Drink more water.

The RDA committee as well as the Food and Nutrition Board Committee on Diet and Health have recommended that people avoid fiber concentrates and supplements. Rather, people should increase fiber in the diet by consuming fruits, vegetables, legumes, and whole-grain cereals. These foods provide not only fiber but also vitamins and minerals.

KEYS TO PRACTICAL APPLICATION

Include more whole-grain cereals and breads in your diet.

When using refined cereal products, be sure they are enriched.

Reduce the amount of all types of sugars you eat; they provide calories but no vitamins and minerals.

Substitute starches for fats and sugars; choose foods that are good sources of fiber and carbohydrate, such as whole-grain breads and cereals, fruits and vegetables, beans, peas, and nuts.

Remember that frequent snacking promotes tooth decay.

Check nutrition labels for sugar content. Remember that the grams of sugar listed represent both naturally occurring and/or added sugar. The ingredients label can help you determine if some or all of the sugar in a product is naturally occurring or added.

Correct misconceptions that carbohydrates are fattening.

Reject diets that severely restrict carbohydrates; they can cause serious harm.

Remember that fiber-rich foods, such as whole grains, fruits, vegetables, legumes, nuts, and seeds, also are nutrient rich.

Increase fiber intake gradually; increase fluid intake as you increase fiber.

KEY IDEAS

Carbohydrates are the chief form of energy for all people.

Starches, sugars, and cellulose are the main forms of carbohydrate in food.

The kind of carbohydrate selected determines the nutritional contribution to the diet. Whole grains, enriched cereal products, and fruits and vegetables provide vitamins, minerals, and fiber; sugars, sweets, and unenriched refined cereals provide little other than energy.

Carbohydrates are classified as monosaccharides (simple sugars), disaccharides (double sugars), and polysaccharides (mainly starches).

The monosaccharides are as follows:

Glucose—Found in some fruits and vegetables; end product of the digestion of starches and sugars; the form of sugar circulating in the bloodstream.

Fructose—Sweetest of all sugars; found in ripe fruits and honey; half of the sucrose molecule.

Galactose—Part of the lactose molecule; found in a few plant foods.

The disaccharides are as follows:

Sucrose—Table sugar.

Maltose—Sugar found in beer and other malt products and produced in the breakdown of starch.

Lactose—Milk sugar.

Mannitol and sorbitol are sugar alcohols used as alternatives to sucrose because they do not raise blood sugar levels or promote tooth decay.

All sugars and sugar alcohols provide about 4 kcal/g, regardless of how sweet they taste.

Important polysaccharides are as follows:

Starch—Main source of food for humans; found in cereal grains and vegetables.

Cellulose—Main form of fiber in plant foods.

Glycogen—Form in which carbohydrate is stored in liver and muscle.

All carbohydrates must be reduced to monosaccharides before they can be absorbed into the bloodstream.

Glucose is the form in which carbohydrates circulate in the bloodstream. All carbohydrate is converted to glucose in the body. Glucose also can be formed from protein, and small amounts can be formed from fat.

The hormone insulin lowers blood sugar and greatly influences the use of carbohydrate and the regulation of the blood sugar level. Some other hormones, notably glucagon, raise the blood sugar level.

Carbohydrate is the body's most economical and efficient energy source.

Carbohydrate spares protein, which then can be used for tissue building and repair rather than energy.

Some carbohydrate is needed for the proper use of fat; in the absence of carbohydrate, fats are not completely burned and ketosis results. Severe restriction of carbohydrates in reducing diets can cause serious health problems.

Carbohydrates are important components of substances needed for regulating body processes; they also encourage the growth of beneficial bacteria, which are involved in the production of certain vitamins and in the absorption of calcium and phosphorus.

Food sources of carbohydrate include cereal grains, fruits, vegetables, nuts, milk, and concentrated sweets.

Milling of cereal grains results in the loss of vitamins and minerals; however, the nutritional quality of milled (refined) cereal products is improved by enrichment—the addition of iron and the vitamins thiamin, niacin, and riboflavin.

Many health authorities recommend increasing carbohydrate to 55% of total calories. Carbohydrates should be eaten regularly and spaced throughout the day.

Aspartame, saccharin, and ACE-K are the three nonnutritive sweeteners approved for use in the United States.

An ADI—the amount determined to be safe to consume daily over a person's lifetime without any adverse effects—has been established for aspartame and ACE-K.

Overconsumption of sugar promotes obesity and frequently leads to a diet poor in nutritional quality.

Diabetes mellitus, lactose intolerance, and galactosemia are examples of diseases in which carbohydrates are not used normally.

Other than its caloric value of 7 kcal/g, alcohol provides no nutrients; the chronic alcoholic frequently is malnourished.

Fiber comprising mostly indigestible carbohydrates is of two general types: soluble and insoluble. Each type functions differently (see Display 8-3).

Fiber promotes normal functioning of the lower intestinal tract, preventing and alleviating constipation and reducing the risk of diverticulosis and hemorrhoids. It may play a role in preventing or treating colon cancer, elevated blood cholesterol levels, high after-meal blood sugar levels in diabetes, and obesity.

The disadvantages of fiber include interference with the absorption of nutrients, intestinal discomfort and gaseousness, and the tendency to constipation and impaction if fluid intake is inadequate.

Fiber is found in whole-grain products; vegetables and fruits that have edible skins and seeds; dry peas, beans, and lentils; and nuts and seeds. Some foods contain primarily soluble fiber, whereas others contain more insoluble fiber (see Displays 8-3 and 8-4).

The dietary fiber content in tables and on labels more accurately represents the total fiber content of foods than the crude fiber content.

A daily dietary fiber intake of 20 mg to 35 mg is recommended. Because the fiber content of the average American diet is low, most Americans would benefit from eating more fiber-rich foods.

KEYS TO LEARNING

STUDY–DISCUSSION QUESTIONS

1. Using the 1-day food diary you kept in Chapter 5, list the foods that supply carbohydrate. Using Appendix E, record the amount of carbohydrate in each food.
2. What is the function of fiber in the diet? What are good fiber sources? What foods in your food diary contain large amounts of fiber? Do you think you are consuming an adequate amount of fiber? Using Display 8-4, estimate the fiber content of the food listed in your diary.
3. If a person's carbohydrate intake is greater than his or her energy needs, what happens to the excess? Explain your answer.
4. Measures have been taken to improve the nutritional quality of refined cereal products. Why has this been necessary? Explain the terms *enriched bread* and *enriched rice*. Why are whole-grain products preferable to enriched products?
5. Discuss in class the overconsumption of refined and processed sugar in the United States. What are some of the harmful effects of this trend? With regard to dental caries, the frequency with which carbohydrate is eaten appears to be more important than the total sugar consumed. Explain.
6. Why are reducing diets that severely restrict carbohydrates dangerous?

Check your answers to questions 7, 8, and 9 by looking up the amount of carbohydrate in each food in Appendix E.

7. Rank the following foods by carbohydrate content, beginning with the food that has the most carbohydrate:
   - One orange
   - One medium baked potato
   - One twelfth of a devil's food cake with icing (made from a mix)
   - One slice of whole wheat bread
   - ½ cup of zucchini, cooked
   - ½ cup of cooked oatmeal
8. Rank the following vegetables by carbohydrate content, beginning with the one that has the most carbohydrate:
   - ½ cup of green snap beans, cooked
   - ½ cup of cooked carrots
   - One baked potato
   - One sweet potato
   - One small stalk of broccoli, cooked
9. Which of the following has the highest fiber content?
   - ½ cup of applesauce
   - 4 oz of sirloin steak
   - One slice of whole wheat bread
   - ½ cup of baked beans

BIBLIOGRAPHY

BOOKS AND PAMPHLETS

DePaola DP, Faine MP, Vogel RI. Nutrition in relation to dental medicine. In: Shils ME, Olson JA, Shike M. Eds. Modern nutrition in health and disease. 8th ed. Philadelphia: Lea and Febiger, 1994:1007.

MacDonald I. Carbohydrates. In: Shils ME, Olson JA, Shike M. Eds. Modern nutrition in health and disease. 8th ed. Philadelphia: Lea and Febiger, 1994:36–46.

National Academy of Sciences, National Research Council, Committee on Diet and Health, Food and Nutrition Board. Diet and health: implications for reducing chronic disease risk (executive summary). Washington, DC: National Academy Press, 1989.

National Academy of Sciences, National Research Council, Food and Nutrition Board. Recommended dietary allowances. 10th ed. Washington, DC: National Academy Press, 1989.

Schneeman BO, Tietyen J. Dietary fiber. In: Shils ME, Olson JA, Shike M. Eds. Modern nutrition in health and disease. 8th ed. Philadelphia: Lea and Febiger, 1994:89–100.

US Dept of Agriculture, Human Nutrition Information Service. The food guide pyramid. Washington, DC: US Government Printing Office, 1992. Home and Garden bulletin 252.

US Dept of Agriculture and US Dept of Health and Human Services. Nutrition and your health: dietary guidelines for Americans. 3rd ed. Washington, DC: US Government Printing Office, 1990. Home and Garden bulletin 232.

PERIODICALS

Caggiula AW. The high fiber diet: practical advice for clients. J Am Diet Assoc 1989;89:1737.

Cooper SG, Tracey EJ. Small bowel obstruction caused by oat-bran bezoar. N Engl J Med 1989;320:1148.

Franz MJ, Maryniuk MD. Position of the American Dietetic Association: Use of nutritive and non-nutritive sweeteners. J Am Diet Assoc. 1993;93:816.

Kurtzweil P. "Nutrition facts" to help consumers eat smart. FDA Consumer (Special Report: Focus on Food Labeling). May 1993. DHHS publication FDA 93-2262.

Warshaw HS. Alternative sweeteners: past, present, pending and potential. Diabetes Spectrum 1990;3:5:335.

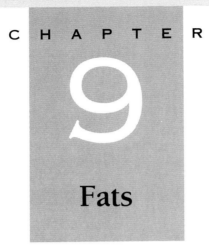

CHAPTER 9 Fats

KEY TERMS

adipose containing fat, as in adipose tissue

atherosclerosis thickening of the inside wall of arteries by atheromas, soft, cellular, fatty deposits that narrow the arteries and hinder blood flow

cholesterol a fatlike compound that occurs in bile, blood, brain and nerve tissue, liver, and other parts of the body; it is found in fatty deposits that line the inner wall of the artery in atherosclerosis; cholesterol occurs in animal foods

chylomicrons small particles in the blood containing fats absorbed from the intestinal tract

fatty acids organic acids that combine with glycerol to form fat; essential fatty acids are those that the body cannot produce and must be obtained in the diet

hydrogenation the addition of hydrogen to a liquid fat, changing it to a solid or semisolid state; generally, the harder the product, the higher the degree of saturation with hydrogen

lecithin a phospholipid containing choline; it is used commercially as an emulsifier; in the body, it has an important role in the absorption and transport of fat and in nerve and brain tissue; it is synthesized by the body

lipid a fat or fatlike substance that is insoluble in water and contains one or more fatty acids in its chemical structure

lipoprotein a combination of a protein with a fat

molecule the smallest quantity into which a specific substance can be divided

phospholipid a lipid that contains phosphorus, fatty acids, and a nitrogenous base; phospholipids are important in fat metabolism and nerve and brain tissue

prostaglandins a group of extremely active hormonelike compounds derived from essential fatty acids and present in many tissues; they are referred to as *local hormones* because they are synthesized within the cell and are metabolically active locally

satiety value the ability of a food to produce a feeling of fullness

saturated filled with hydrogen atoms; describes a fatty acid containing all the hydrogen it can hold; a monounsaturated fatty acid is one in which two carbon atoms are joined by a double bond—hydrogen can be added to each of the carbon atoms at this double bond; a polyunsaturated fatty acid has two or more double bonds—four or more carbon atoms can take up hydrogen atoms

steatorrhea excessive fat in the stool

triglyceride a fat formed by the combination of three fatty acids and glycerol; most animal and vegetable fats are triglycerides

OBJECTIVES

After completing this chapter, the student will be able to:

1. Describe the various forms of fat in food in regard to chain length and degree of saturation and the way in which they affect health.
2. Discuss the important functions of fat in the body.
3. Give the recommendations of authorities regarding fat consumption for the general public and explain why excess dietary fat is a health risk factor.
4. Identify the four types of blood lipids and describe their composition.
5. Identify the food sources of total fat, saturated fat, monounsaturated fat, polyunsaturated fat, and cholesterol.
6. Identify the specific labeling regulations that help consumers meet the dietary guidelines recommending a reduction in fat consumption.
7. Develop an awareness of ingredients used as fat replacers and how they work and an awareness of the impact these fat-modified products have on the overall nutritional quality of an individual's diet.
8. Identify the deficiency disease associated with fat and the conditions under which it is likely to occur.
9. Discuss pros and cons of the use of fish oils and the advice of authorities regarding their use.

Research reports that have linked fat to the development of major chronic diseases have brought more public attention to fats than to any other food group. The controversy over the relation of food fats to cardiovascular disease is now many years old, and technical terms once used only by the biochemist and members of the medical team have become a part of everyday vocabulary. Terms such as *saturated fats, polyunsaturated fats, cholesterol,* and *HDL (high-density lipoproteins) cholesterol* are now familiar to the general public. Misconceptions continue, however. In this chapter, these and other terms are explained, as are the functions and sources of fats.

Fats constituted 32% of the total calories consumed in the United States in the early 1900s. In the 1960s, the level rose to 42%. This change in fat consumption over the years was attributed to increased use of butter, oil, cream, and, particularly, red meats such as beef, lamb, and pork.

In more recent years, the use of fat has begun to decline; the average level of dietary fat intake is presently 36% to 37%. Consumers' demands for changes in the kind and amount of fat in the diet have led to the production of such items as lowfat milk, cheese, and frozen desserts; low-cholesterol egg substitutes; leaner meats; and fat substitutes.

CHARACTERISTICS OF FATS

Fats are essential nutrients comprising carbon, hydrogen, and oxygen atoms in proportions that yield high energy. Fats have a lower ratio of oxygen to carbon and hydrogen and, as a result, provide more energy than either carbohydrate or protein. *Lipid* is the scientific name for fat. It applies to a group of substances, both animal and plant, that have a greasy, oily, or waxy consistency. All lipids are insoluble in water and contain one or more fatty acids in their chemical structure.

Fat is composed mostly of fatty acids. A *fatty acid* is a substance made up of a chain of carbon atoms to which hydrogen atoms and some oxygen atoms are attached. The length of the carbon chain and the number of hydrogen atoms in a fatty acid are factors with nutritional significance. The characteristics of flavor, texture, melting point, and nutritive value depend on the kind of fatty acids a fat contains. A food fat, whether a solid or an oil, contains a mixture of fatty acids. All fats and oils, regardless of their fatty acid content, have the same energy value, yielding 9 calories per gram.

LENGTH OF THE CARBON CHAIN

Fatty acids are grouped according to the length of their carbon chain as follows: short-chain fatty acids: fewer than 6 carbons; medium-chain fatty acids: 6 to 10 carbons; and long-chain fatty acids: 12 or more carbons. The length of the carbon chain affects the ease with which fats are absorbed from the intestinal tract. Long-chain fatty acids require bile salts and must combine with other substances to be absorbed. Short- and medium-chain fatty acids are more readily hydrolyzed, absorbed, and transported. Most natural fats comprise long-chain fatty acids, which pose a problem in diseases in which fats are poorly absorbed. MCT Oil (Mead Johnson, Evansville, IN 47721), an oil comprising medium-chain fatty acids, is a commercial product developed for use in these malabsorption disorders.

DEGREE OF SATURATION WITH HYDROGEN ATOMS

Fatty acids are classified as saturated, monounsaturated, or polyunsaturated, depending on the degree to which hydrogen atoms are attached to the carbon atoms in the molecule (Fig. 9-1). If the carbon atoms in a particular fatty acid are attached to all the hydrogen atoms they can hold, the fatty acid is *saturated.* If some hydrogen atoms are missing and the carbon atoms are joined together by double bonds, the fatty acid is *unsaturated.* Fatty acids with only one double bond in their structure are *monounsaturated.* Those with

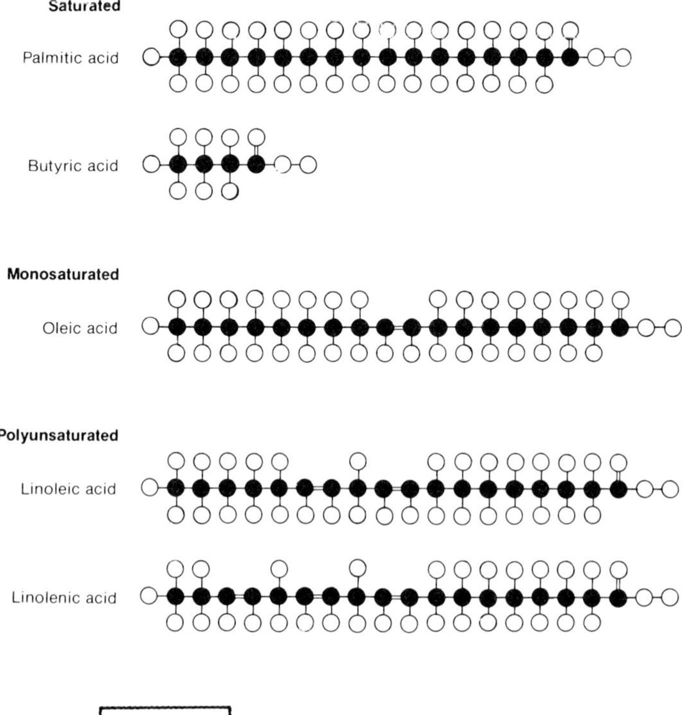

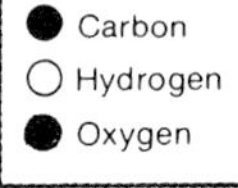

FIGURE 9-1

Chemical structure of fatty acids. *(Adapted from Labuza TP, Erdman JW. Food science and nutritional health: an introduction. St Paul: West Publishing Co, 1984:67.)*

two or more double bonds are *polyunsaturated* fatty acids.

Food fats are complex mixtures of saturated and unsaturated fatty acids. If a food contains mostly saturated fatty acids, it is considered a *saturated fat;* if it contains mostly polyunsaturated fatty acids, it is a *polyunsaturated fat.* Saturated fats tend to be solid at room temperature and are found primarily in animal sources. *Unsaturated fats* occur chiefly in vegetable sources and usually are in soft or liquid form. Oils contain large amounts of unsaturated fatty acids, with the exception of coconut, palm, and palm-kernel oils (the tropical oils), which are highly saturated.

Sometimes unsaturated oils are *hydrogenated,* as in the production of margarines and shortenings. In this process, the fatty acids take on hydrogen and thus become more saturated. The end products are somewhat soft and plastic. Some but not all of the double bonds are hydrogenated and are referred to as *partially hydrogenated* oils. These types of fatty acids have been the focus of interest for some time, especially in regard to their effect on blood cholesterol levels.

SATURATED FATTY ACIDS

Saturated fatty acids cannot take on any more hydrogen; they have a single bond between each carbon atom in the chain. Saturated fats are usually hard, stiff fats. The saturated fatty acids, present in animal and some plant foods (palm-kernel, palm, and coconut oils) have an elevating effect on blood cholesterol. More recent studies, however, have shown that not all saturated fatty acids have the same effect on blood cholesterol. Stearic acid, a saturated fatty acid found in beef, poultry, and cocoa butter, has little effect on blood cholesterol. The greatest cholesterol-raising effect is produced by three saturated fatty acids: myristic, palmitic, and lauric. Palmitic acid is the saturated fatty acid found most abundantly in the food supply. Authorities recommend that saturated fat not exceed 10% of the total caloric intake.

MONOUNSATURATED FATTY ACIDS

Monounsaturated fatty acids can take on hydrogen at only one point in the carbon chain; they have only one double bond between two carbon atoms in the chain. Monounsaturated fat, mainly oleic acid, is found in olive, canola, and high oleic forms of safflower and sunflower oils. It was thought to be neutral in its action on serum cholesterol—neither raising or lowering it. More recently, monounsaturated fats have been found to lower low-density lipoproteins (LDL) or bad cholesterol nearly as much as polyunsaturated fats when substituted for saturated fats in the diet. In addition, they do not lower serum HDL (good) cholesterol levels as do polyunsaturated fats. This is an important characteristic of monounsaturated fats, because HDL cholesterol is a protective factor in heart disease risk.

POLYUNSATURATED FATTY ACIDS

Polyunsaturated fatty acids can take on more hydrogen at two or more points in the carbon chain; therefore, there are two or more double bonds in the carbon chain. The two major families of polyunsaturated fatty acids are omega-6 and omega-3. They are classified according to where the first double bond occurs in their chemical structure. Found in fish oils, omega-3 acids have received much attention in the past few years because of reports that they may protect against heart disease. At high intakes, they substantially reduce serum triglyceride levels. The cholesterol-lowering effect of the major omega-6 polyunsaturated fatty acid—linoleic acid—which is found in vegetable oils such as corn, soybean, and high linoleic forms of safflower and sunflower oils, has been well known. Experts caution against the use of excessive amounts of the omega-6 polyunsaturated fatty acids, however, because they promote obesity, the risk of gallstones, and, in laboratory animals, certain cancers. Also, excess amounts of these fatty acids lower HDL (good) cholesterol in humans. Authorities advise that polyunsaturated fats represent about 7% and not more than 10% of total calories.

TRANS FATTY ACIDS

Hydrogenation is the process that converts vegetable oil to a more solid, more saturated fat such as margarine and shortening. The saturated fat produced is stearic acid, which does not raise serum LDL cholesterol. However, other substances—trans fatty acids—are formed as a result of the partial hydrogenation of unsaturated fatty acids. Although unsaturated, the trans fatty acids have a chemical shape or form different from most polyunsaturated fats found in nature. The safety of trans fatty acids has been questioned because research has indicated that they raise serum LDL cholesterol nearly as much as do cholesterol-raising saturated fats and also may lower HDL levels. People with high serum cholesterol levels are advised to limit intake of hydrogenated fats. See the discussion in the section Hydrogenated Vegetable Oils.

IMPORTANT LIPIDS

TRIGLYCERIDES

Most food fats and the fat stored in the body are known chemically as *triglycerides.* A triglyceride is a compound formed from three (tri-) molecules of fatty acids combined with one molecule of glycerol. The principal difference between fats is the combination of different fatty acids with glycerol. Butter is a complex mixture of 400 to 500 different fatty acids.

PHOSPHOLIPIDS

Phospholipids are lipids that contain fatty acids, phosphoric acid, and nitrogen. The phosphorus–nitrogen part of the molecule makes the phospholipid partially water soluble and gives it emulsifying properties. These properties are useful in the transport of fats in the bloodstream. Phospholipids play a role in cell structure, the formation of certain enzyme systems, and the metabolism of fats. They also are useful in the commercial processing of foods as a smoothing agent.

Lecithin is the most abundant phospholipid in the body and in foods. It is synthesized in the liver in sufficient quantities to meet body needs.

CHOLESTEROL

Cholesterol is a waxlike lipid found only in animal products. It is synthesized by the liver and stored in the livers of humans and animals. Plant foods, regardless of their fat content, do not contain cholesterol.

Cholesterol normally occurs in the blood and in all cell membranes. It is a major part of brain and nerve tissue. Cholesterol is necessary for normal body functioning, as a structural material in body cells, and in the production of bile salts, vitamin D, and a number of hormones, including cortisone and the sex hormones.

Some cholesterol is supplied by food, and some is synthesized by the body. Average levels of dietary cholesterol are 305 mg/day for women and 440 mg/day for men. The body synthesizes several times this amount daily, thus meeting the body's nutritional needs for cholesterol.

Heredity, diet, exercise, and other conditions affect blood cholesterol levels. People with high blood cholesterol levels appear to be more likely than those with desirable levels to develop *atherosclerosis*—a disease in which fatty deposits collect along the inside walls of large- or medium-sized arteries. Unsaturated fats tend to lower blood cholesterol, whereas saturated fat and cholesterol in food tend to raise blood cholesterol (see Chapter 25).

LIPOPROTEINS

Lipoproteins are the form in which fats are transported in the bloodstream. Because fats are insoluble in blood, which is basically water, they combine with protein to form substances that remain suspended in blood plasma. Lipoproteins are composed of triglycerides, protein, phospholipids, and cholesterol. Lipoproteins have been classified according to the amounts of these components they contain (Fig. 9-2).

The four types of lipoproteins are chylomicrons, very low-density lipoproteins (VLDL), low-density lipoproteins (LDL), and high-density lipoproteins (HDL). The blood lipoproteins appear to be important indicators of coronary heart disease risk. Low-density lipoproteins contain 60% to 70% of the cholesterol circulating in the bloodstream. They are considered the most important risk factor for coronary heart disease. High-density lipoproteins carry 20% to 25% of blood cholesterol and are believed to transport cholesterol away from the arteries to the liver, which recycles or disposes of it. For this reason, HDLs are referred to as *good cholesterol.* Low levels of HDL cholesterol are strongly associated with coronary heart disease. Authorities at the National Institutes of Health are now recommending that all adults be tested for both HDL levels and total serum cholesterol every 5 years (see Chapter 25).

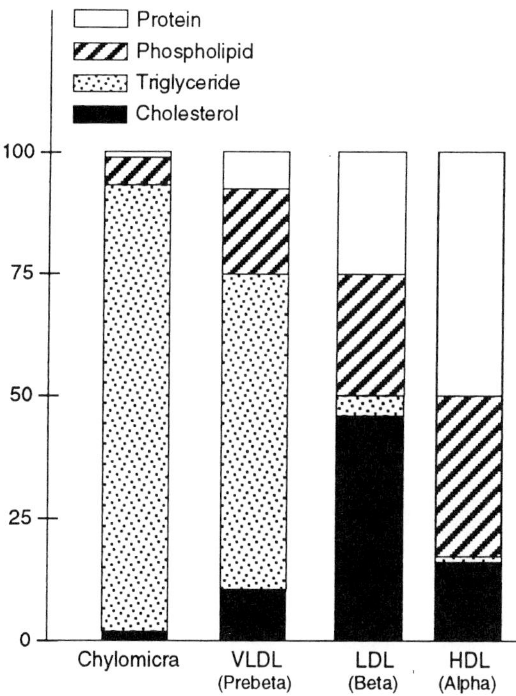

FIGURE 9-2

Composition of Lipoproteins. VLDL = very low density lipoproteins; LDL = low-density lipoproteins; HDL = high-density lipoproteins. *(From: Mahan LK & Arlin M. Krause's Food, nutrition and diet therapy. Philadelphia: WB Saunders Co, 1992:363.)*

DIGESTION, ABSORPTION, AND METABOLISM OF FATS

Before food fats can be absorbed into the bloodstream, they must be reduced to simpler compounds. Only about one third of the fat in the intestine is completely broken down to fatty acids and glycerol; the remainder is absorbed in a partially digested state. Table 9-1 summarizes fat digestion, which is discussed in Chapter 6.

Bile salts attach to digested fat substances and make possible their absorption by the cells of the intestinal wall. When the fatty acids enter the cells of the intestinal mucosa, the bile salt breaks away, and the fatty acids are converted back to triglycerides. These triglycerides, formed from dietary fat, combine with protein in the intestinal wall to form lipoproteins. Lipoproteins so formed are called *chylomicrons.* The chylomicrons then pass into the lymph duct in the center of the villus and are transported by the lymph to the bloodstream. The portal blood system then carries the chylomicrons to the liver, where they are converted to other types of lipoproteins (discussed previously) and then to the cells, where they are burned for energy or used to fulfill the other functions of fat.

Normally, 95% or more of dietary fat is absorbed. When bile is absent, as in gallbladder disease or cystic fibrosis, fat absorption is poor, and fat is lost in the stools (*steatorrhea*).

FUNCTIONS OF FATS

SOURCE OF ESSENTIAL FATTY ACIDS

The essential fatty acids are those that the body cannot synthesize and must be supplied in food. The essential fatty acids are the polyunsaturated linoleic

TABLE 9-1 SUMMARY OF FAT DIGESTION

Site of Activity	Fat	Enzyme	End Products
Mouth	Short-chain triglycerides Medium-chain triglycerides	Lingual lipase	Diglycerides
Stomach	Short-chain triglycerides Medium-chain triglycerides	Gastric lipase	Fatty acids, glycerol, diglycerides, monoglycerides
Small intestine*	Triglycerides, diglycerides	Pancreatic lipase	Monoglycerides, fatty acids, glycerol Resynthesized in intestinal mucosa to form triglycerides ↓ To bloodstream through lymph Smaller portion enters blood capillaries

* Bile salts emulsify fats, allowing enzymes to penetrate more easily.

and linolenic acids. Arachidonic acid was originally thought to be "essential," but now is known to be synthesized from linoleic acid. Linoleic acid, an omega-6 fatty acid, is found in plant foods, especially in vegetable oils produced from seeds such as corn, cottonseed, sesame, safflower, soybean, and sunflower oils. Linolenic acid occurs in plant leaves and a few vegetable oils including rapeseed (canola) and soybean oils. Fish oils are rich in important fatty acids derived from linolenic acid. Fish from deep cold water convert the linolenic acid to eicosapentaenoic acid and docosahexaenoic acid.

Essential fatty acids are needed for the normal functioning of all tissues. They form a part of the structure of each cell membrane, helping transport nutrients and metabolites across the cell membrane. Linoleic acid is involved in the transport and metabolism of cholesterol. Essential fatty acids also are involved in brain development.

The essential fatty acids are required for the transport of other fats and for the synthesis of *prostaglandins*, hormonelike compounds that act as regulators. The prostaglandins are synthesized mainly from arachidonic acid. A deficiency disease results when essential fatty acids are lacking (see the section Essential Fatty Acid Deficiency).

CARRIER OF FAT-SOLUBLE VITAMINS

Fats serve as carriers of vitamins A, D, E, and K. Conditions that interfere with the absorption or use of fat reduce the amount of fat-soluble vitamins available to the body.

ENERGY SOURCE

Fat is the body's most concentrated energy source. Except for the cells of the brain and central nervous system, all cells can use fatty acids directly as an energy source. Fat, in all forms and from all sources, provides 9 kcal/g, more than double the amount of energy provided by an equal weight of carbohydrate or protein. Fat, however, is not as readily available an energy form as carbohydrate because the production of energy from fat is a more complicated process. Fat can be considered a reserve form of energy.

RESERVE FUEL SUPPLY SOURCE

A group of specialized cells called *adipose cells* mainly store fat from excess calories—whether from protein, carbohydrate, or fat. Fat that has been deposited in fatty tissue cannot be excreted; fat stores are reduced only when the caloric value of the food eaten is less than the body's energy needs and fat is released to provide energy. Some fatty tissue is desirable because it serves as a reserve fuel supply for circumstances in which food intake is low, as in illness.

INSULATOR

Fat deposits beneath the skin help insulate the body, protecting it from excessive heat or cold. Fat rounds out the figure and pads joints and other body parts, such as the soles, palms, and buttocks, protecting them from outside pressure. Fat protects the vital organs, such as the heart and kidneys, by holding them in position and protecting them from physical trauma. When there is too much fatty tissue, however, the body cannot work efficiently; heat loss during hot weather is impeded, physical movements are hindered, and various serious health problems result.

PROVIDER OF MEAL SATISFACTION

Fats add flavor and taste to meals. Fats remain in the stomach longer than either protein or carbohydrate because they are digested and absorbed at a slower rate. This prolonged digestion contributes to a feeling of fullness and delays the onset of hunger pangs. Fat is said to have high satiety value.

Because of its high satiety value and concentrated energy, fat reduces the total volume of food eaten. When fat intake is limited, a large volume of nonfat food must be eaten to provide the same amount of energy and satisfy hunger.

AMOUNT OF FAT NEEDED IN THE DIET

In the 10th edition of *Recommended Dietary Allowances,* no recommendation was made for total fat or essential fatty acid intake. Only small amounts of linoleic acid—1% to 2% of total calories—are required to meet the body's need for essential fatty acids. A level of 3 g to 6 g/day of linoleic acid is minimally adequate for adults. The American diet easily meets this level. The major reason given for not establishing a recommended dietary allowance (RDA) for the essential fatty acids is that an essential fatty acid deficiency has not occurred in the general population, but only as a result of medical problems that affect fat intake or absorption. In 1985, the Academy of Pediatrics recommended that infant formulas provide at least 2.7% of total calories as linoleic acid.

In regard to the total fat content of the diet, the National Academy of Sciences Food and Nutrition Board suggested that a reduction of total fat from its present level of 36% to 37% is desirable. *The Surgeon General's Report on Nutrition and Health,* published in 1988, indicated that the reduction of total fats in the diet, especially saturated fat, is the priority for dietary change because of the relation of fat to the development of several chronic diseases. The National Academy of Sciences Committee on Diet and Health in 1989 recommended that total fat intake be reduced to 30% or less of calories, that saturated fatty acid intake be reduced to less than 10% of calories, and that cholesterol be reduced to less than 300 mg/day. These recommendations are similar to those of the American Heart Association, American Diabetes Association, and American Cancer Society, which have been recommending reductions in fat intake for some time. In 1993, the National Cholesterol Education Program in its second report reaffirmed its support of these dietary recommendations. Display 9-1 shows the amount of fat 30% of total calories represents at various caloric levels.

FAT SOURCES

Fats and oils (liquid fats) are sometimes referred to as *visible* or *invisible.* Visible fats are those that can be easily identified, such as butter, cream, oil, margarine, bacon, and the fat seen in some cuts of meat. Invisible fat is hidden, for example, the fat in whole

DISPLAY 9-1 QUANTITY OF FAT REPRESENTING 30% OF TOTAL CALORIES

CALORIE LEVEL	TOTAL FAT (G)
1200	40
1500	50
1800	60
2000	67
2200	73
2500	83
2800	93
3000	100

milk, egg yolk, dark meat of fish and poultry, pastries, nuts, and olives, and fat intermingled with the lean of meat.

Foods that contribute fat to the diet are whole milk and whole-milk products such as cream, butter, and cheese; eggs (yolk only); meat, fish, and poultry; nuts and seeds; and vegetable oil and hydrogenated products. All vegetables and fruits (except olives and avocados), cereal grains (except wheat germ), flour, macaroni products, bread and rolls, and sugars are practically free of fat. Table 9-2 compares the fat content and caloric value of typical portions of various foods.

TOTAL FAT

MILK AND MILK PRODUCTS

Dairy products that contain whole milk or butterfat contribute a considerable amount of fat to the diet. State law sets the minimum fat content of whole milk. The fat content of whole milk is about 3.3% by weight, or 8 g per 8 oz (the equivalent of $1\frac{1}{2}$ tsp of butter). In whole milk, 50% to 60% of the calories come from fat. In 2% milk, there are 5 g of fat per 8 oz (the equivalent of 1 tsp of butter), and 38% of its calories come from fat. An 8-oz portion of skim milk has 1 g or less of fat. Homogenized milk is whole milk processed so that the fat is dispersed in the form of tiny globules suspended throughout the milk. Yogurt is fermented milk that has the same amount of fat as the milk from which it is made.

Butter and margarine are 100% fat. They are equal in caloric content. Whipped butter and whipped margarine have about one third fewer calories than unwhipped products because the whipping process incorporates air into the products. Diet and *light* margarines have about half the calories of regular margarine.

Whole-milk cheeses such as cheddar derive 75% to 90% of their calories from fat. Cheeses made partially from skim milk are lower in fat than those made entirely from whole milk (see Table 9-2). Even the part-skim products, however, contain appreciable quantities of fat. Dry curd, uncreamed cottage cheese, and cottage cheese with 1% fat are low in fat. Consumers need to evaluate each of the many lowfat, reduced fat, and even fat-free cheese products on the market for flavor and fat content. See Display 9-2 for the definitions of labeling terms.

FISH, POULTRY, AND MEAT

The total fat content of fish ranges from 1% to more than 12% by weight. Shellfish such as oysters, clams, shrimp, lobster, and scallops are practically fat free. Mackerel, salmon, tuna, and herring are fatty fish. Even the fish with the highest fat content, however, is low in fat when compared with meat cuts such as ground beef, which may be 28% fat by weight. This represents 76% of total calories from fat. Poultry (without the skin) also is low in fat, ranging from 4% to 8% by weight.

The quantity of fat varies with the animal and with the grade and cut of meat. Prime and choice, the highest grades of beef, contain the most marbled fat (lean interlaced with fat). Because marbled fat cannot be trimmed, it furnishes a significant source of saturated fat and calories.

The fat content of pork and lamb is about equal to that of beef; the range by weight for all meats is from 6% for very lean cuts to 36% for the lean and fat of a rib roast of beef. Veal is much lower in fat. Although pork has been considered a high-fat food, pork from which visible fat has been removed is no higher in fat than other meats. Low-marbled ham is

TABLE 9-2 FAT CONTENT OF COMMON FOODS*

FOODS	FAT CONTENT (G)	TOTAL KCAL†
Milks and Yogurt	Per cup	Per cup
Skim milk (milk solids added)	1	90
Lowfat milk, 1% (milk solids added)	2	105
Lowfat milk, 2% (milk solids added)	5	125
Whole milk, 3.3%	8	150
Lowfat yogurt, plain	4	145
Lowfat yogurt, fruit-flavored	2	230†
Table Fats	Per tbsp	Per tbsp
Butter	11	100
Margarine	11	100
Mayonnaise	11	100
Blue cheese salad dresing	8	75
Creams	Per tbsp	Per tbsp
Half-and-half	2	20
Sour cream	3	25
Whipped topping (pressurized)	1	10
Light cream	5	45
Heavy cream	6	50
Desserts	Per 1/2 cup	Per 1/2 cup
Ice cream, 11% fat	7	135
Ice cream, soft serve	12	188
Ice milk, 4% fat	3	93
Sherbet	2	135†
	Per portion	Per portion
Apple pie, 1/6 of 9-in pie	18	405
Danish pastry, 4 1/4 × 1-in deep	12	220
Doughnut, glazed 3 3/4 × 1 1/4-in deep	13	235
Cheese	Per oz	Per oz
Cheddar	9	115
American processed cheese	9	105
Part-skim mozzarella	5	80
Cottage cheese, 4% fat	5 (1/2 cup)	118
Cottage cheese, 2% fat	2 (1/2 cup)	103
Meat, Fish, Poultry	Per 3 oz serving	Per 3 oz serving
Ham, lean and fat	18	250
Shrimp	1	100
Rib roast, lean and fat	26	315
Ground beef, regular	18	245
Turkey, light meat	3	135

* Source of nutritive values: US Dept. of Agriculture, Human Nutrition Information Service. Nutritive value of food. Washington,DC:US Government Printing Office, 1991. Home and Garden bulletin 72.

† Total kcal represent the kcal not only from fat but also from the protein and carbohydrate the food may contain.

‡ Fat content is relatively low, but sugar content raises total kcal.

DISPLAY 9-2 FAT AND CHOLESTEROL-RELATED FOOD LABELING TERMS: WHAT THEY MEAN

FAT

Fat free: Less than 0.5 g of fat per serving
Saturated fat free: Less than 0.5 g per serving and the level of trans fatty acids does not exceed 1% of total fat
Lowfat: 3 g or less per serving, and, if the serving is 30 g or less or 2 tbsp or less, per 50 g of the food
Low saturated fat: 1 g or less per serving and not more than 15% of calories from saturated fatty acids
Reduced or Less fat: At least 25% less per serving than reference food
Reduced or Less saturated fat: At least 25% less per serving than reference food

CHOLESTEROL

Cholesterol free: Less than 2 mg of cholesterol and 2 g or less of saturated fat per serving
Low cholesterol: 20 mg or less and 2 g or less of saturated fat per serving, and, if the serving is 30 g or less or 2 tbsp or less, per 50 g of the food
Reduced or Less cholesterol: At least 25% less and 2 g or less of saturated fat per serving than reference food

FAT AND CHOLESTEROL

Lean: Less than 10 g of fat, less than 4 g of saturated fat, and less than 95 mg of cholesterol per serving and per 100 g (3½ oz)
Extra lean: Less than 5 g of fat, less than 2 g of saturated fat, and less than 95 mg of cholesterol per serving and per 100 g (3½ oz)

(Stehlin D. A little "Lite" reading. FDA Consumer [Special Report: Focus on Food Labeling], May 1993. DHHS publication FDA 93-2262:29, 32.

considered a lean cut of meat. Roast pork and pork chops are medium-lean cuts. Pork has less saturated fat and more linoleic acid than either beef or lamb.

Luncheon meats, bacon, frankfurters, and sausage are high in fat. Bologna and liverwurst are about 28% fat, cooked link or bulk pork sausage is 44% fat, and bacon is 52% *fat by weight.*

PLANT SOURCES

Vegetable oils are 100% fat and make a significant contribution to our fat intake. We consume vegetable oils in fried foods and in products such as margarine, vegetable shortenings, and salad dressings. Nuts, peanut butter, seeds (e.g., sunflower seeds), and coconut are plant foods with a high fat content. Vegetables and fruits, with the exception of olives and avocados, contain only traces of fat.

BAKED PRODUCTS

Many baked products are a source of hidden fat in the diet. Many types of crackers, chips, croissants, biscuits, muffins, doughnuts, sweet rolls, pies, cakes, and cookies are a source of considerable amounts of fat.

SATURATED FATS

Saturated fatty acids occur mostly in animal products such as meat, poultry, and eggs; in whole milk and whole-milk products such as cream, butter, cheese, and ice cream; and in separated meat fats such as bacon, lard, salt pork, beef tallow, and chicken fat.

However, three plant fats are highly saturated: coconut oil, palm oil, and palm-kernel oil. Coconut and palm oils are more highly saturated than lard. Chocolate fat is equal in saturation to most saturated animal fat. The presence of chocolate in foods is obvious, but the presence of coconut oil or palm oil is not as easily detected and may provide a hidden saturated fat source. The low-cost coconut and palm oils are bland in flavor and do not become rancid as readily as unsaturated fats. Therefore, they have been used widely in commercial foods. Coconut and palm oils are used in the manufacture of most nondairy dessert toppings and coffee lighteners and in many commercial products such as crackers, cookies, muffins, cakes, TV dinners, and microwave popcorn. As a result of public demand, many companies have stopped using these saturated oils.

HYDROGENATED VEGETABLE OILS

Vegetable shortenings and margarines are products produced through hydrogenation, in which hydrogen is added to polyunsaturated vegetable oils, partially saturating the fat and converting some of the polyunsaturated fatty acids to trans fatty acids. People should limit the use of hydrogenated fats such as hydrogenated shortenings, hard margarines, and foods containing these fats because of the presence of these cholesterol-raising trans fatty acids. Soft or liquid margarines have a lower trans fatty acid content than hard margarine and even hard margarine does not have the potential for raising serum cholesterol as much as butter. Therefore, soft and liquid margarines remain better choices than butter.

MONOUNSATURATED FATS

Monounsaturated fats predominate in olives, peanuts, olive oil, canola oil (from rapeseed), peanut oil, and high oleic forms of safflower and sunflower seed oils. Some nuts, such as pecans and Brazil nuts, contain appreciable quantities of monounsaturated fats.

POLYUNSATURATED FATS

Polyunsaturated fatty acids occur in corn, cottonseed, soybean, and sesame oils and high linoleic forms of safflower and sunflower oils; salad dressings that are made from these oils (and that do not contain sour cream or cheese); special margarines that contain a high percentage of liquid oil; and fatty fish, such as mackerel, salmon, and herring.

Special margarines with a high percentage of polyunsaturated fatty acids are available. One can identify these products by carefully reading labels. Those products that list liquid oil as the first ingredient contain more polyunsaturated fat than saturated fat. Total fat and saturated fat must be listed on the label. Polyunsaturated fat and monounsaturated fat, although optional, are usually listed on margarine labels.

CHOLESTEROL

Cholesterol occurs only in animal foods. Organ meats, such as liver, kidneys, heart, and brains are rich cholesterol sources. An average egg yolk contains 213 mg of cholesterol—more than two thirds of the recommended daily cholesterol limit of 300 mg. Some types of shellfish such as shrimp and crayfish are moderately high in cholesterol but low in saturated fat and total fat content.

Other cholesterol sources are meat, fish, poultry, milk, and foods made from milk or butterfat. Lowfat dairy products have less cholesterol than those made with whole-milk products. Plant foods do not contain cholesterol.

FAT-RELATED CONSUMER ISSUES

FIGURING THE PERCENTAGE OF CALORIES FROM FAT

The preceding discussion of fat sources gave, in most cases, the percentage of *fat by weight* of various foods. The purpose was to compare the fat content of one food with another.

Because we usually refer to fat in the diet in terms of *percentage of total calories from fat,* we need to be able to calculate this percentage from the fat by weight figure. It is important for dietary purposes to know, for example, that ground beef labeled 15% fat by weight derives 62% of its calories from fat. Display 9-3 explains how to figure the percentage of calories from fat in a specific food or in the total diet.

LABELING

Labeling regulations that became mandatory in May 1994 make it easier to follow guidelines regarding fat in the diet. Fat-related information that manufacturers must state on the "Nutrition Facts" portion of the label includes

DISPLAY 9-3 HOW MUCH FAT? FIGURING THE PERCENTAGE OF CALORIES FROM FAT

IN A FOOD

You need to know the amount of fat in a portion and the total calories in that portion.

IN A DIET

You need to know the fat content of the diet and the total caloric content of the diet.

THEN

1. Multiply grams of fat in the food or in the diet by 9 (9 kcal/g fat) to obtain calories from fat.
2. Divide the fat calories by the total calories in the food portion or in the diet (whichever applies).
3. Multiply answer by 100 to convert to a percentage.

EXAMPLE

1 oz of cheddar cheese that contains 9 g fat and 110 kcal/oz derives 74% of its calories from fat, figured as follows:

$$9 \times 9 \text{ (kcal/g fat)} \div 110 \times 100$$

$$81 \div 110 = 0.736 \times 100 = 73.6\%$$

calories from fat in one serving.
grams of fat per serving.
grams of saturated fat per serving.
grams of cholesterol per serving.

Other fat-related components of the product that manufacturers may list *voluntarily* are

calories from saturated fat in one serving.
grams of polyunsaturated fat in one serving.
grams of monounsaturated fat in one serving.

Manufacturers must list these optional components if a claim is made about them on the label (see sample label, Figure 5-2).

The regulations also spell out what terms manufacturers can use to describe the level of a nutrient in a food and define what these terms must convey. A list of nutrient content descriptors that relate to the fat content of foods is given in Display 9-2.

Health claims may be used on food labels under specific conditions. In regard to dietary fat, claims for the following relationships are permitted:

fat and cancer.
saturated fat and cholesterol and coronary heart disease.

P:S RATIO

Occasionally, reference may be made to the *P:S ratio*, the proportion of polyunsaturated to saturated fat in a product. You obtain the P:S ratio by dividing the amount of polyunsaturated fatty acids in a food by the amount of saturated fatty acids. For example, a food with 3 g of polyunsaturated fat and 2 g of saturated fat has a ratio of 1.5. A food with 3 g of polyunsaturated fat to every 1 g of saturated fat has a ratio of 3. The higher the number, the more polyunsaturates the food contains.

FAT SUBSTITUTES

The demand for foods low in fat and cholesterol has led to the development of many fat substitutes. The impact of the fat substitutes on the fat content of commonly used processed foods is shown in Table 9-3.

Olestra, developed by Proctor and Gamble, is a *sucrose polyester*, a substance that cannot be digested by intestinal enzymes. It is not absorbed and, therefore, provides no calories. Olestra has the appearance, consistency, and taste of fat. It has been proposed by the manufacturer that Olestra replace 75% of the fat in commercial deep-frying oil, especially for fried snack foods, and 35% of the fat in home cooking oils. If approved by FDA, other uses will most likely follow.

Simplesse, developed by the NutraSweet Co., is made from milk and egg white proteins treated

TABLE 9-3 FAT CONTENT OF FOODS

FOOD	TRADITIONAL RECIPE (G OF FAT)	MADE USING FAT SUBSTITUTE (G OF FAT)
Margarine, 1 tbsp	7–12	0–6
Salad dressing		
Creamy, 2 tbsp	11–21	0–8
Clear, 2 tbsp	5–20	0–6
Mayonnaise, 1 tbsp	11	0–5
Cheese		
Hard, 1 oz	8–11	4–5
Processed, 1 oz	7–9	0–4
Cream cheese, 2 tbsp	9–10	0–5
Sour cream, 1 tbsp	2.5	0–1
Ice cream, ½ cup	7–26	0.3–2

(Pennington JAT. Bowes & Church's food values of portions commonly used. 16th ed. Philadelphia: JB Lippincott Co, 1994; From National Center for Nutrition and Dietetics of The American Dietetic Association. Nutrition fact sheet: Facts about fat substitutes. Chicago: 1994.)

by *microparticulation.* This heating and blending process produces a product that resembles fat. It supplies only 1.3 kcal/g compared with the 9 kcal/g in fat. Because this product is made from protein, heat causes the protein to coagulate and lose its fatlike texture. It is intended for use in cold products such as ice cream, butter, cheese spreads, and mayonnaise. The Food and Drug Administration (FDA) approved Simplesse in February 1990.

Although media coverage has focused on Olestra and Simplesse, many carbohydrate-based fat replacers are now being used to create the fat-free and lowfat foods flooding the supermarkets. The three main categories of fat replacers are carbohydrate based, protein based, and fat based.

Most of the fat replacers that are approved and in use are carbohydrate based. These products contribute to the taste of the food, but also serve as *bulking agents,* which act as fillers and provide the volume lost when fat is omitted. These carbohydrate-based fat substitutes begin either as complex carbohydrates, resulting in such substances as maltodextrins and modified food starch, or as simple sugars, resulting in such products as polydextrose, hydrogenated starch hydrolysate, or sorbitol.

Protein-based fat replacers create a unique texture that provides the creamy feel of fat. Simplesse is the only protein-based fat substitute presently approved; others await FDA approval.

Olestra is an example of a fat-based fat substitute. Other products are in various stages of approval or development. The fat-based fat replacers are not absorbed or only partially absorbed or they are metabolized less efficiently than other fats.

Considerable controversy surrounds the safety and influence that fat substitutes may have on overall nutritional health. Skepticism exists about the beneficial effect of these products on nutritional well-being. The reduction of fat intake due to the use of these products is expected to be modest—only 2% to 4%. Also, it is anticipated that some people will consume more desserts and fried foods made with these fat substitutes, leaving less room for whole grains, fruits, and vegetables. Other authorities feel that fat replacers can play an important role in reducing fat consumption and can have a beneficial effect on health.

FAT INTAKE AND HEALTH

Medical scientists associate the high fat content of the American diet with the major public health problems of coronary heart and blood vessel disease, obesity, and cancer.

OBESITY

Excessive use of fats contributes to obesity. Fats yield $2^1/_4$ times the calories of either proteins or carbohydrates. In addition, fat usually occurs in a concentrated form, whereas carbohydrate foods tend to have a high water content. For example, 1 oz of butter (about 2 tbsp) contains about 200 kcal, whereas 1 oz of snap beans contains 7 kcal. This does not mean that fats should be completely eliminated from the diet. Rather, people must choose fats sparingly and wisely so that they consume those fats that make the greatest nutritional contribution (see Chapter 23).

ATHEROSCLEROSIS

In atherosclerosis, fatty deposits clog or narrow the arterial passageway. If blood clots become lodged in the narrowed vessels, the blood flow to the heart or brain may be partially or completely blocked, resulting in a heart attack or stroke.

The cause of atherosclerosis is unknown. Its development appears to be influenced by many factors, including heredity, obesity, diet, high blood pressure, high serum cholesterol level, cigarette smoking, lack of exercise, hormonal factors, stress, and certain metabolic diseases such as diabetes. High blood cholesterol, high blood pressure, and cigarette smoking appear to be among the most important risk factors in coronary heart disease.

Most authorities consider diet to be the first line of treatment for borderline and high blood cholesterol levels. Many health organizations and agencies, including the surgeon general's office and the National Academy of Sciences Food and Nutrition Board, have recommended reduced fat consumption for the general population as a means of reducing coronary heart disease risk (see Chapter 25).

CANCER

Substantial evidence from both epidemiologic and animal studies has suggested that a strong relation exists between dietary fat intake and increased risk of colon, breast, and prostate cancers. Risk of these cancers is likely to be reduced by a decrease in fat intake.

ESSENTIAL FATTY ACID DEFICIENCY

A deficiency disease resulting from a lack of essential fatty acids may occur in both infants and adults. Symptoms of essential fatty acid deficiency in infants include dry and scaly skin and a slower than normal growth rate. Breast milk contains a generous amount of linoleic acid, four or five times that of evaporated milk. This may account for the low incidence of eczema and other skin conditions in breastfed infants compared with infants fed cow's milk. Commercial infant formulas and precooked infant cereals are good sources of essential fatty acids.

Among the symptoms of essential fatty acid deficiency in adults are dermatitis, infertility, liver and kidney disturbances, and increased susceptibility to infection. Deficiency symptoms in adults were first noted in people who received intravenous feedings totally lacking in fat for several months. The occurrence of essential fatty acid deficiency is now known to be more prevalent than previously thought.

With more sensitive testing techniques, essential fatty acid deficiency has been diagnosed in elderly clients with peripheral vascular disease, in people who have had major intestinal resection, and in those undergoing lowfat, high-protein treatment for kwashiorkor (a severe protein-deficiency disease) and after serious accidents and burns.

GASTROINTESTINAL AND OTHER DISEASES

Fats usually are restricted in diseases that interfere with their digestion or absorption. Examples include gallbladder disease, pancreatitis (inflammation of the pancreas), and cystic fibrosis. Fats usually are not restricted in liver disease unless the bile duct is obstructed (see Chapter 28).

SEIZURE DISORDERS

The *ketogenic diet*, which is high in fat and restricted in carbohydrate and protein, may be prescribed for children with seizure disorders who do not respond to drug therapy. This diet produces a mild ketosis and helps reduce seizures, restlessness, and irritability.

KEY ISSUES

Are Fish Oils Protective or Destructive?

In 1987, the sale of fish oil supplements in the United States reached a peak of $45 million. Offered as a means of preventing heart disease, these capsules contain fat from deepwater fish such as sardines, salmon, and mackerel. The magic ingredient in the fish oil is thought to be a special type of fat called *omega-3 fatty acids:* eicosapentaenoic acid and docosahexaenoic acid. The interest in fish oils was sparked by research reports that indicated the incidence of coronary artery disease is low in areas where fish consumption is high. Fish oils also are popular among the general public because they are available without prescription and are considered a natural substance rather than a medicine.

Sales of fish oil capsules were sparked by claims that they would lower serum cholesterol and triglycerides and prevent blood from clotting, thereby preventing the development of atherosclerosis. In 1988, the FDA warned drug companies to stop making drug claims. As a result, the sales fell dramatically.

Research has continued on the relation of fish oil to disease; there have been many promising developments. The beneficial effects are unrelated to cholesterol lowering but to other factors. Fish oil concentrates, however, are potent substances that affect metabolism in various ways. Doses that are effective in creating beneficial results also have the potential for producing serious adverse side effects. To achieve an intake of omega-3 fatty acids that seems to protect Eskimos from heart disease, one would have to swallow 50 capsules a day. Therapeutic doses range from 8 to 30 capsules a day.

The two major families of polyunsaturated fatty acids are omega-3 and omega-6 fatty acids. The omega-3 fatty acids are found in cold-water marine fish such as salmon, mackerel, herring, and sardines. They are highly unsaturated, containing five or six double bonds in their structure. Linoleic acid, an essential fatty acid, is an omega-6 fatty acid. Found in most vegetable oils, linoleic acid contains only two double bonds and has a well-known cholesterol-lowering effect. The following is a discussion of the beneficial and adverse effects of using omega-3 fish oils.

BENEFICIAL EFFECTS

Reduced blood lipids—Fish oils reduce blood triglycerides. Although they have been widely publicized as reducing blood cholesterol, they do not appear to do so. They may actually increase LDL (bad) cholesterol and decrease HDL (good) cholesterol. Elevated blood cholesterol responds much better to other drugs on the market with proven effectiveness.

Reduced blood pressure—Fish oils cause a modest decrease in both systolic (8 mmHg to 12 mmHg) and diastolic (4 mmHg to 8 mmHg) blood pressure.

Anticlogging effect—It is believed that cholesterol is deposited in an artery after a microscopic injury occurs to the blood vessel wall. The body's response to the injury causes a pileup of material that blocks the blood vessel. Fish oils appear to prevent the accumulation of platelets, smooth muscle cells, and white blood cells, which set the stage for blood clots.

Evidence that fish oil keeps arteries open has come from experience with people undergoing *angioplasty*. In this procedure, cardiologists make an incision in a blood vessel in the leg, through which they thread a small balloon up to the clogged artery. They inflate the balloon and the opening widens. In 25% to 40% of cases, the opening closes within 6 months. Of all the treatments tested, fish oils have been the most effective in keeping the artery open.

Improvement in inflammatory reactions and immune response—Fish oil consumption has resulted in improvement in some inflammatory conditions such as rheumatoid arthritis and lupus erythematosus. It also may reduce inflammation in certain skin disorders such as psoriasis.

ADVERSE EFFECTS

Increased LDL cholesterol—Recent research shows that fish oils may cause a slight rise in LDL (bad) cholesterol rather than a decrease.

Bleeding tendencies—Fish oils inhibit blood clotting and may cause easy bruising. Excessive bleeding may result, especially if taken with other drugs that retard clotting, such as aspirin.

Elevated blood sugar—In people with non–insulin-dependent diabetes mellitus (type II), fish oils appear to raise blood sugar levels because of increased sugar production by the liver.

Weight gain—Each fish oil capsule contains about 10 kcal. The dosage generally prescribed by physicians is 8 to 30 capsules per day. This dosage represents 80 to 300 additional calories daily, or a weight gain of 8 lb to 30 lb/yr.

Excess cholesterol intake—Some fish oil supplements contain about 7 mg of cholesterol per capsule. Based on a dose range of 8 to 30 capsules, this would provide 56 mg to 210 mg of cholesterol daily. Most brands are now lower in cholesterol—less than 5 mg per capsule.

Vitamin A and D toxicity—Fish oil supplements made from cod liver oil could have enough of vitamins A and D to be toxic. People should not use supplements containing these vitamins.

Contaminants—Processing does not remove all of the contaminants in fish oil. Small amounts of polychlorinated biphenyls (PCBs), which are carcinogenic substances, remain. A liberal fish intake (three to four servings a week) would probably supply as much or more PCBs as taking 10 capsules a day, however.

The American Heart Association and many other health authorities do not recommend the use of fish oil supplements because their effectiveness and safety have not been adequately evaluated. Fish oils sometimes are used medically to treat a high level of triglycerides or are prescribed following angioplasty. In these cases, the client is closely monitored. Fish oils should not be self-prescribed. They are potent substances. The regular use of fish in the diet, however, is encouraged.

KEYS TO PRACTICAL APPLICATION

Remember that all fat is high in calories and that excessive fat contributes to obesity.

Be aware of the fat sources—especially hidden fat—in your diet.

Reduce your intake of total fat, saturated fat, and cholesterol. This is a sensible guide for all healthy people.

Read labels carefully to determine the amount and types of fat contained in the food.

Remember: Foods that do not contain cholesterol may, nevertheless, have the potential to raise serum cholesterol levels if they contain coconut, palm, or palm-kernel oils or hydrogenated vegetable oils.

Be an informed shopper by learning the government definitions for terms used on food labels to describe the fat content—such as *lean, extra lean, lowfat,* and *fat free*.

KEY IDEAS

Fatty acids are the basic units of all fats; the physical characteristics and nutritional activity of a fat depend on the kind of fatty acids it contains.

The length of the carbon chain in the fatty acid determines the ease with which fats are absorbed. Short- and medium-chain fatty acids, although in short supply in natural foods, are more readily absorbed than long-chain fatty acids.

A fat is classified as saturated, monounsaturated, or polyunsaturated according to the type of fatty acids that predominate.

P:S ratio refers to the proportion of polyunsaturated to saturated fat in a food. The higher the number, determined by dividing the grams of polyunsaturated fat by the grams of saturated fat in the food, the more polyunsaturates that food contains.

Most food fats and stored body fat are triglycerides, compounds formed from three molecules of fatty acids attached to one molecule of glycerol.

Phospholipids, which comprise fatty acids, phosphoric acid, and nitrogen, are partially soluble in water and have emulsifying properties that are useful in the body and in commercial food processing.

Cholesterol, which is involved in the production of body cells, bile salts, vitamin D, and hormones, is obtained in food and synthesized by the body. High blood cholesterol levels appear to promote atherosclerosis.

Lipoproteins, combinations of fat and protein, are the form in which fats are carried in the bloodstream.

The amount of LDL cholesterol present is considered the most important risk factor for coronary heart disease.

A low amount of HDL cholesterol is also associated with a high risk for coronary heart disease.

Diets rich in saturated fat or cholesterol lead to elevated blood cholesterol levels; unsaturated fats appear to lower blood cholesterol levels.

Trans fatty acids, unsaturated fatty acids produced as a result of hydrogenation, raise serum cholesterol nearly as much as saturated fats.

Fats are a source of essential fatty acids, the most concentrated energy source, a reserve energy supply, a carrier for fat-soluble vitamins, an insulator for the body, and a provider of meal satisfaction.

Linoleic acid must be supplied in the diet in small amounts; a lack of linoleic acid results in a deficiency disease.

No RDA has been established for total fat or essential fatty acids; however, a reduction in total fat is recommended.

Expert health authorities have recommended reducing fat to less than 30% of total calories, saturated fat to less than 10% of calories, and cholesterol to less than 300 mg.

Foods that contribute fat to the diet include whole milk and products containing whole milk or butterfat, such as butter, ice cream, and cheese; egg yolk; meat, fish, and poultry; nuts and seeds; vegetable oils; hydrogenated vegetable fats (shortenings and margarine); and baked goods made with fat.

To figure percentage of calories from fat, multiply the fat content of the portion by 9, divide by total calories in the same portion, and multiply by 100.

Saturated fats are found in whole milk and whole-milk products such as cheese and ice cream, egg yolk, meat and poultry, meat and poultry fat, coconut oil, palm oil, chocolate, and hydrogenated vegetable fats.

Polyunsaturated fat sources are corn, cottonseed, soybean, sesame oils and high linoleic forms of safflower and sunflower oils; salad dressings made from these oils; special margarines that contain a high percentage of liquid oil; and fatty fish such as mackerel, salmon, and herring.

Monounsaturated fat sources are olive oil, canola (rapeseed) oil, high oleic forms of safflower and sunflower oils, peanut oil, peanuts, and other nuts.

Cholesterol is found *only* in animal foods. Organ meats and egg yolk are rich sources; shrimp is a moderately rich source. Other sources include meat, fish, poultry, milk, and foods made from milk or butterfat.

The saturated fat content of food is more important than the cholesterol content in the effect on blood cholesterol.

Labeling regulations, effective May 1994, give substantial information regarding the fat content of foods; descriptive terms used on labels are clearly defined.

Nutrition authorities disagree about the long-range beneficial effects of fat substitutes. Many carbohydrate-based fat replacers are presently in use.

High fat intake in the United States is associated with a high incidence of obesity and coronary heart and blood vessel disease. People with elevated levels of blood cholesterol are more prone to atherosclerosis than those with low levels.

A strong relation appears to exist between high fat intake and increased risk of colon, breast, and prostate cancers.

Fats usually are restricted in diseases that interfere with their digestion or absorption, such as gallbladder disease and pancreatitis. A high-fat diet may be used in the treatment of epilepsy in children who do not respond to drug treatment.

Fish oils rich in omega-3 polyunsaturated fatty acids are the subject of research involving disease, especially coronary artery disease. The effects of fish oils are as follows: *beneficial*—reduce triglycerides, reduce blood pressure, have anticlotting properties; improves inflammatory reactions and immune response; *adverse*—increase LDL cholesterol, cause bleeding tendencies, elevate blood sugar in type II diabetes, possibly cause vitamin A and D toxicity (cod liver oil), and generate weight gain and excessive cholesterol intake.

Fish oils are potent metabolic substances. They should not be self-prescribed.

KEYS TO LEARNING

STUDY–DISCUSSION QUESTIONS

1. Using the 1-day food diary you kept in Chapter 5, calculate your intake of protein, fat, and carbohydrate by referring to Appendix E. Be sure to include (perhaps, estimate) the fat used in cooking and the fat and sugar used for flavoring food. Calculate the percentage of total calories derived from fat. (To do so, first obtain your total daily caloric intake by multiplying the grams of protein and carbohydrate by 4 and the grams of fat by 9. Then divide the fat calories by the total calories for the day). How does this percentage compare with the average fat consumption in the United States and with the recommendation that fat intake be reduced to 30% or less of total calories?

2. Classify the following as saturated, monounsaturated, or polyunsaturated: lamb chops, nondairy whipped topping, mayonnaise, olive oil, regular margarine, scrambled eggs, hamburger patty, vanilla ice cream, baked mackerel, devil's food cake with chocolate icing, corn oil, and butter.

3. Rank the following foods according to fat content, listing the one with the highest fat content first:

   ½ cup of ice cream
   1 cup of whole milk
   3 oz of sirloin steak
   20 large potato chips
   One glazed doughnut
   Two pieces of light-meat turkey (4 × 2.5 inches

   Check your answer with the fat content listed for each food in Appendix E.

4. What are the functions of cholesterol? Is food the only cholesterol source? What component of the diet has the greatest cholesterol-raising effect?

5. Discuss in class the role of fat in the development of atherosclerosis. What is the philosophy of the medical staff (internists and pediatricians) at your hospital concerning fat modification for at-risk people and for the general public? A hospital staff member (physician or dietitian) might be asked to assist you in your discussion.
6. Define the following labeling terms: *cholesterol-free, lowfat, lean, low cholesterol,* and *reduced fat.*

BIBLIOGRAPHY

BOOKS

Linscheer WG, Vergroesen AJ. Lipids. In: Shils ME, Olson JA, Shike M. Eds. Modern nutrition in health and disease. 8th ed. Philadelphia: Lea and Febiger, 1994:47.

National Academy of Sciences, National Research Council, Committee on Diet and Health, Food and Nutrition Board. Diet and health: implications for reducing chronic disease risk (executive summary). Washington, DC: National Academy Press, 1989.

National Academy of Sciences, National Research Council, Food and Nutrition Board. Recommended dietary allowances. 10th ed. Washington, DC: National Academy Press, 1989.

National Center for Nutrition and Dietetics of the American Dietetic Association. Nutrition fact sheet: facts about fat substitutes. Chicago: The American Dietetic Association Foundation, 1994.

National Cholesterol Education Program. Information on "recommended diets" (released June 15, 1993). Bethesda: National Heart Lung and Blood Institute, 1993.

US Dept of Health and Human Services, Public Health Service. The surgeon general's report on nutrition and health (summary and recommendations). Washington, DC: US Government Printing Office, 1988. US Dept of Health and Human Services publication PHS 88-50211.

Woteki CE, Thomas PR. Eds. Eat for life. Washington, DC: National Academy Press, 1992.

PERIODICALS

Farley D. Look for "legit" health claims on foods. FDA Consumer (Special Report: Focus on Food Labeling). May 1993: DHHS publication FDA 93-2262:21.

Kasim S. Is there a role for fish oils in diabetes treatment? Clin Diabetes 1989;7:93.

Kurtzweil P. Good reading for good eating. FDA Consumer (Special Report: Focus on food labeling). May 1993: DHHS publication FDA 93-2262:7.

Kurtzweil P. "Nutrition facts" to help consumers eat smart. FDA Consumer (Special Report: Focus on Food Labeling). May 1993. DHHS publication FDA 93-2262:34.

McBean LD. Health effects of dietary fatty acids. Dairy Council Digest 1992;63:3.

Mela DJ. Nutritional implications of fat substitutes. J Am Diet Assoc 1992;92:4:472.

Powers MA, Warshaw H. Fat replacers: a wide range of choices. Diabetes Spectrum 1992;5:2:72.

Stehlin D. A little "lite" reading. FDA Consumer (Special Report: Focus on Food Labeling). May 1993: DHHS publication FDA 93-2262:29.

Voss AC. Omega-3 fatty acids. Dietetic Currents 1993; 120:2.

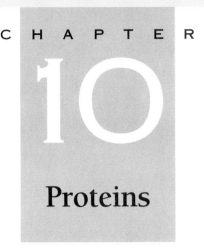

CHAPTER 10 Proteins

KEY TERMS

amino acids compounds containing nitrogen that are the building blocks of the protein molecule

antibody a protein substance produced within the body that destroys or weakens harmful bacteria

biologic value of protein the ability of a protein to support the formation of body tissue

complementary proteins the combination of protein foods that have opposite strengths and weaknesses in their amino acid compositions

complete protein a protein containing all the essential amino acids

edema swelling; a condition in which body tissues contain an excessive amount of body fluid

essential amino acids indispensable amino acids that the body cannot synthesize; they must be provided by food

immobility the condition of being inactive because of disability, such as that experienced by the person confined to bed or a wheelchair

incomplete protein a protein lacking one or more of the essential amino acids or containing some of the amino acids in only small amounts

kwashiorkor a severe protein deficiency disease

lactation the secretion of milk

marasmus a condition characterized by a loss of flesh and strength due to underfeeding; a lack of sufficient calories for a prolonged period

meat analogs foods manufactured from vegetable protein that are similar to animal foods in appearance, texture, and flavor

nonessential amino acids dispensable amino acids that the body can synthesize to meet its needs

textured vegetable protein protein drawn from plant protein, spun into fibers, and manufactured into products that imitate animal protein foods

OBJECTIVES

After completing this chapter, the student will be able to:

1. Discuss how the body uses protein.
2. Explain how amino acid composition affects protein quality and use.
3. Define *essential (indispensable) amino acids* and *nonessential (dispensable) amino acids* and *complete protein* and *incomplete protein.*
4. Explain how the role of protein in energy production compromises its role in tissue building.
5. List the sources of complete protein and incomplete protein; define *complementary proteins* and give examples.
6. Discuss the Recommended Dietary Allowances (RDAs) for protein for adults and how this amount compares with the typical protein consumption in the

United States. Why are authorities recommending a more moderate protein intake?
7. Explain what protein-related information is provided on food labels.
8. Develop an awareness of the profound effect of protein deficiency during illness.
9. Discuss the causes and symptoms of the two major manifestations of protein-calorie malnutrition: nutritional marasmus and kwashiorkor.

The word *protein* originates from a Greek word meaning *of first importance.* It well deserves its name.

In areas where protein quantity and quality are inadequate, the physical characteristics of whole groups of people may be affected. The increased height of the Japanese people in recent generations is an example of the effect of nutrition on stature. The change in stature was a result of an increase in both the total amount of protein and the amount of animal protein in the Japanese diet. Similarly, Japanese Americans who have lived in the United States for a generation or more are taller than their ancestors. Because of a limited diet, the Japanese previously did not reach their hereditary potential. Although it is difficult to assign priorities to the various nutrients, the present study of protein shows that the quality and quantity of protein in the daily diet are of extreme importance.

PROTEIN COMPOSITION

All protein molecules contain carbon, hydrogen, oxygen, and nitrogen. Proteins are the body's only source of nitrogen. Phosphorus and sulfur frequently are present, and some proteins may contain other elements, such as iron (in hemoglobin) and iodine (in thyroxine). The structure of protein is more varied and complex than that of either fats or carbohydrates.

Proteins are large complex molecules made up of amino acids. Amino acids are composed of an amino (nitrogen-containing) group and an acid or carboxyl group attached to the same carbon atom. During the process of digestion, proteins are broken down and released into the bloodstream as amino acids. More than 20 amino acids have been identified. A different grouping (R) attached to the carbon that holds the amino and carboxyl groups differentiates one amino acid from another (Fig. 10-1).

Both animal protein—except gelatin—and plant protein contain some of each of these 20 amino acids. The proportion of the amino acids in each food protein depends on the characteristics of that particular protein. The genetic code within the nucleus of every cell determines the pattern in which the amino acids are arranged to form a specific protein, such as muscle protein or liver protein. Amino acids can join in an almost unending variety of ways to form the estimated 100,000 proteins the body requires. A single protein may contain as few as 23 amino acids and as many as several hundred thousand amino acid units linked together. The amino acids that compose a specific protein are connected by *peptide linkages,* in which the amino group of one amino acid is linked to the carboxyl group of another amino acid.

CLASSIFICATION OF AMINO ACIDS

Amino acids are classified as *essential* or *indispensable,* and *nonessential* or *dispensable* (Display 10-1). Essential (indispensable) amino acids are those that the body cannot synthesize; therefore, they must come from food. Nine amino acids are essential (indispensable): histidine, isoleucine, leucine, lysine, methionine, phenylalanine, threonine, tryptophan, and valine.

Nonessential (dispensable) amino acids are those remaining amino acids that the body can synthesize in sufficient amounts to meet its needs. They are as important as the essential amino acids because they are required for the synthesis of all protein. If adequate amounts are not present when protein is being synthesized, the nonessential amino acids can be formed from essential amino acids or from substances manufactured in the cell.

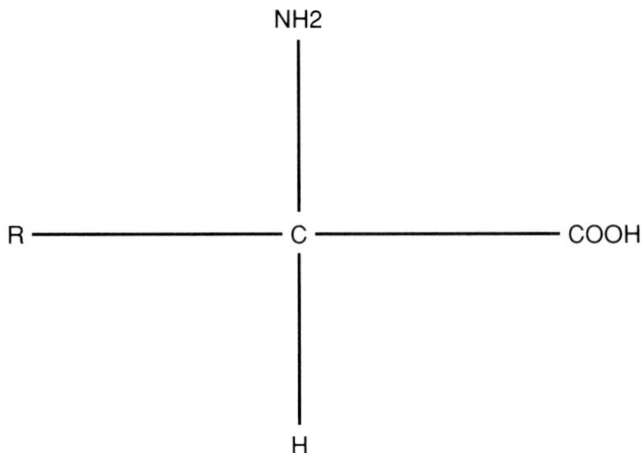

A basic amino group and an acid carboxyl group are attached to the same carbon atom. Amino acids differ from one another by the remainder of the molecule (R), which may contain various groupings.

FIGURE 10-1

Basic structure of an amino acid.

The term *conditionally essential* (indispensable) refers to amino acids that are ordinarily nonessential, but because of impaired metabolism or the individual's physical state, the body may be unable to synthesize them in large enough amounts to meet its needs. Conditionally essential amino acids in premature infants are taurine, cystine, and possibly tyrosine.

PROTEIN QUALITY

Each body cell is composed mainly of protein. Protein makes up the membrane surrounding the cell and also occurs within the cell. During growth periods, such as childhood, adolescence, and pregnancy, the number of cells increases. Protein is required for this cell growth. In all stages of life, tissue protein is constantly being broken down and must be replaced by dietary protein. Proteins also are needed for the formation of enzymes, antibodies, and hormones and other substances that regulate body processes.

Not all dietary protein is used for tissue growth and repair. How much is used depends on its ability to support the formation of body tissue.

A variety of methods can determine the quality of protein foods and food combinations. Two of these methods are the *protein efficiency ratio (PER)* and the *biologic value of protein*. The PER involves feeding a known amount of the test protein to young rats for 4 weeks and determining their weight gain during this period. The PER is calculated by dividing the number of grams of weight gained by the number of grams of protein fed. This ratio is compared to the PER of a high-quality protein such as a milk protein. Proteins of high quality have a PER of 2.5 or better, meaning that the rats have gained 2.5 g or more for every gram of protein fed.

The biologic value method involves determining the amount of nitrogen retained in the body for growth and maintenance. This involves measuring the amount of nitrogen ingested and the amount of nitrogen in urine and feces. The percentage of absorbed nitrogen retained in the body is the **biologic value**. Proteins with a score of 70 or better are considered to be capable of supporting growth.

The nutritional quality of a protein is determined by two factors: its amino acid makeup and how well it is digested and absorbed.

DISPLAY 10-1 CLASSIFICATION OF AMINO ACIDS

ESSENTIAL (INDISPENSABLE)	NONESSENTIAL (DISPENSABLE)
Histidine	Alanine
Isoleucine	Arginine
Leucine	Aspartic acid
Lysine	Cystine*
Methionine	Glutamic acid
Phenylalanine	Glutamine
Threonine	Glycine
Tryptophan	Proline
Valine	Serine
	Taurine
	Tyrosine†

* Cystine can replace 30% of the requirement for methionine.
† Tyrosine can replace 50% of the requirement for phenylalanine.

AMINO ACID COMPOSITION

Proteins that contain all the essential amino acids in the proportions needed by the body have a high biologic value and are sometimes referred to as *complete proteins.* Proteins that supply some of the essential amino acids in limited amounts and are of lower biologic value are *incomplete proteins.*

The production of body protein stops once the supply of just one amino acid is exhausted. This stoppage occurs no matter how generous the amounts of the remaining amino acids. The essential amino acids not used for tissue building are broken down and used for energy. The body cannot store these amino acids for later use.

Animal protein is the best-quality protein because of its similarity to human protein tissue. Egg protein is considered to have the best amino acid pattern of any food; milk protein ranks next. Gelatin is the only animal protein of poor quality. It is completely lacking in two essential amino acids and has inadequate amounts of other amino acids. Animal foods such as meat, poultry, fish, eggs, milk, and cheese provide liberal amounts of complete proteins.

Plant protein, except processed soy protein, is of lower quality than animal protein because it lacks sufficient amounts of one or more essential amino acids. The amino acid that is in short supply is called the *limiting amino acid.* Cereal grains such as wheat and rice are low in lysine; corn is low in lysine and tryptophan; and legumes have limited amounts of methionine. Legumes (beans, peas, lentils, peanuts, and soybeans), nuts, and seeds contain the best-quality plant protein. Although generally of lower quality than animal proteins, plant proteins make an important contribution to the world's protein supply (see the discussion in the next section).

Advances made in processing proteins from soybeans have produced products that are nutritionally equivalent to food proteins of animal origin. These processed soy protein products include soy protein concentrates and isolated soy proteins—soybean products with varying amounts of oil and the water-soluble nonprotein substances removed. Soy protein concentrates are at least 65% protein on a moisture-free basis, and isolated soy protein is at least 90% protein on a moisture-free basis.

COMPLEMENTARITY

Fortunately, plant proteins are not all lacking in the same amino acids. When a variety of foods such as grains, vegetables, legumes, seeds, and nuts are eaten daily, one protein food supplies the amino acids that are limited in another food. A food that provides the amino acids that are in short supply in another is said to complement the other (Display 10-2). For example, legumes are high in lysine and low in methionine, and grains are low in lysine and high in methionine. These foods complement each other and together provide high-quality protein. After absorption, amino acids from food and those from sources within the body combine in the body's protein pool. Because sources of amino acids are available from within the body, it is unnecessary that complementary proteins be precisely matched at each meal, but they should be consumed over the course of the day.

DISPLAY 10-2 COMBINATIONS OF FOODS THAT SUPPLY COMPLEMENTARY AMINO ACIDS

PROTEIN-RICH COMBINATIONS	EXAMPLES
Legumes plus grains	Macaroni and bean soup Beans and rice chili Peanut butter and bread Lentil soup with rice Baked beans with brown bread
Legumes plus seeds plus nuts	Roasted soybeans, sunflower seed, peanut snack mix
Plant protein plus small amounts of animal protein	Cereal and milk Lentil curry (made with yogurt) Bean soup with small pieces of meat Macaroni and cheese Cheese pizza

Another way to improve the quality of vegetable proteins is to serve them with small quantities of animal protein food. Bean soup with small pieces of meat and macaroni and cheese are examples of nourishing combinations. Even small amounts of animal protein that contain all the essential amino acids can provide for the limiting amino acid in the vegetable protein.

Nutrition counselors need to know about complementary proteins. They can put this knowledge to good use in areas where animal protein is scarce; as the world's protein supply diminishes, an understanding of complementarity will become increasingly important. Such knowledge also is important in planning diets for vegetarians. When plant proteins from a reasonable variety of plant sources are consumed in a diet that meets energy needs, adequate amounts of essential and nonessential amino acids are supplied.

The Institute of Nutrition in Central America and Panama (INCAP) has developed a food, Incaparina, based on the principle of protein complementarity. This all-plant product meets the growth needs of small children, even those suffering from severe malnutrition.

DIGESTIBILITY

The degree to which a protein is digested also influences its nutritional value. Animal protein is digested more efficiently than plant protein because digestive enzymes have greater difficulty reaching plant cells, which are surrounded by cellulose and woody substances. Thorough chewing aids protein digestion.

The method of cooking also affects digestibility. Heat alters the structure but not the amino acid content of protein molecules. Overheating, however, may destroy some amino acids or may cause the formation of products resistant to digestive enzymes. Cooking with water improves the digestibility of wheat protein and rice. Cooking may make some protein foods more palatable.

Protein foods spoil more quickly than carbohydrate or fat foods. In the moist state in which they are generally found in foods, proteins decompose readily at room temperature. This breakdown is due to bacterial action, which may lead to the formation of poisonous substances. To prevent or delay spoilage, keep protein foods such as fresh meat, fish, poultry, milk, and eggs in the refrigerator.

PROTEIN DIGESTION, ABSORPTION, AND METABOLISM

Protein digestion involves both the digestion of protein in the diet and also the digestion of cells that have been shed from the intestinal mucosa and the used-up digestive enzymes. The total amount of protein requiring digestion may be double the amount consumed in food. To be absorbed, proteins must be broken down to individual amino acids or small *peptides* (breakdown products of protein digestion composed of only two or three amino acids).

Digestion of protein begins in the stomach through the action of pepsin, which reduces protein molecules to polypeptides. In the small intestine, a series of protein-splitting enzymes reduce the polypeptides to dipeptides and amino acids. Table 10-1 summarizes protein digestion.

The products of protein digestion are released into the bloodstream as amino acids and are transported by the portal vein to the liver and then to all the body cells. Some amino acids stay in the liver to form liver tissue or to produce a variety of plasma proteins. The remaining amino acids circulate in the bloodstream, from which they are rapidly removed and used by the tissues.

When amino acids are broken down, the nitrogen-containing part is split off from the carbon chain. Most of the nitrogen is converted to urea in the liver and excreted by the kidneys. The carbon-containing portion is used for energy.

METABOLIC POOL OF AMINO ACIDS

The body does not store amino acids. Rather, it metabolizes any amount above that needed for the synthesis of tissue and various regulatory sub-

TABLE 10-1 SUMMARY OF PROTEIN DIGESTION

PLACE OF ACTION	PROTEIN	ENZYME	END PRODUCT
Stomach	Protein	Pepsin (in acid environment) →	Large peptides (polypeptides)
Small intestine	Protein, polypeptides	Trypsin, chymotrypsin, carboxypeptidases (secreted by pancreas) →	Polypeptides, dipeptides, amino acids
	Polypeptides, dipeptides	Peptidases (secreted by mucosal cells of small intestine) →	Smaller peptides, amino acids ↓ Enter portal blood ↓ Liver ↓ Body tissues

stances. However, within the body cells, there is a metabolic pool of amino acids in a state of flux that may be called on to meet the demand for amino acids by various cells and tissues.

The body is said to be in a *dynamic state,* that is, the cells are continually being broken down (*catabolism*) and replaced (*anabolism*). The rate of turnover depends on the type of tissue; some cells replace themselves every few days, whereas others, such as those in bone tissue, turn over much more slowly.

Daily protein turnover is several times the normal protein intake. When protein tissue is broken down, amino acids are released into the plasma to be reused for building and repair. It makes no difference whether the amino acids were originally made by the body or obtained from the diet; the body uses them for the same purposes.

This process of recycling is not totally complete. Some amino acids are lost as a result of the metabolism of protein. The end products of protein metabolism—urea, creatinine, uric acid, and others—are excreted in the urine. Additional loss of amino acids occurs in the feces, sweat, and other body secretions and in losses of protein tissue from the skin, hair, and nails. Protein in the diet must replace these losses, even when growth has stopped.

NITROGEN BALANCE

Proteins are the body's only source of nitrogen. Each gram of nitrogen, whether in food, tissue, or urine and feces, represents 6.25 g of protein. Most of the nitrogen resulting from the breakdown of body tissue is excreted in the urine and feces. If 10 g of nitrogen is found in the urine and feces of a person within a specified period, it can be assumed that about 62.5 g of body protein were broken down during that period.

When the quantity of nitrogen from food proteins is about equal to the quantity lost in the feces and urine, the person is said to be in *nitrogen balance.* Nitrogen balance indicates that body tissue is being adequately replaced and repaired and that there is no increase or decrease in total amount of body tissues.

In *positive nitrogen balance,* more nitrogen is taken in than is lost. Positive nitrogen balance is seen when new tissue is being built, as in infancy and childhood, in adolescence, in pregnancy and lactation, and during recovery from an illness or injury in which protein has been lost.

In *negative nitrogen balance*, more nitrogen is lost than is consumed in food protein. Body tissue is breaking down faster than it is being replaced. Negative nitrogen balance is seen when protein intake is too low or of poor quality. Tissue needs for all the essential amino acids are not being met, so nitrogen is being excreted. Negative nitrogen balance also develops when insufficient calories are consumed to meet energy needs. In this case, rather than being used to build body tissue, body protein is broken down to supply energy.

Accelerated breakdown of body tissue due to surgery, injury, severe burns, and fever results in negative nitrogen balance, as does the inactivity imposed on bedridden patients, even when protein intake appears to be adequate. If a sick person does not eat enough protein food to meet the increased needs of his or her illness, the body will lose protein tissue. The same will occur if caloric intake is insufficient. The body will break down body tissue to meet energy needs. Muscles that are not regularly used break down rapidly and are replaced with fatty tissue. During early space explorations, astronauts experienced some breakdown of body tissue, attributed in part to weightlessness in a gravity-free environment. When exercise routines were introduced during subsequent flights, nitrogen loss diminished.

FUNCTIONS OF PROTEIN

TISSUE MAINTENANCE AND GROWTH

Protein is essential for the growth and maintenance of body tissue because it is an essential component of the cells of all living things. Proteins are a major structural component not only of body tissue but also of enzymes, hormones, and body fluids. Only bile and urine do not normally contain protein. Each cell has the ability to synthesize an enormous number of proteins. Normal tissue growth in infancy and childhood and during pregnancy and lactation necessitates amino acids above those needed for tissue maintenance. As many laboratory studies have demonstrated, in the absence of adequate protein, growth is slowed down or even stopped (Fig. 10-2). A sick person's protein needs may be similar to a growing person's protein needs. Additional protein is needed to build new tissue for wound healing and for recovery from surgery, burns, fever, and other conditions that are associated with abnormally high tissue breakdown.

FORMATION OF REGULATORY COMPOUNDS

Hormones, enzymes, and most other regulatory materials in the body are protein substances. Hormones such as insulin, thyroxine, and epinephrine have vital regulatory functions. Every cell contains many different enzymes, each of which is responsible for directing specific chemical reactions necessary to the cell's life processes. Another protein, hemoglobin, is responsible for carrying oxygen to the cells and carbon dioxide to the lungs. Nucleoproteins found in ribonucleic acid (RNA) and deoxyribonucleic acid (DNA) are another example of the regulatory functions of protein.

PROVISION OF TRANSPORT MECHANISMS

Proteins participate in the transport of nutrients and other substances in the body, especially those that are not water soluble. Lipoproteins in the blood transport triglyceride, cholesterol, phospho-

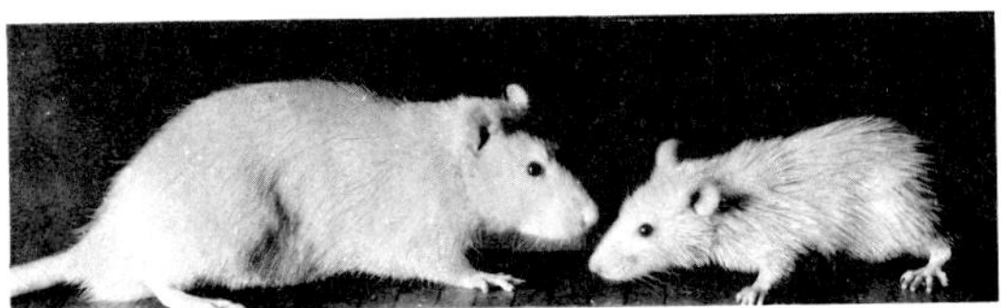

FIGURE 10-2

Adequate and inadequate protein (18% versus 4%) in rats of the same litter. This deficiency produces stunted growth but no deformities.

lipids, and fat-soluble vitamins. Many vitamins and minerals depend on protein for transport. Albumin, the chief protein in the blood serum, carries free fatty acids and acts as a carrier for many drugs.

MAINTENANCE OF FLUID BALANCE

Proteins assist in regulating the fluid balance of cells. Plasma protein molecules are so large that they cannot pass through the capillary membranes; thus they remain in the blood vessels. The presence of these large molecules in the blood vessels creates the pressure needed to draw fluid back out of the cell so that it does not accumulate in the tissues. In a protein deficiency, the number of plasma proteins in the blood is reduced; consequently, the pressure they exert also is reduced. When there is insufficient pressure to remove fluid from the tissues, edema results. Furthermore, hormonal changes interfere with the excretion of fluid. Edema is a symptom of severe protein deficiency.

MAINTENANCE OF BLOOD NEUTRALITY

For normal function, it is essential that the blood be maintained at a nearly neutral, slightly alkaline (or basic) state. A change in pH (acidity or alkalinity) can so alter enzymes that they no longer function. Certain foods can cause acids or bases (alkalies) to form. The presence of protein in the blood prevents the accumulation of too much acid or base. Proteins, because of their structure, can serve as either acids or bases, according to body needs.

PROVISION OF ENERGY

Proteins, like carbohydrate, supply 4 calories per gram. The body's first need is for energy. When calories from fat and carbohydrate in the diet do not meet the body's energy needs, the body breaks down protein to supply energy. This breakdown occurs in the liver, where the amino group is detached from the carbon portion of the molecule. The carbon portion is converted to some of the same substances formed during the breakdown of glucose and fats. Approximately 58% of the protein consumed can be converted to glucose. In starvation, the body uses its protein tissue and fat stores to supply energy. It uses the protein in muscle tissue first, before the protein in vital organs.

Because protein cannot be stored, the excess is converted to energy, which, if not needed, is then converted to fat. The use of protein for energy purposes, however, is expensive in terms of both body needs and economics. If protein is used for energy, it cannot perform its many other vital functions. Proteins also require more energy than carbohydrates for their metabolism. Because protein foods are the most costly foods, using protein for energy is an unnecessary expense.

Most Americans consume more protein than they need. Surveys conducted by the US Department of Agriculture have indicated that protein provides 14% to 18% of the total calories consumed in the American diet. A man aged 25 to 50 years, weighing 174 lb (79 kg), who is consuming the Recommended Dietary Allowance (RDA) for protein of .8g/kg of body weight and the recommended energy intake of 2900 kcal (see Table 7-1), is deriving only about 9% of his total calories from protein.

ANTIBODY FORMATION

Antibodies are proteins that assist the body in fighting infection and other toxic conditions. When the diet does not contain sufficient protein, the production of antibodies is slowed, and susceptibility to infections is increased.

PROTEIN SOURCES

Because protein is a part of cell structure, it occurs in all foods, regardless of the source (Table 10-2). Nevertheless, the protein content of food varies widely.

TABLE 10-2 COMPARISON OF PROTEIN IN SELECTED FOODS*

FOOD	AMOUNT	PROTEIN (G)	BIOLOGIC VALUE OF PROTEIN
Beef round roast	3 oz	25	Complete
Leg of lamb	3 oz	22	Complete
Pork roast	3 oz	21	Complete
Veal cutlet	3 oz	23	Complete
Turkey, light meat	3 oz	25	Complete
Tuna in oil	3 oz	24	Complete
Flounder	3 oz	17	Complete
Spiced ham	3 oz	10	Complete
Frankfurter	1 (1.6 oz)	5	Complete
Peanut butter	1 tbsp	5	Incomplete
Kidney beans	½ cup	7–8	Incomplete
Broccoli	½ cup	3	Incomplete
Carrots	½ cup	1	Incomplete
Applesauce	½ cup	Trace	
Orange	1	1	Incomplete
40% Bran Flakes	¾ cup	4	Incomplete
Bread, white	1 slice (18 per loaf)	2	Incomplete
Egg	1	6	Complete
Nonfat dried milk	1 oz	10	Complete
Milk	1 cup	8	Complete
Cottage cheese	½ cup	14	Complete
Cheddar cheese	2 oz	14	Complete

* Source of nutritive values: US Dept of Agriculture, Human Nutrition Information Service. Nutritive value of food. Washington, DC: US Government Printing Office, 1991. Home and Garden bulletin 72.

Animal sources of protein include milk and milk products (except butter), meat, fish, seafood, poultry, and eggs. Plant sources include cereals (wheat, rye, rice, corn, and barley), legumes (peanuts, dry beans, dry peas, soybeans, and lentils), and nuts and seeds.

ANIMAL SOURCES

MEAT, POULTRY, AND FISH

Meat, poultry, and fish are excellent sources of protein. The protein contents of beef, lamb, pork, fish, and poultry are nearly equal. Beef, the most popular meat in the United States, is wasteful in calories because of its high fat content; a 3-oz piece of rib roast contains about 300 kcal, whereas a 3-oz boneless chicken breast contains about 140 kcal.

Organs and glands (liver, kidney, brain, heart, and sweetbreads, all known as *variety meats*) are richer in vitamins and minerals than muscle meats but, unfortunately, have a high cholesterol content. Liver is high in protein. Luncheon meats, such as spiced ham, liverwurst, bologna, and pressed meat loaves, cold sausages and frankfurters, and cooked pork sausage have about one half to two thirds the protein content of plain meat, fish, or poultry. Although these meats often are considered to be the basis of inexpensive meals, they may be costly sources of protein. For example, a 2-oz portion of bologna or one frankfurter contains only 7 g of protein, whereas a 2-oz portion of ground beef contains 14 g of protein.

MILK AND MILK PRODUCTS

Milk is a less concentrated but valuable source of protein. An 8-oz glass of milk contains about 8.5 g of protein. Two 8-oz glasses of milk provide half the daily protein recommended for a child aged 4 to 6 years. Milk also should help satisfy adult protein needs. Fortified fresh skim milk or fortified reconstituted nonfat dry milk provide the same quantity of protein, calcium, and vitamins as fresh whole milk. Nonfat dry milk is an inexpensive source of milk protein (it costs about one third the price of fresh whole milk); it is the cheapest available source of complete protein. Health workers should encourage its use by people who have limited money to purchase other animal protein foods.

American cheddar cheese contains 21 g of protein in a 3-oz portion, equivalent to the amount of protein in meat. Cottage cheese contains more moisture and is therefore a less concentrated source of protein. A 3-oz portion of cottage cheese provides about 12 g of protein. A 4-oz portion of ice cream provides 4.5 g of protein.

EGGS

Eggs contain excellent-quality protein: one egg provides 6 g. The white is mostly protein and contains no fat or cholesterol.

PLANT SOURCES

Most vegetables contain small amounts of protein: 1 to 3 g per average serving. An exception is legumes, which may contain 4% to 6% protein when fresh and 7% to 9% protein in dried form. Fruits contain little protein: 1 g or less per average serving.

LEGUMES

Legumes—including peas, lentils, kidney beans, navy beans, pinto beans, garbanzos (chick peas), lima beans, soybeans, and peanuts—deposit large amounts of protein in their seeds with the help of bacteria that live in the plant roots. The bacteria are capable of converting atmospheric nitrogen to a form the plant can use. Because legumes provide much protein, they are useful meat substitutes. Lentil soup, split pea soup, chili beans, baked beans, lima bean casseroles, and peanut butter are good, low-cost substitutes for meat. A $\frac{1}{2}$ cup portion of legumes provides 6 to 8 g of protein. Peanut butter contains 5 g of protein per tablespoon. Although the protein of legumes is not as high quality as animal protein, it is an adequate substitute when eaten in combination with other foods, particularly wheat or corn products.

In Eastern Asia, soybeans have been an important part of the diet for centuries; the Japanese obtain 12% to 13% of their protein from soybeans in the form of soy milk, cheese, flour, and sauce and from the beans themselves, either dried or fresh.

NUTS AND SEEDS

Nuts and seeds provide substantial amounts of protein of fairly high quality. They are high in fat and consequently high in calories, however. Because they are expensive, nuts have not become an important source of protein in the diet.

BREADS AND CEREALS

Breads and processed or cooked cereal products provide only small amounts of protein: 2 to 3 g per serving. Use of these foods throughout the day, however, makes a good contribution to the day's protein intake. For example, a serving of cereal and one slice of toast at breakfast, two sandwiches at lunch, and two slices of bread at dinner provide 16 to 20 g of protein.

Cereal grains are the major source of protein for people around the world. Cereals eaten in a mixed diet with legumes and small amounts of animal protein provide all of the essential amino acids.

CONSUMER ISSUES

LABELING

The protein content in grams per serving is a mandatory component of "Nutrition Facts"—the nutrition panel on food labels. In addition, a "% Daily Value" is given for the protein content per serving of the product. The "% Daily Value" for protein is based on 10% of total calories for adults and children older than age 4 years. For labeling purposes, 2000 calories has been established as the reference for calculating "% Daily Value." Therefore, 10% of calories from protein in a daily diet of 2000 kcal represents 50 g of protein ($2000 \times .10 \div 4 = 50$). If the manufacturer uses the option of listing "% Daily Value" for other calorie levels, the Daily Reference Value (DRV) for protein must be based on 10% of calories.

However, the DRV for protein does not apply to certain populations. DRVs for proteins have been established for the following groups: children aged 1 to 4 years: 16 g; infants younger than 1 year: 14 g; pregnant women: 60 g; breastfeeding mothers: 65 g.

Another protein-related regulation requires that manufacturers list on the ingredients label sources of protein hydrolysates used as additives in foods. (*Hydrolyzed proteins* are proteins broken down into amino acids.) Manufacturers may no longer use general terms such as "hydrolyzed vegetable protein." They must now identify the specific protein source such as "hydrolyzed corn protein" or "hydrolyzed casein." This is of importance to consumers who for religious, cultural, or health reasons (e.g., food allergy) need this specific information.

NEW PROTEIN SOURCES

Scientists searching for low-cost, protein-rich foods to extend the lessening protein supply in the world have made progress. One development is *textured vegetable proteins,* manufactured by the extraction of protein from certain oil seeds such as soybeans, peanuts, and cottonseed, which contain no cholesterol and are low in saturated fats. The proteins are combined with colors, flavors, and other ingredients to create food products resembling chicken, beef, tuna, sausage, bacon, and other foods. Textured vegetable proteins are called *analogs* because they resemble other foods. They are useful meat substitutes in vegetarian diets. Textured vegetable proteins provide an inexpensive extender to ground meat.

Single-cell proteins, both microorganisms and algae, are being investigated as potential sources of protein food. Leaf protein, extracted from the leaves of many food crops such as beans and peas, also is the subject of research.

ANIMAL PROTEIN PRODUCTION

Most Americans associate protein with meat. In many developing countries, cereals provide 70% to 80% of the protein in the diet. This near-vegetarian diet is due to economic factors and a scarcity of animal foods. As income increases, the consumption of animal protein also usually increases. The production of animal protein, however, is a wasteful process. Grain must be raised to feed the animals, which humans use for food. Only an estimated 15% of the protein fed to animals is converted to protein that people can eat in the form of meat, milk, and eggs. The amount of grain required to feed the animals that supply the meat, poultry, eggs, and dairy products for one American for 1 year is almost 1 ton—enough to feed many humans directly. More energy is used to produce animal food than is obtained from consuming it.

RECOMMENDED PROTEIN INTAKE

Protein malnutrition is not a common problem in the United States. The average daily intake of protein, about 14% to 18% of total calories, is well above recommended levels. Of this protein, about 60% comes from animal sources such as meat, fish, poultry, eggs, and dairy products (Table 10-3).

TABLE 10-3 PROTEIN CONTENT OF A TYPICAL DAY'S DIET

FOOD	AMOUNT	PROTEIN (G)
Milk	2 cups	16
Meat fish, poultry, egg	6 oz	42
Vegetables		
Potato	1, medium	2
Other vegetables	2 servings	4
Fruits		
Citrus	1 serving	0.5
Other	1 serving	0.5
Bread	4 slices	12
Cereal	1 oz dry or ½ cup cooked	3
Butter, margarine, oil	1 tbsp or more	0
Total		80

Age and body size greatly affect a person's protein needs. The larger a person, the greater amount of living tissue to be maintained and repaired. Age provides an indication of whether more protein than the amount required for maintenance is needed for growth.

In 1989, the National Academy of Sciences Food and Nutrition Board recommended protein allowances ranging from 2.2 g/kg body weight for infants up to age 6 months to .8 g/kg of body weight for males older than age 18 years and for females older than age 14 years. The recommendation is the same for the elderly. The RDA committee felt that research data on this age group was insufficient to establish a separate allowance. The board also recommended an additional 10 g protein per day during pregnancy and an additional 15 g protein per day during the first 6 months of lactation. During the second 6 months of lactation, this allowance would be reduced to 12 g (Table 10-4).

Although not specified by the RDA committee, it is desirable that **at least** one fifth of the daily protein intake for adults and two fifths for children be derived from complete protein foods. Persons consuming diets composed totally of vegetable protein require more total protein than those people consuming diets of mixed vegetable and animal proteins. More protein is required because more of the lower-quality protein will be needed to meet requirements for amino acids and because vegetable proteins are not as completely digested as animal protein and, therefore, are less available. Vegetarian diets are discussed in Chapter 15.

TABLE 10-4 RECOMMENDED ALLOWANCES OF U.S. DIETARY PROTEIN

CATEGORY	AGE (Y) OR CONDITION	WEIGHT (KG)	RDA (g/kg)*	RDA (g/day)
Both genders	0–0.5	6	2.2†	13
	0.5–1	9	1.6	14
	1–3	13	1.2	16
	4–6	20	1.1	24
	7–10	28	1.0	28
Males	11–14	45	1.0	45
	15–18	66	0.9	59
	19–24	72	0.8	58
	25–50	79	0.8	63
	51+	77	0.8	63
Females	11–14	46	1.0	46
	15–18	55	0.8	44
	19–24	58	0.8	46
	25–50	63	0.8	50
	51+	65	0.8	50
Pregnancy	1st trimester			+10
	2nd trimester			+10
	3rd trimester			+10
Lactation	1st 6 months			+15
	2nd 6 months			+12

* Amino acid score of typical U.S. diet is 100 for all age groups, except young infants. Digestibility is equal to reference proteins. Values have been rounded upward to 0.1 g/kg.

† For infants 0 to age 3 months, breastfeeding that meets energy needs also meets protein needs. Formula substitutes should have the same amount and amino acid composition as human milk, corrected for digestibility if appropriate.

(Adapted from National Academy of Sciences Food and Nutrition Board, National Research Council. Recommended dietary allowances. 10th ed. Washington, DC: National Academy Press, 1989:66.)

PROTEIN AND HEALTH

PROTEIN EXCESS

The National Academy of Sciences Committee on Diet and Health has recommended that protein intake be maintained at less than twice the RDA (less than 1.6 g/kg of desirable body weight). This advice is based mainly on epidemiologic studies, which have associated high consumption of meat with atherosclerotic coronary heart disease and certain cancers, especially breast and colon cancer. Whether it is the protein itself or another characteristic of a high-meat diet (e.g., high fat, high cholesterol, few vegetables) that is the offender is unknown. The committee did not recommend eliminating meat from the diet, but suggested that portions be small and that people eat meat less frequently.

High-protein diets also may lead to excessive loss of calcium in the urine, which may be a factor in the development of osteoporosis. Another concern, supported in animal studies, is that excess protein may accelerate a type of kidney disease commonly associated with aging.

PROTEIN DEFICIENCY

Protein deficiency usually accompanies a deficiency of calories and other nutrients. Severe protein deficiency rarely occurs in the United States except as a result of disease and poor nutritional management of acutely ill people.

The effects of protein loss during illness and injury are far reaching. The most evident result is the wasting of muscle tissue and consequent weight loss. Other symptoms include anemia and delayed healing of wounds and fractures. A lowering of serum protein levels and hormonal changes may result in edema, and the reduced production of antibodies makes the affected person susceptible to infection.

Protein losses occur following surgery and during serious illness and injury. The loss of protein is especially acute after bone fractures, burns, and liver surgery. People on bed rest, especially elderly people, lose protein even when their protein intake seems adequate. The ingestion of extra protein during convalescence promotes recovery.

PROTEIN-CALORIE MALNUTRITION

Protein-calorie malnutrition refers to a group of diseases caused by deficiencies of both proteins and calories and frequently accompanied by infections. A vicious cycle develops in which the malnutrition creates a susceptibility to infection and the infection further aggravates the poor nutritional condition. In children who are malnourished, common childhood diseases have serious effects. Protein-calorie malnutrition is the most serious and widespread deficiency disease in developing countries.

The two major manifestations of protein-calorie malnutrition are *marasmus* and *kwashiorkor*. Nutritional marasmus is caused by a diet severely deficient in calories, as well as protein and other nutrients, for a prolonged period. It most frequently is seen in infants and is characterized by muscle wasting, loss of subcutaneous fat, and low body weight. Kwashiorkor primarily results from a protein deficiency. A calorie deficiency is a contributing factor. Associated symptoms include retarded growth, muscle wasting, edema, depigmentation of hair and skin, enlarged liver, mental apathy, and general misery (see Fig. 10-3). The victims are children aged 1 to 3 years whom the mother weans from breast milk abruptly because of the birth of a sibling or because she is pregnant; the children are fed a diet of grains or roots, which are difficult to digest and are poor sources of protein.

Between these two conditions are a variety of disease states that combine some of the features of each. Retarded growth is found in all forms of protein-calorie malnutrition. In general, marasmus is characteristic of urban slums and shantytowns, whereas kwashiorkor most frequently occurs in rural villages.

To prevent and treat these diseases where milk is not readily available, vegetable protein mixtures suitable for infants and young children have been developed. These mixtures comprise locally grown foods. Incaparina is an example.

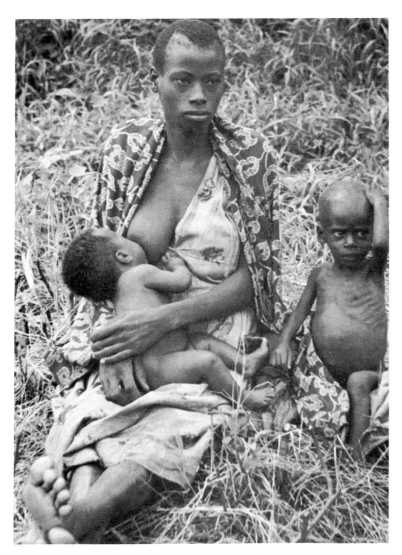

FIGURE 10-3

The older child in this picture shows the protein-calorie deprivation and the malnutrition that occurred when he was deposed, or replaced, at his mother's breast by the new baby. He is subsisting on starchy foods and a few vegetables. *(Courtesy John Bennett, MD, Nutrition Unit, Ministry of Health, Kampala, Uganda.)*

VEGETARIANISM

Vegetarian diets are associated with decreased risk of several chronic degenerative diseases and conditions including obesity, coronary artery disease, hypertension, diabetes mellitus, and some types of cancer. With careful planning, the vegetarian diet can be nutritionally adequate. Whole grains, legumes, vegetables, seeds, and nuts all contain essential and nonessential amino acids. It is important to include a wide variety of plant foods and sufficient caloric intake to meet energy needs. (See Chapter 15 for a more detailed discussion of vegetarianism.)

ABNORMALITIES OF PROTEIN METABOLISM

Some infants are born with the inability to produce the enzymes necessary for the normal metabolism of certain amino acids. In one such disease, *phen-*

ylketonuria, the amino acid phenylalanine and its breakdown products build up in the blood (see Chapter 17).

A person whose digestive system is genetically unable to break down the proteins in specific foods to amino acids develops an allergy to those foods. In an allergic reaction, the body senses the offending protein as foreign and tries to reject it (see Chapter 30).

PROTEIN RESTRICTION

Certain symptoms such as impending hepatic coma in liver disease and uremia in kidney disease may require the restriction of protein. In Parkinson's disease, protein appears to interfere with the action of the drug levodopa used in treatment. Some patients benefit from a reduction of protein in the diet or redistribution of protein intake over the day.

KEYS TO PRACTICAL APPLICATION

Eat moderate amounts of animal protein. Excess protein is wasteful, because the excess is converted to energy and excess energy is converted to fat. Protein food is an expensive form of energy.

Be aware of the wastefulness of using protein supplements under normal conditions. Most Americans consume more protein than they need.

Be aware that protein foods are not low in calories. They provide the same number of calories per gram as carbohydrates. Furthermore, protein foods such as meats and cheese frequently contain many calories from fat.

Eat good-quality protein at each meal to provide a consistent supply of essential amino acids.

At least one fifth of the daily protein intake for adults and two fifths for children should be in the form of animal sources.

Encourage the use of nonfat dry milk as a beverage and in cooking when funds are limited. It is the least expensive source of complete protein.

Plan meals around complementary vegetable protein foods for variety, economy, and increased fiber.

Be aware that meals containing legumes and grains, frequently used by various ethnic groups, are nourishing.

Encourage elderly people to eat sufficient amounts of protein. They need as much as, if not more than, younger adults.

Be aware of the importance of eating sufficient calories as well as extra protein during illnesses that cause excessive breakdown of body tissue. If calories from carbohydrates and fats are insufficient, the body will use protein for energy instead of tissue building and maintenance.

KEY IDEAS

Proteins are composed of carbon, hydrogen, oxygen, and nitrogen; they provide the foundation of every body cell. Proteins are the body's only source of nitrogen.

Proteins are large molecules made up of amino acids joined in long chains.

The amino acids in a specific protein are connected by peptide linkages in which the amino group is linked to the carboxyl group of another amino acid.

Amino acids are classified as *essential (indispensable)*—those the body cannot synthesize and must be obtained from food—and *nonessential (dispensable)*—those the body can synthesize.

Whether a protein food can be used for the growth and repair of tissue depends on its protein quality. Complete proteins contain all the essential amino acids in adequate amounts; proteins of low BV (incomplete proteins) have inadequate amounts of one or more amino acids.

Animal proteins (except gelatin) are complete proteins; vegetable proteins are incomplete.

High-quality protein can result from complementary mixtures of plant proteins, in which one plant protein supplies the amino acid the other plant protein is lacking. Some processed soy products are nutritionally equivalent to animal protein.

Protein provides for growth and maintenance of body tissues; is necessary for the formation of substances needed to regulate body processes, such as hormones and enzymes; is necessary for the formation of antibodies, which help fight infection; assists in regulating fluid balance; helps maintain acid–base balance; provides energy; and provides a transport mechanism for certain nutrients.

Protein in excess of body needs is converted to energy or to carbohydrate and fat; when there is a shortage of total energy, amino acids are used for energy rather than tissue building.

Although the body does not store amino acids, there is a metabolic pool of amino acids in a state of flux that may be called on to meet the demand for amino acids by various cells and tissues.

Body cells are in a dynamic state; they continually are being broken down and replaced. Nitrogen balance studies have compared the amount of nitrogen consumed in food with the amount lost in feces and urine to determine whether there is gain, loss, or maintenance of body tissue. In nitrogen balance, body tissues are adequately replaced and repaired; in positive nitrogen balance, new tissue is built; and in negative nitrogen balance, body tissue is broken down faster than it is replaced.

Animal sources of protein include milk and milk products, meat, fish, poultry, and eggs; plant sources include breads and cereal products, legumes, nuts and seeds, and textured vegetable protein.

Cereal grains are the primary source of protein for the majority of the world population; the production of animal protein is a wasteful process that will become less practical as the world population grows.

The recommended daily protein intake for adults is 0.8 g/kg of body weight, less than the amount ordinarily consumed by Americans. For adults, at least one fifth should be animal protein; good-quality protein should be eaten at every meal.

Listed in the "Nutrition Facts" portion of food labels is the following protein-related information: the grams of protein per serving and the "% Daily Value" based on 10% of total calories for adults and children older than age 4 years.

Protein deficiency rarely occurs alone; it usually accompanies a deficiency of total calories and other nutrients.

Large losses of protein may occur during illness, requiring a substantial increase in protein consumption.

Protein-calorie malnutrition is the most serious and widespread deficiency disease in developing countries. The two major types are nutritional marasmus, due primarily to calorie deficiency, and kwashiorkor, due primarily to protein deficiency.

Vegetarianism requires careful planning so that the vegetarian will consume a variety of complementary plant foods as well as sufficient calories.

Some infants are born with an inability to metabolize phenylalanine, an essential amino acid; mental retardation results if disease is untreated.

The protein in specific foods is considered to be the cause of food allergies.

KEYS TO LEARNING

STUDY—DISCUSSION QUESTIONS

1. Using the 1-day food diary you kept in Chapter 5, calculate your protein intake and compare your consumption of protein with the RDA for your sex and age group given in Table 10-4. Which food items on your record represent the highest quality protein? How many grams of protein do they provide? How many grams of protein are derived from plant sources? How is the protein distributed throughout the day?
2. Each of the foods listed below in the amounts given provides about 18 g of protein. Complete the chart by determining the cost of each item in your supermarket.

   Which item is the least expensive source of protein? The most expensive source?
3. What are essential or indispensable amino acids? What is meant by the term *complementary proteins?* Why is it such an important concept?
4. Protein is said to be an inefficient source of energy from both a physical standpoint and a financial one. Explain.
5. Exchange with your classmates recipes for meatless main dishes that are used in your family meals. Calculate the protein content of the recipes using Appendix E. Divide the total protein by the number of servings to determine the amount of protein in one serving.
6. What are the symptoms of kwashiorkor? In developing countries, what age level is most likely to be affected?
7. Collect and discuss in class newspaper and magazine articles concerning international efforts to solve the problem of worldwide malnutrition.

FOOD	AMOUNT	PROTEIN (g)	COST
Chicken, cooked	2 oz (figure 5 oz raw weight with bone)*	18	
Pork and beans	$1^1/_2$ cups	18	
Flounder, cooked	2 oz (figure 4 oz raw weight)*	18	
Ground beef, cooked	$2^1/_2$ oz (figure $3^1/_2$ oz raw weight)*	18	
Bologna	5 oz	18	
Frankfurters	3 medium	18	
Sirloin steak, cooked	3 oz (figure 4 oz raw weight, boneless)*	18	
Tuna, canned	2 oz	18	

* Raw weight allows for shrinkage and bone, if applicable. Figure the cost of sirloin steak by determining the weight of edible meat (estimate the weight of bone, or weigh the bone and subtract from the total weight of the steak).

BIBLIOGRAPHY

BOOKS AND PAMPHLETS

Crim MC, Munro HN. Proteins and amino acids. In: Shils ME, Olson JA, Shike M. Eds. Modern nutrition in health and disease. 8th ed. Philadelphia: Lea and Febiger, 1994:3–35.

National Academy of Sciences, National Research Council, Committee on Diet and Health, Food and Nutrition Board. Diet and health: implications for reducing chronic disease risk (executive summary). Washington, DC: National Academy Press, 1989.

National Academy of Sciences, National Research Council, Food and Nutrition Board. Recommended dietary allowances. 10th ed. Washington, DC: National Academy Press, 1989.

PERIODICALS

Andres R, Hallfrisch J. Nutrient intake recommendations needed for the older American. J Am Diet Assoc 1989;89:1739.

Havala S, Dwyer J. Position of the American Dietetic Association: vegetarian diets. J Am Diet Assoc 1993;88:1317.

Kurtzweil, P. Daily values encourage healthy diet. FDA Consumer (Special Report: Focus on Food Labeling). May 1993. DHHS publication FDA 93-2262:40.

Kurtzweil P. "Nutrition facts" to help consumers eat smart. FDA Consumer (Special Report: Focus on Food Labeling). May 1993. DHHS publication FDA 93-2262:34.

Lyon RB, Vinci DM. Nutritional management of insulin-dependent diabetes mellitus in adults: review by the Diabetes Care and Education dietetic practice group. J Am Diet Assoc 1993;93:309.

Segal M. What's in a food. FDA Consumer (Special Report: Focus on Food Labeling). May 1993. DHHS publication FDA 93-2262:46.

Slavin J. Nutritional benefits of soy protein and soy fiber. J Am Diet Assoc 1991;91:816.

Young VR. Soy protein in relation to human protein and amino acid nutrition. J Am Diet Assoc 1991;91:828.

CHAPTER

11

Minerals

KEY TERMS

cardiac arrhythmia irregular heart action

cretinism a condition characterized by retarded mental and physical development due to a congenital lack of thyroid secretion

endemic peculiar to a particular locality or population

ferritin an iron–phosphorus–protein complex; the form in which iron is stored in the liver, spleen, and bone marrow

goiter enlargement of the thyroid gland

heme iron iron contained in the red pigment of blood; 40% of the total iron in animal tissue, including meat, liver, poultry, and fish, is heme iron

hemiplegic paralyzed on half of the body

hemochromatosis an iron storage disease

hemosiderin iron-containing pigment obtained from the hemoglobin of disintegrated red blood cells; hemosiderin provides one means of storing iron until it is needed for hemoglobin formation

hypertension high blood pressure

macrominerals minerals found in large amounts in the body and needed in the diet in quantities of 100 mg or more daily

microgram (mcg) 0.000001 g; one thousandth of a milligram

microminerals minerals found in small quantities in the body for which the requirement is a few milligrams or less daily

nonheme iron the form of iron composing 60% of the iron in animal tissue and 100% of the iron in plant foods and iron supplements

osteomalacia a disease in adults in which bones become softened, caused by a deficiency of vitamin D and calcium

osteoporosis a disease in which calcium is lost from bones, which then fracture easily

oxalates substances in some foods, such as spinach and Swiss chard, that combines with calcium, making the calcium insoluble and preventing its absorption

phytates phosphorus compounds found in cereals that form insoluble compounds with some minerals, making them unavailable to the body

resorption removal by absorption

trace elements minerals present in small amounts in the body; also called ***microminerals***

OBJECTIVES

After completing this chapter, the student will be able to:

1. Identify the two basic functions of minerals in the body.
2. Identify the body mechanisms that work to maintain a precise balance of minerals in body fluids.
3. Identify those minerals for which Recommended Dietary Allowances (RDAs) have been established.

4. Identify those essential minerals for which no RDA has been established.
5. Discuss the importance of calcium, iron, sodium, potassium, zinc, fluoride, and iodine. For each, give
   - its function.
   - its RDA or Acceptable Daily Intake.
   - results of deficiency and excess.
   - major food sources.
6. Explain the labeling regulations for each of the following: calcium, iron, and sodium.
7. Appreciate the significance of the interaction between minerals and its relationship to the use of mineral supplements.
8. Discuss the characteristics, risk factors, diagnostic measures, treatment, and prevention of osteoporosis.

GENERAL CHARACTERISTICS OF MINERALS

Minerals are inorganic elements occurring in nature. They are inorganic because they do not originate in animal or plant life but rather from the earth's crust. Although minerals make up only a small proportion of body tissue, they are essential for growth and normal functioning. Minerals are needed in such small quantities that the units of milligram (mg; 0.001 g) and microgram (mcg; 0.000001 g) are used in describing them.

CLASSIFICATION

Mineral elements are classified into two groups on the basis of the amount found in the body. Minerals that occur in large amounts and needed in quantities of 100 mg/day or more are called *macrominerals* (Display 11-1). This group includes calcium, chloride, magnesium, phosphorus, potassium, sodium, and sulfur. Minerals occurring in small amounts and needed in quantities of a few milligrams or less per day are called *microminerals* or *trace minerals.* The essential trace minerals are chromium, cobalt, copper, fluoride, iodine, iron, manganese, molybdenum, selenium, and zinc. As many as 30 other minerals occur in body tissue, among them lead, gold, and mercury. As far as is known, those 30-odd minerals are potentially harmful and are present in the body only as a result of environmental contamination. Some trace minerals formerly thought to be toxic, however, have been found to be essential to normal body function. For example, the toxic effects of selenium were well known before its beneficial effects were discovered.

DISPLAY 11-1 MINERALS

MACROMINERALS*	MICROMINERALS OR TRACE MINERALS†
Calcium	Chromium
Chloride	Cobalt‡
Magnesium	Copper
Phosphorus	Fluoride
Potassium	Iodine
Sodium	Iron
Sulfur**	Manganese
	Molybdenum
	Selenium
	Zinc

* Needed in relatively large amounts.
† Needed in very small amounts.
‡ Human requirement for cobalt met by vitamin B_{12} intake. Appears to function only as an essential part of vitamin B_{12}.
** Human requirement met by essential sulfur-containing amino acids.

FUNCTIONS

The functions of minerals may be broadly divided into two areas: building body tissue and regulating body processes.

BUILDING OF BODY TISSUE

Certain minerals, including calcium, phosphorus, magnesium, and fluorine, are components of bones and teeth. Deficiencies during the growing years cause growth to be stunted and bone tissue to be of poor quality. Adequate intake of minerals continues to be essential for the maintenance of skeletal tissue in adulthood. Potassium, sulfur, phosphorus, iron, and many other minerals also are structural components of soft tissue.

REGULATION OF BODY PROCESSES

Component of Essential Compounds

Minerals are an integral part of many hormones, enzymes, and other compounds that regulate function. For example, iodine is required to produce the hormone thyroxine; chromium is involved in the production of insulin; and hemoglobin is an iron-containing compound. The production of these substances depends on adequate intake of the involved minerals.

Some minerals serve as catalysts. For example, calcium is a catalyst in blood clotting. Some minerals act as catalysts in the absorption of nutrients from the gastrointestinal tract, the metabolism of proteins, fats, and carbohydrates, and the use of nutrients by the cell.

Transmitter of Nerve Impulses and Muscle Contractions

Minerals dissolved in body fluids are responsible for the transmission of nerve impulses and the contraction of muscles. When a nerve is stimulated, the exchange of sodium and potassium particles across the nerve cell membrane creates a change in the electrical charge of the membrane, which passes the impulse along the nerve. Calcium stimulates muscular contractions; sodium, potassium, and magnesium cause muscular relaxation. The normal functioning of muscles requires an appropriate balance between these two forces.

Maintainer of Water Balance

Maintenance of water balance depends on the concentration of minerals in body fluids. (See discussion in Chapter 13.)

Maintainer of Acid–Base Balance

Minerals play an important role in the buffer systems in body fluids that help maintain a normal acid–base balance. (See discussion in Chapter 13.)

INTERACTION

Hundreds of interactions occur among minerals and between minerals and other substances in the diet. For example, fiber and phosphates hinder iron absorption, whereas ascorbic acid, copper, and meat protein promote iron absorption. A high-protein intake appears to increase the excretion of calcium, whereas vitamin D ingestion promotes the absorption and retention of calcium.

SOURCES

In general, minerals are most abundant in unrefined foods. Processed or refined foods such as fats, oils, sugar, and cornstarch contain almost no minerals. Iodine, copper, and other essential trace minerals occur in some soils and drinking water but are lacking in others. Some essential minerals, including potassium, sulfur, chloride, and sodium, are so abundant in the normal diet that deficiencies are unlikely.

Nutrition authorities are concerned about the changes in the nutritional composition of many foods in the American diet. These changes have resulted from advances in food technology and new manufacturing practices. The effects of the increased use of engineered foods, such as textured vegetable protein, egg substitutes, and imitation fruit drinks, on the adequacy of the diet is questioned. The intake of essential trace minerals, some of which may not as yet have been discovered, is threatened by this trend. Excessive as well as inadequate mineral intake may result. For example, increased use of phosphate additives in food processing, although harmless in itself, may result in changes in the calcium/phosphorus ratio, which in turn may adversely affect calcium metabolism. This mineral imbalance is discussed later in this chapter under Factors That Affect Calcium Balance (Solubility Product).

RECOMMENDED ALLOWANCES

Because mineral interactions greatly affect dietary requirements, precise recommendations for mineral intake are not always possible. The 10th edition of *Recommended Dietary Allowances* gives recommendations for calcium, phosphorus, magnesium, iron, zinc, iodine, and selenium. These recommendations appear in Appendix B: Recommended Dietary Allowances summary. General guidelines are provided for five additional minerals. The guidelines given in Table 11-1 are ranges of safe and adequate intakes. Exact recommendations are not given because of incomplete knowledge about the minerals, their interactions with other substances, and their regulation in the body (absorption and excretion). The ranges given appear to be adequate on the basis of current knowledge. The recommendations for the electrolytes sodium, chloride, and potassium are given in terms of minimum requirements of healthy people (Table 11-2).

MACROMINERALS

CALCIUM

Calcium is the body's most abundant mineral. Of all calcium in the body, 99% occurs in the bones and teeth as deposits of calcium phosphate. The remaining 1%, present in the soft tissue and body fluids, has important regulatory functions. Of the calcium in body fluids, 60% is in ionized form, can move freely from one fluid compartment to another, and can be filtered by the kidneys.

FUNCTIONS AND CLINICAL EFFECTS

Bone and Tooth Formation

Together with phosphorus and small amounts of other minerals, calcium provides strength and rigidity to the bones and teeth. Small amounts of magnesium, sodium, carbonate, citrate, chloride, and fluoride are also components of bone.

The two major forms of bone are *trabecular bone* and *cortical bone*. Trabecular bone, which has a porous honeycomblike structure, makes up the inner core of bone and is found in greatest proportion in the vertebrae and at the ends of the bones of the arms and legs. Cortical bone is the dense, compact layer that forms the outer portion of bone.

Despite its hard, solid appearance, bone is active tissue that is constantly being formed and resorbed. In children and adolescents, bone formation exceeds bone loss. Although most bone formation occurs by about age 20 years, some bone formation continues until the mid-20s or even the early 30s, when maximum bone density and strength is achieved. Bone loss begins to exceed replacement at some time after that peak in both men

TABLE 11-1 Estimated Safe and Adequate Daily Dietary Intakes of Selected Vitamins and Minerals*

		Vitamins		Trace Elements†				
Category	Age (Yr)	Biotin (mcg)	Pantothenic Acid (mg)	Copper (mg)	Manganese (mg)	Fluoride (mg)	Chromium (mcg)	Molybdenum (mcg)
Infants	0–0.5	10	2	0.4–0.6	0.3–0.6	0.1–0.5	10–40	15–30
	0.5–1	15	3	0.6–0.7	0.6–1.0	0.2–1.0	20–60	20–40
Children and adolescents	1–3	20	3	0.7–1.0	1.0–1.5	0.5–1.5	20–80	25–50
	4–6	25	3–4	1.0–1.5	1.5–2.0	1.0–2.5	30–120	30–75
	7–10	30	4–5	1.0–2.0	2.0–3.0	1.5–2.5	50–200	50–150
	11+	30–100	4–7	1.5–2.5	2.0–5.0	1.5–2.5	50–200	75–250
Adults		30–100	4–7	1.5–3.0	2.0–5.0	1.5–4.0	50–200	75–250

* Because less information is available on which to base allowances, these figures are not given in the main table of RDA and are provided here in the form of ranges of recommended intakes.

† Because the toxic levels for many trace elements may be only several times usual intakes, the upper levels for the trace elements given should not be habitually exceeded.

(National Academy of Sciences, National Research Council, Food and Nutrition Board. Recommended dietary allowances. 10th ed. Washington, DC: National Academy Press, 1989:284.)

TABLE 11-2 ESTIMATED SODIUM, CHLORIDE, AND POTASSIUM MINIMUM REQUIREMENTS OF HEALTHY PEOPLE

AGE	WEIGHT (KG)	SODIUM (MG)*	CHLORIDE (MG)*	POTASSIUM (MG)†
Months				
0–5	4.5	120	180	500
6–11	8.9	200	300	700
Years				
1	11.0	225	350	1000
2–5	16.0	300	500	1400
6–9	25.0	400	600	1600
10–18	50.0	500	750	2000
>18‡	70.0	500	750	2000

* No evidence suggests that higher intakes confer any health benefit. No allowance has been included for large, prolonged losses from the skin through sweat.
† Desirable intakes of potassium may considerably exceed these values (about 3500 mg for adults).
‡ No allowance included for growth. Values for people younger than age 18 years assume a growth rate at the 50th percentile reported by the National Center for Health Statistics and averaged for males and females.
(National Academy of Sciences, National Research Council, Food and Nutrition Board. Recommended dietary allowances. 10th ed. Washington, DC: National Academy Press, 1989:253.)

and women. The rate of bone loss increases greatly at menopause in women and remains high for several years. The rate of bone loss increases about 10 years later in men. Gradual bone loss is a normal part of aging. Bone loss leads to reduced bone strength and increased risk of fractures. People who achieve a larger bone mass during the years in which bone is being formed have a lower risk of developing fragile bones that fracture easily.

Calcium intake is not the only factor that affects bone health. Vitamin D and other minerals, including sodium, zinc, magnesium, and fluoride, are also involved in bone metabolism. Furthermore, heredity, sex hormones, and physical activity influence bone formation. In women, the rate of decline in bone is closely associated with estrogen status. Estrogen replacement slows the rate of bone loss. Increasing calcium alone has only a small effect on bone loss.

Tooth structure is much more stable than bone structure. There is little exchange of calcium in teeth once they are formed.

Effects of Immobility

The stress of weight bearing stimulates the activity of the bone-forming cells, thus strengthening bone tissue. When an individual is bedridden or inactive for an extended period, the bones no longer receive this stimulation; consequently, there is a loss of calcium, phosphorus, and protein matrix (intercellular material). Osteoporosis (a bone-thinning disease) may occur in a hemiplegic person as early as 2 weeks after a stroke. The person excretes surplus serum calcium in the urine.

The excessive withdrawal of calcium from bone may lead to further problems. If the kidneys are unable to excrete the excess calcium, *hypercalcemia*, or high serum levels of calcium, results. Symptoms of this disorder include nausea, vomiting, gaseousness, headache, and reduced heart rate. In contrast, excretion of the excess calcium in the urine—*hypercalciuria*—may cause the formation of bladder and kidney stones.

Maintenance of Body Function

The remaining 1% of the calcium in the body fluids, in structures within the cell, and in cell membranes plays an important role in maintaining normal body function. The following are some of these functions:

Blood clotting—Calcium in the blood is needed for normal blood clotting. Vitamin K regulates the synthesis of calcium-containing proteins involved in a complex process that results in the conversion of a soluble plasma protein, *fibrinogen,* to a solid mass called *fibrin,* which forms the clot.

Permeability of cell membranes—Calcium regulates the passage of substances across cell membranes.

Transmission of nerve impulses—Calcium plays a role in the transmission of nerve impulses.

Contraction and relaxation of muscles—Calcium is necessary for normal muscle contraction, including that of the heart.

Enzyme activation and absorption of vitamin B_{12}—Calcium is an activator of certain enzymes, including *pancreatic lipase,* which digests fat, and *adenosinetriphosphatase,* which is involved in the release of energy for muscular activity. Calcium also is needed for the absorption of vitamin B_{12}.

FACTORS THAT AFFECT CALCIUM BALANCE

A precise amount of calcium is maintained in the plasma. This need takes priority over bone formation. A number of body mechanisms maintain this crucial balance.

Absorption–Excretion

Absorption of calcium is influenced by several factors: body need, total calcium content of the diet, age and sex, exposure to ultraviolet light, vitamin D intake, and food source. Absorption of calcium increases during periods of increased need when bone formation is occurring. Only 20% to 40% of the calcium consumed is absorbed from the intestinal tract of young adults, whereas as much as 75% is absorbed in children. A higher percentage is absorbed when intakes are low. In adults who consume more than 800 mg/day, absorption of calcium is only about 15% of the total amount consumed. In elderly people, calcium absorption is impaired. Absorption is more efficient in men than in women.

Calcium absorption is aided by adequate intake of vitamin D, an acidic environment in the upper gastrointestinal tract, and normal gastrointestinal motility. Protein, vitamin C, and lactose (milk sugar, which provides lactic acid) increase intestinal acidity, making calcium more soluble and thus more absorbable. The benefits of protein in promoting absorption may be offset by increased urinary excretion of calcium when protein intake is high.

Dietary factors that hinder calcium absorption are *phytates* and *oxalates.* Phytates are phosphorus compounds found in unrefined cereal products such as brown rice and wheat bran. Oxalates are found in certain plant foods such as cocoa, soybeans, spinach, and kale. Phytates and oxalates form insoluble compounds with calcium. These compounds cannot be absorbed and are excreted in the feces. Other factors that decrease calcium absorption include increased gastrointestinal transit time (as in diarrhea), stress, immobilization, reduced gastric acidity, and certain drugs such as anticonvulsive medication, thyrotropin, and hydrocortisone.

Calcium is excreted in the feces, urine, and sweat. Calcium in the feces is mostly unabsorbed dietary calcium. The amount of calcium excreted in the urine is influenced by hormones and the composition of the diet. Protein, sodium, and some carbohydrates increase calcium excretion, whereas phosphorus decreases it. Unless sweating is extreme, little calcium is lost from the skin.

The American diet is high in both phosphorus and protein. Although a high-protein diet increases calcium excretion, this appears to be counterbalanced by the high phosphorus content of the diet.

Calcium Storage in Bone

Calcium in the bone is in a constant state of exchange. If plasma calcium levels are high, calcium is deposited in the bone as the blood passes through it. Bone is the storehouse for calcium, to be drawn on when serum calcium levels are low. Ideally, calcium is drawn from the *trabeculae,* columns of crystalline calcium compounds at the ends of bones. When the diet is adequate in calcium, the trabeculae are well developed. If calcium is lacking over an extended period, however, the trabeculae disappear and calcium is drawn from the dense bone material itself.

Hormones

The interaction of several hormones plays an important role in maintaining blood calcium concentration within normal limits. These hormones include the active form of vitamin D, parathyroid hormone, calcitonin, estrogen, testosterone, and possibly others. These hormones control calcium absorption and excretion and bone metabolism. The hormones respond to changes in serum calcium in the following three ways:

1. Active vitamin D exhibits hormonelike activity, increasing the absorption of calcium from the intestinal tract when the serum calcium level falls. It also controls the deposit of calcium and phosphorus in the bone. Vitamin D is converted to the active form by changes that occur in the liver and kidneys.
2. Parathyroid hormone, secreted by the parathyroid gland, stimulates the following changes when the serum calcium level falls: increased formation of active vitamin D, increased release of calcium and phosphorus from the bone, increased urinary excretion of phosphorus, and decreased excretion of calcium by the kidneys. Disturbances of the parathyroid gland can cause abnormally high or low serum calcium levels.
3. Calcitonin is secreted by the thyroid gland in increased amounts when serum calcium levels rise. This hormone reduces serum calcium concentration by promoting the deposit of calcium in the bones.

Solubility Product

A specific ratio of calcium to phosphorus normally is maintained in the blood serum because of the relative solubility of these minerals. The solubility product of calcium and phosphorus is the result obtained when the concentration of calcium is multiplied by the concentration of phosphorus. An increase in one of the minerals causes a decrease in the other because this product normally remains the same. For example, excess phosphorus in the diet can create a decrease in serum calcium even though recommended amounts of calcium are being consumed. The high phosphate content of processed foods such as carbonated beverages is of concern because it appears to have the potential of disrupting the calcium–phosphorus balance. The low ratio of calcium to phosphorus in the American diet, however, does not appear to have an adverse effect on calcium balance when the diet contains adequate calcium.

Tetany, a condition characterized by uncontrolled muscular contractions (spasms) and pain, results when serum calcium levels fall below normal. Tetany has been seen in newborns fed undiluted cow's milk, which contains a higher ratio of phosphorus to calcium than breast milk. The infant's kidneys are unable to excrete the excess phosphorus, causing the serum calcium level to drop.

SOURCES

More than 55% of the calcium in the American diet comes from dairy products. Milk and hard cheeses such as cheddar, Swiss, and American are the most important sources. All types of milk—whole, nonfat, evaporated, and dry—are good sources of calcium. Including milk in puddings, custards, and creamed foods is a means of increasing calcium intake for people who do not drink sufficient quantities of milk. People who like milk but have difficulty digesting it because they lack the digestive enzyme lactase may be able to tolerate milk that has been treated with the enzyme (see Chapter 28).

Not all dairy products are equally good sources of calcium. Cottage cheese, because of its high water content, is not as good a source of calcium as hard cheese. It takes 1⅓ cups of ice cream (350 calories) to provide the same amount of calcium as 1 cup of skim milk (90 calories). Butter and cream cheese, although made from milk, are fats and are not good sources of calcium.

Dairy products made from whole milk are a major source of saturated fat in the diet. To reduce fat in the diet while reaping the calcium benefits of dairy products, the following are good choices: skim or 1% fat milk and foods such as puddings, cream soups, and creamed foods made from these milks; lowfat cottage cheese; lowfat or nonfat yogurt; and hard cheese containing 5 g or less of fat per ounce.

Other foods that contribute calcium to the diet are leafy green vegetables such as kale, collards, and turnip greens; broccoli; dried peas and beans; lime-processed tortillas; calcium-precipitated tofu; and calcium-fortified foods. The edible bones of canned salmon and small fish such as sardines are rich sources of calcium. Shellfish are fair sources. Table 11-3 shows the calcium content of selected foods.

FOOD LABELING

Labeling regulations require that information on the calcium content of food be included on the "Nutrition Facts" panel of the label. The amount of calcium on the product is given as a percentage of the Daily Value ("% Daily Value"), which is 1000 mg calcium daily regardless of the caloric content of the diet. A product listing 15% calcium means that a serving of the product provides 15% of 1000 mg, or 150 mg of calcium.

Foods containing 20% or more of the Daily Value for calcium (200 mg) per serving may carry a health claim regarding the relationship between calcium and osteoporosis. A food must also have a calcium content that equals or exceeds the phosphorus content of the food and must contain a form of calcium that the body can readily absorb and use.

Whole milk cannot carry the calcium/osteoporosis health claim because it contains too much saturated fat. The labeling law specifies that foods bearing health claims must not contain any nutrient in an amount that increases the risk of a disease or health condition.

RECOMMENDED ALLOWANCES

The recommended calcium level has been raised from 800 to 1200 mg/day for men and women aged 19 to 24 years. Previously, the 1200 mg/day recommendation applied only to 11- to 18-year-olds. This change resulted from scientific evidence that the accumulation of bone tissue does not reach its peak until a person reaches his or her mid-twenties or later. The recommendation for children aged 1 to 10 years is 800 mg/day; for pregnant and breast-feeding women, it is 1200 mg/day.

The National Academy of Sciences Food and Nutrition Board did not change the recommendation for adults older than 25 years, even though people in their forties begin to lose calcium slowly from the bones. The RDA for calcium remains at 800 mg for adults aged 25 years and older. This decision was

TABLE 11-3 CALCIUM AND CALORIC CONTENT OF SELECTED FOODS IN PORTION SIZES TYPICALLY CONSUMED*

FOOD	PORTION SIZE	CALCIUM (MG)	KCAL
Milk, whole	1 cup	291	150
Milk, skim	1 cup	302	85
Cheddar cheese	1 oz	204	115
Cottage cheese, creamed	1/2 cup	68	118
Cottage cheese, 2% fat	1/2 cup	78	103
Ice cream	1/2 cup	88	135
Custard	1/2 cup	149	153
Sardines, Atlantic, canned	3 oz	371	175
Beef patty	3 oz	9	245
Orange	1	52	60
Apple	1	10	80
Bread, white, firm-crumb	1 slice	32	65
Collards, cooked, chopped from frozen	1/2 cup	179	30
Kale, cooked, chopped from frozen	1/2 cup	90	20
Turnip greens, cooked	1/2 cup	125	25
Broccoli, cooked	1/2 cup	89	23
Potato, boiled	1	11	115
Carrots, cooked	1/2 cup	24	35
Dried navy beans, cooked	1/2 cup	48	113
Tofu (soybean curd)	4 oz	108	85
Tortilla, lime processed	1 (1 oz)	42	65

* Source of nutritive values: US Dept of Agriculture, Human Nutrition Information Service. Nutritive value of food. Washington, DC: US Government Printing Office, 1991. Home and Garden bulletin 72.

based on evidence that increased calcium alone has little effect on bone loss after the achievement of peak bone mass. Bone loss in postmenopausal women is influenced mostly by estrogen level. The board believed that the best way to reduce the risk of osteoporosis is to achieve a person's genetic potential to accumulate bone mass during the years bone is being formed. However, the National Institutes of Health and the National Osteoporosis Foundation have recommended higher intakes of calcium for adults. They are 1000 mg/day for adults and 1500 mg/day for postmenopausal women not on hormone replacement therapy.

Throughout life, people should meet the recommended calcium levels. Unfortunately, most women are not meeting these recommendations. The average calcium intake of white women is estimated to be 640 mg/day, and of African American women, only 450 mg/day.

Only a few foods are rich sources of calcium. It is difficult to meet recommended allowances without including adequate amounts of milk in the diet. Preschool and early school-age children should drink 1 to 1½ pt of milk a day; older children, adolescents, and young adults should drink 1½ pt to 1 qt of milk daily; and adults should drink 1 pt. Some calcium may be taken in the form of cheese or other milk products. Foods that contain as much calcium as 8 oz of milk are listed in Display 11-2.

DISPLAY 11-2 FOODS THAT CONTAIN AS MUCH CALCIUM AS 8 OZ OF MILK

1⅓ oz cheddar cheese
1½ oz processed American cheese
1⅓ cups cottage cheese
1 cup cocoa made with milk
1 cup custard
1⅓ cups ice cream
1 cup ice milk, soft serve
¾ cup homemade macaroni and cheese
1 milkshake (made with ⅔ cup milk and ½ cup ice cream)
1 cup oyster stew
1½–1⅔ cup canned cream soup, prepared with equal volume of milk
1 cup unflavored yogurt

DEFICIENCY

The amount of calcium in the soft tissue is maintained at all costs. If calcium intake or absorption is inadequate, the deposit of calcium in bone tissue is slowed in children or calcium is withdrawn from the bone tissue in adults. Calcium deficiency usually goes hand in hand with inadequacies of other nutrients, such as vitamin D and phosphorus, and with other factors that affect calcium absorption and use. If nutrients needed for normal bone formation are insufficient, growth may be stunted; bone growth may continue, but the resulting bones and teeth are of poor quality. The bowed legs, enlarged ankles and wrists, and narrow chest seen in rickets may result. Inadequate intake prenatally when the teeth are being formed may result in poor tooth structure, making teeth less resistant to dental caries. In adults, loss of calcium from the bones results in bones that are porous and weak.

In some parts of the world, *osteomalacia* develops in women who have had repeated pregnancies and periods of breastfeeding. This disease, sometimes called *adult rickets,* is characterized by poor bone calcification and resultant bone softness and flexibility. The bones are then especially susceptible to fracture (see Chapter 12).

Adequate calcium intake throughout life is one of the factors that reduces the risk of osteoporosis, a bone-thinning disease responsible for 1.7 million bone fractures a year. (See the section Key Issues.) In addition to its role in reducing the risk of osteoporosis, new research findings have indicated that calcium may have a protective and therapeutic role in many other diseases and conditions. These include hypertension, colon cancer, kidney stones, control of blood lipid and lipoprotein levels, and the alleviation of symptoms of premenstrual syndrome (see Chapter 13.) More research is needed to confirm these results.

EXCESS

Daily intakes of more than 2000 mg offer no added known benefits to bone health. Excessive calcium may hinder the absorption of iron, zinc, and other essential minerals. High intakes were also thought to increase the risk of urinary stone formation. However, recent studies have suggested that the practice of reducing calcium intake for people prone to stone formation may actually increase the risk of kidney stones, 80% of which contain calcium (calcium oxalate). The authors of these studies believe that oxalate in the urine may be more important than calcium in kidney stone formation and that calcium may bind with oxalate in the intestinal tract, thus decreasing the absorption and urinary excretion of oxalate.

PHOSPHORUS

Phosphorus is a significant component of bones and teeth and an essential factor in regulatory processes. Phosphorus makes up about 1% of body weight. Of all phosphorus in the body, 85% is found in the form of calcium phosphate in bones and teeth.

FUNCTIONS AND CLINICAL EFFECTS

Bone and Tooth Formation

Phosphorus must be available for the formation of calcium phosphate. Poor calcification of bone can result from a lack of phosphorus as well as from a lack of calcium. A lack of phosphorus, however, is most likely to result from excessive excretion of phosphorus in the urine and not from an inadequate supply in the diet. Like calcium, phosphorus is constantly being released from and built into bone tissue as a means of maintaining a normal serum level.

Energy Metabolism

Phosphorus is a component of adenosine triphosphate (ATP) and adenosine diphosphate (ADP), which control energy storage and release in the cell. ATP captures the energy released in the burning (oxidation) of protein, fat, and carbohydrate. As energy is needed, ATP is hydrolyzed (broken down) to ADP, thus releasing the energy needed to fuel reactions of metabolism.

Protein Synthesis and Genetic Coding

Phosphorus occurs in all cells as part of both ribonucleic acid (RNA) and deoxyribonucleic acid (DNA), which are essential for protein synthesis and genetic coding.

Absorption and Transport of Fats and Fatty Acids

Phosphorus combines with insoluble fats so that they may be absorbed from the intestinal tract and transported in the bloodstream.

Enzyme Formation

Phosphorus is a component of enzymes involved in the metabolism of proteins, fats, and carbohydrates.

Acid–Base Balance

The phosphate system is one of the principal buffers in the regulation of acid–base balance.

FACTORS THAT AFFECT PHOSPHORUS BALANCE

The amount of phosphorus in the body is controlled mostly by excretion in the urine rather than by control of absorption. By responding to changes in serum calcium levels, parathyroid hormone and vitamin D hormone indirectly regulate phosphorus balance. Parathyroid hormone regulates the amount of phosphorus reabsorbed by the kidney. Vitamin D promotes the absorption of phosphorus from the intestinal tract.

SOURCES

Phosphorus is widely distributed in food and is unlikely to be lacking. Meats, poultry, fish, eggs, nuts, legumes, whole-grain cereals, and milk are all good sources. Phosphate additives used in a wide variety of products, such as carbonated beverages, processed meats, cheese, dressing, and refrigerated bakery products, contribute significant amounts of phosphorus to the diet.

RECOMMENDED ALLOWANCES

The recommended intake of phosphorus is the same as that of calcium at all ages except in infancy. The recommended calcium/phosphorus ratio in the first 6 months of life is 1.3:1, and in the second 6 months, 1.2:1. The RDA for phosphorus is 300 mg/day from birth to 6 months, 500 mg/day from 6 to 12 months, 800 mg/day from 1 to 10 years, 1200 mg/day from 11 to 24 years, and 800 mg/day beyond 24 years.

In the United States, the phosphorus intake is about 1500 to 1800 mg/day for men and 1000 to 1200 mg/day for women. These allowances are considerably higher than the recommended 1:1 ratio.

DEFICIENCY AND EXCESS

Because phosphorus is widely distributed in food, phosphorus deficiency is rare. Phosphorus deficiency has occurred in small premature infants who received breast milk as their only source of nourishment. Breast milk does not contain enough phosphorus to support the bone growth that is occurring. If additional phosphorus is not provided, rickets caused by a lack of phosphorus may develop.

The prolonged use of aluminum hydroxide antacid has resulted in phosphorus deficiency in adults. The aluminum hydroxide combines with phosphorus, preventing its absorption. Symptoms of phosphorus deficiency are weakness, anorexia, malaise, and pain.

Questions have been raised about the long-term effects of the low calcium/phosphorus ratio in many Americans' diets. No problems related to excessive phosphorus have been noted in the population. Obtaining adequate amounts of calcium and vitamin D can protect against any possible adverse effects.

SODIUM

Although attention usually is drawn to the undesirable effects of high intakes of sodium, this mineral is essential to life, playing a vital role in regulating body processes. About one third of body sodium occurs in bone tissue; most of the remaining two thirds is found in extracellular fluid.

FUNCTIONS AND CLINICAL EFFECTS

Sodium is the principal *cation* (electrolyte carrying a positive charge) of the extracellular fluid. As free ionized sodium, it helps control a number of important body processes.

Water Balance

Sodium acts with other electrolytes, especially potassium in the intracellular fluid, to maintain proper osmotic pressure and water balance (see Chapter 13).

When excretion of sodium is reduced, as in cardiac or kidney failure, water is retained along with the sodium. The water and sodium accumulate in the tissues, increasing the workload of the heart. Accumulation of fluid in the lungs (*pulmonary edema*) and in the extremities (peripheral edema) may then occur. Sodium also is retained when there is excessive secretion of adrenal hormones or when these hormones are given as medication.

Acid–Base Balance

Sodium is a base-forming element. It balances the acidic chloride and bicarbonate ions.

Transmission of Nerve Impulses and Contraction of Muscles

Together with potassium, sodium creates an electrical charge on the nerve cell membrane, which passes impulses along the nerve. It has a relaxing effect on muscle contractions, working to balance those ions that stimulate muscle contraction.

Glucose Absorption and Cell Permeability

Exchange of sodium and potassium across cell walls makes the cell membrane more permeable to other substances.

FACTORS THAT AFFECT SODIUM BALANCE

Reported intakes of sodium in the United States range from 1800 to 5000 mg/day (1.8 to 5 g/day). This probably is an underestimation, inaccurately reflecting the amount of sodium added to food at the table.

This sodium intake is far in excess of body requirements. Most of the sodium consumed is absorbed.

Balance is maintained through excretion by the kidneys. The amount excreted is regulated by the hormone aldosterone, which is secreted by the adrenal gland. When sodium intake is high, urinary excretion increases; when intake is low, excretion decreases. Aldosterone is secreted in response to low sodium levels. It promotes reabsorption of sodium by the kidney.

SOURCES

Table salt (sodium chloride) is the primary source of sodium in the diet. Sodium chloride is 39% sodium by weight; 1 tsp contains about 1950 mg of sodium (usually rounded off to 2000 mg). Other sodium additives such as sodium bicarbonate and monosodium glutamate (MSG) contribute much less sodium to the diet.

In addition to sodium additives, the sodium in foods in their natural state, the water supply, and medications provide sodium. Animal sources such as meat, fish, poultry, eggs, and milk are high in natural sodium content when compared with fruits and most vegetables. In some areas, the water supply is a significant source of sodium. Most community water systems supply water that contains less than 20 mg/liter of sodium. Medications, such as some antacids, may have significant amounts of sodium.

Processed foods contribute large quantities of sodium to the diet (Table 11-4). Diets that have a high proportion of processed food have a high sodium content; those diets that emphasize fresh fruits, vegetables, and legumes have a low sodium content. Most Americans consume excessive quantities of sodium. The source is mostly salt in snacks and other prepackaged foods, not the amount sprinkled on food. See Chapter 26 for a more comprehensive discussion of the sodium content of foods.

TABLE 11-4 EFFECT OF FOOD PROCESSING ON THE SODIUM CONTENT OF FOODS*

FOOD	AMOUNT	SODIUM (MG)
Salmon		
Broiled with butter	3 oz	99
Canned, salt added	3 oz	443
Canned, without added salt	3 oz	41
Cream of Wheat		
Regular	3/4 cup	2
Quick-Cooking	3/4 cup	126
Mix'n Eat	3/4 cup	350
Peanuts		
Unsalted	1/2 cup	4
Dry roasted, salted	1/2 cup	493
Peas		
Fresh, cooked	1/2 cup	1
Frozen, regular, cooked	1/2 cup	100
Canned, regular	1/2 cup	247
Canned, low sodium	1/2 cup	8
Meat		
Beef, lean, cooked	3 oz	55
Pork, fresh, lean, cooked	3 oz	59
Corned beef	3 oz	802
Ham	3 oz	1114
Frankfurters (1 1/2)	3 oz	958
Beef salami	3 oz	1020
Olive loaf	3 oz	1248
Fast Foods		
Fish sandwich	1	882
Jumbo hamburger	1	990
Pizza, cheese	1/4 pie	599
French fries	2 1/2 oz	146

* Source of nutritive values: The sodium content of your food. US Dept of Agriculture, Science and Education Administration. Washington, DC: US Government Printing Office, 1980. Home and Garden bulletin 233.

FOOD LABELING

The sodium content of a product is a required component of the "Nutrition Facts" panel on food labels. The sodium content is given in milligrams per serving of the product and is also expressed as "% Daily Value" for sodium, which is 2400 mg regardless of caloric intake. The 2400 mg value is the uppermost limit considered to be healthy according to current public health recommendations. Definitions have been established for terms such as *sodium free, low sodium,* and so forth. See Display 26-4 for the meanings of the sodium descriptors used on labels to describe the sodium content of a food.

Health claims on labels can be made regarding the link between sodium and high blood pressure. To carry a claim, the food must meet the criteria for the descriptive term *low sodium,* which means that the food has 140 mg sodium or less per serving.

RECOMMENDED ALLOWANCES

In the 10th edition of the Recommended Dietary Allowances, 500 mg/day of sodium is given as a *minimum* intake. An upper limit is not given. The National Academy of Sciences Committee on Diet and Health has recommended that the total daily intake of salt be limited to 6 g, which represents 2400 mg of sodium. Sodium above the minimum allowance is needed during pregnancy and breast-feeding. This requirement is easily met by the usual sodium intake.

DEFICIENCY AND EXCESS

Sodium deficit is as serious as sodium excess. Heavy losses may occur in cystic fibrosis, kidney disease, diseases of the adrenal glands, severe diarrhea and vomiting, with excessive and prolonged sweating, and with the use of diuretics. Symptoms of sodium deficiency include nausea, giddiness, apathy, exhaustion, abdominal and muscle cramps, vomiting, and, finally, respiratory failure if the sodium is not replaced.

Studies have indicated that elevated blood pressure is strongly associated with a high sodium intake. Some people appear to inherit a sensitivity to sodium, making them prone to hypertension. Because susceptible people cannot be identified, some authorities feel that there is a clear advantage to controlling sodium intake. Others are challenging this viewpoint. See Chapter 26 for a discussion of sodium and hypertension.

POTASSIUM

Potassium is an essential component of all living cells. The long-term use of diuretics in the treatment of cardiac disease has focused attention on the body's potassium requirement. Although diuretics are prescribed to prevent the accumulation of sodium and water, the kidneys excrete potassium along with the sodium and water. Potassium lost must be replaced either by a potassium supplement or, preferably, through an increase in dietary potassium.

FUNCTIONS AND CLINICAL EFFECTS

Water Balance and Acid–Base Balance

Potassium is the principal cation (positively charged ion) of the fluid within the cell. It maintains osmotic pressure, water balance, and acid–base balance.

Transmission of Nerve Impulses and Contraction of Muscles

A small amount of potassium in extracellular fluid, together with other ions, influences the transmission of nerve impulses and the contraction of muscles, including the heart.

Energy Metabolism

Potassium is a catalyst for reactions occurring in the cell.

Glycogen and Protein Synthesis

Potassium bound to phosphate is required for the conversion of glucose to glycogen. Potassium is needed for the synthesis of muscle protein.

Maintenance of Blood Pressure

Potassium contributes to the maintenance of normal blood pressure.

FACTORS THAT AFFECT POTASSIUM BALANCE

Potassium is readily absorbed from the gastrointestinal tract. The kidneys maintain potassium balance by excreting excessive amounts. The ability of the kidney to conserve potassium when a deficiency occurs, however, is poor.

SOURCES

Potassium is distributed widely in food. It is found in liberal amounts in meat, fish, and poultry; whole-grain breads and cereals; fruits, especially oranges and grapefruits and their juices, dried fruits, and bananas; and vegetables, especially potatoes, winter squash, tomatoes, and legumes. Display 11-3 lists foods high in potassium.

Unlike sodium, food processing tends to lower the potassium content of foods. Unprocessed foods are the richest sources of potassium.

FOOD LABELING

The potassium content of a product, given in milligrams, **may** be listed on the "Nutrition Facts" panel if the manufacturer so chooses. It

DISPLAY 11-3 HIGH-POTASSIUM FOODS

HIGH (390 MG POTASSIUM)	
Avocado	1/2 cup mashed or 1/2 fruit
Banana, raw	1 medium
Beans, white or red (cooked)	1/2 cup
Molasses, blackstrap	1 tbsp
Orange juice, frozen (diluted)	1 cup
Potato, baked	1 medium
Prune juice, canned	3/4 cup
Squash, winter, all varieties (cooked)	1/2 cup
Tomato juice, canned	1 cup
Vegetable juice, canned	1 cup
MODERATELY HIGH (275–390 MG POTASSIUM)	
All Bran	1/3 cup
Apricot nectar	1 cup
Apricots (canned, raw, or dried)	3 whole
Bran Buds	1/4 cup
Cantaloupe (5-in diameter)	1/6 melon
Honeydew melon (5-in diameter)	1/10 melon
Dates	6 medium
Eggnog	1 cup
Figs	3 medium
Grapefruit juice, canned, unsweetened	1 cup
Lima beans	1/2 cup
Milk (whole, skim, 2%, or buttermilk)	1 cup
Mushrooms (cooked)	1/2 cup
Orange, raw	1 large
Parsnips (cooked)	1/2 cup
Pineapple juice, canned	1 cup
Plums, raw	3 fruits
Potatoes, french fries	15 strips
Potatoes, mashed, hashed brown	1/2–3/4 cup
Prunes, dried	5 medium
Raisins	1/4 cup
Spinach, raw, chopped	1 cup
Tomatoes, raw, whole	1 large
Yams, baked in skin	1 small
Yogurt, 1%–2% fat, unflavored	1 cup

(Adapted from Twin Cities District Dietetic Association. Manual of clinical nutrition. Minneapolis: Chronimed/DCI Publishing, 1994:508.

is a voluntary component of the label. If given, the potassium content will also be expressed as "% Daily Value," which is 3500 mg of potassium regardless of the caloric content of the diet.

RECOMMENDED ALLOWANCES

The estimated *minimum* requirement for adults is 2000 mg/day. Increased amounts are needed during pregnancy and breastfeeding, but these needs are met easily by the usual potassium intake.

The Committee on Diet and Health has recommended that people consume five or more servings of fruits and vegetables daily. This recommendation would increase the potassium intake of adults to 3500 mg/day. This level may help to reduce hypertension and thereby reduce the risk of stroke (see Chapter 26).

DEFICIENCY AND EXCESS

Because potassium is so abundant in the food supply, a deficiency does not occur under normal circumstances. In addition to the use of diuretics, the following may cause a potassium deficiency (*hypokalemia*): severe vomiting, diarrhea, laxative abuse, some forms of chronic renal disease, diabetic acidosis, severe protein–calorie malnutrition, and adrenal gland abnormalities. Symptoms of deficiency include nausea, anorexia, apprehension, muscular weakness, irrational behavior, rapid heart beat, and abnormal heart rhythms (which can be fatal).

High potassium levels in the blood (*hyperkalemia*) also are a health threat. Cardiac arrhythmias (irregular heartbeats), muscular weakness, and numbness of the face, tongue, and extremities are symptoms of hyperkalemia. Death may result from cardiac arrest. Toxic blood levels usually result from abnormal conditions such as kidney failure, abnormal adrenal function, and severe dehydration (see Chapter 26). Hyperkalemia also may be caused by a sudden increase in potassium intake, as with the excessive use of potassium supplements.

MAGNESIUM

Magnesium occurs in the bones and teeth and in soft tissues and body fluids. It activates more than 300 enzyme systems involved in energy metabolism and in the metabolism of other minerals, such as calcium, potassium, phosphorus, and sodium. Together with other minerals, magnesium regulates nerve stimulation and muscle contractions. A deficiency leads to nervous irritability, muscular weakness, nausea, mental derangement, and, if untreated, convulsive seizures. Deficiency occurs in conditions in which magnesium intake or absorption is decreased or excretion is increased, such as chronic alcoholism, diabetes, malabsorption syndrome, kwashiorkor, kidney disease, and glandular disorders.

Magnesium plays an essential role in plant life. It is a component of the green pigment chlorophyll and is abundant in green leafy vegetables. Nuts, whole-grain cereals, and legumes have the highest concentration of magnesium. Cereal grains lose more than 80% of their magnesium when the germ and outer layers of the grains are removed. The RDA for magnesium is 350 mg/day for men, 280 mg/day for women, and 320 mg/day for pregnant and breastfeeding women.

CHLORIDE

Chlorine occurs in the body mainly in the form of chloride, which is the chief anion (negatively charged ion) in extracellular fluid. Chloride helps maintain osmotic pressure, water balance, and acid–base balance. It is a component of hydrochloric acid, which is essential to protein digestion in the stomach. Chloride enhances the carbon dioxide–carrying function of the blood. Sodium chloride (table salt) is the main dietary source of chloride. Processed foods are the major source. The *minimum* requirement for adults is estimated to be 750 mg/day.

SULFUR

Sulfur is part of the protein in every cell. It is a component of several amino acids, several B vitamins, insulin, and other vital body compounds. No

RDA has been set for sulfur. The source of sulfur in the diet is chiefly from sulfur-containing amino acids, and adequacy is dependent on the intake of protein foods.

MICROMINERALS

IRON

The quantity of a nutrient the body requires does not indicate its relative importance. This is well demonstrated by the mineral iron. The body contains less than 5 g of iron, but this small amount performs extraordinarily important functions. About two thirds of the iron is in the blood, and about one third is in the liver, spleen, and bone marrow (as ferritin and hemosiderin). Small amounts of iron are found in muscle myoglobin (an oxygen-carrying protein found only in muscle tissue), in the blood serum, and in every cell as a component of enzymes. (See Table 11-5 on p. 208 for a summary of minerals.)

Absorbed iron combines with protein to form *transferrin,* a transport form of iron in the blood serum. In this form, iron is carried to the bone marrow for hemoglobin synthesis, to the liver or spleen for storage, or to other tissues for their needs.

FUNCTIONS AND CLINICAL EFFECTS

Component of Hemoglobin

Iron is a component of *hemoglobin,* the compound that carries oxygen from the lungs to the cells. The hemoglobin carries some of the carbon dioxide that is produced in the cell back to the lungs, where it is exhaled. The hemoglobin molecule comprises two parts: *globin,* a protein, and *heme,* the iron-containing pigment of the blood that is responsible for its characteristic color. Adequate protein and traces of copper are necessary for hemoglobin synthesis. Other nutrients, including certain vitamins, also promote hemoglobin formation. A red blood cell disintegrates after about 120 days. Its iron is used by the body repeatedly for hemoglobin synthesis.

Component of Cellular Enzymes

In every cell, iron is a component of certain enzymes that are important in energy production.

FACTORS THAT AFFECT IRON BALANCE

The intestinal mucosa regulates iron absorption. Except for about 1 mg/day lost in the urine and through the skin, iron absorbed from the gastrointestinal tract cannot be excreted. Therefore, iron absorption must be regulated so that dangerously high levels of the mineral do not accumulate. Iron is lost mainly through blood loss in hemorrhage, menstruation, blood donations, and parasitic infestations. The amount of dietary iron that is absorbed depends on the food source and the composition of the meal in which that food is eaten. Careful planning can increase or decrease the amount of iron absorbed. Although the main concern is increasing the amount of iron absorbed, a small number of people in whom iron stores accumulate excessively would benefit from a diet low in iron.

The iron in food is divided into two categories: heme and nonheme iron. Heme iron accounts for 40% of the iron in meat, fish, and poultry. A high percentage (23%) of heme iron is absorbed, and absorption is unaffected by other factors in the diet. Nonheme iron accounts for the remaining 60% of the iron in meat, fish, and poultry; for all the iron in other foods; for the iron in compounds added to enrich foods (such as cereals); and for the iron in iron supplements. Only a small amount (as little as 3%) of nonheme iron is absorbed.

The absorption of nonheme iron can be increased to 8% if the mineral is ingested in a meal that includes ascorbic acid or meat, fish, or poultry. The maximum possible amount of nonheme iron is available in a meal that contains more than 90 g (3 oz) of meat, fish, or poultry; more than 75 mg of ascorbic acid (the amount provided by 8 oz of orange or grapefruit juice); or 30 to 90 g (1 to 3 oz) of meat, fish, or poultry plus 25 to 75 mg of ascorbic acid (the amount in 4 oz of orange or grapefruit juice). Thus, meals can be planned so that the

TABLE 11-5 SUMMARY OF MINERALS

Mineral	Function	Deficiency	Sources
Calcium	Bone and tooth formation; blood clotting; cell permeability; nerve stimulation; muscle contraction; enzyme activation	Stunted growth; rickets; osteomalacia; osteoporosis (porous bones); tetany (low serum calcium)	Milk; hard cheese; salmon and small fish with bones eaten; some dark green vegetables; legumes (tofu)
Phosphorus	Bone and tooth formation; energy metabolism—component of ATP and ADP; protein synthesis—component of DNA and RNA; fat transport; acid–base balance; enzyme formation	Stunted growth; rickets (due to excessive excretion rather than to dietary deficiency)	Distributed widely in foods: milk; meats, poultry, fish, eggs; cheese; nuts; legumes; whole grains; processed foods
Sodium	Osmotic pressure; water balance; acid–base balance; nerve stimulation; muscle contraction; cell permeability	Rare: nausea; vomiting; giddiness; exhaustion; cramps	Table salt, salted foods, MSG and other sodium additives; milk; meat, fish, poultry, eggs
Potassium	Osmotic pressure; water balance; acid–base balance; nerve stimulation; muscle contraction; protein synthesis; glycogen formation	Nausea; vomiting; muscular weakness; rapid heart beat; heart failure	Widely distributed in food: meats, fish, poultry; whole grains; fruits, vegetables, legumes
Magnesium	Component of bones and teeth; activates many enzymes, including those involved in energy metabolism; nerve stimulation; muscle contraction	Seen in alcoholism or renal disease; tremors leading to convulsive seizures	Green leafy vegetables; nuts; whole grains; meat; milk; seafood
Iron	Hemoglobin and myoglobin formation; cellular enzymes	Anemia	Liver, lean meats; legumes, dried fruits, green leafy vegetables; whole-grain and fortified cereals
Iodine	Synthesis of thyroid hormones that regulate basal metabolic rate	Goiter; cretinism, if deficiency is severe	Iodized salt; seafood; food grown near the sea
Fluoride	Resists dental decay	Tooth decay in young children	Fluoridated water (1 part per million)
Selenium	Antioxidant—prevents oxidative damage to body tissue	Keshan disease; damage to heart muscle	Fish, meat, breads and cereals
Zinc	Constituent of many enzyme systems, including those involved in protein digestion and synthesis, carbon dioxide transport, and vitamin A use	Delayed wound healing; impaired taste sensitivity. Severe deficiency (rare in the United States): retarded growth and sexual development; dwarfism	Oysters, herring; meat, liver, fish; milk; whole grains; nuts; legumes

TABLE 11-6 IRON CONTENT OF SELECTED FOODS*

FOOD	AMOUNT	IRON (MG)†
Liver, beef‡	3 oz	5.5
Liverwurst‡	3 oz	5.4
Beef patty (10% fat)	3 oz	2.1
Shrimp, canned	3 oz	1.4
Chicken	3 oz	0.9
Frankfurter	3 oz	1.0
Flounder	3 oz	0.3
Infant cereal, dry‡	½ oz	6.7
Bran flakes, fortified	1 cup	10.8
Oatmeal	1 cup	1.6
Cornflakes	1 cup	1.4
Whole-wheat bread	1 slice, 16/loaf	1.0
White bread, enriched	1 slice, 16/loaf	0.8
Split peas, cooked	1 cup	3.4
Peanut butter	2 tbsp	0.6
Spinach, leaf frozen, cooked	½ cup	1.5
Peas, frozen, cooked	½ cup	1.3
Potato, baked, with skin	large	2.7
Snap beans, cooked	½ cup	0.8
Prunes, dried	5	1.2
Raisins	3 tbsp	0.6
Orange	1	0.1

* Source of nutritive values: US Dept of Agriculture, Human Nutrition Information Service. Nutritive value of food. Washington, DC: US Government Printing Office, 1991. Home and Garden bulletin 72.

† The iron in meat, fish, and poultry is more readily available to the body than the iron in plant sources.

‡ Label information.

amount of available iron is increased or decreased according to individual needs.

Some substances in the diet and in medications decrease iron absorption. These include calcium and phosphate salts, edetate (ethylenediamine tetraacetic acid), phytates, fiber, tannic acid (in tea), phosvitin (in egg yolk), and antacid medications.

The amount of iron absorbed also depends on the amount of iron in body stores. When body stores are low, absorption is high; when stores are high, absorption is decreased.

SOURCES

Good sources of iron include lean meat, fish, and poultry; cooked dried peas, beans, and lentils; dark green leafy vegetables; dried fruit; potatoes; whole-grain and enriched bread; fortified cereals; and nuts and nut butters. The iron content of whole-grain products, enriched cereals, and legumes is particularly important for vegetarians and people who must limit purchases of more costly sources of iron, such as meat. Iron-fortified infant formulas and iron-fortified infant cereals are important sources of iron for infants and toddlers.

Liver is an especially rich source of iron. However, its high cholesterol content and poor acceptance limit its usefulness. Foods such as oysters, clams, shrimp, sardines, and dark molasses, although good sources of iron, are not eaten frequently enough or in large enough quantities to be considered important iron sources. The iron in egg yolk, although rich in quantity, is poorly absorbed.

The iron in fibrous vegetable foods, such as bran cereals and leafy vegetables, is not as available to the body as that in meats. For this reason, vegetarians may need to consume considerably more iron to obtain the same amount as would be furnished by animal foods. Table 11-6 gives the iron content of selected foods. Including foods that are sources of ascorbic acid increases the absorption of iron in a meal.

FOOD LABELING

The iron content per serving of a product is a required component of the "Nutrition Facts" panel on food labels. It is expressed as "% Daily Value," which is 18 mg of iron regardless of the caloric content of the diet.

RECOMMENDED ALLOWANCES

The recommended iron allowance for infants to 6 months is 6 mg/day; for infants and children from 6 months to 10 years, adult men throughout life, and postmenopausal women is 10 mg/day; for boys 11 to 18 years is 12 mg/day; and for girls and women of childbearing age, it is 15 mg/day. The high allowance for premenopausal women reflects the need for additional iron during menstruation, pregnancy, and breastfeeding. The loss of iron in menstrual blood flow ranges from 15 to 30 mg or more per month. These allowances are based on the assumption that about 10% to 15% of the iron consumed is available for absorption. The RDA assumes that people consume daily 30 to 90 g (1 to 3 oz) of meat, poultry, or fish or foods containing 25 to 75 mg of ascorbic acid after preparation are consumed daily.

A standard diet that meets nutritional requirements in all other respects contains about 9 mg to 12 mg of iron. The typical American diet does not readily provide the 15 mg/day of iron recommended for menstruating women.

DEFICIENCY: ANEMIA

Poor selection of food, insufficient money to buy adequate food, or lack of appetite during illness may result in deficient iron intake. Iron deficiency anemia occurs when the iron supply is insufficient to support the adequate formation of red blood cells and, consequently, the oxygen needs of the tissues are not met. Although the number of red blood cells is sufficient, their size is inadequate because there is not enough hemoglobin to fill them. In infants and children, symptoms of iron deficiency anemia include irritability, apathy, lethargy, and pallor. Adults are pale and tire easily. Pallor of mucous membranes, especially on the underside of the eyelid and in the interior of the mouth, is a clinical sign of possible anemia. A deficiency of other nutrients, such as protein, also can cause nutritional anemia. Because there are several types of anemia, both nutritional and nonnutritional, a careful diagnosis by a physician is necessary to determine the kind and cause.

Iron intake frequently is inadequate during infancy and other periods of rapid growth when there is an increase in blood volume. In the United States, iron deficiency anemia is the most prevalent deficiency disease of early childhood. The breastfed infant, because of the iron stores the newborn has at birth, can maintain normal hemoglobin levels without any other source of iron for the first 3 months. Thereafter, and for nonbreastfed infants from birth, other sources of iron are required.

If the need for iron is not met, the shortage that begins in infancy usually peaks during the second year of life. The incidence of anemia decreases during later childhood but increases again in adolescence, especially among girls. It also is high in menstruating women and pregnant women, in whom iron intake must meet the needs of the fetus and must replace the iron in the blood that is lost during childbirth.

Poor absorption of iron from the intestinal tract also may produce anemia. In malabsorption syndromes, there usually is poor absorption of several nutrients, including iron. Iron absorption also is reduced in diseases in which there is low gastric acidity. Acid increases the solubility of iron and thus promotes absorption. Both hydrochloric acid and iron supplements may be given in cases of malabsorption.

EXCESS

Hemochromatosis is an inherited disease characterized by excessive iron absorption. It is due to an inability to regulate iron absorption from the intestinal lining. It is a serious condition that gives rise to an accumulation of iron in the liver, spleen, bone marrow, heart, and other tissues.

About 2000 cases of iron poisoning due to the excessive intake of iron supplements occur each year. Most of these cases involve children who consume supplements intended for adults. A dose of about 3 g of ferrous sulfate can be fatal to a 2-year-old.

In recent years, the beneficial effects of an iron-rich diet for the general population has been questioned. A 5-year study of 1900 men conducted in Finland and reported in September 1992 concluded that the amount of iron stored in the body ranks second only to smoking as the strongest risk factor for heart disease and heart attacks. The authors of the study indicated that iron increases heart disease risk by promoting chemical reactions between low-density lipoproteins in the serum and oxygen—reactions that eventually result in blocking the arteries of the heart.

Iron appears to encourage the formation of unstable oxygenated molecules called *free radicals* that have been implicated not only in heart disease but also in cancer, diabetes, arthritis, and the aging process. These free radicals disrupt chemical bonds and can damage DNA molecules. Much more research is needed to substantiate the effects of moderate iron overload in the development of these diseases. Nevertheless, it may be possibly hazardous for people who do not have anemia or are not pregnant to take supplements with iron. Also, the fortification of commercial foods with iron is a practice that will undoubtedly be examined carefully.

IODINE

Normal function of the thyroid gland depends on the availability of adequate amounts of iodine.

The thyroid produces hormones that regulate energy metabolism in the body tissues and are essential for normal tissue growth and development. An adequate supply of iodine is necessary for the production of the hormones thyroxine (T_4) and triiodothyronine (T_3). These hormones are transported in the blood bound to protein and are referred to as *protein-bound iodine.* Some T_4 and T_3 circulate freely. Iodine is easily absorbed from the intestinal tract. About 30% is used by the thyroid gland, and the remainder is excreted in the urine. Thyroid hormone production is controlled by thyroid-stimulating hormone (TSH), which is secreted by the pituitary gland. When the level of thyroid hormones in the bloodstream decreases, TSH stimulates the thyroid to produce more hormones.

Thyroid hormones regulate metabolic rate. Excessive production of thyroid hormones (*hyperthyroidism*) increases the metabolic rate above normal; low production (*hypothyroidism*) reduces the metabolic rate. Measurement of the serum T_3 and T_4 levels and of protein-bound iodine is used to evaluate thyroid function. When thyroid production is low, increased quantities of TSH are found in the bloodstream as the pituitary attempts to stimulate the thyroid to increase hormone production. Without iodine, however, the hormones cannot be produced.

SOURCES

People who live near seacoasts and eat enough seafood receive sufficient iodine. The iodine content of plant foods varies according to the iodine content of the soil in which the plants are grown. Plant foods grown near seacoasts or in the southern states contain more iodine than those grown in the Great Lakes area or in other areas where the surface soil is low in iodine. The use of iodized salt is the most practical way to obtain an adequate amount of iodine.

A considerable amount of iodine finds its way into the food supply accidentally. The iodine content of dairy products is raised above natural levels by the use of iodine-containing disinfectants on cows and milk production equipment and by the addition of iodine-containing substances to animal feeds.

RECOMMENDED ALLOWANCES

The recommended intake for both men and women from age 11 years through adulthood is 150 mcg. The use of iodized salt in noncoastal regions, where iodine levels in the environment and food supply are low, is recommended.

DEFICIENCY AND EXCESS

When the thyroid gland cannot manufacture sufficient hormones, it responds by producing more and larger cells. The result is *goiter,* an enlargement of the thyroid that produces a swelling of the neck. Simple goiter is sometimes called *endemic goiter* because it is common to the inhabitants of a particular region where there is little iodine in the soil. If a goiter goes untreated during pregnancy and if the iodine deficiency is severe, the fetus will not receive enough iodine and is likely to be a *cretin*—a child with arrested physical and mental development. If the child receives treatment immediately after birth, many of the symptoms may be reversible.

High levels of iodine are toxic. Goiter resulting from a high iodine intake has been reported in Japan. There appear to be no adverse reactions to the amount of iodine in the American diet. In the past, concern had been expressed about the increasing amount of iodine due to its use in food processing and to the unintended sources of iodine that enter the food chain. More recently, the use of iodine-containing compounds and the iodine content of the US diet have been declining. The amount of iodine in the diet has declined steadily since 1982. The Food and Nutrition Board has recommended that no additional iodine be introduced into the American diet.

Abnormal thyroxine production can also result from a poorly functioning thyroid gland. See Chapter 30 for a discussion of hypothyroidism (myxedema) and hyperthyroidism (Graves' disease).

FLUORIDE

Fluoride is the term used for the ionized form of the element fluorine as it occurs in drinking water. The two terms are used interchangeably.

Fluoride is a component of bones and teeth; it is especially abundant in dental enamel. The incidence of dental caries is reduced by 50% to 60% in communities in which the water supply has been fluoridated.

Fluoride is found in small amounts in all soils, water, plants, and animals. Consequently, a deficiency severe enough to affect normal growth has not been identified in humans. The Food and Nutrition Board has recommended fluoridation of the water supply where natural fluoride levels are well below 0.7 mg/liter. Where fluoridated water supplies are unavailable, fluoride levels may be increased through the use of sodium fluoride tablets, fluoride toothpastes, and bottled fluoridated water, and by the application of fluoride to the teeth.

Fluoride is toxic in excessive amounts. Years of excessive intake in the range of 20 to 80 mg/day affect bone, kidney, muscle, and nerve function. Excessive amounts in the range of 2 to 8 mg/kg of body weight per day has caused mottling of the teeth in children.

A range of 1.5 to 4 mg/day is an estimated safe and adequate intake of fluoride for adults. Table 11-1 gives the ranges for infants and children. The maximum intake for children and adolescents is 2.5 mg/day to avoid mottling of the teeth.

SELENIUM

Selenium is part of an enzyme, glutathione peroxidase, that prevents oxidative damage to tissues. It is closely related to another antioxidant: vitamin E. Selenium is important for the proper functioning of the heart. Other possible functions are under investigation.

SOURCES

Fish, meat, breads, and cereals are sources of selenium. The selenium content of plant foods depends on the selenium content of the soil in which they are grown. Fruits and vegetables are poor sources of selenium.

RECOMMENDED ALLOWANCES

In 1989, RDAs for selenium were established for the first time. The recommendations are based on studies of Chinese men. The RDA is 70 mcg for men and 55 mcg for women. An increase of 10 mcg during pregnancy and 20 mcg during breastfeeding is recommended.

DEFICIENCY AND EXCESS

In 1979, Chinese scientists reported a connection between low selenium status and *Keshan disease*, a disease of the heart muscle that affects young children and women. Although a virus appears to be involved in the disease, selenium deficiency appears to predispose people to its development. This finding was the first direct evidence that selenium is essential in human nutrition.

Selenium deficiency also has been found in people who have been fed intravenously for long periods. Among the symptoms experienced were muscular discomfort, weakness, and heart muscle abnormalities. These symptoms responded to selenium therapy.

Selenium is highly toxic in excessive amounts. The precise amount needed to cause toxicity is unknown, but as little as 1 mg of selenium daily for more than 2 years has produced toxic symptoms. Symptoms of toxicity include fingernail changes, hair loss, peripheral neuropathy (nerve damage in the extremities), fatigue, nausea, abdominal pain, diarrhea, and irritability.

ZINC

Zinc is a component of many enzyme systems, including those involved in protein synthesis, carbon dioxide transport, and use of vitamin A. Zinc also occurs in insulin.

A condition that responds to zinc therapy has been identified in the Middle East. It occurs in children and adolescent boys and is characterized by dwarfism, an enlarged liver and spleen, delayed sexual development, and anemia. Intestinal parasites, phytates in food, excessive sweating, and clay eating—all of which interfere with zinc absorption—are factors involved in the development of zinc deficiency in these cases.

SOURCES

The zinc in meats and seafood is much more readily available than that in whole-grain cereals, legumes, and nuts. Phytates and dietary fiber hinder zinc absorption. Oysters and herring are the richest sources of zinc. Liver and milk, as well as meat and fish, also are good sources.

RECOMMENDED ALLOWANCES

The RDA of zinc for men and for boys older than age 11 years is 15 mg/day. For women and for girls older than age 11 years, it is 12 mg/day. In pregnancy, 15 mg/day is required; 19 mg/day is recommended in the first 6 months of breastfeeding and 16 mg/day is recommended in the second 6 months.

DEFICIENCY AND EXCESS

Zinc deficiency in adults occurs mainly as a result of diseases that either hinder absorption of zinc or cause excessive excretion of zinc in the urine. Poor taste sensitivity and impaired wound healing have been shown to improve with supplementation.

Zinc supplements in excess of 15 mg/day should not be taken except under close medical supervision. Moderately elevated levels of zinc can impair copper metabolism. More severely elevated amounts also can cause blood abnormalities and impairment of immune responses. See Table 11-5 for a summary of microminerals.

OTHER ESSENTIAL TRACE MINERALS

For the following trace minerals, with the exception of cobalt, Table 11-1 lists estimated safe and adequate daily dietary intakes:

- Manganese is an important mineral in enzyme systems; it functions in blood formation and tendon and bone structure.
- Cobalt, a component of vitamin B_{12}, is necessary for the formation of red blood cells.
- Copper is required for the use of iron in the formation of hemoglobin. It is a component of many enzymes.
- Molybdenum, a component of enzymes, may be involved in the metabolism of fats.
- Chromium is associated with the body's ability to use glucose and is necessary for normal insulin activity.

KEY ISSUES

Osteoporosis: Common and Complex

Osteoporosis, or *porous bone,* is a disease in which bones become excessively fragile. It is the most common bone disease encountered in medical practice. It is a disease of enormous proportions, affecting more than 25 million Americans. One third to one half of all postmenopausal women in the United States have the disease as do nearly half of all people older than age 75 years. Osteoporosis is responsible for an estimated 1.7 million fractures annually. Elderly people with hip fractures have a 12% to 20% greater risk of dying within the first year after the injury than their peers. The estimated cost of osteoporosis and its complications, not including lost earnings, was $10 billion in 1990. With the increase in our elderly population, it will become an increasingly serious public health problem.

GENERAL CHARACTERISTICS

Loss of bone is a natural process of aging, but not all people develop osteoporosis. Osteoporosis is characterized by loss of bone mass, deterioration of bone tissue, and a resulting increase in fracture risk

(Fig. 11-1). Bones may become so fragile that simple movements such as picking up a light package or merely coughing can cause a fracture. Osteoporosis is related to reduced bone mass at maturity, or to excessive bone loss thereafter, or both. Both genetic and environmental factors are involved in its development. Certain risk factors identify those who have an increased tendency to osteoporosis.

RISK FACTORS

Gender

Both men and women can develop osteoporosis. Women are four times more likely to develop osteoporosis, develop it earlier, and have more severe conditions than men. A likely reason is that women have 20% less bone mass than men. Other reasons are the rapid bone loss that occurs at menopause and the longer life span of women.

Thin, Small-Framed Body; Caucasian and Asian Races

White and Asian women who have a small bony frame and low body weight are at greatest risk. Small-boned people have less bone to lose, and decreased muscle and weight stress on bones results in decreased bone formation. African Americans have a higher bone density and lose bone more slowly than whites.

Reduced Sex Hormones

Estrogen deficiency is the main cause of bone loss after menopause; early menopause, either natural or caused by surgical removal of the ovaries, increases the risk of osteoporosis. Younger women who have decreased estrogen production indicated by lack of menstruation or irregular menstruation are also at greater risk. People with anorexia and female athletes who experience menstrual disturbances are prone to bone loss.

The male sex hormone testosterone protects against bone loss. Decreases in sex hormones in both men and women will increase bone loss; however, the results are much more rapid and drastic in women than in men. Some researchers believe that there are different types of osteoporosis, with different causes and treatments. Women are many times more likely to have fractures of the vertebrae than men but only twice as likely to have hip fractures. Hormonal differences between men and women are a possible explanation for the phenomenon. Vertebrae contain mostly trabecular, spongy bone, which is greatly influenced by estrogen. Hip bones are mostly dense, compact cortical bone, which appears to be affected less by hormonal differences.

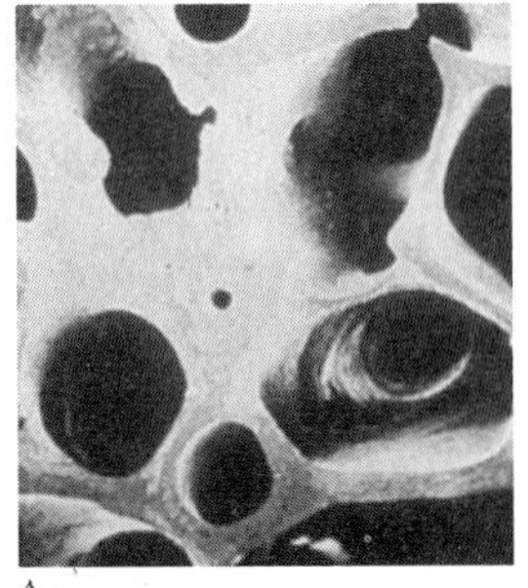
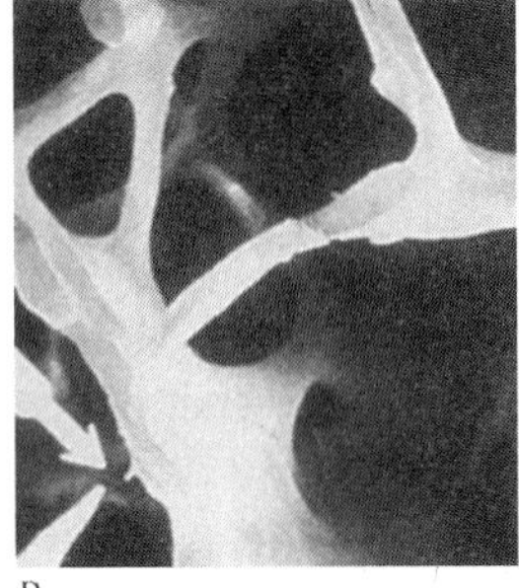

A B

FIGURE 11-1

Photo on right shows loss in bone tissue that occurs in osteoporosis. *(Dempster DW et al. Boning up on osteoporosis. Washington, DC: National Osteoporosis Foundation, 1991:9.)*

Heredity

Research has shown that daughters of women with osteoporosis had lower bone density than daughters of women who did not have the disease. Some researchers have questioned whether this finding is due to genetics or to lifestyle (diet and exercise).

Lack of Calcium and Other Dietary Factors

The amount of calcium consumed from childhood through age 35 years directly affects the attainment of maximal bone density. Despite numerous research studies, many gaps exist in our knowledge of the relationship of dietary calcium to osteoporosis undoubtedly due to the many metabolic as well as dietary factors that affect calcium and bone metabolism. Although important, calcium alone will not protect against osteoporosis.

A study of 225 women 1 year after menopause who were not on estrogen replacement therapy revealed that those who drank milk at each meal during childhood and adolescence had greater bone density than those who drank milk less often. Inadequate vitamin D is another dietary factor that can inhibit bone formation and contribute to bone loss. Vitamin D is needed for the absorption of calcium from the intestinal tract. Among elderly people, vitamin D deficiency is likely to occur due to insufficient exposure to sunlight and inadequate consumption of vitamin D–fortified foods (e.g., milk or cereal).

High levels of caffeine, protein, and sodium in the diet are thought to increase the amount of calcium in the urine. More studies are needed to confirm if these substances cause calcium loss and to establish safe intake levels. Excess intake of phosphate-containing beverages is also linked to reduced bone density, which may predispose to osteoporosis. (See the discussion of calcium–phosphate balance under Calcium Balance [Solubility Product].)

Cigarette Smoking and Alcohol

People who smoke tend to have lower bone densities than nonsmokers. This may be due to lower serum estrogen levels in women who smoke.

People who drink alcohol on a regular basis (2 to 3 oz/day) are also at greater risk of osteoporosis. Alcohol is believed to destroy bone-forming cells and may also interfere with calcium absorption. The poor nutrition that frequently accompanies heavy drinking and the proneness to falls also affect bone health.

Lack of Physical Activity

Bone density is proportional to the amount of exercise a person gets. Weight-bearing exercises such as walking, stairclimbing, running, and tennis play an important role in preventing osteoporosis because the pull of muscle on bone stimulates bone formation. If women exercise to the point of losing their menstrual cycle, however, the benefit of exercise is lost. People who are immobilized or bedridden for long periods or are subject to weightlessness, such as that experienced by astronauts in space, are at high risk of excessive bone loss.

Certain Medications

Glucocorticoids (steroids) can cause significant bone loss if taken for a prolonged period. High doses of antiseizure drugs and excessive thyroid hormone can result in bone loss. The diuretic furosemide and over-the-counter antacids that contain aluminum also interfere with calcium use.

DIAGNOSIS

Ordinary x-rays are not sensitive enough to detect osteoporosis in the early stages. By the time osteoporosis can be detected by x-ray, as much as 25% to 40% of bone tissue has been lost.

In recent years tests, called *bone densitometry* or *absorptiometry*, have been developed that can measure bone mass in various body sites. These safe and painless tests rely on a photon energy source being passed over spine, hips, wrist, or other parts of the skeleton. A computerized tomography (CT) scan, which also can measure the density of bone, exposes clients to higher doses of radiation than the former techniques. These diagnostic tools enable physicians to determine if treatment is needed and, if so, what approach is best. These tests also provide a baseline measurement to which the effectiveness of treatment can be compared.

PREVENTION

Prevention is the best way to deal with osteoporosis. Greater emphasis on education, nutrition, and exercise promises to prevent or delay the onset of the disease. Prevention involves maximizing bone density throughout the years of bone development and reducing bone loss after maturity. Preventive measures to accomplish these two goals are as follows:

- Increase peak bone mass by consuming adequate amounts of calcium-rich foods or a combination of foods and calcium supplements, if necessary. The RDA for calcium should be met throughout infancy, childhood, and young adulthood. The National Institutes of Health and the National Osteoporosis Foundation recommend higher intakes of calcium than the RDAs for adults and postmenopausal women who are not taking hormone replacement therapy, 1000 and 1500 mg, respectively. If enough calcium cannot be consumed in food, a calcium supplement may be needed.
- Take vitamin D supplementation if required. Vitamin D is necessary for both calcium absorption and incorporation in bone. People who are not exposed to sunlight may require a supplement. Supplementation should not exceed 400 IU, unless supervised by a physician.
- Engage in regular weight-bearing exercises such as walking, hiking, stairclimbing, or jogging.

- Avoid or limit alcohol, caffeine, and nicotine use.
- Undergo estrogen replacement at menopause (for high-risk individuals). This is a recommendation of the National Institutes of Health expert panel on osteoporosis. High-risk people include those with premature menopause or surgical menopause, low bone mass (as measured by a bone-density test), family history of osteoporosis, and medical problems associated with osteoporosis. Estrogen replacement is the most important means of improving the condition once it occurs. The use of estrogens, however, has been associated with an increased risk of endometrial and possibly breast cancer. This risk has been reduced by using estrogen in a cycle, with progesterone given at the end of the cycle.

TREATMENT

New methods of diagnosis and treatment can stop or slow the destruction of bone. Treatment consists of a calcium-rich diet, daily exercise, fall prevention, and drug therapy.

Estrogen replacement for women can be used until about age 75 years. Testosterone therapy may be used for men. Calcitonin, a hormone produced by the thyroid gland, is used in the treatment of both women and men. Calcitonin slows down the breakdown of bone tissue. Salmon calcitonin is the only form of calcitonin approved by the Food and Drug Administration (FDA); it is available only by injection at present.

Other drugs, not yet approved by the FDA for the treatment of osteoporosis, are under investigation. These drugs include bisphosphonates, calcitonin by nasal spray, new estrogen preparations, and fluoride.

KEYS TO PRACTICAL APPLICATION

Encourage the consumption of milk at all ages. Calcium is needed throughout life. Remember that nonfat and lowfat milks have just as much calcium as whole milk.

Avoid too much sodium. Add only a little salt in cooking and little or none at the table, and limit your intake of salty foods.

Increase your intake of potassium-rich foods. The relation of sodium to potassium is important; consume the two in about equal amounts. Too much potassium, however, is as bad as too little. Discourage the use of potassium supplements or potassium-containing salt substitutes without a physician's approval.

Discourage the frequent use of antacid preparations without medical supervision. Reducing the acidity of the stomach reduces the absorption of calcium and iron.

Use vitamin C–rich foods at every meal. Vitamin C increases the absorption of nonheme iron.

Encourage the use of iodized salt in noncoastal states. Sea salt should not be used as a substitute, because its iodine is lost during the drying process.

Support community efforts to fluoridate water. Dental decay is reduced 50% to 60% among children in fluoridated communities.

Encourage the use of legumes (dried peas, beans, lentils, and soybeans). They are excellent inexpensive sources of many essential minerals.

Educate your clients on how to use food labels to achieve target levels of calcium and iron and to control sodium.

Make your clients aware of ways to prevent osteoporosis—particularly the need to include adequate calcium in the diet and adequate weight-bearing exercise.

KEY IDEAS

The roles of minerals in the body are interrelated; in some cases, the minerals complement; in other cases, they hinder each other's activities.

Minerals are most abundant in unrefined foods; increased use of processed foods may create deficiencies of trace minerals. See Table 11-5 for a summary of the functions, results of deficiency, and the sources of the various minerals.

The difference between beneficial amounts and harmful amounts of trace elements may be small.

The assumption that if a little is good, more is better is risky when applied to minerals. All minerals are toxic when taken in excessive amounts.

The iron in meat, fish, and poultry is more efficiently absorbed than the iron from other sources, including iron supplements.

Calcium, sodium, and iron are required components of the "Nutrition Facts" panel on food labels; potassium is a voluntary component. Health claims on labels can be made for the relationship between calcium and osteoporosis and sodium and hypertension.

Osteoporosis is a complex disease that involves many factors, including genetics, hormonal levels, calcium intake, and physical activity.

The postmenopausal bone loss is strongly influenced by estrogen status.

The best way to reduce risk of osteoporosis is to maintain calcium intake at a level that allows individuals to accumulate bone mass to their genetic potential; to acquire sufficient vitamin D; to do regular weight-bearing exercise; to avoid or limit alcohol, caffeine, and nicotine; and to undergo estrogen replacement (for women at high risk).

Treatment for osteoporosis includes a calcium-rich diet, daily exercise, fall prevention, and drugs (sex hormones and calcitonin).

KEYS TO LEARNING

STUDY–DISCUSSION QUESTIONS

1. Using the 1-day food diary you kept in Chapter 5, compare your consumption of iron and calcium with the RDAs for your gender and age group given in Appendix B. Which items on your record provide the most calcium? Which provide the most iron?

2. Plan 2 days of meals (including snacks) that meet the RDA for young adults of 1200 mg/day of calcium. Then plan a day's meals without fluid milk. What foods account for most of the calcium in the meals that do not include fluid milk?

3. Rank the following foods according to calcium content, with the richest source of calcium first:

   3 oz of ground beef, cooked
   ½ cup of fresh collards, cooked
   1 oz of cheddar cheese
   1 cup of milk
   ½ cup of carrots, cooked
   3 oz of Atlantic-type sardines, canned

   Check your answers with the calcium content listed for each of these items in Table 11-3.

4. What is the importance of iodine? Where in the United States is there a lack of iodine in the soil and water? What is the most practical means of obtaining an adequate amount of iodine?

5. Discuss in class the importance of a varied diet and how it relates to an adequate intake of minerals. Some authorities have expressed concern about the excessive use of highly processed and synthetic foods. How does this trend threaten the adequate intake of minerals, especially trace minerals?

6. The body has many checks and balances to maintain a state of dynamic equilibrium. Explain the body mechanisms that maintain calcium balance.

7. What factors promote the absorption of iron? How would you use this information to help a client who has iron deficiency anemia?
8. What is the benefit of a fluoridated water supply? Is the water in your community fluoridated? If not, why not?
9. Present a case study of a client with osteoporosis. Include in your presentation the probable risk factors in the case, the treatment plan, the client's progress, and the client's views regarding the disease and its treatment.

BIBLIOGRAPHY

BOOKS AND PAMPHLETS

Allen LH, Wood RJ. Calcium and phosphorus. In: Shils ME, Olson JA, Shike M. Eds. Modern nutrition in health and disease. 8th ed. Philadelphia: Lea and Febiger, 1994:144–163.

Fairbanks VF. Iron in medicine and nutrition. In: Shils ME, Olson JA, Shike M. Eds. Modern nutrition in health and disease. 8th ed. Philadelphia: Lea and Febiger, 1994:185–213.

Jacobus CW. The osteoporosis resource manual: a guide to osteoporosis services in New Jersey. Princeton: The Health, Research and Educational Trust of New Jersey, 1993.

National Academy of Sciences, National Research Council, Committee on Diet and Health, Food and Nutrition Board. Diet and health: implications for reducing chronic disease risk (executive summary). Washington, DC: National Academy Press, 1989.

National Academy of Sciences, National Research Council, Food and Nutrition Board. Recommended dietary allowances. 10th ed. Washington, DC: National Academy Press, 1989.

National Osteoporosis Foundation. Boning up on osteoporosis. Washington, DC: National Osteoporosis Foundation, 1991.

US Dept of Health and Human Services, Public Health Service., The surgeon general's report on nutrition and health (summary and recommendations). Washington, DC: US Government Printing Office, 1988. US Dept of Health and Human Services publication PHS 88-50211.

PERIODICALS

Aloia JF, Vaswani A, Yeh JK, et al. Calcium supplementation with and without hormone replacement therapy to prevent postmenopausal bone loss. Ann Intern Med 1994;120:97.

Duazo F, Khachadurian AK. Prevention and treatment of osteoporosis in the elderly. Top Clin Nutr 1993;8:9:54.

Farley D. Look for "legit" health claims on foods. FDA Consumer (Special Report: Focus on Food Labeling). May 1993. DHHS publication FDA 93-2262:21.

Heaney RP. Protein intake and the calcium economy. J Am Diet Assoc 1993;93:1259.

Herbert V. Everyone should be tested for iron disorders. J Am Diet Assoc 1992;92:1502.

Hernandez-Avila A, Speizer FE, Willett WC. Caffeine, moderate alcohol intake and risk of fractures of hip and forearm in middle-aged women. Am J Clin Nutr 1991;54:157.

Hertzler AA, Frary RB. A dietary calcium rapid assessment method. Top Clin Nutr 1994;9:6:76.

Kurtzweil P. "Nutrition facts" to help consumers eat smart. FDA Consumer (Special Report: Focus on Food Labeling). May 1993. DHHS publication FDA 93-2262:34.

Lloyd T, Andon MB, Rollings JK, et al. Calcium supplementation and bone mineral density in adolescent girls. J Am Med Assoc 1993;270:841.

Massey LK, Roger AL. Modification of dietary oxalate and calcium reduces urinary oxalate in hyperoxaluric patients with kidney stones. J Am Diet Assoc 1993;93:1305.

Rivlin RS. Ed. An update on calcium applications for the 90's. Am J Clin Nutr 1991;54(suppl):1775.

Wardlaw GM. Putting osteoporosis in perspective. J Am Diet Assoc 1993;93:1000.

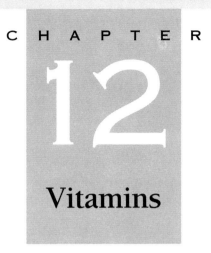

CHAPTER 12 Vitamins

KEY TERMS

anticoagulant a substance that prevents blood clotting
antioxidant a substance that hinders oxidation; oxidation is the combination of a substance with oxygen, causing a breakdown or a change in the substance
antivitamin any substance that interferes with the absorption or functioning of a vitamin; some drugs are antivitamins
avitaminosis a deficiency of a vitamin
carotene a yellow pigment in plants that can be converted to vitamin A in the intestinal wall
cheilosis a condition in which lesions appear on the lips and cracks appear at the angles of the mouth
coenzyme a substance such as a vitamin that attaches to the inactive form of an enzyme, thus forming an active compound or complete enzyme
collagen a gelatinlike protein substance found in connective tissue and bones; a cementing material between body cells
dementia a deteriorated mental state
dermatitis inflammation of the skin
epidemiologic studies research studies that establish relationships between diseases and environmental factors
glossitis inflammation of the tongue
hemolysis destruction of red blood cells, resulting in the appearance of hemoglobin in surrounding fluid
hypervitaminosis a toxic condition due to excessive accumulation of a vitamin in the body
hypochromic cells pale red blood cells lacking hemoglobin
megadose a dose of a vitamin that is 100 or even 1000 times the RDA
myelin a fatlike substance that forms a covering for some nerve fibers
occult hidden or not evident, as in occult blood loss
provitamin or **precursor** a substance that precedes and is converted into a vitamin; for example, beta carotene is the precursor of vitamin A, and tryptophan is the precursor of niacin

OBJECTIVES

After completing this chapter, the student will be able to:

1. Explain the general ways in which vitamins work to support life.
2. Discuss the classification of vitamins according to solubility and compare the general characteristics of fat-soluble and water-soluble vitamins.
3. Discuss the health problems related to inadequate or excessive vitamin intake.
4. Discuss for each of the vitamins
   - its functions in the body
   - food sources
   - the Recommended Dietary Allowance (RDA)
   - symptoms of deficiency

the potential for toxicity when taken in excessive quantity.

5. Explain the labeling regulations regarding vitamins in foods and supplements.
6. Discuss the use of vitamins/mineral supplements, including
   the four basic reasons for caution in the use of supplements
   the pros and cons of antioxidant supplementation
   guidelines in selecting vitamin/mineral supplements

New research pointing toward vitamins as important nutrients in the prevention of chronic disease has all but upstaged the focus on fat in the diet. As one nutrition authority expressed it, "The antioxidant vitamins have become the oat bran of the 1990s." The emphasis on preventive health care and the aging of the US population have fostered great consumer interest in this nutrient group.

The vitamin story began hundreds of years ago with the recognition of a connection between eating habits and certain diseases. Beriberi was described in the 7th century and scurvy in the 13th century. Later, certain foods were identified as cures for specific diseases. Eventually, the specific chemical compounds in these foods that had produced the cures were identified.

In the early 1900s, Casimir Funk, a Polish scientist, discovered a group of substances for which he proposed the term *vitamine,* meaning *vital amine.* An *amine* is a nitrogen-containing compound. When it was later learned that some vitamins could not be classified chemically as amines, the *e* was dropped and the accepted term became *vitamin.*

Vitamins are organic substances needed in small amounts for growth and for the maintenance of life. Some vitamins have hormonelike activity, whereas others are components of enzymes. Many enzymes can function only when combined with certain vitamins and minerals. A main function of many vitamins, especially the B-complex vitamins, is to act as coenzymes in metabolic reactions. A coenzyme is an organic substance that attaches to the inactive form of an enzyme. This combination makes the enzyme an active compound capable of bringing about chemical reactions. Vitamins do not provide calories; however, some vitamins are important in energy metabolism.

The body cannot manufacture vitamins; they must be supplied by foods, through bacterial synthesis, or by vitamin supplements. A serious lack of one or more vitamins will result in one or more deficiency diseases.

GENERAL CHARACTERISTICS

TERMINOLOGY AND MEASUREMENTS

Before their exact chemical nature was known, vitamins were identified by letters of the alphabet. Later, chemical names replaced the letters, although letter names continue to be used to some extent. When what was thought to be one vitamin turned out to be many, each with a different function, numbers were added to the letter name, as in vitamins B_1, B_2, and B_{12}. Sometimes numbers indicate various forms of the same vitamin, such as vitamins D_2 and D_3 (which have similar functions). The active form of a vitamin is the *preformed vitamin.* A compound that can be converted into the active form is called a *precursor* or *provitamin.*

Vitamins occur in small amounts in food. Quantities of most vitamins are measured in either milligrams (0.001 g) or micrograms (0.000001 g). Quantities of some vitamins also may be expressed in international units (IU), a specific measurable amount of vitamin activity. Vitamins A, D, and E were expressed in IU in the Recommended Dietary Allowances (RDAs) before 1980. Since then, other units of measure have been used. Vitamin A now is expressed in retinol equivalents; vitamin D, in micrograms of cholecalciferol; and vitamin E, in milligrams of alpha-tocopherol.

FUNCTIONS

Vitamins are organic substances needed in small amounts for growth and for the maintenance of life. Some vitamins have hormonelike activity, whereas others are components of enzymes. Many enzymes can function only when combined with certain vitamins and minerals. A main function of many vitamins, especially the B-complex vitamins, is to act as coenzymes in metabolic reactions. A *coenzyme* is an organic substance that attaches to the inactive form of an enzyme. This combination makes the enzyme an active compound capable of bringing about chemical reactions.

CLASSIFICATION BY SOLUBILITY

Vitamins are classified according to solubility into two groups: fat soluble and water soluble. Fat-soluble vitamins are found in the fatty parts of cells and foods; vitamins A, D, E, and K are fat-soluble vitamins. Water-soluble vitamins are found in the watery parts of cells and foods; vitamin C and the B-complex vitamins are water-soluble vitamins.

The fat-soluble vitamins are more stable than the water-soluble vitamins and are not lost easily in cooking and storage of food. The water-soluble vitamins are more readily lost in cooking water or destroyed by heat.

RECOMMENDED ALLOWANCES

The quantity of vitamins recommended by the National Academy of Sciences Food and Nutrition Board is sufficient to provide a margin of safety—the RDA is at least several times the quantity needed to prevent deficiency diseases. You should become familiar with the RDAs for each of the vitamins in the various age–gender categories.

Sufficient quantities of all the essential vitamins are supplied by a varied diet containing adequate amounts of fruits and vegetables, milk, grains, bread, poultry, fish, meat, and meat substitutes. Fresh or lightly processed foods are better sources of vitamins than refined, highly processed ones. During critical periods in life, as in infancy, early childhood, and pregnancy, vitamin supplements in amounts equal to the RDA may be prescribed. Requirements above the RDA are also increased for people with deficiency diseases, disorders that interfere with adequate consumption of food or with proper digestion, absorption, or use of nutrients, and when there is increased physical stress as in surgery, fever, burns, and infections.

Many people take megadoses of specific vitamins without medical supervision. These doses may be 50, 100, or even thousands of times greater than the amount needed to prevent deficiency diseases. This is an example of the mistaken belief that if a little is good, more is better. Such people are swayed by false claims that large doses of vitamins will prevent or cure a wide range of physical and emotional ills.

In 1990, a new labeling law gave the Food and Drug Administration (FDA) the authority to limit claims on supplement labels to those claims for which there is substantial scientific agreement in the scientific community. This provision of the law is under fierce attack by the supplement industry (see the discussion in the section Labeling Regulations and Vitamin/Mineral Supplements).

FAT-SOLUBLE VITAMINS

Vitamins A, D, E, and K are absorbed from the intestinal tract in the same manner as fats. Therefore, any disease or condition that interferes with the absorption of fats also may inhibit the absorption of these vitamins. The use of mineral oil in food preparation for reducing diets or as a laxative also interferes with absorption of these vitamins. Mineral oil, a nonfood substance, is not digested but instead passes through the gastrointestinal tract, carrying the fat-soluble vitamins with it.

All fat-soluble vitamins are stored to some extent in the body, mainly in the liver. For example, the liver of a well-nourished person has several months' supply of vitamin A. Thus, signs of deficiency develop more slowly in the case of fat-soluble vitamins than in the case of water-soluble vitamins. See Table 12-3 on p. 241 for summary.

VITAMIN A (RETINOL)

Vitamin A is found in animal foods as the preformed vitamin and in green and yellow plant foods as the provitamin beta carotene. *Vitamin A* is a term used collectively for a group of compounds having similar biologic activity. The parent compound in this group is called *retinol*. The original source of the vitamin A in animal foods, however, is the *carotenoids* in plants—plant pigments that give vegetables and fruits such as carrots, sweet potatoes, and apricots their deep yellow color. Animals and humans can convert a considerable amount of the carotenoids found in food into vitamin A. Dark green plants are also rich in carotenoids, but the yellow color is masked by chlorophyll. Of more than 400 carotenoids found naturally in plants, only a small fraction can be converted to vitamin A. Beta carotene is nutritionally the most active and most plentiful of the carotenoids. The other carotenoids with vitamin A activity have only about half the activity of beta carotene.

Vitamin A activity is sometimes expressed in IU in which 0.3 mcg of retinol or 0.6 mcg of beta carotene is equal to 1 IU. This form of measurement is based on the activity of beta carotene in pure supplement form. It does not account for the poor absorption and inefficient use of the beta carotene in food. It takes about 6 mcg of beta carotene in food to produce the biologic effectiveness of 1 mcg of vitamin A.

The Food and Nutrition Board as well as most nutrition authorities worldwide use *retinol equivalents (RE)* to express the vitamin A activity in food. This system is more precise, accounting for both the incomplete absorption and the inefficient conversion of the carotenes to vitamin A. The equivalents are as follows:

- 1 RE = 1 mcg of retinol
- 1 RE = 6 mcg of beta carotene
- 1 RE = 12 mcg of other carotenes

FUNCTIONS AND CLINICAL EFFECTS

Adaptation to Changes in Light

Vitamin A is necessary for the formation of visual pigments in the eye. Vitamin A combines with the protein opsin to produce rhodopsin in the rods and iodopsin in the cones of the retina. These pigments are responsible for vision in dim and bright light. Some of the vitamin A–containing compound in these pigments is lost when subjected to light. Regeneration of the pigments in darkness depends on the availability of vitamin A.

Maintenance of Epithelial Tissue

Vitamin A is essential for the maintenance of normal epithelial tissue; the skin and mucous membranes, such as the epithelial layer of the eye; and the linings of the respiratory, gastrointestinal, and genitourinary tracts.

Formation of Bones, Teeth, and Soft Tissue

Vitamin A is necessary for the normal growth and development of bones, teeth, and soft tissue. Vitamin A is involved in protein synthesis and cell division and early embryo development, when cells differentiate into tissue-specific cells such as muscle, skin, and nerve cells.

Normal Reproduction

Vitamin A is required for the normal functioning of men's and women's reproductive systems.

Promotion of Immunity

By building and maintaining healthy epithelial tissue, both of the skin and of the inner mucous membranes, vitamin A protects the body from infection. Beta carotene appears to have biologic effects apart from its role as a precursor of vitamin A. Carotenoids have antioxidant properties that have been shown to destroy *free radicals*, substances that can cause abnormal changes in body cells. These antioxidant properties may be responsible for the association between foods rich in beta carotene and reduction of chronic disease risk. See Display 12-1 for foods rich in beta carotene.

SOURCES

Vitamin A is found only in animal foods and is usually associated with animal fats. Liver, whole milk, foods containing milk fat (butter, cream, and whole-milk cheeses), egg yolk, and margarine are good sources. All margarines are fortified with vitamin A and are nutritionally equal to butter in vitamin A content. Many skim and lowfat milks are fortified with vitamin A.

DISPLAY 12-1 FOODS RICH IN BETA CAROTENE

Apricots	Mango
Broccoli	Persimmon
Cantaloupe	Pumpkin
Carrots	Spinach
Chard	Sweet potato
Collards	Turnip greens
Cress	Winter squash
Kale	

Beta carotene and other biologically active carotenoids occur in yellow and dark green vegetables and in some yellow fruits. Good sources are apricot, broccoli, cantaloupe, carrot, chard, collards, cress, kale, mango, persimmon, pumpkin, spinach, sweet potato, turnip greens, and winter squash (Table 12-1). Because many carotenoids and other pigments in plants do not have provitamin A activity, the depth of color of a fruit or vegetable is an unreliable way of judging its provitamin A content. Little vitamin A and carotene is lost in the processing or cooking of food; rather, cooking increases the availability of carotene in vegetables.

Fish liver oils are the richest natural source of vitamin A; they also are rich in vitamin D. These oils are dietary supplements rather than foods. Fish liver oils should be measured carefully and taken only in recommended amounts. Vitamins A and D are stored in the body and excessive intake can be toxic.

RECOMMENDED ALLOWANCES

The recommended daily intake for people aged 11 years through adulthood is 1000 retinol equivalents (RE), or 5000 IU, for males and 800 RE (4000 IU) for females.

DEFICIENCY

When vitamin A is lacking, the formation of visual pigment is slowed. Consequently, the eye has difficulty adjusting to dim light, a condition called *night blindness.* A light-sensitive vitamin A–containing violet pigment in the cones of the retina is responsible for vision in bright light; thus, vitamin A

TABLE 12-1 VITAMIN A CONTENT OF AVERAGE SERVINGS OF SELECTED FOODS

Food	Serving Size	IU*	Retinol Equivalents
Whole milk	1 cup	310	76
Nonfat milk fortified with vitamin A	1 cup	500	145
Butter	1 pat	150	38
Margarine fortified with vitamin A	1 pat	170	50
Liver, beef, fried in margarine	3 oz	30,690	9120
Liverwurst	2 oz	8100	2405
Egg, hard-boiled	1	260	78
Ground beef	3 oz	trace	trace
Carrots, cooked, from fresh	1/2 cup	19,150	1915
Sweet potatoes, baked in skin	1	24,880	2488
Spinach, cooked from fresh	1/2 cup	7370	737
Collards, cooked from fresh	1/2 cup	2110	211
Broccoli, chopped, cooked	1/2 cup	1750	175
Cantaloupe	1/4 melon	4305	431
Peach	1	470	47
Apricots	3	2770	277
Apple	1	110	11
Orange	1	270	27

* Source of nutritive values: US Dept of Agriculture, Human Nutrition Information Service. Nutritive value of food.Washington, DC: US Government Printing Office, 1991. Home and Garden bulletin 72.

deficiency also causes glare blindness. Poor adaptation to changes in light, such as temporary blindness caused by the glare of headlights or entering a darkened theater, is one of the first signs of vitamin A deficiency (Fig. 12-1).

The epithelial cells keratinize (become dry and scaly) because of a lack of vitamin A. The mucous secretions diminish and the mucous membranes lose their soft, moist characteristics that protect the body from bacterial infection. The senses of taste and smell may be affected. The skin becomes rough, dry, and scaly, especially on the arms and thighs, and has a gooseflesh appearance. Adverse changes in the epithelial cells of the genitourinary tract interfere with normal reproductive function.

In the eye, the epithelial tissue becomes dry and thick, the tear ducts fail to secrete, and eventually, in severe vitamin A deficiency, the cells of the cornea become opaque and slough off. This condition, called *xerophthalmia,* leads to blindness if untreated. Vitamin A deficiency is a major nutritional problem in some nonindustrialized parts of the world.

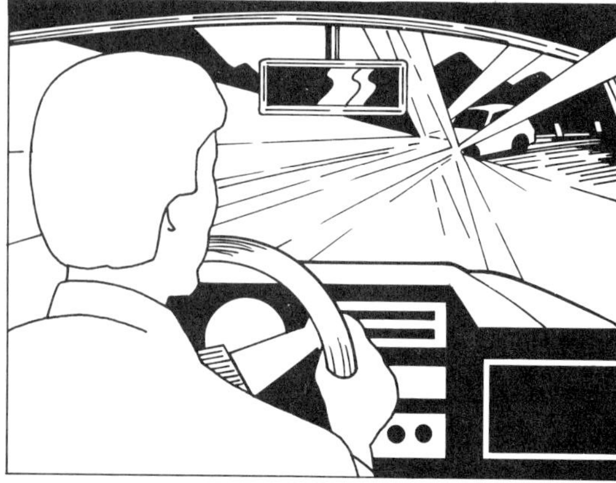

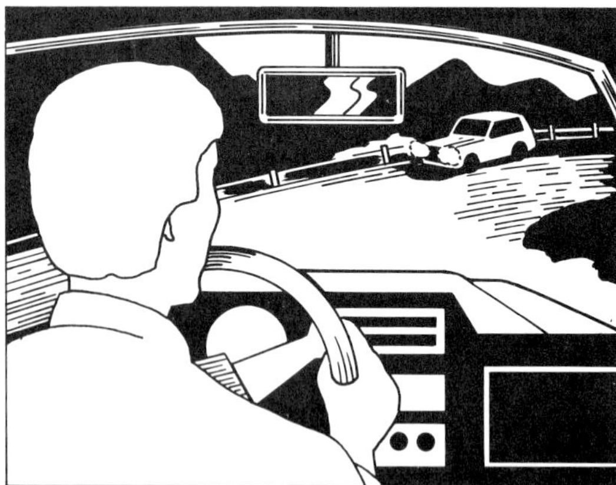

FIGURE 12-1

(*Top*) Glare blindness often is a symptom of vitamin A deficiency. Headlights dazzle the eyes and cause discomfort. The driver is blinded temporarily by oncoming headlights, and the edge of the road is seen with difficulty. (*Bottom*) An adequate intake of vitamin A protects against glare blindness or remedies it. Properly focused headlights no longer dazzle so blindingly, and the road edge can be seen immediately after the headlight glare has passed.

EXCESS

Excessive intakes of vitamin A are toxic. Signs of toxicity appear with prolonged intake, coming from both food and supplements of 15,000 mcg/day of retinol (50,000 IU) in adults and 6000 mcg/day of retinol (20,000 IU) in infants and young children.

Symptoms include nausea, headache, dry skin, dizziness, loss of hair, pain in the long bones, increased bone fragility liver damage and, during pregnancy, birth defects. Excessive intake of carotenes is not toxic but may produce a yellow discoloration of the skin.

BETA CAROTENE AND CHRONIC DISEASE

Beta carotene has been used for many years in the treatment of *erythropoietic protoporphyria,* an inherited light-sensitive disease. Patients treated with beta carotene can better tolerate sunlight.

In recent years, epidemiologic research has discovered a strong relationship between a high intake of food rich in beta carotene and a reduced risk of chronic disease. Beta carotene has been associated with a reduced risk of cancers of the epithelial-cell type, including cancers of the lungs, female reproductive system, gastrointestinal tract, and oral cavity. Beta carotene may also play a beneficial role in preventing cataracts and in the prevention and treatment of heart disease. Randomized clinical research trials are presently being conducted to clarify the specific benefits of beta carotene supplementation.

VITAMIN D (CALCIFEROL)

Calciferol is the general name given to vitamin D, which includes several compounds. From the standpoint of humans, the two most important vitamin D compounds are *ergocalciferol* (vitamin D_2) and *cholecalciferol* (vitamin D_3). These substances, formed from precursors in plants (ergosterol) and in the skin (dehydrocholesterol), are converted to the provitamins D_2 and D_3 by the ultraviolet rays of the sun. The provitamins undergo changes in the liver and kidney. The kidney produces the most active form of vitamin D: calcitriol.

The kidney plays an especially important role in vitamin D metabolism. Its production of calcitriol is regulated by the serum levels of calcium and phosphorus. Parathyroid hormone (PTH), which is released when calcium levels fall, stimulates the production of calcitriol.

How much vitamin D is produced in the body is influenced by several factors: distance from the equator, quantity of exposure to sunlight, environmental conditions such as fog and smoke, and whether the sunlight is filtered through window glass. In some climates, not enough sunlight is available to provide for the needs of infants and children. Vitamin D is stored mainly in the liver; some is stored in the brain, bones, and skin as well.

FUNCTIONS AND CLINICAL EFFECTS

Regulation of Calcium and Phosphorus Metabolism

Vitamin D regulates the absorption and metabolism of calcium and phosphorus so that normal bone calcification can occur and normal serum levels of calcium and phosphorus are maintained. Vitamin D promotes bone formation by providing high levels of calcium and phosphorus.

Vitamin D is necessary for the absorption of calcium and phosphorus from the small intestine. Without it, the amount of calcium absorbed would not meet requirements. Vitamin D activity is directed toward promoting the absorption of calcium; phosphorus absorption follows as an accompanying anion (negatively charged particle).

The presence of vitamin D is essential to the activity of the parathyroid hormone in removing calcium and phosphorus from the bone to maintain normal serum levels of these minerals. Vitamin D also stimulates the reabsorption of calcium by the kidney when serum calcium levels are low.

Hormonal Controls

Vitamin D metabolism is linked to the endocrine systems that control calcium–phosphorus balance. The PTH stimulates the conversion of vitamin D to its active hormonal form in the kidneys when serum calcium levels fall. Calcitonin, secreted by the thyroid gland when serum calcium levels rise, depresses the production of vitamin D hormone.

Calcium loss from bones typically is seen in late stages of chronic kidney failure. This loss is due in part to the inability of the kidney to convert vitamin D to its hormonal form.

SOURCES

Foods in their natural state are not good sources of vitamin D. Fortified foods are the major source of vitamin D in the American diet. Almost all whole milk is fortified with 400 IU of vitamin D per quart; evaporated milk is similarly fortified, as is most lowfat and nonfat milk.

Infant formulas are fortified with the same amount as milk. Breast milk contains little vitamin D. A daily vitamin D supplement is recommended for breastfed infants who are not exposed to sunlight. Eggs, butter, and fortified margarine also contain some vitamin D.

Fish liver oils are rich sources of vitamin D. When used as a vitamin D supplement, the dosage should be carefully measured to avoid excessive intake. Vitamin D in foods and supplements is stable in heat and in storage.

RECOMMENDED ALLOWANCES

Vitamin D is expressed in micrograms of cholecalciferol rather than international units (IU) (2.5 mcg = 100 IU). The RDA is 10 mcg/day (400 IU) of vitamin D from birth through age 24 years; for adults older than age 24 years, the RDA is 5 mcg/day (200 IU), an amount that usually can be obtained through normal exposure to sunlight. Many people in the United States have limited exposure to sunlight, including invalids and people who work nights and sleep during the day. Environmental conditions and clothing also can block the ultraviolet rays of the sun, making sufficient vitamin D unavailable. Consequently, vitamin D must be supplied in the diet in the form of fortified foods or a vitamin supplement.

DEFICIENCY

A deficiency of vitamin D causes *rickets*. This disease was once common among infants and children but rarely is seen today because practically all milk and infant formulas are fortified with vitamin D. In rickets, calcium and phosphorus are lacking in the bones, causing them to become soft and pliable; the long bones bend under body weight. All the bones are affected. Knock knees and bowed legs are seen, the wrists and ankles are thickened, and the teeth erupt late and are of poor quality.

In adults, a severe deficiency of vitamin D, calcium, and phosphorus can lead to *osteomalacia*, sometimes called *adult rickets*. The bones become soft, flexible, and deformed, giving rise to rheumatic pain. The disease is rare in Western countries but is seen in the Middle East and the Orient.

Vitamin D deficiency sometimes is seen in the United States in breastfed infants who have not received supplemental vitamin D or exposure to sunlight. It also may occur as a result of diseases in which there is poor absorption of vitamin D or poor conversion of vitamin D to its active forms. The poor conversion may occur in kidney failure.

EXCESS

Hypervitaminosis D generally results from the excessive intake of vitamin supplements, usually in the form of fish liver oils. Symptoms of hypervitaminosis D include weakness, weight loss, nausea, growth failure, bone deformity, and calcium deposits in the soft tissue, including the blood vessels, heart, and kidneys.

Young children are especially prone to the toxic effects of too much vitamin D. As little as 45 mcg/day (1800 IU) has caused signs of toxicity. Dietary supplements during the warm months when exposure to sunlight is high may be harmful for the child or adult who is consuming at least two glasses of vitamin D–fortified milk daily.

VITAMIN E

A group of closely related compounds exhibit vitamin E activity. Alpha-tocopherol is the most important form. An important characteristic is its ability to accept oxygen and thus prevent oxygen from destroying other substances. Such a substance is called an *antioxidant*.

Vitamin E requires normal bile secretion and pancreatic functioning for absorption. Vitamin E is carried in the blood by lipoproteins. Tissues take up the vitamin E from the lipoprotein.

FUNCTIONS AND CLINICAL EFFECTS

Vitamin E protects fatty acids in cell membranes from oxidative damage and therefore preserves the health of body tissues. It appears to be closely related to the mineral selenium, another antioxidant.

SOURCES

Vegetable oils such as corn, cottonseed, soybean, and safflower, and margarine and shortenings made from these oils are the richest sources of vitamin E in the American diet. Wheat germ also is a rich source. Other good sources are whole-grain cereals, legumes (including peanuts), corn, nuts, and green, leafy vegetables. Except for liver and egg yolk, animal foods are poor sources of vitamin E.

RECOMMENDED ALLOWANCES

The recommended allowance for vitamin E is expressed in alpha-tocopherol equivalents (α-TE). The recommendation is 8 mg α-TE for adult women and 10 mg α-TE for adult men.

There apparently is a greater need than normal for vitamin E when the diet is high in polyunsaturated fats. Because the polyunsaturated fats in the American diet are mostly vegetable oils, which are rich sources of vitamin E, a diet that is high in polyunsaturates is automatically high in vitamin E.

DEFICIENCY

Vitamin E deficiency is rare. It may occur in premature infants because vitamin E is poorly transferred across the placenta and the immature intestinal tract does not adequately absorb dietary vitamin E. Symptoms include *hemolytic anemia,* a condition in which there is an abnormal breakdown of red blood cells.

Vitamin E deficiency also occurs in people who cannot absorb fat normally. In children, poor absorption of vitamin E in such conditions as cystic fibrosis can produce serious neurologic defects. In adults, the malabsorption must be prolonged 5 to 10 years before symptoms, usually neurologic, appear.

A host of vitamin E deficiency diseases have been identified in animals, including muscular dystrophy in rabbits; heart failure in calves; loss of fetuses in female rats, hamsters, mice, and guinea pigs; and brain damage in chickens. In the past, attempts to prevent or cure corresponding diseases in humans by the use of vitamin E have met with failure, however. More recently, research has consistently reported that vitamin E boosts a wide variety of immune responses in the body. Although the body's immune system declines with age, some nutrition authorities have expressed the belief that nutritional intervention can slow down the decline. More research is necessary to clarify the role of vitamin E in disease prevention.

EXCESS

No strong evidence indicates that large doses of vitamin E are harmful. It is advisable to use vitamin E cautiously, however, because it is established that high doses of other fat-soluble vitamins are toxic. Vitamin E appears to have antivitamin K activity, reducing the body's blood clotting ability. People taking anticoagulant drugs should not take large doses of vitamin E because of the danger of hemorrhage. The committee of the Food and Nutrition Board that developed the RDAs does not recommend vitamin E supplementation because supplementation has no known benefits for healthy individuals.

VITAMIN K

A number of compounds have vitamin K activity. One form, *menaquinone,* is produced by bacteria in the intestinal tract. Another form, *phylloquinone,* is found naturally in foods. Some forms are made synthetically; *menadione* is the most potent.

FUNCTIONS AND CLINICAL EFFECTS

Vitamin K has an essential role in the blood clotting process. It is needed for the synthesis of prothrombin and other blood clotting factors in the liver.

Vitamin K also is required for the synthesis of proteins in plasma, bone, and kidney. Vitamin K appears to be closely associated with calcium metabolism in these functions.

SOURCES

Green, leafy vegetables are the best food source, providing 50 to 800 mcg of vitamin K per 100 g (3⅓ oz) portion.

Vitamin K also is found in cauliflower, alfalfa, liver, egg yolk, soybean oil and other vegetable oils, and, to a lesser extent, wheat and oats. Vitamin K is destroyed by strong acids, alkalis, and certain oxidizing agents.

Synthesis by normal bacteria in the intestinal tract has been considered an important source of vitamin K. The extent to which vitamin K produced from bacteria is used is unknown, however.

RECOMMENDED ALLOWANCES

Recommended allowances for vitamin K were set for the first time in 1989. A dietary intake of about 1 mcg/day per kilogram of body weight was determined to be sufficient. Therefore, the RDA for the 79-kg reference man is 80 mcg/day and for the 63-kg reference woman is 65 mcg/day.

DEFICIENCY

Newborn infants are prone to vitamin K deficiency. During fetal life, little vitamin K crosses the placenta, and during the early postnatal period, the intestinal tract is sterile, so that vitamin K cannot be synthesized from bacteria. Prothrombin and other clotting factors are low for about 1 week after birth. A vitamin K supplement usually is given to newborn infants to prevent hemorrhage.

Impaired coagulation due to vitamin K deficiency is rare in adults. It may occur when there is poor absorption of fats or when adults use certain drugs. Any condition that interferes with fat absorption affects vitamin K absorption and may produce a deficiency that makes the affected person prone to hemorrhage. Gallbladder disease, celiac disease, and ulcerative colitis are examples of such conditions. Administration of intravenous vitamin K may be necessary. The use of sulfonamides and antibiotics can depress the production of intestinal bacteria, thereby causing a deficiency of vitamin K, making supplementation necessary.

The coumarin drugs and the salicylates are anticoagulants, which interfere with vitamin K production and thus prevent prothrombin synthesis. In a client who has been given too large a dose of one of these drugs during therapy for certain medical problems, vitamin K is given to correct the problem.

EXCESS

Toxic reactions to large doses of natural vitamin K have not been observed. Overdose of synthetic vitamin K (menadione), however, is toxic in newborns, causing elevation of bilirubin (jaundice), neurologic disturbances, and hemolytic anemia.

WATER-SOLUBLE VITAMINS

ASCORBIC ACID (VITAMIN C)

A lack of ascorbic acid causes *scurvy*, a deficiency disease known for centuries to be caused by a limited food supply and that can be prevented by including fresh foods in the diet. The disease used to be especially threatening to sailors, who existed for long periods on a diet of salted meats and fish and breadstuffs. In the mid-1700s, as prevention against scurvy, limes and lemons were added to the rations of British sailors, who then became known as *limeys*.

FUNCTIONS AND CLINICAL EFFECTS

Collagen Formation

Ascorbic acid plays a vital role in *collagen* formation; collagen is the protein glue that holds the tissue cells together. Collagen consists of insoluble protein fibers, which provide firmness and support to the tissues of the skin, cartilage, tendons, ligaments, blood vessels, bones, and teeth. Collagen is a major component of scar tissue formed during the healing of wounds and bone fractures.

Hemoglobin Formation

Vitamin C increases the absorption of iron from the intestinal tract and promotes its use in the body. It also is needed to convert the inactive form of the vitamin folate (another blood-building nutrient) to the active form.

OTHER FUNCTIONS

Vitamin C appears to have numerous other roles in regulating body processes, many of which have not been clearly defined. It is involved in the metabolism of fats and protein. High concentrations of ascorbic acid in the adrenal gland and its depletion when the gland is stimulated suggest a need for vitamin C during periods of stress. Blood levels of vitamin C decrease during fever, suggesting the body's increased need during this condition. Ascorbic acid may reduce nitrite in food and thus prevent the formation of carcinogenic nitrosamines in the intestinal tract.

SOURCES

Citrus fruits and their juices, whether fresh, frozen, or canned, are excellent sources of vitamin C. Broccoli is another excellent source, as are strawberries, cantaloupe, guava, mango, papaya, and peppers. Other significant sources are tomatoes and tomato juice, cabbage, greens (such as collards, cress, kale, mustard, and turnip greens), and potatoes and sweet potatoes cooked in their jackets. Table 12-2 lists the vitamin C content of selected foods.

Vitamin C is the most unstable of all the vitamins. Care must be taken to conserve it by properly storing and cooking food. Vitamin loss from fresh fruits and vegetables is reduced by storing these foods in the refrigerator. Vitamin C is readily destroyed by alkali; therefore, never add baking soda to vegetables during cooking. Avoid excessive cutting and chopping. Steam vegetables or microwave, if possible, or cook in little water for as briefly as possible. Adding vegetables to boiling water shortens the cooking time. Potatoes have a higher vitamin C content if cooked in their skins.

RECOMMENDED ALLOWANCES

The RDA for ascorbic acid is 60 mg/day from age 15 years through adulthood, 70 mg/day during pregnancy, and 95 mg/day during the first 6 months of breastfeeding and 90 mg/day in the second 6 months. From infancy through age 14 years, the recommendation ranges from 30 to 50 mg/day.

In 1989, the RDA was raised for regular cigarette smokers to at least 100 mg of vitamin C daily. Smokers appear to metabolize vitamin C more quickly than nonsmokers. This recommendation is intended to meet basic needs for vitamin C, so that smokers may have the same serum levels of vitamin C as nonsmokers.

DEFICIENCY

When vitamin C is deficient, the fibers of connective tissue are improperly formed. This improper formation results in skin abnormalities, fragile blood vessels, and poor wound healing (Fig. 12-2).

TABLE 12-2 Ascorbic Acid Content of Average Servings of Selected Foods

Food	Serving Size	Ascorbic Acid (mg)*
Milk, whole or skim	1 cup	2
Cheddar cheese	1 oz	0
Egg	1	0
Beef liver	3 oz	23
Other meat, fish, poultry		0
Broccoli, cooked, chopped, from frozen	½ cup	37
Collards, from fresh, cooked	½ cup	10
Turnip greens, from fresh, cooked	½ cup	20
Cauliflower, from fresh, cooked	½ cup	30
Tomato, raw	1	22
Potato, boiled, peeled after boiling	1	18
Cabbage, cooked	½ cup	36
Carrots, cooked	½ cup	4
Peas, frozen, cooked	½ cup	8
Orange	1	70
Orange juice, frozen, diluted	½ cup	49
Strawberries, whole, fresh	½ cup	42
Grapefruit, fresh	½	41
Grapefruit juice, frozen, diluted	½ cup	42
Banana	1	10
Apple	1	12
Kiwi fruit	1	74

* Source of nutritive values: US Dept of Agriculture, Human Nutrition Information Service. Nutritive value of food. Washington, DC: US Government Printing Office, 1991. Home and Garden bulletin 72.

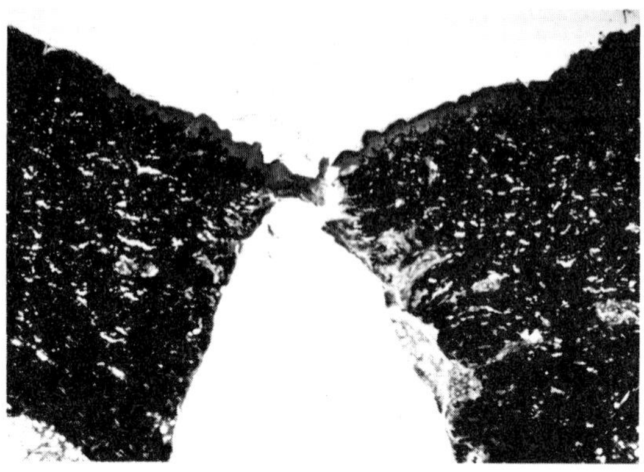

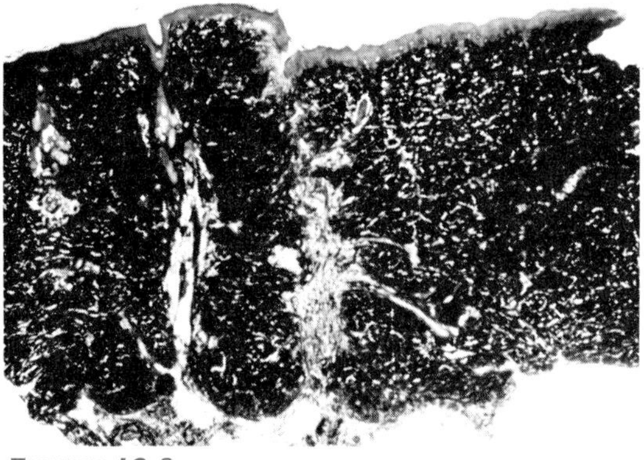

FIGURE 12-2

Role of vitamin C in wound healing. (*Top*) Biopsy specimen 10 days after an experimental wound was made in the back of Dr. John Crandon, who had not consumed any vitamin C for 6 months. No healing is evident except in the epithelium (a gap in tissues was filled with a blood clot). (*Bottom*) After 10 days of treatment with vitamin C, another biopsy specimen of the wound shows healing with abundant collagen formation. *(The vitamin manual. Kalamazoo, MI: Upjohn Co.)*

Skin abnormalities such as adult acne may be the earliest sign of scurvy. Hardening and scaling of the skin surrounding the hair follicles and hemorrhages surrounding the hair follicles also point to scurvy. The hair may be broken and coiled, and some hairs may have a swan-neck deformity. The skin of the forearms, legs, and thighs is most apt to be affected. Other symptoms of scurvy include weakness, fatigue, restlessness, and neurotic behavior; aching bones, joints, and muscles; sensitivity to touch; sore mouth and gums, with bleeding and loosening of the teeth; and bruising and hemorrhaging of the skin. Anemia also may occur. Death results if the deficiency is not corrected.

In the United States, scurvy still may be found among elderly people, who may be eating poorly, or in people on severely restricted diets, such as certain stages of the Zen macrobiotic diet. It also is found in infants exclusively fed cow's milk.

EXCESS

Many people consume 1 g (1000 mg) or more of vitamin C daily without apparent harmful effects. Claims that large doses of vitamin C can prevent or cure the common cold have not been supported by carefully controlled research studies, although colds studied appeared to be less severe when study participants took large doses of vitamin C.

Large doses of vitamin C generally have been considered harmless; however, the safety of megadoses has not been established. Accumulating evidence has indicated that serious harm can result from large doses of vitamin C. Increased risk of kidney stones, destruction of vitamin B_{12}, and interference with anticoagulant drugs are among the harmful effects reported. Because there is no strong evidence that large doses of vitamin C are useful, and because the risk of long-term intake is unknown, large doses of vitamin C are not recommended.

THIAMIN (VITAMIN B_1)

The enrichment of cereal products has almost completely eliminated beriberi, a thiamin deficiency disease, in the United States. Although rare in the West, this disorder is still sometimes seen among alcoholics. Beriberi developed among rice-eating peoples when refined, polished rice began to replace brown rice. The bran layer that is removed during the milling process is rich in thiamin. The disease continues to be a problem in areas where enrichment is not a standard practice.

FUNCTIONS AND CLINICAL EFFECTS

Energy Metabolism

Thiamin is needed for the formation of a coenzyme involved in energy metabolism. Thiamin works with the coenzymes of other B vitamins in key reactions that convert glucose to energy. The roles of the coenzymes are interrelated. Carbohydrates and certain amino acids require thiamin for metabolism. Fats and other amino acids do not.

Synthesis of DNA and RNA

Thiamin also is required for the conversion of some glucose to *ribose,* an essential component of deoxyribonucleic acid (DNA) and ribonucleic acid (RNA), carriers of the genetic code.

SOURCES

Thiamin is found in meats—especially pork and organ meats, wheat germ, whole-grain and enriched breads and cereals, dry peas and beans, peanuts, and nuts. Enriched cereals and grains and bakery products made with enriched grains contribute a large amount of thiamin to the American diet.

If care is not taken in cooking, the thiamin in food may be lost. Because thiamin is water soluble, cook thiamin-containing foods in as little water as possible, at low temperatures, and for as short a time as possible. Whenever practical, use water remaining from cooked foods and meat drippings from which fat has been removed. Alkaline substances, such as baking soda and antacid medications, destroy thiamin.

RECOMMENDED ALLOWANCES

A daily thiamin intake of 0.5 mg per 1000 kcal is recommended for children and adults. Therefore, a man who consumes 2700 kcal/day would require 0.5 mg × 2.7, or 1.4 mg of thiamin. A minimum of 1 mg/day is recommended even for people consuming less than 2000 kcal/day. The allowance for infants is 0.4 mg per 1000 kcal daily.

DEFICIENCY AND EXCESS

Thiamin deficiency affects the gastrointestinal, cardiovascular, and nervous systems, causing symptoms such as loss of appetite, constipation, fatigue, irritability, neuritis, and headaches. These same symptoms, however, can be attributed to many other causes.

A serious deficiency of vitamin B_1 has a devastating effect on the nervous system. The neurologic symptoms are evident in beriberi. In older children and adults, the disease occurs in two forms: dry beriberi and wet beriberi. The dry type is seen mainly among elderly adults and often is associated with long-standing alcoholism. There is a wasting of body tissue and various nervous disorders, including paralysis of the legs. Edema caused by heart failure is the most characteristic symptom of wet beriberi. In both types, there is irritability, confusion, and nausea. Infantile beriberi occurs in infants consuming breast milk low in thiamin. The onset of symptoms is sudden, and the disease is fatal if not treated promptly.

Excessive intake of thiamin has no known effect when taken orally. Large doses may be toxic when given intravenously.

RIBOFLAVIN (VITAMIN B_2)

FUNCTIONS AND CLINICAL EFFECTS

Energy Metabolism

Riboflavin is a component of enzyme systems necessary for the release of energy within the cell. This function involves the energy metabolism of carbohydrates, proteins, and fats.

Tissue Growth and Maintenance

Riboflavin forms enzymes involved in protein metabolism. It is essential for the functioning of vitamin B_6 and niacin.

SOURCES

Milk is a primary source of riboflavin; people who do not drink milk are likely to have a low riboflavin intake. Meats, especially liver and other organ meats; green, leafy vegetables; fish; eggs; and enriched breads, cereals, and bakery products are good sources. Riboflavin is destroyed by ultraviolet light and sunlight, which is why cartons and opaque plastic containers are used for packaging milk.

RECOMMENDED ALLOWANCES

A daily intake of 0.6 mg per 1000 kcal is recommended for infants, children, and adults. The recommendation for the reference woman is 1.3 mg/day and for the reference man, 1.7 mg/day. For adults whose energy intake is less than 2000 kcal, a minimum of 1.2 mg/day is advised.

DEFICIENCY AND EXCESS

Deficiency of riboflavin causes tissue inflammation and breakdown. Lesions appear around the mouth and nose. The lips become cracked and sore, and fissures develop at the corners of the mouth (*cheilosis*). The tongue becomes abnormally smooth and purplish, a condition called *glossitis*. *Seborrheic dermatitis*, a greasy, scaly skin condition, may develop. Cracks and irritation develop around the nose. Skin changes also occur in the scrotum and vulva. Extra blood vessels develop in the cornea, causing the eyes to burn, itch, and tear. Because riboflavin is involved in the functioning of vitamin B_6 and niacin, some symptoms may be due to inadequacies of these vitamins. Excess riboflavin intake has no known effect.

NIACIN

In early efforts to discover a cure for *pellagra* (a disease affecting the skin, gastrointestinal tract, and nervous system), protein foods such as milk, eggs, and meat were found to have a positive effect. Later, it was discovered that niacin is the pellagra-preventive factor. Milk, although curative in pellagra, is low in niacin, however. The connection among these facts became evident when it was learned that niacin can be synthesized from tryptophan, an essential amino acid.

FUNCTIONS AND CLINICAL EFFECTS

Niacin occurs in two forms: nicotinic acid and niacinamide. Niacin affects a number of important metabolic activities needed for the maintenance of healthy skin and the proper functioning of the nervous and digestive systems.

Energy Metabolism

Niacin is a coenzyme in energy metabolism along with the other B-complex vitamins.

Production of Fatty Acids, Cholesterol, and Steroid Hormones

Niacin-containing hormones are involved in the synthesis of fatty acids, cholesterol, and steroid hormones.

SOURCES

Niacin is found in meat (especially liver), fish, poultry, peanuts, peas, beans, and whole-grain and enriched bread and cereal products. Only 30% of the niacin in whole-grain products appears to be available to the body. The synthetic niacin added to fortify refined products is fully available. Milk, eggs, and cheese are poor sources of preformed niacin; as complete protein foods, however, they are good sources of tryptophan, which is converted to niacin in the body. Niacin is not readily destroyed by light, heat, acid, or alkali, but it does dissolve in water and thus may be lost in cooking. To preserve niacin, it is advisable to cook meats at low temperatures to avoid excessive loss of juices and to use the meat juices.

RECOMMENDED ALLOWANCES

The requirement for niacin is met by both the preformed vitamin and its synthesis from the amino acid tryptophan. For this reason, the recommended niacin allowance is expressed in niacin equivalents. One niacin equivalent is equal to 1 mg of niacin or 60 mg of tryptophan. This amount of tryptophan is supplied by about 6 g of protein. Because the typical American diet is high in protein, tryptophan contributes substantially to niacin in the diet. The recommended allowance for adults is 6.6 niacin equivalents for every 1000 kcal consumed daily, but not less than 13 niacin equivalents for caloric intakes under 2000 kcal/day.

DEFICIENCY AND EXCESS

Early signs of niacin deficiency include fatigue, lack of appetite, weakness, mild digestive disturbances, anxiety, and irritability. A prolonged niacin deficiency causes pellagra, an Italian word meaning *rough skin*. The disease is characterized by the four *Ds*: **d**iarrhea, **d**ermatitis, **d**ementia (deteriorated mental state), and, if the disease goes untreated, **d**eath. The skin is dry, scaly, and cracked, and the condition is aggravated by exposure to heat or light. In the acute stages, pellagra resembles severe sunburn; in later stages, the affected areas become darkly pigmented. The lesions occur in the same places on both sides of the body. Gastrointestinal symptoms include soreness of the mouth, swelling of the tongue, and diarrhea. Mental irritability, anxiety, depression, and confusion also may occur.

At one time, pellagra was of great concern in the United States, especially in certain regions of the South. In these areas, the diet consisted mostly of corn, which is deficient in both niacin and protein. The enrichment of breads and cereals has eradicated the disease in the United States. It is now seen only in connection with chronic alcoholism. It continues to be a widespread problem in parts of Africa and Asia.

Niacin is not stored to any significant extent in the body, and any excess is excreted in the urine. High intakes of niacin can damage the liver. Large doses of nicotinic acid, not niacinamide, have been used as a drug to lower serum cholesterol and other blood lipids. Side effects such as skin flushing, gastrointestinal problems, and itching may result.

PYRIDOXINE (VITAMIN B_6)

Vitamin B_6 activity is demonstrated by three closely related compounds: pyridoxine, pyridoxal, and pyridoxamine. These substances form coenzymes that function in many reactions involving amino acids. A few examples follow.

FUNCTIONS AND CLINICAL EFFECTS

Protein Synthesis

Vitamin B_6 is needed for the synthesis of nonessential amino acids.

Synthesis of Regulatory Substances

Vitamin B_6 is involved in producing other compounds from amino acids, such as serotonin from tryptophan. Serotonin causes blood vessels to constrict and is involved in the regulation of brain and other tissue.

Niacin Production

Vitamin B_6 is a catalyst in the conversion of tryptophan to niacin.

Hemoglobin Synthesis

Vitamin B_6 is required for the synthesis of a substance involved in the production of heme. It also is required for the metabolism of folacin.

SOURCES

Good sources of pyridoxine are chicken, fish, kidney, liver, pork, eggs, whole-wheat products, oats, soybeans, brown rice, peanuts, and walnuts. Dairy products and vegetables are poor sources.

A considerable amount of vitamin B_6 is lost in food processing such as freezing, in the production of luncheon meats, and in the milling of grains.

RECOMMENDED ALLOWANCES

The need for vitamin B_6 increases with increased consumption of protein. The RDA is 2 mg/day for men and 1.6 mg/day for women.

About 40 drugs are known to interact with vitamin B_6. Isoniazid, used in tuberculosis therapy, and penicillamine, used in the treatment of Wilson's disease (copper storage disease), inactivate vitamin B_6. Oral contraceptives may increase the vitamin B_6 requirement.

DEFICIENCY AND EXCESS

Vitamin B_6 deficiency usually occurs in combination with deficiencies of other B-complex vitamins. Symptoms include a hypochromic type of anemia, hyperirritability that progresses to convulsions, and dermatitis. Infants fed a formula deficient in vitamin B_6 (the vitamin had been destroyed by overprocessing) became irritable and experienced convulsions. A deficiency of vitamin B_6 occurs in 20% to 30% of alcoholics.

When taken in quantities greater than 200 mg/day for months or years, incoordination and *peripheral neuropathy*—nerve damage that leads to a loss of feeling in the hands and feet—may result. Recovery from symptoms usually occurs in time after discontinuance of the supplements.

FOLATE (FOLACIN)

Folate and folacin are general terms for a group of compounds related to and including folic acid (pteroylglutamic acid). Folate is needed for cell division and protein synthesis.

Folate deficiency is a common disorder in the United States and throughout the world, especially in the tropics. It occurs most frequently in infancy, during pregnancy, and in conditions in which absorption is impaired. Folate has been useful in the treatment of *sprue,* a malabsorption disease characterized by diarrhea, anemia, and general malnutrition, and, more recently, in the prevention of neural tube defects.

FUNCTIONS AND CLINICAL EFFECTS

Protein Metabolism

Folate is necessary for protein metabolism and the synthesis of DNA and RNA. Effects of a deficiency are most evident in rapidly growing tissues or tissues with rapid cell turnover.

Formation of Hemoglobin

The formation of heme, the iron-containing substance in the blood, depends on folate. Folate function is interwoven with vitamins B_{12} and B_6. Vitamin C plays a role in the conversion of folate to its coenzyme form.

SOURCES

Folate is found in green, leafy vegetables, liver, kidney, other meats, fish, nuts, legumes, and whole-grain cereals. It is destroyed easily by poor cooking or storage procedures and by food processing. Folate also is produced by intestinal bacteria.

RECOMMENDED ALLOWANCES

In 1989, the RDA for folate was reduced by half because the Food and Nutrition Board recognized that people consuming half of the previous RDA were able to maintain adequate folate status. The RDA is 200 mcg/day for adolescent boys and adult men and 180 mcg/day for adolescent girls and adult women.

The need for folate is substantially increased during pregnancy and breastfeeding because of the role of folate in cell multiplication. The RDA during pregnancy is 400 mcg/day. This amount can be obtained from the diet. During breastfeeding, the RDA is 280 mcg/day for the first 6 months and 260 mcg/day for the second 6 months. Some authorities have been critical of the 1989 RDA for folate because they feel it may not provide an adequate safety margin for specific at-risk population groups: infants and children, pregnant and breastfeeding women, and elderly people. In 1993, FDA recommended an increase in folate for women of childbearing age. This is discussed in the section which follows under Deficiency.

DEFICIENCY

The outstanding symptom of folate deficiency is *macrocytic anemia,* a condition in which the red blood cells become enlarged and are reduced in number. Glossitis, stomatitis (sore mouth), and gastrointestinal disturbances, including diarrhea, also may be present. Because folate, ascorbic acid, vitamin B_6, and vitamin B_{12} are interrelated in the formation of blood, the anemia of different vitamin deficiency diseases may be similar and may respond to treatment with one or several of these vitamins. All B vitamins are needed, however, and cannot be substituted for one another. Although folate can relieve the anemia of pernicious anemia, it does not cure the neurologic symptoms.

Folate deficiency is associated with the occurrence of spinal bifida and other neural tube defects in newborns. In 1993, the US Public Health Service recommended that all girls and women of childbearing age in the United States who are capable of becoming pregnant consume 400 mcg of folate daily to reduce the incidence of neural tube defects. This recommendation has led the FDA to authorize health claims on labels of food and dietary supplements about the relationship between folate and neural tube defects.

EXCESS

Folate and the anticonvulsive drug phenytoin inhibit each other's uptake by the cells in the intestinal tract and possibly in brain tissue. Large doses of folate may inactivate the drug, causing convulsions in people with epilepsy. Folate supplements also may mask a deficiency of vitamin B_{12}. The maximum amount of folate that does not mask pernicious anemia is about 400 mcg/day; therefore, higher amounts are restricted to prescription formulations. Because early detection of pernicious anemia is necessary to prevent permanent nerve damage, the masking of B_{12} deficiency symptoms by folate could have serious consequences. Because there appear to be no benefits, excessive intakes of folate are not recommended.

COBALAMIN (VITAMIN B_{12})

Vitamin B_{12} is present in all cells and is necessary for their normal functioning. The trace element cobalt is part of the B_{12} molecule. For this reason, the vitamin was named *cobalamin.*

Absorption of vitamin B_{12} from the intestinal tract and its transfer to the bloodstream is a slow and complex process that occurs over a period of hours, in contrast to the seconds required for the absorption of most of the other water-soluble vitamins. Absorption of vitamin B_{12} depends on a protein in gastric juice called *intrinsic factor.* The vitamin B_{12} attaches to intrinsic factor and is carried to the ileum, where it is absorbed.

FUNCTIONS AND CLINICAL EFFECTS

Protein Metabolism

The synthesis of DNA depends on vitamin B_{12}–containing enzymes. Vitamin B_{12} also is necessary for the synthesis of one or more amino acids.

Production of Red Blood Cells

The role of vitamin B_{12} in DNA synthesis is of particular importance in bone marrow, where blood cells are formed. If vitamin B_{12} is lacking, red blood cells do not develop normally. Instead, they become larger than normal and fewer in number. Vitamin B_{12} appears to influence this blood-building process by promoting the functioning of folate.

Normal Functioning of the Nervous System

The exact role of vitamin B_{12} in the health of the nervous system is unknown but appears to be related to carbohydrate metabolism and myelin formation.

SOURCES

Vitamin B_{12} is found only in animal products such as meat, fish, poultry, eggs, milk, and cheese. Soybean milk substitutes, useful in strict vegetarian diets, frequently are fortified with vitamin B_{12}.

It is strongly recommended that children on a vegetarian diet be permitted eggs and milk. Vitamin B_{12} supplements or vitamin B_{12}–fortified foods are necessary for both adults and children who are on vegetarian diets that exclude milk and eggs as well as meat, fish, and poultry.

RECOMMENDED ALLOWANCES

The RDA for vitamin B_{12} is 2 mcg/day from age 11 years through adulthood. Excess vitamin B_{12} is stored in the liver in large amounts.

DEFICIENCY AND EXCESS

A deficiency of vitamin B_{12} usually results from absorption problems rather than from a dietary deficiency. Pernicious anemia, the vitamin B_{12} deficiency disease, is due to a lack of intrinsic factor in gastric juice necessary for the absorption of vitamin B_{12}. In this type of anemia, the red blood cells are abnormally large and are reduced in number. Other symptoms include stomatitis, lack of appetite, neurologic difficulties such as poor coordination in walking, and mental disturbances. A deficiency of vitamin B_{12} also may follow surgery of the stomach or small intestine and diseases that affect nutrient absorption. Injections of vitamin B_{12} must be given throughout the affected person's life. Maintenance dialysis in cases of renal failure also may cause low serum levels of vitamin B_{12} with symptoms of deficiency.

Because vitamin B_{12} is found only in animal foods, a deficiency may develop in people who follow strict vegetarian diets. Children on vegetarian diets are at greatest risk, because they have not accumulated stores of the vitamin.

The body effectively recycles the vitamin from bile and other intestinal secretions. This accounts for its long biologic effectiveness. Vegetarians who eat no animal products develop a vitamin B_{12} deficiency only after 20 to 30 years. The vitamin B_{12} they receive from intestinal bacteria is capable of sustaining them for this period because of reabsorption. In contrast, people with pernicious anemia who cannot absorb the vitamin develop the deficiency in 2 or 3 years.

No toxic effects have been reported due to excessive oral intakes of vitamin B_{12}. Also, no benefits from large intakes have been reported in people who do not have a vitamin B_{12} deficiency.

PANTOTHENIC ACID

FUNCTIONS AND CLINICAL EFFECTS

Pantothenic acid is part of coenzyme A (active acetate), which is essential for many chemical reactions, including the release of energy from protein, fats, and carbohydrates. This vitamin also is involved in the synthesis of amino acids, fatty acids, cholesterol, steroid hormones, and hemoglobin.

SOURCES

The vitamin is distributed widely in foods. Yeast, organ meats, salmon, and eggs are the best sources. Other good sources are broccoli, mushrooms, pork, whole-grain cereals and breads, and legumes. Grains lose half of their pantothenic acid in milling. Synthesis of pantothenic acid by intestinal bacteria is likely, but the quantity and availability from this source is unknown.

RECOMMENDED ALLOWANCES

The requirement for pantothenic acid has not been established. The Food and Nutrition Board has stated that an intake of 4 to 7 mg/day is probably adequate and safe for adults.

DEFICIENCY AND EXCESS

A deficiency is unlikely except in cases of a deficiency of all the B vitamins. A deficiency might result from a diet that consists of highly processed foods, because processing causes large losses of pantothenic acid. Experimental deficiency has produced such symptoms as insomnia, leg cramps, numbness and tingling of the hands and feet, and personality changes.

Naturally occurring deficiencies have not been reported reliably. Pantothenic acid deficiency has been implicated in the *burning feet syndrome* experienced by prisoners of war. The symptoms were relieved by pantothenic acid and not by other B-complex vitamins. Pantothenic acid appears to be nontoxic.

BIOTIN

FUNCTIONS AND CLINICAL EFFECTS

Biotin is involved in the metabolism of proteins, fats, and carbohydrates. Deficiency is rare. *Avidin*, a protein found in raw egg white, combines with biotin and prevents its absorption. Intestinal bacteria synthesize a considerable amount of biotin.

SOURCES

Liver, egg yolk, soy flour, cereals, and yeast are good sources. Information on the biotin content of food is incomplete.

RECOMMENDED ALLOWANCES

No RDA for biotin has been established. A recommended safe and adequate level of 30 to 100 mcg/day has been given.

DEFICIENCY AND EXCESS

Hair loss has been reported in adults and children who have received total intravenous nutrition without added biotin. Seborrheic dermatitis of infants younger than age 6 months has been attributed to biotin deficiency. The condition responds to therapeutic doses of the vitamin. There are no reports of toxicity.

See summary of water-soluble vitamins in Table 12-4.

VITAMINS AND FOOD LABELING

The content of vitamin A and vitamin C are required components of the "Nutrition Facts" panel of the food label. These amounts are expressed as a percentage of the Daily Value ("% Daily Value"), which is 5000 IU for vitamin A and 60 mg for vitamin C regardless of caloric intake. Listing the percentage of vitamin A as beta carotene in the product is optional.

Other essential vitamins may be listed on the label if the manufacturer desires. If the manufacturer makes a claim about any of the optional vitamins, it is mandatory that the manufacturer provide nutrition information about the optional vitamin. The quantity of a vitamin in a product is expressed as "% Daily Value." The "% Daily Value" for vitamins are the Reference Daily Intakes given in Table 5-2.

Health claims on food labels can be made for the relationship between fruits and vegetables and cancer. To carry this claim, a food must meet labeling requirements for "lowfat" (see Ch. 9) and, in addition, must meet labeling requirements for "good source" (without fortification) of at least one of the following: dietary fiber or vitamins A or C. This claim relates diets low in fat and rich in vitamins A and C and dietary fiber to reduced cancer risks.

The FDA has also authorized health claims on food labels and dietary supplements about the relationship between folate and neural tube defects.

LABELING REGULATIONS AND VITAMIN/MINERAL SUPPLEMENTS

In December 1993, the FDA published new labeling regulations to ensure that labeling of dietary supplements is truthful and scientifically valid. The new regulations require that dietary supplements provide the same basic information found on labels of nearly all conventional food and subject to the same standards when making health claims. The ruling does not affect consumers' right to purchase supplements; it only affects the health claims that can be made about them.

The FDA ruling, which became effective July 1994, requires that there be significant scientific agreement among qualified experts before manufacturers can make health claims about dietary supplements (vitamins, minerals, herbs, and other similar nutritional substances). Health claims on supplemental bottles, in catalogs, or implied by the product name require FDA approval. Two health claims for supplements presently approved by FDA are folate and the risk of neural tube defect and calcium and the risk of osteoporosis.

Since July 1995, dietary supplement products must have a nutrition information panel on the label that gives the nutrient content per serving (e.g., tablet, teaspoonful, and packet). The use of nutrient content claims such as *high, low,* and *less* is permitted.

KEY ISSUES

Vitamin and Mineral Supplements: Use or Abuse?

Annual sales of vitamin and mineral supplements in the United States are close to the $4 billion mark. Recent surveys have shown that about 40% of the population is using vitamin supplements. These supplements are mostly self-prescribed and are not based on any known deficiencies.

Traditionally, nutrition scientists have advised the use of vitamin/mineral supplements to treat nutritional deficiencies. In recent years, however, numerous reports have suggested that certain nutrients may help prevent chronic diseases such as cancer and heart disease. Some researchers believe there is sufficient evidence to recommend taking supplements, whereas most hesitate to recommend this route to disease prevention.

ADVERSE EFFECTS

The wisdom of taking megadoses of nutrient supplements is questioned on the following grounds:

Toxic effects—Fat-soluble vitamins are stored in the body. Excess vitamin A and D can be highly toxic—even fatal. Water-soluble vitamins also can be harmful in large quantities. The adverse effects of long-term supersaturation of the tissues with some water-soluble vitamins, which once were considered harmless, have become evident. The toxic effects of vitamin B_6, a water-soluble vitamin, range from mild sensory loss to inability to walk.

Certain nutrients are more likely to be toxic and cause adverse side effects that others. The margin of safety between the amount needed and the toxic level is wide for some nutrients and narrow for others, such as selenium. Those of greatest concern are vitamins A, B_6, C, and D and minerals zinc and selenium. Vitamin A taken at a level of 25,000 IU (only five times the RDA) for 7 to 10 years may cause permanent liver damage.

Interactions with other nutrients or drugs—Nutrients in the body are interrelated. Too much of one nutrient can interfere with the functioning of other nutrients, even in doses that are not considered toxic. For example, an excessive amount of zinc appears to interfere with the absorption of copper and calcium and also reduces high-density lipoprotein (HDL) or good cholesterol. Too much iron may hinder zinc absorption. In the words of Dr. Helene N. Guttman of the US Department of Agriculture Human Nutrition Research Center, "Once you have 100 percent of what you need and you self-prescribe many times more of a nutrient, you force your metabolism to work overtime to rebalance. Some people are successful in this rebalancing act; others are not."

Megadoses of vitamins and minerals may also interact adversely with drugs. For example, large doses of folate can inactivate the anticonvulsive drug phenytoin. Both folate and phenytoin compete for uptake by the cells in the intestinal tract and possibly in brain tissue.

Dependency—In the case of some vitamins, the tissues become dependent on higher levels of the nutrient and symptoms of deficiency may appear when intake is reduced to RDA levels. People on massive doses of vitamin C have been known to have "rebound scurvy" following discontinuance of supplements. They should reduce supplements gradually.

Masking of another disease—The use of iron supplements by people who are not at risk for anemia (men and postmenopausal women) may mask symptoms of occult blood loss due to colon cancer, bleeding ulcers, or other causes. Another example is the masking of pernicious anemia by folate supplements. Folate can correct the macrocytic anemia that accompanies the disease but does not correct the underlying neurologic problems. Because early detection of pernicious anemia is necessary to prevent nerve damage, masking of B_{12} deficiency symptoms could have serious consequences.

TRADITIONAL ADVICE

Nutrition authorities have long believed that the RDAs represent safe and adequate nutrient levels for healthy individuals and that the best source of these nutrients is a diet comprising a variety of foods. Self-supplementation beyond the RDAs has been considered to have no demonstrated benefits and the potential for harm.

Supplementation has been recognized as appropriate in certain special circumstances. These include

- women with excessive menstrual bleeding (iron).
- pregnant and breastfeeding women (folate, iron, and possibly calcium).
- people on very low-calorie diets (all nutrients).
- vegetarians who do not eat eggs or dairy products (calcium, iron, zinc, B_{12}).
- newborns (single dose of vitamin K to prevent bleeding).
- people with certain disorders or diseases or who take medications that interfere with nutrient intake, digestion, absorption, metabolism, or excretion and thus change requirements.

ENTER THE "ANTIOXIDANTS"

Much publicity has surrounded claims that antioxidant nutrients may reduce the risk of cancer, cataracts, and heart disease and may slow down the aging process. Oxidation is a form of deterioration resulting from chemical reactions involving oxygen. Free radicals are continually produced by the body as a result of oxidation, a process that is part of normal metabolism. Free radicals are unstable compounds that are missing an electron, a gap they fill by robbing other tissues and, as a result, damaging these tissues. Antioxidants have extra electrons that they give to free radicals, thus halting cell damage. In the body, nutrients, enzymes, and other compounds normally and automatically neutralize the free radicals.

Nutrients with antioxidant activity include vitamin C, vitamin E, beta carotene, and other carotinoids, some of which do not have vitamin A activity. Proper enzyme formation requires certain trace minerals such as selenium, copper, zinc, and manganese. Except for selenium, these minerals in themselves do not have antioxidant properties.

Nutrition authorities have not disputed the importance of antioxidants. However, much of the evidence supporting the benefits of antioxidants has resulted from *epidemiologic studies,* studies of living patterns associated with the occurrence of disease. There is no way of knowing if study participants have reported their eating habits accurately. After questioning the participants about their eating habits and lifestyle, research scientists follow these participants over a specified period to see what health problems develop. In these types of studies, it is difficult to separate effects of diet from exercise, body weight, and other unidentified factors. Clinical intervention studies are needed that involve two similar groups of people. One group is given a specified amount of antioxidants and both groups are tracked to see if there is a difference in disease rates in the two groups. Several large studies of this type are presently underway in the United States.

The FDA continues to prohibit health claims for the antioxidants on food or supplement packages. Panels of experts convened by the FDA have concluded that no matter what the antioxidant or what the disease, the evidence is too inconclusive to recommend supplements or warrant health claims on packages. Questions remain as to how these nutrients interact, what dosages might be appropriate for various age groups, and for how long a period they should be taken.

The ultimate issue is whether the need for antioxidants can be met by diet alone or are supplements needed. Most authorities agree that modest amounts of beta carotene, vitamin E, and vitamin C in supplement form are harmless. However, there is no evidence at present that healthy people eating fruits, vegetables, and grain products have anything to gain by taking supplements.

GUIDELINES FOR USING SUPPLEMENTS

Food is the best and safest source of nutrients. Improving one's diet gives the most far-reaching benefits. Some people, however, feel more secure with a multivitamin/mineral supplement. The following are 10 guidelines for selecting supplements:

1. Choose supplements that include a mix of essential vitamins and minerals at 100% to 150% of the RDA. Most supplements contain less than the RDA for calcium and magnesium because they add too much bulk to the supplement. Phosphorus is added in small amounts also.
2. Be sure to tell your health care providers about all the supplements you take, including concentrations and amounts.
3. Price is no indication of quality. Supermarkets and major retail chains carry store brands of high quality at a fraction of the cost of some name brands.
4. Do not take calcium that contains bone meal or dolomite. These substances may be contaminated with mercury or arsenic. (Calcium usually is taken as a separate supplement.)
5. Obtain supplements that meet disintegration/dissolution standards proposed by the US Pharmacopeia (USP), the scientific organization that establishes drug standards. The standards require that supplements completely disintegrate within 30 to 45 minutes and that they completely dissolve into a liquid. Some labels will say "proven release" or "release assured."
6. Do not spend extra money for supplements that include substances such as para-aminobenzoic acid (PABA), lecithin, amino acids, bee pollen, and inositol—substances that have never been shown to be essential nutrients for humans. Some are potentially harmful.
7. Choose a supplement that has a substantial percentage of vitamin A in the form of beta caro-

tene. Preformed vitamin A is sometimes referred to on labels as "vitamin A (as acetate)."

8. Unless you have iron-deficiency anemia, do not purchase supplements containing more than 100% of the "% Daily Value" for iron. Men and postmenopausal women do not need an iron supplement, but multivitamin/mineral supplements without iron are hard to find.
9. Ignore claims that "natural" vitamins are superior to synthetic vitamins. The only significant difference between "natural" and synthetic vitamins is the price.
10. Avoid supplements that do not have an expiration date. Store in a cool, dry, dark place. *Keep supplements out of the reach of children.*

Vitamin/mineral supplements should be taken with well-balanced meals. This usually promotes absorption. Above all, do not use supplements as an excuse for eating poorly.

KEYS TO PRACTICAL APPLICATION

When disease conditions interfere with the digestion or absorption of fats, anticipate that fat-soluble vitamins will be poorly absorbed, increasing the risk of deficiency.

Beware of advertisements or articles that promote the benefits of a particular nutrient, such as vitamin C or vitamin E. All of the 50 or more nutrients work together. Adding large amounts of some nutrients may interfere with the functioning of others.

Remember that in normal amounts vitamins are food; in amounts 5, 10, 20 or more times the RDA levels, they are drugs and should be treated as such.

Instruct parents to measure supplements that contain vitamins A or D carefully and use them only in recommended amounts. These vitamins are stored in the body and are toxic in excessive amounts.

Encourage the use of vegetables in both raw and cooked forms. Raw vegetables are not always the better source of vitamins. Cooking reduces the vitamin C content of vegetables, such as tomatoes. Cooked carrots, however, have more available carotene (provitamin A) than raw carrots.

Remember that steaming vegetables for as short a period as possible and microwaving are the best way to preserve water-soluble vitamins. Cooking in large quantities of water, overcooking, excessive cutting and chopping, and the addition of an alkali (such as baking soda) increase the loss of water-soluble vitamins.

To preserve the vitamin content of meats, cook them at low temperatures and do not overcook. Use meat drippings after removing the fat.

Educate your clients on how to use food labels to achieve recommended levels of vitamin A and vitamin C.

Keep abreast of FDA regulations regarding vitamin/mineral supplements and the reasoning behind these regulations.

Know how to advise your clients who are taking vitamin/mineral supplements to use them appropriately.

KEY IDEAS

Vitamins are involved in regulating body processes. Many vitamins function as parts of enzymes; others have hormonelike activity.

Vitamins do not provide energy, but many are involved in enzyme systems needed to convert protein, fat, and carbohydrate to energy.

The body cannot manufacture vitamins; they must be obtained in the diet. A serious lack of one or more vitamins results in one or more deficiency diseases.

Vitamins are needed in minute amounts. They are measured in either milligrams or micrograms.

Vitamins are classified as fat soluble and water soluble.

TABLE 12-3 SUMMARY: FAT-SOLUBLE VITAMINS

VITAMIN	FUNCTION	DEFICIENCY	SOURCES
A (retinol; precursor: carotenes)	Formation of visual purple and visual violet; normal growth of epithelial tissue, especially skin and mucous membranes; normal bone and tooth structure	Night and glare blindness; deterioration of epithelial tissue leading to decreased resistance to infection; dry, scaly skin; eye changes; xerophthalmia leading to blindness	Liver; whole milk and foods containing milk fat, such as butter, cream, cheese; margarine; as carotene in dark green leafy vegetables and some fruits
D (calciferol)	Promotion of absorption of calcium and phosphorus; normal use of these minerals in skeleton and soft tissue	Faulty bone and tooth development; rickets; osteomalacia	Fortified milk; direct exposure of skin to sunlight; fish liver oils
E (tocopherols)	Antioxidation—protection of substances that oxidize readily, such as essential fatty acids, thus prevention of damage to cell membranes	Destruction of red blood cells (hemolysis); deficiency is rare	Vegetable oils and shortening; margarine; green leafy vegetables; whole grains, legumes, nuts
K (menadione)	Normal blood clotting	Prolonged clotting time; hemorrhagic disease in newborns	Synthesis by intestinal bacteria; green leafy vegetables

The fat-soluble group, vitamins A, D, E, and K, are absorbed in the same manner as fats. Because they are stored in the body, deficiencies develop slowly. These vitamins are not readily lost in cooking. See Table 12-3 for a summary of the fat-soluble vitamins.

The water-soluble group, vitamin C and B-complex vitamins, are not stored in the body to any great extent and usually are readily destroyed by heat and in cooking. See Table 12-4 for a summary of the water-soluble vitamins.

The safety of taking large doses of vitamins without medical supervision is questionable; vitamins taken in doses considerably in excess of nutritional recommendations function as drugs and should be treated as such.

KEYS TO LEARNING

STUDY–DISCUSSION QUESTIONS

1. Using the 1-day food diary you kept in Chapter 5, compare your intake of vitamin A, vitamin C, and thiamin with the RDA for your gender and age group given in Appendix B.
2. Rank the following foods in order according to their vitamin content, with the richest source of the specified vitamin listed first:

VITAMIN A

1 cup of milk
½ cup of cooked, chopped broccoli
1 cup of chopped or shredded lettuce
3 oz of beef liver
One peach
1 tbsp of butter
1 tbsp of margarine
½ cup of cooked carrots

TABLE 12-4 Summary: Water-Soluble Vitamins

Vitamin	Function	Deficiency	Sources
Ascorbic acid (vitamin C)	Collagen formation: strong blood vessels, healthy skin, healthy gums, wound healing; formation of red blood cells; absorption of iron, conversion of folacin to its active form	Adult acne; easy bruising; poor wound healing; swan-neck hair deformity; sore gums; hemorrhages around bones; scurvy	Citrus fruit; broccoli; strawberries; cantaloupe; guava, mango, papaya; peppers; tomatoes; greens; potatoes
Thiamin (B_1)	Energy metabolism; synthesis of DNA, RNA	Poor appetite; fatigue; constipation; neuritis of legs; beriberi: wasting, paralysis of legs, heart failure, mental confusion	Meats, especially pork; wheat germ; whole-grain and enriched bread; legumes; peanuts; peanut butter; nuts
Riboflavin (B_2)	Energy metabolism; protein metabolism; essential for functioning of B_6 and niacin	Eye irritation; cheilosis; glossitis; seborrheic dermatitis	Milk; organ meats; meat, fish, eggs; green leafy vegetables; enriched breads and cereals
Niacin (precursor: tryptophan)	Energy metabolism; production of fatty acids, cholesterol, steroid hormones	Fatigue; poor appetite; weakness; anxiety; pellagra: diarrhea, dermatitis, deteriorated mental state	Liver, meat, fish, poultry; peanuts; legumes; whole-grain and enriched breads and cereals; sources of tryptophan: complete protein foods
Pyridoxine (B_6)	Amino acid metabolism involving protein synthesis; synthesis of regulatory substances such as serotonin; niacin production; hemoglobin synthesis	Anemia; dermatitis; irritability; convulsions	Liver, kidney; chicken; fish; pork; eggs; whole-grain cereals; legumes
Folate (folacin, folic acid)	Protein metabolism: synthesis of DNA and RNA, red blood cell formulation	Macrocytic anemia	Green leafy vegetables; liver, kidney, meats, fish; nuts; legumes; whole grains; bacterial synthesis
Cobalamin (B_{12})	Protein metabolism: synthesis of DNA, production of red blood cells; healthy nervous system: carbohydrate metabolism, myelin formation (Intrinsic factor of gastric secretions is required for absorption)	Pernicious anemia: macrocytic anemia, sore mouth, poor appetite, poor coordination in walking, mental disturbances	Found only in animal products: meat, fish, poultry, eggs, milk, cheese; bacterial synthesis
Pantothenic acid	Energy metabolism; synthesis of amino acids, fatty acids, cholesterol, steroid hormones, hemoglobin	Unlikely unless part of a deficiency of all B vitamins; associated with burning feet syndrome	Organ meats; salmon; eggs; broccoli; mushrooms; pork; whole grains; legumes (by bacterial synthesis)
Biotin	Protein, fat, and carbohydrate metabolism	Hair loss; dermatitis; deficiency rare; can be induced by avidin, a protein in raw egg white	Liver, egg yolk, soy flour, cereals; bacterial synthesis

VITAMIN C

½ fresh grapefruit
½ cup of orange juice (from concentrate)
One orange
½ cup of cooked collards (from raw)
One baked potato
½ cup of tomato juice
1 cup of whole milk

NIACIN

3-oz ground beef patty
1 cup of cooked lentils
1 cup of 40% bran flakes
Three slices of whole-wheat bread (16 slices per loaf)
One chicken breast (about 3 oz)
3 oz of beef liver
Three slices of enriched white bread (18 slices per loaf)

Check your answers by recording the vitamin content listed for each of these foods in Appendix C.

3. Define *hypervitaminosis, antivitamin, avitaminosis,* and *provitamin.* Give examples of each.
4. Identify the vitamin involved and explain its relation to each of the following: night blindness, intrinsic factor, scurvy, delayed blood clotting, sunshine, raw egg white, beriberi, isoniazid, cheilosis, pellagra, and tryptophan.
5. Describe ways in which the consumer can conserve the vitamin content of food.

BIBLIOGRAPHY

BOOKS

Food and Drug Administration. Press release and fact sheet. Rockville, MD: Food and Drug Administration, December 29, 1993. Publication no. P93-46 and Supplement.

National Academy of Sciences, National Research Council, Committee on Diet and Health, Food and Nutrition Board. Diet and health: implications for reducing chronic disease risk (executive summary). Washington, DC: National Academy Press, 1989.

National Academy of Sciences, National Research Council, Food and Nutrition Board. Recommended dietary allowances. 10th ed. Washington, DC: National Academy Press, 1989.

Mahan LK, Arlin M. Krause's food, nutrition, and diet therapy. Philadelphia: WB Saunders, 1992:71–108.

PERIODICALS

ADA applauds new FDA labeling rules that regulate health claims on dietary supplements; J Am Diet Assoc 1994;94:146.

A 9-point guide to choosing the right supplement. Tufts University Diet and Nutrition Letter 1993;11:7:3.

Bailey LB. Evaluation of a new Recommended Dietary Allowance for folate. J Am Diet Assoc 1992;92:4:463.

Farley D. Look for "legit" health claims on foods. FDA Consumer (Special Report: Focus on Food Labeling). May 1993. DHHS publication FDA 93-2262:21.

Forman A. Making it through the vitamin maze to choose a suitable supplement. Environ Nutr 1993;16:8:1.

Oeffinger KC. Scurvy: more than historical relevance. Am Fam Physician 1993;48:609.

Salamone LM, Dallal GE, Zantos D. Contributions of vitamin D intake and seasonal sunlight exposure to plasma 25—hydroxyvitamin D concentration in elderly women. Am J Clin Nutr 1994;59:80.

Stephenson MG, Guthrie HA. Positions of the American Dietetic Association: enrichment and fortification of foods and dietary supplements. J Am Diet Assoc 1994;94:661.

Suttie JW. Vitamin K and human nutrition. J Am Diet Assoc 1992;92:585.

US Public Health Service, Communicable Disease Center. Recommendations for use of folic acid to reduce number of spina bifida cases and other neural tube defects. JAMA 1993;269:1233.

Voelker R. Recommendations for antioxidants: how much evidence is enough? JAMA 1994;271:1148.

Werler MM, Shapiro S, Mitchell AA. Periconceptional folic acid exposure and risk of neural tube defects. JAMA 1993;269:1257.

CHAPTER

13

Fluids and Electrolytes

KEY TERMS

electrolyte a form of an element in body fluids that carries an electrical charge; sodium, potassium, and chloride are common electrolytes

homeostasis a stable, balanced state of body fluids that maintains normal body function

hydrostatic pressure pressure created by fluids

insensible unnoticed; something about which one is unaware

interact to act on each other

interstitial pertaining to the spaces between the cells

ions electrically charged molecules; ions with a positive charge are called *cations;* those with a negative charge are called *anions*

medium a substance through which something acts or is done

metabolic water water formed in the body as a result of metabolism

osmolality a measure of the total concentration of particles in a solution

osmosis the passage of a solvent such as water through a semipermeable membrane from a solution of lesser concentration to one of greater concentration

renal referring to the kidneys

semipermeable membrane a membrane that allows the passage of some molecules but not others; a membrane that allows the passage of water but not some of the substances dissolved in it

sensible noticed; something of which one is aware

stimulus something that causes another substance to react

supplementary feedings food provided in addition to meals, usually for therapeutic reasons

OBJECTIVES

After completing this chapter, the student will be able to:

1. State the important functions of water in the body.
2. State the routes of water loss.
3. Give the sources of water and the recommended fluid intake.
4. Describe the body water compartments and how these compartments interact.
5. Discuss the state of dynamic equilibrium (homeostasis) among all parts of the body's fluid environment that is necessary to sustain life.
6. Explain how the various solute particles in body fluids influence internal shifts of water.
7. Describe how a balanced distribution of total body water inside and outside the cell is maintained.
8. Describe how acid–base balance is maintained.
9. Discuss causes of dehydration, preventive measures, and treatment methods.
10. Discuss the present status of the role of nutrition in the cause and treatment of premenstrual syndrome; give diet modifications that appear to be helpful.

WATER

Water, next to oxygen, is the body's most urgent need. It is more essential to life than food. Without water, nutrients are of no value to the body. A person can survive for weeks without food but only days without water.

Failure to understand the role of body water contributes to health problems such as indigestion and constipation and even to needless death. For example, every year during summer training, several athletes die from exposure to heat because they routinely consume salt to replace salt lost in perspiration but also restrict their water intake. Wearing heavy clothing that hinders the loss of body heat from the skin aggravates the problem. Another unhealthy practice among athletes is the restriction of water to control body weight. Water should be freely available to people who have increased water loss due to heavy sweating. Depriving anyone of fluid intake can have serious consequences, unless fluids are restricted for therapeutic purposes, as in some stages of kidney disease.

WATER DISTRIBUTION IN THE BODY

Water makes up half to three fourths of body weight, depending on age and amount of body fat. Infants and children have a greater proportion of water than older people, and obese people have proportionately less water than lean individuals. Water is part of every body cell. This is true even of the cells composing bone tissue, which are one third water. Water forms the basic substance of blood, lymph, and body secretions (Fig. 13-1).

Body fluids are held in compartments separated by semipermeable membranes. These membranes allow water to pass through but prevent the movement of some substances from one side of the membrane to the other. According to new estimates, 40% to 50% of total body water is extracellular; the remaining 50% to 60% is intracellular.

Intracellular water, or cellular water, is located within the cell. It acts as a solvent for nutrients and for waste products produced by the cell, as an activator for biologic reactions within the cell, and as a component of cell structure.

Extracellular water, water outside the cell, is divided into two major body compartments: the blood vessels and the spaces between the cells, called *interstitial spaces.* In the arteries, veins, and capillaries, water, as a constituent of plasma, acts as a solvent for nutrients and for the hormones secreted by the glands. Blood vessels carry these substances to all body parts. Blood vessels also carry waste products such as carbon dioxide and ammonia from the cells to the skin, lungs, and kidneys.

Water fills the interstitial spaces that surround the cells. This interstitial fluid is in close contact with the capillaries, carrying nutrients that have left the plasma through pores in the capillary wall and transporting them to the cell membrane. It also collects waste and hormones secreted by cells, delivering them to the blood vessel membrane. In addition to blood plasma and interstitial fluid, lymph, spinal fluid, synovial fluid, and bodily secretions make up the remaining extracellular water.

FUNCTIONS OF WATER

CHEMICAL REACTANT

Water is the medium in which chemical reactions occur. In some cases, water acts as a catalyst; in others, water takes part in the chemical reaction. As a catalyst, water as a solvent enables substances dissolved in it to interact. For example, some substances develop an electrical charge when dissolved in water. Water also takes part in chemical reactions, as is evident in the digestive process, in the breakdown of starches to monosaccharides, the splitting of glycerol from the fatty acid molecule, and the breakdown of proteins to amino acids. A chemical reaction that requires water for the breakdown of complex compounds is called a *hydrolytic reaction;* the process is called *hydrolysis.*

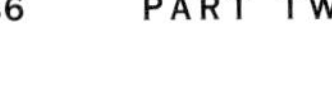

Water intake
Controlled by thirst and appetite
2000–4000 ml.

Water Balance
Some uses of water in the body
(Approximate volumes only)

Water excreted
Controlled by endocrine glands and temperature of environment
2000–4000 ml.

Present in foods
Formed in metabolism
Consumed as fluids

Blood 3500 ml.

By lungs as water vapor
By skin as sweat
In stools
By kidneys as urine

Intestinal juice 3000 ml.
Saliva 1500 ml.
Gastric juice 2500 ml.
Bile and Pancreatic Juice 1500 ml.

Digestive Juices

FIGURE 13-1

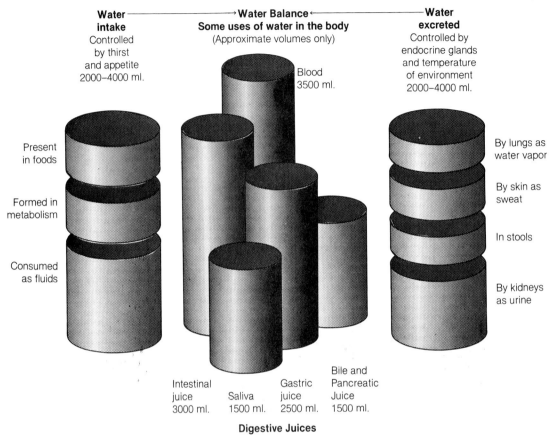

Use and balance of body water. Water intake and output can vary greatly between individuals and in an individual from day to day. Healthy people, however, can maintain water balance over a relatively large range of intakes. The daily use of water by the body greatly exceeds the daily intake. Recycling is possible because of the effective intestinal and renal reabsorption of water that flows through the intestine and the kidneys.

SOLVENT

Because many substances dissolve in water, body fluids are capable of transporting nutrients across the intestinal wall, of carrying nutrients and hormones to all body cells, and of carrying waste products from the cells to the lungs, skin, and kidneys. Acting as a solvent, water allows substances to interact both physically and chemically.

CELL COMPONENT

The intracellular water gives form and shape to the cell. When cells lose water, the cell membranes begin to collapse.

TEMPERATURE REGULATOR

The burning of carbohydrates, fats, and protein for energy provides more heat than is needed to maintain normal temperature. If temperature continued to rise without limit, cellular enzymes eventually would become inactivated and normal function would cease. Excess heat is disposed of primarily through evaporation of water from the skin. Excretion of water in the form of perspiration occurs continuously; normal water loss from the skin accounts for 25% of total water loss. As a rule, we are unaware of this perspiration; perspiration becomes obvious only in a hot environment or after heavy physical exercise.

LUBRICANT

Some body water serves as a lubricant, as in spinal fluid, ocular fluid, synovial fluid, and the mucous secretions of the respiratory, gastrointestinal, and genitourinary tracts.

WATER INTAKE AND OUTPUT

The amount of water consumed is approximately equal to the amount lost. The mechanisms that control this balance are discussed in the section Water Balance.

Water is reused many times for different purposes. For example, the water that carries enzymes to the digestive tract also carries nutrients to the blood and lymph. Although large quantities of water-carrying waste materials circulate through the tubules of the kidneys, most of the water and some of the useful dissolved material is reabsorbed.

WATER INTAKE

Water is consumed in the form of water itself; beverages, such as coffee, tea, fruit juices, and milk; and soups. Solid foods contribute the next largest amount of water, as much as 25% to 50% of water requirements. Some solid foods contain a high percentage of water. Fresh vegetables and fruits are 80% to 90% water; meat is 50% to 60% water; and even bread is about 35% water (Fig. 13-2).

Water formed within the body as a result of metabolism is called *metabolic water*. The burning of 100 g of fat produces 107 g of water, 100 g of carbohydrate produces 56 g of water, and 100 g of protein produces 40 g of water. Thus, the amount of water produced by the burning of fat is considerable. This metabolic water may accumulate periodically, and its presence explains why some people experience a temporary gain in weight during weight reduction programs.

Drinking water in moderate amounts before or during meals aids digestion by stimulating the flow

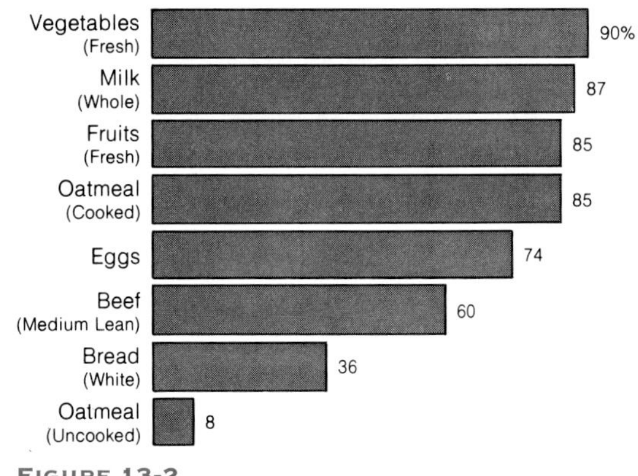

FIGURE 13-2

Percentage of water in common foods.

of gastric juice. However, water should not be used as an alternative to chewing. Water drunk and consumed in solid food is absorbed rapidly from the intestinal tract into the blood and lymph. Some water remains in the gastrointestinal tract and aids in waste elimination by producing a soft stool.

WATER OUTPUT

Under normal conditions, water loss occurs in four ways: from the skin as perspiration, from the lungs as water vapor in expired air, from the kidneys as urine, and from the intestine in feces. Water lost from the lungs and skin is called *insensible* (unnoticed) water loss; water lost in urine and feces is called *sensible* (noticed) water loss. Water is lost mostly in the urine. The daily amount ranges from 600 to 3000 mL/day, depending on fluid intake. A certain amount of water must be excreted to rid the body of metabolic waste products. About 600 mL of urine is required to keep the waste products in solution; this is referred to as the *obligatory water loss*.

Water loss varies from person to person. Table 13-1 indicates the average range of loss. Water loss from the skin and lungs may be 50% to 100% higher than normal in people living in hot dry climates. Strenuous athletic performance or heavy work done in high environmental temperatures may increase water loss from skin and lungs three to ten times. Abnormal conditions such as diarrhea,

TABLE 13-1 TYPICAL DAILY INPUT AND OUTPUT OF AN ADULT

WATER SOURCE	VOLUME (ML)
Intake	
Liquid foods	1300–1500
Moisture from solid foods	500–800
Water derived from oxidation of foods in the body	300–500
Total	2100–2800
Average	2450
Output	
Urine	1080–1650
Feces	100–150
Evaporation from the skin (sweat)	550–600
Expiration from the lungs as moist air	370–400
Total	2100–2800
Average	2450

(Burton BT. Human nutrition. New York: McGraw-Hill, 1976:76.)

vomiting, burns, hemorrhage, and fever may result in large water losses.

RECOMMENDED WATER CONSUMPTION

Because the body cannot store water, the amount lost must be replaced. A person's requirement for water may vary from day to day because of such factors as environmental temperature and physical activity. It is recommended that an adult under average conditions of energy expenditure and environment consume 1 mL of water per calorie expended. Infants have an increased need for water, requiring 1.5 mL/kcal. An adult whose energy expenditure is 2000 to 2500 kcal/day requires about 2 to 2.5 liters of water. Of this quantity, 1.25 to 1.5 liters (5 to 6 cups) should be consumed in the form of fluids; the remainder would come from solid foods and metabolic water. People who work or live in hot environments and those engaged in heavy physical activity in high environmental temperatures or at high altitudes require more water. During breastfeeding, increased amounts of water are needed for milk production.

Water intake is controlled mainly by thirst. The thirst center is located in the hypothalamus (an area of the brain above the pituitary gland). The sensation of thirst usually is a reliable guide to water intake, except in infants and sick people, especially comatose people who cannot respond to the thirst stimulus. Some people seem to lack a thirst stimulus. Elderly people have a depressed thirst sensation. Despite their low physical activity, their water needs may be high, especially during the summer. If losses are not replenished, heat exhaustion and possibly heat stroke may occur.

MAINTAINING A STABLE FLUID ENVIRONMENT

More than half of the body's total weight is water. This continuous body of water, by its chemical nature, maintains balance in its fluid compartments and an environment supportive of life. Despite continual change brought about by the many chemical reactions occurring within it, the healthy body maintains a balanced, stable, internal environment. A constant body temperature, water balance, and acid–base balance are maintained; heart rate, respiratory rate, and blood pressure remain within normal limits. This tendency of the body to maintain a normal state despite opposing forces is known as *dynamic equilibrium* or *homeostasis*.

Practically all illnesses are a threat to this balance. Even in a healthy person, some circumstances can upset the balance, with serious consequences. Heavy physical activity on a hot day, inadequate water intake, or a poorly balanced diet for extended periods can cause fluid and electrolyte disturbances.

PARTICLES IN SOLUTION

Particles dissolved in body water control the water balance and provide an environment that supports the body's chemical reactions. The two main solutes that make up these control mechanisms are electrolytes and plasma protein.

ELECTROLYTES

Electrolytes are compounds that, when dissolved in water, dissociate into separate particles called *ions.* Ions in solution have an electrical charge. Particles that develop positive charges, called *cations,* include sodium, calcium, potassium, and magnesium. Negatively charged particles, called *anions,* include chloride, bicarbonate, phosphate, and sulfate. An electrolyte solution contains equal amounts of anions and cations. Electrolytes are measured in milliequivalents (mEq).

Maintaining precise concentrations of electrolytes in the intracellular and extracellular fluid is a major aspect of homeostasis. The most important electrolytes are sodium, potassium, and chloride. Other major electrolytes are magnesium, calcium, and phosphorus (phosphates). The quantity of each electrolyte in the fluid compartments must be maintained within a narrow range; the amount differs for each electrolyte. An abnormal change in the quantity of any one electrolyte upsets the balance that exists among the other electrolytes, damaging body cells and preventing them from functioning properly.

A number of bodily mechanisms are constantly at work to maintain electrolytes at normal levels. These controls, which differ depending on the electrolyte, include the following:

Release or increased storage of minerals—Changes in mineral storage are regulated by hormones that are highly sensitive to changes in electrolyte concentration. For example, calcium stored in bone is released when serum calcium levels fall; deposits of calcium in the bone increase when serum calcium levels rise.

Excretion by kidneys—Hormones regulate the excretion or reabsorption of water and electrolytes by the kidneys according to need. If sodium intake exceeds body needs, water is reabsorbed and excess sodium ions are excreted.

Increased or decreased absorption from the intestinal tract—The percentage of dietary calcium absorbed from the intestinal tract normally is low. When serum calcium levels fall, a hormone stimulates increased formation of active vitamin D, which in turn increases the intestinal absorption of calcium.

Electrolyte balance is rarely affected by consumption of foods high or low in these minerals. If, however, an imbalance occurs as a result of a problem in the body's control systems, diet may be part of the treatment. For example, if the kidneys are unable to excrete sodium normally, a controlled-sodium diet may be necessary. Each of the electrolytes is discussed in Chapter 11.

PLASMA PROTEINS

Plasma proteins (albumin and globulin) are so large that they cannot pass through the capillary membrane; thus, they remain in the blood vessel. Plasma proteins play a major role in maintaining water balance in the body by exerting osmotic pressure, which controls the movement of fluid in and out of the capillaries (see the section Osmotic Pressure). In a similar manner, cell protein helps to maintain the integrity of water within the cell.

Other dissolved particles, small in size, that also circulate in the bloodstream normally are not present in sufficient quantities to bring about shifts in body water. In abnormal situations in which these compounds accumulate in excessive quantities, water balance is affected. For example, the development of high concentrations of serum glucose and ketones in uncontrolled diabetes brings about excessive water loss.

WATER BALANCE

Under normal conditions, fluid intake and output are in balance. A person does not gain weight or retain fluid as a result of drinking more water. The body gets rid of water it does not need.

OSMOTIC PRESSURE

Exchanges of water among various fluid compartments occur mainly as a result of *osmosis.* In this process, the quantity of a fluid and the direction in which it flows are determined by the quantity of electrolytes and other dissolved particles on either side of the semipermeable membrane. Water moves through the membrane to the compartment with the greater concentration of electrolytes and other dissolved particles.

CELLULAR FLUID/INTERSTITIAL FLUID BALANCE

Water balance between cellular fluid and interstitial fluid is regulated mainly by the potassium concentration within the cell and the sodium concentration in the interstitial spaces. Chloride and phosphate also play a role. If there is a loss or gain of electrolytes in either compartment, the balance is disturbed, and more water passes into the compartment with the higher mineral concentration.

INTERSTITIAL FLUID/CAPILLARY FLUID BALANCE

To nourish the cells, water, nutrients, and oxygen must leave the capillaries and enter the cell. In turn, water and products of cell metabolism including carbon dioxide must be drawn into the capillaries so that cell products can be distributed throughout the body and metabolic waste products can be carried to the lungs and kidneys.

Water exchange between the blood vessels and the interstitial (between the cells) spaces is due to hydrostatic pressure and osmotic pressure. *Hydrostatic pressure* is created by the pumping action of the heart on the fluid in the blood vessels. When the blood first enters the capillaries from the larger blood vessels, the hydrostatic pressure forces fluids and small particles out through the semipermeable membranes of the blood vessel walls into the interstitial spaces to nourish the cells. When fluids and metabolites are ready to reenter the blood circulation, the *initial pressure* exerted by the blood pressure is diminished. Then the greater pressure is the osmotic pressure exerted by the plasma proteins in the blood, which draws the fluids from the interstitial spaces into the blood circulation.

ORGAN SYSTEMS INVOLVED IN WATER BALANCE

In addition to the cardiovascular system, two other organ systems involved in the body's water balance system are the gastrointestinal system and the renal circulation (kidneys).

Gastrointestinal System

The digestive juices and other fluids secreted into the gastrointestinal tract consist of 7 to 9 liters of water daily. Most of these fluids are reabsorbed in the ileum and colon. Water and electrolytes are secreted continually into the gastrointestinal tract to aid digestion of food and absorption of nutrients. Water is constantly moving from the blood, to the secreting cells, to the gastrointestinal tract, and back to the circulating blood. The volume of fluid circulating in the gastrointestinal system is so large—twice that of blood plasma—that any significant loss of this fluid due to vomiting or diarrhea can have serious consequences, especially for infants, young children, and elderly people.

The gastrointestinal circulation is in balance with other extracellular fluid including the blood circulation. This means that the osmotic pressure exerted by one is equal to the osmotic pressure exerted by the other. The *osmolality* of a fluid determines the force or pressure with which it will attract water.

Osmolality. Osmolality is the concentration of particles in a certain volume of fluid. It is expressed in terms of milliosmoles per liter (mOsm/liter). The osmolality of body fluid is between 280 and 295 mOsm/liter.

The osmolality of a liquid depends on the volume of particles and the size of the particles it contains. If two liquids have the same volume of particles, the one having the smaller particles will have a higher osmolality. This occurs because the smaller particles will have a greater total surface area and thus will create a greater attraction for water.

Osmolality has important applications in nutrition and is especially relevant to the fluid balance between the intestinal fluids and the blood. Body fluids will shift to maintain equal osmolality in all the extracellular fluids. If the osmolality of the blood or the intestinal fluid increases, water would move into that area. For example, if a patient fed by tube is fed too concentrated a formula, water would shift from the blood to the intestine to dilute the intestinal contents. This could rapidly reduce

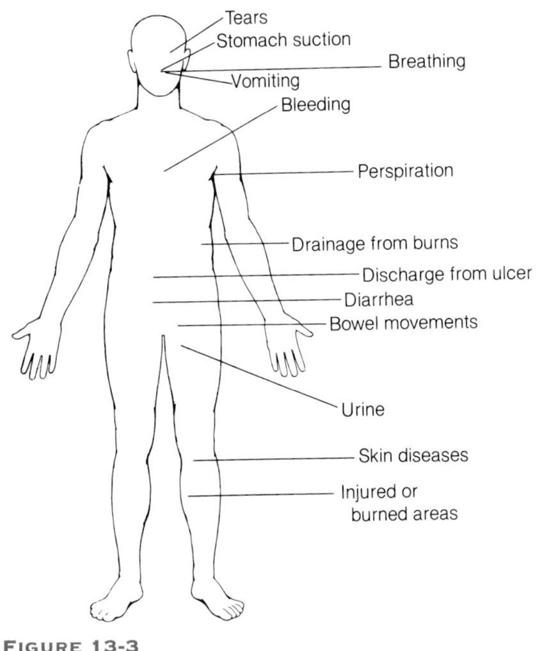

FIGURE 13-3

Ways in which water and electrolytes may be lost from the body.

the volume of circulating blood, resulting in symptoms of shock.

Renal Circulation (Kidneys)

The blood is filtered by millions of minute filters, called *nephrons,* in the kidneys. The filtering process, called *glomerular filtration,* produces a liquid that contains both waste products and vital substances. In a healthy person, the vital substances including some water, electrolytes, and glucose are reabsorbed so that the blood composition remains within normal limits. Waste products such as excess salt and electrolytes are excreted.

Hormones regulate this excretion or reabsorption of water and electrolytes according to body need. The antidiuretic hormone (ADH), produced by the pituitary gland directs the kidneys to reabsorb water. Aldosterone, produced by the adrenal glands when the sodium level of the blood decreases, causes the kidneys to reabsorb sodium. When sodium is reabsorbed, water is reabsorbed with it. Thus, aldosterone indirectly causes water reabsorption.

CLINICAL APPLICATIONS

In many instances, the health worker must give special attention to the client's need for water.

High-Protein Intake

Because the end products of protein metabolism are excreted by the kidneys, additional water is required for infants on high-protein formulas, clients consuming high-protein diets or supplementary feedings, and people who receive concentrated tube feedings or concentrated intravenous solutions. Wastes must be diluted to a certain level before the kidneys can excrete them efficiently.

Dehydration

Excessive loss of water—*dehydration*—may be due to a lack of food and water or to losses of water in heavy perspiration, severe diarrhea, vomiting, hemorrhage, severe burns, or uncontrolled diabetes accompanied by frequent urination (Fig. 13-3). A water loss of more than 10% of body weight is life threatening. Dehydration always is accompanied by electrolyte imbalances. Infants become dehydrated more quickly than older people because their bodies contain a greater proportion of water and because much of this water is outside the cell and therefore is easily lost (Fig. 13-4). Abnormal water loss such as in diarrhea, fever, and vomiting poses a serious threat to infants. Intravenous fluids may be necessary if sufficient fluids cannot be taken by mouth.

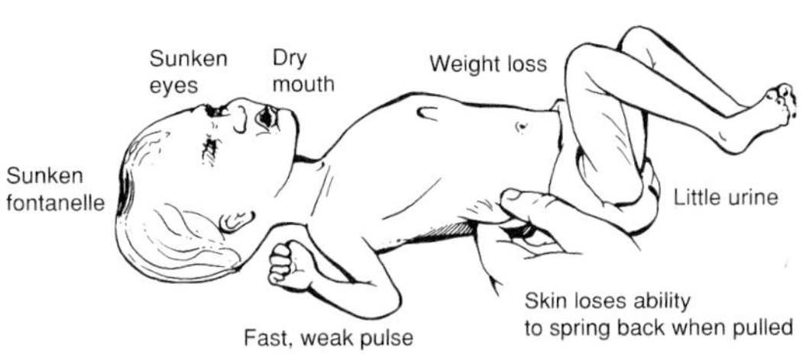

FIGURE 13-4

Symptoms of severe dehydration in an infant.

Dehydration can occur rapidly in comatose clients and in disabled or elderly people with brain impairment who are unable to respond to the sensation of thirst. Bedridden clients urinate frequently because their reclining position promotes urine production. Clients also may perspire freely if heavily covered. Other conditions, such as fever, diabetes mellitus, vomiting, diarrhea, and the use of drugs such as diuretics also increase water need.

Water loss due to excessive perspiration must be corrected by increasing water consumption. Sodium replacement probably is unnecessary, even in heavy sweating. Sodium balance is maintained over a wide range of environmental conditions. Extreme conditions may cause sodium depletion. These conditions include heavy sweating for a prolonged period and diarrhea or renal disease, conditions in which sodium cannot be retained.

Symptoms of heat exhaustion due to dehydration are thirst, fatigue, giddiness, decreased urine output, and fever. Heat exhaustion due to sodium deficiency causes fatigue, nausea, giddiness, and exhaustion, but usually not fever.

Rehydration Therapy

In the hospital, intravenous therapy provides fluid, electrolytes and dextrose. This fluid mixture keeps a stable concentration of electrolytes in the blood. Providing only water without electrolytes would not help to maintain the normal osmotic pressure that is essential to water balance. Providing plain water could have serious consequences.

Several decades ago, the World Health Organization developed oral rehydration therapy (ORT) to treat children and adults with diarrhea in developing countries. A simple solution of clean water, sugar, and electrolytes in specific amounts have saved countless lives.

Today, the prompt use of ORT is recommended for all people with diarrhea. As for very young people, diarrhea can be life threatening for elderly individuals. Dehydration and atherosclerosis in elderly people lead to damage of vital organs. In the United States, commercial ORT products are available that can be given by mouth or by tube. After the rehydration phase, a more dilute solution may be given to maintain hydration. These solutions should be used only under the supervision of a physician or other trained health personnel.

Edema

The spaces surrounding the cells are more susceptible to changes in water volume than are the other fluid compartments. When too much sodium accumulates in the interstitial spaces, as occurs in congestive heart failure, more water is pulled into the interstitial compartment, and the involved area becomes swollen (see Chapter 26). This accumulation of water is called *edema*. Edema also may result from severe protein deficiency, in which the osmotic pressure exerted by proteins in the blood is lessened. Edema is also a symptom in kidney disease and cirrhosis of the liver. Treatment of edema varies depending on the cause. If edema results from sodium retention, sodium in the diet may be restricted.

ACID–BASE BALANCE

Enzymes function only when the fluid within the cell is neutral. Electrolytes play an important role in maintaining this environment. The amount of acid or alkaline (base) in a solution is expressed as *pH*. A pH of 7 is neutral; less than 7 indicates acidity; more than 7 indicates alkalinity. The reaction of the blood is slightly alkaline, with a pH of 7.3 to 7.45.

This precise balance is maintained regardless of the acidic and alkaline substances that result from metabolism. When foods are completely burned, a residue remains. This residue, or ash, is the mineral content of the food. Some ash forms acids when dissolved. Acid-forming substances predominate in meat, fish, poultry, eggs, and cereals; for this reason, these foods are called *acid-forming* or *acid-ash foods*. Minerals that are basic in solution are abundant in most fruits and vegetables and are called *base-forming* or *alkaline-ash foods*. Plums, prunes, and cranberries are the only exceptions. They contain an acid that the body does not metabolize but excretes as such. Citrus fruits, which have an acidic taste because of their organic acids, are alkali-forming foods. The body burns organic acids in citrus fruits, and the mineral ash that remains is alkaline in reaction. Although milk and milk products contain both acid-forming and alkali-forming substances, alkaline substances predominate. Some foods, such as pure fats, sugar, and pure starches, are neutral, because they are not mineral sources.

Most diets contain a surplus of acid-forming minerals. Whether acid-forming or alkali-forming substances predominate, however, a pH of 7.3 to 7.45 must be maintained. The body has several mechanisms through which to maintain this aspect of homeostasis. In the blood are buffers—carbonates, phosphates, and proteins—that react with either excess acid or excess base to prevent changes in pH. The exhalation of carbon dioxide removes carbonic acid. The kidneys remove excessive acid and alkaline substances and produce ammonia, which neutralizes excess acid. Dietary factors alone seldom cause acid–base imbalances.

A condition known as *acidosis* results when the supply of buffers is depleted. Acidosis may be caused by starvation or by a defect in metabolism, as in uncontrolled diabetes and in weight reduction diets that call for low intakes of carbohydrate.

Alkalosis results from the accumulation of alkaline substances or a loss of acid. It is seen in people who have had severe and prolonged vomiting with a heavy loss of hydrochloric acid from the stomach. The regular use of antacid medications is another cause of alkalosis.

KEY ISSUES

Premenstrual Syndrome: Does Diet Help?

Premenstrual syndrome (PMS) has been described as a recurrence of symptoms that begin at ovulation, increase during the premenstrual period, subside at menstruation, and disappear from the time of menstruation to ovulation. More than 100 physical and emotional symptoms have been described for PMS. The cluster of symptoms varies widely among women. The more common symptoms are fluid retention, tension, depression, irritability, crying spells, headaches, breast tenderness, acne, and cravings for chocolate, other sweets, or salty foods. Some women experience symptoms similar to hypoglycemia (low blood sugar). The emotional symptoms cause the most distress. Some women are so severely affected they cannot function normally.

In this chapter, we have seen that hormones are involved in the systems that control water and electrolyte balance. Thus, it is conceivable that, because the hormone levels of women change considerably each month in the 14 days before menses, water and electrolyte balances could be affected. Women often complain they feel bloated and are gaining weight—symptoms of water retention. A woman's ability to metabolize sugar also varies with the phase of the menstrual cycle. Her blood sugar levels are highest at the time of ovulation due to the increase in estrogen levels.

Despite many years of research, the causes of PMS are poorly understood, with conflicting study results of various treatments. Also, studies have been complicated by an unusually high placebo response. That is, a high percentage of study participants who receive so-called "sugar pills" instead of the research drug or supplement reported improvement in symptoms.

TREATMENT THEORIES

Various treatments have been used, including progesterone therapy, stress reduction exercises, dietary modifications, and physical exercise. Various theories about the relation of diet to PMS have led to a number of remedies. Some of these remedies are potentially harmful.

One nutritional theory proposes that a deficiency of vitamin B_6 (pyridoxine) causes PMS. Because vitamin B_6, along with magnesium, is involved in the synthesis of brain chemicals, supplements of these nutrients are thought to be useful in alleviating the psychological changes that occur. Although some evidence has indicated that moderate (50 mg) of B_6 may alleviate emotional symptoms, higher doses can be toxic. Supplements of vitamin B_6 have been prescribed in massive doses, sometimes more than 1000 times the recommended dietary allowance of 1.6 mg. Because B_6 is a water-soluble vitamin, it was assumed that excesses would be excreted and, therefore, could not be harmful. As little as 250 to 500 mg/day, however, has caused nervous system damage. Symptoms include numbness, tingling, difficulty in walking, and spinal problems.

Another remedy is evening primrose oil supplements. The oil, extracted from primrose flower seeds, is believed to raise the body's level of prostaglandins—chemicals thought to be useful in correcting hormonal abnormalities in women with PMS. It has never been proved that a prostaglandin deficiency causes PMS or that primrose oil can correct an existing deficiency. Besides being expensive, primrose oil can cause gastric irritation. The long-term effect of primrose oil on the body is unknown.

Another theory is that some women with PMS have lower levels of magnesium than normal. The magnesium deficiency supposedly occurs because of the high consumption of calcium-rich foods (dairy products). Because the absorption of calcium and magnesium depends on the same carrier, supporters of this theory have claimed that a high calcium intake blocks the absorption of magnesium. They have suggested that women limit their calcium intake. This is surprising advice because many experts believe that, to prevent osteoporosis, women need more calcium than they generally consume. An alternative suggestion is to take a magnesium supplement. Megadoses of magnesium can impair the absorption of calcium. Although magnesium toxicity is rare, people who have poor kidney function could run into problems with high doses of magnesium. Normal intake of calcium has never been proved to interfere with adequate magnesium absorption.

Vitamin/mineral supplements advertised as specifically for women affected with PMS are on the market. The manufacturers of these formulas have claimed that PMS is caused by a deficiency of numerous nutrients. These supplements frequently contain high doses of nutrients, such as vitamin B_6, that can be hazardous.

Women with PMS often suffer the same symptoms as people with hypoglycemia—fatigue, irritability, weakness, and a generally ill feeling. Although symptoms are similar, women with PMS have not been found to have abnormally low blood sugar levels. Nevertheless, many women have found relief from the symptoms of PMS by following these diet guidelines:

- Avoid or severely limit sugar and foods containing concentrated amounts of sugar such as cakes, cookies, candies, ice cream, syrups, and jam. These foods promote insulin production, which may increase feelings of hunger and increase desire for concentrated sweets.
- Increase complex carbohydrates such as whole-grain breads and cereals, pasta, rice, and potatoes.
- Eat small meals and snacks frequently—no more than 3 hours apart.
- Avoid caffeine-containing beverages, chocolate, and medications.
- Reduce consumption of fats—especially saturated fats.
- Reduce sodium intake.
- Avoid alcohol.
- Eat more foods rich in vitamin B_6 and magnesium such as legumes, whole-grain cereals, and green leafy vegetables.

These are healthy eating practices similar to the Dietary Guidelines for Americans. Unlike the remedies discussed earlier, they can make only a positive contribution to health. In combination with regular exercise and stress reduction techniques, these diet guidelines constitute the best advice for treating PMS symptoms.

KEYS TO PRACTICAL APPLICATION

Encourage the drinking of at least 5 or 6 cups of fluid daily. Drinking moderate amounts of water with meals can aid digestion.

Discourage the drinking of water with meals as a substitute for chewing. Chewing and mixing food with saliva is an important step in digestion.

Be aware of the importance of water intake for your clients, especially clients on high-protein diets; comatose clients; disabled or elderly clients with brain impairment; clients with fever, vomiting, or diarrhea; clients with increased urination due to diabetes or usage of drugs that increase urination; clients in hot environments; and infants.

Caution clients who are in danger of upsetting their body pH either by low-carbohydrate fad diets or by the excessive use of antacids.

Encourage people who are discouraged when they fail to lose weight, although they are eating less. Explain that metabolic water temporarily accumulates as a result of the burning of fatty tissue.

Seek prompt treatment for clients experiencing diarrhea. Remember that infants, in particular, become dehydrated quickly. Furthermore, diarrhea in elderly people who also have atherosclerosis can be life threatening.

KEY IDEAS

Water is indispensable to life.

Body fluids are held in body compartments. Of these body fluids, 50% to 60% is within the cells; the remainder is outside the cells in the blood vessels, in the space between the cells and other body fluids (spinal and synovial), and in bodily secretions.

Water is the medium for chemical reactions; a solvent of nutrients, secretions, and waste products; a component of cell structure; a regulator of body temperature; and a lubricant.

Water is lost from skin and lungs and in urine and feces. People consume water in fluids and solid food. Water also is a product of metabolism.

Depriving people, including athletes, of fluid intake can have serious consequences.

Under ordinary conditions, the total water requirement for adults is about 2 to 2.5 liters daily. Of this amount, adults should consume 5 to 6 cups in the form of fluids.

A balanced, stable body environment called homeostasis is required for proper body functioning. Maintaining precise amounts of electrolytes in body fluids is a major aspect. Plasma proteins also play a major role in water balance.

Controls that maintain electrolyte balance include hormonal regulation of the release or storage of minerals, selective excretion of electrolytes by the kidneys, and increased or decreased absorption of minerals, depending on need.

A balance between fluid intake and fluid loss is reached mainly as a result of osmosis.

Water balance between fluid in the cells and fluid surrounding the cells is regulated mainly by potassium within the cells and sodium outside the cells.

Water balance between the blood vessels and spaces around the cells is the result of osmotic pressure due to electrolytes and plasma proteins in the blood and electrolytes in the spaces around the cells. The pumping action of the heart also influences water balance.

In addition to the cardiovascular system, the gastrointestinal and renal systems play major roles in maintaining water balance.

The digestive juices and other fluids secreted into the gastrointestinal tract consist of 7 to 9 liters of water daily, most of which is reabsorbed in the ileum and colon.

If the osmolality of the intestinal fluids is greater than that of the blood, water will shift from the blood to the intestine.

Edema occurs when sodium accumulates in the spaces between the cells or when there is severe protein deficiency, in which case the pressure exerted by proteins in the bloodstream is lower than normal.

Dehydration is life threatening; loss of electrolytes accompanies the loss of water.

Prompt use of ORT is recommended for all people with diarrhea; intravenous rehydration therapy consisting of water, dextrose, and electrolytes is frequently used to maintain water and electrolyte balance in hospitalized clients.

The blood maintains a slightly alkaline reaction, a pH of 7.3 to 7.45, regardless of the acid-forming and alkaline-forming substances produced by metabolism. This acid–base balance is maintained by buffers in blood, exhalation of carbon dioxide, excretion of excess acidic or alkaline substances in the urine, and production of ammonia in the kidneys.

Although there is no proof that PMS is caused by nutritional deficiencies or cured by nutrition intervention, some women find relief in reducing fat, sugar, sodium, caffeine, and alcohol and eating small frequent meals of high-carbohydrate, lowfat foods.

KEYS TO LEARNING

STUDY–DISCUSSION QUESTIONS

1. Estimate the amount of fluid you consumed yesterday. Include water, all beverages, milk, and soup. How does your fluid intake compare with recommended amounts? Why does the requirement for water differ from person to person?
2. How does the nurse provide for the client's need for water? What clients are most likely to require attention in this regard?
3. Most illnesses upset the body's water and electrolyte balance. Discuss in class how this balance is threatened in those clients for whom you are providing care. What measures have you or others taken to maintain or restore balance?
4. What causes edema?
5. What determines whether a food has an acidic or alkaline reaction in the body? What are some of the ways the body maintains a normal blood pH?
6. Discuss any nutritional remedies for PMS that you have heard. Would you recommend these remedies to others? Explain.

BIBLIOGRAPHY

BOOKS

National Academy of Sciences, National Research Council, Food and Nutrition Board. Recommended dietary allowances. 10th ed. Washington, DC: National Academy Press, 1989.

Oh, MS. Water, electrolyte, and acid–base balance. In: Shils ME, Olson JA, Shike M. Eds. Modern nutrition in health and disease. 8th ed. Philadelphia: Lea and Febiger, 1994:112–143.

PERIODICALS

Bennett RG. Oral rehydration therapy for older adults. Dietetic Currents 1992;19:4:1.

Berman MK, Taylor ML, Freeman, E. Vitamin B-6 in premenstrual syndrome. J Am Diet Assoc 1990;90:859.

Can diet affect premenstrual syndrome? Tufts University Diet and Nutrition Letter 1988;6:3.

Fong AKH, Kretsch MJ. Changes in dietary intake, urinary nitrogen and urinary volume across the menstrual cycle. Am J Clin Nutr 1993;57:43.

London RS, Bradley L, Chiamori NY. Effect of a nutritional supplement on premenstrual symptomatology in women with premenstrual syndrome. A double-blind longitudinal study. J Am Coll Nutr 1991;10:494.

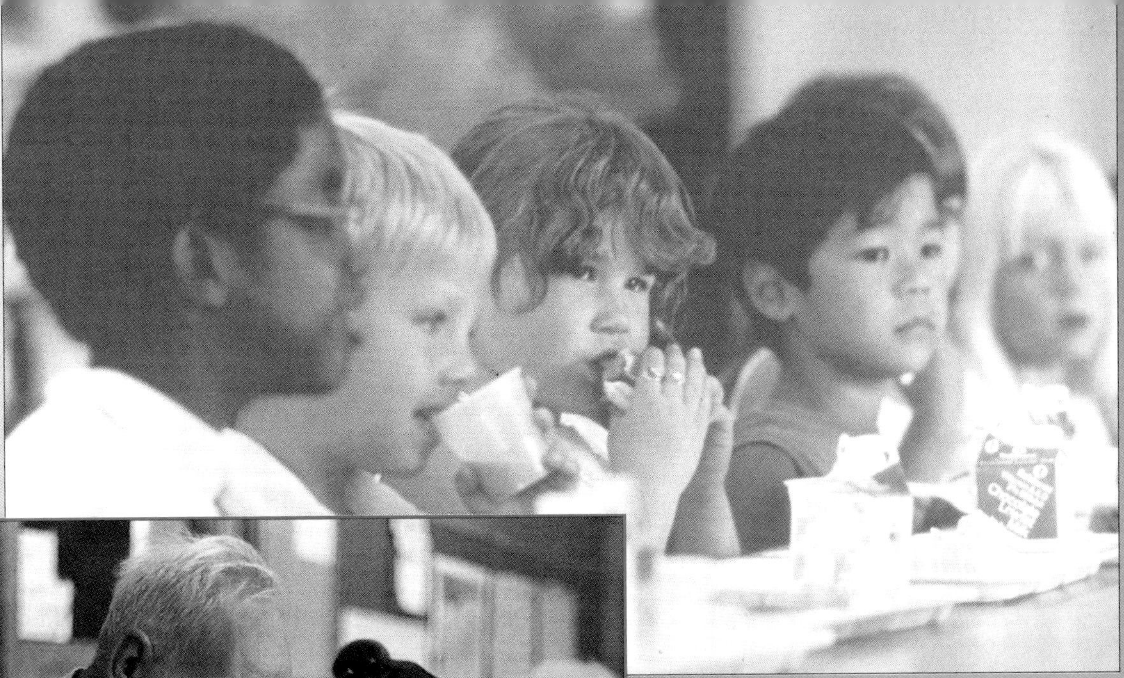

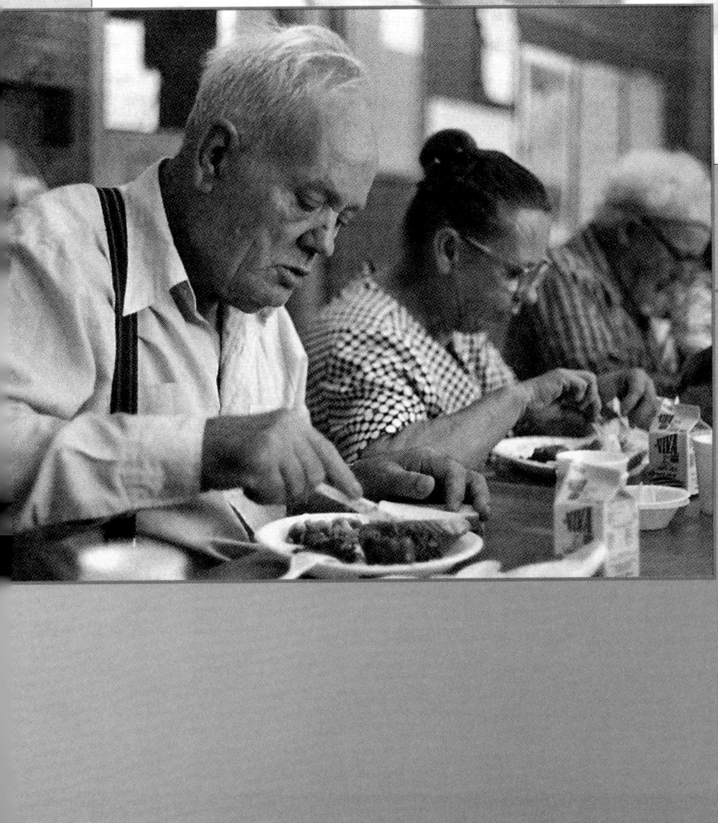

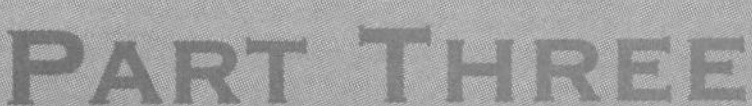

PART THREE

Nutrition in the Life Cycle

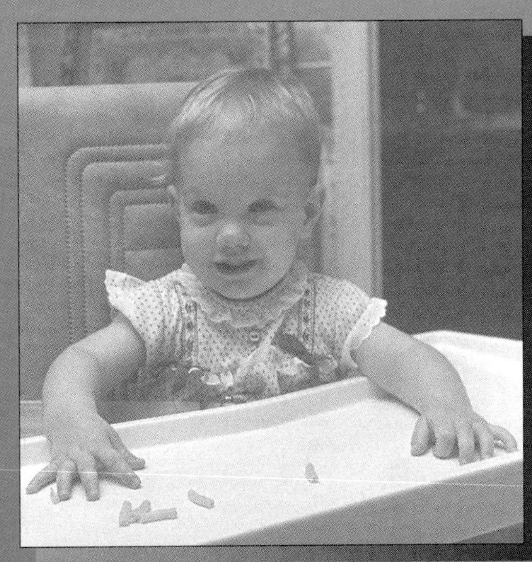

CHAPTER

14

Meeting Nutritional Needs in Daily Meals

KEY TERMS

anesthetic a drug or agent causing loss of feeling, such as pain, touch, or cold

depressant a drug or agent that lowers vital body functions

ferment to undergo a gradual chemical change, becoming sour or alcoholic and giving off gas bubbles

habitual resulting from a constant tendency to act in a certain way, usually acquired by constant repetition

OBJECTIVES

After completing this chapter, the student will be able to:

1. Explain the three components of a nutritious diet: balance, variety, and moderation.
2. Discuss the significance of the US Dietary Guidelines for Americans as a nutrition education message; give the seven guidelines and summarize the recommendations in each.
3. Explain the purpose of food guides.
4. Name the food groups that make up the Food Guide Pyramid, list the number of servings recommended for each group, give examples of serving sizes, and describe the major nutritional contributions of each group.
5. Discuss proportionality and how the pyramid conveys this concept.
6. Explain how the Food Guide Pyramid can be adapted to the needs of all family members.
7. Explain the meaning of "5 a Day for Better Health." What nutrients does this group of foods target?
8. Demonstrate choices from a restaurant menu that are in keeping with the Dietary Guidelines for Americans.
9. Discuss the characteristics of caffeine, its possible adverse effects, and guidelines for its use.
10. Discuss the characteristics of alcohol, its adverse effects, and guidelines for its use.
11. Discuss the benefit that can be derived from advanced meal planning.
12. Discuss how to use shopping aids such as unit pricing, open dating, grade shields, brand names.
13. Name two economical food purchases in each of the food groups.
14. Describe four food preparation techniques that conserve nutrients.
15. Discuss the nutritional pitfalls of eating fast foods and how to make healthful choices.

OBTAINING AN ADEQUATE DIET

A good diet is one that supplies sufficient energy, provides all essential nutrients in adequate amounts, and avoids excesses that predispose individuals to chronic diseases. In the preceding chapters, we studied the essentials of an adequate diet. In this chapter, we put all of the elements of a diet together by addressing how people can select daily foods so that they may achieve an adequate and moderate diet.

One frequently asked question is, How do I know if I am eating a nutritious diet? Three guidelines stand out: balance, variety, and moderation.

BALANCE

Eating an appropriate amount of food daily from each of the five major food groups—grains, fruits, vegetables, milk, and meat and meat substitutes—provides balance. Each of the five food groups contributes different nutrients. Together, they provide all the nutrients the body needs.

VARIETY

A diet that includes a wide variety of foods is more likely to contain all of the 40 essential nutrients than one that includes a limited number of foods. Nutrients are widely distributed in food, and no one food contains all of the required nutrients. Nutrients differ in their concentration in food. For example, milk is high in calcium; a person can obtain adequate calcium by consuming only milk. In contrast, some nutrients, such as iron and the B vitamins, are not highly concentrated in any one food; a wide variety of foods ensures adequate intake.

Eating a wide variety of foods from each food group makes meals more interesting and ensures a diet with adequate amounts of essential nutrients. Foods within the same food group differ in the amount of vitamins and minerals they contain, eg, oranges are a rich source of vitamin C, whereas apricots are a good source of beta carotene.

Variety is important for other reasons, too. Nutrients frequently interact with other nutrients or with nonnutrient substances, sometimes creating a negative effect. For example, too high a protein intake causes excessive calcium excretion, and excessive fiber hinders the absorption of zinc and iron. Variety reduces the likelihood that a person will consume too much of a single nutrient or other food component.

Many substances in food, including nutrients, can be toxic when consumed in excess. Some toxic substances occur naturally in foods, some are added in cooking or processing, and some are introduced by a contaminated environment. Variety protects against the accumulation of toxic levels of these substances by diluting their effects.

MODERATION

Overconsumption of food in general, combined with a sedentary lifestyle, has become a major US public health problem. Too much fat (especially saturated fat), cholesterol, refined and processed sugars, sodium, and alcohol are linked to the development of major chronic diseases. These diseases and disorders include obesity, coronary heart disease, high blood pressure, stroke, diabetes, cirrhosis, dental caries, and some forms of cancer.

Most people, especially those with a sedentary lifestyle, must consume food with a high *nutrient density* if they are to obtain all the nutrients they need without excessive caloric intake. A food of high nutrient density provides the most nutrients for the fewest calories. Fats, sugars, and alcohol provide mainly calories and contribute few, if any, nutrients. Refined, highly processed foodstuffs are less nutritious than unrefined and lightly processed foods. A diet made up primarily of highly processed foods is undesirable.

In the past, the US population was encouraged to eat certain types of foods in specified minimum amounts (the four basic food groups) to meet the Recommended Dietary Allowances (RDAs) for nutrients. The focus was on avoiding nutritional deficiencies. Beginning in the 1960s, nutrition authorities began to express concern about the relation between diet and chronic health problems. A US Senate investigation in 1977 and the Surgeon General's Report on Health Promotion and Disease Prevention in 1979 supported these concerns. Today, recommendations for food selection are based on both the RDAs *and* reports of expert committees that have studied the relation of diet to chronic diseases.

An outgrowth of concern about excesses in the American diet was the publication *Nutrition and Your Health: Dietary Guidelines for Americans,* issued jointly in 1980 by the US Department of Agriculture (USDA) and the US Department of Health and Human Services. The dietary guidelines called for moderation in total calories (to maintain appropriate weight) and in fat, sugar, sodium, and alcohol. The *Dietary Guidelines for Americans* was revised slightly in 1985 and more extensively in 1990. A fourth edition is expected in December, 1995.

In 1988, the first *Surgeon General's Report on Nutrition and Health* reviewed the evidence that linked dietary excesses and imbalance to chronic diseases. Based on the evidence, the report made recommendations, which are discussed in Chapter 5 and summarized in Display 14-1. In 1989, the National Academy of Sciences Committee on Diet and Health issued its first report proposing dietary guidelines for maintaining health and reducing chronic disease risk: *Diet and Health: Implications for Reducing Chronic Disease Risk.* The surgeon general's report and the committee's report were resources used to develop the fourth edition of the Dietary Guidelines for Americans. More recent reviews of the scientific evidence in the World Health Organization's publication *Diet, Nutrition and the Prevention of Chronic Disease* (1990) and a recent review of dietary fat and health, conducted by the U. S. Public Health Service reinforce various sections of the 1995 Dietary Guidelines. The 10th edition of *Recommended Dietary Allowances* and the reports of the National Cholesterol Education Program were among additional resources.

The *Dietary Guidelines for Americans* and the recommendations of the Committee on Diet and Health are compared in Display 14-2.

PRACTICING MODERATION: DIETARY GUIDELINES FOR AMERICANS

Dietary Guidelines for Americans is the central nutrition education message of the federal government. It serves as a basis for nutrition policy in various federal agencies and provides science-based nutrition guidance to healthy Americans in easily understood terms. It is an important publication with which health workers should be familiar.

The basic message in the seven guidelines has remained essentially the same throughout the various revisions (See Display 14-2). The text of the new edition focuses on dietary issues and omits medical advice such as desirable levels of blood cholesterol, blood pressure, and glucose levels. The Food Guide Pyramid is incorporated, and the reader is shown how to use the Nutrition Facts label to make food choices consistent with the Guidelines. For the first time, advice regarding vegetarian diets is included. Tables for food sources of calcium, iron, carotenoids, folate, and potassium have been added. Deliberate efforts have been made to convey positive messages that respect the need to enjoy food and to counteract the impression that many foods are "bad" for health. For copies of the Dietary Guidelines for Americans and the Food Guide Pyramid and related publications contact: The Center for Nutrition Policy and Promotion, USDA, 1120 20th Street, NW, Suite 200 North Lobby, Washington, DC 20036.

DIETARY GUIDELINES: KEY POINTS

Introduction. The Guidelines provide advice about food choices that promote health and prevent diseases and are intended for Americans aged 2 years

DISPLAY 14-1 RECOMMENDATIONS OF THE SURGEON GENERAL'S REPORT ON NUTRITION AND HEALTH

ISSUES FOR MOST PEOPLE

FATS AND CHOLESTEROL
Reduce consumption of fat (especially saturated fat) and cholesterol. Choose foods relatively low in these substances, such as vegetables, fruits, whole-grain foods, fish, poultry, lean meats, and lowfat dairy products. Use food preparation methods that add little or no fat.

ENERGY AND WEIGHT CONTROL
Achieve and maintain a desirable body weight. To do so, choose a dietary pattern in which energy (caloric) intake is consistent with energy expenditure. To reduce energy intake, limit consumption of foods relatively high in calories, fats, and sugars, and minimize alcohol consumption. Increase energy expenditure through regular and sustained physical activity.

COMPLEX CARBOHYDRATES AND FIBER
Increase consumption of whole-grain foods and cereal products, vegetables (including dried beans and peas), and fruits.

SODIUM
Reduce intake of sodium by choosing foods relatively low in sodium and limiting the amount of salt added in food preparation and at the table.

ALCOHOL
To reduce the risk for chronic disease, take alcohol only in moderation (no more than two drinks a day), if at all. Avoid drinking any alcohol before or while driving, operating machinery, taking medications, or engaging in any other activity requiring judgment. Avoid drinking alcohol while pregnant.

OTHER ISSUES FOR SOME PEOPLE

FLUORIDE
Community water systems should contain fluoride at optimal levels for prevention of tooth decay. If such water is unavailable, use other appropriate sources of fluoride.

SUGARS
People who are particularly vulnerable to dental caries (cavities), especially children, should limit their consumption and frequency of use of foods high in sugars.

CALCIUM
Adolescent girls and adult women should increase consumption of foods high in calcium, including lowfat dairy products.

IRON
Children, adolescents, and women of childbearing age should be sure to consume foods that are good sources of iron, such as lean meats, fish, certain beans, and iron-enriched cereals and whole-grain products. This issue is of special concern for low-income families.

(US Dept of Health and Human Services, Public Health Service. The surgeon general's report on nutrition and health (summary and recommendations.) Washington, DC: US Government Printing Office, 1988. US Dept of Health and Human Services publication DHHS (PHS) No. 88-50211.)

and older. While many factors affect food choices, eating is one of life's greatest pleasures. Healthful diets promote growth and development in children, productivity and well-being in adults, and can help prevent chronic disease.

Food is a source of energy, essential nutrients, fiber, and other components important for health. The energy nutrients and alcohol make the following caloric contributions: carbohydrate and protein, 4 kcal/gm; fat, 9 kcal/gm; and alcohol, 7 kcal/gm. Foods high in fat are also high in calories.

Nearly all Americans need to be more physically active. Increasing physical activity helps maintain health and allows people to eat more food, thus more easily meeting their nutrient needs.

Healthful diets provide the essential nutrients and energy to prevent deficiencies and excesses. They also provide the right balance of nutrients to prevent chronic diseases.

DISPLAY 14-2 MODERATION: COMPARING RECOMMENDATIONS

DIETARY GUIDELINES FOR AMERICANS*	RECOMMENDATIONS OF THE NATIONAL RESEARCH COUNCIL COMMITTEE ON DIET AND HEALTH
• Eat a variety of foods.	
Choose foods daily from Food Pyramid.	
Eat calcium-rich and iron-rich food.	Maintain adequate calcium (7).‡
Large dose supplements are harmful.	Avoid taking dietary supplements in excess of the RDA in any one day (8).‡
• Balance the food you eat with physical activity. Maintain or improve your weight.	Balance food intake and physical activity to maintain appropriate body weight (4).‡
Avoid weight gain.	Consider: height/weight ratio; body fat distribution.
Do 30 minutes or more moderate physical activity daily.	
Excess abdominal fat increases health risk.	
• Choose a diet with plenty of grain products, vegetables, and fruits.	Maintain protein intake at moderate levels (3).‡
Select most of calories in your diet from these foods.	Every day eat five or more serving of a combination of vegetables and fruits, especially green and yellow vegetables and citrus fruits (2).‡
Consume 6–11 servings grain products.	
Consume 3–5 servings vegetables.	Increase intake of starches and other complex carbohydrates by eating six or more daily servings of a combination of breads, cereals, and legumes (2).‡
Consume 2–4 servings fruits.	
• Choose a diet low in fat, saturated fat, and cholesterol.	
Total fat should be 30% or less of calories.	Reduce total fat intake to 30% or less of calories.
Saturated fat should be less than 10% of calories.	Reduce saturated fat to less than 10% of calories.
Label standards for cholesterol: 300 mg/daily.	Reduce cholesterol to less than 300 mg daily (1).‡.
• Choose a diet moderate in sugars.	(The committee does not recommend increasing the intake of added sugar.)
Use sparingly if caloric needs are low.	
Avoid frequent snacking on foods containing sugars and starches.	Maintain an optimal intake of fluoride, particularly during the years of primary and secondary tooth formation and growth (9).‡
Adequate fluoride important.	
• Choose a diet moderate in salt and sodium.	
Reference to label standards for sodium: 2400 mg/day (6 g salt).	Limit total daily intake of salt (sodium chloride) to 6 g or less (6).‡
• If you drink alcoholic beverages, do so in moderation.	
Alcohol is not recommended.	The committee does not recommend alcohol consumption. For people who drink alcoholic beverages, the committee recommends limiting consumption to the equivalent of less than 1 oz of pure alcohol in a single day. Pregnant women should avoid alcoholic beverages (5).‡
Moderate drinking is defined as follows: no more than 1 drink (1/2 oz pure alcohol) a day for women; no more than 2 drinks (1 oz pure alcohol) a day for men.	
Alcohol should be avoided by pregnant women or women trying to conceive; people who take medications, plan to drive, or cannot drink moderately; children and adolescents.	

* Adapted from: Dietary Guidelines Advisory Committee. Report of the Dietary Guidelines Advisory Committee on the Dietary Guidelines for Americans, 1995. Hyattsville, MD: US Department of Agriculture, 1995.

† Adapted from National Academy of Sciences, National Research Council, Committee on Diet and Health, Food and Nutrition Board. Diet and health: implications for reducing chronic disease risk (executive summary). Washington, DC: National Academy Press, 1989.)

‡ Numbers in parentheses indicate a descending order of importance as discussed in the report.

TABLE 14-1 THE PYRAMID GUIDE TO DAILY FOOD CHOICES*

This table gives you specific tips for using the Food Guide Pyramid to choose a varied and nutritious diet.

■ Choose foods daily from each of the five major groups. Display 14-3 lists some foods in each group.

■ Include different types of foods from within the groups. As a guide, you can use the subgroups listed below the major food group headings.

■ Have at least the smaller number of servings suggested from each group. Limit the total amount of food eaten to maintain healthy weight.

FOOD GROUP	SUGGESTED DAILY SERVINGS	WHAT COUNTS AS A SERVING?
Breads, Cereals, Rice, and Pasta Whole-grain Enriched 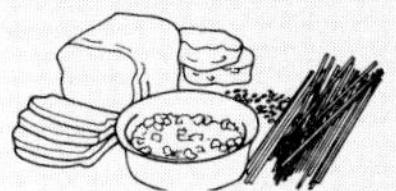	6–11 servings from entire group (include several servings of whole-grain products daily)	1 slice of bread 1/2 hamburger bun or English muffin A small roll, biscuit, or muffin 3–4 small or 2 large crackers 1/2 cup of cooked cereal, rice, or pasta 1 oz of ready-to-eat cereal
Fruits Citrus, melon, berries Other fruits 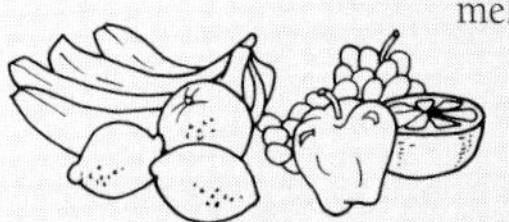	2–4 servings from entire group (include citrus fruits or juices, melons, or berries regularly)	A whole fruit such as a medium apple, banana, or orange A grapefruit half A melon wedge 3/4 cup fruit juice 1/2 cup berries 1/2 cup chopped, cooked, or canned fruit 1/4 cup dried fruit
Vegetables Dark-green leafy Deep-yellow Dry beans and peas (legumes) Starchy Other vegetables 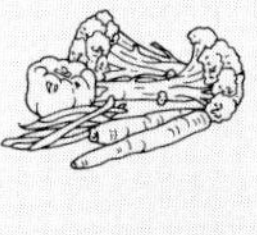	3–5 servings from entire group (include all types regularly; have dark green leafy vegetables and dry beans and peas several times a week)	1/2 cup cooked vegetables 1/2 cup chopped raw vegetables 1 cup leafy raw vegetables, such as lettuce or spinach 3/4 cup vegetable juice
Meats, Poultry, Fish, Dry Beans and Peas, Eggs, and Nuts 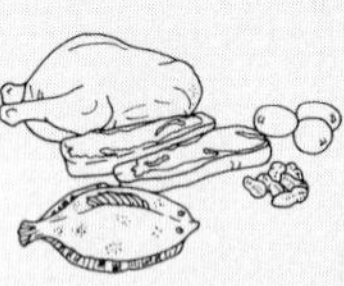	2–3 servings from entire group	Daily amounts should total 5–7 oz of cooked lean meat, poultry without skin, or fish Count 1 egg, 1/2 cup cooked beans, or 2 tbsp peanut butter as 1 oz of lean meat (about 1/3 serving)

(Continued)

TABLE 14-1 *(continued)*

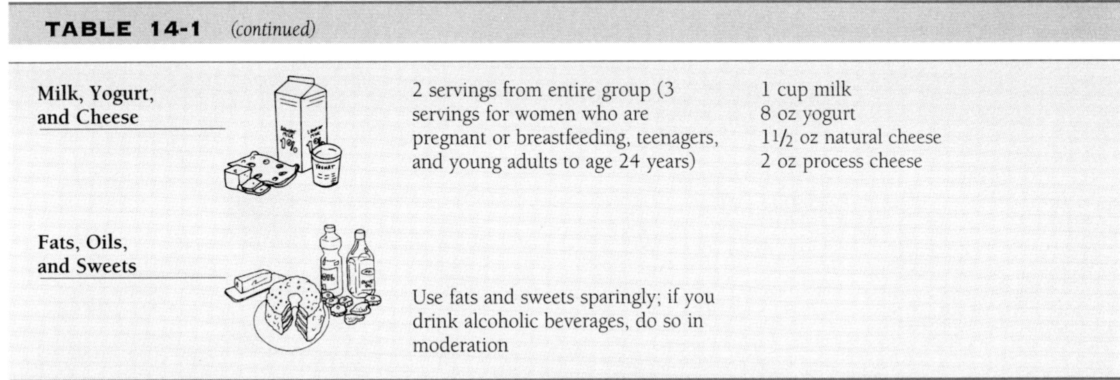

Milk, Yogurt, and Cheese	2 servings from entire group (3 servings for women who are pregnant or breastfeeding, teenagers, and young adults to age 24 years)	1 cup milk 8 oz yogurt 1 1/2 oz natural cheese 2 oz process cheese
Fats, Oils, and Sweets	Use fats and sweets sparingly; if you drink alcoholic beverages, do so in moderation	

* This guide to daily food choices described here was developed for Americans who regularly eat foods from all the major food groups listed. Vegetarians and others may not eat one or more of these types of foods. These people may wish to contact a dietitian or nutritionist for help in planning food choices. (US Dept of Agriculture, Human Nutrition Information Service. Dietary Guidelines for Americans: eat a variety of foods. Washington, DC: US Government Printing Office, 1993. Home and Garden bulletin 253-2.

EAT A VARIETY OF FOODS

Choose foods daily as recommended in the Food Guide Pyramid (See Figure 14-1). The foods from the base of the Pyramid—grains, vegetables, and fruits—should form the foundation of meals. The five food groups, with portion sizes and suggested number of daily servings, are given in Table 14-1, and the nutritional contribution of each group is discussed in detail later in this chapter under Pyramid: Nutritional Contributions of Its Pieces. Choosing a variety of foods within and across food groups is important because foods within the same food group have different combinations of nutrients and other beneficial substances. Display 14-3 gives examples of the variety of foods in each group.

Vegetarian diets can meet the RDAs for nutrients. Special attention should be given to obtaining adequate amounts of iron, zinc, and B-vitamins. Vegetarians who do not eat dairy products and eggs should give additional attention to vitamins B_{12} and D and to calcium.

Women and adolescent girls are advised to eat more calcium-rich roods. Young children, adolescent girls, and women of childbearing age should eat sufficient amounts of iron-rich foods.

Because foods contain many nutrients and other substances that promote health, use of vitamin, mineral and fiber supplements cannot substitute for proper food choices. Sometimes supplements are needed to meet specific needs.

BALANCE THE FOOD YOU EAT WITH PHYSICAL ACTIVITY. MAINTAIN OR IMPROVE YOUR WEIGHT

The high rate of relapse after weight loss suggests that achieving a healthy weight may be impossible for a large number of people. This guideline emphasizes prevention of weight gain, which is an achievable goal for adults at any age.

The amount of energy consumed in food must balance with the amount of energy the body uses. Try to do 30 minutes or more of moderate physical activity on most, preferably all, days.

Eating high-fat foods or eating excessive quantities of lower-fat foods is likely to result in weight gain. Unless part of a daily meal plan, snacking may add many calories to the diet and lead to weight gain. A pattern of binge eating and fasting may also contribute to weight problems.

This guideline provides a chart of healthy weight ranges for men and women (Table 14-2). These weight ranges represent a body mass index of 19 to 25 (Calculation of body mass index is discussed in Chapter 23). The higher weights in the range apply to people with more muscle and bone.

Although achieving a healthy weight remains a major goal, it is secondary to weight maintenance. The idea expressed in the previous edition that people can be somewhat heavier as they grow older

DISPLAY 14-3 MORE VARIETY FROM THE FOOD GROUPS

	WHOLE GRAIN	ENRICHED	GRAIN PRODUCTS WITH MORE FAT OR SUGAR
BREADS, CEREALS, RICE, AND PASTA	Brown rice Buckwheat groats Bulgur Corn tortillas Graham crackers Granola Oatmeal Popcorn Pumpernickel bread Ready-to-eat cereals Rye bread and crackers Whole-wheat bread, rolls, crackers Whole-wheat pasta Whole-wheat cereals	Bagels Cornmeal Crackers English muffins Farina Flour tortillas French bread Grits Hamburger and hot dog rolls Italian bread Macaroni Noodles Pancakes and waffles Pretzels Ready-to-eat cereals Rice Spaghetti White bread and rolls	Biscuits Cake (unfrosted) Cookie Cornbread Croissant Danish Doughnut Muffin Pie crust Tortilla chips

	CITRUS, MELONS, BERRIES	OTHER FRUITS
FRUITS	Blueberries Cantaloupe Citrus juices Cranberries Grapefruit Honeydew melon Kiwifruit Lemon Orange Raspberries Strawberries Tangerine Tangelo Watermelon	Apple Apricot Asian pear Banana Cherries Dates Figs Fruit juices Guava Grapes Mango Nectarine Papaya Passion fruit Peach Pear Plantain Pineapple Plum Prickly pear Prunes Raisins Rhubarb Star fruit

	DARK GREEN LEAFY	DEEP YELLOW	STARCHY
VEGETABLES	Beet greens Broccoli Chard Chicory Collard greens Dandelion greens Endive Escarole Kale Mustard greens Romaine lettuce Spinach Turnip greens Watercress	Carrots Pumpkin Sweet potato Winter squash	Breadfruit Corn Green peas Hominy Lima beans Potato Rutabaga Taro

	DRY BEANS AND PEAS (LEGUMES)		OTHER VEGETABLES			
	Black beans Black-eyed peas Chickpeas (garbanzos) Kidney beans Lentils	Lima beans (mature) Mung beans Navy beans Pinto beans Split peas	Artichoke Asparagus Bean and alfalfa sprouts Beets Brussels sprouts Cabbage Cauliflower	Celery Chinese cabbage Cucumber Eggplant Green beans Green pepper Lettuce	Mushrooms Okra Onions (mature and green) Radishes Snow peas Summer squash	Tomato Turnips Vegetable juices Zucchini
	MEAT, POULTRY, AND FISH			**ALTERNATES**		
MEAT, POULTRY, FISH, AND ALTERNATES	Beef Chicken Fish Ham	Lamb Luncheon meats, sausages Organ meats	Pork Shellfish Turkey Veal	Dry beans and peas (legumes) Eggs	Nuts and seeds Peanut butter Tofu	
	LOWFAT MILK PRODUCTS		**OTHER MILK PRODUCTS WITH MORE FAT OR SUGAR**			
MILK, YOGURT, AND CHEESE	Buttermilk Lowfat cottage cheese Lowfat milk (1% and 2% fat)	Lowfat or nonfat plain yogurt Skim milk	Cheddar cheese Chocolate milk Flavored yogurt Frozen yogurt	Fruited yogurt Ice cream Ice milk	Process cheeses and spreads Puddings made with milk	Swiss cheese Whole milk
	FATS AND OILS		**SWEETS**			**ALCOHOLIC BEVERAGES**
FATS, OILS, AND SWEETS	Bacon, salt pork Butter Cream (dairy, nondairy) Cream cheese Lard Margarine	Mayonnaise Mayonnaise-type salad dressing Salad dressing Shortening Sour cream Vegetable oil	Candy Corn syrup Frosting (icing) Fruit drinks Gelatin desserts Honey	Jam Jelly Maple syrup Marmalade Molasses Popsicles and ices	Sherbets Soft drinks and colas Sugar (white and brown) Table syrup	Beer Liquor Wine

(US Dept of Agriculture, Human Nutrition Information Service. Eat a variety of foods. Washington DC: US Government Printing Office, 1993. Home and Garden bulletin 253-2:6.)

TABLE 14-2 HEALTHY WEIGHT RANGES FOR MEN AND WOMEN

HEIGHT*	WEIGHT IN POUNDS†
4′10″	91–119
4′11″	94–124
5′0″	97–128
5′1″	101–132
5′2″	104–137
5′3″	107–141
5′4″	111–146
5′5″	114–150
5′6″	118–155
5′7″	121–160
5′8″	125–164
5′9″	129–169
5′10″	132–174
5′11″	136–179
6′0″	140–184
6′1″	144–189
6′2″	148–195
6′3″	152–200
6′4″	156–205
6′5″	160–211
6′5″	164–216

* Without shoes.
† Without clothes.
Source: Derived from National Academy of Sciences, National Research Council, Food and Nutrition Board. Diet and health: implications for reducing chronic disease risk. Washington, DC: National Academy Press, 1989.
Taken from: Dietary Guidelines Advisory Committee. Report of the Dietary Guidelines Advisory Committee on the Dietary Guidelines for Americans for Americans, 1995. Hyattsville, MD: US Department of Agriculture, 1995, p. 28.

without risk to health has been rejected by the Advisory Committee. They state: "The health risks due to excess weight appear to be the same for older adults as for younger adults." Older adults should neither lose nor gain weight. Loss of muscle tissue is primarily responsible for weight lost late in life. Physical activity helps to preserve fitness.

Excess weight in the abdomen is associated with greater health risk than in the hips and thighs. Smoking and alcohol increase abdominal fat, rigorous exercise reduces it.

Excessive thinness can occur with anorexia nervosa, other eating disorders, or loss of appetite. Unhealthy behaviors such as excessive exercise, self-induced vomiting, and the abuse of laxatives or other medications can result from excessive concern about weight. Unintentional weight loss can be an early sign of a health problem. See a physician.

If a person is overweight and has excess fat in the abdominal area, weight loss is needed. Overweight is a problem that requires long-term changes. Weight losses of only 5% to 10% of body weight or even less can improve health problems such as high blood pressure and diabetes. If trying to lose weight, do so slowly and steadily at a rate of 1/2 to 1 lb a week.

Helping overweight children achieve healthy weight without jeopardizing normal growth requires caution. Major efforts to change a child's diet should be discussed with a health professional. To prevent obesity, encourage children to eat grains, vegetables, fruits, low-fat dairy and other low-fat protein-rich foods, limit television viewing, and encourage vigorous physical activity.

CHOOSE A DIET WITH PLENTY OF GRAIN PRODUCTS, VEGETABLES, AND FRUITS

This guideline has been elevated to third place in the list of guidelines. The Dietary Guidelines now emphasize not only the starch and fiber content of these foods, but also highlights them as sources of vitamins C, B_6, and folate, carotenoids and other antioxidant nutrients, potassium, calcium, magnesium, and other substances that are important for good health. (Recommended servings and serving sizes are given in Table 14-1.) Grains, vegetables, and fruits are low in fat but can be high in fat if it is added in preparation and/or at the table.

Fiber found only in plant foods is important for proper bowel function, can reduce symptoms of chronic constipation, diverticular diseases and hemorrhoids, and can lower the risk of heart disease and some cancers. Fiber is best obtained from foods rather than supplements because the protective effect of high-fiber foods comes from other components in these foods in addition to fiber.

The importance of folate in reducing the risk of birth defects in infants is noted and a list of folate-rich foods is included. Good sources of carotenes are also provided.

CHOOSE A DIET LOW IN FAT, SATURATED FAT, AND CHOLESTEROL

This guideline emphasizes the continued importance of choosing a diet with less total fat, saturated fat, and cholesterol. Some dietary fat is needed to supply energy, essential fatty acids, and promote absorption of the fat-soluble vitamins. High levels of saturated fat and cholesterol in the diet are linked to increased blood cholesterol levels and greater risk of heart disease. High-fat diets are also linked to overweight and to certain cancers.

The guideline suggests that total fat in the adult diet provides no more than 30% of calories and that saturated fatty acids provide less than 10% of calories. These goals apply to average intake over several days, not to a single meal or food. These goals are not for children younger than age 2 years, who need fat in the diet to obtain sufficient calories. After that age, children should gradually adopt a diet that, by about 5 years of age, contains no more than 30% calories from fat. The text refers the readers to food label standards for cholesterol (300 mg/day) without making a specific recommendation.

CHOOSE A DIET MODERATE IN SUGARS

Sugars, starch, and fiber are carbohydrates. All carbohydrates, except fiber, break down into sugars during digestion. The body cannot tell the difference between naturally occurring and added sugars because they have the same chemical composition.

Research indicates that diets high in sugar do not cause diabetes or hyperactivity. To maintain weight when fat is reduced substitute plant foods from the lower half of the Food Guide Pyramid. Very active people with high caloric needs can use sugar as a additional source of energy; most healthy people should use sugar in moderation, and people with low caloric needs should use sugar sparingly. Eating sugars in large amounts and frequent snacks of sugar-containing foods and beverages supply unnecessary calories and few nutrients.

Sugar substitutes that do not provide significant calories may be useful for persons concerned about caloric intake. Foods containing sugar substitutes are not always lower in calories than similar products that contain sugars.

Both sugars and starches can promote tooth decay. Frequent snacking on foods high in sugars and starches may be more harmful than eating them at meals and then brushing. Adequate intake of fluoride also will help prevent tooth decay.

CHOOSE A DIET MODERATE IN SALT AND SODIUM

Most sodium or salt (sodium chloride) comes from foods to which salt has been added during processing or preparation. Sodium is an essential nutrient involved in regulating fluids and blood pressure. High blood pressure is more prevalent in populations that have a high sodium intake. People at risk of high blood pressure can reduce their chances of developing this condition by consuming less salt or sodium. The relationship between sodium and blood pressure is complicated by the fact that many other substances interact with sodium to affect blood pressure (See Chapter 26 for an in-depth discussion of sodium-controlled diets).

Following other dietary guidelines may also be preventive by addressing other factors that affect blood pressure. Blood pressure rises with weight gain and alcohol consumption. Increased potassium (in vegetables and fruits) and adequate calcium consumption have protective effects on blood pressure.

Most Americans consume more salt and sodium than they need. The Daily Value for sodium on the Nutrition Facts Label is 2,400 mg per day.

IF YOU DRINK ALCOHOLIC BEVERAGES, DO SO IN MODERATION

Alcoholic beverages have been used to enhance meal enjoyment in many societies throughout human history. Alcoholic beverages supply calories but little or no nutrients. Alcohol has drug effects which alter judgement and can lead to dependency and a great many other serious health problems. If adults elect to drink alcoholic beverages, they should drink them in moderate amounts defined as follows: no more than one drink a day for women and no more than two drinks a day for men. One drink is defined as 12 oz of beer, 5 oz of wine, or 1 1/2 oz of 80-proof distilled spirits.

Moderate drinking as defined above is associated with a lower risk of coronary heart disease in some individuals. Higher levels increase the risk for high blood pressure, stroke, heart disease, certain cancers, accidents, violence, suicides, birth defects, and overall mortality. Too much alcohol may cause cirrhosis of the liver, inflammation of the pancreas, damange to the brain and heart, and malnutrition due to poor food intake.

People who should not drink alcohol are:

- Children and adolescents
- Individuals who cannot drink in moderation
- Women who are trying to conceive or are pregnant
- Individuals who plan to drive or engage in other activities that require attention or skill
- Individuals using prescription and over-the-counter medications

Persons who drink alcohol should do so in moderation, with meals, and when consumption does not put the individual or others at risk. Alcohol is discussed in more detail later in this chapter under Alcohol Consumption.

FOOD GUIDES

Food guides have been developed over the years to help individuals translate nutrition recommendations into everyday food choices. These guides use a food group approach involving the grouping of foods similar in composition and nutritive value. Each group contributes specific nutrients—for example, the milk group contributes calcium, the meat group contributes iron, and the fruit group contributes vitamin C.

The first food guide was introduced in the early 1900s. Since then, food guides have been revised to reflect new nutrition knowledge as well as political (war) and social (economic depressions) events.

The focus of food guides in the past has been to promote growth and development (in children and in pregnancy) and to reduce the risk of nutrient deficiency. The food guides accomplished this goal by emphasizing a basic *foundation diet* to which additional food could be added for extra energy. Since the 1970s and 1980s, the focus has changed to a concern with chronic diseases associated with dietary excesses. The contemporary food guides focus on the *total diet*—one that meets nutrient needs but also addresses current concerns about excessive calories, fat, and sugar (See Chapter 5 under Food Guides).

FOOD GUIDE PYRAMID

As a component of the Dietary Guidelines for Americans, the USDA developed a daily food guide to help people make daily food choices in keeping with the suggestions in the guidelines. In 1992, the USDA introduced *The Food Guide Pyramid,* a graphic representation of a daily food guide (Fig. 5-1 and 14-1). The pyramid replaces the Four Food Group Wheel in the federal government's nutrition education program.

The Food Guide Pyramid emphasizes the following five major food groups:

1. breads, cereals, rice, and pasta.
2. vegetables.
3. fruits.
4. meat, poultry, fish, dry beans and peas, eggs, and nuts.
5. milk, yogurt, and cheese.

In addition, the consumer is advised to use fats, oils, and sweets sparingly.

The Pyramid Guide to Daily Food Choices (see Table 14-1) gives the suggested daily servings from each food group and specifies the quantities of foods that count as one serving. The variety of foods

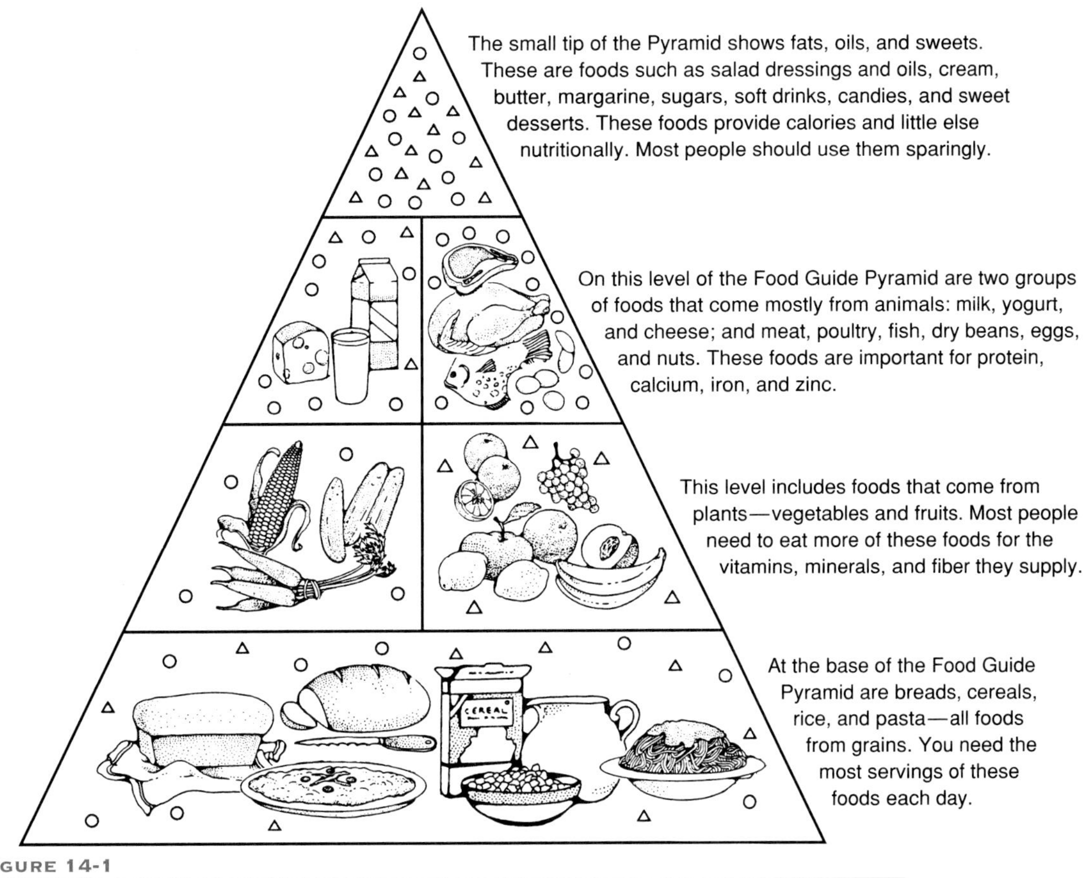

The small tip of the Pyramid shows fats, oils, and sweets. These are foods such as salad dressings and oils, cream, butter, margarine, sugars, soft drinks, candies, and sweet desserts. These foods provide calories and little else nutritionally. Most people should use them sparingly.
On this level of the Food Guide Pyramid are two groups of foods that come mostly from animals: milk, yogurt, and cheese; and meat, poultry, fish, dry beans, eggs, and nuts. These foods are important for protein, calcium, iron, and zinc.
This level includes foods that come from plants—vegetables and fruits. Most people need to eat more of these foods for the vitamins, minerals, and fiber they supply.
At the base of the Food Guide Pyramid are breads, cereals, rice, and pasta—all foods from grains. You need the most servings of these foods each day.
CEREAL

FIGURE 14-1

Looking at the Pieces of the Pyramid. The Food Guide Pyramid emphasizes foods from the five major food groups shown in the three lower sections of the Pyramid. Each of these food groups provides some, but not all, of the nutrients you need. Foods in one group cannot replace those in another. No one food group is more important than another—for good health, you need them all. *(US Dept of Agriculture, Human Nutrition Information Service. The food guide pyramid. Washington, DC: US Government Printing Office, 1992. Home and Garden bulletin 252:4–5)*

contained in each of the food groups is shown in Display 14-3.

PYRAMID AND PROPORTIONALITY

The greatest strength of the Food Guide Pyramid is its ability to illustrate the relative amounts (proportion) of foods recommended from each food group. The size of the food group piece corresponds to the recommended number of daily servings from that food group. The pyramid conveys the following messages:

- Eat plant-based foods—breads, cereals, grains, pasta, fruits, and vegetables—foods that should form the basis of the diet.
- Eat moderate amounts of lower fat foods from the milk and meat groups.
- Use sparingly the foods in the small tip of the pyramid—fats, oils, and sweets.

The circle (fat) and triangle (sugar) shapes concentrated in the tip of the pyramid represent those fats and sugars added to foods at the table or in food preparation and to foods high in sugar such as jelly, candy, sweet desserts, and soft drinks. The circle and triangle shapes scattered throughout the pyramid pieces represent the added and naturally occurring fat and oil in certain foods (i.e., whole milk, sausage, french fries, and peanut butter) as well as added sugars (i.e., fruit in heavy syrup, sweetened cereals, and bakery products).

PYRAMID: NUTRITIONAL CONTRIBUTIONS OF ITS PIECES

BREADS, CEREALS, RICE, AND PASTA

The bread and cereal group is the main provider of B vitamins and iron. If these foods are eaten in large quantities, as in vegetarian diets, they provide generous amounts of protein. Whole-grain breads and cereals also contribute magnesium, folate, and fiber.

The nutritional contribution of this group depends on the use of whole-grain, enriched, or fortified products. Refined breads and cereals that are not enriched provide few vitamins and minerals. Because some products on the market are made with unenriched flour, consumers should read labels carefully.

Whole-grain products contain the entire edible portion of the grain. This portion includes the bran and germ as well as the starchy endosperm. The bran and germ portions contain most of the fiber, vitamins, and minerals. In addition to whole-grain breads and cereals, examples of whole grains include popcorn, brown rice, corn tortillas, scotch barley in soup, and tabouli—a bulgur salad.

FRUITS

Fruits provide many nutrients, including vitamin A, folate, potassium, and magnesium; they are an especially important source of vitamin C and fiber. In addition to citrus fruits (oranges and grapefruit), melons, and berries, kiwi fruit and papaya are good sources of vitamin C. Yellow fruits such as apricots, cantaloupe, and mangos are good sources of vitamin A (Display 14-4).

VEGETABLES

Vegetables are rich sources of vitamins, minerals, and fiber. Vegetables vary, however, in the kind and amount of nutrients they provide. Dark green vegetables are generally good sources of vitamins A and

DISPLAY 14-4 SOURCES OF VITAMINS A AND C IN VEGETABLES AND FRUITS

VITAMIN A	VITAMIN C	
(BETA CAROTENE)	GOOD SOURCES	FAIR SOURCES
Broccoli	Grapefruit or grapefruit juice	Honeydew melon
Carrots	Orange or orange juice	Lemon
Chard	Cantaloupe	Tangerine or tangerine juice
Collards	Guava	Watermelon
Kale	Mango	Asparagus tips
Cress	Papaya	Raw cabbage
Pumpkin	Fresh strawberries	Collards
Spinach	Broccoli	Cress
Sweet Potatoes	Brussels sprouts	Kale
Turnip greens	Green pepper	Kohlrabi
Other dark green leafy vegetables	Sweet red pepper	Mustard greens
Apricots		Potatoes and sweet potatoes cooked in jacket
Cantaloupe		Spinach
Mango		Tomato or tomato juice
Persimmon		Turnip greens

C, riboflavin, folate, iron, calcium, magnesium, and potassium. Deep yellow vegetables are good sources of vitamin A (see Display 14-4). Dry peas and beans are good sources of thiamine, folate, iron, magnesium, phosphorus, zinc, potassium, protein, and starch. Starchy vegetables such as potatoes contain varying amounts of certain vitamins and minerals such as niacin, vitamin B_6, zinc, and potassium.

MEAT, POULTRY, FISH, DRY BEANS, EGGS, AND NUTS

This group provides protein, iron, phosphorus, zinc, niacin, and vitamin B_6. Foods of animal origin in this group provide vitamin B_{12}.

All meat, fish, and poultry contain cholesterol and varying degrees of saturated fat. Organ meats and egg yolks contain the most cholesterol. Shrimp is moderately high in cholesterol and fish is low. A person can reduce the fat content of meats, fish, and poultry considerably by properly selecting and preparing the food, such as choosing lean cuts of meat, trimming visible fat from meat, removing the skin from poultry, and cooking so that fat drains from the food. Most fish and white meat poultry without skin are low in calories and saturated fat.

It is wise to use a variety of foods from this group, because the contributions of nutrients differ considerably. Red meats and oysters are rich sources of zinc, and legumes are a good source of magnesium. The iron in meat, fish, and poultry is more readily absorbed than that in plant products. Lean meat, shellfish, and dried peas and beans are good sources of iron. Cereals, especially whole-grain, in combination with dry peas, dry beans, lentils, and other legumes provide significant amounts of protein, iron, and B vitamins.

MILK, YOGURT, AND CHEESE

The milk group supplies about three fourths of the daily RDA of calcium, as well as significant amounts of riboflavin, and high-quality protein. Milk also is a good source of phosphorus, thiamine, and vitamin B_{12}. Vitamin A occurs naturally in whole milk and is added to lowfat and skim milk. Most commercial milks also are fortified with vitamin D. Because an adequate amount of vitamin D is not found naturally in foods, vitamin D–fortified milk is the main source of this vitamin.

Skim milk and nonfat yogurt are lowest in fat and contain no added sugar. Although other milks, yogurts, and cheeses (except cottage cheese) provide the same calcium, they also contain more fat especially saturated fat, and fruited yogurt contains added sugar. Cottage cheese contains less calcium than other cheeses: 1 cup contains only as much calcium as $^1/_2$ cup of milk.

FATS, OILS, SWEETS, AND ALCOHOL

Foods in this group have a low nutrient density—they are low in vitamins, minerals, and protein in relation to calories. One exception is vegetable oils, which provide vitamin E and essential fatty acids. Polyunsaturated oils, such as corn, safflower, sunflower, sesame, soybean, and cottonseed oils, and wheat germ supply linoleic acid, an essential fatty acid. However, small amounts satisfy the body's requirement for this nutrient. Polyunsaturated oils are used in making commercial mayonnaise, salad dressings, and margarines.

USING THE FOOD GUIDE PYRAMID IN PLANNING MEALS AND SNACKS

Each day's meals should include foods from each of the five major food groups in the pyramid. People should use foods in the sixth group—fats, sugars, and alcoholic beverages—sparingly. Displays 14-5 and 14-6 are examples of how a person might use the pyramid in planning meals and snacks for a single day.

Most of the food groups in the pyramid have suggested ranges of daily servings. The number of servings an individual needs depends on his or her caloric needs. People with lower caloric needs require only the lower number of servings. Some people, such as teenage boys, need the higher number of servings, and very active teenage boys need even more. To obtain the nutrients and fiber needed, meals and snacks

DISPLAY 14-5 A TYPICAL DAY'S MENU FOR AN ADULT: USING THE PYRAMID GUIDE

MORNING	Grapefruit Oatmeal Peanut butter Whole-wheat toast Lowfat milk	**EVENING**	Roast chicken Baked potato Broccoli Cole slaw Whole-wheat bread with margarine Sponge cake Coffee
MIDDAY	Split pea soup Tossed salad with French dressing Enriched hard roll with margarine Pear Lowfat milk	**EVENING SNACK**	Corn flakes with lowfat milk

BREADS, CEREALS, OTHER GRAINS (6–11)*	FRUITS (2–4)*	VEGETABLES (3–5)*	MEAT, POULTRY, FISH, ALTERNATES (5–7 oz)*	MILK, CHEESE, YOGURT (2–4)*
1 cup of oatmeal	$\frac{1}{2}$ grapefruit	Split peas	1 tbsp peanut butter	$2\frac{1}{2}$ cups of milk
2 slices of whole-wheat bread	1 pear	Tossed salad	$1\frac{1}{2}$ cups of split pea soup	
1 enriched kaiser roll	Raisins	Baked potato	3 oz of roast chicken	
2 oz of corn flakes		Broccoli		
		Cole slaw		

FATS, SWEETS, ALCOHOLIC BEVERAGES
French dressing
Margarine
Slaw dressing
Sponge cake
Sugar in coffee

* Suggested servings.

for the day should include at least the lower number of servings from each food group. People who need more food than the pattern provides, such as very active teenagers, should choose more foods from each of the first five food groups and use foods high in sugar and fat sparingly.

Toddlers and young children need less food but should receive the same variety of foods. Caregivers should offer young children smaller amounts from each of the food groups, with the exception of milk. Children need the equivalent of 2 cups of milk daily, which can be offered in small amounts at one time, such as $\frac{1}{2}$-cup portions. Because children have a small capacity for food at one time, they should be offered nutritious foods as snacks.

The lower number of servings from each food group with a moderate amount of fat and sugar added supplies about 1600 kcal, an energy level appropriate for sedentary women and some older adults. Most men can have the middle to upper number of servings in the ranges. The highest number of servings from each food group with moderate amounts of fat and sugar added supplies about 2800 kcal to 3200 kcal, a caloric level appropriate for teenage boys. (See Table 14-3 for sample diets at three calorie levels.)

DISPLAY 14-6 A DAY'S MEALS FOR A LACTOOVOVEGETARIAN DIET: USING THE PYRAMID GUIDE

MORNING	Orange–grapefruit sections French toast Syrup, light Milk, 1% fat	**EVENING**	Meatless chili Rice Creamed spinach Cornbread with margarine Baked apple Tea
MIDDAY	Vegetable soup Cottage cheese-stuffed tomato Whole-wheat bread with margarine Graham crackers Sherbet Milk, 1% fat	**EVENING SNACK**	Peanut butter and whole-wheat crackers Milk, 1% fat

BREADS, CEREALS, OTHER GRAINS (6–11)*	FRUITS (2–4)*	VEGETABLES (3–5)*	MEAT, POULTRY, FISH, ALTERNATES (5–7 OZ)*	MILK, CHEESE, YOGURT (2–4)*
1 slice of toast (enriched) 1 slice of whole-wheat bread 3 squares of graham crackers 1 cube of cornbread ½ cup of rice (enriched) 4 whole-wheat crackers	Orange–grapefruit sections Baked apple	Vegetable soup Tomato Kidney beans Spinach	Egg for French toast ½ cup of cottage cheese 1 cup of meatless chili 1 tbsp of peanut butter	3 cups of skim milk

FATS, SWEETS, ALCOHOLIC BEVERAGES
Syrup Margarine Sugar for tea Sherbert

* Suggested servings.

5 A DAY FOR BETTER HEALTH

The daily minimum of five servings of fruits and vegetables recommended in the pyramid is a challenge to achieve but one that people should take seriously. In 1991, the National Cancer Institute (NCI) began a national *5 a Day for Better Health* program to encourage Americans to eat five or more servings of fruits and vegetables a day. The NCI message also conveys that a healthful diet is also low in fat and high in fiber.

The NCI began the program based on the results of up to 200 studies on diet in cancer. The majority of the results showed that an increased intake of fruits and vegetables is associated with a reduced risk of various cancers. Before beginning the program, a survey of 3000 adult Americans showed that only 23% ate the recommended five or more servings a day and only 8% even thought they should be eating five or more servings daily.

FLEXIBILITY

An attractive feature of The Pyramid Guide to Daily Food Choices (see Table 14-1) is its flexibility. It can be adapted to the eating habits of

TABLE 14-3 SAMPLE DIETS FOR A DAY AT THREE CALORIE LEVELS

FOOD GROUP	ABOUT 1600	ABOUT 2200	ABOUT 2800
	1600 calories is about right for many sedentary women and some older adults	2200 calories is about right for most children, teenage girls, active women, and many sedentary men; pregnant or breastfeeding women may need somewhat more	2800 calories is about right for teenage boys, many active men, and very active women
Bread group servings	6	9	11
Fruit group servings	2	3	4
Vegetable group servings	3	4	5
Meat group	5 oz	6 oz	7 oz
Milk group servings	2–3*	2–3*	2–3*
Total fat (g)	53	73	93
Total added sugars (tsp)	6	12	18

*Pregnant or breastfeeding women, teenagers, and young adults to age 24 years need 3 servings.
(US Dept of Agriculture, Human Nutrition Information Service. Dietary Guidelines for Americans: Eat a variety of foods. Washington DC: US Government Printing Office, 1993. Home and Garden bulletin 253-2:5.)

most cultural and religious groups and to different lifestyles.

If a person's eating pattern does not conform to this food guide, the health worker should not prejudge it as being inadequate. The person must first evaluate it in terms of each essential nutrient according to tables of food composition (see Appendix E). People who omit foods from one or more of the five basic food groups may need assistance in making food choices that provide all of the essential nutrients.

The flexible nature of the food groups does have its pitfalls. A wide choice of foods is available within most of the food groups, and the nutritional values of the foods differ. Knowledge of the nutritional composition of food helps people make the best choices within each group. Such knowledge is especially important for people whose lifestyle involves *grazing*—eating a number of small meals rather than the traditional three meals a day. Such people can have a nutritious diet if they use the pyramid in making selections. If the small meals include mostly snack foods, individuals should be encouraged to investigate the nutrient and caloric value of these foods.

SPACING OF MEALS

Distribution of food throughout the day is important. The body needs a steady supply of nutrients, and it is unwise to overload the mechanisms for digesting, absorbing, and metabolizing food at any one time.

A common pattern of eating in the United States is to have a small breakfast or none, a light to medium lunch, and a heavy dinner. Eating a more substantial breakfast and lunch and a lighter dinner is a much healthier pattern. It makes little sense to skimp on food after a 10- to 12-hour fast, during the period of the day when a person is most active, and to eat heavily when the day's activity is done. Adults and children who eat breakfast have a higher overall nutritious diet than those who do not. Research has suggested that eating breakfast improves cognitive performance, behavior, and learning success.

MODERATION AND BALANCE WHEN EATING OUT

Many Americans frequently eat out. Busy lifestyles and households in which all adults are working contribute to this trend. Adults eat about 30% of their total caloric intake away from home and spend 40% or more of their food dollar on food eaten away from home. This food includes not only meals but snacks eaten at malls, at the movies, and at parties.

The principles for eating in accordance with the Dietary Guidelines for Americans are the same whether a person eats the food at home or away from home. Although people have less control over how foods are prepared outside of the home, they usually can choose appropriate foods in moderate amounts. The challenge is to eat a variety of foods that provide all of the nutrients needed with an appropriate amount of calories while avoiding excessive fats, saturated fats, cholesterol, sugars, sodium, and alcohol.

The effect of eating out on the overall diet depends on what and how much a person orders and the extras added to foods. These factors, in turn, are strongly influenced by where a person eats.

Full-service restaurants offer the greatest variety and flexibility. If foods are prepared to order, the customer has even more control. Snacking on breads or crackers while waiting for prepared-to-order foods to arrive and the oversized portions frequently provided are problems. Cafeterias and restaurant buffets provide some control over portion sizes and condiments but may encourage overeating with all-you-can-eat offers. Fatty side dishes in restaurants specializing in steak or fish can provide greater problems than the entrées. French fries, hush puppies, cole slaw, and fried onion rings frequently accompany the entrées.

Pizza parlors offer variety in crust types and toppings. Toppings differ in their caloric, fat, and sodium content. In sandwich shops, the size of the sandwiches and the use of high-fat cheese and luncheon meats and spreads can be a problem. It is necessary to carefully specify the ingredients desired. Although fast-food restaurant offerings are limited, smaller servings and small orders of side dishes are available. People can request that food preparers omit sauces and other condiments. Vegetables (salad or a baked potato), skim milk, grilled chicken and other lowfat foods are becoming more available in fast-food restaurants (see Key Issues section). Many items offered in convenience stores and vending machines are high in fat, sugar, sodium, and calories, such as hot dogs, sausages, prepackaged sandwiches, pastries, and candy.

Eating at other people's homes is probably the most difficult eating situation to control. Buffets and informal parties provide some opportunity for a person to control what and how much he or she eats.

ORDERING TECHNIQUES

Meeting the demands of health-conscious consumers is a dominant trend in the food industry today. Patronize restaurants that are making an effort to provide healthful foods. Call ahead to find out if a restaurant accepts special requests. Do not hesitate to ask your server questions about the following:

Portion sizes—Ask if small or half-sized portions are available. To reduce portion sizes, order an appetizer as a main dish, order à la carte, share food with your dining companion, order one course at a time and stop when you are full, or ask for a take-home bag.

Preparation methods—Ask how menu items are prepared and what ingredients are used: Are broiled and baked meats, fish, and poultry basted with fat? If so, which fats? Are menu items served with sauces or are they buttered or creamed? Are vegetables fresh or canned? Learn to recognize menu terms that signify foods that are higher in fat and sodium. The following terms signify lower fat: *broiled, stir-fried, roasted, poached,* and *steamed.*

Acceptance of special requests—Ask if you may order foods broiled without the addition of fat, chicken prepared without the skin, dressings and sauces served on the side, and foods prepared without the addition of salt or other ingredients.

Availability of foods not on the menu—Ask if margarine, skim or lowfat milk, lowfat yogurt, fresh fruit, or any other desired item is available.

MAKING HEALTHFUL CHOICES

The following are suggestions for making healthful choices in keeping with the Dietary Guidelines for Americans.

APPETIZERS

Good choices are steamed seafood, raw vegetables or fruits, broth- or tomato-based soups, and fiber-rich soups such as lentil, bean, or split pea. Use rich sauces and dips, batter-fried foods, chips, and nachos sparingly.

BREADS

Choose whole-grain breads and crackers for extra fiber. Avoid breads that are high in fat or sugar, such as croissants, biscuits, hush puppies, sweet rolls, and sticky buns. Use butter and other spreads sparingly, if at all.

ENTRÉES

Choose meat, fish, or poultry that is grilled, broiled, baked, steamed or poached, or stir-fried. Request that food not be basted with fat or request that lemon juice, wine, or only small amounts of fat be used. If fried foods are your only choice, remove the skin or breading. Select lean cuts of meat; order small portions or half-sized portions or ask for a take-home bag. Select vegetarian entrees including vegetables and grain products and/or meat analogs such as veggie burgers but inquire about food ingredients and preparation methods. Avoid those made with excessive amounts of table or cooking fats and other high-fat ingredients such as cheese, nuts, or seeds.

Choose vegetable toppings on pizza. Sausage, pepperoni, anchovies, and olives are high in fat. For sandwiches, choose lean deli meats such as turkey, ham, or lean roast beef instead of bologna or salami; use oil, mayonnaise, and pickles sparingly. Order a half-submarine sandwich or split a whole one with a dining companion.

VEGETABLES AND SALADS

Plain vegetables are good choices because they are high in fiber and nutrients. Butter, margarine, and sauces can increase calories, fat, and sodium considerably. Vegetables seasoned with lemon, herbs, or spices are better choices.

Salads of fresh vegetables and fruits are good choices. Sparingly use salads that contain liberal amounts of mayonnaise, salad dressing, or oil, such as macaroni salad, potato salad, and cole slaw. Have a salad and baked potato in place of french fries or potato chips. Use salad dressings and toppings sparingly.

DESSERTS

Choose fruit for dessert or select a light dessert such as sorbet, fruit ice, or sherbet. If you decide on a rich dessert, share it with your dining companion.

BEVERAGES

Select skim or lowfat milk; use soft drinks and sweetened fruit drinks sparingly. For a nonalcoholic cocktail, have fruit juice mixed with seltzer or mineral water or a glass of tomato juice with a twist of lemon or lime. If you drink alcoholic beverages, limit the number of drinks. Order a glass of wine rather than a carafe. Request liquor mixed with water or seltzer; drink light beer. Regular or decaffeinated coffee and tea have no calories unless you add cream or sugar.

ADD-ONS

The ingredients added to foods in the form of condiments and salad dressings may add a considerable number of calories and amounts of fat or sodium to the diet. A dill pickle strip has only 3 kcal but adds 430 mg of sodium to the diet. Hollandaise sauce (1 tbsp) adds 70 kcal and 65 mg of sodium. Limit amounts of high-fat add-ons such as butter or margarine, cheese spreads, salad dressings, sour cream, bacon bits, and grated processed cheese. Soy sauce, steak sauce, ketchup, and pickles add considerable amounts of sodium.

CAFFEINE CONSUMPTION

Caffeine is a daily ingredient in the diet of most individuals, including children. Although we tend to think of caffeine in terms of coffee consumption, three fourths of soft drinks contain caffeine. Excluding those foods such as coffee, tea, cocoa, and other products in which caffeine is naturally present, most of the 2 million pounds of caffeine added to food annually is in soft drinks.

A 12-oz can of a caffeine-containing soft drink has about the same amount of caffeine as a 5-oz cup of tea (40 mg). Children as young as age 6 months consume excessive amounts of caffeine in soda. Some toddlers consume twice as much caffeine for their body weight as adults. Because drug dosage is related to body size, a small child who drinks one can of cola consumes the amount of caffeine comparable to that amount consumed by an adult who drinks 4 cups of instant coffee. Caffeine is an addictive drug with adverse side effects and has no place in the diet of young children.

Caffeine has been a component of the diet for thousands of years, dating back to 4700 BC when the use of tea originated in China. In recent years, there has been much concern about the health effects of caffeine. Caffeine has been suspected of causing a multitude of disorders ranging from high blood pressure to birth defects. Research has been conflicting, and conclusive evidence to support these accusations has been lacking.

DISPLAY 14-7 CAFFEINE CONTENT OF BEVERAGES AND FOODS

ITEM	CAFFEINE (MG)	
	AVERAGE	RANGE
Coffee (5-oz cup)		
Brewed, drip method	115	60–180
Brewed, percolator	80	40–170
Instant	65	30–120
Decaffeinated, brewed	3	2–5
Decaffeinated, instant	2	1–5
Tea (5-oz. cup)		
Brewed, major US brands	40	20–90
Brewed, imported brands	60	25–110
Instant	30	25–50
Iced (12-oz glass)	70	67–76
Cocoa beverage (5-oz cup)	4	2–20
Chocolate milk beverage (8 oz)	5	2–7
Milk chocolate (1 oz)	6	1–15
Dark chocolate, semi-sweet (1 oz)	20	5–35
Baker's chocolate (1 oz)	26	26
Chocolate-flavored syrup (1 oz)	4	4

(US Food and Drug Administration, Food Additive Chemistry Evaluation Branch, based on evaluations of existing literature on caffeine levels; Lecos CW. Caffeine jitters: some safety questions remain. Washington, DC: US Dept of Health and Human Services, 1993. FDA publication FDA 88-2221.)

CHARACTERISTICS OF CAFFEINE

Caffeine is a drug that stimulates the central nervous system. It is found naturally in more than 63 species of plants and is an added ingredient in more than 1000 nonprescription drugs and many prescription drugs. The most common natural sources of caffeine are coffee beans, tea leaves, cacao seeds (cocoa), and kola nuts (cola). The caffeine content of various beverages and medications is found in Displays 14-7 through 14-9.

Caffeine is absorbed rapidly, and within a few minutes after ingestion, enters all organs and tissues. The metabolic effect of caffeine lasts about 3 hours. There is no day-to-day accumulation because it almost completely disappears from the body overnight. Most of the caffeine is excreted in the urine.

About 200 mg of caffeine is needed to produce its drug-related effects in an adult. Caffeine produces the following effects:

- It stimulates the central nervous system (brain) and prolongs a person's ability to stay awake with alertness.
- It stimulates heart action.
- It relaxes smooth muscles, such as those found in the digestive tract and the blood vessels.
- It increases urination (i.e., acts as a diuretic).
- It stimulates gastric acid secretion.
- It increases muscle strength and the length of time that physically exhausting work can be performed.

A dose of 1000 mg or more usually produces adverse effects such as insomnia, restlessness, excitement, trembling, rapid and irregular heart-

DISPLAY 14-8 CAFFEINE CONTENT OF SOFT DRINKS (per 6-oz serving)

	CAFFEINE (MG)
REGULAR	
Cola, pepper	15–23
Decaffeinated cola, pepper	0–0.09
Cherry cola	18–23
Lemon lime (clear)	0
Orange	0
Other citrus	0–32
Root beer	0
Ginger ale	0
Tonic water	0
Other regular	0–22
Juice added	<0.24
DIET DRINKS	
Diet cola, pepper	0.3
Decaffeinated diet cola, pepper	0–0.1
Diet cherry cola	0–23
Diet lemon lime	0
Diet root beer	0
Other diets	0–35
Club soda, seltzer, sparkling water	0
Diet juice added	<0.24

(Source of caffeine content: National Soft Drink Association, Washington, DC. Amount of fruit juices added varies from 10% to 25%; Lecos CW. Caffeine jitters: some safety questions remain. Washington, DC: US Dept of Health and Human Services, 1993. FDA publication FDA 88-2221.)

beats, increased breathing, increased urination, and ringing in the ears. People who consume moderate amounts (400 mg) of caffeine may develop symptoms of low blood sugar when blood glucose falls into the low normal range. Some people are particularly sensitive to caffeine and experience these unpleasant side effects with much smaller doses. This is one reason why there will always be some uncertainty about the health effects of caffeine. Furthermore, high doses of caffeine—more than 170 mg/kg body weight—can be fatal.

One property that is frequently attributed to caffeine is untrue. Black coffee does not sober up a person who has drunk too much alcohol. It takes about 1.5 hours to metabolize the amount of alcohol in $1\frac{1}{2}$ oz of distilled liquor, 5 oz of wine, or 12 oz of beer. Nothing can speed the process.

DISPLAY 14-9 CAFFEINE CONTENT OF DRUGS

Caffeine is an ingredient in many prescription and nonprescription drugs. It is often used in alertness or stay-awake tablets, headache and pain relief remedies, cold products, and diuretics. When caffeine is an ingredient, it is listed on the product label. Some examples of drugs that contain caffeine follow.

DRUG	CAFFEINE (MG PER TABLET OR CAPSULE)
PRESECRIPTION DRUGS	
Cafergot (migraine headaches)	100
Norgesic Forte (muscle relaxant)	60
Norgesic (muscle relaxant)	30
Fiorinal (tension headache)	40
Fioricet (headache pain relief)	40
Darvon compound (pain relief)	32.4
Synalgos-DC (pain relief)	30
Synalgos-DC-A (pain relief)	30
NONPRESCRIPTION DRUGS	
Alertness Tablets	
No Doz	100
Vivarin	200
Pain Relief	
Anacin, Maximum Strength Anacin	32
Vanquish	33
Excedrin	65
Midol	32.4
Diuretics	
Aqua-Ban	100
Cold/Allergy Remedies	
Coryban-D capsules	30

(Source of caffeine content: US Food and Drug Administration Center for Drugs and Biologics; Lecos CW. Caffeine jitters: some safety questions remain. Washington, DC: US Dept of Health and Human Services, 1993. FDA publication FDA 88-2221.)

HARMFUL EFFECTS OF CAFFEINE

In the early 1980s, various research studies reported a possible association of caffeine with a number of health problems. The Food and Drug Administration (FDA) was particularly concerned about a study that demonstrated the potential for caffeine to cause birth defects in laboratory animals. Since then, numerous studies on the health effects of caffeine have been conducted; the results have somewhat lessened concerns about its adverse effects. Determining the effect of caffeine among humans is not a simple matter, because other factors such as smoking, alcohol consumption, and drug use can also affect health.

According to the Committee on Diet and Health, there is a lack of strong and consistent evidence linking coffee consumption to the risk of coronary heart disease and cancer. In several conditions, however, caffeine may have some serious adverse effects.

MISCARRIAGES, BIRTH DEFECTS

Pregnant and breastfeeding women are of special concern because caffeine enters the bloodstream and reaches the fetus through the placenta and the breastfed infant through the mother's milk. The fetus is unable to metabolize caffeine, so the caffeine may be held in fetal tissue for 3 or 4 days. The caffeine may affect the unborn child's breathing and heart rate.

In 1980, the FDA advised pregnant women to avoid or limit the amount of caffeine they consume. This warning was based on research that showed birth defects in the offspring of rats fed high doses of caffeine. No definite link to birth defects in humans was found in the late 1980s. After subsequent studies, the FDA concluded that the earlier research studies were faulty, inconclusive, or contradicted by later findings and that the concern about caffeine and birth defects had lessened.

In 1993, the National Institutes of Health reported that mothers who drank 3 cups of coffee a day were no more likely to have a miscarriage than those who drank little or none. In 1994, a study conducted in Canada produced conflicting results—that even small amounts of caffeine doubled the possibility of having miscarriages.

In light of these conflicting results, it is wise to exercise caution. Women drinking 3 or 4 cups of coffee or the equivalent caffeine in tea or cola would be wise to cut back to no more than 2 cups of coffee or equivalent amount of caffeine daily.

EXCESSIVE GASTRIC ACIDITY

People with excessive gastric acidity should avoid both regular and decaffeinated coffee. Caffeine is know to stimulate release of acid in the stomach; other substances in coffee also promote acid secretion.

IRREGULAR HEARTBEAT

People who experience irregular heartbeats may find this problem worsened when they drink caffeinated beverages. People with heart rhythm disorders should avoid caffeine or consume it only on the advice of their physicians.

INTERACTION WITH ASTHMA MEDICATION

Caffeine helps expand the airways of the lungs and has been reported to reduce the incidence of asthma attacks. Caffeine may interact with the asthma medication theophylline, however, causing severe symptoms such as nausea, delirium, and seizures. People who take theophylline should discuss caffeine consumption with their physicians.

BENIGN BREAST LUMPS

Caffeine has been linked to the incidence of fibrocystic breast disease (benign breast lumps). The FDA has stated that more recent and reliable studies have failed to show a relation between this disease and coffee consumption.

REDUCING CAFFEINE INTAKE

Aside from the situations described, there appear to be no long-term health problems associated with moderate consumption of caffeine—2 or 3 cups

(5 or 6 oz each) of coffee or the equivalent amount of caffeine in the form of tea or cola. Many people, however, experience unpleasant symptoms from this potent drug and would benefit from avoiding it.

People who desire to stop consuming caffeine should do so gradually. Caffeine is addictive; people who stop consuming it abruptly may experience severe headaches, irritability, restlessness, and fatigue. Gradually reduce the amount consumed over a period of weeks or brew coffee that is half regular and half decaffeinated. Some coffee manufacturers are now selling such mixtures. Gradually increase the amount of decaffeinated and reduce the regular coffee until the caffeine is eliminated. Similarly, replace caffeinated soda with caffeine-free soda gradually.

People who smoke tend to metabolize caffeine more quickly than nonsmokers. When a person quits smoking, it may be advisable to gradually reduce caffeine intake. Otherwise, the coffee may have more of an impact, causing jitters and irritability.

ALCOHOL CONSUMPTION

Anthropologists believe that alcohol was produced by almost every prehistoric society that had fermentable substances—fruits and starches—available in its environment. Only the Eskimos did not have the necessary ingredients to produce alcohol.

The alcohol used in alcoholic beverages is ethyl alcohol or ethanol. It is produced by fermenting sugar or starches such as corn, barley, rye, wheat, rice, and potatoes. The three main types of alcoholic beverages are

1. beers, made from grain by brewing and fermenting; beers contain 2% to 8% alcohol.
2. distilled beverages, such as whiskey, gin, and vodka; these beverages contain 40% to 45% alcohol.
3. wines, made by fermenting grapes and other fruits; wines contain 8% to 12% alcohol.

Because alcohol supplies energy (7 kcal/g), it is considered a food. Other than energy, it does not provide nutrients to any significant extent. The effects of alcohol can occur quickly because it requires no digestion. About 20% is absorbed directly from the stomach and the remainder is absorbed from the small intestine. Alcohol is less intoxicating if consumed after eating. Food decreases alcohol absorption in the stomach because it reduces the contact of the alcohol with the stomach wall. Food delays the passage of alcohol into the small intestine, where most of it is absorbed. Food also appears to stimulate enzymes in the stomach and small intestine that help to metabolize some of the alcohol before it reaches the bloodstream.

The alcohol that enters the bloodstream is metabolized by the liver. Alcohol is metabolized in the body slowly. It takes about 1.5 hours for a man of average size to burn off the 14 g of alcohol in one drink. Alcohol has a greater effect on women because of their typically smaller body size. Nothing can speed the rate of metabolism, including cold showers, black coffee, and brisk walks.

The excess alcohol is carried by the blood throughout the body, where it tends to concentrate in organs that have a high water content. Concentration is high in the brain because of its high concentration of blood and, therefore, its high water content.

Alcohol is a depressant, acting as an anesthetic on areas of the brain. This effect begins in the area of the brain that controls social behavior. Inhibitions are lowered and judgment is affected. If blood alcohol levels continue to rise, other brain centers become depressed, resulting in slurred speech, blurred vision, and walking difficulties. When the entire brain becomes anesthetized, the individual passes out. If enough alcohol is consumed in a short period, the brain centers that control breathing and heart rate are affected and death may result. A person usually passes out before this occurs. It is possible, however, for a person to drink so much alcohol in a such a short period that he or she consumes a deadly dose before becoming unconscious. This tragedy has occurred on college campuses.

Physical conditions can intensify the effect of alcohol, including tiredness, depressed emotional state, premenstrual syndrome, medications such as oral contraceptives, small body size, and drinking on an empty stomach. What causes the morning-after hangover is unknown, but it is probably the alcohol itself and the lactic acid that builds up as alcohol is metabolized. Ways of reducing alcohol intake and its harmful effects include the following:

- Limit alcoholic beverages to one every 1.5 to 2 hours. Sip rather than gulp. Have a glass of water with your alcoholic beverage; this helps slow down liquor consumption. Be aware that carbonated beverages may increase alcohol absorption, especially on an empty stomach.
- Eat protein-rich and starchy foods before and while drinking.
- Measure alcohol when mixing drinks.
- Drink nonalcoholic beverages such as sparkling fruit juices and mineral water, club soda, or nonalcoholic beers and wines.

HARMFUL EFFECTS OF ALCOHOL

Chronic excessive alcohol consumption has dire consequences to physical health, personal functioning, and interpersonal behavior. How much alcohol must be consumed to do lasting physical damage is unknown. Health experts generally agree that limiting drinks to two a day may help reduce the risk of alcohol-related disease. Avoiding alcohol altogether is recommended. The two-drink limit is a means of controlling what could become a devastating habit. The following are the physical effects of excessive alcohol consumption.

MALNUTRITION

People who abuse alcohol are at high risk for malnutrition due to both poor food intake and disturbances in the body's use of nutrients. Excessive drinking causes loss of appetite and irregular eating habits. The empty calories in alcohol displace nutrient-dense calories in food (Display 14-10). Alcohol also adversely affects the digestion, absorption, metabolism, and excretion of nutrients. Alcohol abuse causes changes in the gastrointestinal tract that result in the malabsorption of thiamin, folate, and other nutrients. Protein, fat, and carbohydrate are not metabolized normally, leading to reduced protein synthesis and fatty infiltration of the liver. When thiamin and niacin are deficient, the cells cannot properly use glucose for energy. Brain cells especially are affected because they rely on glucose for energy. Increased urination due to alcohol consumption causes excessive loss of magnesium, potassium, and zinc.

Several alcohol-related neurologic disorders are due to nutritional deficiencies, especially of thiamin. Peripheral polyneuropathy is characterized by weakness, numbness, partial paralysis of the extremities, and pain in the legs. The condition is reversible with an adequate diet and supplements of thiamin and other B vitamins. If untreated, the polyneuropathy may progress to Wernicke's disease. The chief symptoms include paralysis of the eye muscle, involuntary rapid movement of the eyeballs, lack of muscular coordination, apathy, drowsiness, and inability to concentrate. The symptoms usually respond to large doses of thiamin.

Closely associated with Wernicke's disease is Korsakoff's syndrome. It is characterized by disorientation and a memory defect in which the person gives fictitious details about experiences or in answer to questions. These symptoms may not respond to thiamin therapy, indicating that the longstanding nutritional deficiency may have caused structural damage to the nervous system.

HIGH BLOOD PRESSURE

Excessive alcohol intake—more than three drinks a day—causes a rise in blood pressure in most people. Drinking is responsible for 5% to 11% of high blood pressure in men.

HEART DISEASE

Heavy drinking increases the risk of coronary heart disease and may produce changes in the heart tissue of young adults. Although some studies have suggested that moderate drinking may protect against heart disease and stroke, there are safer methods, such as diet and exercise, to achieve such a defense. No one should take up drinking to prevent heart disease.

DISPLAY 14-10 ALCOHOL AND CALORIC CONTENT OF ALCOHOLIC BEVERAGES*

DRINK	SIZE (FL OZ)	ALCOHOL (G)	CALORIES†
BEER			
Beer or ale, regular	12	13	150
Beer, light	12	12	100
Beer cooler	12	12	100
Near beer	12	1	30
BRANDY	1½	14	95
CORDIAL OR LIQUEUR	1½	12	160
WINE			
Dessert—sweet vermouth, port, sherry, etc.	3½	16	160
Dry, table, red or white burgundy, chablis, champagne, dry sherry, etc.	5	13	100
Light	5	9	70
Wine spritzer	7	11	85
Wine cooler	12	14	180
Nonalcoholic	5	0	10
LIQUOR			
Gin, 90-proof	1½	16	110
Rum, vodka, 80-proof	1½	14	95
Whiskey bourbon, rye, scotch, 86-proof	1½	15	105
MIXED DRINKS‡			
Margarita	2½	18	170
Gin and tonic	7½	16	170
Whiskey sour	3	15	125
Daiquiri	2	14	110

* There is a wide range of serving sizes for alcoholic beverages. Those listed are typical servings.
† The number of calories from alcohol may vary due to variation of people's response to alcohol.
‡ Volume of mixed drinks is without ice. Actual serving with ice could be much larger.
(US Dept of Agriculture, Human Nutrition Information Service. Dietary Guidelines for Americans: If you drink alcoholic beverages, do so in moderation. Washington, DC: US Government Printing Office, 1993. Home and Garden bulletin 253-8.)

LIVER DISEASE

The liver becomes enlarged with prolonged heavy alcohol use due to the accumulation of fat in the liver cells. This liver disorder can be reversed by avoiding alcohol and consuming a nutritious diet. More serious consequences are alcohol-induced hepatitis and *cirrhosis,* which is a hardening of liver tissue. These conditions appear to be directly due to the effects of alcohol and may occur even in the presence of an adequate diet. Cirrhosis is irreversible; the survival rate beyond 5 years is only 50%.

CANCER

Heavy alcohol intake increases the risk of cancers of the pharynx, esophagus, and larynx, especially when combined with cigarette smoking. Some evidence has suggested that alcohol consumption is associated with liver cancer, and moderate beer drinking with rectal cancer. The association of alcohol with pancreatic and breast cancer has not been clearly defined.

DECREASED IMMUNITY

People who are heavy consumers of alcohol have a lowered resistance to infections of all types. Alcohol depresses the bone marrow's capacity to produce the white blood cells that fight harmful bacteria.

REPRODUCTIVE SYSTEM DISORDERS

Long-term alcohol abuse in men may lead to decreased levels of male sex hormones and subsequent infertility. Women who abuse alcohol may develop hormonal imbalances that lead to infertility and menstrual disturbances.

HARM TO FETUS; FETAL ALCOHOL SYNDROME

There is no known safe level of alcohol consumption during pregnancy. Drinking alcohol during pregnancy is one of the three leading causes of birth defects in the United States. It may cause low infant birth weight and fetal alcohol syndrome. Common characteristics of fetal alcohol syndrome are stunted growth, mental retardation, malformed facial features, cardiac malformations, and motor dysfunction.

A woman should stop drinking as soon as she is aware that she is pregnant. Women who are trying to become pregnant should not drink alcohol because the early weeks of pregnancy are a critical period for embryonic growth. Women who are breastfeeding should also refrain from alcohol, which is secreted in the milk. Brain cells continue to develop in the child until about age 2 years.

FOOD MANAGEMENT

The topic of food management includes meal planning, food buying, safe storage and handling of food, and food preparation. See Chapter 4 for information on safe food storage and handling. Food management provides techniques for obtaining nutritious meals at an economical price. The following information applies to your personal food management and your professional interaction with clients. As a health worker, you can help educate consumers to eat well at the lowest possible cost. You also can apply this information, for example, in guiding a young pregnant woman in food purchasing and preparation or helping an unemployed client eat healthful foods while living within his or her food stamp allotment.

MEAL PLANNING

Advanced planning is the most important factor in obtaining nutritionally adequate and economical meals. Haphazard meals frequently are unbalanced and costly. Planning what the family will eat for a few days or a week in advance helps one take advantage of local market specials and assures nourishing menus at a lower cost. A guide such as The Pyramid Guide to Daily Food Choices (see Table 14-1) can assist the meal planner in selecting a wide variety of foods to provide good nutrition.

Most Americans could lower their food bills without sacrificing nutritional quality by buying more lowfat milk and lowfat milk products, legumes, vegetables and fruits, and whole-grain and enriched bread and grains, while buying less red meat, fat, oil, sugar, sweets, coffee, tea, soft drinks, and snack foods, which are costly items.

SHOPPING WITH A LIST

A food shopping list based on a planned menu helps prevent impulse buying of unneeded items and trips back to the store for forgotten foods. Shoppers with a list can use coupons wisely to reduce the cost of needed foods.

Families purchasing food at a neighborhood grocery store that gives credit usually pay more for food than they would at a supermarket. They depend on these stores because they are frequently short of cash to buy food. Some families may accept help in managing their finances so that they can eventually buy food in markets where they will receive the greatest value.

UNIT PRICING

Unit pricing is a method some stores use of displaying the price per weight or measure of a particular product, such as the price per ounce or quart. It enables shoppers to compare the costs of two different-sized products or the same size of two different brands to determine the best buy.

OPEN DATING

Open dating is helpful in making food selections based on freshness. Its usefulness, however, is limited because the handling and storage of food have a greater bearing on freshness than time. There are four types of dating: pack date (e.g., Packed Dec. 1996); pull date (e.g., Sell by January 3); quality assurance or freshness date (e.g., Best if used before August 30, 1997); and expiration date (e.g., Do not use after Sept. 15, 1996).

GRADE SHIELDS

Foods that carry USDA grade shields have been graded according to federal quality grade standards. Grading is not required by law. The USDA grade shields are most likely to be found in meats, poultry, eggs, instant nonfat dry milk, and butter. Grade shields help consumers choose food items that are most suitable for their intended use.

Information on USDA grading standards can be obtained from the state or county Agricultural Cooperative Extension Service or from Information Office, Agricultural Marketing Service, US Department of Agriculture, Room 3510, South Agriculture Building, Washington, DC 20250.

BRANDS

A *brand* is a company name or a product identified with a specific company. Some supermarkets also offer products carrying their own labels. These private-label goods are usually well-established products of reliable quality and are less expensive than brand name items. Some chains offer store-brand labels that reflect grades; for example, tomatoes may be packed under three labels comparable to grades A, B, and C.

In recent years, food retailers have introduced *generic labeling* as a means of offering consumers a wider choice in price and quality. These generic or "no-frills" products, which do not carry a brand name or trademark, can save consumers an average of 25% over national brands and 15% over store brands. Most generic food items are USDA grade C, and some are grade B. Brand names and top-label store brands are primarily grade A, with a few grade B.

Health workers should remember that grading does not indicate nutritional value. A low grade does not mean that the nutritional quality is inferior to that of higher grades.

MAKING ECONOMICAL CHOICES

MILK AND DAIRY PRODUCTS

Nonfat dry milk provides excellent nutritional value at a low price. Half a cup of evaporated whole or evaporated nonfat milk mixed with half a cup of water can substitute for 1 cup of whole or nonfat milk in recipes.

Less expensive types of cheese are as good a source of protein and calcium as more expensive types. Grated cheese and individually wrapped slices are more expensive.

MEAT AND MEAT SUBSTITUTES

To reduce their intake of saturated fat and cholesterol, many people are reducing the amount of meat in their diet. The recommended limit for adults is 6 oz per day of cooked meat, poultry, or fish. Macaroni products, rice, and corn make nutritious substitute main dishes when combined with eggs or egg substitutes, milk, lowfat cheese, dried peas, beans, and nuts, or when added to small amounts of meat, poultry, or fish.

Meat and poultry products have USDA inspection seals that indicate that the food is safe and wholesome at the time of inspection. Products produced and sold within a state may be state inspected according to standards meeting those of the federal government.

The USDA grades for beef are prime, choice, select, standard, and commercial. Grades are a guide to tenderness and amount of fat but not to nutritive value. Less expensive cuts of meat are just as nutritious but may need longer cooking. Planning for two or three meals from one large roast can save money, especially if the meal planner uses the leftover meat for sandwiches rather than buying sandwich meats.

The quality and size of eggs determine their price. Grade AA and A eggs are best for poaching and frying. Grade B eggs are suitable for general cooking and baking. Brown eggs and white eggs have the same nutritional value.

Protein Cost

One way to identify good buys among protein foods is to compare costs in terms of the quantity of protein provided. Price per pound or other unit of measure does not necessarily indicate the cost of protein, because the amount of protein in meats and meat substitutes varies. For example, 1 lb of frankfurters provides only half the protein of 1 lb of ground beef. Although the frankfurters may cost less per pound, they actually are a more expensive source of protein than ground beef.

Cost per Serving

The cost per serving can be determined by dividing the cost per market unit (pound, can, or package) by the number of servings the food provides. It may be more economical to pay more per pound for meat that is well trimmed of fat and waste than to select meat on the basis of price alone. A pound of meat that is boneless yields four servings per pound, whereas the same weight of meat with bone yields two to three servings.

VEGETABLES AND FRUITS

Compare the prices of fresh, frozen, and canned fruits and vegetables to determine best buys. Fresh produce usually costs less if purchased in season when the supply is plentiful.

Canned fruits and vegetables sold as cut-up pieces often cost less than the whole or halves in the same-sized can. The nutritive value is the same. Plain frozen vegetables cost less than those prepared in sauces.

The USDA grades for canned and frozen fruits and vegetables are grade A or Fancy, grade B or Choice, and grade C or standard. Grading is related to such product qualities as color, uniformity of size, degree of ripeness, and absence of blemishes. The nutritive value of lower grades is the same as that of more expensive grades.

BREADS AND CEREAL PRODUCTS

Home-cooked cereals are less expensive than ready-to-eat cereals. A person may save money by buying large loaves of bread, large boxes of cereal, and day-old bakery products. Select enriched or whole-grain products. Some breads are colored with molasses to make them look dark, as if they were whole-grain. Read the ingredients label to be sure.

CONVENIENCE FOODS

In most cases, fully or partially prepared food items cost more than unprocessed products. Ingredients are listed in descending order according to the amount in the product. If gravy is listed first and meat last, there is more gravy that anything else. Each consumer must decide how much to pay for convenience. Current labeling regulations that require nutrition information on virtually all food labels have taken the guesswork out of comparison shopping.

Some convenience foods, such as frozen concentrated orange juice, canned orange juice, canned and frozen out-of-season vegetables and fruits, pancake and waffle mixes, and pudding mixes, cost less than unprocessed products.

CONSERVING NUTRIENTS IN FOODS

VEGETABLES

Wash fresh vegetables thoroughly to remove dirt and traces of insecticide spray. Trim sparingly the dark outer leaves of greens, which are rich in iron, calcium, and vitamins. Avoid peeling vegetables and fruits whenever possible because vitamins are concentrated just beneath the skin. Bake or cook potatoes in their skins, even for hashed browns or potato salad. Cook vegetables whole or cut into large pieces to avoid exposing a large surface area.

Cook vegetables in little or no water. Steaming, stir-frying, or microwave cooking preserves vitamins and minerals. Do not add baking soda to cooking water to preserve the green color because it destroys B vitamins and vitamin C.

To retain the nutrients in canned vegetables, pour the liquid from the can into a saucepan and heat it to reduce the liquid. Then add the vegetables to the remaining liquid and heat before serving.

ANIMAL PROTEINS

Meat, poultry, and fish are best cooked at low temperatures to encourage tenderness, reduce shrinkage, and retain nutrients. Eggs are also toughened by high temperatures. Simmer eggs gently, rather than boiling them.

FOOD ASSISTANCE PROGRAMS

You will undoubtedly encounter situations in which an individual or family does not have enough money to purchase food for an adequate diet. You should be acquainted with your community's resources.

The Food Stamp program is intended to increase poor people's power to purchase food. This federal program issues food stamps monthly to families and single people who meet income eligibility requirements. People use the stamps like money to purchase any kind of food (except pet food) and any nonalcoholic beverages and to buy seeds and plants for producing food. The value of the stamps issued depends on the size of the household and its financial resources. For information about the Special Supplemental Food Program for Women, Infants, and Children (See chapter 17), school feeding programs, and child-care food programs, see Chapter 18.

The Nutrition Program for the Elderly is a federal program designed to improve the nutrition of people aged 60 years and older or people with spouses that age. All people who meet the age criterion are eligible; there are no financial or health considerations. A contribution toward the cost of the meals is encouraged but not required. The program provides a noon meal served at least 5 days a week in a church, school, or other community building. The meal must provide at least one third of the recommended dietary allowances for elderly individuals. The program also provides services to increase socialization and self-reliance in the elderly person; these services include transportation, shopping, and recreational activities. A certain percentage of the meals can be home-delivered to homebound elderly individuals.

Meals-on-Wheels is a voluntary program supported by local civic or religious organizations. Volunteers pack and deliver meals to people of any age who are ill and disabled and cannot prepare food for themselves. Many programs provide both a noon meal and a bag supper for the evening meal 5 days a week. The recipient pays only for the cost of the food. People who cannot afford the full cost are usually charged according to their ability to pay.

The Expanded Food and Nutrition Education Program of the USDA Cooperative Extension Service employs program aides to work directly with low-income families to help them improve their diets. (Contact your local Cooperative Extension Service for more information.) In addition, churches and other community organizations often help families or individuals with food purchases on a short-term basis.

KEY ISSUES

Fast Foods: Are They Junk Foods?

The nutritional impact of fast foods is an important consideration because they are an ever-increasing part of the American diet. The nutritional consequences of eating fast foods depends on several factors: how often they are eaten, the nutritional content of the consumer's choices, and the nutritional quality of the consumer's other meals and snacks.

Occasional fast-food meals (once a week or so) have little impact on the nutritive value of a week's diet. Many people, however, eat fast foods every day or almost every day. The expansion of fast-food restaurants on college campuses and the fast-food style menu in schools may encourage people to become dependent on fast foods for one or more meals a day. This is contrary to one of the most important principles of nutrition—variety. Relying on a limited selection of food increases the risk of nutrient deficiency and excess. By knowing the nutritional problems associated with fast-food menus and how to compensate for them, consumers can learn to use fast food without compromising their nutritional well-being.

Fast foods generally do not deserve the junk food label sometimes given them. Many fast-food main dishes supply substantial amounts of nutrients. They also, however, tend to have high levels of calories, sugar, sodium, and fat, which are problem areas in the American diet. These areas are the target of the Dietary Guidelines for Americans and of the expert committees that have studied the relation of diet to chronic disease.

In recent years, the fast-food industry has been responding to consumer interest in lowfat foods by adding such items as cereal, fat-free muffins, lower fat hamburgers, grilled chicken sandwiches (beware of sauces, bacon, and other add-ons), lowfat milk shakes, and lowfat frozen yogurt.

The goal is to obtain all of the essential nutrients and fiber within a framework of moderation in calories, fat, sodium, sugar, and, possibly, protein. Meeting these goals in the fast-food restaurant is a challenge—one that is becoming easier as more lowfat choices become available. The key is to know the food value of the foods you are ordering. The portion sizes and nutritional content of fast foods are consistent. The nutritional composition of all the items offered by fast-food chains are readily available from the chains themselves and from various books that list the nutritional values of foods.

ON THE PLUS SIDE

Fast-food meals provide 50% to 100% of the daily protein recommended for young adults. Hamburgers and roast beef sandwiches contain substantial amounts of iron. Adequate calcium is supplied by pizza or by milk or a milk shake. Typical fast-food meals are good sources of other nutrients, as well, such as thiamin, riboflavin, niacin, vitamin B_{12}, phosphorus, and zinc.

ON THE MINUS SIDE

Fast foods are poor sources of vitamins A and B_6, folate, pantothenic acid, vitamin C, and fiber, nutrients which tend to be below recommended levels in the American diet. Keeping in mind the recommendations to maintain reasonable weight—reduce fat to less than 30% of total calories, reduce sodium to 2400 mg/day, increase fiber, and reduce sugar—let's look at these aspects of fast foods.

Energy

Fast-food meals usually are too high in calories. A typical meal consisting of a quarter-pound cheeseburger, a large serving of french fries, and a vanilla milk shake supplies 1200 kcal. This amount represents 55% of the total daily energy intake recommended for a young woman (2200 kcal). This is too many calories for one meal. For people with lower energy requirements or for those who are dieting to lose weight, this 1200-kcal meal can represent 60% to 100% of their caloric needs for the day. Display 14-11 gives the energy content of other typical fast-food meals.

Fat

Most of the calories in fast-food meals come from fat. The fast-food meal of a quarter-pound cheeseburger, a large serving of french fries, and a vanilla milk shake contains 59 g of fat; fat provides 44% of its total calories. Most fast-food meals derive 40% to 60% of their total calories from fat, most of which is saturated fat. Frying adds a considerable amount of fat and calories to many fast-food items. Although poultry and fish are lower in fat than ground beef, the poultry and fish in fast-food sandwiches usually are breaded and fried. The fat and caloric content of these sandwiches can be as high as or higher than that of a quarter-pound hamburger (Display 14-11). In some cases, beef fat, which is high in saturated fat and cholesterol, is used for frying—adding to the unhealthful qualities of the food. In addition to frying, large portions of meat, as in double or triple burgers, cheese sauces, and toppings add to the fat and caloric content of the food.

Sodium

Most fast-food items provide large amounts of sodium from salt and other ingredients. The fast-food meal of a quarter-pound cheeseburger, a large serving of french fries, and a vanilla milk shake contains 1655 mg of sodium, almost 70% of the 2400 mg of sodium recommended as a daily limit. Salted french fries, onion rings, milk shakes, battered and breaded food, pickles, sauces, and other condiments add considerably to the sodium content of the meal.

Sugar

Soft drinks and milk shakes provide most of the sugar in fast-food meals. A 12-oz can of soda contains 8 to 11 tsp sugar, as does a typical milk shake. The milk shake also contains the equivalent of 2 to 4 tsp of fat. Some chains have lowfat milk shakes available that have less than a ½ teaspoon of fat. Most of the available desserts—pies, danish, and cookies—are loaded with calories, fat, and sugar.

MAKING WISE CHOICES

In recent years, foods lower in calories, fat, and sodium have been introduced in response to consumer demand. Display 14-12 compares some high-fat fast foods with lower fat choices.

Large salads containing a variety of vegetables, fresh fruits, cottage cheese, and reduced-calorie salad dressings are good choices. Avoid add-ons such as bacon, cheese, seeds, regular salad dressings, and items mixed with mayonnaise or oil (such as potato salad). Boxed salads with chicken or shrimp are good choices. They supply protein along with fiber, vitamins, and minerals from the vegetables. Again, beware of salad dressings. A 2.5-oz package of blue cheese dressing available with boxed salads at one chain contains 345 calories (34.5 g fat).

Regular sandwiches are a wiser choice than triple or double hamburgers. Omit extras such as cheese, bacon, and special sauces in favor of lettuce and tomato. A plain hamburger, salad, and diet soda is a low-calorie meal. Use sandwich rolls or pita bread in place of croissants, which are high in calories and fat. Biscuits also are high in fat.

A roast beef sandwich (335 kcal) is a better option than most burgers. Avoid the cheese; it adds another 107 kcal. A roasted chicken breast fillet on a bun, preferably a multigrain bun, is an excellent choice.

DISPLAY 14-11 ENERGY, FAT, AND SODIUM CONTENT OF TYPICAL FAST-FOOD MEALS

FOOD	TOTAL CALORIES (KCAL)	FAT (G)	SODIUM (MG)
Large hamburger with sauces and cheese (706 kcal), regular order of french fries (341 kcal), vanilla milk shake (334 kcal)	1381	66	1529
Fried fish sandwich (440 kcal), regular order of french fries (341 kcal), apple pie (311 kcal), 12-oz diet cola (0 kcal)	1092	53	1602
Two slices pepperoni pizza with thin crust (460 kcal), 12-oz cola (150 kcal)	610	17.5	845
Fried chicken dinner: 2 pieces chicken, biscuit, cole slaw, mashed potato, gravy (854 kcal), 12-oz cola (150 kcal)	1004	43.9	2158
Large hotdog with cheese (580 kcal), large chocolate malt (889 kcal)	1469	55	1909

(Source of food values: Sucher KP, Kittler PG. Fast foods: the current state of affairs. Dietetic Currents 1991;18:4:3–4.)

DISPLAY 14-12 COMPARISON OF FAT IN SELECTED FAST FOODS

FAST FOOD	TOTAL FAT (G)	TOTAL CALORIES (KCAL)
Biscuit/sausage/egg	34.5	520
Hot cakes/butter/syrup	9.2	410
Quarter Pounder with cheese	29.2	520
McLean Deluxe	10.0	310
Quarter Pounder (no cheese)	20.7	410
Roast beef sandwich	14.8	353
Regular (small) hamburger	9.5	260
Chicken sandwich	19.0	430
New Chili	7.0	220
Apple danish	17.9	390
Blueberry muffin (fat free)	0.0	170
Vanilla milk shake	10.0	334
Lowfat vanilla milk shake	1.3	290

(Source of food values: Sucher KP, Kittler PG. Fast foods: the current state of affairs. Dietetic Currents 1991;18:4:3–4.)

Fried chicken and fish, french fries, and pies derive 40% to 60% of their calories from fat, so it is best to avoid them. If you do order fried foods, remove the breading or batter coating. Avoid extra-crispy varieties. Limit french fries to small servings without salt. You can add a small amount of salt, if desired. A tossed salad may take the place of fries.

A plain baked potato with small amounts of sour cream, butter, or margarine is a good choice. A baked potato with all the toppings—bacon, cheese, butter, and sour cream—can have as much as 690 kcal, with more than 50% of its calories derived from fat.

Skim or lowfat milk is preferable to soda or low-fat milk shake. If milk is unavailable, ask for water. Both the soda and milk shake are loaded with sugar.

Skip desserts, which are high in calories, fat, and sugars. Lowfat frozen yogurt is an acceptable choice.

Choices that add fiber to the diet include baked beans, chili, vegetables, fruits, garbanzo or kidney beans at the salad bar, and baked potatoes with the skin. (Avoid potato skins, which are deep-fat fried and are served with melted cheese or other fatty, salty toppings.)

People who eat fast foods regularly must be more careful about their selections than those who eat fast foods occasionally. To control calories, eat fast foods at mealtimes rather than as snacks. Choose foods in other meals carefully to supply the nutrients and fiber that are lacking in fast foods. In other meals, emphasize green leafy and yellow vegetables, fruits, whole-grain cereals and breads, and legumes.

KEYS TO PRACTICAL APPLICATION

Use the Food Guide Pyramid in helping your clients make healthful food choices; know how the pyramid supports the Dietary Guidelines for Americans.

Use the fats–sugar–alcohol group sparingly—this group contains mostly calories and few nutrients.

Encourage your clients to consume “5 a Day for Better Health.” Learn the vegetable and fruit sources of beta carotene and vitamin C.

Distribute your food intake into meals spread throughout the day. The body needs a steady supply of nutrients. Avoid overloading the body with food at any one time.

Select restaurants that provide sufficient variety so that you can make healthful choices.

Do not hesitate to ask your server questions about portion sizes, preparation methods, and availability of foods not on the menu; ask for foods prepared or served in ways that keep fat content to a minimum.

Inform your clients of the effects of caffeine and the wisdom of moderation. Advise people who desire to stop consuming caffeine to do so gradually.

Make parents aware of the caffeine their small children may be consuming in soda. Tell them about the sugar content of sodas—8 to 11 tsp of sugar per 12-oz can.

Avoid alcohol. If you drink alcoholic beverages, limit consumption to a maximum of two drinks (1 oz of pure alcohol) in a single day. Alcohol is the most widely used and destructive drug in the United States.

Plan meals—planning is the key to nutritious and economical eating.

Use unit pricing to find the best buy among a variety of brands in a package size that is most practical for you.

Become familiar with the grading system involved in USDA grades, brand names, store brands, and generic labeling; buy the quality that suits your needs.

Remember that cost per serving, not cost per pound or package, is the key to finding the most economical buy.

Encourage the use of nonfat dry milk. It is the least expensive source of high-quality protein.

Discourage the use of excessive amounts of meat, fish, and poultry. These foods are too expensive to use for energy.

Learn to identify good buys among protein foods by comparing costs in terms of the amount of protein the foods provide.

To conserve nutrients, cook vegetables by steaming, stir—frying, or microwaving, if possible; avoid cutting, soaking, peeling, and overcooking.

Learn to handle and store food at home for maximum freshness (see Chapter 4).

Become familiar with the food assistance programs in your community that can help people who do not have the money to purchase an adequate diet or who, because of disability, cannot obtain an adequate diet.

Enjoy fast foods without abusing them. Make fast-food choices with an awareness of the energy and nutrient value of the foods; choose appropriate foods at other meals to provide nutrients that are lacking in fast foods; use fast foods occasionally and only as a meal, not a snack. Remember the importance of variety.

KEY IDEAS

A good diet is one that controls energy needs, supplies all of the essential nutrients, and avoids excesses in fat, sodium, sugar, and alcohol.

Selecting a diet that provides balance, variety, and moderation best assures a nutritious diet.

In a sedentary society, most people must eat foods of high nutrient density to avoid weight gain without sacrificing nutritional adequacy.

Dietary Guidelines for Americans is the main nutrition education message of the federal government. The new guidelines are as follows: Eat a variety of foods; balance the food you eat with physical activity, maintain, or improve your weight; choose a diet with plenty of grain products, vegetables, and fruits; choose a diet low in fat, saturated fat, and cholesterol; choose a diet moderate in sugars; choose a diet moderate in salt and sodium; and if your drink alcoholic beverages, do so in moderation (Display 14-2).

The recommendations of the surgeon general (see Display 14-1) and the Committee on Diet and Health (see Display 14-2) are similar with the following exceptions: *The Surgeon General's Report on Nutrition and Health* also emphasizes the need for iron; the committee makes additional recommendations regarding the need to moderate protein intake and the cautious use of dietary supplements.

Food guides translate scientific information into practical advice for everyday eating. The Food Guide Pyramid is the food guide being used in the federal government's nutrition education program. It consists of five major groups: breads, cereals, and other grain products; fruits; vegetables; meat, poultry, fish, eggs, and dry beans, peas, and nuts; and milk, cheese, and yogurt. A sixth group consists of fats, sweets, and alcoholic beverages, which provide calories but few nutrients. Minimum servings from each group with moderate amounts of fats and sugars supply about 1600 kcal.

The food guides can be adapted to an individual's caloric needs and to most lifestyles and eating habits.

Each of the major food groups contributes specific nutrients to the total diet.

Nutrient values of foods within each group vary. Knowledge of the nutritional value and composition of foods is necessary to make the best choices within each group.

The National Cancer Institute program "5 a Day for Better Health" recognizes the association of a liberal intake of fruits and vegetables with reduced cancer risk.

Distributing food intake over the day so that the body has a steady supply of nutrients is important; avoid overeating at any one time.

Healthful eating while dining out involves advance planning, good ordering techniques, and a knowledge of healthful food choices.

Caffeine is an addictive drug with stimulating effects. For most adults, a few cups of coffee, tea, or caffeine-containing soda does not appear to cause long-term health problems. People who should avoid or severely limit caffeine are pregnant women, people with ulcers, people with heart rhythm disturbances, people taking theophylline, and people who are particularly sensitive to the effects of caffeine. (See Displays 14-7 and 14-8 for the caffeine content of various foods.)

Many children consume excessive amounts of caffeine in soda.

Habitual drinking of alcoholic beverages, even in moderation, is not good for you. The negative effects of alcohol far outweigh any positive ones. The physical problems associated with excessive consumption of alcohol include malnutrition, cirrhosis, heart disease, cancer, high blood pressure, impaired immunity, reproductive system disturbances, and fetal alcohol syndrome.

Advance planning is the most important factor in obtaining nutritionally adequate and economical meals.

An understanding of unit pricing, open dating, and food grading can result in more efficient food purchasing.

Cost per serving, not cost per pound, can, or package, is important in economical food buying—especially in meat buying.

Most Americans could lower their food bills without sacrificing nutritional quality by buying more milk, vegetables and fruits, and whole-grain and enriched cereals and bread and by buying less meat, fats, oils, sugar, coffee, tea, and snack foods.

Figuring the cost of protein identifies foods that are good buys among protein-rich foods.

A person can reduce the cost of protein by using smaller portions of meat, fish, and poultry; by using lower grades and less expensive cuts of meat; and by using legumes, peanut butter, eggs, and cheese in the place of meat for some meals.

A person should periodically compare the cost per serving of fresh, frozen, and canned fruits and vegetables to determine the best buy at a particular time of year.

Bakery foods and convenience foods usually cost more than the same products made entirely at home.

The excessive use of fast food limits variety, creating the risk of nutritional deficiencies. The high energy, fat, and sodium content of fast foods increases the risk of nutritional excess.

Fast foods tend to provide adequate amounts of protein, thiamin, niacin, riboflavin, vitamin B_{12}, phosphorus, and zinc; calcium and iron contents vary with the food.

Fast foods tend to lack vitamins A and B_6, folate, pantothenic acid, vitamin C, calcium, and fiber.

Guides to using fast foods appropriately include the following: choose lower fat items, eat fast foods as a meal not a snack, choose foods in other meals carefully with an emphasis on fruits, vegetables, and whole-grain cereal products.

KEYS TO LEARNING

STUDY—DISCUSSION QUESTIONS

1. Record your food intake for 3 consecutive days. Include all foods and beverages, including diet beverages. Include 1 weekend day in your record. Compare your daily food intake to the Pyramid Food Guide to Daily Food Choices (Table 14-1) using the format in Display 14-5. Have you eaten foods from all of the food groups in the amounts recommended? Have you included sources of vitamins A and C?
2. In addition to *The Pyramid Guide to Daily Food Choices,* (Table 14-1) what other factors are important in meal planning?
3. Why is the spacing of meals important? Overconsumption of food at the evening meal and excessive snacking in the evening are common problems in the United States. Discuss ways of controlling these habits.
4. Discuss the importance of a varied diet from the standpoint of food safety.
5. Share family recipes for vegetable dishes.
6. What are the long-range harmful physical effects of excessive alcohol consumption? Do you think teenagers and young adults are aware of these consequences?
7. Using your 3-day food diary together with Displays 14-8 and 14-9 calculate the amount of caffeine in your diet. Are you consuming more than 200 mg/day of caffeine?
8. Investigate the food assistance programs in your community. Present a report to the class on one program. Include eligibility requirements, benefits, and location of the enrollment office (if it applies) of the program you have selected.
9. In light of the chapter discussion of fast foods, what changes, if any, will you make in your use of fast foods?
10. Why is the advance planning of meals and snacks an important factor in food management?
11. Using The Pyramid Guide to Daily Food Choices (Table 14-1), plan a low-cost menu for 1 week for a family of four: a mother, 30 years old; father, 32 years; girl, 9 years; and boy, 6 years. Include three meals a day and an after-school snack for the children. Calculate the cost based on current market prices. In class, compare the costs of the various menu plans. What factors account for differences in cost?
12. Define the following and explain their importance in food management: unit pricing, open dating, USDA grade shields, cost per serving, brand name, generic labeling, and cost of protein.
13. Compare the nutrition labeling on the following: homogenized whole milk, 2%-fat milk, 1%-fat milk, nonfat milk, commercial buttermilk, dry nonfat milk powder (reconstituted), plain yogurt, and lowfat plain yogurt. Compare the costs of an 8-oz serving of each of these forms of milk.
14. Assume that you are attempting to encourage a parent of two school-age children to use more milk instead of sweetened fruit-flavored drinks at mealtime. How could you use nutrition labeling in your discussions with the parent?
15. What are the advantages of using low temperatures in cooking meat, fish, and poultry? Discuss food preparation practices that conserve the nutritive value of vegetables.
16. Collect menus from popular local restaurants. Using these menus, select meals that meet the recommendations of the Dietary Guidelines for Americans.

BIBLIOGRAPHY

BOOKS AND PAMPHLETS

Dietary Guidelines Advisory Committee. Report of the Dietary Guidelines Advisory Committee on the Dietary Guidelines for Americans, 1995, Hyattsville, MD: US Department of Agriculture, 1995.

Lecos CW. Caffeine jitters: some safety questions remain. Washington, DC: US Dept of Health and Human Services, 1993. FDA publication FDA 88-2221.

National Academy of Sciences, National Research Council, Committee on Diet and Health, Food and Nutrition Board. Diet and health: implications for reducing chronic disease risk (executive summary). Washington, DC: National Academy Press, 1989.

National Academy of Sciences, National Research Council, Food and Nutrition Board. Recommended dietary allowances. 10th ed. Washington, DC: National Academy Press, 1989.

National Dairy Council. Guide to good eating: leader guide. Rosemont, IL: National Dairy Council, 1992.

US Dept of Agriculture and US Dept of Health and Human Services. Nutrition and your health: dietary guidelines for Americans. 3rd ed. Washington, DC: US Government Printing Office, 1990. Home and Garden bulletin 232.

US Dept of Agriculture, Human Nutrition Information Service. Dietary Guidelines for Americans: choose a diet with plenty of vegetables, fruits, and grain products. Washington DC: US Government Printing Office, 1993. Home and Garden bulletin 253-5.

US Dept of Agriculture, Human Nutrition Information Service. Dietary Guidelines for Americans: dietary guidelines and your diet—an overview. Washington, DC: US Government Printing Office, 1993. Home and Garden bulletin 253-2.

US Dept of Agriculture, Human Nutrition Information Service. Dietary Guidelines for Americans: eat a variety of foods. Washington, DC: US Government Printing Office, 1993. Home and Garden bulletin 253-2.

US Dept of Agriculture, Human Nutrition Information Service. Dietary Guidelines for Americans: if you drink alcoholic beverages, do so in moderation. Washington, DC: US Government Printing Office, 1993. Home and Garden bulletin 253-8.

US Dept of Agriculture, Human Nutrition Information Service. Dietary Guidelines for Americans: maintain healthy weight. Washington DC: US Government Printing Office, 1993. Home and Garden bulletin 253-3.

US Dept of Agriculture, Human Nutrition Information Service. Eating better when eating out using the dietary guidelines. Washington, DC: US Government Printing Office, 1989. Home and Garden bulletin 232-11.

US Dept of Health and Human Services, Public Health Service. The surgeon general's report on nutrition and health (summary and recommendations). Washington, DC: US Government Printing Office, 1988. US Dept of Health and Human Services publication PHS 88-50211.

PERIODICALS

Anderson J. US government dietary guidelines: past review and present opportunity. Nutr Update 1993;3:1:1.

Fortier I, Marcoux S, Beaulac—Baillargeon L. Relation of caffeine intake during pregnancy to intrauterine growth retardation and pre-term birth. Am J Epidemiol 1993;137:931.

Havas S, Heimendinger J, Reynolds K, et al. 5 a day for better health: a new research initiative. J Am Diet Assoc 1994;94:1:32.

Kerr RS, Sherwin F, Pavalkis PB, et al. Effects of caffeine on the recognition of and responses to hypoglycemia in humans. Ann Intern Med 1993;119:799.

McBean LD. The food group approach to eating in the 1990's. Dairy Council Digest, 1993;64:1:1.

Sucher KP, Kittler PG. Fast foods: the current state of affairs. Dietetic Currents 1991;18:4:1.

CHAPTER

15

Meeting Nutritional Needs in Various Cultures and Lifestyles

KEY TERMS

acculturation the process of adopting the cultural traits of another group

botanical a drug or supplement made from part of a plant (e.g., root, leaves, or bark)

food fad any diet concept that is unproved scientifically and that claims exaggerated health benefits

fraudulent misleading information used to gain advantage

hala'l food permitted by law for Muslims to eat

kosher food that is selected and prepared according to the Jewish kashruth dietary laws; the term is derived from a word meaning *right* or *fit*

lacto-ovovegetarian a person who eats foods of plant origin in addition to dairy products and eggs, but does not eat meat, fish, or poultry

staple a basic or necessary item of food

vegan a person who eats only foods of plant origin and does not eat any animal products, including dairy products or eggs

OBJECTIVES

After completing this chapter, the student will be able to:

1. Give examples of how the region in which people live helps to shape their eating habits.
2. Give examples of how meanings attached to food differ among cultures.
3. Explain the following statement: More than a passing knowledge of a particular culture is necessary if health workers are to provide effective nutrition counseling.
4. Discuss the general characteristics of the food patterns, beliefs, and preferences and the potential nutrition-related problems of the following cultures in America:
   - African American
   - Hispanic (Mexican, Puerto Rican)
   - Chinese
   - Filipino
   - Southeast Asian
   - American Indian
   - Alaska Native
   - Jewish
5. Give the components of a well-balanced vegetarian diet and the nutrients that need special attention.
6. Give four examples of nondairy sources of calcium.
7. Discuss the potential danger of taking dietary supplements.
8. Discuss the factors that motivate people to accept the extravagant health claims made by the food supplement industry.
9. Give four clues that can alert an individual to food misinformation and fraud.
10. Give five sources of reliable nutrition information.

CULTURAL DIVERSITY AND NUTRITION-RELATED HEALTH PROBLEMS

The U.S. population is becoming increasingly diverse. One of the three broad national goals expressed in *Healthy People 2000* (see Chapter 1) is to reduce health inequalities among Americans and to finally eliminate health gaps among the nation's different population groups. Nutrition intervention and education play an extremely important role in meeting these national health goals. To achieve these goals, health workers must know and respect cultural values and personal preferences and use culturally sensitive educational methods and materials.

Risk of disease with nutritional implications often varies among different ethnic populations. Some ethnic groups may be genetically predisposed to certain diseases. For example, celiac sprue frequently is found in people of Irish descent; hypertension is prevalent among African Americans; and a high incidence of diabetes exists among African Americans, Hispanics, and American Indians.

Nutritional needs may also differ among various ethnic groups. African American women have lower hemoglobin levels than white women; this finding is not based on iron intake. On the other hand, African Americans have a lower incidence of osteoporosis than whites, even though African Americans have a lower overall calcium intake.

CULTURAL DIVERSITY AND NUTRITION COUNSELING

Each person has a unique cultural background that influences what he or she eats. Peoples' eating habits—what they eat, their pattern of eating, and the cooking methods used—are influenced by ethnic, social, and economic factors.

This chapter describes food behaviors of various ethnic groups. It should not be assumed, however, that members of a particular ethnic group make all (or any) of their food choices according to traditional eating habits. Health workers must find out what an individual actually is eating. Frequently, there is a blending of traditional ethnic food preferences with those of the general population.

Health workers should not prejudge eating habits that are unfamiliar, even when those habits do not seem to fit commonly used food guides. Analysis may show the diet to be perfectly adequate.

REGIONAL INFLUENCES

Eating habits are determined mainly by the foods available in a particular area. Cultural factors such as nation of origin and religious beliefs play a role, too. Near the sea, fish is an important source of protein, whereas inland, fish is used less frequently. Agricultural conditions in the southern states favor the growth of a wheat suited to the preparation of hot breads rather than yeast breads. In the northern central states, the German, Polish, and Scandinavian influences are evident; in the far west, the Oriental culture is influential, and so on. Fried chicken, hot breads, and fat-seasoned greens are associated with the South; tortillas, chili con carne, and enchiladas with the Southwest.

Regional differences are not as pronounced as they once were because of magazine, newspaper, and television advertising, which promotes ethnic and regional food products; the popularity of fast-food chains serving ethnic and regional foods; and the mobility of the American family. Also, foods from all over the world are available throughout the year. Perhaps the greatest influence of ethnicity on food is seen in large cities, where entire sections may be inhabited by people of similar backgrounds.

CULTURAL INFLUENCES

Meanings attached to foods vary greatly among cultures. What is considered acceptable as a food by one culture may be considered inedible by another. For example, some cultures consider dog and cat meat to be acceptable food. Members of other cultures, who view these animals as pets, consider this practice unthinkable.

Religious beliefs in some cultures have a strong influence on eating habits. Some foods are considered sacred, whereas others are forbidden. Some religions have strict observances and rituals involving food (e.g., Jewish dietary laws).

Some cultures attribute opposing qualities to foods. The Hispanic culture classifies foods as *caliente* (hot) or *frio* (cold). These designations have nothing to do with the temperature of the food but rather with the effects these foods are thought to have on the body (Display 15-1). This culture also classifies illnesses according to this system. People treat so-called cold illnesses with hot foods and hot illnesses with cold foods. Similarly, the Chinese have the yin–yang theory involving opposing forces: *yin,* the female force, and *yang,* the male force (Display 15-2). Both the Hispanic and Chinese cultures believe that good health is achieved by a balance between these elements.

DISPLAY 15-1 "HOT" AND "COLD" FOODS IN THE HISPANIC CULTURE

HOT	COLD
Onion	Green beans
Fish	Carrots
Sugar	Peas
Pork	Squash
Turkey	Radish
Wheat bread	Cauliflower
Beans	Lamb
Rice	Beef
Wheat tortillas	Milk
	Lentils

VERY HOT	VERY COLD
Chili pepper	Cucumber
Garlic	Pickles
White beans	Spinach
	Tomatoes
	Breast milk

(Kaufman-Kuzrock DL. Cultural aspects of nutrition. Top Clin Nutr 1989;4:2:2.)

DISPLAY 15-2 YIN AND YANG PRINCIPLE IN RELATION TO FOOD*

YIN (COLD)	YANG (HOT)
White turnips	Gingerroot
Seaweed	Hot water
Bean sprouts	Rooster meat
	Korean ginzen

* There is no complete list of "hot" and "cold" foods. Categorization of these foods often varies from one family to another.

(Kaufman-Kurzrock DL. Cultural aspects of nutrition. Top Clin Nutr 1989;4:2:2.)

Most cultures believe that certain foods have healing properties (see Display 2-4). Some foods are considered appropriate for certain physiologic conditions, such as pregnancy, breastfeeding, and menstruation. In Mexico, people use herbs such as lemon leaves, cloves, and cinnamon bark as medicines.

Social foods are those used for celebrations or entertaining. The meals eaten at the Chinese New Year, Thanksgiving dinner, and the Passover Seder are examples.

NUTRITION COUNSELING

More than a passing knowledge of a particular culture is necessary if health workers are to provide effective nutrition counseling. Unless health workers understand the culture, they may overlook important aspects of the diet. For example, it is important to know that pregnant Hispanic women may avoid some valuable protein foods because they believe these foods mark, or scar, the baby. It also is important to know that tortillas made from corn that has been soaked in lime water and that soups made by soaking bones in acidified broth are significant sources of calcium. In addition to having a thorough knowledge of the culture, nutrition counselors must be able to accurately evaluate the nutrient content of the ethnic diet and then provide practical and thorough recommendations that are culturally appropriate.

Health workers should support the traditional diet of the individual or family no matter how different it is from the American diet. In most cases, the traditional diet is nutritionally adequate. More often, nutritional problems arise through acculturation—when the individual begins adopting some of the food habits of the new culture. Acculturation may lead to the displacement of healthy traditional food with sugar and fats.

The Food Guide Pyramid, commonly used to plan and evaluate diets in the United States, may not be an appropriate guide when working with cultures with quite different eating habits. The United Nations Food and Agriculture Organization has developed a system that is more adaptable to the eating habits of Southeast Asians, Mexican Americans, Filipinos, and others. This classification of foods includes three groups:

1. Staple foods (rice, corn, and so on)
2. Bodybuilding (or protein) foods (legumes, tofu, eggs, seeds, fish, meat, poultry, and nuts)
3. Protective foods (fruits and vegetables)

Figure 15-1 is an example of a culturally sensitive food guide using a three-group format.

People from Cambodia, Vietnam, and other foreign lands may be unable to find or afford in the United States some of the foods they enjoyed in their homeland. They need help finding acceptable substitutes for these foods and learning the economics of food purchasing in the United States—buying fresh and locally grown produce in season. They may need help learning how to retain the nutrients in food and how to improve their nutritive intake by means acceptable to them.

In many foreign countries, raw rice is coated with an inedible substance called *talc*. The rice must be washed several times before cooking to remove this substance. Nutritional counselors should discourage washing of rice produced in the United States because the rice does not contain talc. Most of the rice in the United States is enriched; rinsing, then, would wash away valuable vitamins and iron. Also, because many people of color have a lactose intolerance and do not consume milk, it is important to know the nondairy sources of calcium within the culturally acceptable foods and to encourage their use.

CULTURAL AND RELIGIOUS EATING PATTERNS

AFRICAN AMERICANS

African Americans are the largest minority group—12% of the U.S. population. One third live in poverty. Life expectancy is lower than that of the general population and the gap has widened since the mid-1980s. African Americans experience a higher incidence of hypertension; strokes in men; cancer (especially lung cancer in men); diabetes; and the serious complications of diabetes. Overweight is a serious problem for 44% of African American women older than age 20 years. Obesity plays a major role in the incidence of both hypertension and diabetes. Infant mortality rates are twice those of the white population.

Eating habits usually reflect the part of the country from which a person comes. Although the southeastern United States includes many cultures—Cajun French, Cuban, and others—the cooking style most prevalent in and most associated with this region is the *soul food* of southern African Americans. This term is associated with foods of the South that both poor African Americans and poor whites eat. It represents not only the food but also an atmosphere of warmth, acceptance, and love. Some African Americans who have migrated to other parts of the country continue to prefer this type of food. Many African Americans, however, have the same food preferences as whites who have always lived in the North.

Pork, fish, and chicken generally are popular among African Americans. Meat from every part of the pig is used, including chops, spareribs, sausage, country ham, bacon, salt pork, jowls, neck bones, ham hocks, chitterlings (lining of the pig's stomach, which is boiled and then fried), feet, tail, and ears. Fresh vegetables generally are eaten in large quantities. Greens—mustard, turnip, collard,

(text continues on page 302)

PRENATAL CULTURAL FOOD PLAN
for Caribbeans from the English-speaking Islands

	FOOD/NUTRIENT GROUP	FOOD	SERVING SIZE	SERVINGS/DAY	ALIMENTS
GROWTH	Vegetable Protein	Kidney beans, lentils, cooked	1 c	4 or more	Pois rouge, lentils, cuit
		Pigeon peas, cow peas, cooked	1¼ c		Pois congo, Pois inconnu, cuit
		Split peas, cooked	1 c		Patte d' arachnide (mamba)
		Peanut butter	4 tbsp		Tofu
		Tofu	2 large pieces		
	Animal Protein	Eggs	2		Oeufs
		Beef, goat, pork, lamb	3 oz		Boeuf, cabrit, cochon, mouton
		Chicken, turkey, duck	3 oz		Poulet, dinde, canard
		Codfish, saltfish, mackeral, tuna	3 oz	Liver also counts as one serving of Vitamin A	Morue, poisson salé, mackereau, tuna
		Liver (beef, chicken, goat)	3 oz		Folé, (boeuf, poulet, cabrit)
	Protein/Calcium	Sardines	6 sardines	5	Sardines, poisson rose, Taza, avec les os
		Cheese	2 oz		Fromage
		Milk, yogurt	1 c		Lait, yogurt
		Evaporated milk	4 oz		Lait evaporé
	Vegetable Calcium	Callaloo, green leafy, cooked	1 c	Sardines and these vegetable foods are good for women who cannot tolerate milk products	Cresson (l'oseille), maché
		Spinach, cooked	1 c		Épinard, cuit
		Broccoli, cooked, chopped	1¼ c		Broccoli, cuit, maché
		Collard greens, cooked, chopped	1½ c		Grandes feuilles vertes, cuit, maché
PROTECTION	Vitamin C	Orange, grapefruit juice	1 c	1	Jus d' orange, chadèque, pamplemousse
		Mango, guava nectar	1 c		Jus de mango mûre, guayave
		Mango, sliced	1⅓ c		Mango mûre, morceaux
		Papaya, strawberries	1 c		Papaye, fraises
		Cabbage, shredded	2½ c		Chou, rappé
		Broccoli, cooked	¾ c		Broccoli, cuit
		Green pepper, raw	¾ c		Mandarine
					Piment vert, poivron
	Vitamin A	Dark orange squash, pumpkin	1 c	1	Giromon
		Orange sweet potato	1 medium		Patate douce jaune
		Pak choi, cooked, chopped	2 c		Épinard
		Spinach	¾ c		Carrote, jus de carotte
		Carrots, carrot juice	½ c		Mango mûre, morceaux
		Mango, slices	1½ c		Papaye
		Papaya, paw paw	1½ medium		Melon france
		Cantaloupe melon	½ melon		

Group	Category	Foods			Servings	French	
	Other Fruits & Vegetables 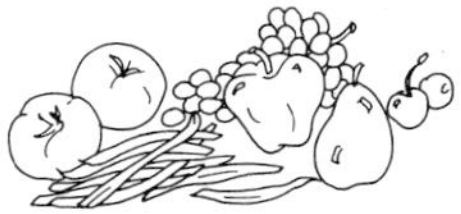	Apples, pears,	Christophine	Corn		Pomme, poires, péches	Mirliton
		peaches	(cho-cho)	Tomato		Quenépe, raisins verts	Berejen
		Guinep, grapes	Eggplant	Cucumber	1	Jus de corosol	Petit pols vert
		Soursop juice	(garden egg)	Beets		Jus de tamarin	Calalou
		Tamarind juice	Green string beans	Lettuce		Anana, melon d'eau	Oignons
		Pineapple	Yellow wax beans	Mushrooms		Aubergine	Mais
		Watermelon	Onions	Green peas			
ENERGY	Staples & Ground Provisions 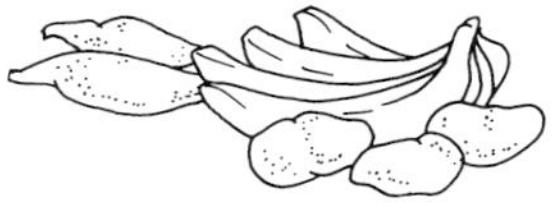	Caribbean yam	1 c			Yam blanc, patate douce	
		Caribbean sweet potato	1 c			Cassave, manioc, noix de coco	
		Cassava, coco	1 c			Banane verte mûre, banane figue mûre	
		Plantain green/ripe	1 fruit			Banane	
		Green/yellow banana	1 fruit			Veritab	
		Breadfruit	1 c			Pomme de terre	
		Irish potato	1 medium-large		4		
	Cereals 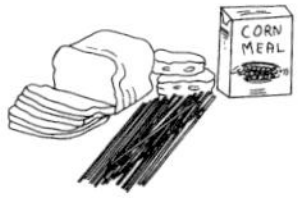	Rice, cooked	1 c			Riz, cuit	
		Bread	2 slices			Pain	
		Macaroni, spaghetti cooked	1 c			Macaroni, spaghetti, cuit	
		Cornmeal, cooked	1 c			Mais mouli, farine, avoine, cuit	
		Crackers	10 crackers			Biscuit soda	
	Fats & Oils	Avocado Butter Margarine Ghee Coconut oil Cream cheese Ackee Pork fat Mayonnaise Cooking oils					
		These fat foods and sugar foods such as Condensed milk add calories to your diet.					

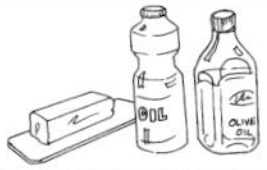

If your doctor has prescribed a vitamin or iron pill, remember to take it according to directions. An average weight gain for pregnancy is approximately 25 lb to 30 lb.

Prenatal women at especially high risk or vegetarians may need to add an extra serving of protein, calcium, and extra calories per day. A mixed and balanced diet of the above is designed to meet or exceed the 1989 US Recommended Dietary Allowances for the standard pregnant woman.

The ideas and procedures in this pamphlet should be used only with a doctor's approval and supervision; the author does not make medical diagnoses or prescribe treatment. The author and publisher make no warranties, assume no responsibility, and disclaim all liability.

(Pictures used with permission from the Caribbean Food and Nutrition Institute, Kingston Jamaica. Layout by Kevin Holder. Nutrition Education Services International, 218 9th St. NE, Washington, DC 20002.)

FIGURE 15–1.

An example of a culturally appropriate food guide using a three-group format. *(Pictures used with permission from the Caribbean Food and Nutrition Institute, Kingston Jamaica. Layout by Kevin Holder. Copyright © 1988, 1990 by Sharon Stowers, R.D. All Rights Reserved. Nutrition Education Services International, 218 9th St. NE, Washington, DC 20002.)*

and kale—are widely eaten. Stewed okra, corn, tomatoes, and cabbage also are well liked. Sweet potatoes and squash are popular pie ingredients. Oranges, melons, bananas, and peaches are favored fruits. Grits, rice, and white and sweet potatoes are the chief sources of carbohydrate. Hot breads, such as cornbread, biscuits, and muffins, take the place of yeast bread at meals. Black-eyed peas and other dried beans provide both carbohydrate and protein.

Frying is the preferred method for cooking meat, fish, and poultry. Stewing is used for some meat–vegetable combinations. Vegetables usually are boiled for a long time with fatty meat, usually some form of pork. Both the vegetable and the cooking liquid (called pot liquor) are eaten.

The intake of sweets in the form of syrups, cakes, pies, candy, soft drinks, and sweetened beverages is high. Furthermore, milk and milk products are used in limited amounts, perhaps partially because of the prevalence of lactose intolerance among this population. Buttermilk, evaporated milk, and ice cream are popular forms of milk.

Health workers should encourage a reduction in sweets, soft drinks, fats, and foods high in sodium. The use of vitamin D–enriched milk should be encouraged for children, especially those who do not frequently eat greens. Health workers should be aware of the possibility of milk intolerance, however. A person who does not use milk may be lacking in calcium and vitamin D.

Hypertension is the most prevalent chronic disease among African Americans; reducing sodium can serve as a preventive measure. This population should reduce the use of salty meats such as salt pork, ham hocks, bacon, and sausage. Furthermore, health workers should encourage consumption of fish, poultry, and dried beans rather than fatty meats and baking and broiling rather than frying. These practices would reduce the high fat level of the diet, which also is associated with cardiovascular disease.

HISPANICS

The Hispanic population is the second largest minority population in the United States—about 8% of the total population, and the fastest growing minority group. It comprises various subgroups: Mexicans, Puerto Ricans, Cubans, and peoples from other countries of Central and South America and the Caribbean. Those of Mexican and Puerto Rican ancestry make up the largest part of the Hispanic population. The health concerns of this group vary from one subgroup to another. Overweight is a common problem among Hispanics, especially among Mexican American women. The incidence of diabetes is high, especially among Puerto Ricans, Mexican Americans, and Cuban Americans.

The Hispanic meal pattern generally includes breakfast, lunch, and dinner and sometimes an afternoon snack—a pattern similar to that in the United States. People of Hispanic background living in the United States tend to maintain a Spanish lifestyle. They often keep the good habits of their country of origin while adopting some of the eating habits of the American culture. Foods eaten daily are simple, home-prepared foods such as rice, beans, soup, and starchy root vegetables.

PUERTO RICANS

Foods that Puerto Ricans frequently eat daily are rice, red kidney beans, and *viandas*. Viandas are a group of 14 or more starchy root vegetables and unripe starchy fruits with a nutritional value similar to that of potatoes. The flavors and textures of viandas vary. Dried salted codfish, lard, and coffee with milk also are part of the daily fare. Puerto Ricans may use other beans, such as garbanzo beans (chick peas) and pigeon peas, although red kidney beans are more popular. *Sofrito,* a sauce made with tomatoes, pepper, onions, garlic, herbs and spices, anato seeds, and lard is used with many foods. It serves as a basis for most cooking.

A beverage called *malta* is popular. It is made from caramel, malt extract, and sugar. Because it is thought to be nutritious, it frequently is provided for pregnant women and children; however, it actually has little nutritional value.

A typical day's meal pattern begins with a breakfast of bread and coffee with milk (half coffee, half milk). Lunch consists of rice, beans, meat, and salad. Supper is similar, usually consisting of leftovers from lunch. If rice and beans are not served, the meal usually consists of viandas served with codfish and oil or a hearty soup. In addition to liberal amounts of sugar in coffee, sweets in the form of fruit preserves are popular. Fruit usually is eaten between meals as a snack. Generally, Puerto Ricans in the United States heavily consume carbonated beverages, fried snacks, and sweets.

The basic Puerto Rican diet provides almost all of the essential nutrients. Greater variety in food selection should be encouraged, including the use of deep yellow and deep green leafy vegetables. More frequent use of lowfat cheese would improve the calcium level. Using milk liberally in coffee and preparing cooked cereals with milk should be encouraged, as well as replacing the use of lard with unsaturated vegetable oil.

Many Puerto Ricans buy food every day in the Spanish stores, which carry familiar foods. Using canned tomatoes and canned or frozen fruits and juices when fresh fruits and vegetables are out of season, using inexpensive cuts of meat, and buying all but the special Puerto Rican foods at the supermarket help to stretch the food budget.

MEXICANS

Dry beans, chili peppers, and corn or wheat *tortillas*—thin, flat, unleavened bread cooked on a hot griddle—are staple items in the Mexican American diet. Pinto, calico, and garbanzo are the varieties of beans most commonly eaten. Chili peppers, from mild to hot, are used as both vegetables and seasoning. Mexican Americans of limited income use meat, fish, and poultry sparingly, combined with peppers and other foods in main dishes. Stewed tomatoes and tomato puree are common ingredients. Most foods are fried. Lard, the preferred fat, is used liberally.

Corn has been the basic cereal. Mexicans make a stiff dough, called *masa,* from dried corn that has been soaked in lime water. From this dough they make tortillas. The lime-treated dough is a source of appreciable amounts of calcium. This is an especially important aspect of the diet, because Mexican Americans drink little milk. Wheat is gradually replacing corn in the making of tortillas, thus reducing the calcium intake.

Enchiladas, tamales, tacos, and chili con carne are popular Mexican-American dishes. Enchiladas are made by rolling tortillas with a filling of cheese, onion, and shredded lettuce. Tacos are tortillas folded with a filling of ground meat in a highly seasoned sauce and shredded lettuce. Tamales are made of corn dough and ground meat wrapped in corn husks and steamed. Chili con carne consists of beef seasoned with garlic, beans, and chili peppers.

Vegetables such as potatoes, pumpkin, greens, onions, and carrots sometimes are used. Bananas, melons, peaches, and canned fruit cocktail are the most commonly used fruits.

Sugar and sweets are used liberally. Candy, soda pop, and sweet rolls are popular. French fries and other deep fat-fried foods add additional fat to a diet already high in fat.

The basic pattern of beans, chili peppers, and breads made of corn is nutritionally good and forms a sound foundation on which to build. Increased use of economical cuts of meat should be encouraged. Tortillas should be retained in preference to sweet rolls.

More milk and lowfat cheese would greatly improve the protein quality and the calcium content of the diet. Calcium is especially important if wheat is used in making tortillas. Health workers should encourage the addition of green and yellow vegetables and increased use of tomatoes, potatoes, and inexpensive sources of vitamin C, such as canned and frozen citrus fruits and juices. The Mexican culture has greatly influenced the diet of Americans living along the Mexican border.

SALVADORANS

Plantains, a bananalike fruit, are a popular food in the diets of people from El Salvador. Plantains usually are fried. Boiling or baking can be suggested as a means of reducing fat in the diet. The Salvadoran diet contains many fried foods and is high in total fat.

GENERAL CONSIDERATIONS

Hispanics tend to prefer soda pop, fruit drinks, and coffee to milk. Health workers should suggest ways of improving calcium intake as discussed earlier.

Greater variety in the selection of vegetables would improve the vitamin A content of the diet.

Dark green and yellow vegetables frequently are lacking. Chilies, carrots, and avocados are well liked and are good sources of vitamin A. Some of the viandas, such as sweet potatoes and yams, also are foods rich in vitamin A.

The Hispanic diet may have a high sugar content. A baked sweet bread called *pan dulce* may be eaten more than once a day. French bread sometimes is an acceptable substitute.

There is a high incidence of obesity in the Hispanic population. Many individuals may be unaware of the large quantity of food they are eating. Sometimes a large quantity of tortillas is consumed at a meal because they are used as utensils, with the food placed or wrapped in the tortilla.

Viandas, such as plantains, are calorically dense, especially when fried. These, also, frequently are eaten in excessive quantities. Obesity is a risk factor for noninsulin-dependent diabetes. This may explain the high incidence of diabetes among Hispanics.

ASIANS AND PACIFIC ISLANDERS

Asians and Pacific Islanders represent the third largest minority group, numbering more than 11 million. This group is diverse, with more than 30 different languages and cultures represented. About three fourths of this population are immigrants, mostly from Southeast Asia. The health status of those who have been in the United States for generations is the same as that of the general population. Furthermore, the median income is higher; however, some subgroups, especially recent immigrants, are extremely poor. Data about the leading causes of death, disease, and disability are lacking for the many subgroups. The incidence of two infectious diseases—tuberculosis and hepatitis B—is high. Hepatitis B is associated with chronic liver disease, cirrhosis, and liver cancer.

CHINESE

The eating habits of Chinese Americans differ according to the part of China from which they came. China is divided into five regions, each with its own style of cooking:

1. *Canton*—Low in fat, uses herbs and thin soy sauce
2. *Szechwan*—Contains many sweet and hot dishes
3. *Hunan*—Contains many sweet and sour dishes
4. *Fukien*—Relies heavily on fish
5. *Shantung*—Uses scallions, leeks, and garlic

Rice is the staple cereal in southern China, whereas wheat, corn, and millet seed are used in the north. These grains and, in some areas, sweet potatoes provide the chief source of calories.

Most of the Americans of Chinese descent in California have eating habits similar to those of Canton, in southern China. The pattern includes three meals a day. Rice is the staple grain. Clients should be advised not to wash or rinse enriched rice before or after cooking to avoid losing water-soluble nutrients. Milk is not widely used. Fruits usually are eaten fresh; desserts are not traditionally a part of the meal.

Meat is eaten in small quantities and usually is mixed with vegetables. Pork, lamb, chicken, duck, fish, and shellfish are favored. Almost every part of the animal is used, including the brain, spinal cord, internal organs, skin, and blood. Blood pudding (coagulated blood) is inexpensive and is eaten frequently. Beef is not commonly eaten. Soybeans are plentiful and are an important source of protein. Eggs are well liked.

In China, soybean milk, soybean cheese, and, in some areas, water buffalo milk are used. Milk consumption is low in all regions of China. There is a prevalence of lactose intolerance among the Chinese. If milk is not drunk, soybean curd or tofu, soybeans, and greens should be eaten to increase calcium intake. Soybean curd contains 128 mg of calcium per 3.5 oz. It can be added to soups or vegetable stir-fries or eaten as is, either raw or fried. A fish soup is prepared that uses the whole fish, including the bone. It has a high calcium content and traditionally is served after pregnancy. Because of the low milk consumption, vitamin D and riboflavin intake also may be low. A vitamin D supplement may be needed for pregnant women, infants, and children.

Generally, foods are cooked quickly on top of the stove by stir-frying, boiling, or steaming.

Although roasting is an acceptable method of food preparation, ovens rarely are used for the traditional diet. Food preparation—trimming, chopping, and slicing meats and vegetables—is time-consuming.

A large variety of vegetables are eaten, including cabbage, cucumbers, greens, bamboo shoots, bean sprouts, mushrooms, and sweet potatoes. Vegetables are prepared in a manner that preserves their nutritional value. They are cooked for a short time in a little oil, and then a bit of water is added. The cooking liquid is served with the vegetable.

Lard and soybean, sesame, and peanut oils are used in cooking. Soy sauce, which is highly salted, accompanies almost every meal. Tea is the most popular beverage.

Because of the seasonings and sauces used, the sodium content of the diet is high (Display 15-3 lists the sodium content of some Chinese condiments). Health workers must address this issue when counseling clients for whom a sodium-controlled diet has been prescribed.

Some Chinese and other cultural groups with roots in Eastern religion or philosophy believe in a yin–yang theory, which requires balancing the intake of foods, as discussed earlier.

DISPLAY 15-3 SODIUM CONTENT OF COMMONLY USED CHINESE CONDIMENTS

CONDIMENT	SODIUM/TSP (MG)*
Dark soy sauce	380
Light soy sauce	429
Hoisan sauce	160
Hot bean sauce	298
Sweet bean sauce	160
Fermented black bean	112
Shrimp sauce	412
Oyster sauce	261
Chinese brown or red vinegar	36

* Source of nutritive values: Chew T. Sodium values of Chinese condiments and their use in sodium-restricted diets. J. Am Diet Assoc 1983:82:398. Values are averages of brands given.

FILIPINOS

Filipino food customs are a blend of Chinese and Spanish influences. The typical meal pattern consists of breakfast, lunch, a light afternoon meal, and dinner. The entire family gathers at the evening meal, which is the heaviest. This pattern is retained in the United States with the exception of the afternoon snack—usually a sweet food and beverage—which may be inconvenient.

The Filipino diet contains a variety of protein foods, vegetables, and fruit. Rice is a staple food, eaten at every meal. Sugar is added to foods liberally. Not much milk is consumed.

The protein foods include fresh and cured meat, fish, eggs, nuts, and legumes. Meat is boiled, fried, or roasted. Organ meats are popular and are the principal ingredients in a traditional dish called *bachoy*. It is made of kidney, tongue, liver, and pork. Eggs are eaten every day. Soy sauce and anchovy sauce are used liberally.

The Filipino diet is high in sodium and cholesterol. When the diet needs to be modified in these components, nutrition counselors must help their clients find acceptable alternatives to favorite foods.

For those who are not lactose intolerant, the consumption of milk should be encouraged. Adding more milk to coffee may be an acceptable means of increasing milk consumption. Many Filipinos begin drinking coffee as children. The excessive use of sugar is a problem, especially if the client has diabetes. The use of a sugar substitute may be an acceptable alternative.

SOUTHEAST ASIANS

Southeast Asians (Hmong, Cambodians, Vietnamese, and Laotians) have eating habits that differ considerably from those of their new country. Two types of meal patterns are followed. In the most common pattern, two meals a day are eaten, the first at 9 or 10 AM and the second at 3 or 4 PM. Other Southeast Asian families eat three meals a day, with breakfast at 6 or 7 AM, dinner at 12 or 1 PM and supper at 6 or 7 PM. The midday meal is the largest and most important meal of the day. The family does not necessarily eat together, especially the morning and evening meals. The food is prepared and family members serve themselves over a period of 1 to 3 hours. Parents are flexible regarding the timing of children's meals. Substantial nutritious snacks for young children should be encouraged.

Rice is the staple food for Southeast Asians. It is the main source of energy in the diet and provides a significant amount of protein. Rice is served at every meal and is eaten in large quantities—1 cup to $1\frac{1}{2}$ cups for children and 1 to 3 cups for adults.

Other rice products that are used include rice noodles, rice sticks, and rice papers wrapped around meats. Cereal products that have been well accepted by Southeast Asians in the United States are French bread, ready-to-eat cereals, and pasta products such as ramen noodles and spaghetti.

Bodybuilding foods that may not have been eaten in any substantial quantity in their homeland because of their high cost and limited availability are well accepted in the United States. These include pork, chicken, eggs, tofu, organ meats, and peanuts. In Southeast Asia, milk rarely is consumed after infancy; therefore, dairy products, including cheese, are not well accepted. Fish and soybean products are good sources of calcium and protein. Fish and many types of seafood were eaten daily by Cambodians, Vietnamese, and some Laotians in their native countries. Other foods contributing calcium include tofu, sardines, mung beans, and soybeans. When milk and cheese are not consumed, the use of traditional foods high in calcium should be encouraged.

The wide variety of fruits and vegetables available in their native countries may be unavailable or unaffordable in the United States. Vegetables that are similar to those of their homeland and are inexpensive are well accepted, including all types of cabbage, dark leafy greens, broccoli, and green beans. Most of these vegetables also contribute significant amounts of calcium. Vegetables are purchased fresh and then chopped or stir-fried with protein foods and seasonings. They are not served as a side dish. To make fruits and vegetables more affordable, clients should be encouraged to buy fruits and vegetables that are in season or locally grown and to start their own garden, if possible.

The style of cooking differs in each region of Southeast Asia because of different cultural influences on the various countries. Vietnamese cooking has been influenced by the Chinese who live in Vietnam and by the French. Every family has a unique cooking style. This is a source of pride among the Vietnamese. In Cambodia, the influence of Indian cuisine is seen in currylike dishes. Cambodian and Vietnamese food is quite spicy, whereas Hmong cooking is relatively plain.

American sweets and snacks are foods Southeast Asians equate with affluence because they were expensive in their homelands. Soft drinks are consumed in large quantities at the expense of more nutritious beverages. Other popular sweets and snack foods are doughnuts, cookies, candy, ice cream, and chips. The differences in the nutritional value of soda pop, fruit drinks, and 100% fruit juice should be explained. Suggestions should be made for nutritious snacks.

ALASKA NATIVES AND AMERICAN INDIANS

The descendants of the original inhabitants of North America now compose the smallest of the defined minority groups in the United States, numbering 1.6 million. This population group comprises numerous tribes and more than 500 federally recognized groups that live on reservations and in small rural communities, each with its own traditions and cultural heritage. In addition, large numbers live in metropolitan areas. Educational levels and income are low, with 25% living below the poverty level. Eskimos, Aleuts, and Indians residing in Alaska are referred to as Alaska Natives. Those living in other states are referred to as American Indians (or Native Americans). Although substantial differences exist, these tribes share such characteristics as a spiritual attachment to the land, a commitment to sharing and hospitality, and a determination to retain their culture.

Health is perceived as a state in which the entire body is in balance. Many continue in the tradition of their ancestors to rely in times of illness on medicine men and women, on herbalists, and on treatments that includes healing and purification ceremonies, teas, herbs, special foods, and therapeutic sings.

This population is young compared with the U.S. population as a whole, undoubtedly because of the shorter life span. Most of the excess deaths—those that would not have occurred if American Indian death rates were comparable to those of the total population—can be traced to six causes. Four of these causes of death—(1) unintentional injuries, (2) cirrhosis, (3) suicide, and (4) homicide—are alcohol related. The other two causes are pneumonia and complications of diabetes. Diabetes is very prevalent. In many tribes, the incidence of diabetes is more than 20%, and among two tribes, it is 40%. American Indians have a higher incidence of diabetes and cirrhosis than the general population. Alcoholism and obesity are the two outstanding risk factors.

ALASKA NATIVES

The diet of the Alaska Native has traditionally been a high-protein, high-fat diet. Traditional foods include fish, sea mammals, and game. Fish eggs and bird eggs also are consumed. Seaweed, wild greens, and berries are some of the few edible plants. Sources of fat, depending on geographical location, include sea mammals, wild game, fish, seal oil, whale blubber, and fish oil. Boiling is the traditional food preparation method. Alaska Natives living in small native communities continue to follow many of the traditional food practices. In the 1700s and 1800s, beef and pork and the use of sugars and starches were introduced by Asians and Europeans.

Alaska Natives presently obtain more of their foods from grocery stores, a trend encouraged by federal programs such as food stamps, school lunch, and the Special Supplemental Food Program for Women, Infants, and Children (WIC). Imported foods are expensive.

Fish and shellfish consumption remains high. Other protein sources include eggs, chicken, frankfurters, ham, and luncheon meats. Not much beef is consumed. Dried peas and beans are unpopular. Game meats are eaten more often in the winter. Frozen dinners and entrees are popular.

Canned vegetables and fruits are eaten more frequently than fresh because of availability. The daily average consumption of fruits and vegetables is only two servings. Sources of carbohydrate include sugar, white bread, rice, *pilot bread* (large round dense crackers), pancakes, and cooked cereals.

Adults consume little milk. When used, milk is usually evaporated or nonfat dry milk. Fresh milk is expensive. Children and young adults consume soda pop, powdered juice mixes, and punch-type drinks. Chips and candies are popular. A high percentage of carbohydrate in the diet comes from sugars. Major sources of fat include fish, *agutuk* (Eskimo ice cream), beef fat, seal oil, whale blubber, chicken fat, butter, and margarine. The ingredients in agutuk are berries, hydrogenated vegetable shortening (or caribou tallow), and sugar.

Meals are not necessarily eaten in a regularly scheduled manner. Midday and evening snacking are common.

The use of fish, lean game, berries, greens, and seaweed should be encouraged. The nutritional content of the diet could be improved by adding more fruits and vegetables, substituting whole-grain breads for white bread, and reducing sweets, fats, and cured meats.

AMERICAN INDIANS

As with the Alaska Natives, foods and methods of preparation differ among the American Indians according to what can be grown, harvested, hunted, or fished in the region in which they live and the proximity to grocery stores and restaurants, including fast-food outlets. Traditional foods, prepared somewhat differently from region to region, include fry bread, mutton stew, corn soup, fish chowder, and beans. Corn is used in many ways—for bread, hominy, in soups and stews, and ground to form a thickener for stews and drinks.

An example of American Indian food habits are those of the Navajos. Their traditional foods consist of corn, mutton, wild vegetables and fruits, nuts and seeds, and some cultivated foods, in addition to corn, such as cantaloupe, watermelon, beans, and squash. Traditional corn products include tortillas or fry bread, corn hominy, dried corn silk, and blue cornbread.

Some Navajo Indians continue to live primarily off the land. Many low-income families receive food stamps or participate in the Food Distribution Program on Indian Reservations. The Food Distribution Program makes available, monthly, such foods as canned meat, canned fruits and vegetables, nonfat dry milk, flour, oil, and corn syrup. Mutton continues to be the preferred meat. Many people eat meat, poultry, or smoked or processed meat at least once a day. Bread in the form of tortillas or fry bread is a staple food. Coffee is popular among adults; soda pop and sugar-sweetened drinks are consumed regularly by all age groups. Other foods consumed year-round include eggs, potatoes, green beans, tomatoes, corn, apples, oranges, and canned fruit. Frying is a common method of preparation. Lard is a frequently used fat.

Reservation communities now have large supermarkets, convenience stores, and restaurants. Greater access to convenience foods has led to increased consumption of foods high in fat, sugar, sodium, and total energy content. The high intake of fats, sweets, and snack foods among children is of particular concern.

JEWS

The dietary laws of Judaism, called the *rules of kashruth,* are based on tradition and the Bible. They date back to biblical times and are complex. Foods prepared and selected in accordance with these rules are called *kosher foods.* Foods that are nonkosher are called *trayf.* The degree to which these regulations are followed by American Jews depends on whether they belong to Orthodox, Conservative, or Reform Judaism. Orthodox Jews greatly value these practices and follow them under all conditions. Conservative Jews usually observe the laws in their own homes but accept changes outside the home. Reform Jews place less importance on the dietary laws.

The dietary laws are concerned with three areas: (1) the selection and slaughtering of animals and fowl, (2) forbidden foods, and (3) the mixing of foods. Only animals that have split hooves and chew their cuds are kosher. This includes cattle, sheep, goats, and deer. Fowl must be known by tradition to be kosher; kosher fowl include chicken, duck, white goose, pigeon, and turkey. Food from pigs, wild game birds, birds of prey, and rabbit are not allowed. Permitted animals and fowl must be slaughtered by a *schochet,* a man trained in the precise methods taught by the code of Jewish law. The procedure must be supervised by a rabbi. The permissible parts of the animals must be *koshered* before cooking, which involves draining the blood from the carcass, soaking the carcass in water with coarse salt, and then draining and rinsing the meat.

Only fish that have both fins and scales are kosher. Shellfish as well as many common fish are not kosher. Fish is not required to undergo the koshering process.

All dairy products must be from a kosher animal. They may contain no nonkosher substances and no meat products, such as renin or gelatin, which may be found in products such as cheese and ice cream.

Meat and dairy products may not be combined. Six hours must elapse after eating meat before eating dairy products, and at least 30 minutes to 1 hour after eating dairy products before eating meat. Separate sets of dishes, pots, and cutlery must be maintained for meat and dairy meals. Foods containing milk products such as whey, lactose, nonfat milk solids, and casein cannot be used with meat products. For example, bread made with whey or nonfat milk solids cannot be used in a meat meal. Usually, two meals a day are dairy meals and one is a meat meal.

Foods that contain no meat or dairy products, or foods made from sources other than meat or dairy are considered *pareve* (neutral). They may be combined with either meat or dairy. Pareve foods include permitted fish, fruits, vegetables, grains, eggs, and most drinks and juices. Eggs must contain no blood spots.

Processed foods, including vegetable oils, are considered kosher only if they have a statement on the label certifying reliable rabbinic supervision. Any beverage containing grape products also must have this certification.

Legumes, fish, and dairy products are well liked. Many favorite foods such as corned beef, smoked meats, herring, lox (salted, smoked salmon), and relishes are highly salted. The Jewish diet may be rich in fats and in sweets such as pastries, cake, and preserves. The use of more green vegetables and fruits should be stressed. In homes in which the dietary laws are strictly observed, children may lack the recommended amount of milk. In such cases, the use of more milk should be encouraged.

A hospital or other health care facility that prepares and serves food according to the Jewish dietary laws requires special facilities and equipment, including two separate kitchens, one for dairy and one for nondairy foods. In other health facilities, the needs of the client who follows the Jewish dietary laws may possibly be met by cooking foods in foil, using disposable dishes and silverware, and using frozen kosher dinners. Health workers should meet with the client and family to determine how best to meet the client's needs.

MUSLIMS

Muslim dietary laws are based on Islamic teachings in the Koran. Food permitted by law for Muslims to eat is termed *hala'l*. The dietary laws of the Muslims apply mainly to meat, pork and pork products, and alcoholic beverages. These laws require that meat be slaughtered in the name of Allah in a prescribed manner. Muslims may choose to eat kosher meat, eliminate the use of meat entirely and possibly substitute fish, or do their own slaughtering. Some Muslims eat meat slaughtered by Jews or Christians and invoke the name of Allah before eating it.

Pork and all pork products as well as alcohol and any product containing alcohol are strictly forbidden. This includes flavoring extracts such as vanilla, which contains alcohol, and any drugs and cosmetics containing either alcohol or a product derived from pigs.

Among the customs of the Muslim people is a 30-day period of prayers and fasting during Ramadan, Islam's holy month. Ramadan is the 9th month of the Islamic lunar year. During Ramadan, Muslims consume no food or drink from dawn to sunset. Pregnant women are exempt from fasting during Ramadan, but must fast later. In a study of 34 pregnant Muslim women in England, 35% chose to fast with their families rather than make up the time later.

VEGETARIANS

In recent years, interest in vegetarian diets has increased. This trend has been an outgrowth of the unprecedented interest in personal health habits, which has led Americans to adopt healthier diets and exercise patterns. A considerable amount of research points to a positive relation between the vegetarian diet and risk reduction for a number of chronic diseases and conditions. These include obesity, coronary artery disease, hypertension, non-insulin–dependent diabetes, and colon cancer. In addition to diet, other lifestyle characteristics of vegetarians, such as maintaining desirable weight, exercise, and abstinence from smoking, alcohol, and drugs, may also be responsible for these beneficial effects. In addition to health benefits, other considerations—ecologic, economic, philosophic, or ethical—may lead individuals to vegetarianism.

The vegetarian diet, like the nonvegetarian diet, can be a healthy, adequate diet when well planned. The greater the variety of foods included, the greater the probability that the diet is adequate. There are various types of vegetarian diets; the most common are as follows:

Semivegetarian—Includes dairy products, eggs, and fish; excludes red meat and possibly poultry

Lacto-ovovegetarian—Includes eggs and dairy products; excludes meat, poultry, and fish

Lactovegetarian—Includes dairy products; excludes meat, fish, poultry, and eggs

Vegan—Excludes all food of animal origin, including dairy products, eggs, meat, fish, and poultry

A variation of the vegan diet is the multistage Zen macrobiotic diet, which progressively excludes animal products, fruits, vegetables, and cereals. At the highest level, the diet consists primarily of a whole grain, usually brown rice. The final stages of the diet are grossly lacking essential nutrients and can lead to severe malnutrition if followed for a prolonged period.

Adequate amounts of high-quality protein are not difficult to obtain in diets that contain dairy products and eggs. The body's need for essential amino acids also can be met by plant sources of protein alone. Plant protein can provide both essential and nonessential amino acids, assuming that there is a reasonable variety of plant sources and that caloric intake is sufficient to meet energy needs. After amino acids are absorbed, they combine with other amino acids in the body's protein pool. These other amino acids come from the continual turnover of protein in the body—tissues being broken down and rebuilt. Although plant proteins contain less of the essential amino acids than an equal amount of animal protein, plant foods provide adequate amounts of essential amino acids when a variety of foods are eaten daily. Proteins from grains, legumes, nuts, seeds, and vegetables complement each other so that the shortcomings in one protein are made up by another. Some soy protein products are equivalent in value to animal proteins and can serve as the sole source of protein in the diet. See Chapter 10 under Amino Acid Composition. Proteins that complement each other should be consumed over the course of the day. It is unnecessary to match precisely complementary proteins at each meal.

Although the vegetarian diet meets the recommended dietary allowance for protein, it usually provides less protein than the nonvegetarian diet. This is not necessarily a disadvantage, because there are no known advantages to the excessive protein intake typical of the American diet. A diet lower in protein usually is lower in fat. Such a diet may decrease the risk of osteoporosis, because protein increases the excretion of calcium and may improve kidney function in people with kidney damage.

A daily food guide for vegetarians (Display 15-4) includes the following food groups: breads, cereals, rice, and pasta; vegetables; legumes and other meat substitutes; and fruits. Dairy products and eggs are optional. Fats and sugars should be used sparingly. A sample vegetarian menu for one day is given in Display 14-6. Legumes are a necessary food in the diet of the strict vegetarian. Legume protein is needed to balance the protein in grains so that all of the essential amino acids are provided (see Chapter 10 under Amino Acid Composition and Complementarity). Some vegetarians use meat analogues. These are products made from textured vegetable protein (frequently soybean) that resemble and taste like various meat, poultry, and fish products.

Vegetarians should use a wide variety of foods, including whole-grain products, nuts, seeds, legumes, lowfat dairy products or fortified soy dairy substitutes, and a limited number of eggs. Foods with a low nutritive value should be kept to a minimum. Whole-grain products should be used instead of refined foods. Including a food rich in vitamin C at each meal enhances iron absorption.

Vegans need to pay closer attention to planning than other vegetarians to avoid deficiencies. Although it is possible to develop a well-balanced vegan diet, a diet that contains no animal foods at all may be low in calories and in some essential vitamins and minerals. This is of greatest concern for people with special needs, such as infants and children, pregnant and breastfeeding women, and people recovering from illness. Consultation with a registered dietitian or other qualified nutrition professional is recommended.

Vitamin B_{12} is found in all animal foods. Vegans should take a supplement or use vitamin B_{12}-fortified foods, such as some brands of soybean milk, commercial breakfast cereals, and some brands of nutritional yeast. The vitamin B_{12} in fortified foods, however, may not be provided in sufficient quantity.

Because milk and cheese are excluded from the vegan's diet, careful planning is necessary to obtain adequate amounts of calcium from vegetable sources. Broccoli, collard greens, mustard greens, and kale are good sources of calcium, as is tofu. Dried beans, oranges, cabbage, and pumpkin contain small amounts of calcium. Calcium absorption appears to be hindered by such substances in plant foods as phytic acid, oxalic acid, and fiber. This action may not be significant, however, because some studies have indicated that vegetarians absorb and retain more calcium than nonvegetarians. Incorporating fortified soybean milk in the diet is recommended, especially for children.

Obtaining enough vitamin D is another concern for the vegan, because fortified milk is the best

DISPLAY 15-4 FOOD GUIDE FOR VEGETARIANS

FOOD GROUP	SUGGESTED DAILY SERVINGS	SERVING SIZES
Bread, cereals, rice, and pasta	6 or more	1 slice bread 1/2 bun, bagel, or English muffin 1/2 cup cooked cereal, rice, or pasta 1 oz dry cereal
Vegetables	4 or more	1/2 cup cooked or 1 cup raw
Legumes and other meat substitutes	2 to 3	1/2 cup cooked beans 4 oz tofu or tempeh 8 oz soy milk 2 tbsp nuts or seeds (these tend to be high in fat, so use sparingly if you are following a lowfat diet)
Fruits	3 or more	1 piece fresh fruit 3/4 cup fruit juice 1/2 cup canned or cooked fruit
Dairy products	Optional—up to 3 servings daily	1 cup lowfat or skim milk 1 cup lowfat or nonfat yogurt 1 1/2 oz lowfat cheese
Eggs	Optional—limit to 3 to 4 yolks per week	1 egg or 2 egg whites
Fats, sweets, and alcohol	Go easy on these foods and beverages	Oil, margarine, and mayonnaise Cakes, cookies, pies, pastries, and candies Beer, wine, and distilled spirits

(Daily food guide for vegetarians. In: Eating well—the vegetarian way. Chicago, American Dietetic Association, 1992.)

source. Vitamin D supplements may be necessary, especially for infants, children, pregnant women, and residents of northern climates.

Zinc is found in nuts, legumes, and grains. Plant sources of iron include legumes, dried fruit, green leafy vegetables, and whole-grain and fortified breads and cereals. The iron in plant foods is not as well absorbed as that in animal foods. Absorption can be improved, however, by including foods rich in vitamin C at all meals.

The feeding of infants in vegan families is of particular concern to health workers. If breastfeeding is impossible, a nutritionally adequate soybean formula should be provided. This formula or soybean milk fortified with vitamin B_{12} should to be given by cup after the child is weaned. A wide variety of foods should be chosen, with emphasis on those that are high in iron and vitamins A, B complex, and C. In addition to soybean milk, mixtures of legumes and cereals are needed to supply sufficient protein.

Overall, vitamin D, calcium, iron, vitamin B_{12}, and possibly zinc need particular attention in diets that contain no animal foods at all. Supplements may be needed to meet recommended levels.

NONTRADITIONAL FOOD CHOICES

FOOD FADS

Food faddism is a strong force involving expenditures of billions of dollars in the United States yearly. Fear makes many people susceptible to faddism—fear of death, fear of mental or physical problems, or fear of losing physical strength. Underlying these motives are needs such as stability, acceptance, independence, and self-worth. To work effectively with persons prone to faddism, health workers must understand and respect these needs.

Food fads fall into four general categories: (1) those claiming that specific foods can prevent or cure disease; (2) those that omit certain foods because of their supposed harmful properties; (3) those emphasizing so-called natural foods; and (4) those involving diets for certain conditions, such as obesity and arthritis. The most acute problem created by food fads is that the false promises of superior health and cures for disease may cause people with serious disorders to delay seeking competent medical care.

Knowing the facts about nutrition can help health personnel recognize misinformation. Food fallacies often are formulated by pseudoscientists, who take bits of information from scientific papers and put them into a context that suits their purposes but changes the original meaning. Health workers should be suspicious of material that presents nutrition as a cure-all for serious disease or makes exaggerated claims for certain nutrients taken in high doses. (See the discussion of nutrition claims in Key Issues at the end of the chapter.)

ORGANICALLY GROWN FOODS

Organically grown foods are foods that are produced without the use of agricultural chemicals, such as pesticides, fertilizers, and herbicides. The Center for Science in the Public Interest, a consumer advocate group, is advising its followers to reduce their risk of harmful chemicals in food by using organically grown foods. This is easier said than done. The federal government has no regulations governing organically grown foods. Some states have enacted organic certification programs; most, however, do not have laws that even define what *organic* means. In states that do have laws, the definition of organic differs. For example, California requires that food cannot be called organic unless 1 year has passed from the last time the field was chemically treated. Minnesota requires a lapse of 3 years. Some states do not specify any time lapse at all.

Even with government protection, organic foods may be contaminated with traces of pesticides. Some pesticide residues remain in the soil for years; pesticides also can be blown by the wind from pesticide-treated fields to organic crops. Another concern is that organic fertilizers may contain pathogenic bacteria. The cost of organically grown foods is 20% to 100% higher than nonorganic foods.

Organically grown foods are not more nutritious or better tasting. To what extent people are protecting their health by using organic foods is unknown. Consumers, however, should have the right to purchase organic foods if they want to and to have some assurance that the food has indeed been produced organically. The establishment of organic certification programs in all states should be supported.

NATURAL FOODS

The term *natural foods* usually refers to foods in their original state or those that have undergone minimal refinement or processing, with no artificial substances added. Raw sugar, honey, brown rice, and stone-ground wheat are examples of so-called natural foods. These foods are good sources of trace minerals. However, they do not possess the miracle or curative properties sometimes attributed to them. Furthermore, the natural food movement has led to an increased demand for certified raw milk; however, this milk may not be absolutely safe from disease-causing organisms.

Many of the so-called natural vitamin preparations are made in part of synthetic vitamins. Synthetic B vitamins may be added to yeast, or synthetic ascorbic acid may be added to preparations made from natural rose hips. Consumers must read labels carefully.

The term *health foods* usually refers to specific foods thought to have special health-giving prop-

DISPLAY 15-5 EXAMPLE OF HEALTH CLAIMS MADE FOR DIETARY SUPPLEMENTS

PRODUCTS	CLAIMS	COMMENTS
Ma huang	Boosts energy; causes weight reduction	Derived from an evergreen plant; reported adverse effects include high blood pressure, rapid heart beat, nerve damage, muscle injury, stroke, memory loss, psychosis
Shark cartilage	Anti-inflammatory agent—reduces inflammation of joints and stiffness due to injury; protects against cancer	Claims never confirmed by clinical tests
Yohimbe	Body building "Enhanced male performance"	Tree bark; kidney failure, seizures and death have been reported to the Food and Drug Administration (FDA); currently under investigation
Ginseng	Increases energy and sexual desire Cures cancer and other diseases	Preparation made from root of ginseng plant; no proven benefits; prolonged use may produce the following symptoms: hypertension, nervousness, insomnia, skin eruptions, edema, and diarrhea

erties. These foods often are purchased in health food stores and may be promoted as preventing or curing disease.

Lecithin, kelp, bee pollen, ginkgo biloba, sea salt, and germanium are examples of health foods. Many of the substances are harmless, but some have potentially toxic properties. Some typical health foods and the claims made about them are given in Display 15-5.

The individual has a choice of what foods to eat; health workers should respect this choice. The public should be protected, however, from claims that health foods are cure-alls for the dreaded diseases of our time.

KEY ISSUES

How Reliable are Health Claims?

Since ancient times, belief in the curative or almost mystical properties of certain foods or substances has existed. This belief has been reinforced recently by reports from highly respected health authorities, such as the surgeon general and the National Academy of Sciences, that certain components of the diet appear to promote chronic diseases, whereas others are protective (see Chapter 14). The current emphasis on health promotion also has attracted those who see this situation as an opportunity for lucrative businesses. The dietary supplement business now exceeds $4 billion. All manner of tailor-made products and systems have been promoted to resist or cure disease, improve overall well-being, or slow the aging process.

Dietary supplements in the marketplace include vitamins; essential minerals; protein; amino acids; botanicals (plant products) such as ginseng and yohimbe; extracts from animal glands; garlic extract; fish oil; fibers such as acacia and guar gum; compounds not generally recognized as foods or nutrients, such as bioflavinoids, enzymes, germanium, nucleic acids, *para*-aminobenzoic acid, and rutin; and mixtures of these substances. These supplements come in capsules, tablets, liquids, or powders. They are sold to prevent or cure whatever disease or condition is eluding the medical profession. Sometimes the product name gives more than a subtle hint about the condition for which it is intended: Fat-Burner, Menstrual-Ease, Immune-Guard.

POTENTIALLY UNSAFE DIETARY SUPPLEMENTS

The potential for danger in the use of vitamin and essential mineral supplements is generally well known because scientists have a considerable amount of knowledge about the toxic effects of these nutrients (see Chapters 11 and 12). However, the general population may not be sufficiently aware of the seriousness of the problem. For example, excessive ingestion of high-potency iron tablets is the most common cause of child poisoning deaths in the United States, resulting in about 2000 poisonings a year. Continuous high intakes of vitamin A can cause liver damage and, during pregnancy, birth defects.

The main concern of the Food and Drug Administration (FDA), however, is the tremendous assortment of other products—such as amino acids, herbs, and botanicals. Little is known about these products and none of them has been evaluated for safety. In many cases, the harmful effects have been discovered only after the fact.

In 1989, the FDA called for the voluntary recall of L-tryptophan, an essential amino acid promoted as a cure for sleeplessness and pain relief. In November 1989, supplements of L-tryptophan were linked to a rare blood disorder, eosinophilia-myalgia (EMS). That same month, the FDA banned the sale of L-tryptophan and any product in which it is the main ingredient. More than 1500 cases including 38 deaths resulted from L-tryptophan ingestion. Although initial studies reported that an impurity in the product caused the blood disorder, the exact cause is uncertain. Cases of EMS have occurred with the use of a compound similar to L-tryptophan but not associated with the impurities in manufacturing. It is now believed that L-tryptophan itself plays a role in causing EMS.

An enormous array of worthless substances have been sold, many of which are potentially harmful. (See Display 15-5 for a list of the more popular dietary supplements, the health claims made about them, and the potential for harm.)

DEATH KNELL FOR FRAUDULENT HEALTH CLAIMS?

In December 1993, the FDA announced regulations setting standards to ensure that the labeling of dietary supplements is truthful and scientifically sound. The regulations state that health claims will be authorized only if there is significant scientific agreement among qualified experts that these claims are valid. The health claim standard took effect in July 1994. (See Chapter 12 on the rules regarding nutrition labeling and nutrient content of dietary supplements, which became effective in July 1995.) The new rules require vitamins, minerals, herbs, or other similar nutritional substances to be subject to the general requirements for health claims that already apply to conventional food. Only two health claims for dietary supplements have been authorized by the FDA: (1) folate and the risk of neural tube birth defects and (2) the claim for calcium and osteoporosis.

The effectiveness of these FDA regulations in halting fraudulent health claims remains to be seen. Some authorities are skeptical. The dietary supplement industry spends $500 million on promotion. The nutrition supplement industry does not need the label to successfully promote its products. Health claims for supplements can be made in newspaper or magazine articles, booklets, pamphlets, lectures, and probably, most effectively, in radio and television talk shows. Within the store, booklets, pamphlets, health magazine articles, and advice by store clerks are effective. How far the FDA can go in regulating these types of promotion is unclear.

SORTING RELIABLE FROM UNRELIABLE

What makes people fall for the extravagant health claims of the supplement industry? Psychological and emotional factors are deeply involved. A small segment of the population seems to find emotional satisfaction in following unusual dietary practices. Reports of nutrition research in the media raise the expectations of the public beyond what medical sci-

DISPLAY 15-6 RELIABLE NUTRITION INFORMATION SOURCES

LOCAL RESOURCES

REGISTERED DIETITIANS
In private practice; in community health facilities and agencies

COLLEGES AND UNIVERSITIES
Departments of: Dietetics
Home Economics
Food Science and Nutrition
Public Health

HEALTH DEPARTMENTS—STATE, COUNTY, CITY
Divisions of: Nutrition
Chronic Disease
Child Health

STATE OR LOCAL CHAPTERS OF PROFESSIONAL ORGANIZATIONS
American Dietetic Association
American Association of Family and Consumer Sciences
Society for Nutrition Education
American Public Health Association

FDA
US government offices in states, some cities

AGRICULTURAL EXTENSION SERVICE (STATE OR COUNTY OFFICE)

NONPROFIT ORGANIZATIONS, STATE AND LOCAL CHAPTERS
American Cancer Society
American Diabetes Association
American Heart Association
American Red Cross
March of Dimes, Birth Defects Foundation

NATIONAL RESOURCES

PROFESSIONAL ORGANIZATIONS

American Association of Family and Consumer Sciences
1555 King Street, Suite 400
Alexandria, VA 22314

American Dietetic Association
216 W. Jackson Blvd. Suite 800
Chicago, IL 60606-6995
Consumer Nutrition Hot Line: (800) 366-1655

American Medical Association
535 N. Dearborn Street
Chicago, IL 60610

American Public Health Association
Food and Nutrition Section
1015 Eighteenth Street, NW
Washington, DC 20036

Society for Nutrition Education
2140 Shattuck Avenue, Suite 1110
Berkeley, CA 94704

FEDERAL HEALTH INFORMATION CENTERS

Center for Nutrition Policy and Promotion
1120 20th Street, NW
Suite 200, North Lobby
Washington, DC 20036
(202) 418-2312

Food and Drug Administration
Office of Consumer Affairs
5600 Fishers Lane, HFE-50
Rockville, MD 20857
(301) 443-3170

Food and Nutrition Information Center
National Agricultural Library, Room 304
10301 Baltimore Blvd.
Beltsville, MD 20705-2351
(301) 504-5719

ODPHP National Health Information Center
Box 1133
Washington, DC 20013-1133
(800) 336-4797
(301) 565-4020

National Maternal and Child Health Clearinghouse
8201 Greensboro Drive, Suite 600
McLean, VA 22102
(703) 821-8955, extension 254 or 265

President's Council on Physical Fitness and Sports
701 Pennsylvania Avenue, NW, Suite 250
Washington, DC 20004
(202) 272-3430

Consumer Information Center (Printed Material)
Pueblo, CO 81009

CONSUMER ORGANIZATIONS

American Council on Science and Health
1995 Broadway
New York, NY 10023

Center for Science in the Public Interest
1755 S Street, NW
Washington, DC 20009

National Council Against Health Fraud, Inc.
Box 1276
Loma Linda, CA 92354

ence now can do. People who are desperately looking for a miracle when medical science has failed to find a cure for serious illness may decide to take treatment into their own hands. Many sensible people are concerned about environmental pollution and have turned to organic and health food products. True and false information can be so skillfully mixed that it is impossible to judge what is valid. Food faddists may quote respected scientific journals but may slant the information or omit important aspects of scientific reports to suit their own purposes.

How can we protect ourselves and our clients from false nutrition claims? The following are some questions to ask:

- Is a diet that contains a variety of foods from the Food Guide Pyramid recommended or is the consumption of food supplements recommended?
- In the case of weight reduction, is a balanced variety of food recommended, or are only a few foods emphasized and entire food groups omitted? Does weight reduction rest solely on consuming a special formula, with no emphasis on physical activity or behavioral change?
- Are the medical claims for the dietary supplements supported by recognized authorities and organizations in the fields of nutrition and health?
- Does the author or promoter claim to be persecuted by health professionals or the government?
- Are anecdotal stories (accounts or experiences of other people) used to support the claim?
- Does the author or promoter have a financial motive?

RELIABLE INFORMATION SOURCES

Where does one find reliable nutrition information? Dietitians, including those in state and local health departments and welfare agencies, public health nursing associations, diet counseling services, hospital clinics, and health centers all can help. Consumer information officers in field offices of the FDA and nutrition and medical faculty members in universities and colleges also can provide assistance, as can state and local chapters of professional associations such as the American Dietetic Association, American Public Health Association, and Society for Nutrition Education. (See Display 15-6 for specific sources of reliable nutrition information.)

KEYS TO PRACTICAL APPLICATION

Remember that there are many good reasons why people eat the way they do. The foods available in a particular region are an important factor.

Respect your clients' eating habits; in many ways, the habits express their way of life.

Accentuate the positive; emphasize the good points in an individual's eating habits.

Find out what clients are actually eating; do not assume that they are eating the traditional foods of their ethnic group.

Avoid judging as inadequate ethnic eating habits that are unfamiliar to you. There may be hidden factors that improve the nutritional quality of the diet. Seek assistance from a dietitian in analyzing the diet.

Avoid attacking the value system underlying unusual eating habits.

Be aware that vegetarian diets can be nutritionally adequate but that careful planning is important.

Try to understand the psychological and emotional factors involved in food faddism.

Be suspicious of claims that specific foods or nutrient supplements taken in large doses can prevent or cure serious disease.

Learn to identify agencies from which you can obtain reliable nutrition information and to which you can refer clients.

Recognize that dietary supplements such as amino acids, herbs, and botanicals may pose the most serious danger because little is known of their safety.

Keep abreast of developments in the enforcement of labeling regulations that are designed to eliminate fraudulent health claims.

KEY IDEAS

Unless health workers understand the cultural influences on eating habits and can translate them into practical, culturally sensitive recommendations, they cannot provide realistic, effective nutrition counseling.

Meanings attached to foods vary greatly from one culture to another.

The availability of foods in a particular region, together with nationality and religious factors, strongly influences eating habits.

The Food Guide Pyramid may not be an appropriate guide when working with cultures that have eating habits that differ considerably from those in the United States.

A three-group classification may be more appropriate when working with some cultural groups. These three groups might include (1) staple or energy-providing foods, (2) bodybuilding or growth foods, and (3) protective foods.

People from other cultures may need help finding substitutes for favorite foods that they cannot obtain or afford in the United States and learning the economics of food purchasing in the United States.

In the United States, rice should not be rinsed either before or after cooking; otherwise, valuable nutrients with which it has been enriched are lost. Rice in the United States does not contain talc.

Nondairy sources of calcium in the culture must be known and encouraged because lactose intolerance is common.

Vegetarian diets can be nutritionally adequate, but careful planning and choice of food is necessary.

Nutritional needs are readily met in vegetarian diets that include dairy products and eggs.

Achieving adequate amounts of nutrients in vegetarian diets that contain no animal products requires considerable knowledge of the nutritional composition of food; nutrients that need special attention are vitamin D, calcium, iron, and vitamin B_{12}.

Health workers must respect the beliefs of those following nontraditional eating habits if their nutrition education efforts are to be successful.

The most serious problem created by food faddism is that false promises may delay people with serious health problems from seeking competent medical advice.

People who promote food faddism distort scientific information to suit their own purposes.

Amino acids, herbs, and botanicals may be among the most dangerous supplements on the market.

Diets that severely limit variety and eliminate complete food groups can be extremely dangerous.

Many sources of reliable nutrition information are available in the community (see Display 15-6).

Recent FDA regulations require that only health claims authorized by the FDA can be used on supplement labels and in product catalogs.

KEYS TO LEARNING

STUDY-DISCUSSION QUESTIONS

1. Prepare a report on the eating habits of a particular ethnic or nationality group. If possible, select the one represented by your own family background. Discuss your report with the class. Include one or two favorite recipes illustrating the eating habits of the group. Compile the recipes of all participants in a booklet for distribution to the class members. The class might

consider having a potluck party in which students singly or in groups of two or three are responsible for preparing and bringing to class a food representative of a particular cultural group. A variety of foods should be encouraged so that all the components of a meal are covered (i.e., entrees, vegetables, salads, breads, and desserts). The amount of money to be spent by each student should be set beforehand and limited to a moderate amount, perhaps the cost of a cafeteria meal.

2. Why is it important to consider a client's regional or cultural eating habits when providing advice on nutrition? Is it wise to assume that a person of a particular ethnic background is following a traditional diet?
3. Can the vegan diet be made nutritionally adequate? What aspects of the diet require special consideration?
4. Collect newspaper or magazine advertisements or articles that represent food misinformation. Discuss the fallacy involved. How is this fallacy psychologically or emotionally appealing? Also collect articles relating to the FDA's attempts to eliminate fraudulent health claims.
5. If you were uncertain about the validity of nutrition books or other types of nutrition information, where would you seek reliable information? What are some clues to food misinformation?
6. Make a directory of reliable nutrition resources in your community. As a class project, obtain the information for the directory by contacting various health and welfare agencies, organizations, and professional associations to determine what nutrition information services are provided.

BIBLIOGRAPHY

BOOKS AND PAMPHLETS

Algert SJ, Ellison TH. Ethnic and regional food practices. Mexican American food practices, customs, and holidays. Chicago: American Dietetic Association and American Diabetes Association, 1989.

Barrett S, Herbert V. Fads, frauds, and quackery. In: Shils ME, Olson JA, Shike M. Eds. Modern nutrition in health and disease. 8th ed. Philadelphia: Lea and Febiger, 1994:1526-1532.

Farley D. Making sure hype doesn't overwhelm science. Washington, DC: US Government Printing Office, 1993. US Food and Drug Administration publication FDA 94-2272.

Farley D. Vegetarian diets. The pluses and the pitfalls. Washington, DC: US Government Printing Office, 1992. US Food and Drug Administration publication FDA 93-2258.

Federal Register, Tuesday, Jan. 4, 1994. Part II. Dept of Health and Human Services, Food and Drug Administration. 21 CFR Parts 20 and 101. Food labeling; general requirements; final rules and proposed rule.

Halderson K. Ethnic and regional food practices. Alaska native: food practices, customs, and holidays. Chicago: American Dietetic Association and American Diabetes Association, 1993.

Ikeda JP. Ethnic and regional food practices. Hmong American food practices, customs and holidays. Chicago: American Dietetic Association and American Diabetes Association, 1992.

Kashruth Committee, Lubavitch Women's Organization. Body and soul: a new look at kashruth. Brooklyn: Lubavitch Women's Organization, n.d.

Ma KM. Ethnic and regional food practices. Chinese American: food practices, customs, and holidays. Chicago: American Dietetic Association and American Diabetes Association, 1990.

Pelican S, Bachman-Carter K. Ethnic and regional food practices. Navajo: food practices, customs, and holidays Chicago: American Dietetic Association and American Diabetes Association, 1991.

Twin Cities Dietetic Association. Manual of clinical nutrition. Minneapolis: Chronimed/DCI Publishing, 1994.

US Dept of Health and Human Services, Public Health Service. Healthy people 2000: national health promotion and disease prevention objectives. Washington, DC: US Government Printing Office, 1990.

US Dept of Health and Human Services, Public Health Service. Prevention '91—'92, federal programs and progress. Washington, DC: US Government Printing Office, 1992.

PERIODICALS

American Dietetic Association. Position of the American Dietetic Association: vegetarian diets. J Am Diet Assoc 1993;93: 1317.

Bronner Y. Cultural sensitivity and nutrition counseling. Top Clin Nutr 1994;9:2:13.

Chew T. Sodium values of Chinese condiments and their use in sodium-restricted diets. J Am Diet Assoc 1983;82:397.

Kahn A. Keeping kosher. Diabetes Self-Management, March/April 1989.

Looker AC, Loria CM, Carroll MD, et al. Calcium intakes of Mexican Americans, Cubans, Puerto Ricans, non-Hispanic whites and non-Hispanic blacks in the United States. J Am Diet Assoc 1993;93:1274.

Pachter LM. Culture and clinical care: folk illness beliefs and behaviors and their implications for health care delivery. JAMA 1994;271:690.

Reeves J. Pregnancy and fasting during Ramadan (letter). Br Med J 1992;304:843.

Short SH. Health quackery: our role as professionals. J Am Diet Assoc 1994;94:607.

Shovic AC. Development of a Samoan nutrition exchange list using culturally accepted foods. J Am Diet Assoc 1994;94:541.

Stowers SL. Development of a culturally appropriate food guide for pregnant Caribbean immigrants in the United States. J Am Diet Assoc 1992;92:331.

Sucher KP, Kittler PG. Nutrition isn't color blind. J Am Diet Assoc 1991;91:297.

Zupke MP, Milner I. Bee pollen, shark cartilage, ginseng: the truth about 10 top supplements. Environmental Nutrition 1993;16:9:1.

CHAPTER

16

Nutrition During Pregnancy and Lactation

KEY TERMS

anomaly abnormality
chronological age age in years
embryo unborn offspring in the early developmental stage, from conception through the third month
fetus unborn offspring from the end of the third month until birth
gestational diabetes diabetes that begins during the second half of pregnancy
gynecologic age years since the onset of menstruation
immature not fully developed
lactation the period during which the infant is breastfed; the secretion of milk
macrosomia very large baby at birth
maturity period of attainment of full growth or development
menarche time when menstruation starts
multipara multiple births
parity the condition of a woman with regard to the number of children she has borne
placenta organ attached to the wall of the uterus through which the fetus receives nourishment and eliminates waste products
postpartum time following childbirth
puberty period during which sexual maturity is attained
teratogen substance or disease state that can cause birth defects

OBJECTIVES

After completing this chapter, the student will be able to:

1. Discuss the vital role of nutrition in pregnancy.
2. Explain the importance of preconception nutrition counseling.
3. State at least five factors that can adversely affect the pregnancy outcome.
4. Explain the importance of adequate weight gain in pregnancy.
5. State the recommended rate of weight gain for the woman whose prepregnancy weight is within normal range.
6. Discuss, giving specific Recommended Dietary Allowances during pregnancy, for

   energy
   protein
   calcium
   iron
   folate
   sodium.
7. Give the number of servings from each food group in the Food Guide Pyramid recommended during pregnancy and during lactation.

8. Describe three practical ways to promote milk consumption.
9. Discuss the potential problems associated with each of the following: pica, skipping meals, vitamin/mineral excesses, alcohol consumption, caffeine consumption, and sugar substitutes.
10. Discuss the traditional and more recent dietary treatment for morning sickness.
11. Discuss the major public health problems created by teenage pregnancy and the challenges that teenage pregnancy presents to the nutritional management of pregnancy.
12. Give the additions to the food guide required during breastfeeding.
13. Discuss the usual pattern of weight loss after pregnancy and the recommended limits for the overweight, breastfeeding woman.

Physical growth occurs through an increase in cell number, cell size, and *intercellular matrix* (the substance between cells). Most tissues, such as bone tissue, grow through increases in cell number and size.

Although growth is a continuous process, its rate is not uniform. Rapid growth occurs during prenatal life, early infancy, and adolescence. Slower and more uniform growth occurs between infancy and adolescence. Critical stages of growth exist for some organs. For example, the number of brain cells increases rapidly prenatally, falls off at birth, and reaches its maximum at about age 2 years.

The period of greatest risk of cellular damage is when the number of cells is increasing. If cell division is disrupted because of a lack of nutrients, the desirable number of cells may never be achieved. Thus, nutritional deficiencies occurring during critical periods may result in permanent damage to a particular organ. The critical periods of development are those stages at which tissues and organs are at risk of permanent damage if the essential nutrients are not provided.

Many factors come together to shape the course of pregnancy. Although this chapter concentrates on the nutritional aspects of pregnancy, the influences on the course and outcome of pregnancy are many and complex. In addition to nutrition, they include genetics, health status, motivation, education, family size and structure, and financial status.

IMPORTANCE OF GOOD NUTRITION DURING PREGNANCY

Nutritional status exerts its greatest influence during prenatal life and infancy. Within 2 months to 3 months of conception, all of the major body systems are formed. Embryonic growth is slow, and the quantity of food required is small; the *quality* of the food supply, however, is critical. The nutritional status of the pregnant woman at the time of conception is extremely important.

In the next 6 months—the fetal period—the fetus undergoes phenomenal growth, increasing 500-fold from a weight of 6 g at 9 weeks to a weight of 3500 g at birth. Skeletal development begins in the second month and continues to the end of puberty. Fatty tissue begins to develop at about the sixth month. Throughout pregnancy, maternal tissue grows in the uterus and the breasts, and the placenta develops.

The United States has a high rate of infant mortality when compared with other developed countries. In 1990, 20 other developed countries had lower rates. Poor maternal nutrition has been identified repeatedly as one of the causes of poor pregnancy outcomes. If maternal nutrition is poor, blood volume does not increase and fat is not deposited normally. A malnourished woman is more likely to have a small baby; a baby weighing less than 5.5 lb (2.5 kg) is more likely to have a birth defect and to have difficulty surviving his or her first year. Evidence also has suggested that adequate nutrition during pregnancy is a factor in mental development. A malnourished baby has fewer brain cells than a healthy infant. Moreover, a dangerous condition called *pregnancy-induced hypertension (PIH)* is seen more frequently in poorly nourished than in well-nourished women.

PRECONCEPTION CARE

Ideally, maternal nutrition should be viewed as a composite of three periods—before conception, during conception, and after delivery. Of these three, the most important may well be the nutritional guidance provided as a part of preconception care. Malformations occur in the first weeks after conception, when body systems are developing, often before most women enter prenatal care. Nutrition care provided during the preconception period allows for preparation of the best possible environment for conception. A woman who is informed of possible risk factors can delay pregnancy until she achieves a healthier state.

The nutrition component of preconception care includes assessment to identify nutrition-related risk factors; nutrition education; and counseling referral and other interventions as needed to solve or reduce identified problems. Preconception care aims to encourage appropriate weight for height and healthy eating habits and to treat identified risk factors.

NUTRITION ASSESSMENT

RISK FACTORS

If preconception counseling has not occurred, the health provider should evaluate the pregnant woman's nutritional status as early as possible in the pregnancy. Women who are at high risk of developing nutrition-related problems should be identified and should receive intensive nutritional guidance. A number of conditions can adversely affect the outcome of pregnancy such as exposure to excessive or inadequate nutrient intake, exposure to drugs that interfere with nutrient metabolism, preexisting diabetes, alcoholism, and eating disorders. Worthington-Roberts and Williams have classified the nutrition-related risk factors into five categories: personal characteristics; personal habits and living situation; chronic preexisting medical problems; obstetric history, and current or potential pregnancy-induced problems (Table 16-1).

DIET

The health care provider must collect data on the kinds and amounts of food consumed, the distribution of food over the day, and the influences on eating habits—such as ethnic, social, financial, and religious factors. A nutrition questionnaire such as the one in Display 16-1 is easy to answer and provides a useful starting point for identifying possible problem areas. Various tools such as a food diary kept by the client enable the health care provider to collect specific information concerning the foods the client is eating. The data obtained are compared with a daily food guide for pregnancy, such as the one in Table 16-2. The difference between the kinds and amounts of food specified in the food guide and the foods actually eaten may identify needed changes. If ethnic food habits are involved, a more in-depth analysis may be required (see Chapter 15).

The client and health care provider should discuss the use of self-prescribed vitamins, minerals, and other supplements. The health provider must discourage the use of any kind of supplement or medication unless approved by a physician who knows that the woman is pregnant or planning a pregnancy. Vitamins, minerals, and other dietary supplements have the potential to produce nutrient imbalances, nutrient excesses, and can introduce the body to toxic substances. Excessive vitamin A, for example, is a *teratogen* (a cause of birth defects).

Furthermore, the health provider must thoroughly investigate socioeconomic factors that may affect nutritional status. These factors include lack of money for food, lack of cooking facilities, cigarette smoking, alcoholism, and drug abuse. He or she also should determine the pregnant woman's intentions regarding breastfeeding. Under ordinary circumstances, breastfeeding is recommended for all infants in the United States. Encouragement and support from health care providers is important.

LABORATORY STUDIES

Because the blood supply of the pregnant woman expands, certain constituents of the blood become diluted, which affects various laboratory values. For this reason, laboratory values of pregnant women should not be compared with values that are considered normal for nonpregnant women. Rather, they should be compared with normal blood values for pregnancy.

TABLE 16-1 High-Risk Pregnancies: Risk Factors in Pregnancy-Induced Complications and Preexisting Chronic Conditions in the Mother

Personal Characteristics (Cannot Change)	Personal Habits, Living Situation (Seek to Change)	Chronic Preexisting Medical Problems (Screen, Treat)	Obstetric History (Screen, Prevent)	Current/Potential Pregnancy-Induced Problems (Screen, Prevent, Treat)
Sex Age Adolescent Older woman Family history Diabetes Heart disease Hypertension Phenylketonuria	Smoking Alcohol/drug use Poor diet Malnutrition Obesity Underweight Sedentary lifestyle	Hypertension Insulin-dependent diabetes mellitus (type I) Non–insulin-dependent diabetes mellitus (type II) Heart disease Pulmonary disease Renal disease Maternal phenylketonuria	Low birth weight Macrosomia Stillbirth Abortion Fetal anomalies High parity Multipara	Anemia Iron deficiency Folic acid deficiency Pregnancy-induced hypertension Gestational diabetes

(Worthington-Roberts BS, Williams SR. Nutrition in pregnancy and lactation. St. Louis: Mosby–Year Book, Inc. 1993:240.)

Nonpregnant women (nonsmokers) who have a hemoglobin below 12 g/dL are considered anemic. Pregnant women (nonsmoker) with a hemoglobin below 11 g/dL in the first and third trimesters or below 10.5 g/dL in the second trimester are considered anemic. The cutoff values for pregnant women who are moderate smokers are 11.3 g/dL in the first and third trimesters and 10.8 g/dL in the second trimester, and for pregnant women who are heavy smokers, 11.5 g/dL and 11 g/dL, respectively. Blood glucose levels in pregnancy also differ from those in the nonpregnant state (see the section Gestational Diabetes).

WEIGHT GAIN DURING PREGNANCY

Infant birth weight is a factor closely related to infant death. Infants who are born too small—less than 5 lb, 8 oz (2.5 kg)—are at highest risk. The greatest influence on the birth weight of full-term infants is the weight gain of the mother because birth weight increases with increasing maternal prenatal weight gain. The second greatest influence on birth weight is the mother's prepregnancy weight. The higher the prepregnancy weight, the higher the weight of the newborn. If the woman is underweight and, in addition, fails to gain adequate weight during pregnancy, the resulting birth weight is even less. Smoking during pregnancy is the third factor that affects birth weight. Smoking appears to affect fetal growth directly. Adding to the adverse effects of smoking is the typically lower prepregnancy weight of smokers, who gain less weight during pregnancy than nonsmokers.

RECOMMENDED WEIGHT GAIN

A wide range of weight gains can support a healthy pregnancy. The average weight gain is about 25 to 30 lb (11.5 kg to 14.0 kg). Weight gain during pregnancy consists of the weight of the fetus and

DISPLAY 16-1 NUTRITION QUESTIONNAIRE

What you eat and the lifestyle choices you make can affect your present and future nutrition and health. Your nutrition can also have an important effect on your baby's health. Please answer these questions by circling the answers that apply to you.

EATING BEHAVIOR

1. Are you frequently bothered by any of the following? (circle all that apply)

   Nausea Vomiting Heartburn Constipation

2. Do you skip meals at least three times a week? No Yes
3. Do you try to limit the amount or kind of food you eat to control your weight? No Yes
4. Are you on a special diet now? No Yes
5. Do you avoid any foods for health or religious reasons? No Yes

FOOD RESOURCES

6. Do you have a working stove? No Yes
   Do you have a working refrigerator? No Yes
7. Do you sometimes run out of food before you are able to buy more? No Yes
8. Can you afford to eat the way you should? No Yes
9. Are you receiving any food assistance now? No Yes
   (circle all that apply):

Food stamps	School Breakfast	School lunch
WIC	Donated food/ commodities	CSFP*

   Food from a food pantry, soup kitchen, or food bank
10. Do you feel you need help in obtaining food? No Yes

FOOD AND DRINK

11. Which of these did you drink yesterday? (circle all that apply):

Soft drinks	Coffee	Tea	Fruit drink
Orange juice	Grapefruit juice	Other juices	Milk
Kool-Aid®	Beer	Wine	Alcoholic drinks
Water	Other beverages (list)		

12. Which of these foods did you eat yesterday? (circle all that apply):

Cheese	Pizza	Macaroni and cheese
Yogurt	Cereal with milk	

   Other foods made with cheese (such as tacos, enchiladas, lasagna, cheesburgers)

Corn	Potatoes	Sweet potatoes	Green Salad
Carrots	Collard greens	Spinach	Turnip greens
Broccoli	Green beans	Green peas	Other vegetables

Apples	Bananas	Berries	Grapefruit
Melon	Oranges	Peaches	Other fruit

Meat	Fish	Chicken	Eggs
Peanut butter	Nuts	Seeds	Dried beans

Cold cuts	Hot dog	Bacon	Sausage
Cake	Cookies	Doughnut	Pastry
Chips	French fries		

   Other deep-fried foods such as fried chicken or egg rolls

Bread	Rolls	Rice	Cereal
Noodles	Spaghetti	Tortillas	

   Were any of these whole grain? No Yes
13. Is the way you ate yesterday the way you usually eat? No Yes

LIFESTYLE

14. Do you exercise for at least 30 minutes on a regular basis (3 times a week or more)? No Yes
15. Do you ever smoke cigarettes or use smokeless tobacco? No Yes
16. Do you ever drink beer, wine, liquor, or any other alcoholic beverages? No Yes
17. Which of these do you take? (circle all that apply):

    Prescribed drugs or medications

    Any over-the-counter products (such as aspirin, Tylenol®, antacids, or vitamins)

    Street drugs (such as marijuana, speed, downers, crack, or heroin)

* Commodity Supplemental Food Program

(National Academy of Sciences Institute of Medicine, Food and Nutrition Board, Committee on Nutritional Status During Pregnancy and Lactation, Subcommittee for a Clinical Application Guide. Nutrition during pregnancy and lactation: an implementation guide. Washington, DC: National Academy Press, (1992:7–8.)

TABLE 16-2 DAILY FOOD GUIDE FOR PREGNANCY AND BREASTFEEDING

Food Group	Pregnancy: Adult Woman	Pregnancy: Adolescent	Breastfeeding Woman
Milk, yogurt, cheese	3–4 servings	4–5 servings	4–5 servings
Meat and meat substitutes	5 oz.–6 oz	6 oz.–7 oz	6 oz.–7 oz
Fruits	2–4 servings	2–4 servings	2–4 servings
Vitamin C–rich	1–2 servings	1–2 servings	2 servings
Vegetables	3–5 servings	3–5 servings	3–5 servings
Vitamin A–rich	1 serving	1 serving	1 serving
Bread, cereals, rice, pasta	6–11 servings	6–11 servings	6–11 servings
Fats, oils, sweets	To meet caloric needs	To meet caloric needs	To meet caloric needs

associated fetal tissue (e.g., placenta), plus the weight increases in maternal tissue (Display 16-2).

Recommendations for weight gain are divided into three categories based on the woman's pre-pregnancy weight. The weight category is determined using body mass index (BMI). Refer to Display 23-1 for the formula for determining BMI. The recommended weight gain for women of normal BMI (19.8 to 26.0) is 25 to 35 lb (11.5 kg to 16.0 kg); for underweight women, 28 to 40 lb (12.5 kg to 18.0 kg); and for overweight women, 15 to 25 lb (7.0 kg to 11.5 kg). Women who have a BMI greater than 29 should gain at least 15 lb (7 kg) during the pregnancy. Young adolescents (less than 2 years after menarche) and African American women should try to gain the weight at the upper end of the range, whereas short women (less than 62 inches [157 cm]) should strive for gains at the lower end of the range (Table 16-3).

Women whose weight gain is less than recommended are more susceptible to complications and are more likely to have low–birth weight babies. Women of ideal weight should avoid excessive weight gain during pregnancy.

A weight gain of 15 lb (7 kg) has been associated with improved pregnancy outcome in the obese woman. Although the obese woman should

DISPLAY 16–2 DISTRIBUTION OF WEIGHT GAIN IN PREGNANCY

Body Part	Weight (lb)	
Full-term baby	7.7	Fetal tissue
Placenta	1.4	
Amniotic and body fluids	1.8	
Uterus	2.0	
Breasts	0.9	Maternal tissue
Blood volume	4.0	
Interstital body fluids	2.7	
Maternal storage fat	3.5–7.5	
Total	24–28	

TABLE 16-3 RECOMMENDED TOTAL WEIGHT GAIN RANGES FOR PREGNANT WOMEN*

Prepregnancy Weight-for-Height Category	Recommended Total Gain (lb)	(kg)
Low (BMI < 19.8)	28–40	12.5–18.0
Normal (BMI 19.8 to 26.0)	25–35	11.5–16.0
High (BMI > 26 to 29)	15–25	7.0–11.5
Obese (BMI > 29)	≥15	≥7

* For singleton pregnancies. The range for women carrying twins is 35 lb to 45 lb (16 kg to 20 kg). Young adolescents (<2 years after menarche) and African American women should strive for gains at the upper end of the range. Short women (<62 inches [<157 cm]) should strive for gains at the lower end of the range.

(National Academy of Sciences, Institute of Medicine, Food and Nutrition Board, Committee on Nutritional Status During Pregnancy, Subcommittee for a Clinical Application Guide. Nutrition during pregnancy and lactation: an implementation guide. Washington, DC: National Academy Press, 1992:44.)

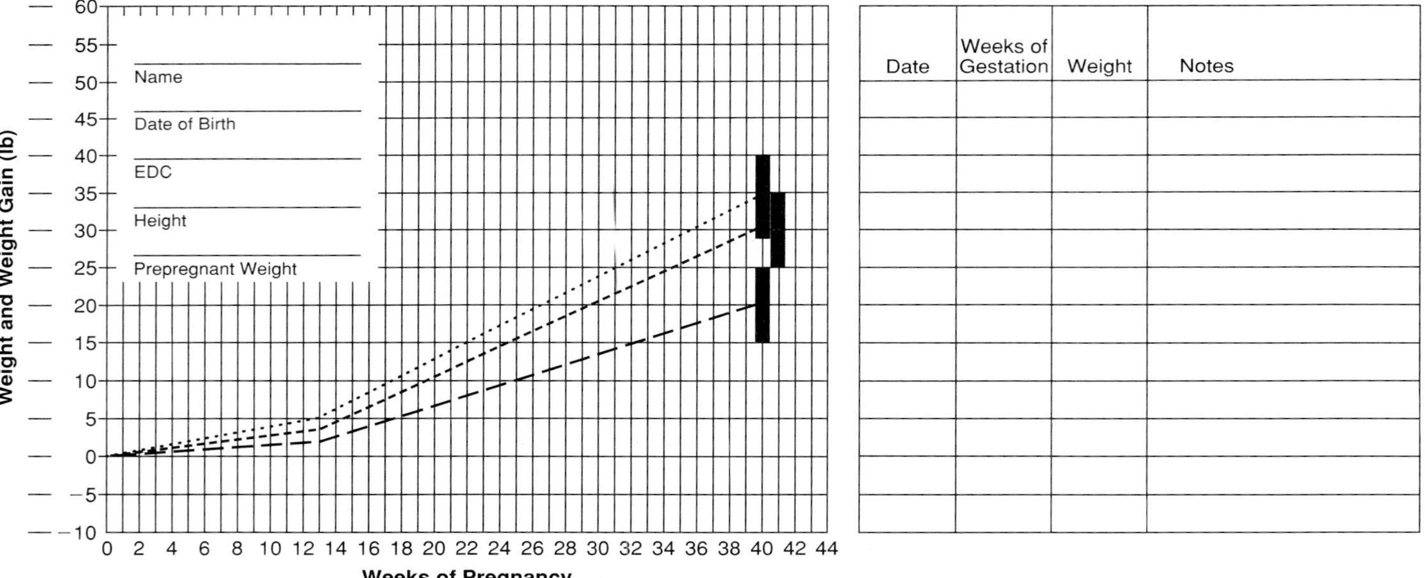

FIGURE 16-1

Prenatal weight gain chart.
(·····) prepregnancy BMI is <19.8, (-----) prepregnancy BMI is 19.8–26.0 (normal body weight), (—–—), prepregnancy BMI is >26.0. EDC is Estimated Date of Conception. Note: The prepregnancy weight rounded to the nearest pound is written on the line to the left of the zero. *(National Academy of Sciences, Institute of Medicine, Food and Nutrition Board, Committee on Nutritional Status During Pregnancy and Lactation, Subcommittee for a Clinical Application Guide. Nutrition during pregnancy and lactation: an implementation guide. Washington, DC: National Academy Press, 1992:15.)*

avoid excessive weight gain, she should not attempt to lose weight during pregnancy. Severe caloric restriction during pregnancy can be harmful to both fetus and mother, depriving them of essential nutrients. Also, when calories are severely restricted, *ketosis* results from the excessive breakdown of fat and can cause neurologic damage to the fetus.

The weight gain recommendations should be discussed with the pregnant woman and a weight gain range agreed on jointly. The woman should understand that adequate weight gain reduces the risk of a low–birth weight baby prone to complications. Use of a weight gain chart such as the one in Figure 16-1 is recommended.

PATTERN OF WEIGHT GAIN

The health provider should closely monitor pattern of weight gain as a means of assessing the adequacy of the pregnant woman's caloric intake. It is important to measure the height and weight of the pregnant woman carefully and with a reliable method initially and to use the same care in measuring her weight at each prenatal visit.

A steady rate of weight gain is the goal. As a general guide, 2 to 5 lb (1 kg to 2.3 kg) is gained during the first trimester. Weight gain during the second and third trimester is about 1 lb (0.5 kg) per week. The recommended weight gain is slightly more for the woman with a low BMI and about $^{2}/_{3}$ lb (0.3 kg) for a woman with a high BMI.

MEETING NUTRITIONAL REQUIREMENTS

Metabolism undergoes tremendous changes during pregnancy. The tasks of the body are three-fold: it must adapt to the pregnancy, which involves changes in the respiratory and circulatory systems and in hormonal secretions; it must prepare for breastfeeding; and it must provide for fetal growth and development. It is not surprising that the requirements for all nutrients increase during pregnancy. Table 16-4 compares the Recommended Dietary Allowances (RDAs) for selected nutrients during pregnancy with those of the nonpregnant woman.

TABLE 16-4 RDAs for Selected Nutrients for Nonpregnant, Pregnant, and Breastfeeding Women

Nutrient	Nonpregnant, 25–50 y	Nonpregnant, 15–18 y	Pregnant	Breastfeeding 1st 6 mo	Breastfeeding 2nd 6 mo
Calories (kcal)	2200	2200	First trimester: +0 Second and third trimesters: +300	+500	+500
Protein (g)	50	44	+10	+15	+12
Calcium (mg)	800	1200	+400	+400	+400
Iron (mg)*	15	15	+15	+0	+0
Vitamin A (mg RE)	800	800	+0	+500	+400
Vitamin C (mg)	60	60	+10	+35	+30
Vitamin B_6 (mg)	1.6	1.5	+0.6	+0.5	+0.5
Folate (folacin) (mcg)	180†	180†	+220	+100†	+80†
Vitamin D (mg)	5	10	+5	+5	+5

* Daily iron supplements are recommended during pregnancy.

† The US Public Health Service in 1993 recommended 400 mcg folate daily for all women of childbearing age.

(Data based on National Academy of Sciences, National Research Council, Food and Nutrition Board. Recommended dietary allowances. 10th ed. Washington, DC: National Academy Press, 1989.)

ENERGY

Sufficient energy is required to achieve the recommended weight gain. Little additional energy is needed during the first trimester. Energy needs increase in the second trimester and remain elevated for the remainder of the pregnancy. During the second trimester, increased energy is needed mainly for maternal tissue growth; in the third trimester, increased energy is needed for fetal tissue growth. The increased need may be partially offset by the woman's decreased physical activity in the latter part of pregnancy.

Although the RDA estimates the increased energy need during the second and third trimesters of pregnancy to be 300 kcal per day, research has indicated that energy needs during pregnancy vary widely among women. Health providers must pay extra attention to the caloric intake of women who have a low prepregnancy weight to reduce their risk of delivering low–birth weight babies. *The rate of weight gain is the best indicator of the adequacy of caloric intake.* Discovering the causes of inadequate weight gain and careful monitoring of weight gain for all women over the course of pregnancy are important.

Generally speaking, the caloric increase during pregnancy is small compared with the increased need for protein, vitamins, and minerals. Pregnant women must carefully choose foods to supply the needed nutrients without excessive caloric intake.

PROTEIN

An increase of 10 g of protein daily is recommended during pregnancy. Protein is essential for the growth of new cells and tissues both in the fetus and the mother (e.g., growth of uterus, placenta, and breasts). Sufficient caloric intake is also needed so that protein can be used for tissue building rather than for energy.

VITAMINS AND MINERALS

The need for all vitamins and minerals increases during pregnancy. Both deficiencies and excesses can create problems: deficiency of iron, folate (folacin, folic acid), or B_{12} can lead to anemia in the mother; deficiency of folate can result in neural tube defects; excessive vitamin A is toxic to the fetus; and excessive vitamin D and calcium may interfere with zinc absorption.

A well-balanced diet is considered to be the best source of all nutrients for most pregnant women, except iron. A daily supplement of 30 mg of ferrous iron is recommended for all women during the second and third trimesters of pregnancy. The adequacy of folate also requires special attention. In 1993, the US Public Health Service recommended that all women of childbearing age consume 400 mcg of folate daily to prevent neural tube defects in newborns. If folate intake is inadequate, a supplement may be necessary. If a woman has had a previous pregnancy involving a fetus or infant affected with a neural tube defect, she should see a physician as soon as she plans a pregnancy. In that situation, a high dose supplement of folate is given from at least 4 weeks before conception through the first trimester of pregnancy.

Women who are intolerant to milk or who will not drink milk may need supplements of calcium, vitamin D, and riboflavin. The RDA for calcium during pregnancy is 1200 mg. Three 8-oz glasses of milk will provide approximately 900 mg of calcium and the remainder of the diet (vegetables, breads, and so forth) will provide an additional 200 to 300 mg. Sources of calcium other than milk are listed in Table 11-3.

The need for sodium increases during pregnancy. Daily sodium intake during pregnancy should not fall below 2 to 3 g. The pregnant woman is advised to salt her food to taste unless advised otherwise by her physician. The moderate edema that may occur during pregnancy is considered to be normal and is no longer treated with diuretics and reduced sodium diets. Severe restriction of sodium during pregnancy may lead to serious complications including damage to the hormone system regulating the resorption of sodium and water and excretion of potassium by the kidney.

MULTIVITAMIN AND MINERAL SUPPLEMENTS

For heavy smokers, women who are vegans (see Chapter 15), women expecting multiple births, and other women whose nutrient intake is inadequate or who are at high risk of developing nutrition-related problems, a low-dose vitamin/mineral supplement is recommended. It is suggested that the supplement comprise the following nutrients: vitamins D, C, B_6, B_{12}, and folate, and the minerals iron, zinc, copper, and calcium.

Depending on need, calcium and higher doses of iron (60 mg to 120 mg) may be given in addition as single supplements. The pregnant woman should take calcium with food to promote absorption and iron supplements at bedtime or between meals with water or juice.

NUTRITION COUNSELING

The pregnant woman, especially one expecting her first child, usually is highly motivated to correct poor eating habits. Nutrition counseling during pregnancy is far reaching if it addresses both family members' usual needs and the additional needs imposed by pregnancy. Nutrition counselors should help parents-to-be to become aware of the influence their eating habits have on their children. Their many questions afford counselors good opportunities for discussion.

The woman who is eating a good diet needs to know that she is doing well and should be encouraged to continue. If a woman's dietary intake is poor, the counselor needs to work closely with her in a positive way to determine the cause and find acceptable alternatives to correct eating problems. The counselor and woman should discuss ways of treating common problems of pregnancy such as heartburn and constipation. In follow-up visits, the counselor plots weight on the prenatal weight-gain grid and reevaluates dietary intake. In the latter part of pregnancy, the counselor and woman discuss the diet during breastfeeding and infant feeding.

It is important to consider cultural factors that may be influencing a woman's eating habits. Ethnic groups frequently have beliefs regarding certain foods and their effect on pregnancy or the unborn child. It is important to know what these beliefs are and to know a client's cultural eating patterns. Although it is unwise to presume that an individual is eating in a certain way, knowing the eating habits of a particular ethnic group can help alert the counselor to problem dietary practices (see Chapter 15).

Counselors should be sensitive to situations in which clients are having difficulty obtaining adequate food. They should refer clients to food assistance programs such as the Special Supplemental Food Program for Women, Infants, and Children (WIC) and the Food Stamp program.

USING FOOD GUIDES

Food guides are available to assist pregnant and breastfeeding women in making food choices that meet their increased nutritional needs. Most food guides for pregnancy meet the RDA for all nutrients except iron, for which a supplement is provided. Daily food patterns based on The Pyramid Guide to Daily Food Choices for both pregnancy and breastfeeding are given in Table 16-2.

The Food Guide Pyramid, which emphasizes increased use of whole-grain breads and cereals, vegetables, and fruits, provides generous amounts of vitamins, minerals, and fiber. Careful attention should be given to good sources of folate and iron.

During pregnancy, the recommendations made in *Dietary Guidelines for Americans* are modified somewhat. No special effort should be made to reduce sodium, high-protein foods should be encouraged, and fats may be used in moderately increased amounts to maintain adequate weight gain, if necessary. The increased fats should come from nutritious rather than empty-calorie foods.

CHOOSING FOODS WISELY

The additional 10 g of protein recommended during pregnancy can be consumed by increasing amounts of protein of high biologic value such as meat, fish, poultry, milk, eggs, and cheese. Each ounce of meat, fish, or poultry adds 7 g of protein to the diet and each additional cup of milk adds 8 g of protein.

Milk also provides calcium and phosphorus, which are needed for the development of fetal bony structure and teeth as well as for the mother. Fortified milk also supplies 400 International Units (IU) of vitamin D per quart. Pregnant women may flavor milk with decaffeinated coffee, fruit purees, or molasses, or take milk in the form of cream soup, puddings, and custards. A $1\frac{1}{2}$-oz serving of cheddar cheese supplies the same amount of protein and calcium as 1 cup of milk. Furthermore, one can reduce the volume of milk consumed by adding $\frac{1}{3}$ cup of dry nonfat milk to every 8 oz of fluid milk. This mixture supplies the nutrients in two glasses of milk.

Women who have a problem digesting lactose (lactase deficiency) should be encouraged to consume milk products on a trial basis because lactose tolerance often improves during pregnancy. Some strategies that may help include

- consumption of small (4 oz) servings of milk with other foods
- use of yogurt containing active, live cultures in place of fluid milk; one may add fruit, sugar, jam, or other flavorings
- use of aged cheeses such as cheddar
- consumption of lactase tablets or drops when drinking milk or using lactase-treated milk and milk products
- use of cultured buttermilk.

Nutrition counselors should encourage the use of nondairy sources of calcium also (see Table 11-3).

Lean meat, prunes and prune juice, dried peas, beans, and lentils, green leafy vegetables, and whole-grain cereals are good sources of iron. Including a vitamin C–rich food with meals increases the absorption of nonheme iron (see Chapter 11).

Meeting folate requirements is essential. Folate is found in leafy green vegetables, organ meats, dried peas and beans, nuts, fresh oranges, green vegetables such as asparagus and broccoli, and whole-grain cereals and breads.

Moderate use of salt is recommended, because the tissues of both the pregnant woman and fetus require salt. The woman should use iodized salt because of the increased need for iodine in pregnancy. The need for water also is increased. The daily diet should include 6 cups to 8 cups of fluid, which the woman can obtain from a variety of beverages.

POTENTIAL DIETARY PROBLEMS

PICA

Pica is the practice of eating nonfood substances such as laundry starch, clay, chalk, cigarette ashes, baking soda, and ice. It is important to inquire about this practice at an early prenatal visit. Pica is prevalent in some cultures; the reasons for these abnormal cravings are unknown. The possible harmful effects of pica include reduction in the intake of nutritious food, interference with the absorption of iron and other nutrients, intestinal obstruction or impaction, and the introduction of toxic substances such as lead. As a result, the mother and infant's health may suffer. Pregnant women with pica are considered to be at risk of developing a nutritional deficiency.

The nutrition counselor should discuss the possible effects with the pregnant woman. Together, they should explore possible substitutions for pica substances and behaviors, such as walking, chewing sugarless gum, and chewing fruit juice cubes in place of ice.

SKIPPING MEALS

The developing fetus requires a continual supply of energy and nutrients. The pregnant woman should avoid long intervals between meals. Breakfast is especially important, because it follows a long period without food. Small- to moderate-sized meals taken at regular intervals throughout the day as well as nutritious snacks should be encouraged.

VITAMIN/MINERAL EXCESSES

Although most essential nutrients can be obtained in recommended amounts with a good diet, most obstetricians prescribe a low-dose prenatal vitamin/mineral supplement on confirmation of pregnancy.

The pregnant woman should take only the amounts prescribed and should avoid overdose.

Supplements of all types, including herbs and other botanicals, should be avoided unless approved by the health care provider. Women considering pregnancy should be cautioned about taking vitamins, minerals, and other supplements. These substances may cause nutrient imbalances, or excesses, and may introduce toxic substances. Supplements containing vitamin A and D are of particular concern because excesses of both are associated with abnormalities in the offspring.

ALCOHOL CONSUMPTION

Women who are planning to become pregnant as well as pregnant women should not drink alcohol—liquor, wine, or beer. Use of alcohol is associated with the risk of birth defects, because alcohol enters both the maternal and the fetal bloodstream. Babies born to alcoholic mothers may develop *fetal alcohol syndrome.* This disorder is characterized by low birth weight, slow growth and development, and, in some cases, permanent mental retardation (see Chapter 14). A safe lower limit for alcohol consumption during pregnancy is unknown.

CAFFEINE CONSUMPTION

Caffeine, a central nervous system stimulant, crosses the placenta and enters the fetal bloodstream. It is considered wise, during pregnancy, to avoid substances that have a druglike effect and can cross the placenta. In 1980, the US Food and Drug Administration issued a statement advising pregnant women to avoid or to use only sparingly foods and drugs containing caffeine. Since then, the concerns about caffeine during pregnancy have lessened, although research continues to report conflicting results. Limiting sources of caffeine (coffee, tea, or cola) to two or fewer servings is recommended. See Chapter 14 for the caffeine content of beverages and other foods and medications.

The use of herbal teas as a replacement for caffeine-containing beverages should be discouraged. The composition and safety of these products is unknown. Women who use herbal teas should be advised to use only those in filtered tea bags and to limit consumption to two 8-oz servings daily.

SACCHARIN AND ASPARTAME INTAKE

Because saccharin has been shown to be weakly carcinogenic in laboratory animals, it seems wise to moderate its use in pregnancy for the safety of both mother and infant. Since 1965, scientific organizations around the world have studied aspartame. No adverse effects have been documented. It is considered safe for use by all people, including pregnant and breastfeeding women. However, people with phenylketonuria should be cautioned about the use of aspartame, which contains the amino acid phenylalanine. People with this rare genetic disease cannot metabolize phenylalanine properly and must monitor the intake of this amino acid from all foods, including those containing aspartame.

DISCOMFORTS AIDED BY DIETARY MEASURES

NAUSEA

At least 50% of pregnant women are afflicted with *morning sickness,* a condition characterized by nausea, vomiting, fatigue, and other symptoms. Contrary to popular opinion, the symptoms are not limited to the morning nor to the first 3 months of pregnancy. The symptoms may persist throughout the day and, for 10% to 20% of pregnant women, they last the entire pregnancy. Another disturbing aspect of morning sickness is the common mistaken belief among both laypeople and health professionals that the cause is basically emotional, possibly an underlying fear or rejection of the pregnancy. Each year severe morning sickness, known as *hyperemesis gravidarum,* results in the hospitalization of about 55,000 women as a result of dehydration and other problems.

Traditional dietary treatment for morning sickness included eating dry toast, dry cereal, or crackers before arising from bed, sipping fluids frequently between meals rather than taking them with solid foods, and avoiding fatty and spicy foods. A new approach to treating this age-old problem has been suggested by Miriam Erick, registered dietitian for the obstetric units of Brigham and Women's Hospital in Boston. This approach is based on the theory that the nausea and vomiting are the body's reaction to a surge of hormones, including estrogen, that occurs naturally in pregnancy. The high level of estrogen increases the sense of smell to the point that subtle odors in the environment become potent and make pregnant women queasy.

As a means of treatment, Erich has recommended that women pay close attention to smells—both food and nonfood odors—that trigger nausea and try to avoid them. The next priority is to find foods that will stay down. Anything that sounds good should be tried. Taste, texture, and temperature seem to be the factors that affect appeal. Erich has found that potato chips and lemonade are one of the most successful food remedies for nausea. The goal is to consume calories regardless of their source to break the cycle of nausea and vomiting. For women who are hospitalized with hyperemesis gravidarum, a private room, to minimize exposure to odors, is recommended.

CONSTIPATION

Diminished peristalsis due to hormonal changes in pregnancy and to the pressure of the fetus on the colon frequently causes constipation. Lack of exercise and the use of iron supplements also may contribute to the problem.

A liberal intake of fluids, 2 qt daily in the form of water, milk, juice, and soup is recommended. Warm or hot liquids taken soon after arising are helpful. Eating high-fiber cereals containing bran and generous amounts of whole grains, legumes, fruits, and vegetables should be encouraged. Physical activity such as walking and swimming will also improve peristalsis. Pregnant women should avoid taking laxatives unless approved by the health care provider.

HEARTBURN

Heartburn, a burning sensation in the chest area, may occur in the later stages of pregnancy due to the pressure of the enlarging uterus on the stomach. The pushing up against the stomach causes the muscle between the stomach and the esophagus to open. The acidic fluid in the stomach regurgitates into the esophagus, causing heartburn. The following are suggestions for preventing heartburn:

Eat small, frequent meals; eat slowly.
Avoid fatty and spicy foods, coffee, and carbonated beverages.
Avoid lying down for 1 to 2 hours after eating. Elevate head when lying down.
Wear loose-fitting clothing.

PREGNANCY COMPLICATIONS

GESTATIONAL DIABETES

Gestational diabetes usually appears between weeks 24 and 28 of pregnancy. Some women may not have a significantly elevated blood glucose level until week 32, when the hormonal stress of pregnancy reaches a peak. Gestational diabetes affects about 2% to 4% of all pregnancies. In certain populations groups with a high risk of diabetes, the prevalence may be as high as 12%. It is the most common medical complication of pregnancy. Of women with gestational diabetes, 98% no longer have diabetes after the baby is born. However, 60% develop non–insulin-dependent diabetes mellitus (type II) later in life. Women who are overweight at the beginning of pregnancy are most likely to develop gestational diabetes.

The diagnosis and treatment of gestational diabetes is important because even a mildly elevated blood glucose level in the pregnant woman can cause adverse effects to the unborn child; however, the infant is not born with diabetes. The condition also creates problems for the pregnant woman. Gestational diabetes is discussed in Chapter 24.

The International Workshop for Gestational Diabetes has recommended that all pregnant women be screened for gestational diabetes at weeks 24 to 28. Screening involves a blood test to determine blood glucose level 1 hour after consuming 50 g of glucose. If the results are higher than 140 mg/dL of glucose, a complete blood glucose tolerance test is given. The glucose tolerance test involves measuring blood glucose levels taken from venous plasma while fasting, and at 1 hour, 2 hours, and 3 hours after consuming 100 g of glucose. The criteria for the diagnosis of gestational diabetes are given in Display 16-3. Normal blood glucose levels during pregnancy differ from those of nonpregnant women because the expansion of blood volume dilutes the blood constituents. Earlier screening for gestational diabetes is recommended for women who have had gestational diabetes in a previous pregnancy, delivery of a baby weighing more than 9 lb (4.05 kg), unexplained stillbirth, malformed infant, and family history of diabetes.

DISPLAY 16–3 GLUCOSE TOLERANCE TEST CRITERIA FOR DIAGNOSIS AND CLASSIFICATION OF GESTATIONAL DIABETES

CLASS A_1

Fasting <105 mg/d: and two or more values above

- 1 hour > 190 mg/dL
- 2 hour > 165 mg/dL
- 3 hour > 145 mg/dL

TREATMENT

Diet therapy. Initiate insulin if normoglycemia is not maintained on diet alone.

CLASS A_2

Fasting >105 mg/dL and two or more values above

- 1 hour > 190 mg/dL
- 2 hour > 165 mg/dL
- 3 hour > 145 mg/dL

TREATMENT

Prescribe diet and insulin therapy to achieve normoglycemia.

(National Diabetes Data Group. Classification and diagnosis of diabetes mellitus and other categories of glucose intolerance. Diabetes 1979;28:1039.)

HYPERTENSIVE DISORDERS

Disorders associated with high blood pressure (hypertension) during pregnancy can seriously threaten both the mother's and fetus's health. The disorders are associated with either chronic high blood pressure that existed before pregnancy or to pregnancy induced hypertension (PIH).

CHRONIC HYPERTENSION

Women with chronic high blood pressure (140/90 mm Hg or higher) before pregnancy may develop symptoms of persistent elevated blood pressure, edema, and protein in the urine in the latter half of pregnancy. If untreated, the condition may progress to convulsions and coma.

PREGNANCY-INDUCED HYPERTENSION

Pregnancy-induced hypertension is a condition that typically occurs at about week 20 of pregnancy. It is characterized by elevated blood pressure, protein in the urine, and edema of the hands, face, and ankles. If uncontrolled, the condition may progress to convulsions and coma, a condition known as *eclampsia.* The cause of PIH is unclear but is associated with poverty and lack of prenatal care. Poor diets, especially low-protein diets, have been implicated. Sometimes women who are well nourished develop PIH. Other factors such as genetics or immune function may be involved in these cases.

Most pregnant women experience a certain amount of edema in the extremities. In PIH, however, the edema is much more severe, and involves the hands, face, feet, and legs. It may be accompanied by dizziness, headache, blurred vision, nausea, and vomiting. Low serum protein levels, not sodium retention, is the cause of the edema. Because many young women normally have prepregnancy blood pressure levels less than 120/80 mm Hg, the use of 140/90 mm Hg to diagnose hypertension in pregnancy is inappropriate. The diagnosis is best made by comparison with an individual's prepregnancy blood pressure levels. The diagnosis of PIH is based on repeated blood pressure measurements of 140/90 mm Hg or higher or an elevation of 30 mm Hg systolic (top number) or 15 mm Hg diastolic (bottom number) above the woman's prepregnancy blood pressure level.

Diet counseling during pregnancy is extremely important, especially for women with poor eating habits. A diet containing optimum amounts of high-quality protein, sufficient calories to achieve desired weight gain, and ample amounts of vitamins and minerals appears to be the best means of decreasing the risk of developing PIH. Salt restriction and the use of diuretics usually are avoided because salt requirements are increased during pregnancy. Normal amounts of salt are recommended. Occasionally, a mild sodium restriction involving no added salt at the table may be used. Severe sodium restrictions *are not recommended* in PIH.

ANEMIA

Anemia is common in pregnancy. For women who are anemic, a therapeutic dose of 60 mg to 120 mg/day of elemental iron is prescribed. In addition, a low-dose vitamin/mineral supplement for use in pregnancy is prescribed to ensure adequate amounts of copper and zinc, also needed to correct the anemia.

Folate is needed for optimal growth of tissues. A diet low in folacin causes *megaloblastic anemia,* a condition in which the red blood cells are large and immature. The RDA of 400 mcg of folate during pregnancy can be met by a well-chosen diet. Supplements of folate are recommended for pregnant women who are not meeting this level of intake.

HUMAN IMMUNODEFICIENCY VIRUS

Woman who are infected with the human immunodeficiency virus (HIV) are at increased risk of developing gastrointestinal problems, anemia, and weight loss. A thorough nutrition assessment and frequent monitoring of the woman's nutritional status are necessary to provide dietary assistance that will promote normal weight gain during pregnancy and the proper functioning of the immune system. Vitamin and mineral supplementation is indicated. Women with HIV also will need information about preventing secondary infections such as foodborne illness.

TEENAGE PREGNANCY

Pregnancy during adolescence is a major US public health problem and is largely responsible for the relatively high infant mortality rate. Teenage pregnancies—those occurring between the ages 11 years and 18 years—are considered to be high risk. More of these infants are born preterm, are of low birth weight, require intensive care, or die at birth than infants of adult mothers. These infants also are twice as likely as infants of adult mothers to have physical problems or to die after the newborn period. The teenager, herself, is more vulnerable than other age groups to PIH, which may possibly lead to cardiovascular and renal complications in later life.

NUTRITIONAL NEEDS

The teenager is in a critical stage of growth, so pregnancy may seriously retard her own growth as well as that of her baby. This is especially true if the pregnant teenager is younger than age 14 years or is within 24 months of her first menstrual cycle. The teenager's physically immature body and the psychosocial problems she faces contribute to the risk of poor pregnancy outcome.

In evaluating the physical needs of the pregnant teenager, *gynecologic age* (the number of years since the onset of menstruation) is more useful than chronological age. A 16-year-old who started menstruating at age 12 years has a gynecologic age of 4 years—complete growth in height is not achieved until 4 years after the onset of menses. Girls who become pregnant at a gynecologic age of less than 2 or 3 years have the greatest nutritional needs and are at greater risk because they are physically immature. A young woman with a gynecologic age of 5 years is not at increased risk.

The nutritional needs of the pregnant adolescent have not been well investigated. Nutrition recommendations are determined by adding the pregnancy RDAs for the adult woman to the RDAs for the nonpregnant teenager (see Table 16-4). Because nutritional status at the time of conception is of utmost importance, the frequently inadequate diets of adolescents pose a particularly serious problem for pregnant teenagers. Meal skipping, poor-quality snacks, eating away from home, limited food choices, and overconcern about weight are common patterns of behavior. Low intakes of calcium, vitamin A, folate, iron, and zinc, likely to be present in adolescent diets, may adversely effect the outcome of pregnancy. The pregnant teenager who is on a vegan diet may have additional deficiencies of protein, riboflavin, vitamin B_{12}, vitamin D, and trace minerals.

NUTRITION COUNSELING

The teenage years are difficult enough without the added stress of pregnancy and the social problems it creates for the teenager. The pregnant teenager requires a comprehensive health care program that includes proper prenatal care, weight gain monitoring, nutrition assessment, counseling and support, family planning, and continued schooling. Parents or other care-givers should be included, if possible, in counseling sessions. A nonjudgmental attitude is essential to establishing open communication. It is important to assess the teenager's state of emotional development and to individualize the counseling approach based on stage of development—the teenager's ability or inability to set realistic goals—rather than chronological age.

Once the health counselor has established rapport and assessed developmental needs, he or she should evaluate dietary intake and make suggestions for improvement that are both practical and acceptable to the adolescent. The weight goal in a teenage pregnancy frequently is higher than the optimal weight gain for adults. If the teenager is underweight, a gain to bring her weight to normal for her height, plus weight associated with gynecologic age, is added to the usual pregnancy weight gain. Because teenagers are usually concerned about body image, some may need special guidance in achieving recommended weight gain goals. A preoccupation with weight, excessive exercise, or dieting may signal an eating disorder.

The pregnancy may be the catalyst for improving the teenager's eating habits. Iron and folate supplementation are recommended for all pregnant teenagers. Additional vitamin and mineral supplementation may be necessary if the quality or quantity of the diet continues to be inadequate. Furthermore, the pregnant teenager should also be informed of the adverse effects of smoking, alcohol, and street drugs.

NUTRITION DURING BREASTFEEDING

NUTRITION NEEDS

As during pregnancy, the breastfeeding woman needs a diet of high nutritional quality. The RDAs for most nutrients are greater during breastfeeding than during pregnancy (see Table 16-4). The RDAs during breastfeeding are provided for the first and second 6-month periods to reflect the differences in the amounts of milk produced: 750 mL/day in the first 6 months and 600 mL/day in the second 6 months, when solid foods are given the infant to supplement milk.

An additional 500 kcal/day is recommended throughout breastfeeding, 200 kcal/day more than the recommendation during pregnancy. The recommendation of an additional 500 kcal/day is based on the assumption that the fat stores of 2 kg (4.5 lb) or 3 kg (6.5 lb) accumulated during pregnancy can provide additional 100 to 150 kcal/day during the first 6 months of breastfeeding. In this way, the extra fat that accumulated during pregnancy is lost gradually. For women who gained less than the recommended weight during pregnancy or those who lose weight while breastfeeding, an additional 650 (500 + 150) kcal/day is recommended. In the second 6 months of pregnancy, milk production decreases to about 600 mL/day. The additional 500 kcal/day in the diet alone is sufficient to cover the energy cost of producing this quantity of milk.

Breastfeeding requires an additional 15 g of protein during the first 6 months of breastfeeding and 12 g during the second 6 months, which is more than the extra 10 g recommended during pregnancy. The breastfeeding woman also needs more of the vitamins A, E, C, thiamin, riboflavin, niacin, and B_{12} and more of the minerals magnesium, zinc, iodine, and selenium than she did during pregnancy. The breastfeeding woman should drink enough fluids to satisfy thirst.

The RDA for iron is the same for the breastfeeding woman as for the nonpregnant woman. Iron losses in breast milk are less than menstrual losses, which are absent during breastfeeding. This differs from previous recommendations that women take iron supplements for 2 or 3 months after delivery to restore iron reserves.

The amounts of certain nutrients in breast milk have been shown to be influenced by the mother's intake, including unsaturated fats, vitamin A, vitamin E, thiamin, riboflavin, niacin, pyridoxine, vitamin B_{12}, manganese and iodine. Also, the quantity of milk may be smaller in a poorly nourished woman.

NUTRITION COUNSELING

A nursing mother can follow the food guide she used when pregnant with the addition of 1 cup of milk a day and an additional ounce or equivalent of food from the meat and meat substitute group. Of the three to five servings of vegetables recommended, at least one serving should be a good source of vitamin A. Of the two to four servings of fruit, two servings of a good source of vitamin C are recommended. See the food guide during breastfeeding in Table 16-2.

Most substances that enter the mother's body are secreted in the milk. Consequently, breastfeeding women must give attention to the use of drugs (over-the-counter, prescription, and street drugs) and alcohol and to smoking habits. If women must take any medication that is secreted in breast milk and is known to affect the infant, they are advised not to breastfeed. The advice for sugar substitutes is the same as that for pregnancy. Breastfeeding women should be advised to avoid alcohol and also be informed that, contrary to popular opinion, beer does not aid breastfeeding. Limits should be strongly recommended for women who choose to consume alcohol—no more than 2 oz to $2\frac{1}{2}$ oz of liquor, 8 oz of table wine, or two cans of beer on any one day—less for small women. Breastfeeding women also should avoid caffeine-containing beverages or limit them to two servings or less per day. Furthermore, they should be alerted to the need to listen for advisories from public health officials regarding contaminants in food or the environment such as mercury or pesticides.

Most women, whether they are breastfeeding or not, are concerned about returning to their prepregnancy weight. They should be informed that most women will gain weight in the first 4 days after delivery and will begin to lose weight by the day 5 postpartum. After a few weeks of rapid weight loss, the average weight loss is about 1 to 2 lb (0.5 to 1.0 kg) per month through the first 6 months after delivery.

For overweight breastfeeding women, the maximum suggested rate of weight loss after the month 1 postpartum is about $4\frac{1}{2}$ lb (2 kg) a month. These women should consume no fewer than 1800 kcal to achieve this weight loss. Lower intakes would not provide adequate amounts of protein, vitamins and minerals. In addition, the use of liquid diets and weight loss medications is not recommended. Physical activity is encouraged.

KEYS TO PRACTICAL APPLICATION

Advise clients who are planning pregnancies of the importance of preconception care.

Help clients understand the importance of adequate weight gain during pregnancy.

Strongly discourage clients who are obese from attempting to lose weight during pregnancy. Weight gain during pregnancy is essential; however, the weight gain goal may be lower than for the normal-weight woman.

Encourage quality in eating habits. Explain that caloric needs increase little compared with increased need for protein, vitamins, and minerals. There is little room for foods with empty calories.

Tell your clients that the Food Guide Pyramid is an excellent basis for diet during pregnancy.

Advise clients that skipping meals is a poor practice, especially for the pregnant woman. The fetus needs a steady supply of nutrients.

Strongly discourage pregnant women from using alcohol and encourage them to limit caffeine intake.

Instruct clients to take only the vitamins and minerals as prescribed. Excessive amounts can be harmful.

Instruct clients of the potential danger involved in using herbs and other dietary supplements without medical approval. Little is known about the effects of these substances.

Advise the woman who has morning sickness of the importance of identifying the odors that trigger nausea. Help her identify foods that "sound good" and will stay down.

Encourage the use of high-fiber foods and plenty of fluids to avoid constipation.

Give priority to helping pregnant teenagers improve their eating habits. Together with the teenager, plan meals and snacks that are nutritious and at the same time acceptable to her.

Take advantage of the client's high motivation during pregnancy to provide nutrition education for the family as well as for the pregnant woman.

Encourage the breastfeeding mother to continue the high-quality diet she consumed during pregnancy and increase the amounts of milk, green leafy and yellow vegetables, and vitamin C–rich foods.

KEY IDEAS

Physical growth occurs by an increase in cell number, in cell size, and in the amount of material between cells.

The rate of growth is not uniform; rapid growth occurs in prenatal life, early infancy, and adolescence.

During critical stages of development, certain tissues and organs of the body are at risk of permanent damage if essential nutrients are not provided.

Major body systems of the embryo are formed in the first 2 months after conception; therefore, the nutritional status of the mother at the time of conception is extremely important. For this reason, preconception counseling is strongly encouraged.

Nutrition is one of many factors that shape the course of pregnancy.

Adequate nutrition is an important factor in the successful outcome of pregnancy; nutrition has its greatest effect on physical and mental growth during prenatal life and infancy.

Low–birth weight infants are more likely to have birth defects and have a higher death rate than normal-weight babies. Birth weight is the factor most closely related to infant death.

Factors that influence birth weight include weight gain during pregnancy, prepregnancy weight, and smoking.

The recommended weight gain during pregnancy is about 25 to 35 lb (11.5 to 16 kg). Women who are underweight are encouraged to gain more and those who are obese may need to gain less.

The obese woman should not attempt to lose weight during pregnancy. The ketosis that may result from caloric restriction may cause neurologic damage to the fetus.

The recommended pattern of weight gain for the woman of normal prepregnancy weight is 2 to 5 lb (.9 to 2.3 kg) in the first trimester and a steady increase of about 1.0 lb (0.5 kg) per week in the second and third trimesters.

Energy needs during pregnancy increase little (300 kcal/day) compared with the increased needs for nutrients; the diet must be chosen carefully to include all of the necessary nutrients without excessive calories. The rate of weight gain is the best indicator of the adequacy of caloric intake.

The use of a food guide during pregnancy should be encouraged; most guides meet all RDAs except iron, for which a supplement is given.

The recommendations made in *Dietary Guidelines for Americans* are modified somewhat during pregnancy: fats may be increased moderately if weight gain is inadequate, sodium should not be limited, and high-protein foods are encouraged.

Iron supplements are recommended for all pregnant women.

A folate intake of 400 mcg is recommended for all pregnant and nonpregnant women of childbearing age.

Women at high risk of developing nutritional deficiencies (see Table 16-1) should be identified and given intensive nutritional guidance.

Weight gain during pregnancy needs to be monitored carefully.

Nutrition education directed toward the pregnant woman may influence the entire family; motivation usually is high at this time.

Serious complications of pregnancy include gestational diabetes, hypertensive disorders, and anemia.

Pregnant women should be screened for gestational diabetes between weeks 24 and 28 of pregnancy.

Pregnancy-induced hypertension is a condition that occurs after week 20 of pregnancy. Symptoms include high blood pressure, protein in the urine, severe edema, and eventually, if treated unsuccessfully, convulsions and coma.

Iron deficiency anemia is common in pregnancy. It requires the use of an iron supplement.

Megaloblastic anemia may be caused by a diet low in folate.

Women with a lactase deficiency may be able to tolerate dairy products by using one or more of the following: small servings at one time, cultured yogurt or cultured buttermilk, aged cheese, lactase tablets or drops, or lactase-treated milk.

Women with pica are prone to the development of nutritional deficiencies.

Pregnant women should avoid long intervals between meals; the fetus requires a continual supply of energy and nutrients.

"Morning sickness" may be a mild condition or it may be so severe that it requires hospitalization. An enhanced sense of smell during pregnancy appears to be a major underlying cause.

Birth defects are associated with the overdoses of vitamin supplements and the use of alcohol. The use of alcoholic beverages of any type is not recommended during pregnancy.

Caffeine-containing beverages should be limited to two servings daily.

The pregnant teenager has growth needs of her own as well as those of the fetus. Complications of pregnancy are high among teenagers. High priority should be given to helping pregnant teenagers meet their nutritional needs.

Teenagers' concern with body image may hinder efforts to achieve weight gain goals.

The counseling approach should be individualized to accommodate the pregnant adolescent's stage of emotional development.

Nutritional needs continue to be high during breastfeeding. For many nutrients, the need is even higher than during pregnancy.

Breastfeeding women who are overweight should not consume fewer than 1800 kcal/day. The maximum rate of weight loss recommended after month 1 postpartum is $4^{1}/_{2}$ lb (2 kg) per month.

KEYS TO LEARNING

STUDY–DISCUSSION QUESTIONS

1. Why is the nutritional status of the woman at the beginning of pregnancy so important? What nutritional problems are involved in teenage pregnancies? What suggestions do you have for encouraging the teenager to

improve her eating habits? What approach would you use? Discuss your answers in class.

2. What is meant by the phrase *critical stages of growth?* How does this concept apply to brain development?
3. Why would it be unwise for an obese woman to attempt to lose weight or to severely limit her weight gain during pregnancy? What would you suggest to a woman who is gaining excessive amounts of weight during pregnancy?
4. Plan 3 days of menus for a pregnant teenager using the food guide in Table 16-2.
5. Priority should be given to providing nutrition education to parents-to-be. Why?

CASE STUDY

Mrs. T, a 25-year-old office manager, went to her physician after she missed her menstrual period. She was delighted to learn that the pregnancy test was positive. Both she and her husband had looked forward to starting a family. She is interested in attending the prenatal classes at the hospital and plans to breastfeed her baby. Her physician found that her hemoglobin level of 10.5 and her hematocrit level of 32% were below the acceptable range. Mrs. T is 67 inches (170 cm) tall and weighs 125 lb (57 kg); she has a medium frame. She is conscious of her weight and is concerned about gaining too much weight during the pregnancy. She attends aerobics classes for 1 hour two times a week and jogs for 1 hour on the other days. She and her husband do not smoke.

Mrs. T says she is too rushed to eat breakfast in the morning, but usually has something to eat at her midmorning break. She eats lunch in one of the nearby luncheonettes or fast-food restaurants. She has about three "light" beers a week. She and her husband eat out once a week, usually Mexican food, and her husband brings home a pizza for dinner once a week.

The following is Mrs. T's 24-hour diet recall:

7:00 AM	6 oz of orange juice
10:30 AM	One jelly doughnut
	Coffee with half and half
12:30 PM	1 cup of chicken and rice soup
	One hot dog with mustard and relish
	Diet soda
3:00 PM	Ice cream sandwich
5:00 PM	Chicken pot pie (frozen)
	Salad
	Two chocolate chip cookies
	One apple
	Diet iced tea
9:00 PM	Popcorn—3 cups
	Diet soda

1. Evaluate Mrs. T's weight status. What might be a reasonable weight goal for her pregnancy?
2. How would you deal with Mrs. T's fear of gaining too much weight?
3. What are some of the positive factors in Mrs. T's history?
4. Using the 24-hour diet recall given above, compare Mrs. T's food intake with the daily food guide for pregnancy (see Display 16-2).
   What nutritional needs are being met?
   What eating practices are good and need to be maintained?
   What aspects of her diet and eating habits need to be improved?
   What practices should be eliminated?
5. What advice would you give Mrs. T for improving the iron content of her diet? (Mrs. T will be given iron supplements during her pregnancy. She should be made aware of the eating habits that are responsible for the iron deficiency anemia, however.) How can the absorption of iron be improved?
6. Mrs. T is not in the habit of drinking milk. It is not one of her favorite foods, but she will drink it. What suggestions can you offer for increasing milk consumption?

BIBLIOGRAPHY

BOOKS AND PAMPHLETS

Barness LA. Ed. Pediatric nutrition handbook. 3rd ed., Elk Grove Village, IL: American Academy of Pediatrics, 1993.

Mahan LK, Arlin MT. Krause's food, nutrition and diet therapy. 8th ed. Philadelphia: WB Saunders, 1992:Chapter 9.

National Academy of Sciences, Institute of Medicine, Food and Nutrition Board, Committee on Nutritional Status During Pregnancy and Lactation. Nutrition services in perinatal care. Washington, DC: National Academy Press, 1992.

National Academy of Sciences, Institute of Medicine, Food and Nutrition Board, Committee on Nutritional Status During Pregnancy and Lactation, Subcommittee for a Clinical Application Guide. Nutrition during pregnancy and lactation: an implementation guide. Washington, DC: National Academy Press, 1992.

National Academy of Sciences, National Research Council, Food and Nutrition Board. Recommended dietary allowances. 10th ed. Washington, DC: National Academy Press, 1989.

US Dept of Agriculture and US Dept of Health and Human Services. Nutrition and your health: dietary guidelines for Americans. 3rd ed. Washington, DC: US Government Printing Office, 1990. Home and Garden bulletin 232.

Worthington-Roberts BS, William SR. Nutrition in pregnancy and lactation. St. Louis: Mosby–Year Book, Inc. 1993.

PERIODICALS

American Dietetic Association. Position of the American Dietetic Association: nutrition care for pregnant adolescents. J Am Diet Assoc 1994;94:449.

American Dietetic Association. Position of the American Dietetic Association: promotion and support of breast feeding. J Am Diet Assoc 1993;93:467.

Erick M. Battling morning (noon and night) sickness. J Am Diet Assoc 1994;94:147.

Gunderson E. Gestational diabetes mellitus: overview. On the Cutting Edge 1992;13:6:1.

Karra MV, Auerbach KG, Olson L, et al. Hospital infant feeding practices in metropolitan Chicago: an evaluation of five of the ten steps to successful breast feeding. J Am Diet Assoc 1993;93:1437.

Pope J, Skinner JD, Carruth BR. Cravings and aversions of pregnant adolescents. J Am Diet Assoc 1992;92:1479.

Skinner JD, Carruth BR, Pope J. Food and nutrient intake of white pregnant adolescents. J Am Diet Assoc 1992;92:1127.

Springer NS, Bischoping K, Sampselle CM, et al. Using early weight gain and other nutrition-related risk factors to predict pregnancy outcomes. J Am Diet Assoc 1992;92:217.

CHAPTER

17

Meeting Nutritional Needs During Infancy

KEY TERMS

allergen substance capable of producing an allergic reaction

colostrum thin, yellow fluid secreted from the breast for 2 or 3 days after childbirth, before the secretion of milk begins; colostrum contains mainly serum and white blood corpuscles

extrusion reflex protrusion of tongue when spoon is placed in the infant's mouth; the infant unable to transfer food to the back of the mouth

failure to thrive seriously retarded growth in infants younger than age 18 months; term also applied to older children and adolescents

let-down reflex reflex that moves milk out of the glands and into the nipple

rooting reflex infant's reflex movement to seek the nipple

wean to stop breastfeeding when the infant can take substantial food from other sources; usually accomplished gradually

OBJECTIVES

After completing this chapter, the student will be able to:

1. Explain the advantages of breastfeeding for both mother and infant.
2. Explain how the nutritional needs of the breastfed infant and of the formula-fed infant are met in the first 4 to 6 months of life.
3. List specific ways in which the health care team can promote the success of breastfeeding.
4. Describe the intervals of feeding for both breastfed and bottle-fed babies.
5. Describe the differences between commercial infant formula and home-prepared cow's milk formula; explain why cow's milk formula is not recommended.
6. Describe the introduction of supplemental foods, including the schedule for their introduction and the rationale behind it.
7. List four infant feeding practices that are unwise or dangerous.
8. Explain the dangers of heating formula and baby food in the microwave and describe what precautions should be taken.
9. Describe and discuss the following nutrition-related problems of infants: failure to thrive, iron deficiency anemia, acute diarrhea, phenylketonuria, and galactosemia.
10. Explain the benefits and eligibility requirements of the Special Supplemental Food Program for Women, Infants, and Children (WIC program).

Adequate nutrition is essential to support the newborn's growth during the early months—growth that is more rapid than at any other time of life. The infant's birth weight doubles by about age 4 to 6 months. After that, weight gain slows down somewhat, but by the age of 10 to 12 months, birth weight has tripled and length has increased about 10 inches. The body of the newborn contains more water than that of an older child; however, the amount of subcutaneous fat increases during the first year.

The first months of life are a critical period in the growth and development of the brain and central nervous system, skeleton, teeth, kidneys, and gastrointestinal system. The brain and nervous system develop rapidly during fetal life and early infancy. Protein, emulsified fat, and simple carbohydrates can be readily digested by the newborn's gastrointestinal tract. As the infant's body increases its production of digestive enzymes, the ability to digest other fats and starches improves. The infant's skeleton is soft; it becomes hard during childhood and adolescence. Teeth begin to appear at age 5 or 6 months, and by the end of the first year, the baby has five to ten teeth. Kidneys reach their full functional capacity by the end of the first year.

The full-term infant is born with a store of iron in the liver and with a high hemoglobin level: 17 to 20 g/dL. This is nature's way of providing an iron supply for the first few months of life, when the infant's diet consists of milk, a poor source of iron. The infant's iron store gradually becomes depleted unless iron supplements or iron-fortified foods are given. Even with adequate iron intake, the hemoglobin level drops to 11 to 12 g/dL in the second 6 months.

NUTRITIONAL NEEDS

Because of the infant's extremely rapid growth rate, the requirements for energy and nutrients per unit of body weight are higher in infancy than at any other time of life. The Recommended Dietary Allowances (RDAs) for the first 6 months of life are based on the amount of nutrients in the average volume of breast milk consumed by a healthy infant. The RDAs for the second 6 months are based on a slightly lower volume of breast milk or of formula supplemented by solid foods.

ENERGY

The caloric requirement during the first 6 months is three times that of the adult requirement per unit of body weight. As the infant's growth rate gradually decreases, so too does the caloric requirement. Both breast milk and commercial infant formulas supply about 20 kcal/oz. Energy needs vary widely from infant to infant. Under normal circumstances, infants will consume amounts equal to their needs.

CARBOHYDRATE AND FAT

No recommendation is made for carbohydrate and fat. Lactose is the main carbohydrate in human milk and is the infant's source of carbohydrate for the first 6 months of life.

The fat content of human milk varies from woman to woman. The average fat content of human milk is higher than that of cow's milk. Almost half the calories of human milk are supplied by fat. Human milk also has more of the essential fatty acid, linoleic acid, and more cholesterol than cow's milk.

PROTEIN

It is not surprising that the protein requirement per unit of body weight is higher in infancy than at any other time of life. The recommendation is 2.2 g/kg during the first 6 months of life, decreasing to 1.6 g/kg during the second 6 months.

FLUIDS

The infant's need for fluids is satisfied by breast milk or formula. When an unusual loss of fluid occurs because of hot weather, fever, or diarrhea, water also should be given. Water may be necessary when supplemental foods are given, especially if these foods are high in protein, sodium, or potassium. The body needs extra water to excrete the end products that result from the metabolism of these nutrients.

VITAMINS

All newborns should be given a single dose of vitamin K to prevent against hemorrhagic disease of the newborn. This treatment is now required by law in many states.

Breast milk provides all the vitamins the infant needs for the first 4 to 6 months of life, except possibly vitamin D. Vitamin D supplementation is recommended for breastfed infants who are dark skinned or who have limited exposure to sunlight. If the breastfeeding woman is a vegan, a B_{12} supplement is recommended for her infant. Multivitamin supplements are recommended for breastfed infants in malnourished mothers. Commercial infant formula consumed in adequate amounts provides all the vitamins needed for the first year of life.

MINERALS

To increase resistance to dental decay, fluoride supplement is recommended for breastfed infants beginning shortly after birth. Some physicians prefer to start fluoride supplementation at 6 months.

Fluoride supplements also are recommended for infants given ready-to-use commercial formulas because they are made with water low in fluoride. When powdered or concentrated commercial formulas that must be mixed with water are used, fluoride supplements are unnecessary unless the water supply contains less than 0.3 part per million of fluoride.

The amount of iron in human milk is adequate to supply the infant's needs for the first 6 months of life. After 6 months, the RDA for iron increases, and all breastfed infants should be given a supplement or iron-fortified cereal. The American Academy of Pediatrics has recommended that all formula-fed infants be given iron-fortified formulas. Research has not supported the belief that iron supplementation causes constipation and other feeding problems.

BREASTFEEDING

The committees on nutrition of both the American Academy of Pediatrics and the Canadian Paediatric Society have strongly endorsed breastfeeding as the best means of feeding infants. The number of women breastfeeding peaked in the early 1980s, following a decline from 1955 to 1970. Since then, the numbers have fallen. National health goals for the year 2000 aim to increase to at least 75% the proportion of mothers who breastfeed their babies in the early postpartum period and to at least 50% the proportion who breastfeed until their babies are 5 to 6 months old. In 1990, 56% of infants received commercially prepared formula in the hospital. By the time the infants were 5 to 6 months old, 85% were formula fed. Unfortunately, the decline of breastfeeding is most prevalent among women who are in lower socioeconomic circumstances.

During pregnancy, the health care provider should discuss feeding plans with the woman. If she chooses to breastfeed, they should discuss breast care. The woman needs to learn as much as she can about the techniques of successful breastfeeding before giving birth. The health care worker can provide information and resource materials and can refer the client to supportive community organizations, such as nursing mother's councils or chapters of the La Leche League. The Special Supplemental Food Program for Women, Infants, and Children (WIC program) supports breastfeeding.

After delivery, professional personnel should provide support and counseling because the early days of breastfeeding are important to establishing a good milk supply and effective *let-down reflex*. This reflex moves the milk out of the mammary glands and into the nipple (Fig. 17-1). Because hospital stays for new mothers are so short, they should make arrangements for telephone contact with the physician or breastfeeding instructor and possibly a return visit in 10 to 14 days. New mothers may also make arrangements with hospital-provided or private lactation consul-

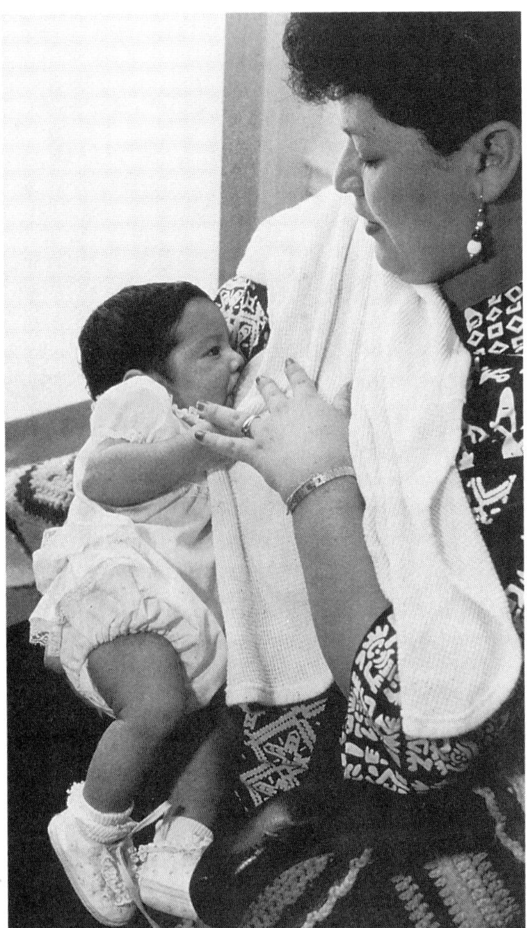

FIGURE 17-1

Leading authorities have strongly endorsed breastfeeding as the best means of feeding infants. *(Courtesy of the US Dept of Agriculture)*

tants who make home visits and are available on a 24-hour basis for phone advice. La Leche League has a telephone support system in many areas.

ADVANTAGES FOR THE INFANT

The composition of breast milk is specifically suited to the infant's nutritional needs. Human milk is composed of nutrients, enzymes, and hormones that differ from other types of milks. The forms of protein and sugar in breast milk are more easily digested and absorbed than those supplied by cow's milk. Breast milk is higher in cholesterol than the commercial infant formulas made with vegetable oils. Cholesterol is needed for the child's developing nerve and brain tissue. Breast milk contains more vitamin C than cow's milk, which loses much of its vitamin C content during processing and storage.

Colostrum, a watery, yellowish fluid, is the first secretion to come from the breast a day or so after delivery. It is rich in body-building proteins and appears to be the ideal food for infants in the first 3 or 4 days of life. Both colostrum and the breast milk that follows provide infants with antibodies and other factors that protect against infectious disease. Breastfeeding appears to provide immunity against gastroenteritis, certain kinds of diarrhea, and respiratory infections.

Breastfeeding often is recommended when there is a strong family history of allergy. Early exposure to cow's milk and solid foods is believed to be related to allergic conditions that develop later. Protection against obesity is another advantage of breastfeeding; there is a tendency to overfeed when infants are bottle-fed. Some research has suggested that breastfeeding may reduce the risk of some chronic diseases such as celiac disease.

ADVANTAGES FOR THE MOTHER

Breastfeeding has advantages for the mother. It may help her lose the extra weight she gained during pregnancy because the production of milk requires more energy than the pregnancy required. Breastfeeding also helps the uterus return to its normal size because nursing stimulates the hormones that cause the uterus to contract. Breastfeeding is the most economical and convenient form of infant feeding. Even when the cost of the extra food the mother needs is considered, breastfeeding is less expensive than infant formula.

Breast milk always is available, it is at the proper temperature, and it is sterile; it also saves the time required for bottle washing. Women who must leave their baby for extended periods can manually express or pump breast milk into bottles. The milk may be stored in the refrigerator for use within 24 to 48 hours.

CONTRAINDICATIONS AND PRECAUTIONS

Although breastfeeding offers many benefits, it is not always practical, and a mother should not be pressured to breastfeed or made to feel guilty if she decides against it. Breastfeeding is contraindicated for women with tuberculosis, human immunodeficiency virus (HIV) or acquired immunodeficiency virus (AIDS), and hepatitis B and for infants who cannot tolerate milk because of genetic disorders, such as lactase deficiency or galactosemia.

Because most drugs pass from the mother's blood to her milk, nursing women should only take medications, even over-the-counter varieties, under medical supervision. Drugs that are contraindications to breastfeeding include those that suppress immune function, radioactive isotopes, some antithyroid drugs and sulfonamides, and also drugs that suppress breastfeeding such as chlorathizide. Also, the mother's body may concentrate toxic chemicals from the environment. These, too, may appear in the breast milk and may present a risk to the infant. An example is the presence of higher levels of the toxic chemical benzene hexachloride and polychlorinated biphenyls (PCBs) in women who consume freshwater fish from contaminated areas. Mothers also should avoid excessive caffeine and other stimulants from coffee, tea, soda, and herbal teas.

FEEDINGS

Breastfeeding is begun as soon after delivery as possible. The mother and infant should not be separated for the first 24 hours except for assessment or treatment. The mother should be helped to position herself comfortably and to assist the infant so the child will grasp the breast properly. Stroking the infant on one cheek will cause the child to turn his or her head in that direction and open the mouth. This automatic seeking of the breast is called the *rooting reflex*.

Once the mouth is open, the mother should guide the nipple into the infant's mouth with as much of the areola as possible to facilitate the act of sucking. The infant's proper grasp of the breast and subsequent ability to suck the breast milk is referred to as "latching on." To accomplish this activity with some infants may take a considerable amount of time and patience. After a 3- or 4-minute suckling period, the mother breaks the suction by gently slipping her clean finger into the corner of the infant's mouth and the brief feeding is repeated on the second breast. Breastfeedings continue when the infant is awake and hungry (i.e., on demand), at least every 4 to 5 hours or as frequently as every 2 hours to stimulate milk production. The act of sucking signals the let-down reflex, which begins milk production.

The length of the feeding is gradually increased until, by postpartum day 3, the infant is taking each breast for about 10 minutes or more at a feeding. Each feeding should include nursing on both breasts. After about 10 minutes, the infant has probably taken all the available milk in one breast.

The infant is breastfed on demand and not according to a set schedule. During the first few weeks of life, the infant usually requires a feeding every 2 or 3 hours—a minimum of 6 to as many as 12 feedings a day. After the initial period, the infant breastfeeds about every 3 or 4 hours. By about the second month, the infant sleeps through the 2 AM to 3 AM feeding and about 2 to 3 months later, the child sleeps through the late evening (10 PM to 11 PM) feeding.

Frequent nursing assures an adequate supply of milk. For this reason, supplemental bottles of water or formula are discouraged for the first few weeks of breastfeeding. The baby also may become confused because of the differences in the breast and bottle nipples. The sucking action involved with a standard nipple is different than that required for breastfeeding. The baby must work harder to obtain milk at the breast.

If the newborn is sleeping 2 or 3 hours between feedings and regains his or her birth weight by age

3 weeks, the quantity of milk is sufficient. If the baby continues to lose weight after 10 days of life, the intake is inadequate and the situation needs to be evaluated.

BONDING

One major benefit of breastfeeding is that it promotes bonding—a strong interaction between mother and infant. Bonding begins soon after birth when the baby is cuddled while being fed. Close physical contact with the mother gives the infant a sense of warmth and security. The mother feels a special closeness and a sense of accomplishment in fulfilling the infant's needs. This close relationship is thought to have lasting emotional and psychological effects. When bottle-fed babies are held as they are fed, they can be given just as much love and attention as the breastfed infant, thus developing a bond of closeness between mother and infant and father and infant. The father of the breast-fed infant may also share this closeness by feeding the infant expressed breast milk in a bottle on a limited basis (e.g. one feeding a day).

WEANING

Weaning from breast milk is best accomplished gradually, sometimes taking 2 or 3 months to totally discontinue breastfeeding. One bottle a day is given as a replacement for one breastfeeding. After about 1 week, a second bottle is given. The bottles should be given at the same time each day to help the mother's body begin to produce less milk at that particular time. If breastfeeding is discontinued at or after age 8 months, the infant may be weaned directly from the breast to the cup. Infants weaned before age 1 year should consume an iron-fortified commercial formula by bottle or cup instead of cow's milk, which is unsuitable for infants until after age 1 year. Many cultures and the La Leche League encourage the idea of baby-led weaning (baby loses interest in breastfeeding), which may occur after the first year.

FORMULA FEEDING

COMMERCIAL FORMULAS

Commercial milk-based formula is recommended when breastfeeding is not adopted or if it is stopped before the infant is 1 year old. Commercial formulas consist of cow's milk that is modified to resemble breast milk. The changes may include the treatment of protein to produce a digestible curd and the replacement of butterfat with vegetable oil. The American Academy of Pediatrics has developed standards for these formulas. These standards form the basis of the mandatory Food and Drug Administration regulations for the composition of infant formulas that specify the minimum levels of 29 nutrients and maximum levels of 9 nutrients.

Commercial formulas are available in powdered, concentrated liquid, ready-to-use, and ready-to-feed forms. Powder is the least expensive form and ready-to-feed (sold in nursing bottles) is the most expensive. The powder and the liquid concentrate must be diluted with water.

Directions for use should be followed carefully, and the mother or other care-giver should be instructed in preparation. When the care-giver uses powdered or concentrated forms of formula, it is important that he or she use the proper dilution. For sanitary reasons, feedings should be prepared one at a time rather than 24 hours in advance.

Standard commercial formulas are available with a soy protein base as well as a cow's milk base. The soy protein–based formulas and cow's milk–based lactose-free formulas such as Lactofree (Mead Johnson) are used for infants who are lactose intolerant (see Chapter 28), or who have galactosemia (see the section Enzyme Deficiencies). Vegans may also give soy formulas to their infants who are not breastfed. Specialized commercial formulas also are available for infants who have extraordinary problems such as severe allergy to intact protein, low birth weight, or phenylketonuria (PKU; see the section Enzyme Deficiencies).

HOME-PREPARED COW'S MILK FORMULA

Cow's milk or home-prepared formula made from whole or evaporated milk is not recommended until after age 1 year when at least two thirds of the infant's caloric requirements are being met by supplemental foods. Although a home-prepared formula is considerably less expensive than a commercial formula, it has a number of disadvantages for the infant: it contains high concentrations of certain nutrients (e.g., protein, calcium, and sodium) that place a greater burden on the kidneys and increases the infant's risk of dehydration; is low in iron and contains a form of iron not readily absorbed by the infant; may cause occult gastrointestinal blood loss in a small number of infants; has limited amounts of essential fatty acids, vitamins C and E, zinc, and other trace minerals; and increases risk of milk allergy.

Reduced fat milk (2%, 1%, or skim) are not recommended for infants or children younger than age 2 years. These milks have a higher protein-to-calorie ratio than whole milk, breast milk, or commercial formula. The infant must consume more to obtain sufficient energy, and this additional protein metabolism and subsequent excretion of protein end products burden the kidneys and increase the risk of dehydration.

FEEDINGS

As in breastfeeding, the infant is fed when he or she is hungry and not according to a set schedule. Formula should be fed at room or body temperature.

The capacity of the infant's stomach is only 30 mg to 90 mg (1 oz to 3 oz) at birth. During the first week, 6 to 12 feedings daily are required to meet the infant's needs. The stomach grows larger as the child grows, and the feedings stay in the stomach longer. As the amount taken at a feeding increases, the number of feedings decreases. At age 3 to 5 months, the infant usually is taking 5 oz to 8 oz at each of four or five feedings.

The infant should be held as though being breastfed. This physical closeness helps meet the infant's need for love and physical contact. The bottle should not be propped. Putting a child to bed with a bottle should be strongly discouraged. This practice promotes dental decay and may promote ear inflammation. The infant also may become psychologically dependent on the bottle.

INTRODUCTION OF SUPPLEMENTAL FOODS

The American Academy of Pediatrics describes the periods of infant feeding as three overlapping stages: (1) the nursing period in which breast milk or formula is the sole source of nutrients; (2) a transitional period in which specially prepared solid foods are introduced; and (3) a modified adult period in which most nutrients come from table foods. The rate of progression through these stages is individualized according to the infant's maturity level. See Display 17-1 for a discussion of food practices to avoid in infants.

TRANSITIONAL PERIOD

The addition of food other than breast milk or formula should be delayed until the baby is at least age 4 to 6 months. Before then, the gastrointestinal tract and kidneys are not equipped to handle food other than milk. During the first 2 or 3 months, the infant's natural response to solid food is to push the food out of the mouth when placed on the tongue—the *extrusion reflex*. Furthermore, waiting until age 4 to 6 months to feed solid food can prevent overfeeding and, possibly, allergic conditions in later childhood. By this time, the infant has lost the extrusion reflex, can lean forward with mouth open to invite food, and can lean back and turn the head away to reject it.

The first supplementary food to be introduced usually is infant cereal, which has been enriched with iron in a form that is easily absorbed. Rice cereal, which contains no gluten, is usually well tolerated. Breast milk or formula is added to the cereal to thin its consistency and it is then fed with an infant spoon.

Thereafter, other single-ingredient foods are added at intervals of 1 week or more, giving the infant a chance to become accustomed to the food and allowing time to observe allergic reactions to

DISPLAY 17-1 FOOD PRACTICES TO AVOID

- Do not force or encourage the infant to finish all available food. Allow the infant to indicate when he or she is full.
- Avoid the following foods, which present a choking hazard: hot dogs, nuts, grapes, raw carrots, popcorn, corn, celery, raw peas, fish with bones, potato chips, apple pieces, raisins, seeds, and round, hard, or sticky candies.
- Discourage daily intake of sweets such as cookies, candy, soft drinks, fruit-flavored drinks, and sugar-coated cereal.
- Never fill nursing bottles with sugar-containing liquids, such as sugar water, sweetened gelatin, soft drinks, or juice, because this practice can lead to nursing bottle caries (see the section Nursing Bottle Caries). Juices should be given when the infant can drink from a cup. Also, do not dip the infant's pacifier in sweetened liquid.
- Do not put the infant to sleep with a nursing bottle filled with carbohydrate-containing liquid (formula, milk, or juice). This practice promotes tooth decay. It also may lead to ear infection because the liquid may pool in the mouth and flow through the eustachian tube to the ear.
- Do not put solid foods such as cereal in a nursing bottle. This practice deprives the infant of social contact during feedings. Also, the infant needs to learn the distinction between drinking and eating, how to chew, use a spoon, and handle different textures.
- Do not use honey or corn syrup in preparing formula or food for children younger than age 1 year. These sweeteners may be contaminated with *Clostridium botulinum,* which causes food poisoning.

it. A small amount of the new food should be given at first and then gradually increased. New foods include pureed vegetables, fruits, and meats. The order in which foods are introduced is not important. To prevent the development of nursing bottle caries, give juices in a cup when the infant can drink from a cup (see the section Nursing Bottle Caries.) If the infant refuses the new food, the care-giver should reintroduce it in a week or two. The person feeding the infant should not convey a personal preference or dislike for the food.

Foods that commonly cause allergic reactions should be introduced later in the first year. These foods include egg white, citrus juice, wheat, chocolate, and nut butters. Slow introduction of new food will help to identify allergic reactions (Table 17-1).

Salt and sugar should not be added to foods for infants. Although single-ingredient commercially prepared infant foods do not have salt and sugar added, many combined dinners or desserts have added sugar, salt, or both. Care-givers should be instructed to read labels carefully and to select those baby foods that have the least amount of unnecessary ingredients added.

HOME-PREPARED INFANT FOODS

Baby foods made at home are just as acceptable as commercial infant foods as long as high-quality ingredients are used and sanitary practices are observed when the foods are prepared and stored. All equipment, including blender jars, should be scrubbed in hot water and soap and rinsed well. Fresh or frozen foods that do not have salt, sugar, or other unnecessary ingredients added should be used. Food prepared from salted canned food or in salted water are higher in sodium than commercial baby foods. Foods should be freshly prepared and then blended or pureed. Food not used immediately may be frozen in serving-size portions in ice cube trays or paper cupcake liners.

Home-prepared spinach, beets, turnips, carrots, or collard greens should not be fed to infants during early infancy because these foods may contain sufficient nitrate to cause *methemoglobinemia.* This poisoning causes changes in hemoglobin formation and symptoms of cyanosis, dizziness, headache, diarrhea, and anemia.

INTRODUCTION OF TABLE FOODS

At about age 8 to 10 months, the modified adult period begins. The physiologic mechanisms involved with eating have matured to almost an adult level. Tender table foods need only to be cut into small pieces. When table foods are used, no fat or

TABLE 17-1 SUGGESTED FEEDING SCHEDULE FOR THE FIRST YEAR OF LIFE

AGE	FOOD ITEM	AMOUNT*	RATIONALE
Birth–6 mo	Human milk or iron-fortified formula	Daily totals 0–1 mo 18–24 oz 1–2 mo 22–28 oz 2–3 mo 25–32 oz 3–4 mo 28–32 oz 4–5 mo 27–39 oz 5–6 mo 27–45 oz	Infants' well-developed sucking and rooting reflexes allow them to take in milk and formula Infants do not accept semisolid food because their tongues protrude when a spoon is put in their mouths They are unable to transfer food to the back of the mouth Human milk needs supplementation
	Water	Not routinely recommended	Small amounts may be offered under special circumstances (e.g., hot weather, elevated bilirubin, or diarrhea)
4–6 mo	*Iron-fortified infant cereal;† begin with rice cereal (delay adding barley, oats, and wheat until 6th mo)	4–8 tbsp after mixing	At this age, there is a decrease of the extrusion reflex; the infant is able to depress the tongue and transfer semisolid food from a spoon to the back of the pharynx to swallow it
	*Unsweetened fruit juices;† ‡ plain, vitamin C–fortified	2–4 oz	Cereal adds a source of iron and B vitamins; fruit juices introduce a source of vitamin C
	Dilute juices with equal parts of water		Delay orange, pineapple, grapefruit, or tomato juice until the 6th mo
	Human milk or iron-fortified formula	Daily totals 4–5 mo 27–39 oz 5–6 mo 27–45 oz	Do not offer water as a substitute for formula or breast milk, but rather as a source of additional fluids
	Water	As desired	
7–8 mo	*Fruits, plain strained; avoid fruit desserts	1–2 tbsp	Teething is beginning; thus, there is an increased ability to bite and chew
	*Yogurt†		
	*Vegetables,† plain strained; avoid combination meat and vegetable dinners	5–7 tbsp	Vegetables introduce new flavors and textures
	*Meats,† plain strained; avoid combination or high-protein dinners	1–2 tbsp	Meat provides additional iron, protein, and B vitamins
	*Crackers, toast, zwieback†	1 small serving	
	Iron-fortified infant cereal or enriched cream of wheat	4–6 tbsp	
	Fruit juices‡	4 oz	
	Human milk or iron-fortified formula	24–32 oz	Iron-fortified formula or iron supplementation with human milk continues to be needed because the infant is not consuming significant amounts of meat
	Water	As desired	May introduce a cup to the infant

(Continued)

TABLE 17-1 *(continued)*

AGE	FOOD ITEM	AMOUNTS*	RATIONALE
9–10 mo	*Finger foods†—well-cooked, mashed, soft, bite-sized pieces of meat and vegetables	In small servings	Rhythmic biting movements begin; enhance this development with foods that require chewing
	Iron-fortified infant cereal or enriched cream of wheat	4–6 tbsp	Decrease amounts of mashed foods as amounts of finger foods increase
	Fruit juices‡	4 oz	
	Fruits	6–8 tbsp	
	Vegetables	6–8 tbsp	
	Meat, fish, poultry, yogurt, cottage cheese	4–6 tbsp	Formula or breast milk consumption may begin to decrease; thus, begin other sources of calcium, riboflavin, and protein (e.g., cheese, yogurt, and cottage cheese)
	Human milk or iron-fortified formula	24–32 oz	
	Water	As desired	
11–12 mo	Soft table foods† as follows:		Motor skills are developing; enhance this development with more finger foods
	Cereal: iron-fortified infant cereal; may introduce dry, unsweetened cereal as a finger food	4–6 tbsp	
	Breads: crackers, toast, zwieback	1–2 small servings	Rotary chewing motion develops; thus, child is able to handle whole foods, which require more chewing
	Fruit juice‡	4 oz	
	Fruit: soft, canned fruits or ripe banana, cut up; peeled raw fruit as the infant approaches 12 mo	½ cup	Infant is relying less on breast milk or formula for nutrients; a proper selection of a variety of solid foods (fruits, vegetables, starches, protein sources, and dairy products) will continue to meet the young child's needs
	Vegetables: soft cooked, cut into bite-sized pieces	½ cup	
	Meats and other protein sources: strips of tender, lean meat, cheese strips, peanut butter	2 oz or ½ cup chopped	Delay peanut butter until the 12th month
	Mashed potatoes, noodles		
	Human milk or iron-fortified infant formula	24–30 oz	
	Water	As desired	

* Amounts listed are daily totals and goals to be achieved gradually. Intake varies depending on the infant's appetite.

† New food items for age group.

(Adapted from: Twin Cities District Dietetic Association. *Manual of clinical nutrition* with permission from its publisher Chronimed Publishing) 13911 Ridgedale Dr, Minneapolis, MN 55343, 1994;54–56.)

‡ Author note: The Committee on Nutrition of the American Academy of Pediatrics recommends that fruit juices be introduced when infant can drink from a cup.

seasoning should be added to the infant's portion. When infants begin reaching for objects and putting them in their mouths, finger foods should be encouraged. In addition to cooked vegetables, finger foods such as melba toast, teething biscuits, graham crackers, soft canned fruit, ripe banana, and cooked tofu cubes may be offered.

Strained meats should be replaced by finely chopped meats without fat or gristle. Strips of chicken, tender lean meat, or ground meat patties may be given the baby to suck or chew. Cooked fish from which all bones have been removed can be offered (see Table 17-1).

WATER

When breast milk or commercial formula is the sole source of nutrients, infants require no supplemental water, except in hot weather. When solid foods are begun, additional water may be necessary especially if infants are given foods high in protein and electrolytes such as meats, egg yolk, and meat dinners. Water should be offered as part of a feeding. Additional water is needed when fluid losses are increased, such as during illness.

MICROWAVE PRECAUTIONS

Formula should be fed at room or body temperature. Heating infant formula in the microwave is not recommended because of the risk of burning the infant's mouth. The formula may heat unevenly, and, although the bottle may feel only warm to the touch, the formula itself may be hot.

Commercial baby foods that contain substantial amounts of protein should not be heated in a microwave oven. Protein foods include plain meats and poultry, meat dinners, egg yolks, and meat sticks. These foods also heat unevenly in the microwave oven, resulting in the possibility of explosion. Other baby foods may be heated in the microwave oven, but extreme caution is advised. After heating, the food should be thoroughly mixed and tested before it is given to the infant. Follow manufacturer's directions at all times.

NUTRITION-RELATED HEALTH PROBLEMS IN INFANTS

NURSING BOTTLE CARIES

Nursing bottle caries is decay of the upper front teeth resulting from the ingestion of carbohydrate-containing liquids from a nursing bottle for prolonged periods such as at bedtime or naptime (Fig. 17-2). Carbohydrate-containing fluids include milk, juice, and sugar-containing fluids. This practice also may encourage ear infections. When the infant falls asleep with the bottle, the liquid that pools in the mouth can flow into the *eustachian tube*—an open passageway extending from the ear to the throat—and up into the ears, where it can cause infection.

Juices should not be fed in a nursing bottle. Juices should be given when the infant can drink from a cup. Putting an infant to bed with a bottle as a pacifier should be strongly discouraged.

FAILURE TO THRIVE

Failure to thrive is a condition involving an infant or young child whose weight is below the third percentile or who weighs less that 80% of the median

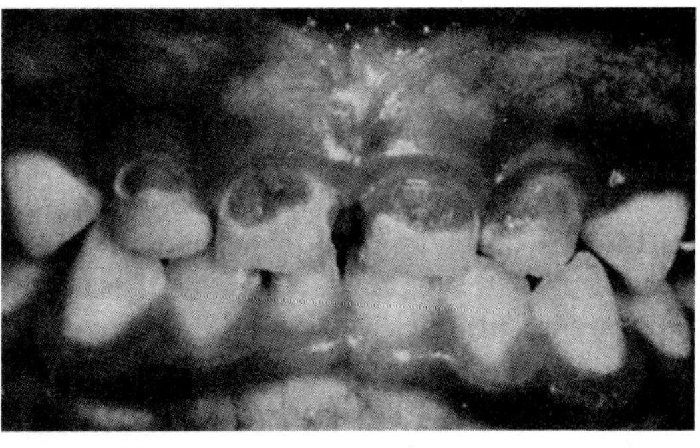

FIGURE 17-2

Baby bottle tooth decay. *(From Levine N [ed]. Current treatment in dental practice. Philadelphia: WB Saunders, 1986:447.)*

for his or her age group, or whose growth curves drop two or more percentile ranks. A National Center for Health Statistics (NCHS) chart used to monitor physical growth is shown in Figure 17-3. The long-term consequences of failure to thrive include retarded growth into the school-age years, psychomotor delay, emotional disturbances, and delayed reading age. Failure to thrive is caused by insufficient caloric and protein levels to meet the growth needs and may be either organic or inorganic.

Organic causes of growth failure are physical disorders such as gastrointestinal malabsorption, recurring infections, and chronic diseases. Inorganic causes may be environmental, such as poverty, famine, abuse, neglect, or parental ignorance of the infant's food needs. Frequently, poor feeding practices are uncovered: making the infant formula too dilute, overfeeding soft drinks and juices, or giving foods with a low caloric density.

Increasing cases of failure to thrive are being attributed to feeding practices of health-conscious parents, who are giving skim milk and other lowfat foods to prevent heart disease. Although these parents are well intentioned, guidelines that are appro-

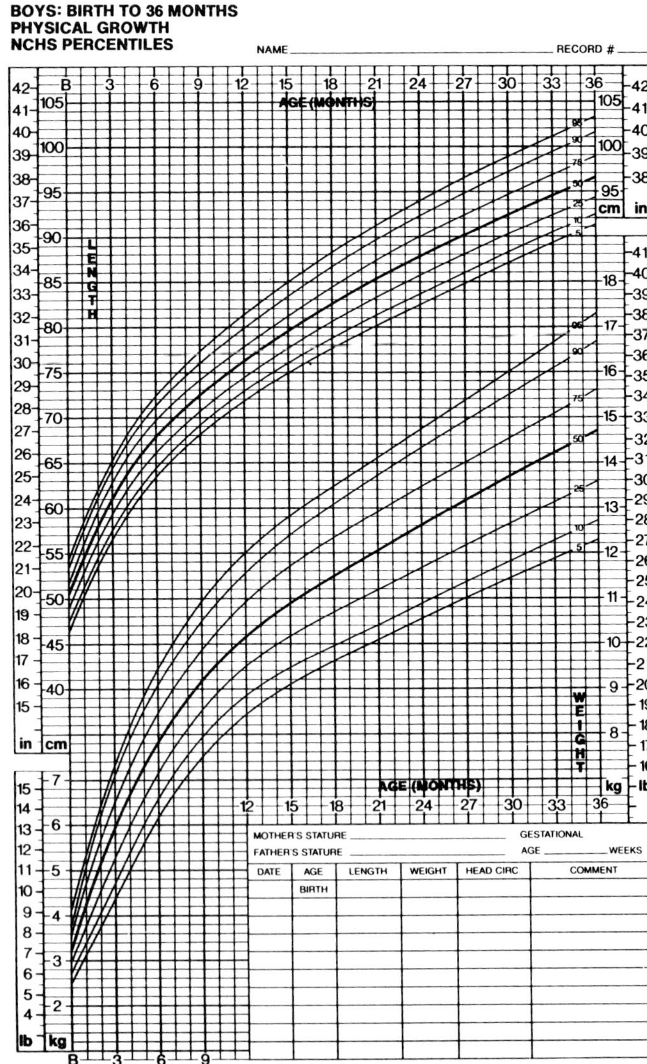

FIGURE 17-3

Example of NCHS chart for boys and for girls from birth through age 18 years that is commonly used to monitor physical growth of infants, children, and adolescents. *(Hamill PW, et al. Physical growth: National Center for Health Statistics. *Ross Laboratories, Columbus, OH. Am J Clin Nutr (1979;32:607–629.) Data from NCHS, Hyattsville, MD.)*

priate for adults are inappropriate for rapidly growing infants and children younger than age 2 years.

TREATMENT

The child usually is hospitalized for an initial refeeding period. The child needs to begin to grow again and to catch up to the normal growth for his or her age. Because failure to thrive in infants involves malnourishment and one or several other problems, it is treated by a team comprising a physician, dietitian, nurse, and social worker. Nutritional management involves providing sufficient energy and protein to achieve catch-up growth; individualized, practical nutrition instruction for the family; and long-term follow-up.

ANEMIA

Iron deficiency anemia occurs commonly among infants of low–birth weight, full-size infants between ages 6 and 24 months. Preventive measures include the use of iron-fortified formula, iron-fortified infant cereal, or iron supplements. Once iron deficiency anemia occurs, iron supplements are necessary to correct the deficiency.

DIARRHEA

Moderate to severe diarrhea in infants is extremely serious and sometimes fatal. Dehydration and fever can damage the developing nervous system. Because diarrhea is a symptom of disease, the cause must be determined and treated.

The first need is restoration of fluid and electrolyte balance. In infants, this may be accomplished by using a commercial oral electrolyte–glucose solution that can be given by bottle. If sufficient fluid cannot be taken by mouth, hospitalization is required.

Food is reintroduced as soon as possible. A significant amount of food consumed during acute diarrhea is absorbed, and because fasting further reduces the body's ability to digest food, the reintroduction of food usually should not be delayed more than 24 hours.

Breast milk is frequently well tolerated. Breastfed infants usually can continue to be breastfed during all phases of therapy for acute diarrhea. Infants on formula are frequently started on dilute formula and the concentration is gradually increased. Sometimes lactose-free infant formulas may be necessary for a short time.

Solid foods appropriate to the infant's age are added gradually. Rice cereals, banana, potatoes, and other carbohydrate-rich foods are usually well tolerated.

The health worker should ensure that the care-giver understands directions for the use of commercial oral rehydration preparations and is advised about the kinds of fluids the care-giver should offer the infant. The diet should be restricted no longer than necessary. (See Chapter 13, Rehydration Therapy.)

CONGENITAL HEART DISEASE

Increased metabolic rate and difficulty in sucking and swallowing contribute to growth failure in the infant with congenital heart disease. These infants tire easily and it is difficult for them to consume normal quantities of food.

The nutrition care of these infants is complex and must be managed with great diligence. Specialized infant formulas may be necessary. For example, respiration may be improved by increasing the fat content of the diet because the metabolism of fat produces less carbon dioxide than carbohydrate.

Sodium control is frequently necessary. When solid foods are added, unsalted strained vegetables and unsalted strained meats are appropriate. (Salt and other sodium compounds are no longer added to single-ingredient commercial baby foods.) The sodium-controlled diet is discussed in Chapter 26.

Nutrition care provided in the home must be adjusted to the abilities of the family. Feeding an infant with congenital heart disease is time-consuming, because the infant needs to rest frequently while eating. The parents may need help arranging the family's schedule.

Providing adequate calories and other nutrients increases the child's strength and promotes growth, hastening the day that corrective surgery can be performed. Surgery usually is delayed, if possible, until a specific weight goal is reached.

ENZYME DEFICIENCIES

Phenylketonuria and galactosemia are among a group of inherited diseases called *inborn errors of metabolism*. These disorders involve the absence or defective functioning of an enzyme needed for normal metabolism. Nutrition therapy used to treat and control many of these disorders is provided in metabolic centers, where physicians and dietitians who specialize in treating these diseases are available.

PHENYLKETONURIA

Phenylketonuria is an inherited disease in which phenylalanine, an essential amino acid, cannot be metabolized normally because of the lack of a liver enzyme that is needed to convert phenylalanine to tyrosine. As a result, phenylalanine and some if its breakdown products accumulate in the blood and are excreted in the urine. These toxic substances interfere with the normal development of the central nervous system, causing mental retardation, personality changes, and other neurologic disturbances.

If the disease is detected and a phenylalanine-controlled diet is started in the first few months of life, damage to nerve tissue can be prevented, and normal physical and intellectual development follows. If the disorder is detected only later, mental retardation cannot be prevented, but the child's behavior can still be somewhat improved by nutrition therapy. The disease occurs in 1 in 10,000 to 15,000 live births. All states now require that a blood test for PKU be performed on all newborns.

The need for a phenylalanine-controlled diet appears to continue throughout life. Loss of intelligence quotient (IQ), poor school achievement, behavior problems, and neurologic deterioration have occurred after the diet is discontinued.

Infants born to women with PKU—women who did not have normal blood phenylalanine levels at conception and during pregnancy—have a high incidence of birth defects. If a woman with PKU discontinues the use of a phenylalanine-controlled diet, she should resume the diet if she is planning to become pregnant and continue it during the pregnancy.

Treatment

The purpose of diet therapy in PKU is to limit phenylalanine to the amount required to maintain an adequate blood level (2 to 16 mg/dL). Phenylalanine cannot be completely eliminated from the diet because it is an essential amino acid and is necessary for the production of body proteins. In addition, all other nutrients must be provided in amounts that promote growth and development. This includes the amino acid tyrosine, which becomes an essential amino acid in PKU and must be supplied in the diet.

The amount of phenylalanine required depends on enzyme activity, age, sex, growth rate, and monitoring of blood phenylalanine level. All proteins contain 4% to 6% phenylalanine. Because all foods except oils and sugars contain some protein, the diet is extremely limited. It is impossible to plan a diet that is restricted in phenylalanine and adequate in protein and calories with the use of natural foods alone.

Special products have been developed that are either low in or free of phenylalanine. These formulas are available for different age groups ranging from those for infants to those suitable for older children and adults. Lofenalac (Mead Johnson) is low in phenylalanine and is used for infants and young children. Maximum XP (Ross Laboratories) is free of phenylalanine and is intended for people aged 8 years to adult and during pregnancy. Experienced metabolic dietitians and physicians prescribe and monitor product use. Diets that incorporate these special formulas can be adequate in all nutrients. It is important to provide adequate calories to avoid protein breakdown, which can elevate blood phenylalanine levels.

Controlled amounts of phenylalanine must be added to the diet to meet total phenylalanine requirements. Specific amounts of infant formula, breast milk, or solid foods are added to the infant's diet. For older children and adults, low-protein foods such as fruits, vegetables, and special low-protein breads, cereals, and pastas in prescribed amounts fulfill the phenylalanine requirements. High-protein foods (e.g., meat, fish, poultry, eggs, legumes, and nuts) are excluded from the diet. Foods and beverages containing the sweetener aspartame are excluded also because it is derived from phenylalanine. Foods containing aspartame must carry the following warning label: "PHENYLKETONURICS: CONTAINS PHENYLALANINE."

An exchange system has been developed for use in the phenylalanine-restricted diet. The lists are composed mainly of fruits, vegetables, cereals, and fats; there are no lists for meat, eggs, or milk. Another method consists of using phenylalanine equivalents in which one equivalent equals 15 to 20 mg of phenylalanine.

Care-givers of the infant or child are instructed by the dietitian. The cooperation of the entire family is essential because they play a major role in controlling the disease. The dietitian maintains close contact with the parents through visits, correspondence, and by telephone. The parents receive instruction about the preparation of special formulas. They must carefully measure or weigh all ingredients and foods and must keep an accurate record of the child's food intake.

GALACTOSEMIA

Galactosemia is a disorder in the metabolism of galactose, a simple sugar. In this disease, enzymes needed for the normal conversion of galactose to glucose are lacking. Galactose thus reaches abnormal blood levels and is excreted in the urine (*galactosuria*). If untreated, one type of galactosemia causes failure to thrive, cataracts, mental retardation, liver failure, and death. These problems can be prevented if treatment is started within the first few days of life. Galactosemia, an inherited disorder, occurs in 1 in 25,000 to 50,000 births in the United States.

Treatment

Treatment is to eliminate galactose from the diet. The main source of galactose is lactose, or milk sugar, which is broken down to glucose and galactose in the intestinal tract. Therefore, milk, milk products, cheese, butter, and dry milk powder are avoided. Commercial products and medications made with lactose-containing ingredients must be excluded; these ingredients include lactose, whey, milk solids, casein, calcium caseinate, sodium caseinate, lactalbumin, and curds. Products containing lactate and lactic acid do not contain galactose and can be used. Careful reading of food labels is necessary. Breads, candies, cold cuts, prepared and processed foods, commercial sauces and gravies, monosodium glutamate extenders, and alternate sweeteners such as Equal (Nutra Sweet Consumer Products, Inc.) and Sweet'n Low (Cumberland Packing Corp.) are likely sources of lactose.

It is difficult to completely eliminate galactose from the diet because it is found widely in nature and as lactose in processed foods. Some fruits and vegetables contain significant amounts of galactose. Sources of galactose include organ meats, peas, lima beans, soybeans, lentils, and dried beans.

Soy formula or fortified soy milk is used as replacement for milk. If the child refuses these milk replacements, supplements of calcium and vitamin D may be needed.

A galactose-free diet presents little difficulty during infancy, when lactose-free commercial formulas are used. As the child grows older, the diet becomes more complex. Galactose must be completely avoided, especially in the first few years of life. How strict the diet must be after early childhood is controversial. If the older child's diet is liberalized to include foods that contain small quantities of milk, his or her condition should be monitored.

WIC PROGRAM

The federally funded WIC program provides monthly food packages of infant formula, milk, cereal, eggs, cheese, and juice for pregnant, breastfeeding women and postpartum women and for infants and children age 5 years and younger. Participants receive vouchers they can use like money in a grocery store to purchase the designated foods. Eligible applicants must be at nutritional risk because of a poor or inadequate diet, previous history of miscarriages or premature birth, nutritional anemia, or abnormal growth pattern, *and* low income. Nutrition education is included in this program.

KEYS TO PRACTICAL APPLICATION

Encourage and support breastfeeding as the best means of feeding infants.

Advise parents to avoid overfeeding from birth.

Encourage parents to follow their pediatrician's advice about introducing supplementary foods.

Do not feed cereal or other semisolid food from a bottle.

Discourage propping a bottle or putting an infant to bed with a bottle.

Emphasize to parents that lowfat, high-fiber diets are inappropriate for infants.

Avoid giving infants foods that may cause choking. Always supervise infants when they are eating.

Caution parents and other care-givers about the dangers of heating formula and infant foods in the microwave.

Become familiar with the benefits, eligibility requirements, and referral process for the WIC program.

KEY IDEAS

RDAs for first 6 months of life are based on nutrients in breast milk.

Requirements for energy and nutrients per unit of body weight are higher during infancy than at any other time of life.

Commercial infant formulas are formulated to resemble breast milk. These formulas meet standards developed by the American Academy of Pediatrics.

Home-prepared cow's milk formulas are not recommended.

Breast milk provides all of the nutritional needs of the infant for 6 months, except fluoride and vitamin D.

Infants fed commercial iron-fortified formula do not need any supplements except fluoride.

The formula-fed infant is at risk of having a low hemoglobin level by age 6 months unless an iron supplement or an iron-fortified formula is used.

Breastfeeding provides better nutrition than bottle-feeding and promotes bonding, immunity against infection, and protection against allergy and obesity.

Breastfeeding helps the mother lose extra fat deposited during pregnancy and helps the uterus return to its normal size.

Incidence of breastfeeding has been declining since the early 1980s.

Health team members have an important role in the success of breastfeeding.

Breastfeeding is a learned skill; the breastfeeding woman benefits from guidance.

Both breastfed and bottle-fed infants are fed when hungry, not according to any set schedule. Infants may have 6 to 12 feedings per day during the first weeks of life.

Putting a child to bed with a bottle promotes tooth decay, ear infections, and psychological dependence on the bottle.

Early introduction of solid foods may promote overeating and allergies.

New foods should be added gradually, one at a time, and in small amounts beginning at about age 4 to 6 months.

Iron-fortified infant cereal is usually the first solid food introduced, followed by single-ingredient pureed foods (fruits, vegetables, and meats). New foods are added at intervals of 1 week or more.

Salt, sugar, and fat should not be added to foods for infants.

Late in the first year of life, the infant progresses from strained to chopped food and from breast or bottle to cup. Breast and bottle feeding may continue beyond the first year.

When feeding solid foods is begun, water should be offered as part of a feeding.

Infants should be closely supervised to prevent choking; hazardous foods should be avoided.

It is unwise to feed the older infant excessive amounts of milk, because this extra milk tends to be given at the expense of iron-rich foods.

Extreme precaution must be taken when microwaving foods for infants to prevent burning. Heating formula in microwave is not recommended.

Reduced-fat milk is not recommended for children younger than age 2 years.

Inorganic failure to thrive is caused by some psychosocial disturbance in the infant or small child's environment.

There is an increased incidence of failure to thrive caused by the feeding practices of health-conscious parents who feed lowfat, high-fiber diets to children younger than age 2 years.

Anemia in infancy is prevented by the use of iron-fortified formula, iron-fortified cereal, or iron supplements.

In acute illness involving diarrhea, restoring fluid and electrolyte balance is the first priority; a careful record of fluid intake and output is important.

Nutrition care of chronically ill infants and small children is time-consuming and must be adjusted to the abilities of the family.

Phenylketonuria is an enzyme deficiency disease in which phenylalanine, an essential amino acid, is not metabolized normally. Phenylalanine is controlled in the diet to amounts needed to maintain adequate blood levels. The special formulas specifically developed for use in people who have PKU are the main source of protein and calories; other foods are added in amounts required to achieve caloric balance and maintain a normal blood phenylalanine level.

Galactosemia is an inherited disease caused by a lack of enzymes needed to convert galactose to glucose in the body; beginning in the first few days of life, foods that contain lactose and galactose are avoided as a means of preventing severe mental retardation, cataracts, and other serious consequences.

WIC program provides infant formula, milk, cereal, eggs, cheese, and juice for infants and children aged 5 years or younger who are both at nutritional risk and in low-income families.

KEYS TO LEARNING

STUDY–DISCUSSION QUESTIONS

1. What are the benefits of breastfeeding? What factors may hinder successful breastfeeding?
2. What advice would you give parents who favor the early feeding of supplemental foods because it helps their infant sleep through the night?
3. What instruction should parents be given about the use of commercial formula? Why should the propping of a nursing bottle be discouraged?
4. During the second half of the first year and during the toddler stage, there is a tendency for parents to give their children a lot of milk. Why should this practice be discouraged?
5. It is recommended that fruit juice be fed by cup and not in a nursing bottle. Why?
6. What measures should be taken during infancy to prevent iron deficiency anemia?
7. Invite a representative from the WIC program or the social worker in the outpatient department of your hospital to speak to the class about the benefits of WIC, the eligibility requirements, and referral procedures.

BIBLIOGRAPHY

BOOKS AND PAMPHLETS

Barness LA. Ed. Pediatric nutrition handbook. 3rd ed., Elk Grove Village, IL: American Academy of Pediatrics, 1993.

Chicago Dietetic Association and the South Suburban Dietetic Association. Manual of clinical dietetics. 4th ed. Chicago: The American Dietetic Association, 1992.

National Academy of Sciences, Institute of Medicine, Food and Nutrition Board, Committee on Nutritional Status During Pregnancy and Lactation. Nutrition services in perinatal care. Washington, DC: National Academy Press, 1992.

National Academy of Sciences, National Research Council, Food and Nutrition Board. Recommended dietary allowances. 10th ed. Washington, DC: National Academy Press, 1989.

Twin Cities District Dietetic Association. Manual of clinical nutrition. Minneapolis: Chronimed Publishing, 1994.

Worthington-Roberts BS, William SR. Nutrition in pregnancy and lactation. St. Louis: Mosby–Year Book, Inc. 1993:Chapter 10.

PERIODICALS

Barnes GP, Warren WA, Lyon TC, et al. Ethnicity, location, age, and fluoride factors in baby bottle tooth decay and caries prevalence of Head Start children. Public Health Reports 1992;107:2:167.

Freed GL. Breastfeeding: time to teach what we preach. JAMA 1993;269:243.

Greve LC, Wheeler MD, Green-Burgeson DK, et al. Breastfeeding in the management of the newborn with phenylketonuria: a practical approach to dietary therapy. J Am Diet Assoc 1994;94:305.

Gropper SS, Gross AC, Olds SJ. Galactose content of selected fruit and vegetable baby foods: implications for infants on galactose-restricted diets. J Am Diet Assoc 1993;93:328.

Jason J. Breastfeeding in 1991. N Engl J Med 1991;325:1036.

Koch R, Levy HR, Matalon R, et al. The North American collaborative study of maternal phenylketonuria: status report 1993. Am J Dis Chil 1993;147:1224.

Nicklas TA, Webber LS, Koschak ML, et al. Nutrient adequacy of low fat intakes for children: the Bogalusa heart study. Pediatrics 1992;89:221.

Ris MD, Williams SE, Hunt MM, et al. Early-treated phenylketonuria: adult neuropsychologic outcome. J Pediatr 1994;124:388.

Sullivan SA, Birch LL. Infant dietary experience and acceptance of solid foods. Pediatrics 1994;93:271.

CHAPTER

18

Meeting Nutritional Needs During Childhood Through Adolescence

KEY TERMS

food jag usually refers to a young child's insistence on eating only one or a few foods to the exclusion of a normal variety; considered a normal part of child development; may last several days to a week or more

purge to cleanse, flush out, get rid of

OBJECTIVES

After completing this chapter, the student will be able to:

1. Give five suggestions for developing good eating habits in toddlers and preschoolers.
2. Discuss the changing nutrient needs, problem eating behaviors, and guidelines for developing good eating habits among children.
3. Discuss the nutritional needs, variations in needs, and major food problems of adolescents.
4. Give suggestions for promoting good food habits among adolescents.
5. Appreciate the emotional and nutritional significance of having a meal together as a family.
6. Describe and discuss the following nutrition-related childhood problems: failure to thrive, obesity, dental caries, iron deficiency anemia, and nutrition misinformation and athletic performance.
7. Identify and describe community programs that provide food assistance.
8. Describe the characteristics and nutrition therapy for cystic fibrosis.
9. Discuss the characteristics, treatment, and prognosis of anorexia nervosa and bulimia nervosa.

Socioeconomic changes in US society are also having a significant effect on children's diets and nutritional status. These changes include the growing number of mothers working outside the home, the increase in children requiring day care, and the increase in the number of children living in poverty. Recognizing that the growth, health, and ability to learn of many children are being jeopardized because of poor nutrition, the federal government has designated several of its Healthy People 2000 objectives to improving the nutritional status of young children (See Display 1-1). These objectives include reducing growth retardation, iron deficiency, anemia, and dietary fat intake and increasing physical activity and nutrition education.

Reports of the relationship between diet and chronic diseases are another factor affecting nutrition recommendations for children. Parents are concerned about these reports and are confused about how this information affects their decisions about what food to feed their children. Some experts are concerned that attitudes about feeding children are becoming too negative and restrictive.

TODDLERS AND PRESCHOOLERS

Nutritional guidance for the child aged 1 to 5 years aims to promote optimal growth and to meet the child's developmental and behavioral needs. This period is not without its frustrations for parents. The likes and dislikes of this age group change rapidly and unpredictably from day to day and the appetite level can vary considerably from rather large on one occasion to nearly nothing on another.

NUTRITIONAL NEEDS

ENERGY

During the second year of life, the child's growth rate slows. The average weight gain for the year is 8 to 10 lb. The child's weight is about four times the birth weight at 2 years, and at 4 years, the child is two times the birth length.

Energy estimates of the National Academy of Sciences Food and Nutrition Board are 1300 kcal/day for 1- to 3-year-olds and an additional 500 kcal/day for 4- to 6-year-olds. However, energy needs may vary considerably according to the child's level of physical activity. The child's growth rate should be monitored regularly to determine if energy intake is adequate. If sufficient food is available and the psychological environment is positive, the child will consume just enough food to satisfy energy requirements. This balance occurs despite the wide differences in quantity of food the child consumes from one meal to another.

CARBOHYDRATES

More than half of the child's energy intake is provided by carbohydrate, preferably natural sugars such as fruit and milk and complex carbohydrates such as cereals, breads, grains, legumes, and starchy vegetables. Excessive amounts of fibrous foods, however, may cause gastrointestinal problems for very young children and should be avoided.

Although parents and teachers have attributed overactivity and other disruptive behavior to the consumption of candy and other high-sugar foods, well-controlled research studies have not substantiated this theory. Diets high in sugar content should be strongly discouraged because of other reasons: They are detrimental to the overall nutritional quality of the diet and to dental health.

PROTEIN

The recommended daily intake of protein is 1.2 g/kg body weight for children aged 1 to 3 years and 1.1 g/kg body weight for children aged 4 to 6 years. Diets of most American children more than meet these recommendations. Risk of inadequate intake may occur for children on strict vegan diets or those who have limited access to food because of poverty or neglect.

FAT

The committees on nutrition of both the American Academy of Pediatrics and the American Heart Association have agreed that fat and cholesterol in the diet should not be restricted during the first two years of life. For children older than age 2 years, it is recommended that no more than 30% of total calories be consumed as fat, less than 10% as saturated fat, and no more than 10% as polyunsaturated fat. Cholesterol should be limited to less than 300 mg/day. These recommendations are averages that should be achieved over a period of several days and do not refer to a single meal or food.

Concern has been expressed that lowfat diets may be too low in energy level and essential nutrients to adequately promote growth and development. See the discussion in the section Failure to Thrive.

VITAMINS AND MINERALS

Most young children consume adequate amounts of vitamins and minerals. Minerals likely to be inadequate for some children are iron, calcium, and zinc.

The recommendation of 10 mg/day of iron is not easily met. Children between ages 1 and 3 years are at high risk of developing iron deficiency anemia. Iron-rich roods such as lean meat as well as whole-grain and iron-enriched breads and cereals and other grain products should be emphasized. Consuming vitamin C–rich foods at a meal will increase the absorption of iron from foods with a less available form of iron (e.g., vegetables, breads, cereals, and eggs).

Adequate calcium is necessary for the optimal growth and maintenance of bone tissue. If calcium is inadequate in the early years, the child's growth potential may not be reached and bone tissue may be weaker and more prone to osteoporosis in later life. Children who consume limited amounts of milk and dairy products are at risk for calcium deficiency. The Recommended Dietary Allowance (RDA) for calcium for children aged 1 year to 10 years is 800 mg/day. Children who have difficulty digesting lactose (milk sugar) may be able to tolerate milk in small quantities at one time or in the form of yogurt or aged cheese. Lactose-reduced and lactose-free milks are available, as well as calcium-fortified foods such as some commercial varieties of orange juice. Some nondairy sources of calcium are given in Table 11-3.

Milk is also the main dietary source of vitamin D, which is necessary for the absorption of calcium and for the deposit of calcium in the bones. Most milks are fortified with vitamin D. Yogurt and cheese are usually not made from vitamin D–fortified milk.

Mild zinc deficiency has been linked to low height-for-age in young children. Children who have low intakes of meat, poultry, and seafood that contain a readily absorbed form of zinc are more prone to zinc deficiency. Phytates and fiber hinder absorption of zinc in plant sources such as whole-grain cereals, legumes, and nuts. Children on vegan diets may require zinc supplements.

MEAL PLANNING

The Pyramid Guide to Daily Food Choices (see Chapter 14) is a good food guide for toddlers and preschoolers. The portion sizes, however, should be smaller than those for older children and adults. For example, the portion size for milk is 4 oz rather than 8 oz and the portion sizes for fruits and vegetables are about half that of an adult. One pint of milk and 1 or $1\frac{1}{2}$ oz of meat or meat substitutes meets the toddler's daily needs for protein, calcium, phosphorus, and magnesium. Table 18-1 gives a food guide for toddlers and preschoolers.

The child should be offered as wide a variety of food as possible both for nutritional reasons and to acquaint the child to different textures and tastes. Care must be taken to avoid the overuse of milk at the expense of other foods higher in iron. One pint to 3 cups of milk a day is adequate at this age. Vegetables and fruits that are good sources of vitamins C and A should be served each day (see Chapter 14). A vitamin D supplement may be necessary if the amount consumed in fortified milk and other fortified foods (e.g., cereal) does not meet the RDA.

The best way to achieve a nutritious food intake is to plan set mealtimes and snack times—three meals plus two or three snacks each day. This way, the parent can closely watch what the child is eating. If the child is permitted to eat small amounts of food indiscriminately throughout the day, the parent can easily lose track of what the child has eaten.

Because toddlers and preschoolers have great energy needs for growth and a small stomach capacity for food, snacks are important. It is difficult to meet the child's energy needs with three meals alone. Snacks supply about 20% to 25% of the energy needs and should be composed of foods that enhance the quality of the diet, such as yogurt, milk, fruits, cereals, and whole-grain breads (Display 18-1).

During the preschool years, the family begins the challenge of coping with outside pressures—especially television—concerning food selection. These pressures must not be permitted to influence the child's eating habits.

EATING HABITS AND THE FEEDING RELATIONSHIP

Good eating habits are established early in life. Developing positive eating habits involves more than just providing nutritious food. The social and emo-

TABLE 18-1 GUIDELINES FOR FOOD SELECTIONS: TODDLER AND PRESCHOOL YEARS

FOOD GROUP	RECOMMENDED DAILY SERVINGS	SERVING SIZE GUIDELINES 1–3 y	4–5 y
Meat, poultry, fish, eggs, dry beans and peas, nuts and seeds	≥2 servings		
	Lean meat, fish, poultry	2–3 tbsp or 1–2 oz	4–5 tbsp or 2–3 oz
	Eggs	1	1
	Dry peas and beans	1–3 tbsp	2–4 tbsp
Milk, cheese, yogurt	3–4 servings	$\frac{1}{2}$ cup or $\frac{1}{2}$ oz cheese	$\frac{3}{4}$ cup or $\frac{3}{4}$ oz cheese
	Milk, yogurt, cheese (whole milk and whole milk products should be given to children younger than age 2 y)		
Breads, cereals, rice, pasta	≥6 servings		
	Breads, buns, pizza	$\frac{1}{4}$–$\frac{1}{2}$ slice	1 slice
	Plain crackers	2–3	4–6
	Cereal (whole-grain or enriched)	$\frac{1}{4}$–$\frac{1}{3}$ cup	$\frac{1}{2}$ cup
Vegetables	≥2 servings		
	Raw (for older children)	2–3 pieces (if tolerated)	$\frac{1}{4}$–$\frac{1}{2}$ cup
	Cooked	$\frac{1}{4}$ cup	$\frac{1}{3}$–$\frac{1}{2}$ cup
Fruits	≥2 servings	$\frac{1}{4}$ cup or $\frac{1}{4}$–$\frac{1}{2}$ piece	$\frac{1}{4}$–$\frac{1}{2}$ cup or $\frac{1}{2}$ piece
	Juice*	$\frac{1}{3}$ cup	$\frac{1}{2}$ cup
Fats and oils	3–4 servings	1 tsp	1 tsp
	Margarine, butter, or oil		

* Include daily one serving of citrus juice or fruit or vegetable that is a good source of vitamin C and 1 serving dark green or orange vegetable or fruit rich in vitamin A.

(Adapted from Chicago Dietetic Association and the South Suburban Dietetic Association. Manual of clinical dietetics. 4th ed. Chicago: The American Dietetic Association, 1992:164.)

tional environment parents or other care-givers provide is important.

A respect for the division of responsibility between parent and child is key to establishing positive eating habits. Parents have the responsibility of providing food that is nutritious and developmentally appropriate for the child. They determine what, where, and when food is offered to the child. The child decides how much to eat.

LACK OF APPETITE

In children between ages 6 and 12 months, the appetite begins to lessen, reaching a low point at about age 3 or 4 years. This decrease in appetite is to be expected because the growth rate slows down and the child becomes increasingly interested in his or her surroundings. Health care workers must help parents understand that these changes in appetite are normal. If parents become overly concerned and react by urging or forcing the child to eat or bribing the child with sweets as a reward for eating, more serious appetite problems may result. The child may become tense and may tend to eat less or to overeat. Parents may have unrealistic expectations about the amount of food a toddler should eat. Table 18-1 provides a guide to portion sizes for a young child. Parents should be encouraged to create an environment that is conducive to enjoyment in eating—to have a relaxed atti-

DISPLAY 18-1 EXAMPLES OF NUTRITIOUS SNACKS

TODDLERS AND PRESCHOOLERS

Whole-wheat crackers or whole-wheat bread (quartered) with small pieces of cheese, lean meat, or poultry, or peanut butter
Apple or banana slices, plain or with peanut butter
Graham crackers, animal crackers
Low-sugar cereals
Orange wedges
Cooked vegetables such as cooked whole green beans or cooked carrot strips
Plain yogurt with unsweetened fruit (or packed in fruit juice)
Custard or puddings
Hard-cooked egg, quartered

SCHOOL-AGE CHILDREN AND ADOLESCENTS

Fruit, fresh, or canned (unsweetened or packed in its own juice)
Frozen fruit-juice pops
Whole-grain bread, whole-wheat English muffins
Fruit and vegetable juices
Pita or whole-grain crackers; bagels
Part-skim string cheese; reduced-fat cheese
Whole-wheat waffles and whole-wheat pancakes topped with yogurt or fruit
Low-sugar whole-grain cereals
Homemade sandwich spreads such as bean, cottage cheese, egg, tuna
Peanut butter (in moderation)
Mixtures of whole-grain cereals with dried fruits and nuts
Soups, preferably homemade or reduced-sodium varieties
Air-popped corn with parmesan cheese (spray popped corn lightly with nonstick oil spray so that cheese will adhere)
Fresh vegetables such as cherry tomatoes; carrot, celery, and cucumber sticks; pepper slices (with lowfat yogurt dip, if desired)
Plain yogurt or cottage cheese with unsweetened fruit
Salads made with salad greens and other raw vegetables with nonfat dressings
Tortilla with melted lowfat cheese

tude and resist the tendency to control how much their young children eat.

FAMILY MEALTIME

The importance of having a mealtime together as a family cannot be overemphasized. The structure and reliability of family mealtimes not only promotes good eating habits but also helps to secure a child's emotional health at all age levels. The young child learns about appropriate eating habits at the family table. The family mealtime provides a sense of unity and togetherness and establishes family relationships. Also, children who are involved in mealtime food-related activities in the home, such as setting the table, planning menus, and preparing simple foods, have a greater awareness of nutrition.

A family mealtime is not an easy feat to accomplish in many households, especially if it is a single-parent household or if both parents work. Nevertheless, the family mealtime is an important parental responsibility.

Physical activity should be encouraged. Snacking and eating while watching television should be discouraged. Suggestions for establishing good eating habits for young children are given in Display 18-2.

Children learn to feed themselves at between ages 1 and 2 years. Self-feeding is messy until about age 18 months (Fig. 18-1). Parents need to respect

DISPLAY 18-2 GUIDELINES FOR PROMOTING GOOD EATING HABITS IN TODDLERS AND PRESCHOOLERS

- Encourage the child to try new foods by involving him or her in meal planning, food shopping, and food preparation.
- Arrange food attractively; serve foods in a variety of colors, textures, and interesting shapes.
- Be sensitive to the child's preferences: does the child prefer food warm or hot, moist or dry, served separately, or mixed together in a casserole or sandwich?
- Offer small servings using smaller plates and cups; allow the child to ask for more.
- Encourage a young child to begin learning how to feed herself or himself by offering foods in easy-to-handle forms: meat, vegetables, fruit, bread, and cheese in small strips or finger sandwiches.
- Provide eating utensils that accommodate the child's stage of development when he or she is ready to use them: utensils with short, straight, broad, and solid handles; spoons with a wide bowl; and fork with blunt tines. The child should learn to use a spoon before attempting a fork.
- Serve meals at consistent times.
- Allow the child to eat with other family members. The child learns table manners and is encouraged to try new foods by imitating others.
- Do not use desserts and sweets as a reward for finishing a meal because this practice teaches that dessert is the most desirable part of a meal.
- Give sweets and other high-calorie, low-nutrient foods occasionally if they do not displace more nutritious foods.
- Introduce a new food at a meal that includes a favorite food. Without force or bribery, encourage the child to try at least one bite. If rejected, reintroduce it at another time.
- Plan a rest or quiet time before meals.
- Make mealtime a happy, social time.
- Allow the child sufficient time to finish the meal; a child who plays with food probably has had enough to eat and should be allowed to leave the table rather than disturb others.
- Avoid encouraging the child to eat all the food on his or her plate when no longer hungry. This practice can lead to overeating or to an aversion to food.
- Supervise the child during meals and snacks because of the risk of choking. A child who is coughing may be removing an obstacle naturally; allow the child to cough out the food before intervening. Foods that pose a choking risk are nuts, seeds, some raw fruits, vegetables, popcorn, hotdogs, and round hard candies.
- Offer small and satisfying snacks but not too often or too close to mealtime. Provide a variety of nutritious snacks (see Display 18–1). Reserve cakes, cookies, and so forth for occasional use.
- Avoid providing sweet, sticky foods that remain in the mouth for a long time because this practice will increase chances for tooth decay.

(Adapted from Chicago Dietetic Association and the South Suburban Dietetic Association. Manual of clinical dietetics. 4th edition. Chicago: The American Dietetic Association, 1992:164–161.)

that developing eating skills and food acceptance is a slow and difficult process for the child.

FOOD JAGS

Preschoolers are prone to food jags and food rituals. A child may not eat one food if it touches another food on the plate. Children in this age group frequently have strong preferences and dislikes for food. It is easy to understand a parent's concern when children will eat only a handful of foods. Parents are advised to remain calm and patient, meet the child's demands, as long as they are reasonable, avoid calling attention to the monotonous diet, and continue to offer other foods, allowing the child to refuse them. Most children outgrow these jags and suffer no ill effects from them.

SCHOOL-AGE CHILDREN

The school years bring about many changes in a child's life. The daily schedule changes, more meals are eaten outside the home, and the child makes

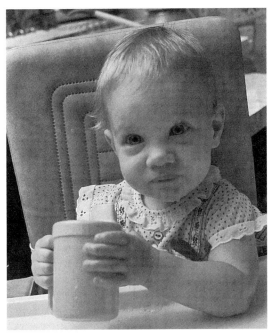

FIGURE 18-1

Children learn to feed themselves between ages 1 year and 2 years. *(Courtesy of the US Dept of Agriculture.)*

more choices for himself or herself. Television and peers increase their influence. After-school and social activities compete with family meal time. The child encounters new foods. During this period, it is critical that parents not only promote good eating habits, but also emphasize physical activity and educate the child about the negative effects of alcohol, nicotine, and other drugs.

NUTRITIONAL NEEDS

The period of age 6 to 10 years is one of steady growth and few feeding problems as compared with the preschooler. Height usually increases by 2 to 2.5 inches/year, with an average annual weight increase of 4.5 lb from age 6 to 8 years and an annual increase of 9 or 10 lb as the child approaches puberty. Each child has an individual pattern of growth and development, with growth occurring in spurts. The diet should supply adequate energy for growth and increased physical activity and adequate nutrients to be stored for the growth that will occur in adolescence.

ENERGY

Energy needs of school-age children are influenced by sex, age, body size, onset of puberty, and physical activity. In this age group, the RDA for energy and other nutrients is the same for both sexes. Until about age 10 years, differences in body composition between boys and girls is small. The RDA for energy for this age group is 2000 kcal/day, but varies considerably depending on growth rate and physical activity.

PROTEIN

The RDA for protein for the school-age child is 1 g/kg body weight. This recommendation is readily met in the United States.

CARBOHYDRATES AND FATS

Energy needs should be met mostly by complex carbohydrates and naturally occurring sugars such as whole-grain breads and cereals, dried peas and beans, vegetables, and fruits. The National Cholesterol Education Program has recommended that children's intake of total fat be limited to no more than 30% of total calories, with less than 10% as saturated fat, no more than 10% polyunsaturated fat and dietary cholesterol limited to less than 300 mg/day.

VITAMINS AND MINERALS

The RDAs for some vitamins and minerals are higher for 10-year-olds than for 6-year-olds, whereas the RDAs for others, such as vitamins D, E, and C and the minerals calcium, iron, phosphorus, zinc, and selenium, remain the same (see Appendix B). The child's intake of calcium and iron warrants special attention. The consumption of soda, fruit-flavored drinks, and juices to the exclusion of milk may result in a low calcium intake in some school-age children. Inadequate calcium intake can adversely affect bone growth and bone quality and the child may fail to develop his or her genetic potential for peak bone mass.

Failure to meet iron needs can lead to learning difficulties. Children with iron deficiency have difficulty concentrating and tend to do poorly on tests. They may be irritable, lack physical stamina, and be more prone to infection. A well-chosen diet can fulfill the iron requirements of children between ages 2 and 10 years. When there is an excessive use of milk and other dairy products or when a high percentage of the calories in the diet are provided by unenriched bakery goods, candies, and soft drinks, the iron content of the diet is likely to be low.

MEAL PLANNING

The Pyramid Guide to Daily Food Choices (see Tables 14-1 and 18-2) provides guidelines for establishing a meal pattern for the school-age child. At least three meals should be provided with between-meal snacks as needed. Time should be allotted for breakfast, which children often skip because of bus schedules, working parents, and so forth. The after-school snack should not be so large that it replaces the evening meal. School breakfast and lunch programs contribute significantly to the diets of many school-age children. Table 18-2 gives a food guide for the school-age and adolescent years.

According to a survey conducted between October 1991 and January 1992, more than 1.6 million American children through age 14 years are unsupervised each day after school until a parent returns home. Of this number, half a million are younger than 12 years old. These latchkey children may select and prepare their own snacks and, sometimes, meals. These snacks and meals will be of high nutritional value if the home is stocked with a variety of well-liked nutritious foods (see Display 18-1).

Among school-age children, eating fast foods is less common than among teenagers. The impact of these foods on nutritional status depends on what foods the children choose and how frequently they eat them. If they eat fast foods frequently, nutrition problems can develop if the nutrient excesses (fat, sodium, and sugar) and deficiencies (vitamins A and C) are not counterbalanced at other meals during the day (see Chapter 14).

EATING HABITS

Once the child is in school, the parent or care-giver loses control over the child's diet. Children swap lunches, throw food away, or eat only foods they

TABLE 18-2 GUIDELINES FOR FOOD SELECTION: SCHOOL-AGE AND ADOLESCENT YEARS

FOOD GROUP	NO. OF SERVINGS	SUGGESTED SERVING SIZES*
Milk, cheese, yogurt	≥2 ≥3 for adolescents	1 cup lowfat milk or yogurt 1 1/2 oz lowfat cheese
Meat, poultry, fish, eggs, dry beans and peas, nuts and seeds	2–3 (for a total of 6 oz/day)	3 oz cooked meat The following count as 1 oz of lean meat: 1 egg 1/2 cup cooked dried beans or peas 2 tbsp peanut butter
Breads, cereals, rice, pasta	6–11	1 slice of bread 1 oz or 3/4 cup dry cereal 1/2 cup cooked cereal, rice, or pasta 3–4 small crackers or 2 large
Vegetables	3–5	1/2 cup cooked or chopped raw vegetables 3/4 cup vegetable juice
Fruits	2–4	1 whole medium-sized fruit 1/2 cup cooked or canned fruit 3/4 cup fruit juice

* Younger children may require smaller portion sizes.

like. Thus it becomes even more important to see that nutritious foods are eaten when the child is at home. *Having regular family meals is one of the most important factors in promoting good eating habits and enhancing nutritional status.*

Parents must continue to set limits. They should establish firm mealtimes and snack times. A child who is allowed to have chips or cookies whenever he or she desires will not have an appetite for more nutritious foods at mealtimes.

Sufficient time should be allotted for breakfast. The child or parent's busy schedule should not be permitted to interfere with eating properly at any meal.

A variety of nutritious foods and snacks should be offered. Snacks of low nutritional value should be limited to occasional use. The child's food preferences and appetite level should be respected. The child decides how much to eat; parents should never force, bribe, or cajole the child to eat. However, parents should continue to offer refused foods periodically.

Mealtimes should be pleasant and relaxed. They are not a time to scold children for previous misbehavior or to nag about what or how they eat. Family mealtimes are for socialization with family and friends and when parents set the example of good eating habits that they want their children to emulate.

Parents whose children become involved early in competitive sports should be alert for altered eating habits. Questionable nutrition advice and regimens that may be permissible to older children or professional athletes should not be imposed on young children. A high-carbohydrate diet with plenty of fruits, vegetables, breads, grains, and other starches, adequate calories, and plenty of extra fluids is the best way to enhance athletic performance.

ADOLESCENTS

Adolescence is a period of rapid growth and physical maturation. The rate of growth during this period of life is second only to that of the fetal period. The growth involves increases in height and weight, alterations in body composition and the enlargement of many organ systems. The adolescent is also developing on psychosocial and intellectual levels. Health professionals must consider all of these aspects—rapid growth, maturation, and psychosocial changes—when assisting with the nutritional management of each adolescent.

Until about age 9 years, girls and boys grow in height and weight at about an equal rate. The tremendous growth spurt of adolescence usually occurs in girls between ages 10 and 13 years and in boys between ages 12 and 15 years. From ages 13 to 16 years, the growth rate for girls decreases, whereas boys continue to grow into their late teens. The age of sexual maturity varies widely, and at age 10 years, some girls may have already entered puberty. Nutritional needs are related to sexual growth rate and to maturity and not to chronological age.

Girls gain more fat tissue than boys in specific areas. Boys gain mostly lean muscle tissue. The growth in height is about 3 inches/year for girls and 4 inches/year for boys.

NUTRITIONAL NEEDS

The RDAs are given separately for boys and girls starting at age 11 years (see Appendix B). The guidelines for energy and other nutrients are divided into two age periods: 11 to 14 years and 15 to 18 years.

ENERGY

Energy allowances are based on the median energy intakes of children who do light activities. The median daily energy intake for aged 11 to 14 years is 2500 kcal for boys and 2200 kcal for girls and for aged 15 to 18 years is 3000 kcal for boys and 2200 kcal for girls. Beginning at about age 11 years, girls need an average of about 550 kcal/day less than boys. Thus, girls must select foods more carefully than boys so that they can meet their nutrient needs without consuming too many calories.

The timing and size of the adolescent growth spurt and the level of physical activity vary widely.

Energy allowances must be adjusted for the individual child depending on body weight, activity, and growth rate. At all age levels, the child's individual growth pattern is the most important consideration. Because growth charts can be misleading, both skinfold measurements and weight-for-height determinations should be used to assess adequacy of energy intake. For example, an adolescent in the 90th percentile for weight and triceps skinfold in the lower percentiles would be considered muscular, not obese.

PROTEIN

Protein requirements represent the amount needed for maintenance of protein tissue plus the amount needed for the growth of new tissue. The recommended amounts of protein are 1 g/kg of body weight for both girls and boys aged 11 to 14 years and .8 g/kg for girls and .9 g/kg for boys aged 15 to 18 years. Most adolescents consume more than the recommended amount of protein. However, some teenagers who restrict food to lose weight or are living in poverty may be at risk of inadequate protein intake. If the amount of calories consumed are inadequate, protein may not meet bodily needs because it is used to supply energy rather than to build tissue.

CARBOHYDRATES AND FATS

Many adolescents' diets are high in both total fat and saturated fat. The National Cholesterol Education Program has recommended that adolescents consume diets containing no more than 30% of total calories from fat, less than 10% from saturated fat, no more than 10% as polyunsaturated fat, and less than 300 mg/day of dietary cholesterol. Carbohydrates, preferably complex carbohydrates and naturally occurring sugars, should be the major energy source.

VITAMINS

Adolescents need vitamins to support the growth spurt and their increased energy needs. Intake of vitamin A, which is required for vision, cell growth, reproduction, and a healthy immune system, is likely to be low. Vitamin D is involved in the mineralization of bone and vitamin C is needed for collagen (connective tissue) synthesis. Smoking and the use of oral contraceptives may increase requirements for vitamin C.

Folate (folacin) is important for its role in deoxyribonucleic acid (DNA) synthesis during this period of rapid growth. Adequate folate intake is especially important for teenage girls because of the association of folate deficiency with birth of infants with neural tube defects.

The rapid cell growth during adolescence increases the need for vitamins B_{12} and vitamin B_6. Vitamin B_6 is involved in several enzyme systems associated with protein metabolism. Riboflavin, niacin, and thiamin are involved in energy metabolism.

MINERALS

Calcium, iron, and zinc are especially associated with the growth of new tissue and need special attention during adolescence. The RDA for calcium increases from 800 mg/day for children aged 6 to 10 years to 1200 mg/day for adolescents and young adults through age 24 years. This increased calcium is necessary because 45% of the adult skeletal mass is formed during the adolescent years. Consuming adequate amounts of calcium promotes bone growth and also increases bone mass, or density. Deposit of calcium in bone tissue continues until at least age 25 years. A high peak bone mass may protect against the development of osteoporosis later in life (see Chapter 11).

Meeting calcium requirements is especially important for girls because women are more prone to osteoporosis. Three to four servings from the milk, cheese, and yogurt food group in The Pyramid Guide to Daily Food Choices (see Chapter 14 and Table 18-2) meets the recommendations for calcium. Unfortunately, many adolescents consume soft drinks to the exclusion of milk.

The RDA for iron increases substantially from 10mg/day for 6- to 10-year-olds to 15 mg/day for adolescent girls and 12 mg/day for adolescent boys. This increase is necessary to supply iron for the expanding blood volume and the increase in blood cell mass and muscle mass in both sexes. Girls need more iron because of losses during menstruation.

Iron supplements may be necessary for some adolescent girls.

Zinc is involved in protein synthesis and is an important factor in the growth process and in sexual maturation. The RDA for zinc is 12 mg/day for adolescent females and 15 mg/day for adolescent males. Adolescents who are growing rapidly are at high risk of zinc deficiency. Zinc-rich foods such as poultry, lean meats, legumes, lowfat dairy products, and whole grains should be encouraged.

MEAL PLANNING

A variety of foods chosen from the five food groups of The Pyramid Guide to Daily Food Choices can meet the adolescent's needs. Snacking is characteristic of teenage eating habits. If the teenager chooses snacks wisely and consumes snacks in moderation, snacks can make a substantial nutritional contribution to the adolescent diet.

EATING HABITS

Parents must continue to encourage good eating habits by continuing to have regular family meals and by having nutritious snack foods on hand (see Display 18-1). Badgering teenagers to make better choices probably will make them more resistant to change. The parents' good example is probably the best teacher at this point.

Many teenagers are at nutritional risk. Because they are growing rapidly and maturing physically, their nutritional needs are high. A number of eating behaviors characteristic of this age group threaten the nutritional quality of the diet. These behaviors include skipping meals, snacking on foods of poor nutritional quality, excessively using fast foods, and following fad diets. Psychosocial issues behind these eating behaviors include emerging independence, busy schedules, difficulty in accepting existing values, dissatisfaction with body image, search for self-identity, desire for peer acceptance, and need to conform to the adolescent lifestyle. Some teenagers may adopt fad diet practices and the use of unnecessary diet supplements as a means of enhancing body-building and athletic performance (see Chapter 7). Others may become preoccupied with being slim and, as a result, consume nutritionally inadequate diets. Some may develop eating disorders such as bulimia nervosa and anorexia nervosa (see the section Key Issues: Anorexia Nervosa and Bulimia Nervosa). Nutrition problems are further compounded by teenage pregnancy (see Chapter 16).

FOOD MISINFORMATION AND ATHLETIC PERFORMANCE

Young athletes, eager to improve their performance, are susceptible to misinformation on nutrition. They are bombarded with advice about dietary supplements that promise to improve stamina and strength. Pressure to "make weight" or to reduce weight to an abnormally low level can lead to unhealthy practices such as use of diuretics, laxatives, and diet pills, as well as starvation and excessive sweating. These unhealthy practices can lead to other problems including more difficulty controlling weight after repeated bouts of weight loss and regain, and eating disorders such as bulimia nervosa. A high-carbohydrate diet with plenty of fruits, vegetables, starches, and grains, adequate calories, and plenty of extra fluids is the best diet for children who participate in competitive sports.

NUTRITION EDUCATION

Although many teenagers have an awareness of desirable eating habits, this is not necessarily translated into healthy eating habits. Teenagers know the importance of eating breakfast, but many teenagers are not motivated to make time for breakfast. On the other hand, their knowledge may be incomplete and they may lack the information to make healthy choices. Teenagers may know the health problems associated with excessive dietary fat and sodium but they may not know which foods are high in fat and sodium and in other target dietary components such as sugar and fiber.

The health team can play an important role in helping teenagers adopt healthy eating and exercise habits by providing teenagers with reliable and useful information and helping them identify circumstances in which they are motivated to make good choices. Nutrition education should be relevant to their interests such as physical development, appearance, and sports performance.

FOOD PROGRAMS THAT AFFECT CHILDREN

The health care worker should know about community programs that can improve the nutritional status of children, keep abreast of changes in those programs, and promote their use by eligible people. The US Department of Agriculture, with the cooperation of state agencies, administers most of these programs. Family-oriented programs such as the Food Stamp program are described in Chapter 14. See Chapter 17 for information on the Special Supplemental Food Program for Women, Infants, and Children (WIC program). The following are programs geared specifically to children.

SCHOOL AND CHILD CARE PROGRAMS

The National School Lunch Program provides a federal subsidy toward lunches served to all children and a larger subsidy for meals served to needy children. Children from low-income families may receive the lunches free or at reduced prices. The school lunch is designed to provide about one third of the RDA for children. The similarly designed School Breakfast Program also is available in some schools (Fig. 18-2). The Child Care Food Program assists public and nonprofit child care facilities in providing nutritionally sound meals.

In June 1994, the US Department of Agriculture announced new school lunch regulations effective in the 1996–1997 school year. To meet those regulations, schools have to ensure that no more than 30% of lunch calories come from fat and no more than 10% come from saturated fat. Sodium and cholesterol are to be reduced but specific levels have not been set. The nutrient goals are based on meals during a 1-week period. Some meals may be higher in fat than the regulations require, whereas others may be lower. The average for the week will have to meet the regu-

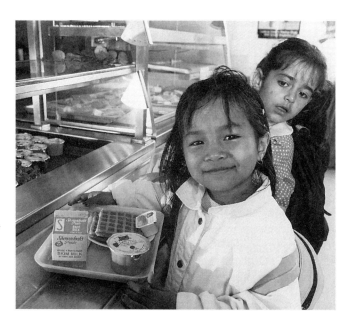

FIGURE 18-2

The School Breakfast Program makes low-cost breakfasts available to more than 5 million children in nearly 55,000 schools and institutions each school day. *(US Dept of Agriculture. Nutrition: eating for good health. Washington, DC: US Government Printing Office, 1994. Agriculture Information bulletin 685:102.)*

lations. Schools will no longer be restricted by specific "meal patterns." The menu must continue to supply one third of the daily calories, carbohydrate, protein, vitamins, and minerals, but the schools will have more flexibility in how to achieve this nutrient level.

NUTRITION-RELATED HEALTH PROBLEMS IN CHILDREN AND ADOLESCENTS

FAILURE TO THRIVE

Failure to thrive in children and adolescents may result from the same organic and inorganic causes that lead to growth failure in infants (see Chapter 17). These causes include diseases, poverty, abuse, and misinformation. Additional factors occurring in this age group are psychological stresses, such as those caused by parental divorce or other family crisis. Other causes may be eating disorders such as anorexia nervosa and bulimia nervosa, excessive exercise, and athletic programs.

If young children and toddlers are severely malnourished, as in some developing countries, they may never reach their full growth potential. In less severe cases, calories and protein in excess of the normal recommendations must be supplied for the child to catch up to the normal growth for the age group. In adolescents with eating disorders, more extensive treatment is required (see the section Key Issues: Anorexia Nervosa and Bulimia Nervosa).

OBESITY

In the United States, 15% to 25% of children are significantly overweight and the incidence of obesity is increasing. Whether obesity in infancy and early to middle childhood leads to adult obesity is the subject of controversy. Overweight teenagers are at greatest risk of becoming overweight adults. Many obese children become obese adults and tend to have more severe obesity than people who become obese as adults.

Obesity in childhood is a serious problem because it affects physical and mental health. Obesity is the major cause of hypertension in children and adolescents. Obese children have higher cholesterol and blood sugar levels. The psychological effects also are serious. The discrimination and ridicule obese children frequently endure may destroy their self-esteem for a lifetime.

Educating parents to the dangers of overfeeding deserves high priority. Breastfeeding and delayed use of solid foods are useful in preventing overfeeding. Children of all ages should not be pressured to eat every last spoonful of food on their plates. Ellyn Satter, family therapist and dietitian, and other authorities in childhood nutrition have indicated that children are able to regulate their own energy intake and that everyone is born with an internal mechanism for regulating the amount of food needed. Parents should not focus on how much the child eats but, rather, on the healthfulness and nutritional quality of the food they are offering the child. The parents decide on what, where, and when food is offered; the child decides how much. When parents focus on quantity of food, a conflict in the feeding relationship between child and parent may develop. Both denying the child food to avoid obesity and overfeeding the child may have the same result.

Another important factor in childhood obesity is a lack of physical activity. The average American school-age child watches television 25 hours/week. The amount of time spent watching television has been shown to be directly related to the degree of obesity in this age group. Television viewing not only takes away from participation in more physical activity but it also is associated with snacking on high-calorie, low-nutrient foods, such as snack chips and candy.

The changing lifestyle of the American family has contributed to obesity. The time constraints of single parents or of two working parents have placed greater reliance on school lunches, fast foods, and restaurant meals. The well-balanced, home-cooked family meal is a thing of the past for many families.

TREATMENT

It is important to identify the cause of the problem. Obesity may arise from family problems or disorganization, depression, lack of activity, or a conflict in the parent–child feeding relationship. The family must be involved in the treatment and must be willing to make changes. The health care worker and the family should encourage intense physical activity and emphasize sports the child can continue to enjoy as an adult, such as hiking, swimming, and tennis.

Health care specialists are recommending that overweight children not be subjected to weight loss diets but, rather, to healthy attitudes toward food. Parents and care-givers should make healthful eating a priority, and avoid applying negative pressure about the quantity of food eaten. Parents are advised to treat overweight children the same as normal weight children in the household with respect to food and feeding.

Group weight loss programs designed specifically for children of various age levels have been developed in the past years. These programs, run by a team of qualified professionals, include nutrition education, exercise, and image building. Family members are involved in the program.

EATING DISORDERS

Adolescents and even school-age children are influenced by our culture's preoccupation with thinness. Some children have such a fear of obesity that they restrict food to the point where growth failure and delayed physical development result. This fear of obesity syndrome in children may be a precursor of anorexia nervosa. Anorexia nervosa is a serious eating disorder, usually affecting adolescent girls, in which severe dieting and compulsive exercise are used as a means of achieving thinness. In extreme cases, this disorder is fatal (see the section Key Issues: Anorexia Nervosa and Bulimia Nervosa for more information on eating disorders).

Early detection of the fear of obesity is important. Growth patterns of children should be monitored regularly so that changes in growth rate can be noted and investigated. Girls should be helped to understand the changes in body contour that occur before and early in puberty. These body changes should not be mistaken for obesity.

DENTAL CARIES

Dental caries is the progressive decay of teeth caused by destruction of the outer tooth surface. It is the most prevalent disease for all age levels after infancy. Carbohydrates promote caries by encouraging the growth of the harmful bacteria that produce the tooth-eroding acids (see Chapter 8). Consuming fluoridated water throughout lifetime can reduce the risk of dental caries by 50% to 60% in permanent teeth (see Chapter 11).

ANEMIA

Iron deficiency anemia in children and adolescents usually is caused by insufficient iron intake. Iron deficiency anemia can occur when the majority of calories are derived from milk, soft drinks, sweets, and juices, at the expense of other nutritious foods. Adolescent girls are especially at risk because of iron loss during menstruation. When anemia is present, children and adolescents require iron supplements.

To prevent iron deficiency anemia emphasis is placed on iron-rich foods. Meat and foods rich in ascorbic acid promote the absorption of nonheme iron sources when eaten with a meal (see Chapter 11).

MALABSORPTION DISORDERS

CYSTIC FIBROSIS

Cystic fibrosis is an inherited disease of the exocrine glands, the glands that excrete to the outside of the body. Occurring in 1 in every 2000 births, it is the most common potentially fatal genetic disorder in Caucasians. Characteristic of this disease is the secretion of an abnormally thick mucus, which blocks the air passages in the lungs and may plug the ducts of the liver, pancreas, and gallbladder.

The sweat glands produce sweat higher in sodium and chloride than normal, and this loss, especially in hot weather, may be so extreme it causes death. Lung problems, especially repeated infections, are the greatest threat to life. It is likely that nutritional deficiencies contribute greatly to the occurrence of infection.

The malnutrition associated with cystic fibrosis is caused by malabsorption due to the blockage of pancreatic enzymes and frequent respiratory tract infection. The malabsorption in turn causes steatorrhea (excessive amounts of fat in the stool) and poor absorption of nutrients, especially fat-soluble vitamins and essential fatty acids. Abdominal cramps, flatulence (gas in the intestinal tract), and diarrhea are common. The affected child's growth and development are retarded.

The nutritional needs of a child with cystic fibrosis are much greater than normal. Energy needs are 20% to 50% and protein needs are as much as 200% or more above normal requirements. Adequate caloric intake is essential to spare protein for growth and repair.

Nutrition therapy aims to provide a high-calorie and high-protein diet with liberal amounts of fat and sodium chloride. To meet the high caloric requirements, fats contribute 40% to 50% of the total caloric intake. Pancreatic enzymes are increased as extra fat is added. Liberal use of table salt is encouraged. Supplementation of fat-soluble vitamins is also indicated.

The introduction of enteric-coated pancreatic enzymes in the early 1980s has permitted more liberal amounts of fat in the diet. Before, clients were advised to eat lowfat diets to decrease steatorrhea and gastrointestinal symptoms. Clients can now consume foods that they previously omitted.

The tolerance for various foods differs greatly from one client to another. The diet must be adapted to individual needs, likes, dislikes, and tolerance for fats. Nutritious snacks in addition to three meals each day are required. Creative approaches are sometimes necessary to increase the caloric density of preferred food—adding fats to cooked cereal, dried fruit to breadstuffs, and padding foods with nonfat milk powder. Sometimes nutrition supplements such as Carnation Instant Breakfast (Carnation Co.), Pediasure or Ensure (Ross Laboratories), or Sustacal (Mead Johnson) may be added.

In some cases, special dietary products that are more readily absorbed than regular food may need to be considered. Medium-chain triglycerides are better absorbed than dietary fats. For infants, protein hydrolysate infant formulas may be used. Semisynthetic, fiber-free formulas (see Chapter 29) may also be used for older children and adults. If nutritional status does not improve, tube feedings or parenteral nutrition may be necessary.

CELIAC DISEASE

Celiac disease is described in Chapter 28. Affected infants receive rice cereal and other baby foods free of gluten. Older children are given the gluten-free diet described in Chapter 28. Care must be taken both in the hospital and at home to see that other children or well-meaning adults do not offer the affected child foods that contain gluten.

ELEVATED BLOOD CHOLESTEROL

See the discussion Elevated Cholesterol Levels in Children and Adolescents in Chapter 25.

KEY ISSUES

Anorexia Nervosa and Bulimia Nervosa

The desire for thinness has developed into a national obsession over the past several decades. This trend has been accompanied by an epidemic rise in two eating disorders—anorexia nervosa and bulimia nervosa. These illnesses usually occur during adolescence and young adulthood. Anorexia nervosa was described as an illness as early as 1668. Bulimia was first included as a distinct syndrome in the *Diagnostic and Statistical Manual of the American Psychiatric Association* in 1980.

ANOREXIA NERVOSA

Anorexia nervosa is a life-threatening psychological disorder characterized by deliberate self-starvation. It has a high mortality rate of 9% to 21%. People with anorexia nervosa are obsessed with food but because of emotional problems refuse to permit themselves to eat.

Some people use extreme dieting and strenuous exercise to achieve weight loss, whereas others combine food restriction with even more dangerous behaviors such as self-induced vomiting, high doses of laxatives, and misuse of diuretics and appetite suppressants.

Anorexia nervosa most frequently occurs in Caucasian adolescent females (90% female, 10% male); the age of onset appears to peak at age 13 to 14 years and again at age 17 to 18 years. Of girls between ages 12 and 18 years, 1 in every 250 will develop the disorder. There is an especially high incidence among dance and modeling students.

The person who develops the eating disorder is frequently a female overachiever who is described as a model child eager to please. She strives for perfection in everything she does. She cannot accurately perceive her body size and feels she would be more attractive if she could only lose more weight.

Fear of new responsibilities of adolescence (forming peer relationships and increasing independence from family) may be overwhelming. The extreme dieting allows her to delay biologic maturity and its new responsibilities. As she continues to restrict her eating, she begins to experience a new sense of control and confidence.

The family dynamics appear to influence the development of this disorder. The parents usually are educated, conscientious people who are high achievers. The environment in the family frequently is overprotective, behavior is tightly controlled, communication is poor, and expectations placed on the children are unrealistically high. One of the parents may be overly concerned about eating patterns and is likely to be a perfectionist. The self-starvation becomes a weapon against the over-controlling parents. The behavior dominates the family as the parents react with hopelessness, anger, and guilt.

Behavioral Symptoms

The most common behavioral symptom is the irregular consumption of meals of poor nutritional quality. Dieting and weight loss continue and the teenager becomes preoccupied with food. She becomes expert at counting calories and frequently limits herself to 600 to 900 kcal/day or less. This dieting is coupled with a high level of physical exercise and hyperactivity. Some people hoard, hide, or dispose of food. Occasionally, the anorectic person may gorge and then either vomit or fast. Self-induced vomiting occurs in one fourth to one half of all cases. Usually food idiosyncrasies are present including vegetarianism, avoidance of red meat, and avoidance of or preference for sweets.

Even after the teenager becomes emaciated, she continues to fear weight gain and to express feeling of fatness. Dieting, excessive exercise, and other behaviors associated with maintaining weight loss become her way of life.

Physical Symptoms

The most striking physical symptom is a loss of 20% to 25% of body weight. A wide range of associated physical symptoms reflects the body's way of adapting to starvation. These symptoms include lack of a menstrual period (amenorrhea), excessive constipation, loss of hair, growth of fine body hair (lanugo), intolerance to cold, low blood pressure, low pulse rate, decreased immunity, and hyperactivity. If the individual also engages in binge eating, vomiting, and purgative abuse, many additional distressing complications may be present (Display 18-3). All body systems are affected. When malnourishment is extreme, apathy, confusion, and social isolation occur. Cardiac complications are the most common cause of death in anorectic clients.

Psychological Symptoms

The main psychological symptoms include a distorted body image, confusion of the self-image, a sense of being incompetent or ineffective as a per-

DISPLAY 18-3 MEDICAL COMPLICATIONS ASSOCIATED WITH ANOREXIA NERVOSA

STARVATION	VOMITING*	BINGE EATING	PURGATIVE ABUSE*
Amenorrhea	Cardiac arrhythmias	Acute stomach dilation	Diarrhea
Bradycardia	Tetany and paresthesias	Painless salivary gland enlargement	Steatorrhea
Constipation	Seizures		Dehydration
Cold intolerance	Dehydration		
Hypotension	Dental enamel erosion		
Kidney stones	Hoarse voice		
Lanugo hair	Gastrointestinal reflux		
Dry skin			
Osteoporosis			

(Opremcak C. Anorexia nervosa in adolescence: an overview. Pediatr Perinat Nutr 1987;1:1:13.)

* Author note: Complications associated with vomiting, binge eating, and purgative abuse also occur in bulimia nervosa.

son (low self-esteem), fear of maturing and becoming an independent individual, depression, and withdrawal from others. The isolation increases as the disease progresses. Some of these characteristics are hidden by the client's negative, defiant, and stubborn outward behavior. For the person with anorexia nervosa, being thin is the predominant standard for establishing self-worth. She works hard to maintain control despite intense hunger pains and takes pride and pleasure in being able to do something so difficult.

Treatment

Convincing the client that treatment is necessary is usually the first challenge. The steps in the treatment of anorexia nervosa are given in Display 18-4. Treatment is best when conducted in inpatient or outpatient units of hospitals or other health facilities that specialize in treating anorexia nervosa. These units are staffed by a multidisciplinary team that is skilled in dealing with anorectic behaviors.

The first priority is to treat the medical complications and restore a normal state of nutrition. Clients need to gradually return to a normal weight, which is determined by scientific norms. The weight goal is nonnegotiable. Bed rest after meals is usually required to prevent vomiting (in secret) or strenuous exercise. Some programs incorporate a supervised exercise program for people who are physically able. Clients who are allowed to exercise tend to accept weight gain better; the exercise program also provides guidance on healthy levels of activity.

Long-term psychotherapy is an essential component of treatment. This treatment is supple-

DISPLAY 18-4 SEVEN ESSENTIAL STEPS IN THE TREATMENT OF ANOREXIA NERVOSA

1. Diagnose and treat the medical complications of starvation and the behaviors that have induced them.
2. Restore a normal state of nutrition by encouraging the client to eat a normal, balanced diet.
3. Use behavioral techniques, when necessary, that reward weight gain.
4. Provide sound guidance about nutrition and exercise.
5. Alter anorexic attitudes and thinking by cognitive therapy.
6. Optimize support by family counseling and education.
7. Enhance autonomy, facilitate identity formation, raise self-esteem, and prevent invalidism by psychotherapy.

(Beumont PJV, Russell JD, Touyz SW. Treatment of anorexia nervosa. Lancet 1993;341:1635.)

mented by psychological counseling and mental health education for the client and her family. Participation in a self-help group often is a useful aid.

The dietitian is an essential part of the treatment team. The dietitian plans the refeeding program and assists in its implementation. Initially, nutritional status is improved while a low weight is maintained, and then gradual weight gain through self-feeding is encouraged. Intravenous and tube feedings are usually unnecessary. The aim is to guide the client to eating in a normal and relaxed way.

Nutrition intervention involves establishing a trusting relationship with the client so that food-related fears and eating behaviors can be openly and honestly discussed. Within this trusting relation, change gradually can be implemented. The client is helped to understand how the psychological and medical aspects of the illness relate to eating and weight behaviors.

BULIMIA NERVOSA

Bulimia nervosa is characterized by recurrent episodes of binge eating followed by self-induced vomiting or other means of getting rid of (purging) the food calories, such as laxatives, diuretics, and exercise. (Weight loss that follows laxative use most likely is due to dehydration and electrolyte disturbances, as it is with the use of diuretics.)

Bulimia nervosa occurs most often in women in their late teens to mid-thirties. Binge eating tends to begin in late adolescence and frequently follows a period of dieting for weight loss. Self-induced vomiting or laxative abuse usually follows about 1 year later. Periods of binge eating often are separated by periods of severe dieting. The person with bulimia is usually within 15% of normal weight.

Behavioral Symptoms

Binge eating usually involves consumption of large quantities of high-calorie, easily digested foods such as pastries, bread, ice cream, or candies. The person with bulimia usually binges on food perceived to be high-calorie, forbidden foods. Binges may last 15 minutes to several hours and occur in a secretive and frenzied manner. They usually occur when the individual is alone and may be planned or spontaneous. The episodes increase during periods of stress. A minimum average of two binge eating episodes a week for at least 3 months is one criteria for the diagnosis of bulimia nervosa.

Physical Symptoms

Physical problems caused by bulimia include menstrual irregularities, swollen glands, and significant weight fluctuation. The fasting, vomiting, and use of laxatives and diuretics may cause dehydration, electrolyte imbalances, and malnutrition. The frequent vomiting causes esophageal irritation, extensive erosion and decay of teeth, and glandular and metabolic disturbances. Other possible complications include pancreatitis, narrowing of the esophagus, acute expansion of the stomach, and calcium malabsorption.

Psychological Symptoms

The condition appears to be triggered by binge eating that results from strict and prolonged dieting. The bulimic person, typically a female, is overly concerned with body shape and weight, but she does not usually have a distorted body image. Food may be an outlet for feelings of frustration, disappointment, anger, loneliness, or boredom. She is usually aware of the abnormal nature of her eating patterns and fears that she will be unable to stop eating.

Various theories have suggested the cause of bulimia nervosa. One such theory, the biopsychosocial model, suggests that young women with biologic tendencies to overweight, depression, and metabolic disturbances become vulnerable to social pressure for thinness.

Treatment

Treatment is best conducted by a team of health professionals specially trained to work effectively with bulimic clients. Medical treatment and both psychotherapy and counseling for client and family members are involved.

Diet therapy involves educating the client to the principles of good nutrition, establishing regularity in meals, and developing a clear understanding of the dangers of purging. The goal is to maintain a weight that is appropriate for the individual. A realistic weight goal, one that considers the client's previous weight history, should be identified. A well-balanced diet that includes a moderate amount of fat has been suggested. Fat provides satiety and may reduce binge eating between meals.

Health workers should be aware of the characteristics of these disorders and the population at risk so that they can identify and treat people with these illnesses as soon as possible. The public also must be educated about the dangers of fad diets and about healthy weight ranges and healthy means of controlling weight.

Two national organizations provide information and assistance. They are as follows: National Association of Anorexia Nervosa and Associated Disorders (ANAD), PO Box 271, Highland Park, IL 60035, and American Anorexia/Bulimia Association, Inc., 418 East 76 Street, New York, NY 10021.

KEYS TO PRACTICAL APPLICATION

Advise parents that toddlers and young children will consume enough energy to meet their needs. Parents should determine what, where, and when the child eats; the child determines how much.

Instruct parents that lowfat, high-fiber diets are inappropriate for toddlers and young children.

Avoid giving children food that may cause choking (see Display 17-1). Always supervise young children when they eat.

Make parents aware of the effects of overtiredness, excitement, and strange surroundings on a child's appetite. Instruct them not to bribe, force, or coax a child to eat.

Provide nutritious between-meal snacks such as fruit, vegetables, cheese, cereal, cold meat, whole-wheat bread, pudding, custard, yogurt, and milk.

Encourage active play by the young child and intense physical activity by the older child. Limit children's television viewing.

Encourage food choices from The Pyramid Guide to Daily Food Choices for people of all ages including children and adolescents.

Emphasize the importance of family meals for both their nutritional and emotional significance.

Counsel parents that having nutritious meals and snacks available and providing a good example are the best ways to influence teenagers' food habits.

Educate about the dangers of fasting and fad diets.

Be alert to the symptoms of anorexia nervosa and bulimia nervosa.

KEY IDEAS

Changes in appetite are normal during the toddler stage. Parents should not resort to forcing or bribing the child to eat.

Having set mealtimes and snack times for children is a good way to achieve a nutritious diet and monitor what is being eaten.

Extreme caution must be taken when microwaving foods for small children to prevent burning.

After age 2 years, recommendations for fat intake are as follows: no more than 30% of total calories from fat, less than 10% as saturated fat, and no more than 10% as polyunsaturated fat, and cholesterol limited to less than 300mg/day.

See Display 18-2 for ways of promoting good eating habits in young children.

The Pyramid Guide to Daily Food Choices is a good food guide from the toddler to the adult stages. Portion sizes are smaller for the young child.

Because of the small capacity for food, a young child needs nutritious snacks in addition to three meals a day.

Parents determine what, where, and when food is offered the child. The child decides how much to eat.

Having regular family meals is one of the most important factors in promoting good eating habits and enhancing emotional health.

Making available nutritious snacks for children and adolescents can improve their nutritional status. Stocking the home with nutritious foods is important.

During ages 4 to 10 years, growth slows down and becomes more uniform; RDAs are the same for boys and girls.

During adolescence, growth is rapid; nutritional needs are related to sexual maturity, not chronological age.

Adolescent girls must select foods carefully so that they can meet their nutritional needs without consuming too many calories. Boys have higher caloric needs and are more likely to meet their requirements because of the volume of food they consume.

Meeting the increased calcium recommendations during adolescence is important, especially for girls.

Good example is probably the best way to enhance good eating habits in adolescents.

Inorganic failure to thrive is caused by some disturbance in the infant or child's environment.

Prevention of obesity in childhood deserves high priority; both eating habits and physical activity should be considered.

Both denying the child food to avoid obesity and overfeeding may promote obesity.

Diets are not recommended as treatment for childhood obesity.

Frequent snacking on carbohydrate foods promotes the development of dental caries; the use of fluoridated water reduces the incidence of caries by 50% to 60%.

Iron deficiency anemia is a common problem in childhood and adolescence, especially among adolescent girls.

See Chapter 25 for a discussion of elevated cholesterol levels in children and adolescents.

Malnutrition, which frequently accompanies cystic fibrosis, is due to poor absorption of nutrients caused by a lack of pancreatic enzymes and frequent respiratory infections. Maintaining adequate caloric intake is essential. The use of enteric-coated pancreatic enzymes permit more liberal amounts of fat in the diet.

A well-balanced diet that contains sufficient calories and fluids is the best way to enhance athletic performance.

Immediate professional attention should be obtained for people exhibiting symptoms of anorexia nervosa or bulimia nervosa, both of which are serious eating disorders. Both of these psychological disturbances can result in serious physical deterioration.

KEYS TO LEARNING

STUDY–DISCUSSION QUESTIONS

1. A mother is concerned about her toddler's lack of interest in food and occasional refusal to eat at mealtimes. What advice would you give her?
2. Discuss the importance of active play and its relation to a child's nutritional well-being.
3. What measures should be taken during infancy, childhood, and adolescence to prevent iron deficiency anemia?
4. Make posters comparing the nutritional value of commonly used snack foods. Compare the costs of what you would consider good snacks and poor snacks.
5. Discuss the role of nutrition in the prevention of dental caries.
6. One of the basics of parenting is setting limits. Discuss how you would relate setting limits to promoting good eating habits in children.
7. Discuss the importance of nutrition care for the client with cystic fibrosis. Why are pancreatic enzymes given as medication? Increased amounts of salt may be necessary.

Why? Despite a high caloric intake, a child with cystic fibrosis may be undernourished. Why?

8. Plan a day's menu for a 4-year-old child on a gluten-free diet. (See Chapter 28 for a discussion of the gluten-free diet.)

9. What are the potential consequences of anorexia nervosa and bulimia nervosa? Discuss in class the prevalence of these eating disorders in the adolescent and young adult population. Invite a mental health professional who specializes in treating eating disorders to speak to the class.

BIBLIOGRAPHY

BOOKS AND PAMPHLETS

American Psychiatric Association, Diagnostic and statistical manual of mental disorders. rev. 4th ed. Washington, DC: American Psychatric Association, 1994.

Barness LA. Ed. Pediatric nutrition handbook. 3rd ed., Elk Grove Village, IL: American Academy of Pediatrics, 1993.

Chicago Dietetic Association and the South Suburban Dietetic Association. Manual of clinical dietetics. 4th ed. Chicago: The American Dietetic Association, 1992.

Gong EJ, Heald FP. Diet, nutrition, and adolescence. In: Shils ME, Olson JA, Shike M. Eds. Modern nutrition in health and disease. 8th ed. Philadelphia: Lea and Febiger, 1994.

National Academy of Sciences, Institute of Medicine, Food and Nutrition Board, Committee on Nutritional Status During Pregnancy and Lactation. Nutrition services in perinatal care. Washington, DC: National Academy Press, 1992.

National Academy of Sciences, National Research Council, Food and Nutrition Board. Recommended dietary allowances. 10th ed. Washington, DC: National Academy Press, 1989.

Satter EM. How to get your kid to eat . . . but, not too much. Palo Alto: Bull Publishing, 1987.

Twin Cities District Dietetic Association. Manual of clinical nutrition. Minneapolis: Chronimed Publishing, 1990.

US Dept of Health and Human Services, Public Health Service, National Cholesterol Education Program. Highlights of the report of the expert panel on blood cholesterol levels in children and adolescents. Bethesda, MD: National Institutes of Health, National Heart, Blood, and Lung Institute, 1991. NIH publication 91-2731.

US Dept of Health and Human Services, Public Health Service. Health people 2000: national health promotion and disease preventon objectives. Washington, DC: US Government Printing Office, 1988.

PERIODICALS

Albertson AM, Tobelmann RC, Engstrom A. Nutrient intakes of 2 to 10 year old American children: 10 year trends. J Am Diet Assoc 1992;92:1492.

Anliker JA, Laus MJ, Samonds JW, et al. Mothers' reports of their three-year-old children's control over foods and involvement in food-related activities. J Nutr Educ 1992;24:285.

Beumont PJV, Russell JD, Touyz SW. Treatment of anorexia nervosa. Lancet, 1993;341: 1635.

Briley ME, Gray CR. Nutrition standards in child care: technical support paper. J Am Diet Assoc 1994;94:324.

Campbell MK, Kelsey KS. The PEACH survey: a nutrition screening tool for use in early intervention programs. J Am Diet Assoc 1994;94:1156.

Cannella PC, Bowser EK, Guyer LK, et al. Feeding practices and nutrition recommendations for infants with cystic fibrosis. J Am Diet Assoc 1993;93:297.

Centers for Disease Control. Selected tobacco-use behaviors, dietary patterns among high school students—United States, 1991. JAMA 1992;268:448.

Clark N. Counseling the athlete with an eating disorder: a case study. J Am Diet Assoc 1994;94:656.

Emerson EN, Stein DM. Anorexia nervosa: empirical basis for restricting and bulimic subtypes. J Nutr Educ 1993;25:329.

Graves KL, Farthing MC, Smith SA, et al. Nutrition training, attitudes, knowledge, recommendations, responsibility, and resource utilization of high school coaches and trainers. J Am Diet Assoc 1991;91:321.

Himes JH, Dietz WH. Guidelines for overweight in adolescent preventive services: recommendations from an expert committee. Am J Clin Nutr 1994;59:307.

Klesges RC, Shelton ML, Klesges LM. Effects of television on metabolic rate: potential implications for childhood obesity. Pediatrics 1993;91:281.

Marcos A, Varela P, Santacruz I, et al. Evaluation of immunocompetence and nutritional status in patients with bulimia nervosa. Am J Clin Nutr 1993;57:65.

Nicklas TA, Webber LS, Koschak ML, et al. Nutrient adequacy of low fat intakes for children: the Bogalusa heart study. Pediatrics 1992;89:221.

Reiff DW, Reiff KKL. Position of the American Dietetic Association: nutrition intervention in the treatment of anorexia nervosa, bulimia nervosa, and binge eating. J Am Diet Assoc 1994;94:902.

Thomas LF, Long EM, Zaske JM. Nutrition education sources and priorities of elementary school teachers. J Am Diet Assoc 1994;94:318.

CHAPTER

19

Meeting Nutritional Needs During Adulthood and Older Adulthood

KEY TERMS

dysgeusia impaired sense of taste
dysosmia impaired sense of smell
dysphagia difficulty in swallowing
hyperthermia above-normal body temperature
hypothermia subnormal body temperature
xerostomia mouth dryness due to decreased secretion of saliva

OBJECTIVES

After completing this chapter, the student will be able to:

1. Discuss the changing energy needs of adults in early, middle, and older adulthood.
2. Interpret meal planning guidelines for adults using The Pyramid Guide to Daily Food Choices and offer suggestions to counteract negative concepts concerning a "healthful diet."
3. Discuss the role of nutrition and sex differences in the nutrition-related health concerns of adults.
4. Explain why standards and methods used for assessing nutritional status are less reliable for the older person compared with the younger adult.
5. Give three anthropometric data and/or laboratory values that may indicate malnutrition.
6. Explain why the health care worker should carefully investigate rapid involuntary weight loss.
7. Discuss five factors that may affect the older adult's nutritional status.
8. Explain the following statement: "As people get older, there is a lessening relationship between age in years and physical age."
9. Discuss the nutritional recommendations for the older adult with regard to fat, fluid, vitamins A, D, and B_{12}, and calcium.
10. Discuss the purpose of the Nutrition Screening Initiative and explain the use of its centerpiece checklist and warning signs in the DETERMINE format.
11. List five ways of increasing food intake in older adults who have lost interest in eating and give suggestions for encouraging adequate fluid intake.
12. Discuss the impact of eating alone on the older adult and provide suggestions for overcoming associated problems.
13. Explain the statement, "Some of the physical changes that occur with advancing age can be attributed, in part, to a decrease in physical activity." Describe the benefits of exercise for middle-aged and older adults.
14. Recognize the warning signs of alcoholism among older adults; be more aware of its prevalence in the elderly population.

The process of aging is a gradual one, starting at birth and continuing over many decades. We have discussed previously the nutritional needs and food-related psychosocial issues associated with infancy and the various stages of childhood and adolescence—all periods of physical growth. In this chapter, the discussion focuses on the nutritional needs of the adult—the person who has reached physical maturity.

The average life expectancy for people born in 1990 in the United States is 75.4 years. The proportion of older people in the US population is increasing; by 2030, 20% of the population (one in every five people) will be older than age 65 years. People 85 years old and older compose the fastest growing segment of the population. As life expectancy increases, health promotion and disease prevention become more important than ever so that the added years are quality years.

In our discussion, adulthood is divided into three stages: early adulthood (18 to 40 years), middle adulthood (40 to 65 years), and older adulthood (65 and older). The 10th edition of the *Recommended Dietary Allowances* divides adulthood into three age categories: 19 to 24 years, 25 to 50 years, and 51 or more years.

EARLY AND MIDDLE ADULTHOOD

NUTRITIONAL NEEDS

Growth does not come to an abrupt halt at age 18 years. Physical growth may continue until the early twenties and bone growth continues until the mid-twenties to early thirties. For this reason, the Recommended Dietary Allowances (RDAs) for adolescents of 1200 mg/day of calcium and 10 mcg (400 International Units [IU]) of vitamin D have been extended to the 19- to 24-year-old group. The RDA for calcium drops to 800 mg/day and vitamin D drops to 5 mcg/day (200 IU) after age 25 years. With the cessation of physical growth in early adulthood, nutritional needs decrease to just the amount needed to maintain and repair body tissue. Maintenance needs remain substantially the same throughout adulthood, except for calories and, in women, iron.

Metabolically active tissue and activity pattern vary with age. After age 21 years, energy needed for metabolism slowly decreases. After early adulthood, lean body mass declines at a rate of 2% to 3% per decade and the resting energy expenditure declines to the same extent. Activity level, however, probably has a greater effect on total energy needs than resting energy expenditure. Because the RDA for the B vitamins thiamin, niacin, and riboflavin are based on caloric intake, the recommended levels of these nutrients decrease in proportion to energy expenditure.

Iron requirements decrease for women after menopause, dropping from 15 mg to 10 mg/day. Nutritional needs during early and middle adulthood have been emphasized throughout this book. See Chapters 7 through 14.

NUTRITION-RELATED HEALTH ISSUES AND SEX DIFFERENCES

Health needs change as an individual progresses through the decades of adult life. Sex also affects health concerns. A startling finding has been that women have more advanced cardiovascular disease at the time of diagnosis than men and are at greater risk of dying within 1 year of their first heart attack. Because previous medical research tended to exclude women, scientific knowledge about sex differences is limited. Several long-term studies are being conducted to clarify the special needs of women and of men. A 14-year study being conducted by the National Institutes of Health (NIH) involves 150,000 women aged 50 years and older.

Women of child-bearing age require emphasis on iron because of the risk of iron deficiency anemia and on folate (folacin) to prevent neural tube defects in newborns. Women in their twenties and thirties need to continue to build calcium stores to protect against osteoporosis—a disease that is four times more prevalent in women than in men—in later life.

Cardiovascular disease is the leading cause of death in both sexes. However, the age of onset differs and the relative importance of risk factors may differ. Cardiovascular disease occurs about 10 to 12 years later in women than in men. Although a high total blood cholesterol level is a strong risk factor in men, a low high-density lipoprotein (HDL) level appears to be a greater predictor of heart disease in women. Nutrition intervention for the prevention and treatment of cardiovascular disease is discussed in Chapters 25 and 26.

Authorities have estimated that dietary factors contribute to one third of cancer deaths each year. Appearing to have the greatest influence are fat as a promoter and fiber as a protector. Certain nutrients known as antioxidants—vitamins C, E, and beta carotene (a precursor of vitamin A) and the mineral selenium—may also play a protective role.

Lung cancer due almost entirely to smoking is the number one cause of cancer deaths in both men and women. Breast and colon cancers rank second and third, respectively, for women; colon and prostate cancers rank second and third, respectively, for men. High-fat intake and obesity, especially upper body obesity, has been linked to an increased risk of breast cancer. Colon cancer has been firmly associated with a high-fat intake, obesity, and lack of dietary fiber. The diet of the American male tends to be low in fiber. Cancer is discussed in Chapter 30.

Obesity is also a risk factor in hypertension, cardiovascular disease, and diabetes. More women than men are overweight and seriously overweight. Also, men are more likely to be successful at weight loss using traditional means of increasing exercise and decreasing caloric intake. Obesity is discussed in Chapter 23.

EATING HABITS

Americans are more concerned about their eating habits than they have been in the past. They are aware of the recommendations to eat a varied diet, control calories, increase fiber, and limit total fat, saturated fat, cholesterol, salt, and sugar. Recent food consumption surveys, however, have indicated that people are eating more processed foods, more partially prepared foods, more microwaveable convenience foods, and more gourmet treats. Moreover, studies have indicated that people who do reduce the fat in their diets are not maintaining the overall nutritional quality of their diets. Adults are not choosing foods that are both lowfat and high in nutrients. Most Americans are not putting their knowledge of nutrition into practice.

MEAL PLANNING

One possible explanation for failure to act on nutrition recommendations is that many adults view a balanced diet negatively. They frequently perceive a balanced diet as a rigid diet, devoid of foods they like and one that involves more sacrifices than they are capable of making. Most adults label foods as either good or bad and many think that all fat in the diet must be eliminated.

Fat is an essential nutrient. Fat carries the fat-soluble vitamins throughout the body and helps maintain the function of cell membranes as well as other functions (see Chapter 9). Although it is recommended that the diet contain less than 30% fat calories, this does not mean that every item in the diet should be less than 30% fat. Rather, the diet as a whole should have less than 30% of its calories from fat. This means combining small amounts of high-fat foods with lowfat foods such as fruits, vegetables, pasta, breads, and cereals. Lean red meats need not be eliminated; rather, serve them in smaller portions and less frequently—two to three times a week rather than every day. Daily consumption of eggs is also not recommended; but consuming up to three eggs (213 mg cholesterol each) per week is unlikely to cause the average intake to exceed the recommended 300 mg/day of cholesterol.

A balanced diet, according to our current knowledge of nutrition, is one that includes more plant foods, fewer animal foods, and two to three servings of milk products (preferably lowfat or nonfat varieties) daily. Special emphasis should be given to eating more fruits and vegetables.

The Pyramid Guide to Daily Food Choices and *Nutrition and Your Health: Dietary Guidelines for Americans* on which the pyramid is based are excellent guides for achieving a balanced diet. Both these US government publications form the basis of meal planning recommendations discussed in detail in Chapter 14. Sample menus are given in Displays 14-5 and 14-6.

OLDER ADULTHOOD

ROLE OF NUTRITION

Malnutrition in the older person can have devastating consequences–physical, social, psychological, and economic. Physical effects include increased risk of infection, respiratory difficulties, skin breakdown, poor wound healing, musculoskeletal weakness, prolonged postoperative complications, and cardiac abnormalities. Psychological symptoms frequently associated with aging such as apathy, irritability, memory loss, and confusion can be nutrition related. The remainder of this chapter is devoted to the nutritional needs of the older adult.

NUTRITION ASSESSMENT OF THE OLDER ADULT

Nutrition standards and methods used for assessing nutritional status (Chapter 2) have been developed from younger adults and are not necessarily reliable for an older person. For example, changes in skin compressibility, thickness, and elasticity due to aging alter skinfold measurements. Anthropometric, biochemical, immunologic, and clinical parameters are all affected by the aging process, yet no standards exist for older people. Perhaps the best assessment is a comparison of the older person with himself or herself over time. This assessment involves taking repeated measurements at regular intervals and signifying any changes as a percentage of previous measurements.

Measuring the height of older adults may be difficult due to kyphosis or scoliosis or because they are bedridden. Display 19-1 gives equations based on knee height, which can be used to estimate height.

DISPLAY 19-1 ESTIMATING HEIGHT OF DIFFICULT-TO-MEASURE ADULTS

Men:
$64.19 (0.04 \times \text{age}) + (2.02 \times \text{knee height})$

Women:
$84.88 - (0.24 \times \text{age}) + (1.83 \times \text{knee height})$

Height estimate: Measure knee height (inches) from the bottom of the foot to the anterior of the knee with the ankle and the knee at 90°; measure age in years. These standards probably do not apply to non–Caucasians.

(Chumlea WC, Roch AF, Mukherjee D. Nutritional assessment of the elderly through anthropometry. Columbus, OH: Ross Laboratories, 1984.)

People at greatest risk of malnutrition have low values for serum cholesterol, albumin, hematocrit, hemoglobin, body mass index (BMI), and triceps skinfold measurement. Serum cholesterol below 160 has been associated with increased mortality in elderly populations. High total blood cholesterol levels above 240 have been identified as high risk by the National Cholesterol Education Program. Table 19-1 gives anthropometric data and laboratory values that are major indicators of malnutrition.

Weight changes should be carefully investigated. Rapid weight loss could be a sign of serious undiagnosed illness. Excessive weight gain could indicate fluid retention, possibly due to kidney or heart failure, electrolyte imbalances, or medication problems.

The symptoms of nutritional deficiencies frequently are vague and often are mistaken for the results of aging or are attributed to disease. It is important that the food intake of elderly people be monitored and that their nutritional status be evaluated on a continuing basis.

An additional assessment should be made of the individual's ability to perform the tasks of daily living. The skills of the entire medical team are needed to assess the client's capacity to acquire and consume adequate amounts of food.

TABLE 19-1 Major Indicators of Malnutrition That Require Medical Intervention

Indicator	Description
Weight	>10% weight loss in 6 mo 5% weight loss in 1 mo 7.5% weight loss in 3 mo BMI <24 or <80% ideal body weight BMI >27 or >120% ideal body weight
Triceps skinfold	<10th percentile >95th percentile
Midarm muscle circumference	<10th percentile
Serum albumin	<3.5 mg/dL
Serum cholesterol	<160 mg/dL* >240 mg/dL
Change in functional status	Change from independent to dependent in activities of daily living, especially those pertaining to eating and obtaining food
Inappropriate food intake	Failure to consume a diet that meets the Dietary Guidelines for Americans for more than 3 months
Presence of nutrition-related disorders	Osteoporosis Osteomalacia Folate deficiency B_{12} deficiency

* Serum cholesterol below 160mg/dL has been associated with increased mortality in the elderly.

(Adapted from: Nutrition Screening Initiative. Nutrition screening manual for professionals caring for older Americans. Washington, DC: Greer, Margolis, Mitchell, Greenwald, and Associates, 1991.)

NUTRITION SCREENING INITIATIVE

Although eating well preserves health and enhances the quality of life, the focus often has been on correcting problems after they occur. To identify people at nutritional risk before their health deteriorates significantly, the American Academy of Family Physicians, American Dietetic Association, and National Council on the Aging have undertaken the *Nutrition Screening Initiative.*

The main tool of the initiative is a *checklist* that is designed to make people aware of nine key factors that adversely affect nutritional health among older Americans. These factors are disease (both physical and mental), poor eating habits, tooth loss or mouth pain, economic hardship, reduced social contact, multiple medications, involuntary weight loss or weight gain, needing assistance with self-care, and being older than age 80 years. A brief discussion of each key risk factor accompanies the checklist. Both the checklist and the warnings signs in the DETERMINE format are given in Display 19-2. The word DETERMINE is composed of the first letter of each of the warning signs listed with the checklist and was designed to be useful in helping people remember the warning signs.

FACTORS THAT AFFECT NUTRITIONAL STATUS

Genetic and environmental factors contribute to the decline in body function associated with aging. It is difficult to determine how much each factor contributes to the process of aging. Because life events of individuals differ, the older people become, the more unalike they are. The life events and environmental factors that influence the rate at which a person ages include smoking, illness, physical ac-

(text continues on page 388)

DISPLAY 19-2 DETERMINE YOUR NUTRITIONAL HEALTH

This checklist and explanation of warning signs in the DETERMINE format are the main tools of the Nutrition Screening Initiative.*

The Warning Signs of poor nutritional health are often overlooked. Use this checklist to find out if you or someone you know is at nutritional risk.

Read the statements below. Circle the number in the *yes* column for those that apply to you or someone you know. For each yes answer, score the number in the box. Total your nutritional score.

	YES
I have an illness or condition that made me change the kind or amount of food I eat.	2
I eat fewer than two meals per day.	3
I eat few fruits, vegetables, or milk products.	2
I have three or more drinks of beer, liquor, or wine almost every day.	2
I have tooth or mouth problems that make it hard for me to eat.	2
I don't always have enough money to buy the food I need.	4
I eat alone most of the time.	1
I take three or more different prescribed or over-the-counter drugs a day.	1
Without wanting to, I have lost or gained 10 pounds in the past 6 months.	2
I am not always physically able to shop, cook, or feed myself.	2
	TOTAL

TOTAL YOUR NUTRITIONAL SCORE. IF IT'S—

0–2 **Good!** Recheck your nutritional score in 6 months.

3–5 **You are at moderate nutritional risk.** See what can be done to improve your eating habits and lifestyle. Your office on aging, senior nutrition program, senior citizens center, or health department can help. Recheck your nutritional score in 3 months.

6 or more **You are at high nutritional risk.** Bring this checklist the next time you see your doctor, dietitian, or other qualified health or social services professional. Talk with them about any problems you may have. Ask for help to improve your nutritional health.

Remember that warning signs suggest risk, but do not represent diagnosis of any condition. Read the following to learn more about the warning signs of poor nutritional health.

(Continued)

DISPLAY 19-2 DETERMINE YOUR NUTRITIONAL HEALTH *(Continued)*

The Nutrition Checklist is based on the following warning signs. Use the word DETERMINE to remind you of the warning signs.

DISEASE

Any disease, illness, or chronic condition that causes you to change the way you eat, or makes it hard for you to eat, puts your nutritional health at risk. Four out of five adults have chronic diseases that are affected by diet. Confusion or memory loss that keeps getting worse is estimated to affect one out of five or more older adults. This loss can make it hard to remember what, when, or if you've eaten. Feeling sad or depressed, which happens to about one in eight older adults, can cause big changes in appetite, digestion, energy level, weight, and well-being.

EATING POORLY

Eating too little and eating too much both lead to poor health. Eating the same foods day after day or not eating fruit, vegetables, and milk products daily will also cause poor nutritional health. One in five adults skips meals daily. Only 13% of adults eat the minimum amount of fruit and vegetables needed. One in four older adults drinks too much alcohol. Many health problems become worse if you drink more than one or two alcoholic beverages per day.

TOOTH LOSS/MOUTH PAIN

A healthy mouth, teeth, and gums are needed to eat. Missing, loose, or rotten teeth or dentures that don't fit well or cause mouth sores make it hard to eat.

ECONOMIC HARDSHIP

As many as 40% of older Americans have incomes of less than $6000 per year. Having less—or choosing to spend less—than $25 to $30 per week for food makes it very hard to get the foods you need to stay healthy.

REDUCED SOCIAL CONTACT

One third of all older people live alone. Being with people daily has a positive effect on morale, well-being, and eating.

MULTIPLE MEDICINES

Many older Americans must take medicines for health problems. Almost half of older Americans take multiple medicines daily. Growing old may change the way we respond to drugs. The more medicines you take, the greater the chance for side effects such as increased or decreased appetite, change in taste, constipation, weakness, drowsiness, diarrhea, nausea, and others. Vitamins or minerals, when taken in large doses, act like drugs and can cause harm. Alert your doctor to everything you take.

INVOLUNTARY WEIGHT LOSS/GAIN

Losing or gaining a lot of weight when you are not trying to do so is an important warning sign that must not be ignored. Being overweight or underweight also increases your chance of poor health.

NEEDS ASSISTANCE IN SELF-CARE

Although most older people are able to eat, one of every five has trouble walking, shopping, buying, and cooking food, especially as that person gets older.

ELDER YEARS ABOVE AGE 80

Most older people lead full and productive lives. But as age increases, risk of frailty and health problems increase. Checking your nutritional health regularly makes good sense.

* These materials were developed and distributed by the Nutrition Screening Initiative, a project of the American Academy of Family Physicians, The American Dietetic Association, and the National Council on the Aging.
The Nutrition Screening Initiative, 2626 Pennsylvania Avenue, NW, Suite 301, Washington, DC 20037.
The Nutrition Screening Initiative is funded in part by a grant from Ross Laboratories, a division of Abbott Laboratories.

tivity, nutrition, pregnancies, occupation, socioeconomic status, accidents, and war.

PHYSICAL CHANGES

Aging causes many body changes that affect food intake and the way the body processes food (Display 19-3). The progressive reduction in body organ functioning affects the digestion, absorption, metabolism, and excretion of nutrients.

Body Composition

A gradual decrease in height and a change in body composition occur. Muscle mass and total body water decrease with age and the proportion of body fat increases. Fat deposits around the internal organs and in the trunk of the body increase. The decrease in metabolically active muscle tissue coupled with reduced physical activity result in a lower energy requirement and can lead to excessive weight gain if caloric intake is not reduced accordingly. The basal metabolic rate decreases 20% between ages 30 and 90 years due mostly to lean body mass reduction.

DISPLAY 19-3 BIOLOGIC FUNCTION CHANGES BETWEEN AGES 30 YEARS AND 70 YEARS

BIOLOGIC FUNCTION	CHANGE
Work capacity (%)	↓ 25–30
Cardiac output (%)	↓ 30
Maximum heart rate (beats/min^{-1})	↓ 24
Blood pressure (mmHg)	
Systolic	↑ 10–40
Diastolic	↑ 5–10
Respiration (%)	
Vital capacity	↓ 40–50
Residual volume	↑ 30–50
Basal metabolic rate (%)	↓ 8–12
Musculature (%)	
Muscle mass	↓ 25–30
Hand grip strength	↓ 25–30
Nerve conduction velocity (%)	↓ 10–15
Flexibility (%)	↓ 20–30
Bone (%)	
Women	↓ 25–30
Men	↓ 15–20
Renal function (%)	↓ 30–50

(Physician Sports Med 1983;11:92.)

Bodily Senses

Decreases in taste, smell, and thirst sensations may lead to anorexia and dehydration. The number of taste buds drops from 245 in children to 88 in adults aged 74 to 85 years. The diminished sense of smell (dysosmia) is also strongly associated with the reduced sense of taste. Sensitivity to sweet and salty taste declines with age. Some medications also can dull the sense of taste (*dysgeusia*). Treatment and nutrition therapy for people with dysgeusia are discussed in Chapter 21.

Chewing and Swallowing

Chewing difficulties and pain resulting from loss of teeth, periodontal disease, and ill-fitting dentures may cause individuals to avoid certain nutritious foods. Diminished saliva secretion decreases the ability to masticate and swallow. Certain medications such as antihypertensive drugs cause mouth dryness (*xerostomia*), which contributes to chewing and swallowing difficulties (*dysphagia*). Treatment and nutrition therapy for people with xerostomia and dysphagia are discussed in Chapter 21.

Gastrointestinal

Reduced saliva and reduced secretion of hydrochloric acid and enzymes may reduce the absorption of nutrients such as calcium and iron. Reduced secretion of hydrochloric acid may also lead to bacterial overgrowth in the stomach. Some bacteria can attach to nutrients such as vitamin B_{12}, making them unavailable to the body.

Changes in peristalsis frequently result in constipation and, ultimately, a decrease in appetite. Inactivity, fatigue, and the eating of soft foods due to dental problems make the condition worse. Changes in gastrointestinal tract function also may result in chronic diarrhea and loss of appetite. Treatment and nutrition therapy for people with gastrointestinal disorders are discussed in Chapter 28.

Other Body Systems

Changes in other body systems indirectly affect nutritional status. With age, the ability of the body to use glucose is reduced. Blood vessels become less elastic, leading to increased pressure and hypertension. Kidney function can diminish 50% between ages 30 and 80 years. Immune function declines and there is a diminished ability to fight infection.

Chronic Diseases

About 85% of older adults have one or more chronic diseases, such as cardiovascular disease, diabetes, cancer, hypertension, arthritis, and osteoporosis, and deficiencies in mental function. Chronic diseases can impair appetite, reduce physical activity, and promote attitudes that adversely influence food intake and, consequently, nutritional status. Physical disabilities that make food shopping and food preparation difficult frequently result in the adoption of unhealthy eating patterns.

MENTAL DISORDERS

Mental disorders can seriously affect food intake. This is especially true in depression, in which anorexia is a major symptom. Other symptoms, such as apathy and withdrawal, further interfere with adequate food intake.

Older people who suffer from dementia (mental deterioration) also may fail to eat adequately due to social deterioration, isolation, and inability to select, purchase, and prepare food properly. They may forget to eat and may be at risk of malnutrition, especially if they have swallowing difficulties or other feeding problems.

Although mental disorders have a significant effect on eating habits, the effect of nutrition on their development is less clear. Some well-known mental disorders are caused by nutritional factors, for example, the mental disorders caused by alcohol-related deficiency diseases or deficiencies of specific nutrients such as thiamin. More research is needed, however, to determine the effects of marginal deficiencies on the development of mental disorders.

MEDICATION

Older adults are the greatest consumers of prescription and over-the-counter drugs. Aging affects the distribution of drugs in the body and also their metabolism and excretion.

Drugs can affect nutritional status adversely by altering food intake and the digestion, absorption, and use of nutrients. Food can also alter the effectiveness of some drugs. See Chapters 21 and 30 for more detailed discussions. Examples of drug nutrient interactions are given in Table 21-1 and Display 30-6.

LIFESTYLE FACTORS

Eating Alone

In Chapter 18, we discussed the important influence that family meals have on a child's nutritional, social, and emotional well-being. Eating alone also has a significant impact on adults—putting people at risk for consuming poor diets and creating a sense of isolation. Almost 9½ million people live alone—more than ever before.

Food is more than nourishment for the body; it conveys many deeply felt human emotions and experiences. Shared meals are an expression of unity, caring, and acceptance. People who live alone are less likely to prepare complete meals when they are feeding no one but themselves.

For older adults, eating meals alone may be the greatest hindrance to good eating. Who they eat with may be just as important as what they eat. Older people who live alone, especially those who have recently lost a spouse or loved one, simply eat less and are more likely to skip meals. Seniors who have an extensive friendship network are more likely to have better diets.

Social contact can be increased by joining a congregate feeding program supported by social services agencies (Fig. 19-1) or by joining luncheon clubs that have been developed in some areas for people who are too disabled or weak to travel to senior citizen centers. Sharing meals with other single neighbors is another means of having companionship at meals.

Exercise

Bodily changes formerly thought to be a natural part of aging, such as decreased aerobic capacity, muscle mass, muscle strength, flexibility, and balance, may be due, in part, to a decrease in physical activity. Exercise can prevent or reverse several

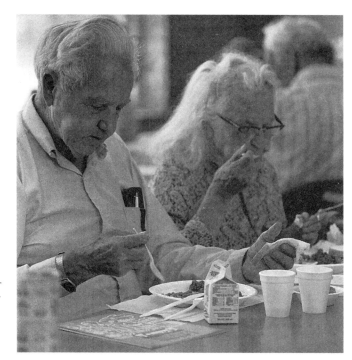

FIGURE 19-1

The Nutrition Program for the Elderly provides nutritious meals in a social setting. Congregate feeding programs address the problem of social isolation among many older Americans. *(Courtesy of the US Dept of Agriculture.)*

chronic conditions associated with aging such as non–insulin-dependent diabetes mellitus (type II), obesity, osteoporosis, cardiovascular disease, and mild hypertension.

People who keep physically active after age 45 years have a much better chance of reaching and living through old age in an independent and healthy way (Fig. 19-2). Exercise benefits all people, even those in their eighties and nineties. However, once the exercise is stopped, the benefits are quickly lost. Regular exercise is a lifelong process.

Exercise programs should include both aerobic and resistance exercises (see Chapter 7). The American College of Sports Medicine has recommended that all men older than age 40 years and all women older than age 50 years should have a medical exam before beginning a vigorous exercise program.

Alcohol Consumption

An estimated 4% to 8% of older adults abuse alcohol. Although many of these people have longstanding histories of alcohol abuse, one third do not start drinking excessively until they are in their sixties, seventies, and eighties. Most of the late-onset alcohol abusers have recently lost a spouse; another large segment are those who have not adjusted well to retirement and are bored and lonely.

Older adults drink smaller amounts of alcohol and drink more frequently than younger people addicted to alcohol. The 65-year-old is more sensitive to the effects of alcohol than the 45-year-old, and requires less alcohol to achieve the same effect. This is because of physiologic changes in metabolism and body composition that are part of aging. Increased organ dysfunction and the use of medications that accentuate the effects of alcohol are additional factors that increase the risks of alcohol abuse.

The problem tends to be hidden in the older adult because it is less socially disruptive and less likely to come to the attention of employers, police, and other authorities. Another reason is that many of the symptoms associated with al-

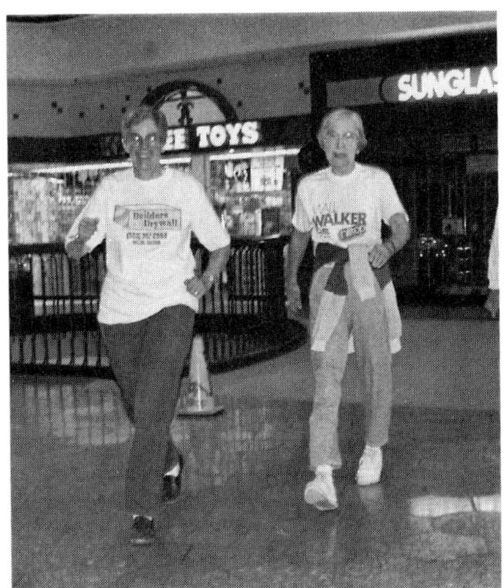

FIGURE 19-2

Regular exercise benefits all—even people in their eighties and nineties. *(Nursing: a human needs approach. Philadelphia: JB Lippincott, 1994:345.)*

coholism—depression, memory loss, confusion, and so forth—are confused with signs of aging. Display 19-4 gives symptoms associated with alcohol abuse in the older person. Early identification of alcohol abuse is important, especially for people who develop the disease late in life. These people tend to respond well to treatment programs.

NUTRITIONAL REQUIREMENTS OF THE OLDER ADULT

The RDAs developed by the National Academy of Sciences Food and Nutrition Board group all people older than age 50 years in one nutrient category. The main reason for this inappropriate situation is the lack of research regarding the nutritional requirements of older people. Although it is recognized that much change occurs between ages 50 and 90 years, data are lacking to specify at what age levels other groupings should be made.

It is difficult to develop nutritional standards for older adults because as people get older, there is a lessening relationship between age in years and physical age. Elderly people have widely differing capabilities and levels of functioning. There are frail 65-year-old people and there are 85-year-olds who play tennis. Also, the RDAs do not consider the effect of factors such as chronic disease states and drug therapy on nutritional status. Despite these uncertainties, the following discussion gives generally accepted recommendations.

ENERGY

The average energy intake given in the 1989 RDAs for people aged 51 years and older is 2300 kcal for the 77 kg (170 lb) male and 1900 kcal for the 65

DISPLAY 19-4 SIGNS ASSOCIATED WITH ALCOHOL ABUSE IN THE OLDER ADULT

MEDICAL PROBLEMS	SYMPTOMS; BEHAVIOR
Anemia	Confusion
Cardiac arrhythmias	Memory loss
Gastrointestinal bleeding	Dementia
Weight loss	Chronic fatigue
Malnutrition	Falls and accidents
Trauma	Sleep impairment
Hypertension	Seizures when alcohol has been withheld
Edema	Self-neglect
Osteoporosis	Concern by friends or relatives about alcohol abuse
Pain and numbness	Anxiety, panic
	Isolation and withdrawal

kg (143 lb) female. Although energy needs decline, the needs for other nutrients remain the same. Wise food choices are necessary if adequate amounts of nutrients are to be included in a smaller caloric framework. Increasing physical activity, if possible, permits increased intake of energy nutrients and other nutrients as well.

PROTEIN

The RDA for protein for adults aged 51 years and older is .8 g/kg of body weight—the same as for younger adults. Because of the possibility of less efficient use of protein as a person ages, 1 g/kg body weight is frequently recommended for older adults.

Elderly people recovering from surgery, burns, infections, and bone fractures require extra protein to meet increased metabolic and wound healing requirements. Clients with renal disease may need to reduce their protein intake.

FAT

There is no RDA for fat. Reducing fat intake is the best way to reduce calories with the least harmful effect on the nutritional value of the total diet. It is widely believed that a diet with 30% or less of calories as fat and no more than 10% as saturated fat may be just as important for older adults as for younger adults for preventing or improving chronic disease such as heart disease and cancer.

CARBOHYDRATE

There is no RDA for carbohydrate. Carbohydrate is the main source of calories in the American diet. The American Heart Association and the American Cancer Society have recommended that 55% to 60% of calories come from carbohydrate. Complex carbohydrates that are good sources of nutrients and fiber should be emphasized. Fiber-rich foods may play a role in the prevention of chronic diseases such as colon cancer and are useful in the management of diverticulosis and constipation, common chronic conditions in elderly people. When fiber is increased, adequate amounts of fluid must be taken.

FLUID

Total body fluid declines with age. The body of a newborn is 80% water, whereas that of an older adult is 60% or less. Loss of body fluid results in less thirst, mouth dryness, less efficient temperature regulation (more prone to hypothermia or hyperthermia), increased proneness to toxicity of water-soluble medications, and increased risk of dehydration as a result of diuretic therapy. Fluid intake should not be left to chance; it should be scheduled into the client's daily routine. The recommended intake of fluid is 30 ml/kg body weight.

Fluid and electrolyte imbalances caused by dehydration can result in confusion, nausea, and death. Factors that contribute to severe dehydration include renal disease, incontinence, mental confusion, immobility, multiple drug therapy, and severe nausea, vomiting, or diarrhea.

VITAMINS

Low intake of vitamins is likely. In addition, physical changes associated with aging may increase or decrease vitamin absorption. The adequacy of the RDAs for the older adult has been questioned by some authorities. The RDAs for vitamin D, B_6, and B_{12} are thought to be too low, whereas the RDA for vitamin A may be too high.

Vitamin D

The lack of exposure to sunlight, the reduced synthesis of vitamin D in the skin, and the impaired conversion of vitamin D to its active form in the kidney suggest that the need for vitamin D in the older adult may be higher than the RDA of 5 mcg (200 IU). A supplement of 10 mcg (400 IU) of vitamin D has been recommended for elderly people who are homebound or in nursing homes.

B Vitamins

The requirements for vitamin B_6 may be too low because of changes in absorption or metabolism with age. Some researchers have indicated that a significant number of people older than age 60 years may lack vitamin B_{12}. The lack of B_{12} is not due to an inadequate intake but to atrophic gastritis that develops in a significant number of people that age. Because of this condition, their stomachs do not produce enough hydrochloric acid for the body to use vitamin B_{12}. Without an acid environment, the enzyme that separates the vitamin from the protein to which it is attached in food does not function and vitamin B_{12} cannot be absorbed. Furthermore, a lack of acid in the stomach promotes an overgrowth of certain bacteria that use whatever amount of vitamin B_{12} is separated from the protein.

Symptoms of B_{12} deficiency are similar to those often thought to be the natural result of aging: tingling sensations, inability to coordinate muscular movements, weakened limbs and lack of balance, memory loss, mood changes, and disorientation. If these symptoms appear in an older adult and other causes have been ruled out, the health care provider should screen for a B_{12} deficiency.

Vitamin A

Tolerance for preformed vitamin A (not beta carotene) appears to decrease with age because of increased absorption of vitamin A and decreased uptake by the liver. It is suggested that more of the vitamin A requirement be obtained from carotene-containing fruits and vegetables.

MINERALS

Calcium

Calcium absorption decreases with age, possibly due to a reduction of hydrochloric acid in the stomach and low intake of vitamin D. There is some disagreement, however, regarding the appropriate recommended intake for the older adult. The RDA for calcium of 800 mg/day is considered by some experts to be inadequate. The National Academy of Sciences Committee on Diet and Health, Food and Nutrition Board, has stated that it is not well documented that there is any benefit to taking more than the RDA in an effort to prevent osteoporosis or hypertension and that the use of calcium supplements above 800 mg/day is unjustified. The National Institutes of Health have recommended 1000 mg of calcium for all adults and 1500 mg of calcium for postmenopausal women who are not taking estrogen.

Iron

The RDA for postmenopausal women and for men is 10 mg of iron. Iron deficiency anemia in men and postmenopausal women is most often caused by blood loss due to chronic disease or medication rather than inadequate intake.

Potassium

Potassium needs to be monitored carefully because it can be depleted easily. Many medications affect its absorption, use, and excretion.

Sodium

Blood levels of sodium are affected by medications and fluid balance. Severe restriction of sodium in people taking diuretics is not advised. Excessive sodium intake can contribute to hypertension and edema, however.

MEAL PLANNING FOR THE OLDER ADULT

The Pyramid Guide to Daily Food Choices (Table 14-1) is as excellent a guide for the older adult as it is for the younger adult. If the older adult consumes at least the minimum number of servings from each food group and eats a variety of foods, there is reasonable assurance that the diet is balanced and adequate. These minimums are three servings of vegetables; two servings of fruit; six servings of bread, cereals, and pasta; two servings of milk, yogurt, or cheese; and two servings of meat, poultry, fish, dried beans and peas, eggs, and nuts. Special emphasis may need to be placed on consuming the minimum recommended servings of fruits and vegetables. For people whose sense of taste and smell have diminished and who have lost interest in eating, suggestions for enhancing mealtimes are provided in Display 19-5.

COMMUNITY NUTRITION PROGRAMS

Many communities sponsor programs to improve the nutritional status of elderly people. Group meals and home-delivered meals are examples (see

DISPLAY 19-5 IDEAS FOR ENHANCING MEALTIME PLEASURE FOR THE OLDER ADULT

Eat the largest meal when your appetite is at its peak.
Plan ahead; cook several meals at one time and freeze foods for the days you do not feel like cooking.
Set the table attractively: use colorful cloths, placemats, and napkins. Add flowers, candles, and seasonal accents.
Play pleasant music on the radio or stereo system.
Combine foods in attractive color combinations. Colorful garnishes such as chopped fresh herbs or chopped colorful vegetables can brighten colorless foods such as potatoes, rice, pasta, fish, and chicken.
Add texture to soft foods by adding diced fresh fruit to pudding or frozen yogurt and chopped cooked vegetables to mashed potatoes, rice, and pasta.
Counteract diminished senses of taste and smell as follows:

- Season foods with herbs and spices (avoid salt or use sparingly).
- Use onion and garlic powders (if fresh onions and garlic cause stomach upset).
- Sprinkle foods lightly with grated cheese.
- Use flavor extracts such as almond or vanilla in milk drinks.
- Chew food well to obtain maximum flavor.

Use fruit juices, vegetable, and chicken broths thickened with cornstarch to moisten and flavor foods.
Use smaller food packages and single-serving products to avoid having leftovers. Even though the cost per serving is higher, it avoids having to eat the same food for several days until it is finished.
Invite a friend to share a meal.
Have a standing weekly date with a friend to eat out together.

Chapter 14). Home health or neighborhood aides are made available by certain community agencies to help disabled people with food shopping and preparation of meals. The aides are trained and supervised by nurses. Health care workers should be informed of the services available in their locality.

KEYS TO PRACTICAL APPLICATION

Emphasize the need for calcium throughout life. Remember that bone growth is occurring even into the early thirties.

Counteract negative views about current dietary recommendations to reduce fat. Remember that the diet as a whole, not all of the individual foods, should contain less than 30% of the calories from fat. Avoid labeling foods as "good" or "bad."

Remember that, except for energy, the nutritional needs of elderly people are just as high as, if not higher than, those of younger adults.

Be aware of the impact of emotional factors and drugs on the nutritional well-being of elderly people.

Become familiar with the checklist of the Nutrition Screening Initiative and the nine key risk factors that underlie the questions. Use this information to identify adults at nutritional risk.

Help your clients who have inadequate fluid intakes schedule fluid into their daily routine.

Become aware of the community nutrition programs that serve elderly people in your community.

Encourage physical exercise at all stages of life.

Become aware of the signs of alcoholism among elderly people.

KEY IDEAS

By the year 2030, 20% of the population will be older than age 65 years; the 85 years and older age group is the most rapidly growing age group.

Increased life expectancy makes health promotion and disease prevention more important than ever.

Physical growth may continue into a person's early twenties; accumulation of bone mass continues into the mid-twenties to the early thirties. The RDAs for calcium and vitamin D for the 19- to 24-year age group are the same as for adolescents. The RDA for calcium drops to 800 mg/day and vitamin D drops to 5 mcg/day (200 IU) after age 25 years.

Resting energy expenditure declines at a rate of 2% to 3% per decade in adulthood; activity level probably has a greater effect on total energy needs.

The RDA for the B vitamins thiamin, niacin, and riboflavin decrease as energy expenditure decreases.

Heightened concern about eating habits has not necessarily resulted in improved eating habits; people reducing fat are not maintaining the overall nutritional quality of their diets.

A balanced diet is often perceived as incompatible with eating enjoyment.

The total diet, not every food consumed, needs to be 30% fat or less.

Current diet recommendations advise consuming more plant foods, fewer animal foods, and two to three servings of milk or milk products, and using fats and added sugars sparingly. The Dietary Guidelines for Americans and the Food Guide Pyramid provide excellent detailed information for achieving recommendations.

Health needs change as individual ages; gender also affects health concerns.

Standards and methods of nutrition assessment are not necessarily reliable for older people because of age-related changes.

The best assessment may be comparing an older person against himself or herself over time through repeated measurements at regular intervals.

People at greatest nutritional risk have low values for serum cholesterol (below 160), albumin, hematocrit, hemoglobin, BMI, and triceps skinfold measurements.

Rapid weight loss can be a sign of serious undiagnosed illness.

The Nutrition Screening Initiative aims to identify older adults who are at nutritional risk; a checklist designed to make people aware of nine key risk factors is the centerpiece of the initiative.

Physical factors affecting the nutritional status of the older adult include loss of teeth, reduced sense of smell and taste, diminished secretion of saliva and other digestive juices and enzymes, decreased peristalsis, physical disabilities, and chronic diseases.

Emotions such as worry, loneliness, and fear greatly influence the nutritional well-being of older adults.

Physiologic changes due to aging adversely affect the digestion, absorption, metabolism, and excretion of nutrients.

Nutrition is a factor in both the development and treatment of a number of chronic diseases.

Mental disorders, especially depression, can seriously interfere with an adequate food intake. The role of nutrition in the development of mental disorders is less clear.

Medications can adversely affect nutritional status by altering food intake and the digestion, absorption, and use of nutrients.

Social factors such as living alone, changes in living arrangements, poverty, and reduced ability to shop and prepare food have a profound effect on nutritional status.

Eating alone puts people at risk of eating poorly and becoming isolated.

Group meals, home-delivered meals, and home health aide services are among the community programs available to promote the older adult's nutritional status.

People who keep physically active after age 45 years have a much better chance of reaching and living through old age in an independent and healthy way.

Some of the bodily changes associated with aging may be due, in part, to decreased physical activity.

Alcoholism tends to be hidden in the older adult because it is less socially disruptive and symptoms are mistaken for signs of aging.

As people get older, their age in years and their physical age differ.

Nutrition care of older people must be individualized.

Adults older than age 65 years are the single largest group at risk of malnutrition.

Because of a lack of research regarding nutritional requirements of the older adult, the RDAs group all people older than age 50 years into one nutrient category.

The adequacy of the RDAs for the older adult has been questioned for certain nutrients—the RDAs for calcium and vitamins D, B_6, and B_{12} may be too low and the RDA for preformed vitamin A may be too high.

Adequate fluid intake is important and should be carefully monitored; many factors contribute to high risk of dehydration in elderly people.

The Food Guide Pyramid is as excellent a meal planning guide for the older adult as it is for the younger adult; fluid intake should be scheduled into the daily routine.

KEYS TO LEARNING

STUDY–DISCUSSION QUESTIONS

1. In your opinion, what are the obstacles to following current recommendations regarding eating less fat, cholesterol, and sodium, and more fiber? How can each of these obstacles be overcome?
2. Discuss sex differences in health needs during adult life.
3. Discuss two physical factors that affect the older adult's nutritional status.
4. Discuss the psychological factors affecting elderly people's nutritional well-being.
5. The older people become, the more they differ from each other. Explain. What are some generalizations about the eating habits of the older adult that you have found to be false?
6. What feeding programs for older adults are available in your community? Investigate one of these programs and report your findings to the class. Include in your description the services provided, eligibility requirements, and acceptance by the recipients.

BIBLIOGRAPHY

BOOKS AND PAMPHLETS

Ausman LM, Russell RM. Nutrition in the elderly. In: Shils ME, Olson JA, Shike M. Eds. Modern nutrition in health and disease. 8th ed. Philadelphia: Lea and Febiger, 1994:770–780.

Dwyer JT. Screening older Americans' nutritional health: current practices and future possibilities. Washington, DC: Nutrition Screening Initiative, 1991.

Holloszy JO. Health benefits of exercise in middle-aged and older people. In: Kotsonis FN, Mackey MA. Eds. Nutrition in the 90's: current controversies and analysis. Vol. 2. New York: Marcel Dekker, 1994:81.

National Academy of Sciences, National Research Council, Food and Nutrition Board, Committee on Diet and Health. Diet and health: implications for reducing chronic disease risk (executive summary). Washington, DC: National Academy Press, 1989.

National Academy of Sciences, National Research Council, Food and Nutrition Board. Recommended dietary allowances. 10th ed. Washington, DC: National Academy Press, 1989.

US Dept of Health and Human Services, Public Health Service. Prevention '91—'92, federal programs and progress. Washington, DC: US Government Printing Office, 1992.

PERIODICALS

Ahmed FE. Effect of nutrition on health of the elderly. J Am Diet Assoc 1992;92:1102.

Bass KM, Newschatter CJ, Klag MJ, et al. Plasma lipoprotein as predictors of cardiovascular death in women. Arch Intern Med 1993;153:2209.

Denke MA, Sempos CT, Grundy SM. Excess body weight: an unrecognized contributor to dyslipidemia in white American women. Arch Intern Med 1994;154:401.

Hankin JH. Role of nutrition in women's health: diet and breast cancer. J Am Diet Assoc 1993;93:994.

Kicklighter JR. Characteristics of older adult learners: a guide for dietetics practitioners. J Am Diet Assoc 1991;91:1418.

Kinsella KG. Changes in life expectancy. Am J Clin Nutr 1992;55:1196S.

Kris-Etherton PM, Krummel D. Role of nutrition in the prevention and treatment of coronary heart disease in women. J Am Diet Assoc 1993;93:987.

Morley JE, Solomon DH. Major issues in geriatrics over the last five years. J Am Geriatr Soc 1994;42:218.

Rosenberg IH, Miller JW. Nutritional factors in physical and cognitive functions of elderly people. Am J Clin Nutr 1992;55:1237S.

Russell RM, Suter PM. Vitamin requirements of elderly people: an update. Am J Clin Nutr 1993;58:1005.

St. Jeor, ST. The role of weight management in the health of women. J Am Diet Assoc 1993;93:1007.

Walker D, Beauchene RE. The relationship of loneliness, social isolation, and physical health to dietary adequacy of independently living elderly. J Am Diet Assoc 1991;91:300.

Wardlaw GM. Putting osteoporosis in perspective. J Am Diet Assoc 1993;93:1000.

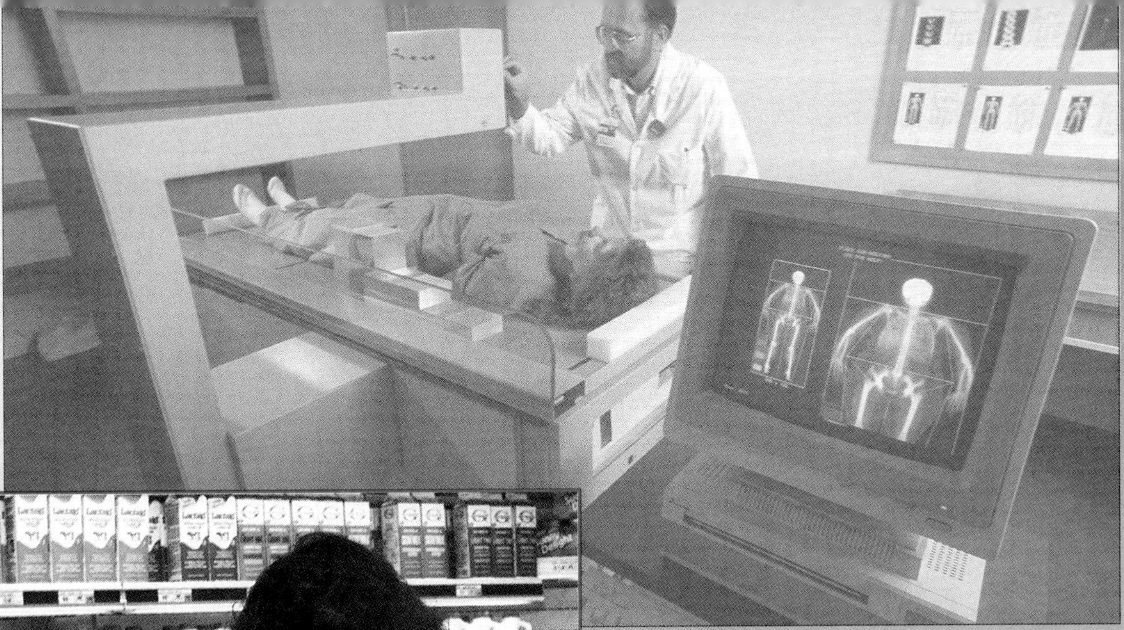

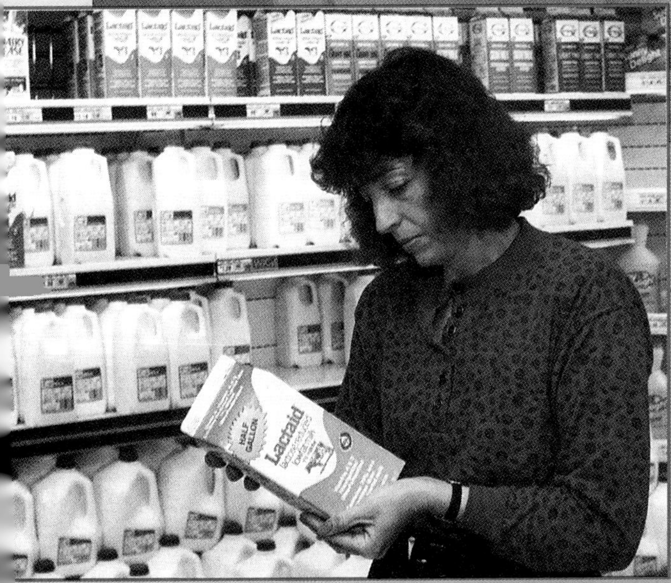

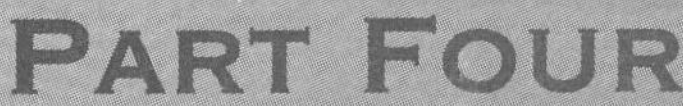

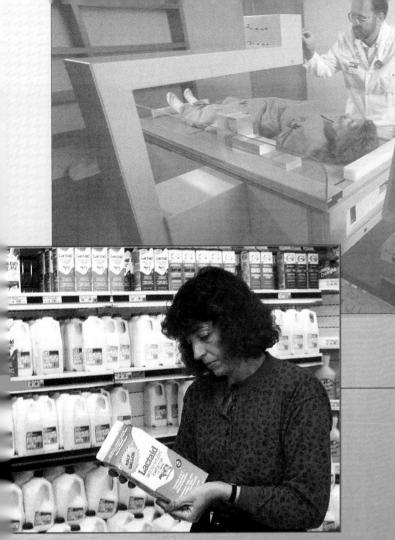

PART FOUR

Nutrition Therapy in Illness

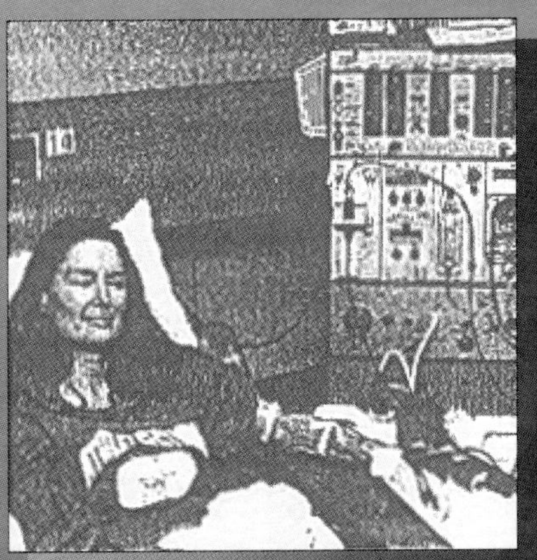

CHAPTER

20

Providing Nutrition Care and Counseling

KEY TERMS

compliance acting in accordance with the advice of health care providers

document to make a written record of important events, activities, and impressions as they occur in the course of providing health care

empowered to feel in control of one's life; having social, psychological, intellectual, and spiritual resources to solve one's problems and achieve goals

evaluation measuring an outcome against an objective or standard

goal aim or end result desired; the change necessary to solve a nutritional problem

implementation putting into practice; steps taken to achieve an objective

medical nutrition therapy nutrition therapy for conditions or diseases that respond to nutrition intervention; it includes assessment of nutritional status and also nutrition therapy, which involves diet modification and counseling or the use of specialized nutrition therapies (using medical foods, tube feedings, and nutrients delivered intravenously)

nutrition care plan meeting nutritional needs of an individual by using the scientific problem-solving approach, which comprises assessment, planning, implementation, and evaluation

objective steps a person must accomplish to meet a goal

prioritize to place in descending order of need; to determine what needs to be done first, second, and so forth

OBJECTIVES

After completing this chapter, the student will be able to:

1. Give and describe each of the four components of the nutrition care process.
2. Explain the client's role in the "planning" component of the nutrition care plan. Explain the following statement: "The client's involvement in the goal-setting process is crucial to the success of nutrition care."
3. Give four physical conditions requiring nutrition intervention.
4. Explain the four basic ways in which diet or meal planning can be changed to accommodate conditions that require nutrition therapy.
5. Demonstrate interviewing techniques that promote the exchange of information between the client and health care worker.
6. Explain what is meant by a *compliant client* and an *empowered client*. Discuss the role of health care providers in helping clients become empowered.

In the previous chapters, we followed a study sequence that began with a look at what is going on in the 1990s that affects how and what we eat and the changes occurring in the health care field. Next, we considered why a nutritionally adequate diet is important and what steps the health care worker must take to determine if an individual is poorly nourished. In addition to the physiologic aspects of nutrition, we also discussed how food affects us from a psychological and emotional standpoint. Our study has progressed to the nutrients and their roles in maintaining good health and to the selection of foods that will meet nutritional needs throughout the life cycle. In Part Four, we consider the role of nutrition intervention in illness, currently referred to as *medical nutrition therapy* (see the section Key Terms.)

Basic food service procedures and techniques of nutrition care in the clinical setting are given in Chapter 3.

PROBLEM SOLVING: THE NUTRITION CARE PROCESS

The problem-solving approach is applied to nutrition care just as to other aspects of health care. It consists of four elements: (1) assessment and identification of the client's needs and problems; (2) planning, in which a plan is developed for correcting these problems; (3) implementation, in which care is provided; and (4) evaluation, in which progress toward correcting the problem is determined.

ASSESSMENT AND PROBLEM IDENTIFICATION

The first step in providing nutrition care is to collect data that has nutritional implications so that the health care worker can identify the client's nutrition problems. These data include the client's body measurements, medical history, diet history, medications, physical examination, laboratory tests, and sociocultural history. In Chapter 2, the tools and procedures used to evaluate an individual's health status were discussed. Sources used to obtain this information include the client's chart, laboratory reports, consultation with other members of the health team, and interviews with the client and the family.

Once the significant data are collected, the health care worker carefully studies the information with respect to nutrient deficiencies or excesses, underlying disease, eating impediments, drug–nutrient interactions, and personal needs and goals. The health worker identifies and prioritizes any problems or needs.

At this point, the nurse makes a *nursing diagnosis,* a statement of a condition that can be treated legally and independently by nurses. Three specific nursing diagnoses related to nutrition have been offered by Carpenito: Nutrition, Altered: Less than Body Requirements; Nutrition, Altered: More than Body Requirements; Nutrition, Altered: Potential for More than Body Requirements. Nutrition intervention is implicated in many other nursing diagnoses such as those relating to effective breastfeeding, impaired swallowing, altered growth, and constipation.

PLANNING

The next step is to formulate a plan for correcting or treating each of the identified problems or needs. The objectives, specific activities, priorities, and means for evaluating progress are established. The establishment of goals and strategy used to be an authoritarian process—the health care team decided what the client needed. Now, however, the client is considered an essential member of the team and has the opportunity to contribute to the planning process. It ideally is a client-oriented process in which the health professional guides the client in goal setting. The client's involvement in the goal-setting process is crucial to the success of nutrition care. Without the client's cooperation, little can be accomplished. In the case of the client who is confused or otherwise unable to communicate, the health care provider must involve family members or significant others in the planning process. The health care professional guides the client in setting his or her own goals and objectives that reflect what the client wants and what the client is willing to do to achieve the desired results.

The goals and objectives should be realistic and should describe measurable results that are acceptable to both the client and the health professional. Goals express the desired results or outcomes in general terms. The goals in the nutrition care plan are aimed at resolving or treating the problems identified in the assessment. Objectives are specific statements that identify what needs to be done to achieve the goals (resolve identified problems). They are written in behavioral form, stating what the client will achieve and how it will be done. For example: "To resolve the problems of late afternoon hypoglycemia, the client (with insulin–dependent diabetes mellitus [type I]) will take a snack consisting of 30 g of carbohydrate at approximately 3 PM daily."

The nutrition care plan is a written statement that outlines specific activities to meet the goals and objectives (Display 20-1). Staff members responsible for carrying out each activity are designated. The plan is coordinated with other components of the client's overall care plan and usually is developed with the guidance of a nutrition specialist (i.e., a dietitian or dietary consultant). The plan may be shared among all members of the health team or may be intended for a particular group, such as the nursing staff or dietary staff.

IMPLEMENTATION

The next step is to put the plan into action. Two functions are involved. The first is to provide an adequate normal or modified diet or other form of nutritional support for a client in a hospital or other

DISPLAY 20-1 NURSING HOME NUTRITION CARE PLAN

Nutrition problem: Client is a 72-year-old woman with rheumatoid arthritis; she is about 25 lb under normal weight because of inadequate caloric intake.

Nutrition goal: Gradual weight gain until desirable weight is attained.

Objective: Weight gain of 4 lb in 1 mo by the addition of 500 kcal/day to meals and snacks.

ACTION	RESPONSIBLE STAFF
Obtain diet history. List favorite foods in dietary client card file.	Food service supervisor
Post caloric values for favorite foods and additional food supplements in kitchen and nursing station.	Consultant dietitian
Determine time of day when client is most hungry and alert and inform charge nurse.	Nursing assistant
Add sufficient food to meals to increase intake by 200 kcal/day.	Food service supervisor
See that foods for between-meal feedings are delivered to floor kitchen.	Food service supervisor
Prepare client for mealtime and transport client to solarium in wheelchair so that he or she may have lunch and support in company of other clients; record food intake.	Nursing assistant
Select foods to be offered to client at three between-meal feedings totaling 300 calories.	Charge nurse
Weigh client at same time on same day of each week.	Nursing assistant

health care facility. The second is to provide nutrition education and counseling and referral to nutrition and food resources in the community, if necessary. In a health care facility, both components may be involved, whereas in the outpatient setting, only the educational and counseling component is needed.

PROVIDING AN ADEQUATE, NORMAL DIET

In the healthy adult, *catabolism* (breakdown) and *anabolism* (building) of body tissue are balanced; in the sick person, especially one who is confined to bed, catabolism is greater than anabolism. The sick person thus has a greater-than-normal need for nutrients that promote tissue building: proteins, vitamins, and minerals. Inactivity or immobilization for a long period causes alterations in the body functions of digestion, metabolism, and elimination. These alterations influence nutritional requirements.

When achieving an adequate food intake is a problem, specific measures need to be taken. For example, a client who is anorectic because he or she is depressed may not be consuming adequate quantities of food. The objectives of nutrition care for this client are to increase the quality of the diet and to create an environment that promotes appetite. Bulky, low-calorie foods such as salads, soups, and tea may be reduced, and low-volume, high-calorie foods such as meats, starches, and fortified milk beverages may be emphasized. Small, frequent meals may be more appealing to the client than three large meals a day. Arranging for the client to eat with other people also may be listed in the care plan.

PROVIDING MEDICAL NUTRITION THERAPY

Medical treatment may require changes in the normal diet. Changes in the diet are made necessary by the following conditions:

- caloric imbalance resulting in overweight or underweight
- poor or abnormal use of nutrients (e.g., poor use of carbohydrates in diabetes mellitus; retention of sodium in congestive heart failure)
- abnormalities in digestion of food or absorption of nutrients, which occur in diseases of the gastrointestinal tract such as celiac disease, colitis, and lactose intolerance
- nutritional deficiencies, including iron deficiency anemia, and severe malnutrition due to emotional disturbances
- the requirement for rest for the body or an organ (e.g., in gallbladder disease, rest may be afforded the organ by a restriction of fat; in the acute phase of coronary heart disease, a liquid diet may be prescribed to conserve the client's strength)
- abnormal laboratory findings indicating an increased risk of developing health problems, such as abnormal serum cholesterol and triglyceride levels.

The normal diet is the basis of most modified diets. Despite the seemingly large number of diets, changes are limited to the following categories:

Texture—The consistency and fiber content may be altered; liquid diets, soft diets, and high-fiber diets are examples of this type of modification.

Amount of nutrients—Certain nutrients may be increased or decreased in amount. A client who suffers from renal failure may require a diet restricted in protein, whereas one recovering from extensive burns requires greatly increased amounts of protein.

Frequency of meals—The usual three meals a day may be replaced by six small meals to reduce stress to the body.

Selection of foods—Products normally included in the diet may be eliminated; for example, wheat products are eliminated for clients who are allergic to wheat.

Every effort is made to adjust the diet to the client's needs. The diet is planned to be as similar as possible to the customary family diet, with as wide a range of choices as possible. Of course, the client's condition may require a drastically different diet from what he or she is used to, and it is up to the health care team to help the client accept the recommended changes.

PROVIDING NUTRITION EDUCATION AND SELF-MANAGEMENT TRAINING

Education is an essential part of health care. Clients want to know, and have a right to know, how they can achieve and maintain good health. Increasingly, health care personnel are involved in managing chronic illness. Clients must manage these conditions on a day-to-day basis for the remainder of their lives. Clients require not only knowledge, but also skills and a self-awareness that enables them to find ways to remain motivated. Physical, emotional, and spiritual influences must be considered.

People do not learn by memorizing. Acquisition of information must be accompanied by a change in attitude and behavior. A person who has learned something about nutrition demonstrates this knowledge with a change in attitude toward food, a change in eating pattern, and an increased understanding of how diet influences health. The following are important points to remember:

1. Treat your clients as individuals with personal eating habits, knowledge about nutrition, and the ability to learn. Be a good listener so you can learn about their eating habits. Involve clients in the educational process. Clients should understand their problems and what they can do to correct them. Without a client's active participation, your efforts will be fruitless.
2. Help your clients see how good nutrition can help them meet their personal goals. These goals may not necessarily be health related, especially for a young person, who may be more interested in sports activities or in peer group acceptance.
3. Build on strengths of the client's eating habits rather than emphasize shortcomings. Set realistic goals. Offer suggestions for improving nutritional well-being or following a modified diet that are within the client's reach.
4. Have your client demonstrate to you his or her acquisition of the skills needed to accomplish the set objectives. The client might write menus, choose foods in accordance with a specific meal plan, use a blood glucose meter correctly, and identify foods on a restaurant menu that are appropriate for a lowfat diet.
5. Give careful attention to timing. Periods of stress may not be the best time for changing long-standing eating habits. The client may be too upset to concentrate or to understand what is being taught. Return visits or referral to a community agency after discharge from the hospital may be necessary.
6. Avoid teaching too much at one time. Try to concentrate on one or two points during a 15- to 30-minute period rather than trying to cover the entire topic in 1 hour.
7. Help clients see the progress they are making no matter how little it may be.

Informal Teaching

There are many opportunities for informal teaching, which usually is carried out on the spot as the need arises. For example, a client may have questions regarding the food served on his or her tray or may need help making correct choices from a selective menu. You can encourage discussion by pointing out, for example, which foods on the tray are of particular importance to the client's health.

You are not expected to know all the answers about nutrition. When confronted with a question you cannot answer, consult the nurse in charge or the dietitian.

Formal Teaching

Diet counseling and group instruction are examples of formal teaching situations.

Diet Counseling. Diet counseling is the process of helping a client develop the ability to manage his or her own nutrition care. It is based on the development of a trusting relationship between the client and the counselor. The counselor provides information, encouragement, and support as the client gradually makes changes in eating behavior. Counseling that involves behavioral change should be conducted by psychologists, nurses, and dietitians who have been trained in behavior change skills.

Group Instruction. In hospitals and clinics and in group medical practice, it often is possible to bring together groups of people with common needs. Besides receiving information and guidance from the nutrition instructor, the members can help each other face common problems. The health care worker assists by providing instruction, giving demonstrations, and preparing visual aids.

EVALUATION

Evaluation is measurement of the client's progress. Has the client gained or lost the appropriate amount of weight? If the client has diabetes, is the blood glucose level under control? If the client is hypertensive, has a sodium-controlled diet caused a reduction in blood pressure? Above all, is the client learning to be in control of his or her own nutritional status?

If progress has not been made, determine the cause and revise the care plan. The client's needs may change, and a new plan may be required. In any case, once you have determined the reason for failure, develop a new plan aimed at correcting the problem.

COMMUNICATION TOOLS THAT PROMOTE NUTRITION CARE

CLEAR, PRECISE DIET ORDERS AND TERMINOLOGY

The diet order is an important communication tool. It usually is written by the physician, but it may be written by dietitians, nurse practitioners, or clinical nurses working closely with physicians. The diet ordered may be either normal or modified.

The term *therapeutic* or *modified* is preferred in reference to diets that deviate from normal, and the description of the diet should be specific and accurate. *Low-calorie diet* could refer to a 1200 kcal/day diet or to a 1700 kcal/day diet; *low-sodium diet* could apply to severe restriction (500 mg/day of sodium) or to moderate restriction (1500 mg to 2000 mg/day of sodium). The level of control should be specified in the diet, e.g. 2000 mg/d sodium diet.

MEDICAL RECORD

All elements of the client's treatment, including nutrition care, are recorded in the medical record. The chart is a communication tool for all members of the health care team—physician, nurse, dietitian, and others. These professionals write progress notes on the client's chart describing the care being given, the progress being made toward solving the client's problems, and follow-up plans. Nutrition education activities also are documented in the client's medical record (see Chapter 3).

GOOD INTERVIEWING TECHNIQUES

An interview is a planned conversation aimed at obtaining specific information and ideas from a client. It is a component of the assessment phase of care. Its purpose is to help determine the client's nutritional needs or to determine what progress is being made toward goals. The interview may be formal or informal. Taking a diet history is an example of a formal interview. Display 20-2 gives examples of the type of information that may be obtained in a diet history and how the questionnaire may be adapted for clients of different ages. An informal interview is a meaningful conversation occurring in a hospital or clinical setting or on the telephone in which the health worker tries to learn how the client is getting along, what his or her needs are, and what progress is being made.

An exchange of information is promoted in an atmosphere of mutual trust and respect (Fig. 20-1). The health care worker's attitude is important in establishing such an atmosphere. Successful interviewers display interest, friendliness, kindness, and open-mindedness. They accept the information the client provides without judgment, recognizing that the client's behavior has meaning and purpose for him or her.

Eating habits are personal because they reflect ethnic background, family customs, philosophy, economics, and other aspects of a person's lifestyle. Health care workers who are aware of the factors

DISPLAY 20-2 DIET HISTORY QUESTIONNAIRES

QUESTIONNAIRE I. ADULT (DIRECTED TO CLIENT OR PRIMARY CARE-GIVER)

BACKGROUND INFORMATION

Name, age, sex, family and occupational roles, general health status, dietary restrictions (past or present)

FOOD PURCHASE AND PREPARATION

Who purchases and prepares food?
What factors influence kinds of foods purchased?
Is budgeting a matter of concern when buying food?
Where is food purchased?
How often do you shop?
What facilities are available for food storage and preparation?
What foods are served most frequently?
Do you participate in community food programs?

RELATIONSHIP OF FOOD TO LIFESTYLE

Food likes and dislikes
Favorite foods when growing up
Special family foods for celebrations
Atmosphere at mealtime
Foods your body needs
Food supplements (vitamins, minerals)
Sources of information about nutrition

QUESTIONNAIRE II. INFANT/TODDLER (DIRECTED TO PARENTS OR PRIMARY CARE-GIVERS)

Who feeds? What foods does an infant need?
Breastfeeding or formula feeding: approximate amount and frequency?
If breastfeeding: pattern and duration of feeding?
If formula: type? Iron-fortified? Preparation?
Supplemental feedings: fluids, solids? Preparation? How liked?
Weaning? Teething? Self-feeding?

QUESTIONNAIRE III. YOUNG CHILD (DIRECTED TO PARENTS OR PRIMARY CARE-GIVER)

What foods does your child need? When does he or she eat?
Appetite? Likes, dislikes? Food jags?
Frequency of snacking? Types?
Vitamin and mineral supplements?
Method of rewarding and punishing child?
With whom does child eat?
Arrangements for eating away from home (school)?

QUESTIONNAIRE IV. ADOLESCENT (DIRECTED TO ADOLESCENT)

What is nutritious? Foods body needs?
Where are meals eaten? When is food eaten?
How much snacking?
How does eating affect appearance?
What do you do when you're unhappy or upset?
Does anyone comment about your eating habits?

QUESTIONNAIRE V. ELDERLY PERSON (DIRECTED TO CLIENT OR PRIMARY CARE-GIVER)

Amount of income budgeted for food?
Where client lives? Where he or she eats?
With whom he or she eats?
Who prepares meals? Purchases food?
Dentures or own teeth? Effect on eating?
Recent changes in food habits?
How does food taste?
Likes, dislikes?
Use of alcohol?
Dietary restrictions?
Amount of normal activity?

(Suitor CW, Hunter MF. Nutrition: Principles and application in health promotion. Philadelphia: JB Lippincott, 1984:227)

that have influenced their own eating habits will be more understanding of other people's eating habits (see Chapter 2).

Straightforward techniques may encourage the client to talk freely. Open-ended questions require the client to respond clearly; for example, When do you eat or drink for the first time in the day? In contrast, asking, Do you eat breakfast? requires only a *yes* or *no* answer. Direct questions—How? What? Why? How much?—require responses that provide the information needed to assess the client's eating habits. The interviewer must avoid questions that suggest answers, such as, You eat vegetables, don't you?

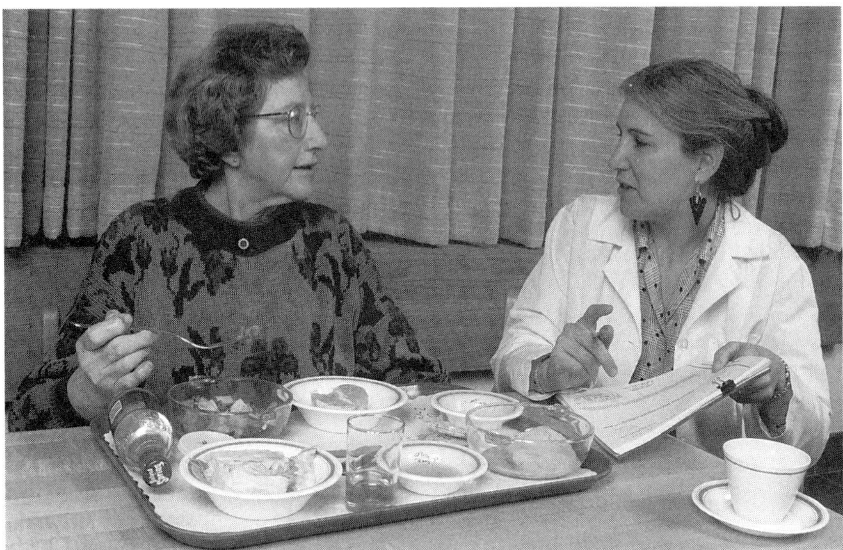

FIGURE 20-1

An exchange of information is promoted in an atmosphere of mutual trust and respect. *(Courtesy of the US Dept of Agriculture.)*

To be useful, the information obtained must be specific: What kind of bread? How much margarine? What is added to vegetables in cooking? What method do you use for cooking chicken? Fish?

The health care worker should not try to teach while conducting an interview. It is best not to comment either positively or negatively about the information the client provides. If the interviewer lectures the client or indicates that he or she disapproves of what the client is saying, the client may hesitate to answer subsequent questions.

COMPLIANCE VERSUS EMPOWERMENT

Until recently, the success of health counseling was considered to be dependent on the degree of compliance—whether or not the client followed the advice and directions dictated by health care professionals. The "good client" was the compliant client. The *American College Dictionary* defines *compliance* as "an act of yielding to others; base subservience." In effect, clients have been advised to follow lifestyles not of their choosing. It is no wonder that they experience a loss of power and a loss of positive quality of life.

An alternative approach, *empowerment,* has been offered in recent years. It is a holistic, client-centered approach to the management of chronic illness. Anderson and Feste in their manual *Empowerment: Facilitating a Path to Personal Self-Care* gave the following basic concepts in the empowerment philosophy:

- Humans have physical, intellectual, emotional, social, and spiritual components to their lives that interact in a holistic and dynamic fashion.
- To be healthy, humans must be able to actualize the physical, intellectual, emotional, social, and spiritual components of their lives.
- Humans have the inherent right and responsibility to make the major decisions regarding the conduct of their own lives.

Empowered people feel that they are in control of their lives. They have learned to use their social, psychological, intellectual, and spiritual resources to make decisions, achieve goals, and maintain an overall sense of well-being in the presence of a chronic health condition. Anderson and Feste presented Albert Schweitzer, noted physician and humanitarian, as one who believed strongly in the healing power within each client. Schweitzer believed that health professionals should awaken this healing power within their clients.

The purpose of the empowerment approach is to empower people to take responsibility for their self-care (including the care of their illness) and live a fulfilling life. To accomplish these goals, the individual must become self-aware of his or her values, needs, and goals in addition to specific knowledge of the disease and its management. Health care personnel require appropriate attitudes, knowledge and skills to incorporate the empowerment approach in chronic disease management and client education. With the increasing older population and the increasing need to manage chronic disease, alternative and nontraditional approaches to nutrition counseling and other types of health counseling undoubtedly will receive greater emphasis.

KEYS TO PRACTICAL APPLICATION

Become informed of the nutrition care plan for each of your clients. Learn how you can support the objectives.

Take advantage of opportunities to find out how your clients are getting along as far as nutrition is concerned. Are they eating well? If not, why not? Do they foresee any problems when they go home from the hospital?

When gathering information, learn to ask questions that require more than a *yes* or *no* answer. Questions about how, what, why, where, and who encourage clients to give information.

Avoid criticizing or showing disapproval of the information your clients provide. Recognize that their eating behavior has meaning and purpose for them. Emphasize the good things they are doing.

When the client is not meeting goals, seek to learn the reasons and do what you can to remove the obstacles or initiate the development of new objectives.

Learn as much as you can about the techniques of empowerment. Strive to awaken the healing power within your clients.

KEY IDEAS

Providing good nutrition care involves four basic elements: identifying the client's problems, developing a plan for correcting the problems, providing care as planned, and evaluating the results.

The nutrition care plan is a written statement that describes the steps to be taken to meet the goals of nutrition care. All team members, including the client, should be involved in planning.

The client's involvement in goal setting is crucial to the success of nutrition care.

Goals should be realistic and objectives should describe results that can be measured.

Nutrition care involves providing an adequate normal or modified diet for clients in a health care facility and providing nutrition education and counseling so that clients can manage their own nutritional needs.

All diets, whether normal or modified, contribute to the individual's health care.

Catabolic body processes are increased in the ill person, especially one confined to bed; greater than normal amounts of nutrients that promote tissue building—protein, vitamins, minerals, and adequate caloric intake—are required. The hospital diet usually exceeds recommended allowances of these nutrients.

Modified diets are those that are changed from normal because of one or more of the following conditions: caloric imbalance, poor use of nutrients by cells or organs, abnormal digestion or absorption, nutritional deficiency or excess, the need to rest an organ or conserve body strength, and abnormal laboratory findings indicating increased risk of developing chronic disease.

The normal diet forms the basis of most modified diets. Changes may be made in texture, amounts of certain nutrients, frequency of meals, and exclusion of substances normally found in the diet.

The modified diet should be as similar as possible to the usual diet of the client and his or her family, providing as wide a range of food choices as possible.

Good communication among members of the health care team is essential to good nutrition care. Accurate diet orders and the documentation of nutrition care on the client's medical record are tools that promote good communication.

Clients have a right to know how to manage their own nutrition care. Education is an essential part of health care.

Clients with chronic conditions need knowledge, skills, and self-awareness to manage their conditions on a day-to-day basis and remain motivated.

Learning is not simply the acquisition of facts; a change in attitude and behavior also must be accomplished.

Good listening skills help in determining a client's individual needs.

Success depends on the willingness of the client to accept change. Clients must be included in setting goals and in other aspects of the educational process.

Behavior change is difficult, especially when it involves long-standing eating habits. What appear to be small changes in behavior may represent a great accomplishment.

Good interviewing techniques are important skills for the health care worker; the interviewer's attitude should be nonjudgmental.

Many opportunities arise while providing health care to strengthen, reinforce, and support nutrition teaching the client has already received.

Nutrition counseling is the total process of helping clients manage their own nutrition care. Group instruction, another type of formal teaching, enables group members to help each other.

Self-awareness and choice are the core concepts in the empowerment process, which aims to empower clients to take responsibility for their self-care and live a fulfilling life.

KEYS TO LEARNING

STUDY–DISCUSSION QUESTIONS

1. With the help of your instructor, select a client who is on a modified diet. How would you evaluate the client's progress? Are the goals of nutrition care being met? Observe the client's reaction to the food served him or her. If the client is considered to have a feeding problem, try to determine the reason behind the behavior. Discuss your findings with the class. What are some possible solutions to this problem?
2. In what ways can the normal diet be changed to treat disease? Give a medical condition or disease state in which each of the modifications might be used. For example, in congestive heart failure, a sodium-restricted diet (nutrient decrease) is likely to be prescribed.
3. Why is it so important to involve the client in the educational process, including the setting of goals?
4. Using the diet history form used in your hospital, role-play a formal interview with a classmate. Have the class evaluate the interview.

What techniques encourage the client to provide information? What hinders the exchange of information?

5. Imagine that you have been assigned to assist an older adult male in improving the nutritional quality of his diet. He is a 68-year-old retired police officer who is living on instant oatmeal, hamburgers, chips, pretzels, cookies, iced tea, and coffee with nondairy creamer. He eats well-balanced meals on weekends when he visits his daughter and her family.

Prepare an outline for your counseling session using the following format:

OBJECTIVES	CONTENT	TEACHING AIDS (VISUAL, HANDOUTS, ETC.)	EVALUATION

BIBLIOGRAPHY

BOOKS AND PAMPHLETS

Anderson RM, Feste CC. Empowerment: facilitating a path to personal self-care. Elkhart, IN: Miles, Diagnostics Division, 1991.

Carpenito LJ. Nursing diagnosis: application to clinical practice. Philadelphia: JB Lippincott, 1993.

PERIODICALS

Anderson RM, Funnell MM, Barr PA, et al. Learning to empower patients: results of professional education for diabetes educators. Diabetes Care 1991;14:584.

Feste C. A practical look at patient empowerment. Diabetes Care 1992;15:922.

Foltz MB, Schiller MR, Ryan AS. Nutrition screening and assessment: current practices and dietitians' leadership roles. J Am Diet Assoc 1993;93:1385.

Johnson CC, Nicklas TA, Arbeit ML, et al. Behavioral counseling and contracting as methods for promoting cardiovascular health in families. J Am Diet Assoc 1992;92:479.

McGinn N. Patient-centered care: opportunities for health care professionals to work together. Dietetic Currents 1993;20:3:1.

Roach RR, Pichert JW, Stetson BA, et al. Improving dietitians' teaching skills. J Am Diet Assoc 1992;92:1466.

Warpeha A, Harris J. Combining traditional and non-traditional approaches to nutrition counseling. J Am Diet Assoc 1993;93:797.

CHAPTER

21

Nutrition Care of the Ill Older Adult

KEY TERMS

achlorhydria absence of free hydrochloric acid in the stomach
atrophy reduction in size of an organ or cell
autoimmune disease disease in which the body's immune system produces antibodies against normal parts of the body
cachexia weakness and emaciation caused by serious disease
clinical relating to direct treatment and care of clients
decubitus ulcers bedsores
involuntary occurring without conscious control
myasthenia gravis disease characterized by muscle weakness
pallor paleness, especially of the skin and mucous membranes
pedal edema swelling of the ankles and feet
Sjögren's syndrome chronic autoimmune disorder that affects a number of body systems; reduced secretions of the exocrine glands, including those that produce saliva, are one symptom of this disease

OBJECTIVES

After completing this chapter, the student will be able to:

1. Explain how each of the following conditions frequently encountered in ill older adults relate to nutritional status: infection, decubitus ulcer, psychological disorders, multiple medications, and dehydration.
2. Give the possible causes and explain the treatment for each of the following: protein-calorie malnutrition, osteoporosis, and iron deficiency anemia in the older adult.
3. Give four causes of constipation in *each* of the following categories: causes due to physical conditions and disorders, causes due to medication, and causes due to lifestyle factors. Give five lifestyle changes that can promote healthy bowel function.
4. Explain and give three methods of treating each of the following feeding problems: changes in sensations of taste and smell, xerostomia, and dysphagia.
5. Discuss nutrition care and medical nutrition therapy of the older adult with respect to the concept of treating the whole person.

The increase in the older population has important implications for the health care worker. The health professions as a whole will eventually spend an estimated three fourths of their time with elderly people. It is imperative, therefore, that we learn all we can about the special needs of this population and acquire the knowledge and develop the attitudes and skills to meet these needs.

The role of nutrition in maintaining health, preventing disease, facilitating recovery from illness, and improving the elderly person's quality of life is increasingly recognized. The factors that affect nutritional status of older adults and the nutrition recommendations are discussed in Chapter 19. The focus in this chapter is the nutrition care of the ill older adult.

COMMON DISEASES AND DISORDERS THAT AFFECT NUTRITION

INFECTION

Infections of various kinds afflict a high percentage of older clients, including infections of the urinary, gastrointestinal, or respiratory tracts or skin or eye infections. A vicious cycle develops between malnutrition and infection—the infection causes weight loss, physical weakness, and loss of appetite that, in turn, makes it difficult for the older person to voluntarily eat enough food to replace energy and protein stores. Consequently, the individual is more prone to a new infection.

Depressed immunity with advanced age is a factor in the prevalence of infection. Increased intake of zinc, vitamin C, protein, and energy can improve immune function.

DECUBITUS ULCERS

Decubitus ulcers, or *pressure sores,* tend to develop in clients confined to bed or a wheelchair. Although pressure sores do not develop if pressure is relieved, nutritional factors are important in preventing them. In a study of 200 nursing home clients, those who developed pressure sores had lower intakes of calories, protein, iron, copper, and thiamin than those who did not. Low serum albumin levels are most closely associated with the development of pressure sores.

Healing requires not only treating the wound itself but also raising the client's nutritional status to a level that promotes tissue growth and repair. To promote healing of decubitus ulcers, a high-calorie diet with adequate amounts of protein, vitamin C, zinc, and other nutrients is needed. Both the total calories and the protein intake must be adequate for the diet to be effective. In addition, the use of multivitamin/mineral supplements is recommended.

PSYCHOLOGICAL DISORDERS

Dementia and depression, common psychological disorders among older adults, strongly influence nutritional status. A high percentage of clients with dementia are malnourished. In dementia, various symptoms affect food intake including a lack of interest in eating, memory loss, impaired judgment, psychosis, and agitation. People with dementia such as Alzheimer's disease have eating behavior that ranges from refusal to eat to the hoarding of food. The energy requirements of people who walk, pace, or wander may be quite high. As many as 50% suffer from protein and energy deficits. Reduced food intake frequently accompanies depression; in some cases, a client may refuse to eat, using food to express a subconscious death wish. Food intake usually increases with the treatment of depression.

ADVERSE DRUG–NUTRIENT INTERACTIONS

Many older adults are taking as many as eight or more medications. This high drug use is the result of multiple medical problems and treatment by more than one health care provider.

The older adult is more prone to adverse drug–nutrient interactions than younger people. As serum albumin declines with age, drugs that bind serum proteins have less protein to bind to, leading to the release of more free drug into the circulation and a subsequent increase in the risk of adverse reactions. Reduced kidney function causes poor drug excretion. As a result, the half-life of certain drugs is extended, thus increasing the risk of toxic effects.

Some drugs can adversely affect nutritional status. Drugs can reduce food intake by depressing appetite, altering taste and smell, and causing gastrointestinal disturbances. Some drugs can stimulate appetite and lead to weight gain. Others may interfere with the digestion, absorption, or metabolism of nutrients. Table 21-1 gives the nutritional side effects of commonly used drugs.

Self-medication with vitamins, minerals, and other nutrition supplements is a common practice among older adults. When taken in doses substantially exceeding the Recommended Dietary Allowances, vitamin and mineral supplements may act as drugs and interact adversely with other nutrients and with bodily processes. Other supplements such as herbs and amino acids may also have serious harmful effects. Clients should be questioned about the nutrition supplements they are taking; these supplements should be listed in the client's medical chart.

GASTROINTESTINAL DISORDERS

Three major problems of the older person are achlorhydria, constipation, and diarrhea.

ACHLORHYDRIA

One of the most detrimental physical changes associated with aging is the diminished secretion of hydrochloric acid (*achlorhydria*) in the stomach,

TABLE 21-1 Drugs Commonly Used by Elderly People and the Nutritional Side Effects

Drug	Nutritional Side Effect
Drugs Influencing Appetite and Food Intake	
Antipsychotics and sedatives	Somnolence; disinterest in food
Digoxin	Marked anorexia; nausea; vomiting; weakness
Cancer chemotherapies	Nausea, vomiting; aversion to food
Drugs Affecting Absorption of Nutrients	
Laxatives and cathartics	Malabsorption of fat-soluble vitamins; fluid and electrolyte loss
Corticosteroids	Decreased vitamin D activity
H_2 receptor blockers	Vitamin B_{12} malabsorption
Aluminum or magnesium antacids	Phosphate depletion
Cholestyramine	Decreased absorption of lipids, folate, iron, vitamin B_{12} and fat-soluble vitamins; gastrointestinal side effects
Drugs Affecting Metabolism of Nutrients	
Isoniazid, hydralazine, L-dopa	Vitamin B_6 antagonists
Salicylates	Iron loss secondary to gastrointestinal bleeding
Anticoagulants	Vitamin K antagonists
Drugs Affecting Excretion of Nutrients	
Thiazides	Loss of potassium, sodium, magnesium, and zinc
Furosemide	Loss of potassium, magnesium, chloride, sodium, and water
Spironolactone	Potassium sparing; hyperkalemia; fluid and electrolyte changes

(Kerstetter JE, Holthausen BA, Fitz PA. Malnutrition in the institutionalized older adult. J Am Diet Assoc 1992;92:1113)

which occurs in 15% to 25% of older adults. This condition interferes with digestion and absorption of folate, vitamin B_{12}, calcium, and iron. Also, people who have abnormally low gastric acid are more prone to foodborne illness because gastric acid protects the body from harmful bacteria.

CONSTIPATION

Constipation is a symptom caused by a number of disorders, conditions, and lifestyle factors associated with aging, including dental problems, immobility, decreased peristalsis, medication, failure to respond to the urge to defecate, laxative abuse, and inadequate intake of food, fiber, and fluid (Display 21-1). Normal bowel habits in healthy adults range from three times a day to three times a week. Individuals who do not experience bloating, pain, or straining in moving bowels are not constipated. Many people who actually have normal bowel habits complain of constipation because they do not have bowel movements as often as they think they should. Use of laxatives may compound the problem because it may eventually destroy the neurologic control of the large intestine.

Constipation itself is usually not serious. However, it may be a symptom of a serious underlying disorder such as cancer. Constipation can lead to hemorrhoids, fissures, and diverticulosis. Fecal impaction may occur in older adults. Clients should consult a physician if symptoms are severe; last more than 2 weeks; are accompanied by complications such as bleeding, hemorrhoids, or fissures; or if a significant and prolonged change in usual bowel habits has occurred.

Treatment

If an underlying disorder or medication is found to be causing the constipation, the cause is treated. If no underlying disease is found, attention is directed to several diet and lifestyle changes.

- Know that a daily bowel movement is unnecessary. Avoid reliance on laxatives. Prunes are a good source of fiber and contain a natural substance that stimulates peristalsis. However, habitual use of prunes can create a reliance on their laxative effect and can cause rebound constipation when the person stops eating them.
- Eat a well-balanced diet that includes high-fiber

DISPLAY 21-1 CAUSES OF CONSTIPATION

LIFESTYLE FACTORS

Poor diet
Imaginary constipation
Poor bowel habits
Laxative abuse
Travel
Inadequate fluids
Lack of exercise

MEDICATIONS

Pain medications, especially narcotics
Aluminum-containing antacids
Antispasmodic drugs
Antidepressants
Tranquilizers
Iron supplements
Potassium supplements
Anticonvulsants

PHYSICAL CONDITIONS AND DISEASES

Hormonal disturbances such as hypothyroidism or hypercalcemia
Anal fissures and hemorrhoids
Pregnancy
Specific disease such as irritable bowel syndrome, multiple sclerosis, Parkinson's disease, gastric cancer, stroke, scleroderma, lupus
Loss of body salts through the kidneys, vomiting, or diarrhea
Nerve damage due to spinal cord injuries or tumor

foods such as wheat bran, whole-wheat breads and cereals, legumes, fruits, and vegetables. Increase fiber gradually to at least 20 to 30 g/day. (Increase fiber cautiously in the diets of older people; plenty of fluids should always accompany increased fiber intake.)
- Drink adequate amounts of fluids: eight 8 oz glasses daily. A cup of *hot* liquid (coffee, tea, or water) first thing in the morning can initiate the gastrocolic reflex, which stimulates the colon and induces a bowel movement.
- Exercise regularly, if capable. Exercise promotes peristalsis.
- Establish good bowel habits. Do not ignore the urge to have a bowel movement. Toileting needs of clients who require assistance should be responded to immediately.

DIARRHEA

Chronic diarrhea may be caused by loss of circular muscle tone in the colon. Diarrhea can also be the result of various diseases and conditions including lactose intolerance and can be a complication of tube feedings that are too highly concentrated.

Treatment depends on the cause. For chronic diarrhea, fluid replacement, vitamin and mineral supplements, and a high-protein, high-calorie diet are used. Medications may be prescribed to slow intestinal motility.

DEHYDRATION

Fluid and electrolyte imbalances caused by dehydration can result in confusion, nausea, and death. Factors that contribute to severe dehydration include renal disease, incontinence, mental confusion, immobility, multiple drug therapy, and severe nausea, vomiting, or diarrhea.

Adequate fluid intake is important and should be monitored carefully. Monitoring is especially important because elderly people have a reduced sense of thirst that cannot be relied on to stimulate adequate fluid consumption. Daily fluid requirements can be estimated as follows: 1 mL for every kilocalorie (i.e., 1500 kcal × 1 mL = 1500 mL fluid) or 30 mL for each kilogram of body weight (120 lb ÷ 2.2 × 30 = 1636 mL).

COMMON FEEDING PROBLEMS

All the knowledge and planning in the world are of no value unless the person consumes the food on his or her plate. In the light of problems with appetite and other symptoms that prevent adequate food intake, getting the elderly client to eat is no small task. The health care worker needs to understand the factors that affect food intake and food preferences. The following are physical conditions that hinder the consumption of adequate amounts of food.

CHANGES IN SENSATIONS OF TASTE AND SMELL

It generally is accepted that the senses of smell and taste declines with age. Some causes of the changes in taste (*dysgeusia*) and smell (*dysosmia*) sensitivity are reduction in the sharpness of the chemical receptors, nutritional deficiencies, mouth dryness, decline of mental functions, smoking, use of dentures, and medication. Diseases such as cancer or hepatitis, metabolic changes or disorders, and nerve damage due to injury or surgery also may alter the sense of taste. Many drugs can alter taste or odor sensitivity. Some drugs are secreted into the mouth and produce an unpleasant taste or travel in the bloodstream and suppress sensory receptors. Deficiencies of zinc and copper also may cause changes in taste.

TREATMENT

Special attention must be paid to increasing the palatability of the food served to a client with impaired senses of taste and smell. The use of flavor enhancers in food preparation is a method for increasing food intake. Flavor can be amplified by the use of spices, herbs, and flavorings. Commercially prepared flavor packets are available. It may be necessary to somewhat relax restrictions of salt and sugar due to medical problems or to use acceptable substitutes for these flavor enhancers.

XEROSTOMIA

Xerostomia is the mouth dryness felt when there is a severe reduction in saliva. It is a common problem among older people. The most frequent causes are drugs that inhibit saliva flow, autoimmune diseases such as rheumatoid arthritis and Sjögren's syndrome (see Key Terms), and irradiation to the salivary glands. Although the secretion of saliva is thought to decrease with age, some experts have indicated that this cause alone would not be severe enough to result in xerostomia.

When saliva is reduced, the lips, teeth, and mouth become coated with dead cells, food products, and dried mucus; if not cleaned, they become infected. Also, with insufficient saliva, the acidity produced by bacteria in the mouth is not controlled, and the client is at high risk for developing severe dental caries. In addition to the feeling of dryness, other symptoms associated with xerostomia include burning and soreness of the mouth, especially the tongue; difficulty in chewing, swallowing, and speaking; impaired taste; painful ulcers; difficulty wearing dentures; increase in dental caries; and an increased intake of fluids.

More than 400 drugs are capable of reducing saliva flow. Among them are antidepressants, sedatives, antihistamines, drugs for Parkinson's disease, antihypertensives, and diuretics. Certain psychogenic factors, such as fear and mental stress, also may reduce the secretion of saliva.

Mastication (chewing) plays an important role in the production of saliva by stimulating nerves in mouth and gum tissues. In clients who have been on liquid diets, the salivary glands atrophy, consequently contributing to xerostomia in susceptible people.

TREATMENT

The purpose of treatment is to increase saliva flow, or, when the flow cannot be increased, to provide moisture to the oral tissue by other means.

If the glands can be stimulated to produce saliva, the following measures are suggested:

- Eat foods that require chewing. Frequent sips of water may make chewing easier.
- Have smaller but more frequent meals.
- Chew sugarless gum between meals.
- Use sugar-free lozenges and sugar-free hard candies. Sugarless lemon drops are particularly effective.
- Sip water throughout the day.
- Drink acidic beverages such as lemon juice and effervescent drinks.
- Avoid alcohol.

For clients who do not secrete saliva, even after stimulation, commercial saliva substitutes are used. These products are designed to keep the mouth moist and may be especially helpful during the night. Keeping the air at an optimum level of humidity may help keep the oral tissues moist.

If xerostomia is due to medication, several approaches can be used, including

- elimination or reduction of the drug
- change in dosage schedule so that peak blood levels do not coincide with the times of the day when mouth dryness is most severe
- substitution of another drug.

Regular dental care is important for all clients with dry mouth. Saliva protects teeth from decay. When it is lacking, there is an increased incidence of dental caries.

DYSPHAGIA

The average person swallows 600 times a day without conscious effort. However, 6 to 10 million Americans have swallowing difficulties, or *dysphagia.* Dysphagia is a symptom of diseases that affect any part of the swallowing function. Its effect can be devastating, causing bouts of aspiration pneumonia, and can lead to death from choking. Swallowing difficulties can occur as a result of neck or laryngeal surgery, following a stroke, and in diseases such as myasthenia gravis (see Key Terms) and Alzheimer's disease, in which the person forgets how to chew and swallow.

People with swallowing difficulties may compensate by changing what and how they eat. When the condition becomes more severe, symptoms such as regurgitation, coughing, and choking may occur. Milder symptoms include clearing the throat, speaking as if one has a cold, retaining solid particles in the throat, and abnormal speech. Esophageal dysphagia, which occurs in the second phase of swallowing, sometimes produces a feeling that food is sticking farther down in the sternum area.

TREATMENT

Some causes of dysphagia can be treated medically or surgically. With other causes, the client must be retrained to swallow. Most people with swallowing problems can be helped. Techniques for rehabilitating people with dysphagia include exercises for the tongue and lips, changes in posture while the person is eating, and changes in the way food is given (e.g., through a straw or syringe). Another strategy is to modify the physical properties of the food—temperature, pH, viscosity, volume, shape, and size. All of these factors can affect how safely food passes during the swallowing process.

One method of modifying food for people with swallowing disorders is gelling it. Some neurologically impaired people cannot swallow water or thin liquids but can swallow thicker, jellylike substances. Thus, clients can manage to swallow gelled lemonade. Commercial products such as Thick-it (Alberto-Culver USA, Inc.) are available; when added to foods and beverages, these products give them a jellylike consistency.

Another technique involves bottle-feeding, used to retrain the swallowing reflex. Some clients who have lost the ability to swallow can suck a bottle with a nipple. After a short period of bottle-feeding, the clients gradually progress to some ability to chew and swallow. This technique appears to be most useful in clients with amyotrophic lateral sclerosis, stroke, neck injuries, and, possibly, Alzheimer's disease.

A multistage diet for clients with dysphagia has been developed. The diet consists of five solid food stages and two liquid stages. Clients who are unable to manage regular liquids are given the thickened liquids. Main features of the diet are given in Display 21-2.

COMMON NUTRITION PROBLEMS

PROTEIN-CALORIE MALNUTRITION

Elderly people who are at greatest risk of developing protein-calorie malnutrition are those who are hospitalized for more than 2 weeks, experience involuntary loss of more than 10% of usual body weight, undergo surgery, or are diagnosed as having cancer. Protein-calorie malnutrition may be caused by an inadequate intake of both calories and protein or by a sufficient caloric intake in the form of carbohydrate and fat but an insufficient protein intake. Symptoms of protein-calorie malnutrition include weight loss, pallor, flaky dry skin, and loss of muscle mass. If calories remain adequate despite a lack of protein, fat stores may be preserved.

Decreased protein intake leads to low serum albumin levels and a depressed immune system, which can predispose the client to infection and delay wound healing. Anemia often is present. Due to these physiologic changes, the client may experience fatigue, shortness of breath, and pedal edema.

If the client can consume at least two thirds of his or her nutritional needs, the balance can usually be supplied by the use of liquid supplements such as milk shakes, instant breakfasts, or commercial liquid supplements. If the client is unable to consume adequate amounts of food by normal means to correct the deficiency of energy and protein, tube feedings may be used. As long as the gastrointestinal tract in functioning, tube feeding rather than intravenous nutrition therapy is the method of choice. See Chapter 29 for a discussion of alternative feeding methods and Chapter 30 for a discussion of nutrition therapy in cancer.

DISPLAY 21-2 MAIN FEATURES OF DYSPHAGIA DIET CATEGORIES

SOLID FOODS

Five categories that progress in swallowing difficulty from easiest to most difficult.

Stage 1—All pureed foods, smooth hot cereals, strained soups thickened to pureed consistency, creamed cottage cheese, smooth yogurt, and puddings

Stage 2—All foods in previous stages plus soft moist whole foods such as pancakes; finely chopped tender meats, fish, and eggs bound with thick dressing; soft cheeses (e.g., American); noodles and pasta; tender cooked leafy greens; sliced ripe banana; soft breads; soft moist cakes

Stage 3—All foods in stages 1 and 2 plus eggs any style, tender ground meats bound with thick sauce, soft fish, whole soft vegetables, drained canned fruits

Stage 4—All foods in stages 1, 2, and 3 plus foods with solids and liquids together (e.g., vegetable soup), all whole foods except hard and particulate foods such as dry breads, tough meat, corn, rice, apples

Stage 5—Regular diet

LIQUIDS

Two categories that are unrelated in ease of swallowing

Thin—Water, all juices thinner than pineapple, Italian ice, other clear liquids except gelatin desserts

Thick—All other liquids including milk, any juice not classified as a thin liquid, sherbet, ice cream

THICKENED LIQUIDS

Liquids thickened with starch to pureed consistency for people who cannot tolerate any other liquids

(Pardoe EM. Development of a multistage diet for dysphagia. J Am Diet Assoc 1993;93:570.)

ANEMIA

Anemia is a common disorder among older adults, usually diagnosed as a result of laboratory tests (a complete blood count). A number of different types of anemia exist, ranging from iron deficiency anemia to less common types such as *aplastic anemia* (resulting from a bone marrow defect). Treatments differ depending on the cause of the anemia. Three common nutrition-related anemias are due to iron, B_{12}, and folate deficiencies.

IRON DEFICIENCY ANEMIA

Iron deficiency anemia results when there is not enough iron in the body from which to make sufficient hemoglobin. Among older adults, the most common cause is *occult blood loss*—slow persistent bleeding from the intestinal tract due to an ulcer, polyps, cancer, or drugs such as aspirin that cause irritation of the gastric mucosa. Although iron deficiency anemia caused by an iron-deficient diet is possible, it is unlikely in the older adult because most iron in red blood cells is recycled to make new ones. This type of anemia is treated by correcting the cause of the blood loss and having the client use iron supplements until the hemoglobin returns to normal. If poor diet is the cause, nutrition counseling should be provided.

B_{12} DEFICIENCY ANEMIA

Pernicious anemia caused by a vitamin B_{12} deficiency usually becomes evident in middle adulthood and beyond. It results from the impaired ability of the digestive tract to absorb vitamin B_{12} in the diet because the intrinsic factor in gastric juice, necessary for the absorption of vitamin B_{12}, is missing. Anemia due to poor absorption of vitamin B_{12} may also occur after a gastrectomy or surgery of the ileum, in achlorhydria, or in malabsorption diseases that affect the ileum. Because vitamin B_{12} is vital for the maintenance of the nervous system as well as for red blood cell production, a deficiency causes neurologic problems in addition to the anemia. Symptoms include numbness and tingling of the hands and feet, change in walking gait, and mental disturbances. Pernicious anemia is treated by lifelong monthly injections of vitamin B_{12}. (A lack of vitamin B_{12} in the diet may occur among strict vegetarians. In this case, the anemia can be treated by oral B_{12} supplements.)

FOLATE DEFICIENCY ANEMIA

A type of anemia can also result from folate (folic acid) deficiency caused by an inadequate intake of folate. It may occur among older adults who have a poor diet and is especially common among people who consume alcohol excessively. It is treated with folate supplements and improvement in diet.

OSTEOPOROSIS

A prolonged deficient intake of calcium is one of several factors contributing to *osteoporosis* (reduction in bone mass). This disease affects 90% of women older than age 75 years and is a major cause of bone fractures. An adequate intake of calcium throughout life is thought to protect against osteoporosis in later life. The progression of osteoporosis can be slowed by increased calcium intake, exercise, and estrogen replacement (see the section Key Issues in Chapter 11).

MINERAL DEFICIENCY AND TOXICITY

The clinical signs of mineral deficiencies are listed in Table 11-5. Elderly people commonly experience many of these symptoms. The actions of many of the trace elements are complicated; they interact with each other and with vitamins. For example, excessive intake of zinc can interfere with the metabolism of copper. Indiscriminate use of mineral supplements can cause such problems. Laboratory tests to measure whether the individual is deficient in a particular mineral are necessary.

VITAMIN DEFICIENCY AND TOXICITY

Elderly people are at greatest risk of deficiencies in the water-soluble vitamins: folate, vitamin C, pyridoxine (vitamin B_6), and vitamin B_{12}. Medications commonly used by the older person may interfere with the metabolism of B vitamins.

Fat-soluble vitamins, which can be stored, are less likely to be deficient. Vitamin K deficiency, however, may result from drugs such as sulfa drugs, antibiotics, and anticoagulants.

Vitamin D deficiency is widespread among older people who are not receiving vitamin supplements. It is caused by a low intake of dairy products that are fortified with vitamin D, minimal exposure to sunlight, and a decline in the ability to metabolize vitamin D. Some drugs such as prednisone and phenobarbital may interfere with the metabolism of vitamin D. Symptoms such as bone pain, fractures, and loss of height may be due to *osteomalacia* (softening of the bones), which results from lowered calcium absorption due to vitamin D deficiency, not from aging or osteoporosis (see Chapter 12).

Toxicity related to excessive intake of vitamins also presents a risk to elderly adults. Many elderly people take vitamin and mineral supplements. Use of such supplements frequently is overlooked when a medical history is taken because the client rarely considers them to be drugs. Although toxicity related to the fat-soluble vitamins A and D is most common because they are stored by the body, excessive intake of water-soluble vitamins can also cause problems. For example, large doses of vitamin C may interfere with the absorption of vitamin B_{12} and also may promote the formation of kidney stones.

TREATING THE WHOLE PERSON: CONSIDERATIONS FOR PROVIDERS OF NUTRITION CARE TO THE OLDER ADULT

Nutrition intervention must be tempered by an awareness of the important role food and eating play in fulfilling a person's psychological and emotional needs. Eating is one of the greatest pleasures of life as a person grows older and one of the most important ties to life. It gives structure to the day, increases self-esteem, provides enjoyment, and provides for social interaction.

Health care workers frequently may overlook the relation between food and feelings. Each person is unique and has developed over a lifetime a unique set of eating habits. These habits represent family traditions, ethnic or religious background, and ties to loved ones. The older person in a health care facility experiences a sense of loss when food no longer conveys these meanings. Clients who lose their motivation to eat may not so much be unwilling to accept the new as be reluctant to give up the old.

Food is a means of expressing hospitality and friendship. Disabling conditions reduce interest in food and, as a result, reduce social contacts. Purchasing and preparing food may not seem to be worth the effort to the person with severe arthritis or heart disease. Older people become embarrassed by their lack of teeth, disabling conditions, and distorted appearance. They sense the rejection of friends, family, and health care workers and withdraw from social situations. When eating ceases to be a social situation, food loses its importance as a source of nutrition and a means of emotional support. The health care worker needs to help clients deal with physical limitations and make them aware that making meals a social experience promotes better nutrition and emotional health as well.

The cultural and religious heritage of the older adult must be considered also. Many find great comfort in the continuation of cultural and religious dietary practices whether they are at home or in a health care facility. An example is the older Jewish person who has always observed the Jewish dietary laws. Observance of these practices is part of his or her daily existence. When a person is ill,

DISPLAY 21-3 ENHANCING THE PSYCHOLOGICAL COMFORT OF FOOD

The following are suggestions that care-givers can use to enhance the psychological comfort of food to elderly people.

- Preserve the individual's self-esteem. Allow food choices. Don't argue.
- Know that the quality of the relationship between the client and care-givers affects the patient's compliance.
- Preserve the client's dignity.
- Do outreach—find out the client's food likes and dislikes, identify any loss in taste, find out how the client likes food presented.
- Match the behavior of the client to establish rapport.
- Allow the client to ventilate.
- Talk to the client during feeding.
- Be flexible and individualize your approach.
- Do not infantilize (treat the client like a child).
- Do not feed the client unless he or she is absolutely unable to feed himself or herself. Use finger foods or feeding aids whenever possible.
- Manipulate the environment to include other clients.
- Include protein in desserts to make every part of the meal nutritious.
- Consider clients' levels of functioning and eating habits when arranging seating in dining areas. The elderly person can become frightened by the behavior of clients who function at a lower level.
- Keep treatment simple and consider costs, traditions, and availability of foods.
- Use concentrated sweets in moderation.
- Arrange nutrition education experiences for older people according to their level of understanding.
- Be aware that when a client is under stress, his or her ability to follow a prescribed program is reduced.
- Involve the client and family in the care plan and in the decision-making process.
- Remember the spouse is at greatest risk in dementia.
- Determine a sleep history with total time in bed to ascertain if the amount of sleep is affecting the client's appetite.

(Adapted from: Kaplan S, Tuckman TB. Considerations for those providing nutritional care to the elderly. J Nutr Elderly 1986;5:57.)

observance of religious beliefs takes on even greater significance.

For the person who has survived to old age, unless there are signs of poor nutrition, it may be best to avoid changing well-established eating habits. Older adults frequently are reluctant to change eating habits. The term "diet" if used in the client's situation may convey the negative meanings of control or restriction. If the client objects to prescribed dietary modifications and begins to lose appetite, the beneficial effects must be weighed against the emotional distress. If the client becomes depressed because he or she is being deprived of food he or she enjoys, the depression could be more crippling to total health than the benefits that can be expected from the diet. The health care worker must consider the whole person and weigh all aspects of care.

Clients are most cooperative when they are involved in making decisions about their treatment. Clients' food preferences should be considered, as well as other aspects of their eating habits. Listen to the clients' objections and frustrations about their diets. The client frequently knows best what he or she can eat. Treating clients with understanding, concern, and dignity is more likely to gain their cooperation (see Display 21-3).

Whether a client is at home or in a health care facility, his or her strengths and capabilities should be emphasized. A person should be encouraged to have meals at the table with family or friends even if they must eat with their fingers or with a utensil attached to their hand. In a health care facility, it is important to seat clients together who are at the same level of functioning. Otherwise, the client who is not functioning well may be verbally abused by other clients. Also, other clients may be frightened or become upset in the presence of serious disabilities.

When food intake is poor, investigate the cause. Do not assume that this is a natural result of aging. A healthy appetite is possible even in advanced age. Remember that food feeds the whole person—body and spirit.

KEYS TO PRACTICAL APPLICATION

When your client does not eat enough food, find the cause. Do not blame old age.

Remember that the time and effort you spend on feeding older clients contributes not only to their health status but also to their quality of life.

Do not assume that clients who have no teeth require pureed foods. Be guided by what they tell you they can eat.

Monitor your clients' fluid intake. Encourage them to drink more water and ensure that water is available and that they receive assistance in drinking it, if needed.

When serious feeding problems such as dysphagia are encountered, seek assistance. Remember that there are numerous ways of overcoming or improving feeding problems. See Displays 21-2 and 21-3.

When taking medical histories, be sure to ask your clients about vitamins, minerals, and other nutritional supplements they may be taking.

Be aware of and learn to use techniques that increase mealtime pleasure for your client (see Display 21-3).

KEY IDEAS

Nutrition is a factor in both the development and treatment of a number of chronic diseases.

Malnutrition in the older adult can have devastating physical, social, psychological, and economic consequences.

Lack of gastric acidity in many older adults and the inability of some older adults to consume enough food are serious problems.

Infections of various kinds afflict a high percentage of institutionalized older people; sometimes a vicious cycle of infection and malnutrition develops.

Low serum albumin levels are closely associated with the development of decubitus ulcers.

Mental disorders, especially depression, can seriously interfere with an adequate food intake.

Medications can adversely affect nutritional status by altering food intake and the digestion, absorption, and use of nutrients.

Older people who have been hospitalized for more than 2 weeks, have involuntarily lost 10% or more of their usual body weight, have had surgery, or have cancer are at greatest risk of protein-calorie malnutrition.

Protein-calorie malnutrition predisposes the client to infection and delayed wound healing, as in the case of decubitus ulcers.

Iron deficiency anemia in the older adult is most likely to be the result of occult blood loss rather than an iron-deficient diet.

An adequate intake of calcium throughout life is thought to protect against osteoporosis in later life. Progression of osteoporosis can be slowed by increased calcium, exercise, and estrogen replacement.

An excessive intake of vitamin/mineral supplements by elderly people can result in toxic reactions; information regarding supplement use should always be included in a medical history.

Achlorhydria, constipation, and chronic diarrhea are major gastrointestinal problems of elderly people.

The use of flavor enhancers may be helpful for people who have impaired senses of taste and smell.

The treatment of xerostomia involves techniques that stimulate saliva production, such as chewing, or, if no saliva is being produced, the use of saliva substitutes.

When swallowing difficulties cannot be treated medically or surgically, emphasis is placed on retraining the client to swallow. This retraining may involve exercises, changes in posture, changes in the way food is given (e.g., through a straw or in a bottle), and changes in the physical properties of food, such as gelling.

For elderly people who are in reasonably good health, changes in diet should be avoided or undertaken cautiously.

Poor food intake is not the natural result of aging; the cause must be investigated.

Eating is one of the greatest pleasures of life as a person grows older and one of the most important ties to life.

Nutrition intervention must be tempered by an awareness of the important role food and eating play in fulfilling psychological and emotional needs.

See Displays 21-2 and 21-3 for techniques to increase food acceptance and mealtime pleasure.

KEYS TO LEARNING

STUDY–DISCUSSION QUESTIONS

1. Discuss two of the factors that affect nutritional status of older people.
2. Discuss the effect of depression on food intake. How often have you encountered depression among your elderly clients? What approaches or techniques have you found useful in getting clients to eat?
3. What changes would you make in the usual hospital or nursing home environment to improve the food intake of the elderly client? Do you think sufficient attention is paid to what and how much older clients eat?
4. Decubitus ulcers are a common problem in older adults confined to bed or a wheelchair.

Discuss this condition in relation to nutrition care.

5. Give four causes of constipation that are not related to diet and lifestyle factors. If no underlying disease is found, what diet and lifestyle changes would you recommend.

6. Give three practical ways of treating each of the following feeding problems: decreased sensations of taste and smell, xerostomia, and dysphagia.

7. Discuss the concept of "food as one of the most important ties to life" for the older person.

BIBLIOGRAPHY

BOOKS AND PAMPHLETS

Dwyer JT. Screening older Americans' nutritional health: current practices and future possibilities. Boston: Johanna Dwyer, 1991.

Schiffman SS. Taste and smell in aging and obesity. In: Gaull GE. Ed. Nutrition in the 90's: current controversies and analyses. New York: Marcel Dekker, 1991:51.

PERIODICALS

Bennett RG. Oral rehydration therapy for older adults. Dietetic Currents 1992;19:4:1.

Davies L, Knutson KC. Warning signals for malnutrition in the elderly. J Am Diet Assoc 1991;91:1413.

Kaplan S, Tuckman TB. Considerations for those providing nutritional care to the elderly. J Nutr Elderly 1986;5:57.

Keller HH. Malnutrition in institutionalized elderly: how and why? J Am Geriatr Soc 1993;41:1212.

Kerstetter JE, Holthausen BA, Fitz PA. Malnutrition in the institutionalized older adult. J Am Diet Assoc 1992;92: 1109.

Livingston J, Reeves RD. Undocumented potential drug interactions found in medical records of elderly patients in long-term-care facility. J Am Diet Assoc 1993;93:1168.

Morley JE, Kraenzle D. Causes of weight loss in a community nursing home. J Am Geriatr Soc 1994;42:583.

Nelson KJ, Coulston AM, Sucher KP, et al. Prevalence of malnutrition in the elderly admitted to long-term-care facilities. J Am Diet Assoc 1993;93:459

Pardoe EM. Development of a multistage diet for dysphagia. J Am Diet Assoc 1993;93:568.

Schlettwein-Gsell D. Nutrition and the quality of life: a measure for the outcome of nutritional intervention. Am J Clin Nutr 1992;55:1263S.

Towers AL, Burgio KL, Locher JL, et al. Constipation in the elderly: influence of dietary, psychological and physiological factors. J Am Geriatr Soc 1994;42:701.

Varma RN. Risk for drug-induced malnutrition is unchecked in elderly patients in nursing homes. J Am Diet Assoc 1994;94:192.

Zaher LP, Holdt CS, Gates GE, et al. Nutritional care of ambulatory residents in special care units for Alzheimer's patients. J Nutr Elderly 1993;12:4:5.

CHAPTER

22

Tools and Teaching Aids in Nutrition Therapy, Including Exchange Lists

KEY TERMS

exchange lists lists of foods that have the same nutritional composition for the nutrients being controlled; any food on the list in the amount given can be exchanged in the diet for any other specified portion of food on the same list in the amount given

literacy the ability to read and write

standard measure a level measure using standard measuring cups and spoons

target nutrients nutrients being controlled or emphasized in the diet

OBJECTIVES

After completing this chapter, the student will be able to:

1. Discuss the choice of strategies in the management of nutrition-related conditions and the value of giving the client a choice.
2. Discuss the use of teaching aids in nutrition education and counseling and describe three aids other than written materials.
3. Explain the use of client-kept records such as food diaries and exercise diaries.
4. Describe two techniques or methods that promote communication of health messages to the low-literate reader.
5. List four ways in which nutrition labeling can be used in nutrition education.
6. Plan a day's menu using a specific meal plan and the exchange lists.
7. Explain the importance of educating the client about portion sizes and suggest educational techniques he or she (the student) can use.

PERSONAL APPROACH

How clients are taught about diet may have greater significance than what is taught. The primary focus is not the disease, but the client as a person. Instruction about nutritional needs and medical nutrition therapy must be adapted to the individual client's lifestyle. An educational approach must be selected to suit the client's educational level and personality characteristics. The business professional who is nervously tapping a foot and frequently glancing at his or her watch requires a different approach than the individual who comes to the health care worker with detailed food diaries and numerous questions about food shopping and preparation. Likewise, the illiterate disabled elderly woman requires a different approach than the 40-year-old school teacher.

There is no right or wrong method for teaching meal planning and other aspects of the nutritional management of disease as long as the goals of treatment (e.g., lowered blood pressure or weight loss) are achieved. Meal plans and exchange lists represent one approach used in nutrition counseling. These tools are used in conditions in which the energy nutrients need to be controlled as in diabetes and weight reduction.

In diabetes and in most other conditions, there are various approaches to achieving a particular goal. For example, a person who needs to reduce caloric intake might use a structured meal plan and exchange lists *or* monitor total calories *or* monitor total grams of fat in the diet to achieve the desired goal, which is weight loss. The client should be given a choice of methods or approaches from which to choose (see the section Problem Solving: The Nutrition Care Process in Chapter 20).

TEACHING AIDS

PURPOSE AND USE

Teaching aids reinforce the education and counseling provided by the dietitian or other health care provider. Clients are usually provided with written or printed guidelines that summarize the nutrition information and related information provided during the educational program or counseling session. Display 22-1 is an example of take-home guidelines for a client who has been advised to increase the fiber content of his or her diet. The meal planning guidelines are individualized to meet the client's needs. In this case, the dietitian might suggest a stepwise approach indicating what high-fiber food the client might add and at what intervals. In a future counseling session, the dietitian might show the client how to count the amount of fiber in the foods and record the number on the food diary the client has kept. Other printed materials provided might include shopping tips, recipes, and lists of specialized recipe books.

Many other teaching aids can be used to reinforce nutrition education in both normal nutrition and in medical nutrition therapy. These aids include videotapes, audiotapes, computer-assisted programmed instruction, games, role-playing, supermarket tours, and demonstrations (e.g. cooking, measuring portions, or monitoring blood glucose).

RECORD KEEPING

Awareness is a key factor in changing behavior. In the course of nutrition counseling, clients are asked to keep food intake, weight, or exercise records. These records are an important means of maintaining awareness of eating and exercise habits. Also, they are useful in evaluating the client's understanding of the information provided and in determining the influences on eating and exercise behaviors.

The record keeping should be as simple as possible, requiring only the essential information. Display 22-2 gives an example of a food intake record. Careful instruction on keeping the records should be given to the client. Foods eaten should be recorded as they are eaten and not at the end of the day. Accurate estimation of portion sizes is also very important.

Many clients find record keeping tedious and difficult to accomplish. It may take time to develop the discipline required, but the results are worth the effort. The client should be encouraged to have patience and to continue to make the effort to keep records. Clients who keep records are the most successful in achieving their goals.

LOW-LITERACY TEACHING AIDS

About 20% of the US population reads at or below a fifth grade level. Although the *average* literacy level is at or below an eighth grade level, nutrition education materials are usually written at a tenth-grade reading level or higher. These

DISPLAY 22-1 EXAMPLE OF A TEACHING AID: HIGH FIBER DIET

WHY FOLLOW A HIGH-FIBER DIET?

By incorporating a high-fiber diet into your lifestyle, you can help prevent and treat constipation. For some people, it may also help to lower blood cholesterol and control blood sugar levels. A high-fiber diet provides 20g to 35g of fiber per day.

SAMPLE MENU FOR A HIGH-FIBER DIET

BREAKFAST
Grapefruit half
Whole-grain cereal* with raisins*
Whole-grain toast* with margarine and jam
Milk
Coffee or tea

LUNCH
Split pea soup* with whole-wheat crackers*
Hamburger with mustard, ketchup, sliced tomato,* onion,* and lettuce
Fresh fruit salad*
Ice water

SNACK
Bran muffin*
Milk

DINNER
Tossed salad with vinegar and oil dressing
Broiled chicken breast
Herbed brown rice*
Steamed broccoli*
Whole-grain roll* with margarine
Lowfat frozen yogurt with fresh blueberries*
Iced tea with lemon

* Good source of fiber.

IMPORTANT POINTS TO KEEP IN MIND

- The foods that supply the most fiber are whole-grain breads and cereals, grains, fruits, and vegetables.
- As you add more fiber to your diet:

  Do it gradually—too much fiber added too quickly may cause gas, cramping, bloating, or diarrhea.
  Drink plenty of fluids—at least 8 cups every day.

(Continued)

materials are too difficult for low-literate readers and, therefore, fail to communicate the practical and relevant information about nutrition that is needed.

Low-literate readers tend to skip over words they do not know and tend to take words at their face value. These characteristics can profoundly affect the meanings that these readers derive from nutrition education materials. The Doaks have suggested the following techniques in preparing written materials: use conversational style, limit objectives and focus on action, give many examples, include an interactive checklist, and conclude by listing the benefits to the reader.

DISPLAY 22-1 EXAMPLE OF A TEACHING AID: HIGH FIBER DIET *(Continued)*

FOOD CATEGORIES	FOODS RECOMMENDED	TIPS
BREADS, CEREALS, RICE, AND PASTA		
6–11 servings daily Serving size = 1 slice bread, 1 cup ready-to-eat cereal, 1/2 cup cooked cereal, rice, or pasta	Whole-grain breads, muffins, bagels, or pita bread Rye bread Whole-wheat crackers or crisp breads Whole-grain or bran cereals Oatmeal, oat bran, or grits Wheat germ Whole-wheat pasta and brown rice	Scan food labels for bread and cereal products listing whole-grain or whole-wheat as the first ingredient. Look for cooked and ready-to-eat cereals with at least 2 g of fiber per serving.
FRUITS		
2–4 servings daily Serving size = 1 medium size, 1/2 cup chopped, 1/4 cup dried	All fruits; in particular, apple, banana, berries, grapefruit, nectarine, orange, peach, pear	Eat raw fruits and vegetables; they have more fiber than cooked or canned foods, or juice. Dried fruits are also good sources of fiber.
VEGETABLES		
3–5 servings daily Serving size = 1 cup raw leafy, 1/2 cup cooked or chopped	All vegetables; in particular, asparagus, broccoli, cabbage, carrots, cauliflower, celery, corn, greens, green beans, green pepper, onions, peas, potatoes (with skin), snow peas, spinach, squash, sweet potatoes, tomatoes, zucchini	Remember the peelings on fruits and vegetables contribute fiber.
MEATS, POULTRY, FISH, DRY BEANS AND PEAS, EGGS, AND NUTS		
2–3 servings or total of 6 oz daily Serving size = 2 oz to 3 oz cooked; count 1 egg, 1/2 cup cooked beans, or 2 tbsp peanut butter as 1 oz of meat	All beans and peas; in particular, garbanzo beans, kidney beans, lentils, lima beans, split peas, and pinto beans All nuts and seeds; in particular, peanuts, Brazil nuts, cashews; sesame, sunflower, and pumpkin seeds All meat, poultry, fish, and eggs	Increase fiber in meat dishes by adding pinto beans, kidney beans, black-eyed peas, bran, or oatmeal. If you are following a lowfat diet, use nuts and seeds only in moderation.
MILK, YOGURT, AND CHEESE		
2–3 servings each day Serving size = 1 cup milk or yogurt, 1 1/2 ounces cheese	All	Dairy foods provide little fiber. Boost fiber by adding fresh fruit, whole-grain or bran cereals, nuts, or seeds to yogurt or cottage cheese.
FATS, SNACKS, SWEETS, CONDIMENTS, AND BEVERAGES		
	Popcorn, whole-wheat pretzels, or trail mix made with dried fruits, nuts, and seeds Cakes, breads, and cookies made with oatmeal, fruit, and nuts	

(From patient education materials available from the American Dietetic Association, 216 W. Jackson Boulevard, Suite 800, Chicago, IL 60606.)

DISPLAY 22-2 EXAMPLE OF A FOOD DIARY*

FOOD RECORD

NAME Mary Clark

DAY Tuesday **DATE** 1/30 **FAT GRAM GOAL:** 50

TIME	AMOUNT	FOOD	FAT GRAMS
7:30 AM	1/3	Cantaloupe	0
	1	Whole-wheat English muffin	1
	1 tbsp	Jelly	0
	1/4 cup	Egg substitute	0
12:00	1	Taco Supreme (Taco Bell)	15
	1	Vegetable salad	0
	2 tbsp	Low-calorie salad dressing	4
	1	Pear	0
3:30 PM	1 oz	Potato chips	10
	12 oz	Cola beverage	0
6:00 PM	1/2	Chicken breast, roasted—no skin	3
	1	Chicken thigh, roasted—no skin	6
	1 cup	Mashed potato	5
	1/2 cup	Peas	0
	1 slice	Bread	1
	1 tbsp	Light margarine	6
	8 oz	Skim milk	trace
9:30 PM	4 oz	Frozen yogurt, nonfat	0
		TOTAL	**51**

* Client-kept records facilitate behavior change.

Forms of communication other than written materials may be better ways to communicate with low-literate clients. Examples are short, simple messages printed on or taped to items used every day; picture messages; messages in comic books, cartoons, and rap songs; and peer-helper programs.

NUTRITION LABELING: A VITAL EDUCATION TOOL

In recent years, the demand for high-fiber foods and foods that are low in total calories, fat, sodium, or sugar has increased tremendously. The food industry

DISPLAY 22-3 "CORE TERMS" FOR NUTRIENT CONTENT CLAIMS ON FOOD LABELS

CORE TERM	APPLIES TO	(DEFINITION) PER SERVING
Free	Calorie-free	<5 kcal
	Sugar-free	<.5 g
	Fat-free	<.5 g
Low	Lowfat	≤3 g
	Low saturated fat	≤1 g
	Low-sodium	<140 mg
	Very low-sodium	35 mg
	Low-cholesterol	<20 mg
	Low-calorie	≤40 calories
High		Contains 20% or more of the Daily Value for that nutrient
Good source		Contains 10% to 20% or more of the Daily Value for that nutrient
Reduced	Nutritionally altered product	Contains 25% or less of a nutrient or of calories than the reference product
Less	May be nutritionally altered or unaltered	25% or less of a nutrient or calories than the reference food
Fewer	Applies to calories Altered or unaltered product Comparison to similar or dissimilar products	Must include percentage difference and identify reference food
Light	re: calories	$^1/_3$ fewer than reference food
	re: fat	$^1/_2$ the fat of reference food
	re: sodium content of low calorie, lowfat food	Reduced at least 50%
	re: "light in sodium"	At least 50% less sodium than reference food
More	Altered or unaltered product	Contains a nutrient that is at least 10% of the Daily Value more than the reference food
Lean	Applies to meat, poultry, seafood, and game meats	<10 g fat, <4 g saturated fat, and <95 mg cholesterol per 100 g ($3^1/_2$ oz)
Extra lean	Applies to meat, poultry, seafood, and game meats	<5 g fat, <2 g saturated fat, and <95 mg cholesterol per 100 g ($3^1/_2$ oz)

(Adapted from Stehlin D. A little "lite" reading. FDA Consumer (Special Report: Focus on Food Labeling), May 1993. DHHS publication FDA 93-2262:29.)

is meeting this demand by introducing many new foods that claim to meet one or more of these characteristics. It is important to evaluate these products carefully or to seek advice about them from a dietitian.

Evaluation of foods has been greatly simplified by the Nutrition Labeling and Education Act of 1990. Regulations requiring nutrition labeling on most foods became effective in May 1994. In addition, only health claims authorized by the Food and Drug Administration may be made on the label. The label regulations also spell out which nutrient content claims are allowed and under what circumstances they can be used (See Ch. 5). There are 11 core terms that can be used on labels to describe nutrient content claims. These core terms and their definitions are given in Display 22-3. Other more specific labeling regulations relating to sugar, fat, cholesterol, and sodium are given in Chapters 8, 9, 11, 23, 24, 25, and 26.

Nutrition labeling is a vital education tool. Food labels can be used to help a person budget total calories or target nutrients such as fat, saturated fat, cholesterol, and sodium. Good sources of vitamins, minerals, and fiber can be easily identified. Nutrition labeling is useful in counting approaches such as calorie counting, fat counting, and carbohydrate counting (used in diabetes). Because portion sizes given on nutrition labels are now more uniform, it is easier to compare the nutrient content of foods (Fig. 22-1).

EXCHANGE LISTS

Nutrition therapy frequently involves control of calories or of the quantities of one or more nutrients—such as fat, carbohydrate, protein, sodium, or potassium. Calculating foods consumed daily to see that they meet the prescription for calories or specific nutrients would be time-consuming and impractical.

A practical and rapid method for planning diets involves the concept of *exchange lists.* Exchange lists are foods listed together because they have a similar composition with respect to the nutritional factors being controlled; for example, foods with similar protein, fat, and carbohydrate composition may be grouped together. Measured amounts of foods in a single exchange group are equal to each other with respect to the nutrients being controlled and may be exchanged for one another. Exchange lists simplify meal planning for clients and make possible a wide choice of foods. The system originally was developed for planning meals for people with diabetes. The basic idea has been adapted for use in other modified diets, such as sodium-controlled and weight-reducing diets.

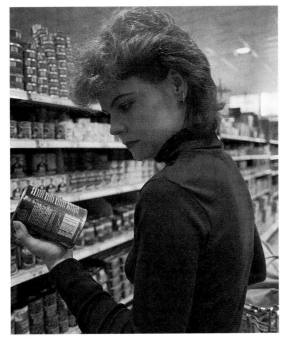

FIGURE 22-1

Nutrition labeling is a vital education tool. *(Courtesy of USDA)*

Exchange lists are not diets in themselves. They are only lists of foods that have a similar nutritional composition in regard to calories or the target nutrients. The exchange lists are used together with a meal plan that indicates the number of servings the client may have from each exchange group for each meal and snack for the day. For example, if two starch exchanges are permitted for dinner, the client may choose two slices of bread, one slice of bread and $^1/_2$ cup of mashed potatoes, or any two choices from the starch exchange list. The meal plan is the part of the exchange list system that constitutes the diet. The meal plan should be specifically designed to meet the individual's nutritional and therapeutic needs as well as his or her lifestyle and food preferences. Display 22-4 is an example of a meal plan developed using the Exchange Lists for Meal Planning described in the section which follows. In Display 22-5, the calculation of this 1800-kcal meal plan is demonstrated.

Exchange lists can also be used without a specific meal plan in fat counting or carbohydrate counting systems. See Chapters 23 and 24.

USING "EXCHANGE LISTS FOR MEAL PLANNING"

The health care worker should be familiar with the most widely used exchange lists, the Exchange Lists for Meal Planning, developed jointly by the American Diabetes Association and the American Dietetic Association. The first edition, published in 1950, has been revised several times. The Exchange Lists for Meal Planning presented in this book is the 1995 edition.

DISPLAY 22-4 DAILY MEAL PLAN FOR AN 1800-kcal DIET USING EXCHANGE LISTS*

DAILY MEAL PLAN

NUTRITIONAL COMPOSITION		AMOUNT	KIND OF FOOD
Protein	84 g	9	Starch exchanges
Carbohydrate	249 g	5	Meat exchanges (lean–medium fat)
Fat	55 g	3	Vegetable exchanges
		5	Fruit exchanges
		2	Skim milk exchanges
		6	Fat exchanges (unsaturated)

MEAL PLAN	SAMPLE MENU
BREAKFAST	
1 fruit exchange	1/2 cup of orange juice
3 starch exchanges	3/4 cup of cornflakes
2 fat exchanges	2 slices of whole-wheat toast
1 skim milk exchange	2 tsp of margarine
	1 cup of skim milk
LUNCH	
2 meat exchanges (lean–medium fat)	Turkey sandwich
2 starch exchanges	2 slices of rye bread
1 vegetable exchange	2 oz of turkey
1 fat exchange	1 tbsp of mayonnaise, reduced fat
2 fruit exchanges	1/2 sliced tomato
1 skim milk exchange	1 pear, large
	1 cup of skim milk
DINNER	
3 meat exchanges (lean–medium fat)	3 oz of pot roast
3 starch exchanges	1/2 cup of mashed potatoes
2 vegetable exchanges	1/2 cup of green beans
3 fat exchanges	1/2 cup of pickled beets
1 fruit exchange	1 slice of whole-wheat bread
	3 tsp of margarine (for bread and vegetables)
Coffee or tea, if desired	1/2 cup of sugar-free pudding†
	1/3 cantaloupe
	Tea
	Noncaloric sweetener
EVENING SNACK	
1 starch exchange	3 squares graham crackers
1 fruit exchange	1/2 cup of pineapple chunks, canned
1 skim milk exchange	1 cup of skim milk

* Used with exchange lists in Display 22-6.

† Food choices from the Other Carbohydrates List can be substituted for starch, fruit, or milk exchanges in the meal plan, but should be done in the context of a balanced meal.

DISPLAY 22-5 CALCULATION OF 1800-KCAL DAILY MEAL PLAN USING EXCHANGE LISTS*

EXCHANGE LIST	NO. OF EXCHANGES	CARBOHYDRATE (G)	PROTEIN (G)	FAT (G)
Milk, skim	2	24	16	—
Vegetable	3	15	6	—
Fruit	5	75	—	—
		114		
Starch	9	135	27	
			49	
Meat, lean-med. fat	5	—	35	25
Fat	6	—	—	30
Total		249	84	55
Calories per gram		×4	×4	×9
Total calories: 1827		996	336	495
% calories		55%	19%	28%

* Used with exchange lists in Display 22-6. Nutritional composition is as follows: carbohydrate, 250 g; protein, 84 g; fat, 55 g.

The most significant change in this latest edition is the organization of the exchange lists into three main groups based on their nutrient content:

Carbohydrate group—includes the starch, fruit, milk, other carbohydrates and vegetable lists.

Meat and meat substitutes group—includes the very lean, lean, medium-fat, and high-fat meat and substitutes lists. These four meat lists provide the major source of protein in the exchange lists.

Fat group—includes the monounsaturated, polyunsaturated, and saturated fat lists.

New features of the 1995 edition are the inclusion of the "Other Carbohydrates List" and the ad-

(text continues on page 443)

TABLE 22-1 NUTRIENT VALUES OF THE EXCHANGE LISTS

GROUP/LISTS	CARBOHYDRATE (GRAMS)	PROTEIN (GRAMS)	FAT (GRAMS)	CALORIES
Carbohydrate Group				
Starch	15	3	1 or less	80
Fruit	15	—	—	60
Milk				
Skim	12	8	0–3	90
Low-fat	12	8	5	120
Whole	12	8	8	150
Other carbohydrates	15	varies	varies	varies
Vegetables	5	2	—	25
Meat and Meat Substitute Group				
Very lean	—	7	0–1	35
Lean	—	7	3	55
Medium-fat	—	7	5	75
High-fat	—	7	8	100
Fat Group	—	—	5	45

DISPLAY 22-6 EXCHANGE LISTS FOR MEAL PLANNING*

CARBOHYDRATE LISTS

STARCH LIST

One starch exchange equals 15 grams carbohydrate, 3 grams protein, 0–1 grams fat, and 80 calories.

BREAD

Bagel	½ (1 oz)	Pita, 6 in. across	½
Bread, reduced-calorie	2 slices (1 ½ oz)	Roll, plain, small	1 (1 oz)
Bread, white, whole-wheat, pumpernickel, rye	1 slice (1 oz)	Raisin bread, unfrosted	1 slice (1 oz)
Bread sticks, crisp, 4 in. long × ½ in.	2 (⅔ oz)	Tortilla, corn, 6 in. across	1
English muffin	½	Tortilla, flour, 7–8 in. across	1
Hot dog or hamburger bun	½ (1 oz)	Waffle, 4 ½ in. square, reduced-fat	1

CEREALS AND GRAINS

Bran cereals	½ cup	Kasha	½ cup
Bulgur	½ cup	Millet	¼ cup
Cereals	½ cup	Muesli	¼ cup
Cereals, unsweetened, ready-to-eat	¾ cup	Oats	½ cup
Cornmeal (dry)	3 Tbsp	Pasta	½ cup
Couscous	⅓ cup	Puffed cereal	1 ½ cups
Flour (dry)	3 Tbsp	Rice milk	½ cup
Granola, low-fat	¼ cup	Rice, white or brown	⅓ cup
Grape-Nuts	¼ cup	Shredded Wheat	½ cup
Grits	½ cup	Sugar-frosted cereal	½ cup
		Wheat germ	3 Tbsp

STARCHY VEGETABLES

Baked beans	⅓ cup	Plantain	½ cup
Corn	½ cup	Potato, baked or boiled	1 small (3 oz)
Corn on cob, medium	1 (5 oz)	Potato, mashed	½ cup
Mixed vegetables with corn, peas, or pasta	1 cup	Squash, winter (acorn, butternut)	1 cup
Peas, green	½ cup	Yam, sweet potato, plain	½ cup

CRACKERS AND SNACKS

Animal crackers	8	Pretzels	¾ oz
Graham crackers, 2 ½ in. square	3	Rice cakes, 4 in. across	2
Matzoh	¾ oz	Saltine-type crackers	6
Melba toast	4 slices	Snack chips, fat-free (tortilla, potato)	15–20 (¾ oz)
Oyster crackers	24	Whole-wheat crackers, no fat added	2–5 (¾ oz)
Popcorn (popped, no fat added or low-fat microwave)	3 cups		

(Continued)

DISPLAY 22-6 EXCHANGE LISTS FOR MEAL PLANNING *(Continued)*

DRIED BEANS, PEAS, AND LENTILS

(Count as 1 starch exchange, plus 1 very lean meat exchange.)

Beans and peas (garbanzo, pinto, kidney, white, split, black-eyed)	1/2 cup
Lima beans	2/3 cup
Lentils	1/2 cup
Miso*	3 Tbsp

STARCHY FOODS PREPARED WITH FAT

(Count as 1 starch exchange, plus 1 fat exchange.)

Biscuit, 2 1/2 in. across	1
Chow mein noodles	1/2 cup
Corn bread, 2 in. cube	1 (2 oz)
Crackers, round butter type	6
Croutons	1 cup
French-fried potatoes	16–25 (3 oz)
Granola	1/4 cup
Muffin, small	1 (1 1/2 oz)
Pancake, 4 in. across	2
Popcorn, microwave	3 cups
Sandwich crackers, cheese or peanut butter filling	3
Stuffing, bread (prepared)	1/3 cup
Taco shell, 6 in. across	2
Waffle, 4 1/2 in. square	1
Whole-wheat crackers, fat added	4–6 (1 oz)

FRUIT LIST

One fruit exchange equals 15 grams carbohydrate and 60 calories. The weight includes skin, core, seeds, and rind.

FRUIT

Apple, unpeeled, small	1 (4 oz)
Applesauce, unsweetened	1/2 cup
Apples, dried	4 rings
Apricots, fresh	4 whole (5 1/2 oz)
Apricots, dried	8 halves
Apricots, canned	1/2 cup
Banana, small	1 (4 oz)
Blackberries	3/4 cup
Blueberries	3/4 cup
Cantaloupe, small	1/3 melon (11 oz) or 1 cup cubes
Cherries, sweet, fresh	12 (3 oz)
Cherries, sweet, canned	1/2 cup
Dates	3
Figs, fresh	1 1/2 large or 2 medium (3 1/2 oz)
Figs, dried	1 1/2
Fruit cocktail	1/2 cup
Grapefruit, large	1/2 (11 oz)
Grapefruit sections, canned	3/4 cup
Grapes, small	17 (3 oz)
Honeydew melon	1 slice (10 oz) or 1 cup cubes
Kiwi	1 (3 1/2 oz)
Mandarin oranges, canned	3/4 cup
Mango, small	1/2 fruit (5 1/2 oz) or 1/2 cup
Nectarine, small	1 (5 oz)
Orange, small	1 (6 1/2 oz)
Papaya	1/2 fruit (8 oz) or 1 cup cubes
Peach, medium, fresh	1 (6 oz)
Peaches, canned	1/2 cup
Pear, large, fresh	1/2 (4 oz)
Pears, canned	1/2 cup
Pineapple, fresh	3/4 cup
Pineapple, canned	1/2 cup
Plums, small	2 (5 oz)
Plums, canned	1/2 cup
Prunes, dried	3
Raisins	2 Tbsp
Raspberries	1 cup
Strawberries	1 1/4 cup whole berries
Tangerines, small	2 (8 oz)
Watermelon	1 slice (13 1/2 oz) or 1 1/4 cup cubes

(Continued)

DISPLAY 22-6 EXCHANGE LISTS FOR MEAL PLANNING *(Continued)*

FRUIT JUICE

Apple juice/cider	1/2 cup	Grape juice	1/3 cup
Cranberry juice cocktail	1/3 cup	Grapefruit juice	1/2 cup
Cranberry juice cocktail, reduced-calorie	1 cup	Orange juice	1/2 cup
Fruit juice blends, 100% juice	1/3 cup	Pineapple juice	1/2 cup
		Prune juice	1/3 cup

MILK LIST

One milk exchange equals 12 grams carbohydrate and 8 grams protein.

SKIM AND VERY LOW-FAT MILK (0–3 GRAMS FAT PER SERVING)

Skim milk	1 cup	Plain nonfat yogurt	3/4 cup
1/2% milk	1 cup	Nonfat or low-fat fruit-flavored yogurt sweetened with aspartame or with a nonnutritive sweetener	1 cup
1% milk	1 cup		
Nonfat or low-fat buttermilk	1 cup		
Evaporated skim milk	1/2 cup		
Nonfat dry milk	1/3 cup dry		

LOW-FAT (5 GRAMS FAT PER SERVING)

2% milk	1 cup	Sweet acidophilus milk	1 cup
Plain low-fat yogurt	3/4 cup		

WHOLE MILK (8 GRAMS FAT PER SERVING)

Whole milk	1 cup	Goat's milk	1 cup
Evaporated whole milk	1/2 cup	Kefir	1 cup

OTHER CARBOHYDRATES LIST

One exchange equals 15 grams carbohydrate, or 1 starch, or 1 fruit, or 1 milk.

FOOD	SERVING SIZE	EXCHANGES PER SERVING
Angel food cake, unfrosted	1/12th cake	2 carbohydrates
Brownie, small, unfrosted	2 in. square	1 carbohydrate, 1 fat
Cake, unfrosted	2 in. square	1 carbohydrate, 1 fat
Cake, frosted	2 in. square	2 carbohydrates, 1 fat
Cookie, fat-free	2 small	1 carbohydrate
Cookie or sandwich cookie with creme filling	2 small	1 carbohydrate, 1 fat
Cupcake, frosted	1 small	2 carbohydrates, 1 fat
Cranberry sauce, jellied	1/4 cup	2 carbohydrates
Doughnut, plain cake	1 medium (1 1/2 oz)	1 1/2 carbohydrates, 2 fats
Doughnut, glazed	3 3/4 in. across (2 oz)	2 carbohydrates, 2 fats
Fruit juice bars, frozen, 100% juice	1 bar (3 oz)	1 carbohydrate
Fruit snacks, chewy (pureed fruit concentrate)	1 roll (3/4 oz)	1 carbohydrate

(Continued)

DISPLAY 22-6 EXCHANGE LISTS FOR MEAL PLANNING *(Continued)*

FOOD	SERVING SIZE	EXCHANGES PER SERVING
Fruit spreads, 100% fruit	1 Tbsp	1 carbohydrate
Gelatin, regular	1/2 cup	1 carbohydrate
Gingersnaps	3	1 carbohydrate
Granola bar	1 bar	1 carbohydrate, 1 fat
Granola bar, fat-free	1 bar	2 carbohydrates
Hummus	1/3 cup	1 carbohydrate, 1 fat
Ice cream	1/2 cup	1 carbohydrate, 2 fats
Ice cream, light	1/2 cup	1 carbohydrate, 1 fat
Ice cream, fat-free, no sugar added	1/2 cup	1 carbohydrate
Jam or jelly, regular	1 Tbsp	1 carbohydrate
Milk, chocolate, whole	1 cup	2 carbohydrates, 1 fat
Pie, fruit, 2 crusts	1/6 pie	3 carbohydrates, 2 fats
Pie, pumpkin or custard	1/8 pie	1 carbohydrate, 2 fats
Potato chips	12–18 (1 oz)	1 carbohydrate, 2 fats
Pudding, regular (made with low-fat milk)	1/2 cup	2 carbohydrates
Pudding, sugar-free (made with low-fat milk)	1/2 cup	1 carbohydrate
Salad dressing, fat-free*	1/4 cup	1 carbohydrate
Sherbet, sorbet	1/2 cup	2 carbohydrates
Spaghetti or pasta sauce, canned*	1/2 cup	1 carbohydrate, 1 fat
Sweet roll or Danish	1 (2 1/2 oz)	2 1/2 carbohydrates, 2 fats
Syrup, light	2 Tbsp	1 carbohydrate
Syrup, regular	1 Tbsp	1 carbohydrate
Syrup, regular	1/4 cup	4 carbohydrates
Tortilla chips	6–12 (1 oz)	1 carbohydrate, 2 fats
Yogurt, frozen, low-fat, fat-free	1/3 cup	1 carbohydrate, 0–1 fat
Yogurt, frozen, fat-free, no sugar added	1/2 cup	1 carbohydrate
Yogurt, low-fat with fruit	1 cup	3 carbohydrates, 0–1 fat
Vanilla wafers	5	1 carbohydrate, 1 fat

VEGETABLE LIST†

One vegetable exchange equals 5 grams carbohydrate, 2 grams protein, 0 grams fat, and 25 calories.

Artichoke
Artichoke hearts
Asparagus
Beans (green, wax, Italian)
Bean sprouts
Beets
Broccoli
Brussels sprouts
Cabbage
Carrots
Cauliflower
Celery
Cucumber
Eggplant
Green onions or scallions
Greens (collard, kale, mustard, turnip)
Kohlrabi
Leeks
Mixed vegetables (without corn, peas, or pasta)
Mushrooms
Okra
Onions
Pea pods
Peppers (all varieties)
Radishes
Salad greens (endive, escarole, lettuce, romaine, spinach)
Sauerkraut*
Spinach
Summer squash
Tomato
Tomatoes, canned
Tomato sauce*
Tomato/vegetable juice*
Turnips
Water chestnuts
Watercress
Zucchini

* = 400 mg or more sodium per exchange.

† = 1 exchange is 1/2 cup cooked vegetables or vegetable juice or 1 cup raw vegetables.

(Continued)

DISPLAY 22-6 EXCHANGE LISTS FOR MEAL PLANNING *(Continued)*

MEAT AND MEAT SUBSTITUTES LIST

VERY LEAN MEAT AND SUBSTITUTES LIST

One exchange equals 0 grams carbohydrate, 7 grams protein, 3 grams fat, and 55 calories. One very lean meat exchange is equal to any one of the following items:

Poultry: Chicken or turkey (white meat, no skin), Cornish hen (no skin)	1 oz
Fish: Fresh or frozen cod, flounder, haddock, halibut, trout; tuna fresh or canned water	1 oz
Shellfish: Clams, crab, lobster, scallops, shrimp, imitation shellfish	1 oz
Game: Duck or pheasant (no skin), venison, buffalo, ostrich	1 oz
Cheese with 1 gram or less fat per ounce:	
Nonfat or low-fat cottage cheese	¼ cup
Fat-free cheese	1 oz
Other: Processed sandwich meats with 1 gram or less fat per ounce, such as deli thin, shaved meats, chipped beef*, turkey ham	1 oz
Egg whites	2
Egg substitutes, plain	¼ cup
Hot dogs with 1 gram or less fat per ounce*	1 oz
Kidney (high in cholesterol)	1 oz
Sausage with 1 gram or less fat per ounce	1 oz

Count as one very lean meat and one starch exchange.

Dried beans, peas, lentils (cooked)	½ cup

* = 400 mg or more sodium per exchange.

LEAN MEAT AND SUBSTITUTES LIST

One exchange equals 0 grams carbohydrate, 7 grams protein, 3 grams fat, and 55 calories.
One lean meat exchange is equal to any one of the following items:

Beef: USDA Select or Choice grades of lean beef trimmed of fat, such as round, sirloin, and flank steak; tenderloin; roast (rib, chuck, rump); steak (T-bone, porterhouse, cubed), ground round	1 oz
Pork: Lean pork, such as fresh ham; canned, cured, or boiled ham; Canadian bacon*; tenderloin, center loin chop	1 oz
Lamb: Roast, chop, leg	1 oz
Veal: Lean chop, roast	1 oz
Poultry: Chicken, turkey (dark meat, no skin), chicken white meat (with skin), domestic duck or goose (well-drained of fat, no skin)	1 oz
Fish:	
Herring (uncreamed or smoked)	1 oz
Oysters	6 medium
Salmon (fresh or canned), catfish	1 oz
Sardines (canned)	2 medium
Tuna (canned in oil, drained)	1 oz
Game: Goose (no skin), rabbit	1 oz
Cheese:	
4.5%-fat cottage cheese	¼ cup

(Continued)

DISPLAY 22-6 EXCHANGE LISTS FOR MEAL PLANNING *(Continued)*

Grated Parmesan	2 Tbsp
Cheeses with 3 grams or less fat per ounce	1 oz
Other:	
Hot dogs with 3 grams or less fat per ounce*	1 ½ oz
Processed sandwich meat with 3 grams or less fat per ounce, such as turkey pastrami or kielbasa	1 oz
Liver, heart (high in cholesterol)	1 oz

MEDIUM-FAT MEAT AND SUBSTITUTES LIST

One exchange equals 0 grams carbohydrate, 7 grams protein, 5 grams fat, and 75 calories. One medium-fat meat exchange is equal to any one of the following items:

Beef: Most beef products fall into this category (ground beef, meatloaf, corned beef, short ribs, Prime grades of meat trimmed of fat, such as prime rib)	1 oz
Pork: Top loin, chop, Boston butt, cutlet	1 oz
Lamb: Rib roast, ground	1 oz
Veal: Cutlet (ground or cubed, unbreaded)	1 oz
Poultry: Chicken dark meat (with skin), ground turkey or ground chicken, fried chicken (with skin)	1 oz
Fish: Any fried fish product	1 oz
Cheese: With 5 grams or less fat per ounce	
Feta	1 oz
Mozzarella	1 oz
Ricotta	¼ cup (2 oz)
Other:	
Egg (high in cholesterol, limit to 3 per week)	1
Sausage with 5 grams or less fat per ounce	1 oz
Soy milk	1 cup
Tempeh	¼ cup
Tofu	4 oz or ½ cup

HIGH-FAT MEAT AND SUBSTITUTES LIST

One exchange equals 0 grams carbohydrate, 7 grams protein, 8 grams fat, and 100 calories.

Remember these items are high in saturated fat, cholesterol, and calories and may raise blood cholesterol levels if eaten on a regular basis. One high-fat meat exchange is equal to any one of the following items.

Pork: Spareribs, ground pork, pork sausage	1 oz
Cheese: All regular cheeses, such as American*, cheddar, Monterey jack, Swiss	1 oz
Other: Processed sandwich meats with 8 grams or less fat per ounce, such as bologna, pimento loaf, salami	1 oz
Sausage, such as bratwurst, Italian, knockwurst, Polish, smoked	1 oz
Hot dog (turkey or chicken)*	1 (10/lb)
Bacon	3 slices (20 slices/lb)

Count as one high-fat meat plus one fat exchange.

Hot dog (beef, pork, or combination)*	1 (10/lb)
Peanut butter (contains unsaturated fat)	2 Tbsp

* = 400 mg or more sodium per exchange.

(Continued)

DISPLAY 22-6 EXCHANGE LISTS FOR MEAL PLANNING *(Continued)*

FAT LIST

MONOUNSATURATED FATS LIST

One fat exchange equals 5 grams fat and 45 calories.

Avocado, medium	1/8 (1 oz)
Oil (canola, olive, peanut)	1 tsp
Olives: ripe (black)	8 large
green, stuffed*	10 large
Nuts	
almonds, cashews	6 nuts
mixed (50% peanuts)	6 nuts
peanuts	10 nuts
pecans	4 halves
Peanut butter, smooth or crunchy	2 tsp
Sesame seeds	1 Tbsp
Tahini paste	2 tsp

POLYUNSATURATED FATS LIST

One fat exchange equals 5 grams fat and 45 calories.

Margarine: stick, tub, or squeeze	1 tsp
lower-fat (30% to 50% vegetable oil)	1 Tbsp
Mayonnaise: regular	1 tsp
reduced-fat	1 Tbsp
Nuts, walnuts, English	4 halves
Oil (corn, safflower, soybean)	1 tsp
Salad dressing: regular*	1 Tbsp
reduced-fat	2 Tbsp
Miracle Whip Salad Dressing: regular	2 tsp
reduced-fat	1 Tbsp
Seeds: pumpkin, sunflower	1 Tbsp

* = 400 mg or more sodium per exchange.

SATURATED FATS LIST†

One fat exchange equals 5 grams of fat and 45 calories.

Bacon, cooked	1 slice (20 slices/lb)
Bacon, grease	1 tsp
Butter: stick	1 tsp
whipped	2 tsp
reduced-fat	1 Tbsp
Chitterlings, boiled	2 Tbsp (1/2 oz)
Coconut, sweetened, shredded	2 Tbsp
Cream, half and half	2 Tbsp
Cream cheese: regular	1 Tbsp (1/2 oz)
reduced-fat	2 Tbsp (1 oz)
Fatback or salt pork, see below‡	
Shortening or lard	1 tsp
Sour cream: regular	2 Tbsp
reduced-fat	3 Tbsp

† Saturated fats can raise blood cholesterol levels.

‡ Use a piece 1 in. × 1 in. × 1/4 in. if you plan to eat the fatback cooked with vegetables. Use a piece 2 in. × 1 in. × 1/2 in. when eating only the vegetables with the fatback removed.

(Continued)

DISPLAY 22-6 EXCHANGE LISTS FOR MEAL PLANNING *(Continued)*

FREE FOODS LIST

A *free food* is any food or drink that contains less than 20 calories or less than 5 grams of carbohydrate per serving. Foods with a serving size listed should be limited to three servings per day. Be sure to spread them out throughout the day. If you eat all three servings at one time, it could affect your blood glucose level. Food listed without a serving size can be eaten as often as you like.

FAT-FREE OR REDUCED-FAT FOODS

Cream cheese, fat-free	1 Tbsp
Creamers, nondairy, liquid	1 Tbsp
Creamers, nondairy, powdered	2 tsp
Mayonnaise, fat-free	1 Tbsp
Mayonnaise, reduced-fat	1 tsp
Margarine, fat-free	4 Tbsp
Margarine, reduced-fat	1 tsp
Miracle Whip®, nonfat	1 Tbsp
Miracle Whip®, reduced-fat	1 tsp
Nonstick cooking spray	
Salad dressing, fat-free	1 Tbsp
Salad dressing, fat-free, Italian	2 Tbsp
Salsa	$^1/_4$ cup
Sour cream, fat-free, reduced-fat	1 Tbsp
Whipped topping, regular or light	2 Tbsp

SUGAR-FREE OR LOW-SUGAR FOODS

Candy, hard, sugar-free	1 candy
Gelatin dessert, sugar-free	
Gelatin, unflavored	
Gum, sugar-free	
Jam or jelly, low-sugar or light	2 tsp
Sugar substitutes§	
Syrup, sugar-free	2 Tbsp

§ Sugar substitutes, alternatives, or replacements that are approved by the Food and Drug Administration (FDA) are safe to use. Common brand names include:

- Equal (aspartame)
- Sprinkle Sweet (saccharin)
- Sweet One (acesulfame K)
- Sweet-10 (saccharin)
- Sugar Twin (saccharin)
- Sweet 'n Low (saccharin)

DRINKS

Bouillon, broth, consomme*	
Bouillon or broth, low-sodium	
Carbonated or mineral water	
Cocoa powder, unsweetened	1 Tbsp
Coffee	
Club soda	
Diet soft drinks, sugar-free	
Drink mixes, sugar-free	
Tea	
Tonic water, sugar-free	

CONDIMENTS

Catsup	1 Tbsp
Horseradish	
Lemon juice	
Lime juice	
Mustard	
Pickles, dill*	1 $^1/_2$ large
Soy sauce, regular or light*	
Taco sauce	1 Tbsp
Vinegar	

(Continued)

DISPLAY 22-6 EXCHANGE LISTS FOR MEAL PLANNING *(Continued)*

SEASONINGS

Be careful with seasonings that contain sodium or are salts, such as garlic or celery salt, and lemon pepper.

Flavoring extracts
Garlic
Herbs, fresh or dried
Pimento
Spices
Tabasco or hot pepper sauce
Wine, used in cooking
Worcestershire sauce

* = 400 mg or more of sodium per choice.

COMBINATION FOODS LIST

Many of the foods we eat are mixed together in various combinations. These combination foods do not fit into any one exchange list. Often it is hard to tell what is in a casserole dish or baked food item. This is a list of exchanges for some typical combination foods. This list will help you fit these food meal plan. Ask your dietitian for information about any combination foods you would like to eat.

FOOD	SERVING SIZE	EXCHANGES PER SERVING
ENTREES		
Tuna noodle casserole, lasagna, spaghetti with meatballs, chili with beans, macaroni and cheese*	1 cup (8 oz)	2 carbohydrates, 2 medium-fat meats
Chow mein (without noodles or rice)	2 cups (16 oz)	1 carbohydrate, 2 lean meats
Pizza, cheese, thin crust*	1/4 of 10 in. (5 oz)	2 carbohydrates, 2 medium-fat meats, 1 fat
Pizza, meat topping, thin crust*	1/4 of 10 in. (5 oz)	2 carbohydrates, 2 medium-fat meats, 1 fat
Pizza, meat topping, thin crust*	1/4 of 10 in. (5 oz)	2 carbohydrates, 2 medium-fat meats, 2 fats
Pot pie*	1 (7 oz)	2 carbohydrates, 1 medium-fat meat, 4 fats
FROZEN ENTREES		
Salisbury steak with gravy, mashed potato*	1 (11 oz)	2 carbohydrates, 3 medium-fat meats, 3–4 fats
Turkey with gravy, mashed potato, dressing*	1 (11 oz)	2 carbohydrates, 2 medium-fat meats, 2 fats
Entree with less than 300 calories*	1 (8 oz)	2 carbohydrates, 3 lean meats
SOUPS		
Bean*	1 cup	1 carbohydrate, 1 very lean meat
Cream (made with water)*	1 cup (8 oz)	1 carbohydrate, 1 fat
Split pea (made with water)*	1/2 cup (4 oz)	1 carbohydrate
Tomato (made with water)*	1 cup (8 oz)	1 carbohydrate
Vegetable beef, chicken noodle, or other broth-type*	1 cup (8 oz)	1 carbohydrate

* = 400 mg or more sodium per exchange.

(Continued)

DISPLAY 22-6 EXCHANGE LISTS FOR MEAL PLANNING *(Continued)*

FAST FOODS†

FOOD	SERVING SIZE	EXCHANGES PER SERVING
Burritos with beef*	2	4 carbohydrates, 2 medium-fat meats, 2 fats
Chicken nuggets*	6	1 carbohydrate, 2 medium-fat meats, 1 fat
Chicken breast and wing, breaded and fried*	1 each	1 carbohydrate, 4 medium-fat meats, 2 fats
Fish sandwich/tartar sauce*	1	3 carbohydrates, 1 medium-fat meat, 3 fats
French fries, thin	20–25	2 carbohydrates, 2 fats
Hamburger, regular	1	2 carbohydrates, 2 medium-fat meats
Hamburger, large*	1	2 carbohydrates, 3 medium-fat meats, 1 fat
Hot dog with bun*	1	1 carbohydrate, 1 high-fat meat, 1 fat
Individual pan pizza*	1	5 carbohydrates, 3 medium-fat meats, 3 fats
Soft-serve cone	1 medium	2 carbohydrates, 1 fat
Submarine sandwich*	1 sub (6 in.)	3 carbohydrates, 1 vegetable, 2 medium-fat meats, 1 fat
Taco, hard shell*	1 (6 oz)	2 carbohydrates, 2 medium-fat meats, 2 fats
Taco, soft shell*	1 (3 oz)	1 carbohydrate, 1 medium-fat meat, 1 fat

* = 400 mg or more of sodium per serving.

† Ask at your fast-food restaurant for nutrition information about your favorite fast foods.

The Exchange Lists are the basis of a meal planning system designed by a committee of the American Diabetes Association and The American Dietetic Association. While designed primarily for people with diabetes and others who must follow special diets, the Exchange Lists are based on principles of good nutrition that apply to everyone.

dition to the various exchange lists of many of the fat-modified commercial food products that have flooded the market in recent years. These products include fat-free chips, fat-free or reduced fat cheeses, luncheon meats, salad dressings and margarines. Other important changes are the addition of vegetarian foods and fast foods to the exchange lists.

The Other Carbohydrates List shows the client how to exchange a food such as tortilla chips, fat-free frozen yogurt or chocolate milk for a starch, fruit, or milk exchange in their meal plan. The aim is to make meal planning more flexible. This supports the 1994 nutrition recommendations of the American Diabetes Association, which focus on the importance of the total carbohydrate in meal plans for people with diabetes rather than on the type of carbohydrate consumed. The grouping together of all the carbohydrate-containing exchange lists will also facilitate *carbohydrate counting,* an alternative method of meal planning being used in diabetes mellitus (discussed in Chapter 24).

In Exchange Lists for Meal Planning (Display 22-6)foods with a similar composition with respect to protein, fat, and carbohydrate are listed in various groups. One exchange represents an average serving of each food (e.g. 1 slice bread, 8 oz milk, 1 tsp margarine), except meat. One meat exchange represents 1 oz of meat or its protein equivalent (e.g. $^{1}/_{2}$ cup cooked dry beans).

When developing a meal plan for a certain caloric level or for a specific protein, fat, and carbohydrate composition, the dietitian frequently uses the nutrient values of the exchange lists given in

Table 22-1 on page 433. Anyone who has used food composition tables to calculate diets can readily see what a timesaver this method can be.

Descriptions of each of the exchange lists in Display 22-6 follows.

CARBOHYDRATE GROUP

STARCH LIST

The starch list is composed of cereals, grains, pasta, breads, crackers, snacks, starchy vegetables, and cooked dry beans, peas, and lentils. One starch exchange averages 15 g of carbohydrate, 3 g protein, 1 g of fat or less and 80 kcal. The client is encouraged to choose mostly those starches which are made with little fat and is cautioned to check the size of muffins and bagels, 1 oz being equivalent to 1 starch exchange. Muffins and bagels can be 2, 3, or 4 oz in size and, therefore, count as 2, 3, or 4 starch choices. Starch foods prepared with fat are listed separately within the exchange and count as one starch and one fat serving for a total of 125 kcal.

FRUIT LIST

Fresh, frozen, canned, and dried fruits and fruit juices are on the fruit list. Canned fruits on the list are based on those that are labeled unsweetened, no sugar added, or in extra-light syrup. Those fruits packed in extra-light syrup have the same amount of carbohydrate per serving as the other two packs. One fruit exchange is composed of 15 g carbohydrate and 60 kcal. Portion sizes are for the fruit and a small amount of juice. Whole fruit is suggested as a better choice than juice.

MILK LIST

One milk exchange equals 8 fluid ounces and contains 12 g carbohydrate and 8 g protein. Milk exchanges are divided according to their fat content: skim or very low fat, 0-3 g fat, 90 kcal-100 kcal per serving; low fat, 5 g fat, 120 kcal per serving; and whole milk, 8 g fat, 150 kcal per serving. The client is encouraged to use lower fat varieties.

Dry milk, yogurt, and evaporated milk are additional choices in the milk list. (Rice milk is listed on the Starch List and soy milk is listed on the Medium-fat Meat List.)

OTHER CARBOHYDRATES LIST

This lists cakes, cookies, pudding, syrups, jelly, snack chips, frozen desserts, and other desserts and snacks that have added sugar or fat. Chocolate milk, canned spaghetti sauce, and fat-free salad dressings are also on this list. One exchange contains 15 g of carbohydrate and can be substituted for a starch, fruit, or milk exchange. Some foods on this list also count as one or more fat choices. The client is advised that the foods on this list are not as nutritious as choices on the Starch, Fruit, or Milk list, and, if chosen should be part of a balanced meal. Portion sizes of foods on the Other Carbohydrates List may be very small because many of the foods are concentrated sources of carbohydrate and fat. The client is referred to the Nutrition Facts panel on the food label as the most accurate source of information regarding the carbohydrate and fat content of a specific commercial product.

VEGETABLE LIST

Those vegetables containing small amounts of carbohydrates and calories, averaging 5 g carbohydrate, 2 g protein, and 25 kcal per ½ cup cooked or as vegetable juice or 1 cup raw vegetable are on this list. One or two vegetable choices may be eaten at a meal without counting their carbohydrate or caloric content, because only small amounts of carbohydrate are involved. Starchy vegetables such as corn, peas, and potatoes are found in the Starch List.

MEAT AND MEAT SUBSTITUTE GROUP

The lists in this group are divided according to fat content to inform the client of the fat and caloric content of protein foods and to encourage the use of choices from the very lean and lean meat lists. In general, one meat exchange consist of 1 oz meat, fish, poultry or cheese or ½ cup cooked dry beans. Meat substitutes listed include eggs; egg substitutes;

dry cooked beans, peas, lentils; tofu, tempeh, and soy milk; and peanut butter.

VERY LEAN MEAT AND SUBSTITUTES LIST

The foods on this list average 7 g protein, 0–1 g fat, and 35 kcal per ounce. In addition to white meat poultry (no skin), fish, shellfish, and game, the following meat substitutes are listed: nonfat and low-fat cottage cheese, fat-free cheese, egg whites, plain egg substitutes, and cooked dry peas, beans and lentils.

LEAN MEAT AND SUBSTITUTES LIST

One lean meat exchange averages 7 g protein, 3 g fat, and 55 kcal. This list contains lean, trimmed cuts of beef, pork, lamb, and veal; poultry; fish and game; and hot dogs and processed sandwich meats with 3 g or less fat per ounce. Also included are cheeses with 3 g fat or less per ounce, small amounts of grated parmesan (2 tbsp), and 4.5% cottage cheese.

MEDIUM-FAT MEAT AND SUBSTITUTES LIST

The foods on this list average 7 g protein, 5 g fat, and 75 kcal per ounce. Medium-fat cuts of beef, pork, lamb, veal, and poultry and fried fish products are listed. Cheese with 5 g or less fat per ounce, eggs, soy milk, tempeh, and tofu are also on this list. The client is advised to limit eggs to 3 per week.

HIGH-FAT MEAT AND SUBSTITUTES LIST

The client is advised to limit choices from this list to 3 times per week or less because these items are high in saturated fat, cholesterol, and calories and may raise serum cholesterol if eaten on a regular basis. One exchange from this list averages 7 g protein, 8 g fat, and 100 calories. This list includes fatty cuts of pork, regular cheeses (e.g. American, cheddar, Swiss, Monterey jack), processed sandwich meats, and turkey or chicken hot dogs. Beef, pork, and combination hot dogs and peanut butter (contains unsaturated fat) count as one high fat meat plus one fat exchange.

FAT GROUP

FAT LIST

Fats are divided into three groups: monounsaturated, polyunsaturated, and saturated. One fat exchange, regardless of the kind of fat, contains 5 g fat and 45 kcal. Typically, one fat exchange is 1 tsp regular margarine or vegetable oil or 1 tbsp of regular salad dressings. The client is advised that saturated fats are linked to heart disease and cancer.

OTHER LISTS

FREE FOODS LIST

Exchange Lists for Meal planning provides a list of free foods. A free food is any food that contains less than 20 kcal per serving. Some foods on the list have insignificant calories, such as sugar-free carbonated drinks, and may be used as desired. Foods that are almost 20 kcal per serving, such as ketchup or low-calorie salad dressing, are limited to three servings per day.

This list includes fat-free or reduced fat creamers, salad dressings, toppings and margarines; condiments, seasonings, and sugar substitutes. Also included are some sugar-free products such as candy, gelatin dessert, jam, jelly, and beverages.

COMBINATION FOODS LIST

Average values are given for a typical combination or mixed foods that fit into more than one category or exchange list. These foods include homemade casseroles, pizza, chili, macaroni and cheese, soups, frozen entrees, and fast foods.

In addition to those given with the Exchange List, exchange equivalents are available from fast-food restaurants and food manufacturing companies. Exchange values of recipes also appear in cookbooks for people with diabetes and in some low-calorie cookbooks.

USING NUTRITION LABELS WITH EXCHANGE LISTS

Nutrition labels are especially helpful to people on controlled-calorie or diabetic meal planning. They indicate the number of calories and amount of protein, fat, and carbohydrate in one serving of food. This information can be compared with exchange lists; by estimating how many exchanges are represented in a serving of food, it is possible to include that food in the meal plan.

COUNTING CALORIES WITH EXCHANGE LISTS

The exchange list system provides a quick way of estimating the caloric content of a diet. Using the calories for each of the exchanges, summarized in Table 22-1, the health care worker can estimate the calories in the basic foods in the diet. The caloric value of 90% of the processed foods on the market can be determined using the nutrition labels. A calorie counting book may be useful for caloric values of combination dishes, fast foods, and restaurant foods.

ESTIMATING PORTION SIZES

When a diet involves the control of calories or specific nutrients, such as fats or sodium, accurate estimation of portion sizes is important to achievement of treatment goals. A "bowl of cereal" or a "glass of milk" is an inaccurate description of portion size. Each food should be estimated in terms of standard household measures, such as 3 oz of meat, $^1/_2$ cup of applesauce, or 1 tsp of margarine. The client must learn how to estimate portions accurately. It generally is recommended that the client measure all foods for 1 week or so and then measure them periodically thereafter.

All measures are based on standard measuring cups and spoons and are level measure. Liquids and some solid foods (e.g., cottage cheese and canned fruits) can be measured with a measuring cup. Measuring spoons are used for measuring margarine, oil, salad dressings, peanut butter, and other foods used in small amounts. A scale is useful for measuring meat, fish, or poultry and some starch exchanges such as French and Italian bread, bagels, and pretzels.

Clients should weigh or measure all food after cooking unless the food is eaten uncooked, such as fruit or raw vegatables. Some foods, such as meats, weigh less after cooking; starches increase in volume after cooking.

KEYS TO PRACTICAL APPLICATION

Be aware that there usually are a variety of ways to achieve a nutrition-related goal. Suit the approach to the client; give him or her a choice.

Think of ways to reinforce the nutrition education you provide, such as using pictures, posters, and food labels.

Give your client a take-home written or printed summary of the information and concepts you have presented.

Encourage your clients to persevere in their efforts to keep food and exercise records—they are important tools for changing behavior.

Be aware of your clients' literacy levels—try to find or develop your own appropriate teaching aids.

Remember that handing a client a diet sheet is not diet counseling.

Study the lists in *Exchange Lists for Meal Planning* (Display 22-6) carefully. You will undoubtedly encounter the use of exchange lists many times.

You may need to help clients make menu selections that fit into their meal pattern.

Study the nutrition labeling regulations so that you can use food labels effectively in nutrition education (See Ch. 5).

Reinforce the need for clients to portion foods accurately, as specified in their meal plan. Check to see that clients understand the use of standard measure.

KEY IDEAS

Diet counseling involves adapting information about nutritional needs and the nutrition therapy itself to the client's lifestyle. It also means providing information and influencing eating behavior with an approach that suits the client's educational level and personality.

There are usually a variety of different approaches to achieving a particular goal.

Teaching aids reinforce the education and counseling provided to the client.

Teaching aids need to be modified to reach low-literacy clients.

Client-kept records help maintain awareness of eating and exercise behavior.

The exchange system simplifies meal planning and provides clients on a modified diet with a wide choice of foods. Foods with similar composition with respect to the nutrients being controlled are grouped into various lists. A food within a list may be exchanged for any other food within the same list.

In the exchange system used in diabetic and calorie-controlled meal planning, foods with similar protein, fat, carbohydrate, and energy compositions are grouped in various lists.

Accurate portion sizes are extremely important when calories or other nutrients are to be carefully controlled. Measuring food for the first week or so and then periodically thereafter provides good training.

Food labels can be used to budget or count total calories or target nutrients, determine good sources of nutrients and fiber, and compare the nutrient content of foods.

KEYS TO LEARNING

STUDY–DISCUSSION QUESTIONS

1. As a class, prepare a notebook of teaching aids used in nutrition education and counseling in your hospital. Classify these materials based on the type of nutrient being modified or the condition being treated.
2. Develop one teaching aid of your own that could be used to reinforce or illustrate the concepts of a particular aspect of nutrition therapy (e.g. sodium control, fat control).
3. Keep a food record for 2 days. Count the calories of all the foods and beverages you have eaten using exchange list values and food label information. What were the advantages of this exercise? What difficulties did you encounter?
4. The following food exchanges represent the total amount of food permitted on a particular diet for 1 day: seven starch exchanges, six lean meat exchanges, two vegetable exchanges, three fruit exchanges, two skim milk exchanges, five fat exchanges. Using the food values given for the exchange lists in Table 22-1, determine the amount of protein, fat, and carbohydrate and the number of calories the diet contains. Divide these exchanges into three meals. Using the exchange lists in Display 22-6, provide a menu for each meal. Be sure to include the amount of each food permitted.

BIBLIOGRAPHY

BOOKS AND PAMPHLETS

American Diabetes Association/ American Dietetic Association. Exchange lists for meal planning. Rev. ed. Alexandria, VA: American Diabetes Association; Chicago: American Dietetic Association, 1995.

American Diabetes Association/ American Dietetic Association. Healthy food choices. Alexandria, VA: American Diabetes Association; Chicago: American Dietetic Association, 1986.

Barry B, Castle G. Carbohydrate counting: adding flexibility to your food choices. Minneapolis: International Diabetes Center, 1994.

Doak CC, Doak LG. Teaching patients with low literacy skills. Philadelphia: JB Lippincott, 1985.

PERIODICALS

Busselman KM, Holcomb CA. Reading skill and comprehension of the Dietary Guidelines by WIC participants. J Am Diet Assoc 1994;94:622.

Doak CC, Doak LG. The literacy challenge in diabetes education: "so that clients may understand." On the Cutting Edge 1993;14:2:9.

Hartman W, Jacobs N. Keeping records: a challenge for clinicians and clients. Weight Control Digest 1991;1:5:75.

Maryniuk MD. Being creative. On the Cutting Edge 1990;11:2:2.

McCarthy P. Innovative nutrition education approaches to reach persons with low-literacy skills, 1993. On the Cutting Edge. 1993;14:2:13.

Plimptom S, Root J. Materials and strategies that work in low literacy health communication. Public Health Reports 1994;109:86.

Reeves RS, Bolton MP. Fat budgeting: a useful alternative. Weight Control Digest 1991;1:7:110.

Ruud J, Betts NM, Dirkx J. Developing written nutrition information for adults with low literacy skills. J Nutr Educ 1993;25:1:11.

Stehlin D. A little "lite" reading. FDA Consumer (Special Report: Focus on Food Labeling), May 1993. DHHS publication FDA 93-2262:29

Trenkner LL, Achterberg CL. Use of focus groups in evaluating nutrition education materials. J Am Diet Assoc 1991;91:1577.

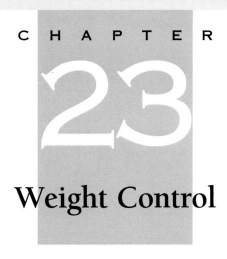

CHAPTER 23

Weight Control

KEY TERMS

adipose tissue fatty tissue
android having male characteristics
apnea temporary suspension of respiration
behavior modification a teaching technique in which learned habits are changed
gross obesity extreme fatness up to two to three times the ideal weight
gynecoid having female characteristics
restrained kept in check, held down

OBJECTIVES

After completing this chapter, the student will be able to:

1. Discuss the complex nature of the causes of obesity and its treatment.
2. Appreciate the baseless nature of discrimination against persons who are obese and verbalize the health worker's role in helping the client develop a more positive self-image.
3. Describe the benefits and the adverse effects of weight loss.
4. Discuss the impact of America's obsession with thinness on physical and mental health. Describe the hazards of weight loss efforts among people of healthy weight.
5. Discuss the basis for changes that are evolving in the treatment of obesity.
6. Describe each of the following components in the traditional treatment of obesity: diet, exercise, behavior modification, drugs, and surgery.
7. Give examples of the lure and fallacy of novelty diets and the clues to fraudulent claims.
8. Describe three components of a weight control program that focuses on positive health habits.
9. State the essential characteristics of binge eating disorder.
10. Give five guidelines for promoting weight gain in underweight people.

Probably no other aspect of health is as much a topic of conversation as weight. At any one time, an estimated 50% of adult women and 25% of adult men are trying to lose weight. Sadly, the number of people dieting is far greater than the number classified as obese. This is especially true among adolescent girls, many of whom are dieting even though they are at or below a normal weight. Although obesity in the United States is much more prevalent than underweight, both represent malnutrition and both can have far-reaching effects on physical and mental health.

Weight control is a matter of balancing the energy value of foods eaten with the body's energy needs. When more calories are provided than are needed, the extra energy is stored as fat (positive energy balance). When caloric intake is less than is needed, the body uses up stored fat, and weight is lost (negative energy balance). When all fat deposits are used up, muscle and other body tissues are drawn on for energy.

One pound of body fat represents about 3500 kcal. Consumption of an excess of only 100 kcal/day means an excess of 3000 kcal/month, or 10 lb/year (and 20 to 30 lb in 2 or 3 years). This 100 kcal can be supplied by 2 tbsp of sugar, one large creme-filled cookie, 2 tsp of butter or margarine, or 2 tbsp of jelly. Many people become obese not by eating huge amounts of food but by eating small amounts of extra food over a period of years.

Although the basic cause is an imbalance between energy intake and energy expenditure, why this occurs is not well understood. In recent years, it has become evident that overweight is not simply a matter of will power, but a complex disorder involving many factors. A discussion of childhood obesity can be found in Chapter 18.

DEFINING OBESITY

One fourth to one third of adults in the United States are classified as being overweight, depending on the definition of overweight being used. The highest rates are found among women, poor people, and some ethnic groups. The prevalence of obesity increases with age.

Stunkard, an authority in the field of obesity, classified obesity as follows: mild obesity, 20% to 40% overweight; moderate obesity, 41% to 100% overweight; and severe obesity, greater than 100% overweight. The terms *obesity* and *overweight* frequently are used interchangeably. Although in a strict sense *overweight* refers to excessive weight for height and *obesity* is the excessive accumulation of adipose tissue, most individuals who are overweight have accumulated excess fat. On rare occasions, we may encounter individuals who may be overweight without being overfat—for example, an athlete who has above-average muscular development.

There are several ways of measuring body fat. The skinfold thickness test provides a useful means of determining degree of fatness or leanness because more than half of body fat is deposited under the skin (see Chapter 2). The amount and distribution of fat changes with age and differs by sex. Because the way in which fat is distributed differs even among adults of the same sex, some authorities feel that a sum of four skinfolds (biceps, triceps, subscapular, and suprailiac) will better reflect total body fat.

A more recent method of assessing body fat involves computerized instruments that detect interactive light waves. In research, various other methods including underwater weighing may be used to assess body fat.

BODY MASS INDEX VERSUS HEIGHT–WEIGHT TABLES

What constitutes "ideal" or "desirable" weight is controversial. For years, life insurance height–weight tables were the standard for determining ideal weight for height. The height–weight table of the Metropolitan Life Insurance Company (see Appendix) gives those weights associated with the lowest mortality rate. Data from 25 insurance companies representing 4 million individuals were used in developing the tables. The weights in the Metropolitan Life tables are no longer labeled *desirable* or *ideal.* See Displays 2-1 and 2-2 for methods for estimating body frame size.

Body mass index (BMI) is currently a widely used means of assessing body weight. The BMI is derived by dividing the individual's weight in kilograms by height in meters squared. This formula corresponds well with body fat percentage. Display 23-1 gives formulas for determining the BMI using both kilograms and meters and pounds and inches. Table 23-1 gives the BMI for people of various heights and weights. Suggested desirable BMI ranges extend from 19 to 27 for adults through middle age. People with a BMI of 28 to 30 or higher are classified as overweight or obese (Table 23-2).

After studying the research on the effect of body weight on health and mortality, the National Academy

DISPLAY 23-1 CALCULATING BMI

Example: Calculate the BMI for an individual with a weight of 150 lb and height of 62 inches.

Using the metric system, calculate as follows:

$$\text{BMI} = \frac{\text{Weight in kilograms}}{\text{Height in meters squared}}$$

$$\text{BMI} = \frac{150 \text{ lb} \div 2.2^{*}}{(62 \text{ in} \div 39.37)^{2}\dagger} = \frac{68}{2.46} = 27.6$$

Using pounds and inches, calculate as follows:

$$\text{BMI} = \frac{\text{Weight in pounds}}{\text{Height in inches squared}} \times 705$$

$$\text{BMI} = \frac{150}{3844} \times 705 = .039 \times 705 = 27.5$$

(Conversion formula developed by Stensland and Margolis: Stensland SH, Margolis S. Simplifying the calculation of body mass index for quick reference. J Am Diet Assoc 1990;90:856.)

* 1 kg = 2.2 lb. To convert pounds to kilograms, divide by 2.2.

† 1 m = 39.37 in. To convert inches to meters, divide by 39.37.

of Sciences Committee on Diet and Health has concluded that people can be somewhat heavier as they grow older without an adverse effect on health. The Dietary Guidelines Advisory Committee on the Dietary Guidelines for Americans, 1995 has rejected this concept. Their report states: "The health risks due to excess weight appear to be the same for older as for younger adults." Most adults should not gain weight as they grow older. Acceptable weight ranges for adults are given in Table 14-2. The Advisory Committee also recommends that maintaining weight is equally important for older people, who tend to lose weight as they age. Since some of this weight loss is due to muscle loss, maintaining muscle tissue through regular activity is stressed.

OBESITY AND HEALTH

The complications of obesity have long been associated with a shortened life span. It is now apparent that the relationship between weight and mortality differs at various times of life and also differs depending on the cause of death. Generally speaking, there is a relationship between obesity and mortality at a young age and no such relationship at an older age. As people grow older, risk factors other than obesity have increased importance. New research has indicated that the adverse effects of obesity occur at much higher weights than was previously thought.

Obesity is associated with elevated serum cholesterol, hypertension, and non–insulin-dependent diabetes mellitus (type II). Excessive weight also increases risk for gallbladder disease, gout, coronary heart disease, and some types of cancer and has been implicated in the development of osteoarthritis of the weight-bearing joints. Grossly obese people are poor risks for surgery because their reactions to anesthesia are impaired and they heal slowly. Often, obese people have accompanying psychological and social problems, although it may be difficult to determine whether these are the cause or effect of obesity.

BODY FAT DISTRIBUTION

Where body fat is deposited in the body seems to strongly influence the medical complications of obesity. Increased fat in the upper body or abdominal area, called *android* (male-like) or *apple-shaped obesity,* appears to carry an increased risk of chronic diseases. In contrast, increased fat in the hips and thighs, called *gynecoid* (female-like) or *pear-shaped obesity,* is not associated with increased risk (Fig. 23-1). Upper-body obesity can be determined by dividing the waist measurement by the hip measurement. A number higher than 0.95 for men and 0.80 for women indicates increased risk.

BENEFITS OF WEIGHT LOSS

Weight loss reduces the severity of type II diabetes and hypertension. In fact, diet and exercise programs leading to weight loss can prevent the onset of type II diabetes and hypertension. Weight loss also improves blood lipids, lipoprotein levels, sleep apnea and, in very obese people, weight loss in-

TABLE 23-1 Body Weights in Pounds According to Height and BMI*

Height (in)	Body Mass Index (kg/m^2)													
	19	20	21	22	23	24	25	26	27	28	29	30	35	40
	Body Weight (lb)													
58	91	96	100	105	110	115	119	124	129	134	138	143	167	191
59	94	99	104	109	114	119	124	128	133	138	143	148	173	198
60	97	102	107	112	118	123	128	133	138	143	148	153	179	204
61	100	106	111	116	122	127	132	137	143	148	153	158	185	211
62	104	109	115	120	126	131	136	142	147	153	158	164	191	218
63	107	113	118	124	130	135	141	146	152	158	163	169	197	225
64	110	116	122	128	134	140	145	151	157	163	169	174	204	232
65	114	120	126	132	138	144	150	156	162	168	174	180	210	240
66	118	124	130	136	142	148	155	161	167	173	179	186	216	247
67	121	127	134	140	146	153	159	166	172	178	185	191	223	255
68	125	131	138	144	151	158	164	171	177	184	190	197	230	262
69	128	135	142	149	155	162	169	176	182	189	196	203	236	270
70	132	139	146	153	160	167	174	181	188	195	202	207	243	278
71	136	143	150	157	165	172	179	186	193	200	208	215	250	286
72	140	147	154	162	169	177	184	191	199	206	213	221	258	294
73	144	151	159	166	174	182	189	197	204	212	219	227	265	302
74	148	155	163	171	179	186	194	202	210	218	225	233	272	311
75	152	160	168	176	184	192	200	208	216	224	232	240	279	319
76	156	164	172	180	189	197	205	213	221	230	238	246	287	328

* Each entry gives the body weight in pounds (lb) for a person of a given height and BMI. Pounds have been rounded off. To use the table, find the appropriate height in the left hand column. Move across the row to a given weight. The number at the top of the column is the BMI for the height and weight.

(Bray GA, Gray DS. Obesity. Part 1: pathogenesis. West J Med 1988;149:429–441.)

creases the ability to function, reduces absenteeism, and improves social interaction.

ADVERSE EFFECTS OF WEIGHT LOSS

Very low-calorie diets are associated with a number of adverse effects (see the section Very Low-Calorie Diets). Changes in the composition of the commercial formulas being used have largely eliminated these short-term complications, although little is known about the long-term effects of these diets. A serious complication of severe calorie restriction is the increased risk for gallstones and acute gallbladder disease.

Weight cycling (repeated weight loss and regain) has been associated with increased risk of disease and premature death. Studies on this subject have produced conflicting results. Weight cycling may initially result in a fast regaining of weight; how-

TABLE 23-2 Assessment of Body Weight Using BMI

Category	BMI
Normal	19–27
Overweight	28–30
Obese	30–40
Morbidly obese	>40

ever, the long-term effects on mental and physical health are unknown. Although even moderate weight loss leads to the loss of muscle tissue, severe calorie restriction (less than 1200 kcal) can result in excessive loss of lean body mass.

Depression tends to decrease in obese people who lose weight, but returns when weight is regained, which occurs in most cases. Self-esteem, self-confidence, and the general level of happiness are poorly affected by weight regain. Some evidence has indicated that women who are mildly or moderately overweight and who are dieting are at risk for binge eating (bulimia) without vomiting or purging. Whether well-designed weight control programs increase the risk of bulimia is unknown. Another concern is the wide use of over-the-counter weight-reducing drugs by adolescents and young adults because the long-term safety of this practice is unknown.

PEOPLE OF NORMAL WEIGHT TRYING TO LOSE WEIGHT

Many Americans who are not overweight, particularly young women, are trying to lose weight for reasons of appearance, fitness, or self-image. This practice should be discouraged because it can have adverse physical and psychological consequences. These adverse effects include poor nutrition, weight cycling, and possible development of eating disorders and other serious psychological consequences due to repeated failed attempts to lose weight.

INDICATIONS FOR WEIGHT LOSS

Weight loss is indicated for all people with health problems that can be improved by weight loss. These problems include hypertension, type II diabetes elevated blood lipids, and sleep apnea. The higher the weight, the greater the need for weight reduction. Also, intervention to control weight should be strongly encouraged for people who are at the upper end of a healthy weight range to prevent any further weight gain.

Supervision of weight loss by a physician or other health professional trained in the field of weight control is necessary for people who are severely overweight, children, people older than age 65 years, pregnant and breastfeeding women, and people with medical conditions that would make weight loss efforts dangerous. Although weight loss is not recommended for pregnant women, a supervised nutrition management program can promote nutritional status and appropriate weight gain during pregnancy. It is important that the health professional screen the client for preexisting eating disorders or underlying psychological problems.

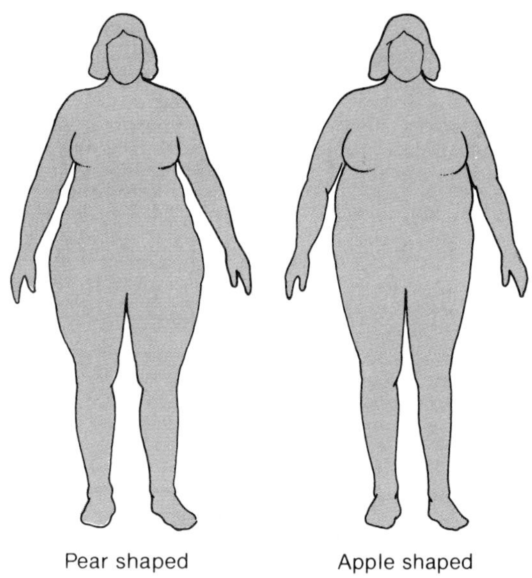

FIGURE 23-1

Gynecoid (*left*) and android (*right*) distribution of body fat. *(Beebe CA. Obesity management in people with diabetes. Diabetes Spectrum 1988;1:19.)*

CAUSES OF OBESITY

Of the patients who lose weight, 80% to 90% regain it. Although body weight is simply a balance between caloric intake and energy expenditure, the causes and treatment are complex. Environmental, cultural, socioeconomic, hereditary, metabolic, and emotional factors and activity levels all are involved in its development.

Why people gain weight and why they have so much difficulty losing weight and keeping it off has been the subject of much research. A number of myths about obesity have been dispelled. Obese people do not necessarily consume more calories than people who are not obese, and not all cases can be attributed to a lack of physical exercise. Obesity is not totally a psychological problem manifested by lack of willpower. Evidently there are different types of obesity and different causes.

PHYSICAL FACTORS

More scientists are investigating physical factors that effect changes in the body's energy-regulating system as a cause for obesity. The following are theories concerning the physical causes of obesity.

GENETICS

Heredity appears to have a strong influence on weight. In a study conducted in Denmark of 540 adults who had been adopted as infants, the participants' weights were found to be more like those of their biologic parents than their adoptive parents. Genes appear to influence body type, body size, and distribution of body fat and to affect energy-regulating processes. Environmental factors also contribute to obesity; it is difficult to separate the effects of environment from those of genetics. Although there apparently is a genetic predisposition to obesity, an individual is not powerless to control weight. A person who is predisposed to obesity, however, may have more difficulty keeping weight at a desirable level.

FAT CELL NUMBER

Obesity can develop through an increase in the size and number of fat cells. If energy intake exceeds energy expenditure, the fat cells will increase in size to a maximum of about 1.0 mcg. When this point is reached, the size of the fat cell cannot increase further. If positive energy balance continues, new fat cells are formed. Because the ability to increase the number of fat cells is virtually unlimited, fat storage can reach enormous proportions if caloric intake remains high.

The periods in life when an increase is cell number is likely to occur is a controversial subject. Evidence has indicated that fat cells in humans increase in size during the first year of life and in number beyond the first year. Typically, the number of fat cells increases five times from age 1 year to 22 years. Fat cells may continue to increase in number as long as excessive caloric intake occurs. Once fat cells are formed, the number appears to remain fixed, even with weight loss. When weight loss occurs, the size of fat cells, not the number, is reduced toward normal or eventually below normal.

A child who is obese at age 3 years is not necessarily destined to become an obese adult. The child may have more fat cells than other 3-year-olds, but fewer cells than a lean adult. The child can outgrow the obesity by not excessively increasing the cell number as he or she grows older.

One theory has suggested that adipose tissue regulates energy intake and balance. If people with excessive fat cell numbers lose weight, this weight loss must be accomplished by reducing cell size to below normal, a condition that cannot be maintained. This theory requires further research.

LIPOPROTEIN LIPASE

Lipoprotein lipase is an enzyme synthesized by the fat cell that determines the rate at which fat cells take up fat circulating in the bloodstream. Lipoprotein lipase is elevated in obesity. It has been suggested that lipoprotein lipase rises above previous levels when people who have been on low-calorie diets begin to increase their food intake.

EFFICIENT METABOLISM

Many obese adults consume no more calories than normal-weight adults. They, however, may be more efficient in using energy or in releasing energy as heat. Differences in metabolic rate for people of the same age, sex, and muscle tissue can be as high as 30%. Therefore, on a fixed caloric intake, one individual may gain weight and the other may not.

Metabolic rate differs among individuals of the same sex and between men and women. Women have a lower basal metabolic rate (BMR) than men, partly because they have a lower percentage of muscle tissue. The BMR decreases with age. People who do not adjust food intake to the slower metabolic rate can gain unwanted weight.

SET-POINT THEORY

According to this theory, each individual has a set-point for body weight. Internal factor such as fat cells, hormones, and enzymes program an individual's body weight and amount of fatty and lean body tissues. This theory holds that, because of genetic factors, the vast majority of people who lose weight are unable to avoid regaining the weight without severe restriction of calories or dramatic increases in exercise for the rest of their lives. Some people can lose and maintain limited amounts of weight by decreasing fat intake, increasing exercise, using certain drugs, or using a combination of these approaches.

WEIGHT CYCLING (YO-YO DIETING)

Results of research on the effect of repeated weight fluctuations on the BMR have been conflicting. Although reducing caloric intake causes a drop in the BMR, recent studies have suggested that this depression in BMR is temporary and that the BMR rises once the caloric restriction ends. The drop in BMR appears to be very small in diets that provide at least 1200 kcal/day. Also, the drop in BMR while dieting can be lessened by increasing physical activity.

DIET COMPOSITION

It is well known that fat yields more calories than protein or carbohydrate. In the past 10 years, however, research has indicated that, calorie for calorie, fat has a greater potential for increasing body fat than does carbohydrate. Once absorbed into the bloodstream, carbohydrate goes through different metabolic pathways than fat. When excess carbohydrate is converted to body fat, about 23% of the calories are burned off. When dietary fat is converted to body fat, only 3% of the calories are burned off. The *thermic effect* of food—the increase in metabolism after a meal is eaten—also is greater for carbohydrate than for fat. The body can make fat more readily from fat than from carbohydrate or protein.

PSYCHOSOCIAL FACTORS

A family eating pattern that emphasizes meats, starches, sweets, and fats to the exclusion of fruits and vegetables obviously encourages weight gain. People whose professions require that they frequently attend luncheons, cocktail parties, and dinners often find it difficult not to eat too much. Food has a social role in the celebration of happy occasions, as a demonstration of welcome and hospitality, and in mourning activities. Most of us have at one time or another eaten too much because we felt frustrated, angry, or anxious. Some people tend to fall back on food habitually as a release from their problems.

Parental attitudes play a part in obesity. An overanxious parent may make a habit of overfeeding a child. A parent who uses food as a reward may create an emotional dependence on food.

Some obese people use their obesity as a defense mechanism—it becomes an excuse for their failure to get a certain job or a way of avoiding contact with the opposite sex. In some cases, attempts to lose weight give rise to severe psychological problems. When this occurs, the person is advised to discontinue weight control efforts. Once underlying emotional problems are treated and stabilized under the care of mental health professionals, weight control efforts may possibly resume.

LACK OF PHYSICAL ACTIVITY

Lack of physical activity contributes to the development of obesity. Modern technology has created many labor-saving devices that have greatly reduced energy expenditure. With lessened activity, food intake has decreased, but not enough to compensate for the lowered activity level. Obese people, especially children and adolescents, often do not eat more than people of healthy weight, but gain weight because they are inactive and slow-moving.

CLASSIFICATION OF BINGE EATING AS AN EATING DISORDER

In the fourth edition of the *Diagnostic and Statistical Manual of the American Psychiatric Association* published in 1994, binge eating was listed for the first time as an eating disorder. The primary symptom of this disorder is recurrent episodes of binge eating, commonly referred to as compulsive eating, *without* the regular use of laxatives, self-induced vomiting, or fasting. Binge Eating Disorder is listed in the manual under the category of Eating Disorder Not Otherwise Specified. See Display 23-2 for the diagnostic criteria.

A considerable number of people who seek help for weight control meet the criteria for binge eating disorder. Clients who appear to meet this criteria should be referred for psychotherapy and more complex nutrition care. Clients may need to be made aware that psychological and emotional issues underlie their inability to stop bingeing. See Chapter 18 for a Discussion of two other eating disorders: anorexia nervosa and bulimia nervosa.

DISCRIMINATION AND OBESITY: THE ROLE OF THE HEALTH WORKER

The bias against obesity is everywhere in our culture. Even young children rate children who are obese as less likable than children with physical disabilities. Obese people have been discriminated against in college admissions and employment.

What should health workers' attitudes be toward obese people? Their attitude is important because they may play a key role in helping resolve the problem. Obese people should never be made to feel that their obesity is their own fault, nor should they be made to feel that they are wasting time and space in the health care facility by just being there. Most obese people have been the butt

DISPLAY 23-2 DIAGNOSTIC CRITERIA FOR BINGE EATING DISORDER

BINGE EATING DISORDER

Diagnostic criteria for binge eating disorder:

A. Recurrent episodes of binge eating. An episode of binge eating is characterized by both of the following:
   1. Eating, in a discrete period of time* (e.g., within any 2-hour period), an amount of food that is definitely larger than most people would eat in a similar period under similar circumstances; and
   2. A sense of lack of control over eating during the episode (e.g., a feeling that one cannot stop eating or control what or how much one is eating).

B. The binge eating episodes are associated with at least three of the following:
   1. eating much more rapidly than normal
   2. eating until feeling uncomfortably full
   3. eating large amounts of food when not feeling physically hungry
   4. eating alone because of being embarrassed by how much one is eating
   5. feeling disgusted with oneself, depressed, or feeling very guilty after overeating.

C. Marked distress regarding binge eating.

D. The binge eating occurs, on average, at least 2 days* a week for 6 months.

E. The binge eating is not associated with the regular use of inappropriate compensatory behaviors (e.g., purging, fasting, excessive exercise) and does not occur exclusively during the course of anorexia nervosa or bulimia nervosa.

* Method of determining frequency differs from that used for bulimia nervosa; research should address whether counting the number of days on which binges occur or the number of episodes of binge eating is the preferred method of setting a frequency threshold.

(American Psychiatric Association. Diagnostic and statistical manual. 4th ed. Washington, DC: American Psychiatric Association, 1994.)

of ill-considered jibes or jokes. Do not add to these insults—the obese client already has suffered keenly. A person's fatness or lack of fatness does not define that person. Accept obese people as they are and offer your sympathetic support to their efforts to lose weight. Be a good listener, too, so they come to know that you are on their side. If they sense your support, they will be more receptive to the information you give about nutrition and exercise. Encourage clients who have symptoms of the binge or compulsive eating disorder to seek psychological counseling.

Undoubtedly, the best way to treat obesity is to prevent it. Health care workers can play a key role in their interactions with families and individuals. They can help the family see that physical activity, as appropriate to various ages and stages of development, is a good health habit. They can help parents understand that children benefit from being fed appropriate amounts of food, not from overeating (See discussion of childhood obesity in Chapter 18). They may be able to help identify people at risk of becoming obese, such as the baby who is gaining weight too rapidly, the child of obese parents, or the person who experiences an abrupt increase in appetite.

TRADITIONAL APPROACHES TO TREATMENT

The treatment of obesity is in a state of transition. The traditional approaches of diet, exercise, and behavior modification, no matter how well supervised and managed, have failed to produce permanent weight loss in the vast majority of people who enter weight control programs. Even more disturbing is that the obsession with thinness and the repeated attempts to lose weight appear to play a part in the alarming incidence of eating disorders.

New strategies for dealing with what is now recognized as a complex disorder (or group of disorders) are beginning to emerge. The following is a discussion of both traditional methods and new approaches to treating obesity.

A number of approaches have been and continue to be used to treat obesity. These include diet, exercise, behavior modification, drugs, and surgery.

DIET

Dietary modification is a major part of most weight loss programs. A variety of dietary programs are available to the general public. These programs include popular self-prescribed diets, self-help commercial groups, self-help noncommercial groups, community programs (through hospitals or nutrition counseling services), and work site programs. The diet approaches used in these programs usually fit into one of the following classifications: popular or novelty diets, which include formula diets and diets restricting macronutrients (carbohydrate or fat), very low-calorie diets, and balanced diets with modest caloric control.

Popular Diets

Periodically, dietary manipulation promoted in a new "diet" book and by its authors in the media as a quick and painless way of losing weight gains widespread popularity. These popular self-prescribed diets promote certain nutrients, foods, or combinations of foods as having magical qualities. The success of the diet usually is attributed to some unproven scientific theory. Weight loss is achieved, not by the unique aspects of the diet, but by the limits placed on food selection, which cause the person to eat less food. Because the limits are so extreme, consumers follow them for only a short time, and therefore the effect on health is minimal. People who follow restricted diets for long periods are at risk of nutritional deficiencies. People with increased nutritional needs, such as pregnant women, children, and adolescents, are especially at risk.

Some popular diets severely restrict carbohydrate as a means of rapid weight loss. The initial rapid weight reduction is due to water loss, not fat loss, and is accompanied by the loss of electrolytes. If carbohydrate consumption is less than 100 g, ketosis develops. Nausea, low blood pressure, fatigue, and excessive excretion of uric acid may occur. Excessive production of uric acid can create problems for people predisposed to gout. The high fat content of the low-carbohydrate diet increases the risk of atherosclerosis.

The Atkins and Scarsdale diets are examples of popular diets that severely restrict carbohydrate.

Liquid formula diets are attractive because the consumer is relieved of making decisions about food and of having to prepare food. Product information usually advises consumers to eat one or two small meals in addition to the formula. If the liquid diet program is severely limited in calories, the adverse effects associated with the very low-calorie diet (discussed in the following section) would apply here. Very low-calorie formula diets should not be followed without medical supervision. Herbalife, Slimfast, and the Cambridge Diet are examples of this diet approach.

Losing weight and keeping it off is hard work. Contrary to the claims made by the promoters of the "quick fix" route to weight loss, there are no easy answers to the problem. Clients should be made aware of fraudulent claims (Display 23-3). Long-term success depends on a gradual transition to a lifelong pattern of healthful **restrained** eating and physical activity.

DISPLAY 23-3 CLUES TO FRAUD

It is important for consumers to be wary of claims that sound too good to be true. When it comes to weight-loss scheme, consumers should be particularly skeptical of claims containing words and phrases such as

- Easy
- Effortless
- Guaranteed
- Miraculous
- Magical
- Breakthrough
- New discovery
- Mysterious
- Exotic
- Secret
- Exclusive
- Ancient

(US Dept of Health and Human Services, Public Health Service/Food and Drug Administration. The facts about weight loss products and programs. Bethesda, MD: US Dept of Health and Human Services, 1992. DHHS publication FDA 92–1189.)

Very Low-Calorie Diets

For people who are 40% or more above ideal weight, more aggressive approaches under close medical supervision sometimes are used. Total fasting is no longer an accepted method of weight reduction because of its adverse side effects. In recent years, the very low-calorie diet, also known as the protein-sparing modified fast, has been widely used. The very low-calorie diet is a near fast comprising about 70 g of protein plus essential vitamins and minerals. It provides less than 800 kcal/day. The protein is given as small portions of meat, fish, or poultry or as supplements that are consumed as a liquid diet. The very low-calorie diet was developed to prevent the loss of lean body tissue that occurs during total fasting. It is effective in bringing about large weight losses.

Cardiac arrhythmias and sudden death have been associated with very low-calorie diets. These deaths have been attributed to poor quality protein in the initial commercial formulas, a situation that has been corrected by the use of high-quality protein and the addition of vitamins and minerals. The very low-calorie diet should be followed for no longer than 2 to 3 months and only under close medical supervision. Side effects that may occur include fainting, dehydration, cold intolerance, hair loss, dry skin, and menstrual irregularities.

Maintaining weight loss is as much of a problem in this approach as it is in others. Most people regain lost weight within 2 years. The reduced metabolic rate that occurs with severe caloric restriction may promote rapid weight gain when caloric intake increases. Also, the very low-calorie diet appears to make some people more prone to binge eating. The inclusion of behavior modification techniques helps improve the long-range outcome. Unfortunately, many people are unwilling or unable to put as much effort and finances into the maintenance phase as the weight loss phase of these programs. Optifast and Medifast programs are examples of this very low-calorie diet approach.

BALANCED REDUCING DIETS

Diets that moderately restrict calories to achieve an energy deficit of about 250 to 500 kcal/day, when combined with exercise and behavior modification, promote retention of muscle tissue while bringing about gradual weight loss. Of the traditional diet approaches, this one offers the greatest chance for success. These diets, which range from 1200 to 1800 kcal/day or more, are nutritionally adequate, except for energy.

Balanced reducing diets are most successful when they are part of a planned program that includes exercise and behavior changes. Unless both poor eating habits and poor activity patterns are corrected, the likelihood that weight loss will be long lasting is small. A detailed discussion of moderate calorie control is discussed later in this chapter.

EXERCISE

Exercise is a vital component of weight control. It helps counteract some of the undesirable effects of reduced caloric intake, such as a decrease in metabolic rate, more easily regained weight, and loss of muscle tissue. It enhances psychological factors.

A program that includes both aerobic exercise and strength training is ideal. Aerobic exercise increases the heart rate and burns calories. Examples of aerobic exercise are walking, cycling, swimming, jogging, running, cross-country skiing, and aerobic dance. Strength-building (resistance) exercises help to spare muscle tissue and improve muscle tone. Strength-training exercises require the use of resistance equipment, the use of which is best learned in a supervised setting with qualified instructors. The benefits of exercise in a weight control program are as follows:

- Exercise permits a more liberal caloric intake because exercise burns calories. Exercising is similar in effect to eating less. With exercise, a person does not need to reduce caloric intake to dangerously low levels to lose weight. A low caloric intake may be harmful because it may not provide all of the required nutrients.
- Exercise improves muscle tone. Because muscle tissue requires more energy than fat, the more muscle tissue a person has, the more calories the body burns.
- Exercise increases the metabolic rate during exercise. Contrary to previous reports, the BMR appears to return to normal within 1 hour after mild exercise. The BMR may remain elevated longer after strenuous or prolonged exercise.
- Exercise promotes the loss of body fat and the retention of muscle tissue. Even with a well-balanced diet, some muscle tissue is lost during weight loss. By combining diet and exercise, the loss of body weight is increased and the loss of body protein is decreased.
- Exercise reduces stress and tension and improves adherence to a weight control program. The psychological effects of exercise may be the most important ones—enhancing self-esteem and leading to a better control of food intake.
- Exercise helps prevent the regaining of weight. People who exercise are most likely to maintain the weight loss.

In addition to these benefits directly related to weight loss, exercise contributes to general health by promoting better sleep patterns and reducing the risk of chronic illness such as heart disease, hypertension, and diabetes.

To be effective, the exercise program must be carried out on a regular basis. Clients should check with their physicians before beginning an exercise program (see section Exercising Safely in Chapter 7).

Moderate Versus Intense Exercise

Moderate levels of exercise (below 60% of maximum heart rate) are sufficient for improved health and weight control. Some authorities have suggested that the typical cardiovascular fitness formula for exercise (frequency, intensity, and duration) be avoided with overweight people. Low to moderate levels of exercise are associated with better adherence and greater psychological benefit than vigorous exercise for the overweight person. It appears better to increase the duration of exercise rather than the intensity as the individual progresses.

It also is important to incorporate more physical activity into the daily routine. Brisk walking instead of driving whenever possible and climbing a few flights of stairs instead of taking the elevator are simple forms of exercise most people can follow. These forms of physical activity are of great value in maintaining weight loss and should not be underestimated.

BEHAVIOR MODIFICATION

Behavior modification for weight control is a method of teaching that focuses on behavior change rather than on food or weight loss. A *habit* is a persistent behavior that is automatic and not a result of thought. Behavior modification is based on the theory that bad eating habits are learned behaviors and that they can be replaced by other, better behaviors. Thus, if the problem is obesity and the person changes his or her eating habits, weight loss follows.

Behavior modification programs have been expanded to include other aspects of weight loss, including physical activity, nutrition education, control of negative thought patterns, and techniques for prevention of relapse. Behavior modification programs for weight control are directed by health professionals who are specially trained in the techniques. They may be conducted on an individual or group basis.

Clients begin the program by collecting information about their eating habits. They keep a food diary that describes not only the foods and amounts eaten but also the circumstances: how long it takes them to eat, where they eat and with whom, what they do while eating, and so on (see the sample food diary form in Display 2-3). From this information, clients identify those factors that promote excessive caloric intake. Clients also may keep a diary for physical activity. Once problem behaviors are identified, specific steps are taken to deal with them. In some programs, no specific diet is recommended and no particular food is prohibited; however, recommendations for food selection and preparation are presented. Clients continue to maintain a record to monitor change.

The following are eight practical approaches that help build better eating habits:

1. Eat slowly and concentrate on the smell, taste, and texture of what you are eating.
2. Plan a pause midway through the meal so you can assess what you have already eaten.
3. Celebrate or reward yourself with treats other than food, such as a movie, a manicure, some time to yourself, or a new necktie.
4. Serve food directly onto your plate. Do not place serving dishes of food on the table.
5. Choose food that requires some preparation and has to be eaten slowly, such as a whole orange rather than orange juice.
6. Ask family members to get their own snacks, especially desserts. Many calories are consumed over the course of a year in snacks.
7. Limit the number of places in the house where you eat. For example, eat only at the kitchen or dining room table.
8. Separate eating from other activities. Do not eat while doing other activities such as reading or watching television.

DRUGS

Drugs used to promote weight loss usually are agents that reduce appetite or increase satiety. Amphetamine, a drug that induces anorexia, was the first appetite suppressant and one that was widely used. Because of its harmful side effects including insomnia, dizziness, hypertension, rapid heart beat, and potential for addiction, its usefulness is limited. Also, although the drug may promote rapid weight loss at first, the weight is quickly regained once discontinued. In some people, discontinuing the drug seems to promote the onset of depression.

Other anorectic drugs that have fewer side effects and are less addictive than amphetamine are diethylpropion, mazindol, fenfluramine, phentermine, and phenylpropanolamine. Phenylpropanolamine is a less potent derivative of amphetamine and is available over-the-counter. Some clients may benefit from the use of these drugs, which they should take only under close medical supervision. These drugs are used in combination with control of food intake and exercise.

Bulking (fibrous) agents, which are supposed to expand in the stomach, have not been effective in reducing appetite. Furthermore, thyroid preparations, digitalis, and human chorionic gonadotrophin (a hormone extracted from the urine of pregnant women) should not be used in the treatment of obesity.

Both diuretics and laxatives promote weight loss; however, the weight loss is due to water loss, not to a decrease in fatty tissue. Physicians prescribe diuretics only for clients who are retaining abnormal amounts of water. People who use laxatives habitually to decrease absorption of food cause the disruption of normal nutrient absorption and fluid and electrolyte balance.

SURGERY

Surgery occasionally is performed on people who are grossly obese—more than 100% above desirable weight—and whose obesity is seriously interfering with their health. There are two types of surgery: jejunoileal bypass (bypass of a part of the small intestine) and gastroplasty.

In intestinal bypass, the length of the functioning small intestine is reduced drastically, to about 25 inches. Weight loss occurs by decreased intake of food because of extremely unpleasant gastrointestinal symptoms and the reduced absorption of food. The intestinal bypass is a drastic measure that has been discontinued because of its severe side effects.

Gastroplasty is the most common form of gastric surgery now performed. It involves stapling across the top of the stomach, creating a small 50-mL to 60-mL pouch and a small 1-cm outlet to the rest of the stomach. In another procedure, two longitudinal staple lines form a stomach pouch with a capacity of 20 to 30 mL. Teflon mesh may be used to keep the pouch from expanding and the opening from the pouch to the rest of the stomach from becoming wider. Following both of these procedures, the quantity of food that is eaten must be greatly reduced because of the small storage capacity and weight loss results. Although the complications are considerably less than in the intestinal surgery, both of these procedures are hazardous. Clients must be selected carefully for this form of treatment.

MODERATE CALORIC CONTROL

SETTING REALISTIC GOALS

The poor success rate for correcting obesity may be due in part to the setting of unrealistic goals. For example, a woman weighing 200 lb whose desirable weight is 130 lb is consuming 2600 kcal or more every day. Putting her on a 1200-kcal/day diet would cut her food intake by more than half; this is setting a goal that the client unlikely will achieve.

The caloric level of a reducing diet frequently is based on the person's desirable weight; however, it is far more realistic to begin where the person is and calculate an appropriate caloric level from that point. A man who is maintaining his weight on 2600 kcal/day will lose about 1 lb/week on a 2100-kcal/day diet and about 2 lb/week on a 1600-kcal/day diet. As he loses weight, the calorie content of his diet is reduced because his decreasing body size requires fewer calories.

The grossly obese man of 350 lb who has been overweight from childhood is unlikely to reach a weight of 160 lb and maintain it for the rest of his life; his weight is more likely to fluctuate between 160 lb and 350 lb. It may be healthier for him to reduce to 250 lb and stay there.

Rather than set goals based on desirable or ideal weight, it may be more appropriate to set a goal based on reasonable weight. The reasonable weight goal is based on the person's present weight and past weight history. Setting goals that are unachievable is defeating and demoralizing.

Weight loss of $\frac{1}{2}$ to 1 lb/week is a reasonable goal. A diet that provides 500 kcal/day below energy needs should result in a weight loss of 1 lb/week; 1000 kcal/day below energy needs should result in a loss of about 2 lb/week. A 1000-kcal deficit, however, would be excessive and possibly dangerous for some women who may require only about 1800 kcal or less to maintain their current weight. A loss of more than 2 lb/week is not recommended, because it does not represent a moderate approach.

PROVIDING ESSENTIAL NUTRIENTS

In a diet of less than 1800 to 2000 kcal/day, there is little room for sugar and alcohol. Even when the diet entirely comprises nutritious foods, intake of minerals, such as iron, zinc, and magnesium, and vitamins E and folate are likely to be below recommended levels. A vitamin/mineral supplement may be prescribed for people on such a diet.

In a typical reducing diet, 15% to 20% of total calories are from protein. On this basis, a 1500-kcal/day diet provides 56 to 76 g of protein. Fats and carbohydrates are restricted, but an appropriate balance between the two is maintained. A distribution of 30% or less of calories from fat and 50% to 55% of calories from carbohydrate are common. Water and other noncaloric fluids are not restricted unless there are complicating factors.

CHOOSING COUNSELING METHODS

Calories can be controlled by a variety of methods, such as calorie counting, reducing caloric content of meals and snacks usually eaten (as recorded in a food diary), and using a meal plan and exchange lists. Clients must be actively involved in choosing a system or process with which they feel comfortable. They must be helped to accept that success depends not on the magic of the diet or process but on their own efforts and mind-set.

Using Exchange Lists. The exchange list system frequently is used as a means of controlling caloric intake (Table 23-3). The client is given a meal plan, a sample menu, and a set of exchange lists (see Display 22-6). A 1200-kcal/day diet plan and sample menu are given in Table 23-4. The exchange list system is discussed in detail in Chapter 22.

Using Calorie Counting. For the client who is not on a specific meal plan but is counting calories, the exchange list system offers a simplified calorie-counting system for the basic foods being consumed (Display 23-4). The caloric content of commercial products is readily available on the "Nutrition Facts" label of virtually all products. Calorie counting books are available to assist in estimating the caloric value of mixed dishes and restaurant foods.

TABLE 23-3 REDUCING DIETS BASED ON FOOD EXCHANGE LISTS

FOOD EXCHANGES*	NUMBER OF EXCHANGES	
	1200 kcal	1500 kcal
Milk, skim	2	2
Vegetable	2	2
Fruit	3	4
Starch	4	6
Meat, lean/med-fat	5	6
Fat	3	4
Nutrient Content		
Protein	67 g	80 g
Fat	40 g	50 g
Carbohydrate	139 g	184 g
kcal	1184	1506

* Based on Exchange Lists for Meal Planning, 1995 edition. See Display 22-6.

SELECTING A WEIGHT CONTROL PROGRAM

People who wish to lose weight have a choice of dieting on their own, getting private counseling, or joining a group. Dieting alone works best when only a few pounds are involved. Reducing portion sizes, limiting alcohol and foods that contain mostly fat or sugar, and increasing physical activity can bring about the desired weight loss. Crash dieting or the use of restrictive fad diets should be avoided. Foods should be chosen from all of the food groups. Periodic checkups with the physician are important. Moderate, gradual weight loss resulting from permanent changes in eating and exercise habits is the goal.

Nutrition counseling services and team-managed weight control programs are available in the outpatient facilities of hospitals and other community health agencies or in private practices established by registered dietitians. In light of the new philosophy of weight management (see the section that follows) and the possible adverse effects of weight loss efforts, it is recommended that clients use the weight control programs managed by a team of health professionals who are trained in the field of weight management.

TABLE 23-4 1200-KCAL MEAL PLAN AND SAMPLE MENU

MEAL	FOOD EXCHANGE	NO. OF EXCHANGES	SAMPLE MENU
Breakfast	Fruit	1	1/3 cantaloupe
	Starch	1	1 slice of whole-wheat toast
	Fat	1	1 tsp of margarine
	Milk, skim	1	1 cup of skim milk
			Coffee
Lunch			Tuna salad plate
	Meat, lean/med-fat	2	2 oz water-packed tuna
	Vegetable	1	Cucumber slices marinated in herb vinegar
			Tomato wedges
			Salad greens
	Starch	1	6 rye rounds
	Fat	1	1 tbsp of reduced-fat mayonnaise
	Fruit	1	2 medium-sized fresh plums
			Tea
Supper	Meat, lean/med-fat	3	3 oz of baked chicken
	Starch	1	1/2 cup of cooked rice boiled in chicken bouillon
	Vegetable	1	1/2 cup of broccoli with 1 tsp of margarine
	Fat	1	Green salad with 1 tbsp of oil-free dressing
	Fruit	1	1/2 small banana in sugar-free gelatin
			Seltzer water
Bedtime snack	Milk, skim	1	1 cup of skim milk
	Starch	1	3 ginger snaps

* Based on Exchange Lists for Meal Planning, 1995 edition. See Display 22-6.

A NEW MODEL OF TREATMENT

NEW PHILOSOPHY REGARDING WEIGHT LOSS

Both commercial and well-designed medical treatment programs for obesity have failed to promote permanent weight loss in all but a small percentage of their clients. Although many of the participants in these programs lose weight, most of them regain the weight in a relatively short period. This situation has led authorities in the field of weight control to conclude that the traditional methods of the past have been rigid, unrealistic, and have perpetuated the feelings of failure among people who are obese.

In a position paper issued by the American Dietetic Association in 1994, dietitians were advised to explain to *all* clients who seek weight loss treatment the following realities:

- Most people who lose weight by dieting are unable to maintain substantial weight loss because of their biologic set-point, without dramatically restricting caloric intake and/or increasing exercise on a permanent basis. Some people can lose and maintain small amounts of weight loss by decreasing fat intake, increasing exercise, or using certain medication (e.g., fenfluramine).
- Some people have psychological issues underlying their overeating behavior. They may need to resolve these issues in psychotherapy before considering the possibility of substantial weight loss.

A new model for the treatment of obesity is evolving gradually. In this model, "ideal" weight is not the treatment goal but, rather, a "reasonable" weight that will improve the quality of life and lead to permanent weight control at a reasonable level. *Reasonable weight* is the weight that the individual is capable of achieving and maintaining. Small amounts of weight loss—as little as 10 to 20 lb—can have a significant impact on glucose tolerance (type II diabetes), blood pressure, and cholesterol levels.

The client is an integral part of the treatment plan. People involved in setting their own goals and in developing their own eating and exercise plans are more successful at achieving long-term weight control than people who follow programs prescribed by others.

STRUCTURED DIETS ARE INEFFECTIVE

In general, structured, reduced-calorie diets have not been effective in achieving long-term weight control. It is recommended, instead, that emphasis be placed on the quality of the diet rather than the quantity of food. The quality approach can reduce health risks and is likely to promote long-term weight control. Improving the quality of the diet is easier and more realistic to maintain than severe and rigid restriction of calories.

FOCUS ON HEALTH BENEFITS

At a conference on weight control convened by the National Institutes of Health in 1992, authorities concluded that the best way to improve the physical and psychological health of obese Americans is to focus on treatment approaches that can produce health benefits whether or not the individual can lose weight. The essential characteristic of a weight control program is the maintenance of a stable weight or of a reduced weight. Weight maintenance involves adopting new eating and exercise behaviors on a lifelong basis, which can be a slow and difficult process.

Components of a program that focuses on positive health habits include

- an emphasis on resulting health benefits
- increased physical activity, which will increase muscle tissue and, consequently, increase BMR and also improve cardiovascular health
- a gradual reduction in fat intake, which will reduce the risk of cardiovascular diseases and some cancers, bring about weight loss, and prevent reaccumulation of fat
- an increased awareness of internal cues for food—distinguishing physical hunger from emotional hunger
- a focus on uncovering and treating psychosocial issues that are creating barriers to change.

DISPLAY 23-4 COUNTING CALORIES WITH EXCHANGE LISTS*

EXCHANGE LIST	AMOUNT	KCAL
Starch	Varies†	80
Fruit	Varies†	60
Milk		
Skim	8 oz	90
Low-fat	8 oz	120
Whole	8 oz	150
Vegetables	½ cup cooked 1 cup raw	25
Meat		
Very lean	1 oz	35
Lean	1 oz	55
Medium-fat	1 oz	75
High-fat	1 oz	100
Fat	Varies†	45

* Food labels and a calorie-counting book can be used for calorie counts of commercial foods and mixed dishes.

† Portion sizes given in *Exchange Lists for Meal Planning,* 1995 edition (Display 22–6.)

Comprehensive long-term programs are necessary to effectively treat obesity. A team approach conducted by trained practitioners in the fields of medicine, psychology, nutrition, and exercise physiology is needed to address all aspects of the problem.

FAT BUDGETING: AN ALTERNATIVE TO THE STRUCTURED CALORIE-CONTROLLED DIET

Fat budgeting is a method that can help improve the quality of the diet without having to count food servings or exchanges. Clients are given a daily fat gram allowance based on their estimated average caloric intake. Clients can choose any foods they want as long as they do not exceed the fat allowance. Because clients can choose the foods they desire, they feel less deprived and take more responsibility for their choice of food.

Clients keep a daily food record recording the fat content of each food portion (see Display 22-2). They will require training in estimating portion sizes accurately. After several weeks of weighing or measuring their food, most clients are reasonably accurate at estimating portion sizes. If portion sizes are estimated inaccurately, the calculation of fat in the food consumed will also be inaccurate. The fat content of foods is readily available in lists provided by health organizations (e.g., the American Heart Association), paperback fat-counting books, and especially food labels.

The fat allowance is usually based on current recommendations of limiting fat intake to 30% or less of total caloric intake. Caloric requirements are estimated based on whether weight maintenance or weight loss is desired. Generally, caloric levels for men range from 2000 to 2500 kcal for weight maintenance and 1600 to 2000 kcal for weight loss. For women, the calorie range is 1600 to 2000 kcal for weight maintenance and 1200 to 1600 kcal for weight loss. The fat allowance for each of the calorie levels is given in Table 23-5. It is important for health professionals to monitor not only the accuracy of the fat counting but also the overall quality of the diet.

TABLE 23-5 Fat Allowance Based on Estimated Caloric Intake

Caloric Level	Fat Budget* (g of Fat/Day)
1200	40
1300	43
1400	47
1500	50
1600	53
1800	60
2000	67
2200	73
2500	83
2800	93
3000	100

* Represents 30% of total calories

PRACTICAL SUGGESTIONS FOR REDUCING FAT AND CALORIC INTAKE

PLANNING AHEAD

Planning meals is of great importance to the dieter. Haphazard eating habits, skipping of meals, and impulse eating are the enemies of weight control. People living alone, whether in their twenties or their seventies, are especially likely to have irregular meal patterns. Half an hour or so a week devoted to planning meals and making a shopping list based on these meals will reap many benefits. Planning ahead makes it easier to stick to a diet, results in more balanced meals, and reduces the impulse buying of snacks and sweet desserts, which sabotage weight control effort as well as the food budget.

FLAVORING FOOD

Clients may need guidance in preparing flavorful foods without using fat. Meat, fish, and poultry are kept moist if baked in aluminum foil. Clients may cook foods with fat-free broth, tomato juice, wine, lemon juice, or vinegar, to which they may add onion, garlic, spices, and herbs (fresh and dried). A mixture of tomato juice and flavorings such as grated onion, celery, garlic, horseradish, and spices and herbs to taste can be used hot or cold to add flavor and moisture.

Flavored vinegar such as raspberry, balsamic, red wine, and tarragon can add interesting flavors to a variety of foods. Evaporated skim milk can be substituted for cream, and plain nonfat yogurt adds moisture to baked goods and can be substituted for mayonnaise in salads and dressings.

Clients can use meat and poultry juices for soup or gravy. However, they should remove the fat by refrigerating the drippings overnight; the fat rises to the top and hardens, and can easily be removed. If it is inconvenient to refrigerate drippings, clients should remove as much fat as possible by spoon after the liquid is allowed to set. Then they should add one or two ice cubes to the drippings so they can easily remove the fat droplets that will rise to the surface.

HIGH-CALORIE FLUIDS

Clients need to be made aware that fluids may be high in calories. An 8-oz glass of canned fruit punch supplies 120 kcal, so three or four glasses contribute 360 to 500 kcal (Table 23-6).

FOOD LABELING

Food labeling regulations require that total calories, calories from fat, total grams of fat, and total grams of saturated fat per serving appear on the label of virtually all packaged foods. Labeling terms such as *low-calorie, light,* and *fat-free* are clearly defined in the regulations. See Display 22-3 for the definitions of these "core terms" for nutrient content claims on food labels. If a food is labeled *diet* or *dietetic,* it must be truthful and not misleading and the food has to be labeled a *low-calorie* or *reduced-calorie* food or bear a comparison to the food that is not a "diet" food.

TABLE 23-6 Caloric Value of Selected Liquids

Fluid	Amount (oz)	kcal
Cola-type soda	12	160
Fruit-flavored soda (grape)	12	180
Club soda	12	0
Sugar-free soda	12	0–5
Beer	12	150
Wine, dry, white	$3\frac{1}{2}$	80
Wine, sweet	$3\frac{1}{2}$	140
Gin, vodka, whiskey (80 proof)	$1\frac{1}{2}$	95
Manhattan cocktail	$3\frac{1}{2}$	164
Tomato juice	8	40
Grapefruit juice, unsweetened	8	100
Lemonade	8	107
Fruit punch, canned	8	113
Fruit-flavored drink from mix	8	95
Coffee, black	6	5
Coffee with 1 heaping tsp of sugar	6	25
Coffee with 1 heaping tsp of sugar plus 1 tbsp of half-and-half or liquid creamer	6	45
Water	8	0

(US Dept of Agriculture, Human Nutrition Information Service. Nutritive value of food. Washington DC: US Government Printing Office, 1991. Home and Garden bulletin 72; Pennington, JAT. Bowes and Church's Food values of portions commonly used. 16th ed. Philadelphia: JB Lippincott, 1994).

UNDERWEIGHT

The plight of people who are severely underweight can be just as desperate as that of grossly obese people. This is especially true of people whose extreme thinness is the result of heredity. They lack the normal number of adipose cells that can accumulate fat and, as a result, quickly feel full when they eat.

Underweight resulting from prolonged illness is a frequent problem. Symptoms such as lack of appetite, vomiting, diarrhea, and high fever can cause serious weight loss. An endocrine disorder such as hyperthyroidism is another cause of underweight. Underweight due to anorexia nervosa is discussed in Chapter 18.

Underweight is defined as 10 to 20 lb under the desirable weight for height and bone structure. The underweight person is susceptible to infection, particularly tuberculosis. Underweight also may complicate pregnancy. Nevertheless, thin people are the least affected by so-called degenerative diseases—heart, liver, and kidney diseases and diabetes.

Psychological harm may be a consequence of underweight. People who have inherited their thinness may suffer from an inadequate self-image; for example, a very thin man may feel that he looks weak and unimpressive and an extremely thin woman may feel that her flat body is unattractive.

TREATMENT

To treat underweight, a diet increased in calories with supplements of vitamins and minerals is prescribed. Regular exercise and plenty of rest are advised.

People who have inherited their thinness usually fail in their efforts to increase caloric intake. Probably the best thing for them to do is to forget their thinness and keep physically fit, engage in plenty of outdoor activities, maintain good posture, and wear clothing and hairstyles that complement their slimness.

Setting a goal for weight gain must take into consideration the individual's age, height, and previous weight status. The following are eight suggestions for nutrition therapy:

1. The Pyramid Guide to Daily Food Choices (Table 14-1) should form the basis of the client's food intake.
2. Calories must be increased gradually to a level above the client's needs. This may be accomplished by increasing the amount of food eaten at each meal, increasing carbohydrate and fat intake, and providing more frequent feedings. A sudden increase in food intake may discourage the client and further depress the appetite. Every effort should be made to prepare foods the client likes and to serve them attractively.
3. Because protein tissue as well as fat is lost, a liberal protein level of 1 to 1.5 g/kg of body weight is recommended.
4. Vitamins and minerals, especially thiamin, must be adequate.
5. There should be reduced consumption of foods that have little caloric value (e.g., broth, salads, coffee, and tea) but that may reduce the appetite for other, more concentrated foods.
6. Foods rich in carbohydrate are easily digested and quickly converted to body fat. They should be eaten liberally. Although fatty foods offer the most calories, they must be eaten cautiously because they may depress the appetite. Butter, margarine, cream, and salad oils usually are better tolerated than fats in fried foods.
7. In some cases, liquid nutrition supplements such as Carnation Instant Breakfast (Clintec), Ensure (Ross), or Sustacal (Mead Johnson) may be useful. Start with small portions (4 oz) and gradually increase, if tolerated. Two 8-oz servings of these supplements add approximately 500 kcal to the diet.
8. The frequency of meals depends on the client. For some, it may work best to concentrate on increased intake at regular meals and a substantial bedtime snack. For others, small, frequent meals rather than large meals may work best.

KEYS TO PRACTICAL APPLICATION

Focus on improved quality of life and the health benefits of a healthy lifestyle regardless of whether weight loss is achieved.

Inform your client that, because of biologic factors, most people are unable to maintain a substantial weight loss without lifelong, dramatic changes in food intake and exercise.

Encourage your clients with such conditions as hypertension, elevated cholesterol, type II diabetes, and sleep apnea to choose modest weight loss goals of 5 to 20 lb and lose weight gradually.

Remember that obesity is a complex problem. Accept obese people as they are, apart from their ability to lose weight. Helping them develop a more positive self-image is probably the greatest contribution you can make toward helping them with their weight problem.

Focus on improving the quality of your client's food intake—less fat and more fruits, vegetables, and whole-grain breads and cereals. Remember that rigid, calorie-controlled diets have generally been ineffective on a long-term basis.

Encourage a physically active lifestyle, at all stages of life, as a vital component of healthy living; weight control is virtually impossible without it. Remember that, for the obese person, duration of exercise is more important than intensity.

Be alert to symptoms of eating disorders. Remember that, in addition to anorexia nervosa and bulimia nervosa, bingeing (compulsive eating) is an eating disorder requiring psychotherapy.

Be assured that calories do count. Regardless of the type of diet or other treatment method, a person loses weight only when caloric intake is lower than caloric expenditure.

Be suspicious of programs that offer quick solutions to obesity. Successful treatment is long range and requires changes in eating habits, activity patterns, or both.

Keep an eye on fatty foods, fats added to foods, and

liquid calories. They frequently are responsible for excessive caloric intake.

Emphasize planning. Haphazard eating habits make caloric control difficult.

Evaluate carefully the client who needs to gain weight. The approach varies depending on the cause of the underweight condition.

KEY IDEAS

Weight control is a matter of balance—when energy intake (food) is greater than energy output (energy used by the body), the excess food energy is stored as fat; 3500 kcal represent 1 lb of body fat.

Skinfold thickness measurements are a more accurate means of determining fatness or leanness than height–weight tables.

Obesity has been classified as follows: mild: 20% to 40% overweight; moderate, 41% to 100% overweight; and severe, greater than 100% overweight.

The BMI is the preferred means of assessing weight status; it corresponds well with body fat percentage.

New guidelines have suggested that people can be somewhat heavier as they grow older without adverse effects on health.

The relationship between weight and mortality differs at various times of life and also differs depending on the cause of death.

Excess fat in the abdominal area (apple-shaped obesity) carries an increased risk of chronic diseases; excess fat in the hips and thighs (pear-shaped obesity) is not associated with increased risk.

Obesity is strongly associated with elevated serum cholesterol, hypertension, and type II diabetes.

Weight loss improves glucose tolerance, reduces hypertension, and improves blood lipids, and sleep apnea.

Weight cycling has been associated with increased risk of disease and premature death; research in this regard has been conflicting.

Some lean body tissue (muscle) is lost during weight loss; the loss is greater in severe calorie restriction.

Dieting may promote binge eating in some mildly or moderately obese women.

The common practice of dieting for purposes of appearance, fitness, or self-image among women can have serious adverse physical and psychological consequences.

Obesity is a complex problem that involves physical, psychosocial, behavioral, and physical activity factors; permanent weight reduction is difficult to achieve.

The set-point theory holds that, because of biologic factors, each individual has a set-point for body weight and will be unable to avoid regaining weight to that set-point without substantial restriction of calories and increase in exercise.

Prevention of obesity must begin in infancy and childhood; parents must be informed of the dangers of overfeeding and inactivity.

Binge eating is now classified as an eating disorder; clients who meet the criteria should be referred for psychotherapy and more complex nutrition care.

Grossly obese clients need to be accepted as they are, apart from their ability to lose weight; a person's weight does not define that person.

Treatment of obesity is in a state of transition; past efforts have failed to produce permanent weight loss; new strategies are emerging.

Traditional approaches used to treat obesity include calorie-controlled diet, exercise, behavior modification, drugs, and surgery.

Diet approaches include popular self-prescribed diets, which include formula diets and diets that severely restrict carbohydrate or fat, very low-calorie diets, and balanced diets with moderate caloric restriction.

When exercise is part of a weight control program, the diet need not be so severely restricted, muscle tone is improved, more muscle tissue is retained, the BMR is increased, adherence to the diet is improved, and weight lost is less likely to be regained.

Low to moderate levels of exercise are associated with better adherence and greater psychological benefit than vigorous exercise for the obese person.

Careful planning is necessary to include all of the essential nutrients in calorie-controlled diets of less than 1800 to 2000 kcal/day; there is little room for foods such as fats, sugars and other sweets, and alcohol, which are high in calories for the nutrients they provide.

Behavior modification focuses on behavior change rather than on diet. It is based on the belief that weight loss will result if problem eating habits are changed.

In behavior modification, clients analyze their eating habits and evaluate their progress by means of carefully kept records of their eating behavior.

Anorectic drugs taken under medical supervision have been useful for some clients; they are used in combination with diet control and exercise.

Gastroplasty occasionally is performed on people who are severely obese and whose obesity is seriously interfering with their health.

People seeking weight loss treatment should be informed that permanent, substantial weight loss requires lifelong dramatic restriction of caloric intake and increased exercise because of their biologic set-point.

Losing and maintaining small amounts of weight loss are more achievable goals.

Achievable weight, not ideal weight, should be the treatment goal.

Clients should be involved in setting their own goals and in developing their own eating and exercise plan.

In general, structured, reduced-calorie diets have not been successful in achieving long-term weight control.

The new therapy emphasizes the quality of the diet rather than the quantity of food, health benefits of changing eating and exercise habits, and uncovering and treating psychosocial issues that are creating barriers to change.

Fat budgeting can improve the quality of the diet without rigidly controlling quantity.

Planning ahead, using lowfat flavoring techniques, and using food labeling wisely can help in improving the quality of the diet.

The diet for the underweight person requires a gradual increase in calories to a level greater than energy needs. This may be achieved by increasing the amount of food eaten at each meal, emphasizing carbohydrate-rich foods with some increase in easily digested fats, and eating more frequent and smaller meals.

KEYS TO LEARNING

STUDY–DISCUSSION QUESTIONS

1. Compare the following approaches to reducing caloric intake:

   For 2 days, limit your fat intake to 50 g fat/day. There is no other restriction on what you eat. Keep a diary of the foods you eat and their fat content. What problems did you encounter in doing this assignment?

   Develop for yourself a day's meal plan and sample menu based on 1500 kcal/day reducing diet given in Table 23-3 and the exchange lists in Table 22-6. Make the meal plan as close to your own eating pattern as possible. Follow this meal plan for one day. What problems did you encounter?

   Which approach—fat budgeting or caloric control—do you think you could maintain for an indefinite period?

2. Discuss the social problems the grossly obese person faces. How important is the attitude of health personnel toward the obese client? Why? What approach do you think would be most helpful to the client?

3. What is your opinion of the statement, "Losing weight only takes willpower." Why do you feel this way? Has your opinion changed recently?

4. Obtain a copy of a currently popular fad diet. In light of what you have learned about obesity, present to the class an evaluation of the diet.

5. Assume that you are a parent with three children—two between the ages of 6 and 10 years and one teenager. What measures would you take to prevent the development of obesity in the entire family, parents included? See Chapter 18 for a further discussion of childhood obesity.
6. How would you increase the caloric intake of an underweight person recovering from a severe illness?

BIBLIOGRAPHY

BOOKS AND PAMPHLETS

American Psychiatric Association. Diagnostic and statistical manual of mental disorders. 4th ed. Washington, DC: American Psychiatric Association, 1994.

National Academy of Sciences, National Research Council, Committee on Diet and Health, Food and Nutrition Board. Diet and health: implications for reducing chronic disease risk (executive summary). Washington, DC: National Academy Press, 1989.

Pi-Sunyer FX. Obesity. In: Shils ME, Olson JA, Shike M. Eds. Modern nutrition in health and disease. 8th ed. Philadelphia: Lea and Febiger, 1994:984–1006.

US Dept of Health and Human Services, Public Health Service/Food and Drug Administration. The facts about weight loss products and programs. Bethesda, MD: US Dept of Health and Human Services, 1992. DHHS publication FDA 92-1189.

PERIODICALS

Abernathy RP, Black DR. Is adipose tissue oversold as a health risk? J Am Diet Assoc 1994;94:641.

Anderson RE. Making exercise fun. Weight Control Digest 1992;2:164.

Brownell KD, Rodin J. Medical, metabolic, and psychological effects of weight cycling. Arch Intern Med 1994;154:1325.

Brownell KD, Wadden TA. Matching weight control programs to individuals: how to find the best fit. Weight Control Digest 1991;1:65.

Grilo CM, Wilfley DE, Brownell KD. Physical activity and weight control: why is the link so strong? Weight Control Digest 1992;2:153.

Hall SM, Tunstall CD, Vila KL, et al. Preventing weight gain after smoking cessation. Am J Public Health 1992;82:799.

Kabatznick R. Toward a new psychology of dieting. Nutrition Update 1992;2:3.

Kanders BS, Ullman-Joy P, Foreyt JP, et al. The Black American Lifestyle Intervention (BALI): The design of a weight loss program for working class African American women. J Am Diet Assoc 1994;94:310.

National Institutes of Health, Technology Assessment Conference. Methods for voluntary weight loss and control. Ann Intern Med 1992;116:942.

Orphanidou C, McCargar L, Birmingham CL. Accuracy of subcutaneous fat measurement: comparison of skinfold calipers, ultrasound, and computer tomography. J Am Diet Assoc 1994;94:855.

Parham ES. Nutrition education research in weight management among adults. J Nutr Educ 1993;25:258.

Reeves RS, Bolton MP. Fat budgeting: a useful alternative. Weight Control Digest 1991;1:110.

Reiff DW, Reiff KKL. Position of the American Dietetic Association: nutrition intervention in the treatment of anorexia nervosa, bulimia nervosa, and binge eating. J Am Diet Assoc 1994;94:902.

Robinson JI, Hoerr SL, Strandmark J, et al. Obesity, weight loss, and health. J Am Diet Assoc 1993;93:445.

Shattuck DK. Mindfulness and metaphor in relapse prevention: an interview with G. Alan Marlatt. J Am Diet Assoc 1994;94:846.

Stensland SH, Margolis S. Simplifying the calculation of body mass index for quick reference. J Am Diet Assoc 1990;90:856.

Weigley ES. The body mass index in clinical practice. Top Clin Nutr 1994;9:6:70.

CHAPTER

24

Nutrition Therapy in Diabetes Mellitus

KEY TERMS

autoimmunity condition in which antibodies are produced against the subject's own tissues

classic (symptoms) typical symptoms of a particular disease or condition

continuous subcutaneous insulin infusion an insulin pump

coxsackievirus B_4 virus that has been shown to damage the cells of the pancreas

fructosamine test blood test that indicates the average blood glucose level for the previous 1 to 3 weeks

gestational related to pregnancy

glucagon hormone made by the alpha cells of the pancreas that raises the glucose level in the blood; glucagon can be injected when a person is in insulin shock

glycosuria presence of glucose in the urine

glycosylated hemoglobin (A_{1c}) type of red blood cell that has bonded with glucose; the quantity of this cell present in the blood indicates how well blood sugar has been controlled over the previous 8 to 10 weeks

hyperglycemia excessive amount of glucose in the blood

hypoglycemia abnormally low amount of glucose in the blood

insulin hormone made by the beta cells of the pancreas that helps the body use glucose for energy

insulin receptors areas on the outer surface of a cell that allow the cell to bind with insulin that is in the blood

insulin resistance failure of tissues to use insulin normally

Islets of Langerhans special groups of cells in the pancreas that produce and secrete the hormones insulin, glucagon, and somatostatin

ketonuria presence of ketone bodies in the urine

macrosomia abnormally large body

nephropathy renal (kidney) disease

neuropathy disease of the nerves

perineal pertaining to the genital area

physiologically based based on normal physical processes

polydipsia excessive thirst

polyphagia excessive desire to eat

polyuria passage of an excessive quantity of urine

postprandial after a meal

preprandial before a meal

random (blood glucose level) nonfasting; the blood glucose level as measured any time after a person has eaten

renal threshold concentration at which a substance in the blood that normally is not excreted by the kidney begins to appear in the urine

retinopathy disease of the retina

somatostatin hormone made by the delta cells of the pancreas that may control the secretion of insulin and glucagon

sulfonylureas pills containing sulfur that are used to lower the level of glucose in the blood

vascular relating to blood vessels

OBJECTIVES

After completing this chapter, the student will be able to:

1. Explain how a diagnosis of diabetes is made and explain the problems associated with the terms *mild diabetes* or *borderline diabetes.*
2. Describe the cause or causes, symptoms, and complications of both insulin-dependent and non–insulin-dependent diabetes.
3. Give three ways in which hyperglycemia adversely affects the body.
4. Explain the significance of the Diabetes Control and Complications Trial.
5. Explain how the interrelationship of food, insulin, and activity affect diabetes management and describe the role of self-monitoring of blood glucose.
6. Describe intensive insulin therapy and conventional insulin therapy.
7. Describe the use of oral glucose–lowering medication in the treatment of type II diabetes.
8. List the overall goals of nutrition therapy in the treatment of diabetes mellitus.
9. Explain the two major philosophical changes in the American Diabetes Association's nutrition recommendations of 1994.
10. Describe the American Diabetes Association's recommendations regarding each of the following:
    protein
    fat
    carbohydrate
    sucrose
    nutritive (caloric) sweeteners
    nonnutritive (noncaloric) sweeteners
    fiber
    sodium
    vitamins and minerals
    alcohol
11. Explain the meal planning priorities in type I diabetes and in type II diabetes.
12. Demonstrate ability to plan menus when given a meal plan and exchange lists using information provided in this chapter and in Chapter 22.
13. Explain how carbohydrate counting is used to control blood glucose.
14. Appreciate the many challenges faced by children with diabetes and their families and the need to achieve good control in an atmosphere of flexibility, compromise, and respect for the goals of the child and family members.
15. Explain the importance of "tight control" during pregnancy in diabetes and of avoiding hypoglycemia.
16. Give the symptoms, causes, and treatment of diabetes ketoacidosis and hypoglycemia.
17. State the policy regarding food replacement for clients with diabetes in the student's clinical setting.
18. Discuss the implications of including comprehensive training in self-management as a necessary component of *basic medical care* for people with diabetes (as defined in standards of medical care issued by the American Diabetes Association).

More than 13 million Americans—6% of the US population—have diabetes. By 2000, the number of people with diabetes is expected to approach 20 million. Diabetes is the fourth leading cause of death by disease (when excluding accidents, pneumonia, and influenza) and the seventh cause of death overall. It is the number one cause of new blindness in adults aged 20 to 74 years, increases the risk for heart disease two to four times, causes half of all leg and foot amputations annually, and is the single leading cause of kidney disease. Although there presently is no known cure for the disease, great strides have been made through research in understanding and treating diabetes.

Diabetes was described in an Egyptian manuscript as early as 1500 BC. The Greek physician Aretaeus (150 to 200 AD) named the disease *diabetes,* meaning "to siphon or flow through," a reference to the large amount of urine produced in people with the disease. The Latin word *mellitus,* meaning "honeyed," was added later to indicate the presence of sugar in the urine. It also distinguishes diabetes mellitus from *diabetes insipidus,* a rare disease that also is characterized by excessive urination but without the presence of sugar. Diabetes insipidus in caused by a defect in the pituitary gland.

In 1921, a major breakthrough occurred in the treatment of diabetes mellitus with the discovery of insulin by Canadian researchers Frederick Banting and Charles Best. Before the discovery of insulin, children and young adults who had diabetes lived only a few weeks or months. As the life span increased, however, the long-term complications of the disease began to surface. In the 1950s, scientists learned how to measure the amount of insulin in the blood. They discovered that not all people with diabetes have an insulin deficiency.

In 1993, another major breakthrough occurred with the completion of the Diabetes Control and Complications Trial (DCCT), a randomized controlled 10-year study of 1441 people with insulin-dependent diabetes mellitus (type I). The results revealed that more strict control (intensive management) of blood glucose levels dramatically decreased the overall risk of long-term complications by 60%.

TYPES OF DIABETES MELLITUS

Diabetes mellitus is a group of disorders characterized by an abnormally high blood glucose (sugar) level. There are two major types, which are the focus of this chapter:

Insulin-dependent diabetes mellitus (type I)—An estimated 500,000 children and young adults have type I diabetes. The onset is usually during youth. People with this type of diabetes must take insulin daily to stay alive.

Non–insulin-dependent diabetes mellitus (type II)—Type II diabetes occurs most frequently in adults older than age 40 years. Most people in this category are obese and have a family history of diabetes. In this form of diabetes, insulin injections are not required to sustain life but may be needed during periods of physical stress or to correct elevated blood glucose levels that resist other forms of treatment.

Other classifications of diabetes mellitus that occur less frequently are as follows:

Secondary diabetes—This form includes diabetes caused by drugs or chemicals or resulting from diseases such as pancreatic or endocrine disease.

Gestational diabetes—Pregnant women, most of them obese, may suffer from gestational diabetes. The cause may be the complex metabolic and hormonal changes that occur during pregnancy. Blood glucose levels usually return to normal after delivery. The woman who experiences gestational diabetes has an increased risk of developing diabetes within 5 to 10 years after the pregnancy.

DIAGNOSIS OF DIABETES MELLITUS

The diagnosis of diabetes is made on the basis of blood glucose levels. In nonpregnant adults, a diagnosis of diabetes is made if the person has the classic symptoms of diabetes (excessive thirst, excessive urination, excessive hunger, and weight loss) and a random blood glucose level of 200 mg/dL or greater. A fasting plasma glucose level of 140 mg/dL or greater on at least two occasions also indicates diabetes. When the blood glucose level is suspect but not high enough to definitely establish the presence of diabetes, an oral glucose tolerance test may be done. In this test, the client, who has been fasting for at least 10 hours, has a fasting blood sample drawn and then is given a solution to drink that contains 75 g of glucose. Blood samples are collected at 30-, 60-, 90-, 120-, and 180-minute intervals. If the 2-hour sample and at least one other sample between the start of the test and 2 hours is 200 mg/dL or greater, and if these results are duplicated during at least two oral glucose tolerance tests, a diagnosis of diabetes is made. Clients should be properly prepared to take the glucose tolerance test. The test is invalid if done on people who are chronically malnourished or who have restricted carbohydrate intake to less than 150 g/day for 3 days or longer before the test.

People whose blood glucose level falls between normal (Table 24-1) and diabetic have what is called *impaired glucose tolerance*. They are not classified as having diabetes; however, about 25% of people with impaired glucose tolerance eventually develop diabetes mellitus. A person has or does not

TABLE 24-1 INDICATORS OF BLOOD GLUCOSE CONTROL IN DIABETES*

BIOCHEMICAL INDEX	NORMAL	GOAL	ACTION SUGGESTED†
Preprandial fasting glucose (mg/dL)‡	<115	80–120	<80 >140
Bedtime glucose (mg/dL)	<120	100–140	<100 >160
Hemoglobin A_{1C}** (%)	<6	<7	>8

* For nonpregnant individuals.

† Depending on the individual client's circumstances.

‡ Au note: Fasting and before meals.

** Referenced to Hemoglobin A_{1c} nondiabetic range (4% to 6%).

(American Dietetic Association, Diabetes Care and Education Practice Group. Maximizing the role of nutrition in diabetes management (program manual). Alexandria, VA: American Diabetes Association, 1994:7.)

have diabetes based on the criteria described. The terms *borderline diabetes, mild diabetes,* and *chemical diabetes* should not be used because they are misleading.

BLOOD GLUCOSE CONTROL

SOURCES OF BLOOD GLUCOSE

Glucose circulating in the bloodstream is the primary source of fuel for the body. The sources of blood glucose are carbohydrate, protein, and fat from food. Of these three energy-producing nutrients, carbohydrates are the main source of glucose. All digestible carbohydrate is converted to glucose. Only 10% of dietary fat is converted to glucose; as much as 58% of protein is available for glucose production, depending on the body's needs.

Some of the blood glucose is stored in the liver and muscle as glycogen. Glycogen is converted back to glucose when the body needs it. Although a limited amount of glucose is stored as glycogen, glycogen is constantly being produced and provides a readily available source of glucose when blood sugar levels drop.

FACTORS AFFECTING CONTROL

In people who do not have diabetes, blood glucose levels rarely fall below 60 mg/dL or rise above 150 mg/dL, no matter how much food they consume. *Insulin,* a hormone produced by the pancreas, is a major factor in maintaining this blood glucose control. Insulin is produced by groups of cells scattered throughout the pancreas. These cell clusters are referred to as islets of Langerhans, named after the German physician who discovered them. These islets contain beta cells that make, store, and release insulin.

The conversion of glucose to energy occurs inside the body cells. Getting glucose into the cell requires insulin and insulin receptors. After eating, the amount of glucose in the blood rises. Under normal conditions, the pancreas detects this increase and sends out insulin. Insulin circulates in the blood and attaches to special receptors on the surfaces of fat and muscle cells. This binding of insulin with the cell causes pathways to open that allow glucose to enter the cell, where it can be converted to energy. As the glucose is taken up by the cells, the blood glucose level in the blood begins to drop. When the blood glucose level gets low, the pancreas stops sending out insulin (Fig. 24-1).

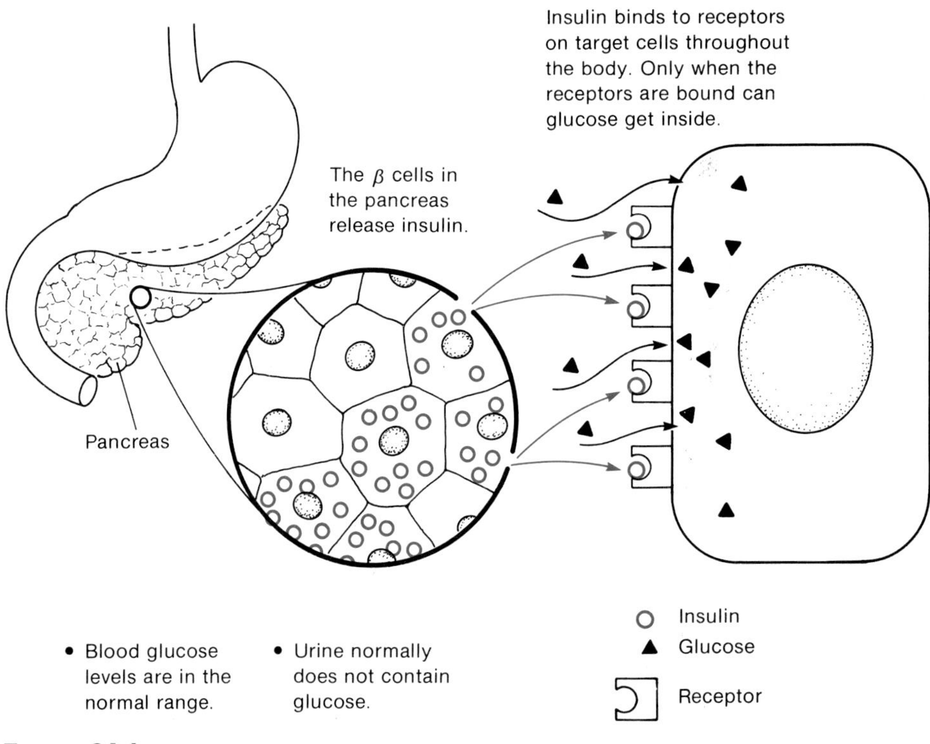
Insulin binds to receptors on target cells throughout the body. Only when the receptors are bound can glucose get inside.
The β cells in the pancreas release insulin.
Pancreas
• Blood glucose levels are in the normal range.
• Urine normally does not contain glucose.
Insulin
Glucose
Receptor

FIGURE 24-1

Diagram of normal glucose metabolism. Converting glucose to energy requires insulin and insulin receptors.

Islets of Langerhans also contain alpha cells, which produce another hormone, *glucagon,* which raises blood glucose. Glucagon causes glycogen stored in the liver to be converted to glucose when the blood glucose level begins to dip too low. *Somatostatin,* a hormone produced by the delta cells of islets of Langerhans inhibits the secretion of both insulin and glucagon and inhibits the release of growth hormone.

CHARACTERISTICS OF DIABETES

In diabetes, the body does not make enough insulin or does not use the insulin properly. In either case, the blood glucose cannot enter the cells. This causes blood glucose to accumulate in abnormal amounts in the blood.

Another result of the abnormal metabolism of foods in diabetes is the elevation of blood fat levels (cholesterol and triglycerides) that tends to occur. Elevated blood glucose levels and elevated blood fat levels are toxic and frequently result in serious complications if uncontrolled. Although all types of diabetes mellitus affect the metabolism of body fuels, the cause, nature, and treatment differ for the two major types.

INSULIN-DEPENDENT DIABETES MELLITUS (IDDM) (TYPE I)

Of all people with diabetes mellitus, 5% have type I, or insulin-dependent, diabetes. Although it occurs mostly in children (the peak age is 6 to 11 years) and young adults who have a lean body type, it can occur at any age. Evidence has suggested that the cause is both hereditary and environmental. People with certain genes have a defect in the immune system that, when challenged by environmental factors such as viruses (especially rubella, mumps, and coxsackievirus B_4), may cause antibodies to develop against the insulin-producing beta cells in the islets of Langerhans. This autoimmune attack results in the inability of the beta cells to produce insulin.

When insulin is lacking, glucose cannot be used for energy. The body looks for other sources of fuel—protein and fat. It is harder for the body to use these substances for fuel. The body cannot burn protein and fat completely, and some of the unused substances, called *ketones,* which are acidic in nature, build up in the blood. The accumulation of these unused acidic substances causes a condition known as *ketoacidosis.* People with type I diabetes require insulin injections to avoid ketoacidosis or ketosis, which, if untreated, can cause death.

Classic symptoms often associated with diabetes are those of type I diabetes. The increase in blood sugar levels followed by excretion of glucose and ketones in the urine (glycosuria and ketonuria) produce the most common symptoms: polyuria and polydipsia. Because people with diabetes do not receive full benefit from the food they eat, they are constantly hungry (*polyphagia*) and lose weight rapidly. Other symptoms include fatigue, weakness, irritability, nausea and vomiting, and perineal itching and irritation.

NON–INSULIN-DEPENDENT DIABETES MELLITUS (NIDDM) (TYPE II)

About 95% of people with diabetes have non–insulin-dependent, or type II, diabetes. Most are obese and are older than age 40 years. The primary cause in people who have a hereditary tendency to the disease is obesity. The genetic link is stronger in type II than in type I diabetes. Among identical twins, if one twin has type II diabetes, the other twin almost always develops it eventually. In contrast, fewer than half of identical twins of people with type I diabetes develop the disease.

Type II diabetes is characterized by several defects in insulin action and secretion, including a blunted insulin secretion, insulin resistance in muscle and fat cells, and an excessive output of glucose by the liver. The beta cells of the pancreas may not respond normally to the sugar signal, which causes a delay in the release of insulin after meals. Although the initial release of insulin after eating is inadequate, increased amounts of insulin may be released later. Many people with type II diabetes make more than enough insulin. There are too few insulin receptors, however, resulting in a delay in insulin action because the hormone cannot attach to the cells fast enough. Without enough insulin receptors to accept the insulin, insulin builds up in the blood and blood sugar continues to rise. Oddly enough, the abnormally elevated insulin levels cause a further shutdown of insulin receptors, possibly as a protective mechanism. Abnormal glucose metabolism within the cell is thought to be another defect involved. This abnormal use of insulin by the tissues is called *insulin resistance.* In addition, the liver may fail to store and release sugar normally, which causes the body to be flooded with glucose.

Type II diabetes is called *non–insulin-dependent* because there is enough effective insulin for survival. The amount of insulin activity, because of resistance, is insufficient to keep blood glucose levels normal, but is sufficient to prevent ketoacidosis. Some people with type II diabetes need insulin injections to avoid symptoms of hyperglycemia, and most require insulin temporarily during periods of stress, such as surgery or severe infections.

The onset of type II diabetes often is gradual. Many people do not become aware that they have the disease until they develop one of the serious complications—heart disease, renal disease, or eye problems. Some people with type II diabetes have the classic symptoms of the disease. Usually, however, the symptoms are less dramatic than they are in type I diabetes. They include blurred vision; tingling or numbness in the legs, feet, or fingers; frequent infections (e.g., skin or vaginal infections); slow healing of cuts and bruises; and drowsiness.

Type II diabetes can be undiagnosed for years and often is discovered through routine examination. People older than age 40 years who are overweight and have relatives with diabetes should be aware that they have a high risk of developing diabetes.

MANAGEMENT OF DIABETES

GOALS

The main purposes of treatment are to restore the body's ability to use carbohydrates properly (which, in turn, results in normal fat and protein metabolism) and to prevent the vascular complications of the disease. Hyperglycemia, due to whatever cause, is toxic to the entire body if left untreated. Effects of hyperglycemia include

- the failure of young people to grow and develop normally
- an increased number of stillbirths and birth defects in infants of women whose diabetes is poorly controlled
- thickening of the walls of the small blood vessels (capillaries)
- an alteration of the blood clotting process, causing the platelets to become stickier and more likely to clot
- abnormal fat metabolism, probably promoting *atherosclerosis,* disease of the large blood vessels
- a reduced ability to fight infection.

The person with diabetes is particularly susceptible to diseases of both the small and large blood vessels. Disease of the small blood vessels, referred to as *microvascular complications,* may result in *nephropathy* (kidney disease), *neuropathy* (nerve disease), or *retinopathy* (eye disease). Atherosclerosis is the major cause of death among people with diabetes in the United States. People with diabetes are at least twice as prone to coronary artery disease as nondiabetic individuals.

THE DCCT: THE VALUE OF "TIGHT CONTROL"

In 1993, the results of a landmark 10-year research study conducted by the National Institute of Diabetes and Digestive and Kidney Diseases were published. The study (DCCT) showed that strict control of blood glucose levels could dramatically slow the onset and progression of diabetic complications. The study put to rest a 50-year controversy over whether long-term complications were the result of the diabetes itself or of the excess glucose in the blood due to inadequate control.

The DCCT consisted of 1441 people with type I diabetes at 29 clinical centers throughout the United States and Canada. The study compared two treatment methods. People in the control group received standard treatment: daily blood glucose tests, one or two insulin injections daily, and a program of diet and exercise. People in the "tight control" group performed blood glucose tests four or more times each day and used three or four insulin injections daily or an insulin pump to keep blood glucose levels as near normal as possible. Study participants in the intensive treatment group adjusted insulin doses according to food intake, exercise, and blood glucose test results.

The average blood glucose level of people in the "tight control" group was 155 mg/dL compared with 231 mg/dL for the control group. (Average normal blood glucose level is 110 mg/dL.) Study results showed that intensive treatment reduced retinopathy by 76%, prevented or delayed the progression of nephropathy by 35% to 56%, and prevented neuropathy by 60%. The overall reduction in risk for the development and progression of these three complications of diabetes was 60%. Cardiovascular disease, another major complication of diabetes mellitus, was not studied in the DCCT.

"Tight control" does pose risks. People in the "tight control" group were three times more likely to have serious episodes of *hypoglycemia* (abnormally low blood glucose levels) and they also experienced significant weight gain. People for whom tight control may be inappropriate are discussed in the section Elements of Control (Medication: Insulin).

Although people with Type II diabetes were not included in the DCCT, authorities believe the results of the study also apply to people with type II diabetes. The goal for most people with diabetes mellitus should be to achieve blood glucose levels as close to normal as possible.

ELEMENTS OF CONTROL

Treatment of diabetes aims to lower and maintain blood glucose to normal or near-normal levels for all people with diabetes, regardless of the type of diabetes. Achieving this goal requires thorough training in self-management and, for most individuals, an intensive treatment program. In June 1994, the American Diabetes Association issued its revised "Position Statement: Standards of Medical Care for Patients With Diabetes Mellitus." The standards list the components of such a training and treatment program as follows:

- frequent self-monitoring of blood glucose
- meticulous attention to meal planning
- physiologically based insulin regimens (i.e., multiple daily injections of short-acting and longer acting insulin or continuous subcutaneous insulin infusion) in type I diabetes and some type II diabetes clients
- less-complex insulin regimens or oral glucose–lowering agents in some type II diabetes clients
- instruction in the prevention and treatment of hypoglycemia and other acute and chronic complications
- continuing education and reinforcement
- periodic assessment of treatment goals.

A normal blood glucose level reflects a balance between factors that reduce blood glucose—physical activity and insulin—and factors that increase blood glucose—food intake and physical stress (Fig. 24-2) The management of diabetes, therefore, involves achieving a balance among three elements: food, physical activity, and insulin (either injected or made by the body).

FOOD

The nutritional management of diabetes involves developing a way of eating that controls blood glucose and blood fats. It is best viewed not as an on-again, off-again diet, but as a way of eating that will foster the goals of diabetes treatment, provide all the nutrients needed for good health, and accommodate as much as possible the individual's lifestyle and food preferences. Nutrition therapy is covered in detail later in the section Nutrition Intervention in Diabetes.

MEDICATION

Insulin

People with type I diabetes require daily injections of insulin to maintain life. Insulin cannot be taken by mouth because it is a protein and would be digested or broken down in the gastrointestinal tract.

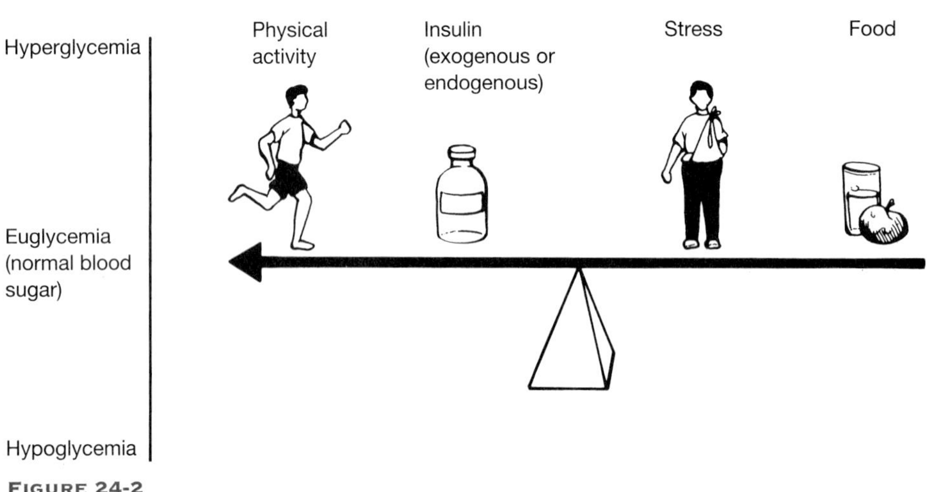

FIGURE 24-2

Factors that must be balanced to maintain normal blood glucose level.

The physician determines the kind and amount of insulin to be used.

Insulin differs in its source and in its action. Beef, pork, a combination of beef and pork, and human insulin are available on the market. The most ideal type of insulin is identical to insulin made by the human body. Eli Lilly & Company has created human insulin in a process in which genes of bacteria are instructed to make human insulin molecules. This process is called *recombinant DNA* (deoxyribonucleic acid), meaning the formation of new combinations of genes. This insulin is called Humulin. The Novo-Nordisk Company also produces human insulin, called Novolin, by DNA technology.

The animal insulin comes from the pancreases of cows and pigs. Pork insulin is more similar to human insulin than is beef insulin. In general, insulin that is most like human insulin is less likely to cause problems.

Insulin that is released by the body is immediately available for use by the cells. This is not so with injected insulin. There are three action times of injected insulin: rapid, intermediate, and long acting. Injected insulins differ in the length of time required to take effect (onset), the time of their greatest glucose-lowering effect (peak action), and how long they continue to work (duration). Table 24-2 shows the general action patterns of the various insulins. The different action patterns are due to the addition of protein or zinc to regular insulin, which is the most rapid acting.

Insulin analogs are a new class of drugs expected to be marketed in the mid-1990s. Recombinant DNA technology allows scientists to design insulin with different properties. Eli Lilly & Company is awaiting FDA approval of Lyspro, an insulin analog that is absorbed and acts more quickly than regular insulin.

Intensive Insulin Therapy. Because the DCCT results have shown conclusively that tight control of blood glucose prevents or at least delays diabetes-related complications, tight control has become the new standard of care. How this is achieved may differ for each person. Some people inject insulin three times a day, whereas others may use four to five injections. Others may use an insulin pump and others may use as many as three different types of insulin.

TABLE 24-2 PHARMACOLOGY OF INSULIN

ANIMAL INSULIN			
ACTION TIME	**ONSET (H)**	**PEAK (H)**	**USUAL EFFECTIVE DURATION (H)**
Regular (rapid acting)	0.5–2	3–4	4–6
Intermediate acting (NPH and Lente)	4–6	8–14	16–20
Long acting (Ultralente)	8–14	Minimal	24–36
HUMAN INSULIN			
ACTION TIME	**ONSET (H)**	**PEAK (H)**	**USUAL EFFECTIVE DURATION (H)**
Regular (rapid acting)	0.5–1	2–3	3–6
Intermediate acting (NPH and Lente)	2–4	4–12	10–18
Long acting (Ultralente)	6–10	?	18–20

(American Dietetic Association, Diabetes Care and Education Practice Group. Maximizing the role of nutrition in diabetes management (program manual). Alexandria, VA: American Diabetes Association, 1994:8.)

Intensive insulin therapy is recommended for most people with type I diabetes and some people with type II diabetes. Tight control may be inadvisable for people with a history of severe hypoglycemia reactions or *hypoglycemia unawareness* (absence of early warning signs of a low blood glucose level); children younger than age 6 or 7 years; older people for whom tight control may not be worth the risks and costs after a certain age; and people with advanced kidney and heart disease.

Conventional Insulin Therapy. Conventional insulin therapy usually involves two injections—one before breakfast and one before the evening meal. The injection usually is a combination of intermediate-acting insulin (e.g., NPH) and regular insulin (rapid-acting). This approach is recommended for most people with type II diabetes who require insulin and for those people with type I diabetes for whom intensive therapy is inappropriate.

Oral Hypoglycemic Drugs

First and Second Generation Sulfonylureas. In 1955, pills were developed that improve insulin secretion and action. These drugs, derived from sulfur, are called *sulfonylureas* and are useful only if the body is producing some insulin. For this reason, they cannot be used in type I diabetes. Also, the sulfonylureas should not be used by pregnant or breastfeeding women.

The sulfonylurea drugs have played a major role in treating type II diabetes. If, after 2 to 3 months of dietary control, blood glucose levels remain elevated, the sulfonylurea drugs are added. These oral agents are not a substitute for, but rather always a supplement to, dietary control. If blood glucose control is not achieved in 3 to 6 months, insulin injections are prescribed.

The first sulfonylureas to be marketed are called the first generation of oral agents (Table 24-3). These have been largely replaced by a second generation of sulfonylureas that are 100 to 200 times stronger and can be given in smaller doses. The two second generation drugs are glipizide (Glucotrol) and glyburide (Diabeta, Micronase, and Glynase). The usual daily dosage and action times of the various drugs differ (Table 24-3).

Third Generation Oral Agents. New oral agents that are not sulfonylureas are currently entering the US market. In 1995, metformin, under the name Glucophage (Bristol-Myers Squibb Co.), became available for use in the United States. Metformin has been used in the treatment of type II diabetes in other countries for more than 30 years. Metformin lowers blood glucose by inhibiting the release of stored glucose by the liver. Insulin resistance may also be lowered. Because metformin does not increase the secretion of insulin as the sulfonylureas do, there is no risk of hypoglycemia. Because met-

TABLE 24-3 ORAL HYPOGLYCEMIC DRUGS

GENERIC	DAILY DOSAGE RANGE (MG)	DURATION OF ACTION (H)
First Generation		
Tolbutamide (Orinase)	250–3000	6–12
Chlorpropamide (Diabinese)	100–500	60
Acetohexamide (Dymelor)	250–1500	12–18
Tolazamide (Tolinase)	100–1100	12–24
Second Generation		
Glipizide (Glucotrol)	2.5–40	Up to 24
Glyburide (Diabeta, Micronase)	1.25–20	Up to 24
Micronized glyburide (Glynase)	0.75–12	Up to 24

(American Dietetic Association. Diabetes Care and Education Practice Group. Maximizing the role of nutrition in diabetes management (program manual). Alexandria, VA: American Diabetes Association, 1994:9.)

formin and sulfonylureas work differently, they are frequently used together. Metformin may be especially useful for obese people.

Awaiting Food and Drug Administration approval is Acarbose (Bayer Corp.), an alpha-glucosidase inhibitor, a drug that affects the digestion and absorption of carbohydrate. The drug aims to slow the passage of glucose through the intestine and into the bloodstream.

Combination Oral Hypoglycemic Drugs and Insulin. The combined use of insulin and oral hypoglycemic drugs is a treatment method that has been introduced for certain clients with type II diabetes. Some clients, after time, lose their sensitivity to the oral agents and require insulin to maintain an acceptable blood glucose level. One way in which these two medications are combined involves the use of an intermediate-acting insulin in the late evening to bring down the overnight rise in blood glucose that occurs frequently in type II diabetes, and the use of oral hypoglycemic pills during the day. In those clients who respond to this therapy, blood glucose control is achieved on a lower insulin dose than if insulin were used alone.

EXERCISE

Physical activity improves the body's ability to use glucose, decreases insulin resistance, lowers cholesterol, lowers blood pressure, and reduces body fat. It also improves circulation and muscle tone and provides a sense of well-being, reducing stress and increasing self-confidence. For people with type II diabetes, exercise, when combined with nutrition therapy, is an effective means of improving blood glucose control and cardiovascular fitness.

The person with type I diabetes also derives cardiovascular benefit and may be able to reduce insulin needs with exercise. Exercise tends to make type I diabetes more difficult to control, however, because it promotes hypoglycemia and the extent of its blood glucose–lowering effects are somewhat unpredictable. Blood glucose control can be achieved more easily if the individual exercises at the same time and for the same duration each day. Adjustment can be made in the meal plan or insulin dosage to accommodate the effects of the exercise. If the exercise is of light to moderate intensity and of short duration (up to 1 hour or so), a snack before and after exercise may be required, depending on blood glucose level. During prolonged strenuous exercise, the equivalent of a fruit or starch exchange (about 15 g of carbohydrate) may be needed every 30 to 60 minutes and insulin dosage may need to be reduced.

Blood glucose levels may continue to decrease after exercise, causing a hypoglycemic reaction several hours after the exercise ends. It is important for clients to know that this decrease may occur and to be alert for symptoms. It can take the body up to 24 hours to replenish the carbohydrate stored in the muscles and liver. Doing self-monitoring of blood glucose before, during, and after exercise helps clients understand how their body reacts to exercise. With the help of the health care team, guidelines for exercise can then be established. It is important to have a source of carbohydrate available during and after the exercise and to exercise with other people who are aware of the diabetes and know what to do if help is needed.

People who have blood glucose levels of more than 240 mg/dL and ketones in the urine should not exercise. Ketonuria indicates a serious deficiency of insulin; increased exercise only increases the blood glucose level. In addition, people with diabetes should consult their physician before beginning an exercise program. The physician will prescribe the type and amount of exercise based on the individual's physical condition. Some types of exercise increase the risk of complications such as retinopathy and foot injuries.

SELF-MONITORING OF BLOOD GLUCOSE

Self-monitoring of blood glucose is an indispensable tool in diabetes management. Clients can be taught how to monitor their blood glucose daily. A single drop of capillary blood is placed on a chemical reagent pad or sensor strip, causing a reaction that indicates the blood glucose level (Fig. 24-3). The test strips are read by a meter, which provides a specific glucose value. The procedure used differs

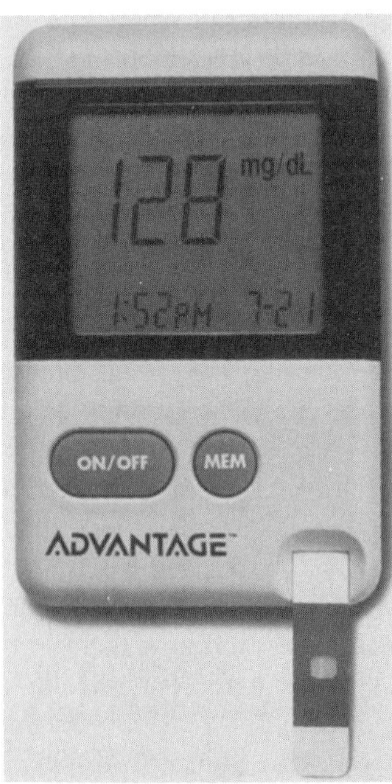

FIGURE 24-3

An example of a commercially available blood glucose meter that electronically measures the amount of glucose in the blood. Self-monitoring of blood glucose is an indispensable tool in diabetes self-management. *(Courtesy of Boehringer Mannheim Corporation, Indianapolis, IN.)*

with the brand and type of equipment, but the manufacturer's instructions must be followed exactly to obtain accurate results. The capillary blood usually is obtained from a finger using an automated finger-sticking device.

Blood values taken before (*preprandial*) and after (*postprandial*) meals provide important information for evaluating how well the meal plan, medication, and exercise program are working. Achieving a near-normal blood glucose level would be impossible and unsafe without self-monitoring of blood glucose. With tight control, the risk of hypoglycemia increases, especially in type I diabetes. The incidence of hypoglycemia can be reduced by regular self-monitoring.

In addition to its use in evaluating treatment, self-monitoring of blood glucose provides clients with feedback. They can see the effects of food and physical activity on blood glucose levels. Self-monitoring of blood glucose increases clients' involvement and promotes a sense of control over their treatment. All people with diabetes, whether treated with insulin or not, benefit from self-monitoring of blood glucose.

Using urine tests to evaluate blood glucose control is not recommended because the amount of glucose in the urine is not a good indicator of blood glucose levels. The level at which the kidneys remove excess glucose from the blood—the renal threshold—varies considerably among individuals. Whereas most individuals spill glucose into the urine when the blood sugar is about 180 mg/dL, others do not spill glucose until blood glucose is much higher, sometimes as high as 300 mg/dL or more. Making adjustments in treatment based on urine tests is inaccurate.

Urine testing for the presence of ketones is important, however. People with type I diabetes should test for ketones in the urine when they are ill or when the blood glucose level is 240 mg/dL or higher. Ketonuria is an early sign that ketoacidosis may be developing.

LABORATORY TESTS

The physician supplements the client's daily blood glucose monitoring with periodic tests to evaluate how well blood glucose is being controlled. The physician usually assesses glucose control with a plasma glucose test (either fasting or postprandial) and a glycosylated hemoglobin test. The *plasma glucose test* (as well as self-monitoring of blood glucose) reflects the metabolic control at the time of the test but does not indicate what it has been over the past weeks or months. The *glycosylated hemoglobin test,* also called *hemoglobin* A_{1c} or *glycohemoglobin,* measures the percentage of total red blood cells that have bonded with glucose in the bloodstream. The higher the blood glucose level, the higher the percentage of glycosylated hemoglobin. Because the bonding remains for the life of the red blood cell, which is about 60 to 90 days, the glycosolated hemoglobin gives a picture of what the average blood sugar control has been for an 8- to 10-week period. This is a valuable test and is performed at least twice a year.

The *fructosamine test* measures average blood glucose control over a 1- to 3-week period. It is useful in clients who need strict blood glucose control, as in pregnancy, and for those who have had a recent major change in their insulin prescription. Fructosamine is a protein in the bloodstream to which sugar becomes attached.

A *C-peptide profile* is a two-stage blood test that measures the amount of insulin produced by the body. It allows the physician to determine which clients truly require insulin therapy. In the case of the person with type II diabetes, this is not always a clear-cut decision.

Lipid profiles and blood and urine tests that evaluate kidney function are other tests important in nutrition assessment. They also are important in the evaluation of people with diabetes mellitus.

DIABETES SELF-MANAGEMENT TRAINING

Diabetes self-management training is an essential part of diabetes management because clients themselves are responsible for day-to-day management of the disease. Obviously, the more clients understand about their disease, the better care they can provide for themselves. Motivation and ability to cope with the many details of managing diabetes differ from client to client. Progress is made when clients are involved in setting their own goals. Health care professionals guide clients in making realistic decisions.

The physician, nurse, and dietitian work together to educate clients. Clients learn about the nature of their disease and how it can be controlled. They are taught how to manage their daily care, including insulin injection, blood testing, urine testing, treatment for insulin reaction and ketoacidosis, personal hygiene, and care of the feet (prone to infection or diabetes). The dietitian, in consultation with the physician and nurse, provides dietary instruction and counseling and helps clients integrate food intake with medication and exercise.

Education is best provided in stages that are appropriate to the client's needs. Basic, or survival, information is given at first. This information includes the basics of meal planning, guidelines for days when the client is ill, and instructions for dealing with hypoglycemic reactions. Once this essential information has been learned, more in-depth education is provided in the second stage. Information includes topics such as increasing fiber and reducing sodium in the diet and guidelines for dining out. The third stage of nutrition counseling involves periodically monitoring the client's nutritional status and updating the previously provided nutrition information. Family members are included in the educational plan. The support of knowledgeable family members is important.

Diabetes Forecast, the monthly magazine of the American Diabetes Association that is written for people with diabetes, contains the latest information in diabetes management. It is an excellent educational tool for both the client and the health care worker. The following are useful resources for people with diabetes:

American Diabetes Association
1660 Duke Street
Alexandria, VA 22314
800-ADA-DISC (800-232-3472)

Canadian Diabetes Association
78 Bond Street
Toronto, Ontario M5B 2J8

National Diabetes Information Clearinghouse
P.O. Box NDIC
9000 Rockville Pike
Bethesda, MD 20892

Juvenile Diabetes Association
23 E 26th Street
Suite 1014
New York, NY 10010

NUTRITION INTERVENTION IN DIABETES

GOALS

Because diabetes is basically a disease in which the body has problems metabolizing food normally, it is understandable that nutritional factors play an important role in its management. The overall goal of nutrition therapy is to assist people with diabetes in making changes in nutrition and exercise habits that will enable them to

- maintain as near-normal blood glucose levels as possible
- achieve recommended serum blood lipid levels
- provide sufficient or appropriate energy intake
- prevent and treat acute and long-term diabetes-related complications
- enhance overall health through optimal nutrition.

To achieve a near-normal blood glucose level, the food eaten must be in balance with the insulin in the body (whether that insulin is produced by the body or whether it is injected) and with physical activity. Once blood glucose levels are normalized, symptoms of diabetes subside and long-term complications of the disease can be prevented or delayed, a factor confirmed by the DCCT. Blood glucose control is the most important factor in preventing or delaying chronic complications. The aim is to achieve blood glucose levels similar to those given in Table 24-1. Nutrition therapy must also address short-term complications such as hypoglycemia, short-term illnesses, and problems of blood glucose control during and following exercise.

Keeping blood fat to ideal levels is as important a goal as maintaining good blood glucose levels because people with diabetes are at least twice as prone as people without diabetes to die from coronary artery disease. Goals for serum cholesterol and triglycerides are given in Table 24-4.

The energy content of the diet must meet the individual's specific needs. Children and adolescents must consume enough calories to achieve their potential for growth and to promote normal development. Pregnant and breastfeeding women who have diabetes need enough calories to provide for their increased metabolic needs. Adults require adequate energy to maintain or achieve a *reasonable weight*— weight that both the client and health care providers determine can be achieved and maintained.

Healthful eating for people with diabetes is the same as that for all Americans. The Dietary Guidelines for Americans and Food Guide Pyramid provide guidelines and a framework for achieving good nutritional health.

GUIDELINES FOR NUTRITION THERAPY

In 1994, The American Diabetes Association issued revised "Nutrition Recommendations and Principles for People with Diabetes Mellitus," superseding the previous 1986 guidelines (Table 24-5). The 1994 recommendations challenge long-standing beliefs about food and diabetes and encourage profound changes in the nutrition management of diabetes.

Two major changes in the philosophy of nutrition care are as follows:

1. Nutrition management of diabetes requires an individually developed prescription based on the individual's metabolic needs (blood glucose levels, serum cholesterol, serum triglycerides, blood pressure, renal status, and so forth) and personal lifestyle considerations. The previous dietary prescription for people with diabetes, often referred to as the *ADA diet,* which was based on specific percentages of protein, fat, and carbohydrate, is obsolete. The "one size fits all" philosophy no longer applies to the nutrition management of diabetes.
2. In the nutrition management of type II diabetes, emphasis is on achieving metabolic goals (optimal blood glucose, lipid, and blood pressure levels) and not primarily on weight loss as it was in the past. Weight loss is viewed as one means among a variety of ways to achieve metabolic goals.

The dietitian uses the four-step approach (Chapter 20) in providing nutrition therapy and diabetes self-management training. An important step is to assess what the client is willing and able to do. Sensitivity to the client's goals is crucial to success.

TABLE 24-4 LIPID LEVELS FOR ADULTS

	RISK LEVEL		
	ACCEPTABLE	BORDERLINE	HIGH
Cholesterol (mg/dL)	<200	200–239	≥240
LDL-C (mg/dL)	<130*	130–159	≥160
HDL-C (mg/dL)	—	—	≤35
TG (mg/dL)	<200†	200–399	≥400

LDL-C: low-density lipoprotein cholesterol; associated with high risk

HDL-C: high-density lipoprotein cholesterol; associated with low risk

TG: triglycerides

* Clients with known coronary heart disease ≤ 100 mg/dL

† Clients at high risk for coronary heart disease should maintain TG ≤ 150 mg/dL.

(American Diabetes Association. Consensus statement. Diabetes Care 1993;16:2:106–112.)

RECOMMENDATIONS REGARDING DIETARY COMPONENTS

PROTEIN

A protein intake of 10% to 20% of the total caloric intake is recommended. This represents the amount of protein generally consumed by the US population. There is no scientific evidence that people with diabetes need higher or lower amounts except for people with nephropathy. At the onset of nephropathy, maintaining a lower intake of .8 g/kg of body weight or approximately 10% of daily energy intake is recommended. These recommendations represent a more liberal approach than the 1986 guidelines.

TOTAL FAT AND CARBOHYDRATE

Specific goals for both carbohydrate and fat are not given in the 1994 recommendations. The total amount of each of these nutrients depends on the metabolic needs and, also, cultural and ethnic factors.

The following are examples of how metabolic needs might influence total fat and carbohydrate intake. Recommendations of the Dietary Guidelines for Americans of 30% or less of energy intake from fat and less than 10% from saturated fat are appropriate for people with diabetes who have normal lipid values and a reasonable weight. Obese people may benefit from a reduction of total fat to 20% of total calories. However, people who have moderately elevated serum triglyceride levels may benefit

TABLE 24-5 COMPARISON OF NUTRITION RECOMMENDATIONS IN DIABETES, 1986 AND 1994

	DISTRIBUTION OF CALORIES		
YEAR	CARBOHYDRATE (%)	PROTEIN (%)	FAT (%)
1986	50–60	12–20	30
1994	Based on assessment	10–20	Total fat: Based on assessment less than 10% saturated fat

from a reduction in carbohydrate and an increase in total fat to 35% to 40% of calories by increasing monounsaturated fats in the diet.

SATURATED FAT AND CHOLESTEROL

Because diabetes is a strong risk factor for cardiovascular disease, a reduction of saturated fat to less than 10% of total energy intake and restriction of cholesterol to 300 mg or less is recommended.

CARBOHYDRATE AND SWEETENERS

No specific goal is given for carbohydrate. Carbohydrate levels are individualized according to glucose and lipid goals and the client's eating habits. The new guidelines emphasize total carbohydrate rather than the specific type of carbohydrate. This emphasis is a change from the previously held position that simple sugars should be avoided and replaced with complex carbohydrates. That viewpoint was based on the assumption that sugars are more rapidly digested and absorbed than starches and, therefore, raise blood glucose levels more rapidly and to a higher level. Many research studies conducted over the past 10 years have failed to support those assumptions.

The effect of various carbohydrate foods on blood glucose levels varies widely. Early research into the topic resulted in the development of the *glycemic index,* which ranks foods according to their effect on blood sugar level. Contrary to previous thinking, the effect of a carbohydrate on blood glucose level does not depend on whether it is a complex or simple carbohydrate, but depends on many other factors. These factors include the nature of the starch granule (corn versus rice versus potato); the food form (whole, cut up, mashed); substances in the food or meal that slow digestion; and the protein, fat, and fiber content of the food. Fruits and milk that contain carbohydrate in the form of simple sugars have been shown to raise blood glucose less than most starches, and sucrose (table sugar) affects blood glucose in a manner similar to bread, rice, and potatoes.

Sucrose

Sucrose and sucrose-containing foods do not have any more of an impact on blood glucose than starchy foods do when substituted for other carbohydrate foods. Sucrose does not impair blood glucose control *when it is used as part of an established carbohydrate allotment for a particular meal.*

The use of sugar requires caution as it does for all people—whether or not they have diabetes. Foods high in sugar are frequently high in fat and also tend to be of poor nutritional quality, that is, low in vitamins, minerals, and fiber.

Fructose

Fructose does not produce as high a rise in blood glucose level as sucrose and most starches. However, large amounts of fructose may raise serum cholesterol and low-density lipoprotein levels; people with serum lipid abnormalities should avoid fructose. It is unnecessary to restrict fruits and vegetables in which fructose occurs naturally or moderate use of fructose-sweetened foods.

Other Calorie-Containing Sweeteners

Other calorie-containing sweeteners in addition to sucrose and fructose include corn sweeteners such as corn syrup, fruit juice or fruit juice concentrate, honey, molasses, dextrose, and maltose. These sweeteners are all considered to provide as many calories and to affect blood glucose in the same manner as sucrose, and are covered by the same recommendations as those that apply to sucrose.

Sorbitol, mannitol, and xylitol are sugar alcohols (polyols) that do not cause as rapid a rise in blood glucose as sucrose and other carbohydrates. Starch hydrolysates used widely in commercial foods are also polyols. They are formed by the hydrolysis and hydrogenation of starches. The caloric value of the polyols is difficult to determine because they are poorly absorbed. There apparently is no significant advantage of using polyols over other caloric-containing sweeteners. Excessive amounts tend to have a laxative effect.

Nonnutritive (Noncaloric) Sweeteners

The American Diabetes Association has found the use of the three FDA-approved nonnutritive sweeteners to be acceptable for use by all people with diabetes. These sweeteners are saccharin, aspartame, and acesulfame-potassium (ACE-K or acesulfame-K). They are called nonnutritive because they are calorie free or provide only minimal calories in the small amounts needed for sweetness. Each packet of a sweetner supplies about 4 kcal due to the use of dextrose or lactose as fillers.

The American Diabetes Association has taken the position that the evidence linking the use of saccharin (Sweet'n Low, Sugar Twin, Sweet-10, Sprinkle Sweet) with cancer of the lower urinary tract is not strong enough to warrant a ban on the product. Because saccharin can cross the placenta during pregnancy, some authorities, including the American Dietetic Association, advise cautious use of saccharin during pregnancy.

Aspartame (Equal, NutraSweet and NatraTaste) is said to be identical in taste to sugar and to leave no bitter aftertaste. Its use in products is limited because it is unstable in heat and acid and loses its sweetness when used in cooking or baking. Aspartame contains phenylalanine, an amino acid, so it cannot be used by phenylketonurics (see Chapter 17), including pregnant women with phenylketonuria.

ACE-K (Sweet One, Sunette, and Swiss Sweet) has the advantage of being stable when heated and thus can be used in cooking. FDA approval is pending for three nonnutritive sweeteners: sucralose, alitame, and cyclamate (See discussion of nonnutritive sweetners in Chapter 8).

FIBER

Fiber recommendations are the same as for the general public: 20 to 35 g daily of dietary fiber from a variety of plant sources. This is a change from the 1986 recommendations, which focused on fiber as a means of lowering blood glucose and cholesterol levels. It has been found that the quantity of fiber needed to achieve these effects is difficult to consume without using fiber supplements. All Americans, including those with diabetes, should be encouraged to increase their consumption of dietary fiber. Fiber is beneficial in preventing several gastrointestinal disorders such as diverticulosis, constipation, and colon cancer, and soluble fiber has a lowering effect on serum cholesterol.

SODIUM

Recommended sodium levels for the general population range from 2400 to 3000 mg/day. These recommendations also are suitable for the person with diabetes. A sodium intake of 2400 mg/day or less is recommended for people with mild or moderate hypertension.

VITAMINS AND MINERALS

There is no evidence of any special need for vitamins and minerals among most people with diabetes. Although chromium is part of a complex that stimulates the action of insulin, most people with diabetes are not chromium deficient and, therefore, supplementation with chromium is of no benefit. Its usefulness has been demonstrated in only one circumstance in which people were deficient as a result of long-term chromium deficient parenteral intravenous nutrition.

Magnesium supplements are recommended only for people who are deficient in magnesium. Magnesium deficiency may play a role in insulin resistance and glucose intolerance.

Potassium supplementation may be necessary for clients who are taking diuretics. Dietary potassium may need to be limited in clients who have renal insufficiency, other diseases, or drug therapy in which excessive potassium is retained.

ALCOHOL

In most cases, a moderate amount of alcohol can be consumed without adverse effects when diabetes is well controlled. The American Diabetes Association has recommended that alcohol consumption be limited to 1 oz/day, the equivalent of two alcoholic drinks. One drink is defined as a 12-oz beer, 5-oz glass of wine, or $1\frac{1}{2}$ oz shot of 80-proof spirits, each of which contains approximately $\frac{1}{2}$ oz or 12 g of alcohol.

Alcohol consumption, however, presents potential problems for the person with diabetes. In addition to warnings regarding alcohol use that apply to everyone, people with diabetes who take insulin or glucose-lowering pills risk having a hypoglycemic reaction if they consume alcohol on an empty stomach. This reaction occurs because glycogen stores in the body may be depleted. When the liver is metabolizing alcohol, it does not convert other sources of glucose, such as protein, to glucose. **Clients should always take alcohol with food**. A hypoglycemic reaction while consuming alcohol could have tragic results if the person's strange behavior or loss of consciousness is mistaken for drunkenness. People with diabetes should wear a visible form of identification that clearly indicates they have diabetes, especially when they are drinking away from home.

Another effect of alcohol on a person with diabetes is the relaxing effect that may make the person careless about eating meals on time and selecting appropriate foods. Alcohol also may make an individual less sensitive to signs of a hypoglycemic reaction.

The person with type I diabetes should not omit any food from the meal plan to make up for the alcohol. The person with type II diabetes who is overweight should substitute alcohol for fat exchanges because the metabolism of alcohol is similar to that of fat. The equivalent of $\frac{1}{2}$ oz of alcohol should be counted as two fat exchanges. The carbohydrate content of drinks with a high-sugar content such as liqueurs, sweet wines, sweet mixes such as Tom Collins mix, soda, tonic water, and cocktail mixes must be considered. Beer and ale contain malt sugar. Light beer is recommended because it contains 3 to 6 g of carbohydrate per 12-oz can compared with 15 g in regular beer. The carbohydrate in beer should be substituted for carbohydrate-containing exchanges in the meal plan or considered as part of the carbohydrate count for that meal.

The oral hypoglycemic agents, especially chlorpropamide (Diabinese), may interact with alcohol to cause the disulfiram reaction. Symptoms include deep flushing, nausea, rapid heart beat, and impaired speech.

Because alcohol may increase plasma triglyceride levels, it is best for people with high triglyceride levels to avoid alcohol. Alcohol should also be avoided in pregnancy and by people with a history of alcohol abuse; limitation of alcohol may also be advised if pancreatitis, neuropathy, or other problems are present.

PRIORITIES FOR MEAL PLANNING

Although the overall goal of nutrition therapy and the dietary recommendations are the same for both type I and type II diabetes mellitus, the priorities for meal planning differ.

TYPE I DIABETES AND INSULIN-REQUIRING TYPE II DIABETES

With *conventional insulin therapy* (usually two injections of a mixed dose of intermediate-acting and short-acting insulins), daily consistency in the timing of meals and snacks and consistency in the quantity and quality of food (especially with regard to carbohydrate content) are the most important priorities. A meal plan is developed based on usual food intake and diabetes management goals. Insulin therapy is integrated into this plan. With a consistent eating pattern and the self-monitoring of blood glucose levels, the insulin dosage is adjusted until good blood glucose control—a good match between food and insulin—is achieved.

Snacks are frequently included in the plan at times of peak insulin action so that hypoglycemia (low blood glucose) can be prevented. These snacks should be viewed as necessary components of the plan and not as extras. People who wait until they experience signs of hypoglycemia before taking a snack tend to consume excess food, more than they would if they ate their planned snack. This excess food leads to high blood glucose levels, which lead to increased doses of insulin that may result in hypoglycemia; as a result a vicious cycle of high and low blood glucose levels is established. This pattern of events frequently leads to excessive weight gain.

With *intensive insulin therapy* that usually consists of one or more injections of long-acting or intermediate-acting insulin and injections of regular insulin before each meal, more flexibility in the timing and the quality and quantity of food eaten is possible. Even with intensive therapy, a period of consistency in eating is useful in determining how much regular insulin is required before each meal to match the food usually eaten. This can lead to establishing a ratio between carbohydrate and insulin, which can be useful in providing more flexibility (see the more detailed discussion in the section Carbohydrate Counting).

TYPE II DIABETES

The priority in type II diabetes is the achievement of glucose, lipid, and blood pressure goals. In the past, emphasis was placed on weight loss because weight loss is useful in achieving those metabolic goals. However, traditional weight loss methods consisting of reduced-calorie diets and exercise and even very low-calorie diets have been ineffective in achieving *long-term* weight loss for most overweight people.

Various strategies can be useful to achieve metabolic control; weight loss is only one of these. An initial step might be overall improvement in the quality of the diet with a gradual reduction in total fat and saturated fat. The way in which food is divided and spaced over the day also is important in achieving blood glucose control in type II diabetes. Clients should spread calories as evenly as possible over the day to avoid a large amount of food at any meal, which tends to overwhelm the body's ability to metabolize it. Meals spaced at least 4 or 5 hours apart allow adequate time for the blood glucose level to return to the premeal level before more food is eaten. Self-monitoring of blood glucose is essential to determine which strategies are useful in achieving blood glucose goals.

Weight loss, if it appears to be an achievable goal, is another strategy that can be pursued. Even small losses in weight of 10 to 20 lb can substantially improve the body's ability to use glucose, even though the individual may remain substantially overweight. Gradual weight loss of $\frac{1}{2}$ to 1 lb/week, requiring a caloric restriction of 250 to 500 kcal less than is required to maintain present weight is recommended.

Regular exercise is another important strategy for achieving metabolic goals. Exercise increases the body's sensitivity to insulin and has many other benefits, both physical and psychological. Furthermore, self-monitoring of blood glucose and monitoring of glycated hemoglobin (glycosylated hemoglobin test), serum lipids, blood pressure, and kidney function by the medical team are essential components of a plan to achieve metabolic control in type II diabetes as they are in type I diabetes.

INDIVIDUALIZED MEAL PLANNING

Nutrition therapy is the most important element of control in the management of all types of diabetes. Clients need an individualized nutrition plan and self-management training appropriate for their educational level, socioeconomic needs, degree of motivation, and nutritional requirements. The meal plan should target metabolic goals and accommodate the individual's food preferences and lifestyle as much as possible.

To individualize meal planning, the dietitian must make a careful nutrition assessment that considers the client's medical needs and factors such as work or school schedules, social needs, food attitudes, eating habits, and family support. Based on the data collected, the client, with the dietitian's guidance, decides how to fit the nutritional goals in diabetes management within his or her lifestyle.

FORMULATING THE MEAL PLAN

On the basis of information obtained during the nutrition assessment, a diet prescription is developed. Three steps are involved: determining an appropriate weight goal, estimating the calories needed to maintain or achieve that body weight, and distributing protein, fat, and carbohydrate within this caloric framework, taking into consideration the client's metabolic needs and usual eating habits.

In children, caloric intake should be sufficient to achieve growth equal to that of children who do not have diabetes. Weight for height is compared with acceptable patterns of growth for children, such as the National Center for Health Statistics growth charts (See Figure 17-3). How well the child progresses is the most reliable guide.

In adults, various methods are used to determine the desirable weight goal. One frequently used method is as follows:

Female: 100 lb for the first 5 ft of height; add 5 lb for each additional inch

Male: 106 lb for the first 5 ft of height; add 6 lb for each additional inch
Small frame: Subtract 10%
Large frame: Add 10%

Other methods include body mass index and various height and weight charts (see Chapter 23).

In most cases of type II diabetes, desirable weight is not considered. In people with a long history of obesity, it is realistic and often reassuring to the client to set a reasonable weight loss goal of 10 to 20 lb rather than to set an unattainable goal of 50 lb or more. Small losses in weight can improve diabetes control in type II diabetes, even if the client remains substantially overweight. In some cases of obesity, the goal may be to maintain the present weight and avoid further weight gain.

Once the weight goal is determined, caloric requirements are estimated based on activity level. The weight goal is multiplied by 10 to get the basal caloric requirement. Additional calories are added for physical activity: 20% to 30% of the basal requirement for sedentary individuals, 50% for moderately active people, and 100% for people who engage in strenuous physical activity.

The energy-producing nutrients—protein, fat, and carbohydrate—are distributed according to metabolic needs within the daily caloric level that has been established. The total caloric level is multiplied by the percentage of calories allotted to each nutrient. This amount is divided by 4 for protein and carbohydrate and by 9 for fat to determine the amount of each. The diet prescription is translated into a meal plan or guidelines or various other approaches. Calculation of an 1800 kcal meal using exchange lists is demonstrated in Display 22-5.

In many cases, the client's usual eating pattern is used as the basis for developing the meal plan. Exchanges are then added or subtracted in order to achieve caloric and metabolic goals.

NUTRITION COUNSELING STRATEGIES

The dietitian also uses the assessment process to decide what educational approach is most appropriate. The dietitian can use any strategy that will help clients achieve normal blood glucose levels, optimum serum lipid levels, and a nutritionally adequate intake. The nutrition intervention must be individualized to meet the client's lifestyle, motivation, ability to grasp information, diet history, and medication (insulin or oral agents), if any. For example, an elderly person might find exchange lists confusing. As an alternative, a plastic plate divided into three sections might be used and the client taught what kind of food and how much to put in each section. A client who resists following a specific diet pattern might be willing to keep a food diary. The diary and the results of blood glucose monitoring could show the client where he or she might want to make changes to meet blood glucose and lipid goals. A college student who needs more flexibility in regard to the timing and composition of meals may find adjusting insulin dose to the carbohydrate composition of each meal to be a useful strategy.

A variety of meal planning approaches are being used. These include basic nutrition guidelines such as the Food Guide Pyramid; individualized menus; the exchange lists; simplified exchange lists designed for a sixth-grade reading level; carbohydrate counting; fat counting; calorie counting; and total available glucose (a system that uses the glucose contribution of carbohydrate, protein, and fat).

Two of these meal-planning approaches are discussed in more detail in the section that follows. The exchange list system is the most frequently used method for meal planning. With the present emphasis on intensive insulin therapy, however, alternative approaches are gaining in popularity. Carbohydrate counting is one such approach.

EXCHANGE LIST SYSTEM

The exchange list system, introduced in the American Diabetes Association and the American Dietetic Association *Exchange Lists for Meal Planning,* simplifies meal planning. The 1995 edition of these exchange lists are found in Chapter 22. It affords a variety of choices and maintains the consistency in composition needed to achieve blood glucose control and a balanced diet.

Health care workers should be thoroughly familiar with the exchange lists and how to use them in planning meals. Nurses frequently are called on to help clients interpret their diets and may help them plan meals or make menu choices using the exchange lists. A meal plan and sample menu are given in Table 24-6. Exchange lists for meal planning are found in Display 22-6. There are some differences among various exchange lists used by physicians and community health agencies; health workers should become familiar with the one their client is using.

In addition to blood glucose control, emphasis is on the control of fat and cholesterol because of the high risk of cardiovascular disease in diabetes. Display 24-1 shows how to use the exchange lists to achieve lowfat, low-cholesterol meals.

The exchange lists can be adapted to various cultural eating patterns. Such lists are available from the American Dietetic Association, state and city health agencies, social welfare agencies, and visiting nurse services in large cities.

Mixed dishes such as beef stew, French toast, and baked macaroni and cheese can be made by combining exchanges. *Exchange Lists for Meal Planning* provides a Combination Foods List that gives average values for typical combination foods such as homemade casseroles, commercial chili with beans, and soups. A series of cookbooks entitled *The American Diabetes Association and the American Dietetic Association's Family Cookbooks* provide hundreds of recipes for which exchange values are given. Clients can obtain these books in libraries, bookstores, or from local chapters of the American Diabetes Association. The exchange value of a commercial food can be determined by using the "per serving" information on the "Nutrition Facts" panel of the food label.

CARBOHYDRATE COUNTING

Carbohydrate counting is a meal planning approach that focuses on the amount of carbohydrate consumed. It is based on the assumption that the amount of carbohydrate in a meal, both complex carbohydrates and simple sugars, is the major factor determining how high blood glucose will rise after a meal. Carbohydrate counting is the most frequently used method of meal planning in the United Kingdom.

Carbohydrate counting can be used in both type I and type II diabetes. For people with type I diabetes, it can be used to determine the dosage of regular insulin needed before each meal to achieve normal blood glucose levels. People with type II diabetes who do not take insulin can use carbohydrate counting to learn how much carbohydrate their body can use without raising blood glucose excessively after meals.

The first step is to establish a carbohydrate quota for the day based on the client's food preferences and metabolic goals (blood glucose, serum lipids, and so forth). The amount of carbohydrate for the day is then divided into quotas for each meal. The final step is to identify the ratio (relationship) between the number of grams of carbohydrate a person eats and the number of units of insulin he or she requires to metabolize them.

The amount of insulin required to cover a specific amount of carbohydrate differs from on person to another. Some people may require one unit of insulin for every 5 g of carbohydrate, whereas another may require one unit of insulin for each 10 to 15 g of carbohydrate in a meal.

The insulin/carbohydrate ratio must be individually determined for each person. The physician or dietitian will provide an estimated insulin to carbohydrate as a starting point (i.e., one unit for every 12 g of carbohydrate). The client will check the blood glucose $1^1/_2$ to 2 hours after the meal and compare it to the blood glucose level before the meal. A rise in blood glucose of 40 to 50 mg/dL or a blood glucose level of no lower than 140 mg/dL and no higher than 180 mg/dL after meals are typical goals that may be set. If the rise is higher than the goal, the insulin to carbohydrate ratio is increased; if lower, the insulin to carbohydrate ratio is reduced. Too low a rise in blood glucose after a meal may result in a low blood glucose reaction within an hour or two. The amount of regular insulin required to use a specific amount of carbohydrate frequently will differ from meal to meal. Usually more insulin is required at the breakfast meal than at the supper meal.

Once the client has determined the insulin/carbohydrate ratio at each meal, he or she can have

TABLE 24-6 2000-KCAL DIABETES MEAL PLAN AND SAMPLE MENU*

	GRAMS	CALORIES (%)
Carbohydrate	279	56
Protein	93	19
Fat	55	25

EXCHANGE LIST*	NO. OF EXCHANGES	PROTEIN (G)	FAT (G)	CARBOHYDRATE (G)
Starch	12	36		180
Meat, lean/med-fat	5	35	25	
Vegetable	3	6		15
Fruit	4			60
Milk, nonfat	2	16		24
Fat	6		30	
Total		93	55	279

TIME	MEAL PLAN EXCHANGES	SAMPLE MENU
Breakfast (7:30 AM)	3 starch 0 meat, lean, med-fat 0 vegetable 1 fruit 1 milk 2 fat	1½ cup of puffed wheat 1 English muffin ½ grapefruit 1 cup of skim milk 2 tsp margarine
Lunch (12:00 noon)	3 starch 2 meat, lean, med-fat 1 vegetable 1 fruit 0 milk 2 fat	1 sandwich: 2 oz lean roast beef 1 tbsp reduced fat mayonnaise Salad with ½ cup of chick peas 1 tbsp French dressing 1 peach
Snack (3:30 PM)	1 starch 1 fruit	3 graham crackers 1 apple
Supper (6:30 PM)	3 starch 3 meat, lean, med-fat 2 vegetable 1 fruit 0 milk 2 fat	3 oz baked chicken ⅔ cup of brown rice Broccoli Carrot sticks 2 sm fat-free cookies† ⅓ cantaloupe 2 tsp margarine
Snack (10:30 PM)	2 starch 1 milk	6 saltine-type crackers ¾ oz salt-free pretzels 1 cup of skim milk

* Based on Exchange Lists for Meal Planning, revised 1995. See Display 22-6.

† Food choices from the Other Carbohydrates List can be substituted for starch, fruit, or milk exchanges on the meal plan, but should be done in the context of a balanced meal.

DISPLAY 24-1 MODIFYING THE EXCHANGE LISTS FOR LOW FAT, LOW CHOLESTEROL MEAL PLANNING

Starch List	Avoid those foods with added fat (e.g., muffins, biscuits, fatty crackers, croissants) unless made with unsaturated oils and egg whites or egg substitutes. Count fat in breadstuff as part of fat allowance.
Fruit List	All fruits may be used, but avoid in cream or custard.
Milk List	Choose skim or 1% fat milk. Also may choose lowfat buttermilk, evaporated skim milk, nonfat dry milk powder, and plain nonfat yogurt.
Other Carbohydrates List	Choose those foods that have no fat or minimal amounts of fat, such as angel food cake, frozen yogurt, or gingersnaps.
Vegetable List	All vegetables may be used, but avoid in cream, butter, and cheese sauces. If sauteed, use oil sparingly; count as part of fat allowance.
Meat List	Choose from Very Lean and Lean Meat lists. Trim visible fat. Use lowfat cooking techniques. Use meatless dishes made with legumes (e.g., dried peas, beans, lentils). Note that 1 cup cooked legumes equals 2 starch and 2 lean meats. Use only amounts indicated on meal plan. Usual limit 5–7 oz/day.
Fat List	Choose from monounsaturated and polyunsaturated lists. Use margarine that lists liquid oil as first ingredient; choose soft and liquid margarines. Use only in amounts indicated on the meal plan.
Free Foods List	All are permitted, except low-calorie salad dressing (use as fat exchange) and whipped topping.
Combination Foods List	Prepare at home with fat-modified recipes. Most commercially prepared entrees are high in fat and sodium. Refrigerate broth-type soups and remove congealed fat. Avoid cream soups. Use skim or 1% fat milk to prepare sugar-free pudding.

more flexibility in the size and quality of meals by adjusting the dose of regular insulin to the amount of carbohydrate the client plans to eat (see the example given in Display 24-2). This approach is more accurate in terms of matching food and insulin, easier to teach, and more flexible than the exchange system. However, some means of monitoring protein and fat intake should also be developed so that protein is adequate and fat and cholesterol are not excessive.

Clients who are familiar with the exchange system have a good basis for learning the grams of carbohydrates in various portions of breads, starches, fruits, starchy vegetables, and milk. Other sources of the carbohydrate content of foods are the nutrition labels on virtually all commercial foods and reference books that list the carbohydrate value of foods. These references are widely available in bookstores.

FOOD LABELING

Nutrition labeling regulations, which became effective in May 1994, are especially helpful for people with diabetes. The label provides the total calories, percentage of calories from fat, and the amount of the following nutrients in a serving of the product: total fat, saturated fat, cholesterol, sodium, total carbohydrate, dietary fiber, sugars, protein, vitamins A and C, calcium, and iron—information that can help the client choose healthy foods and meet the guidelines of nutrition therapy in diabetes. People who are carbohydrate counting or fat counting will find the label information especially useful.

DISPLAY 24-2 ESTIMATING PREMEAL DOSE OF REGULAR INSULIN USING CARBOHYDRATE COUNTING

EXAMPLE

Client	27-year-old male, 165 lb
Estimated ratio	12 g carbohydrate per unit insulin
Planned meal	$1\frac{1}{2}$ turkey sandwiches = 43 g carbohydrate
	Bean soup, 8 oz = 22 g carbohydrate
	Green salad = 5 g carbohydrate
	12 oz lowfat milk = 18 g carbohydrate
	2 homemade cookies = 14 g carbohydrate
Total carbohydrate	102 g
Estimated bolus	102 g carbohydrate ÷ 12 g carbohydrate per unit of insulin = 8.5 units insulin

(Brackenridge BP. Carbohydrate gram counting: a key to accurate mealtime boluses in intensive diabetes therapy. Practical Diabetology 1992;11:2:24)

The grams of sugar listed on the nutrition label include the total of both naturally occurring sugar (sugar in milk, fruit, and vegetables) and added sugar. Added sugar includes not only sucrose but also corn syrup, fructose, honey, fruit juice, maltose, and other simple carbohydrates added during processing or packing.

Special foods are not needed in diabetes, although those reduced in calories and fat may be useful. The meaning of descriptive terms on labels such as *sugar-free, fat-free,* or *reduced-fat* have been clearly defined (these definitions are given in Display 22-3).

CIRCUMSTANCES THAT REQUIRE DIETARY CHANGES

DELAYED MEALS

An unavoidable situation occasionally may result in a delayed meal. People with diabetes who are taking insulin or an oral hypoglycemic agent may experience a serious hypoglycemic reaction if they do not eat, regardless of the circumstances. They should always carry a readily available source of carbohydrate, such as a lump of sugar, hard candy, glucose tablets, or a tube of concentrated glucose. If they anticipate that a delay may occur, as when going to a dinner party or a restaurant, they should eat a snack beforehand. In situations such as banquets and holiday meals, it may be helpful to rearrange meals and snack times to accommodate meals that are served at unusual times. The diabetes management team can assist the client in making these decisions.

STRENUOUS EXERCISE

When people taking insulin increase their physical activity, they may need extra food to avoid a hypoglycemic reaction. No extra food is required if the exercise is mild and of only a short duration, such as walking $\frac{1}{2}$ mile at a moderate pace. If the activity is more intense, such as jogging or swimming, a snack such as a starch exchange and a milk exchange before the exercise and 15 g of carbohydrate (1 fruit or starch exchange) per hour of activity are recommended. Intake of 15 to 30 g of carbohydrate every 30 minutes may be advisable during strenuous activity to reduce delayed hypoglycemia, which may occur hours after the exercise. The client should also eat a hearty snack following the exercise.

If the activity is planned in advance, it may be advisable to reduce the insulin dosage. The insulin that is effective at the time of the exercise is the one the client should reduce.

ILLNESS

A decrease in appetite often accompanies illness or emotional upset. Sometimes the usual diet plan can be followed by substituting foods that are readily tolerated, such as cooked cereal, eggs, crackers, soups, and tender meats. If the client is too ill to eat solid foods, sugar-containing liquids and other easily tolerated foods such as regular carbonated beverages, juices, sherbet, popsicles, custards, puddings, regular gelatin desserts, and sweetened tea or other foods on the "Other Carbohydrates" exchange list (1995) may be used. For each missed meal, about 50 g of carbohydrate should be taken in small, frequent feedings over a period of 3 or 4 hours.

People with type I diabetes should not omit their insulin when they do not feel well, because illness usually causes a rise in blood sugar. More frequent blood testing and urine testing for ketones are necessary during illness.

CARBOHYDRATE REPLACEMENT FOR THE HOSPITALIZED CLIENT

When a hospitalized client receiving insulin or an oral hypoglycemic medication fails to eat a significant portion (usually 10 g or more) of the carbohydrate on his or her tray, a replacement should be given. The hospital usually has a policy that indicates what replacements should be offered. If the client requires replacements repeatedly, the dietitian should be notified.

DIABETIC ACIDOSIS AND COMA

Diabetic acidosis, sometimes called *ketoacidosis* or *ketosis,* is a critical condition that can lead to coma and even death. Immediate medical treatment is required, and the client usually is hospitalized. Insulin and intravenous fluids are given. Diabetic acidosis may result from failure to take insulin or from infection or another stressful condition that requires increased insulin. Symptoms include nausea, vomiting, severe abdominal pain, deep and rapid breathing, drowsiness, and sometimes coma. The symptoms appear gradually, over a period of days, in adults. In children, symptoms usually appear over a period of hours.

HYPOGLYCEMIA

Hypoglycemia, or insulin shock, results from too much insulin, which causes the blood glucose level to fall below normal. The underlying cause may be too large a dose of insulin or oral hypoglycemic medication, too little food or a delayed meal, or too much strenuous exercise without increases in food intake. The symptoms, which develop quickly, include hunger, trembling, sweating, nervousness, drowsiness, headache, and nausea. The client may give the appearance of being drunk or of having a stroke. If untreated, the person lapses into unconsciousness.

At the first sign of a hypoglycemic reaction, 10 to 15 g of a quickly absorbed carbohydrate-containing food should be taken. Appropriate foods that contain about 10 to 15 g of carbohydrate are ½ cup of regular soda, two large sugar cubes, ½ cup of any fruit juice, six or seven Lifesaver candies, and 15 g of carbohydrate from glucose tablets or gel, or another form of glucose available at a pharmacy. The treatment should be repeated every 15 to 20 minutes if symptoms continue and until the blood glucose level is at least 80 mg/dL.

If unconscious, the client is given an intravenous glucose solution or an injection of glucagon. The intravenous glucose solution must be administered by a member of the medical team; a family member can be taught to inject glucagon.

HYPEROSMOLAR, HYPERGLYCEMIC, NONKETOTIC COMA

Hyperosmolar, hyperglycemic, nonketotic coma is a condition that develops in adults with undiagnosed or mild type II diabetes who experience some type of physical stress such as infection, injury, or gastroenteritis. Ketones are normal; blood glucose rises to more than 600 mg/dL, causing extreme water loss due to osmotic diuresis. It usually occurs in elderly people who are not consuming adequate amounts of fluid and whose high blood glucose level has been unrecognized. If permitted to progress, the condition results in cerebral dehydration and coma. The mortality rate is high. Fluid and electrolyte replacement and insulin are used to treat the condition.

DIABETES IN CHILDREN

Type I diabetes is one of the most prevalent chronic diseases of childhood. Of all the newly diagnosed cases of type I diabetes, three fourths occur in people younger than age 18 years; onset peaks between the ages of 6 and 11 years. The American Diabetes Association has recommended that diabetes care for this age group be managed by a diabetes care team that can deal with the special medical, emotional, educational, and behavioral issues involved.

The goals of management are normal growth and development, control of blood glucose, prevention of acute and chronic complications, and achievement of optimal nutritional status. These goals need to be firmly established and diabetes self-management training begun upon diagnosis. Blood glucose goals for children younger than age 6 or 7 years need to be made more liberal because young children lack the capacity to recognize and respond to hypoglycemic symptoms. Pediatric dietitians Connell and Thomas-Dobersen have suggested that "the important considerations should be to guide the child/adolescent to a meal plan that fits the individual lifestyle, promotes optimal compliance, and advances goals of management, and to offer ongoing education and support."

The ideal composition of a meal plan for children is unknown because of inadequate research. Generally, when establishing an energy level, the child's usual food intake when allowed to eat to appetite is a better guide than theoretical formulas. Newly diagnosed children who have lost weight because of the onset of diabetes need additional calories for catch-up growth. Parents have to be cautioned against withholding food when blood glucose levels are high. Parents must be informed that normal growth requires adequate energy and that insulin has to be adjusted to allow for more food.

Liberal amounts of both complex carbohydrate and simple carbohydrate in the form of fruit and milk are included. The use of sucrose should be individualized depending on metabolic control and adherence to the meal plan. It is realistic to expect children to desire sweets; they need to be taught how to include sweets in their meal plan in an appropriate manner. The Other Carbohydrates List in the 1995 edition of the exchange lists is a useful resource.

Protein should be moderate—no more than 1.5 times the Recommended Dietary Allowance (RDA) instead of the 2 to 2.5 times the RDA of protein commonly eaten in the United States. For adolescents with microalbuminuria (very small amounts of albumin in urine, a sign of early kidney disease), protein restricted to about 1 g/kg is recommended.

Because of the high risk of cardiovascular disease in adults with type I diabetes, lowering saturated fat and cholesterol is an important preventive measure. Moderation in the use of sodium is also advisable.

Consistency in the timing of meals and in the quality and quantity of the food eaten as well as consistency in the timing of injections is important. Meals and snacks have to be matched with the action patterns of injected insulin. Meal and snack timing have to be individualized. Most children on conventional insulin therapy need three snacks—midmorning, midafternoon, and before bed—in addition to their meals. Children in middle school and beyond tend to resist the midmorning snack because of wanting to conform to their peers, in which case morning insulin can be reduced. Older children and adolescents who may be on intensive therapy can be more flexible about the timing of meals. Food and insulin adjustments related to spontaneous activity, planned exercise, and participation in team sports must also be addressed.

Each stage in the child's life presents its own special problems, for example, poor appetite during the toddler years, childrens' parties and outings during the school years, and alcohol consumption and eating disorders during adolescence. The parents, child, and health care team must work together to resolve these issues. Compromises often are necessary.

Diabetes nutrition education and self-management training is an ongoing process. After the initial instruction and counseling period, follow-up visits should be scheduled every 2 to 3 months for the first 6 months, then every 3 to 6 months.

DIABETES AND PREGNANCY

Two types of diabetes exist among women who are pregnant: diabetes acquired before the pregnancy and gestational diabetes, which usually develops during weeks 24 to 28 of pregnancy. Gestational diabetes as a complication of pregnancy is discussed in Chapter 16. Both situations increase the risks to the baby, including birth defects, premature delivery, stillbirth, macrosomia (birth weight of more than 9 lb), hypoglycemia of the infant at birth, and jaundice at birth. Macrosomia and newborn hypoglycemia occur because the mother's high blood glucose level (if not properly controlled) stimulates the infant's pancreas to produce excessive amounts of insulin, which in turn promote excessive fat deposit in the infant's body and hypoglycemia at the time the infant is delivered. Risks to the mother include diabetic ketoacidosis, hypoglycemia, and accelerated microvascular complications, such as retinopathy.

In recent years, the chances of a successful pregnancy for the woman with diabetes have tremendously improved. This improvement is due to recognition of the importance of strict blood glucose control, development of the technique of self-monitoring blood glucose as a means to maintain this control, and new techniques in obstetric care.

NUTRITION FOR THE PREGNANT WOMAN WHO HAS DIABETES

The pregnancy is more likely to be successful if the woman who currently has diabetes or who had gestational diabetes in a previous pregnancy prepares for the pregnancy before conception and if she has intense and coordinated medical care and counseling during pregnancy. Strict control of maternal blood glucose is the aspect of care that is most closely associated with a successful pregnancy. However, care of pregnant women with diabetes requires balancing blood glucose control of the mother with the nutritional needs of her fetus. Self-monitoring of blood glucose is essential to achieve the degree of control required. Blood glucose goals during pregnancy are as follows: fasting, 60 to 90 mg/dL, and 2 hours after meals, less than 120 mg/dL. Normal blood glucose goals during pregnancy are lower than those of the nonpregnant woman because the expansion of blood volume dilutes the blood constituents.

Planning the pregnancy is important because a pregnancy complicated by diabetes requires more time, effort, and expense than the pregnancy of a woman who does not have diabetes. Because the baby's organs are formed in the first 10 weeks of pregnancy, it is important that glucose control be established as early in the pregnancy as possible, ideally before conception.

Although nutrition management is similar for pregnant women with type I and type II diabetes and gestational diabetes, each client requires careful and ongoing nutritional counseling and individualized assessment and treatment. In diabetes, the woman's nutrient requirements during pregnancy are the same as those of the pregnant woman who does not have diabetes. Generally speaking, the diet is slightly higher in calories, slightly lower in carbohydrate, higher in protein, and higher in fat (30% to 35% of total calories) than is recommended for a nonpregnant woman with diabetes. Nutrient intake must be distributed so that tight blood glucose control can be achieved. Factors to be considered in planning the diet and the distribution of calories and carbohydrate over the day include the type of insulin used, the number and timing of injections, the severity of morning blood glucose levels (which tend to be high during pregnancy), the extent to which blood sugars rise after meals, the occurrence of hypoglycemia during the night, and the mother's eating habits. Frequently, three meals and three between-meal snacks are planned. Usually, the breakfast meal and morning snack are lighter because blood glucose levels tend to be higher at that time due to hormonal activity. Women with type II diabetes usually require insulin during pregnancy. Oral hypoglycemic agents (sulfonylureas) are discontinued, preferably before conception.

For the pregnant woman who is taking insulin, consistency—consuming the same amount of carbohydrate and calories at the same time each day—

is the key to gaining tight control of blood sugar levels. Carbohydrate counting can provide some flexibility.

NUTRITION IN GESTATIONAL DIABETES

The woman with gestational diabetes also must achieve normal blood glucose goals during pregnancy. Self-monitoring of blood glucose is essential.

Although most women with gestational diabetes are overweight, weight loss should not be attempted during the pregnancy, but excessive weight gain should be avoided. Simple modifications of eating and exercise habits can have a significant effect in lowering blood glucose levels. These include controlling carbohydrate intake, reducing saturated fat, improving the overall quality of the diet, eating a smaller breakfast that includes a source of protein, avoiding constant snacking, and doing light exercise such as walking.

If blood glucose levels continue to exceed goals, insulin may be added. (Oral hypoglycemic drugs are not recommended during pregnancy.) The dietary guidelines would then be the same as those described for type I and type II diabetes during pregnancy.

Women with a history of gestational diabetes should consider preconception counseling to develop good eating habits and weight control, with the hope of eliminating the development of gestational diabetes during the new pregnancy.

KEYS TO PRACTICAL APPLICATION

Inform your client of the DCCT results. Promote the benefits of "tight control."

Encourage people with type II diabetes to take care of themselves. Some tend to neglect their disorder because they mistakenly believe that they have a mild form of the disease.

Inform clients of the importance of regular moderate meals and physical activity. Oral hypoglycemic drugs are not a substitute for diet and exercise.

Explain to people on conventional insulin therapy the relation of insulin to the timing of meals and snacks and the importance of eating at the time specified on their meal plan. Clients should know when to expect the greatest sugar-lowering effect from the insulin they are using.

Emphasize the importance of maintaining good control of blood glucose, serum lipids, and hypertension in the obese person with diabetes. If it appears achievable, encourage the client to set small weight loss goals. Even small losses (10 to 20 lb) can have a significant impact.

Check trays of clients with diabetes after meals to see how well they are eating. If a client taking insulin or a hypoglycemic drug refuses food, a carbohydrate replacement is given, according to hospital policy.

Ensure that hospitalized people with diabetes receive the between-meal snacks included in their meal plan. People with type I diabetes who are on conventional insulin therapy usually have one or two such feedings.

Use clients trays to reinforce dietary instruction. Help them relate the food on the tray to the exchange lists, carbohydrate counting, or other approach being used. Encourage them to be aware of portion sizes.

Be alert to misconceptions clients may have about so-called dietetic foods. Special foods are unnecessary. People with diabetes should learn how to identify those modified foods (lowfat, reduced calorie, and so forth) that may be useful and how to exchange them for regular foods in their meal plan. The 1995 edition of Exchange Lists for Meal Planning lists many of these new food items.

KEY IDEAS

Diabetes mellitus is a group of diseases in which there is an abnormally high blood sugar level.

The person with diabetes is unable to use or store glucose normally because of a deficiency of insulin, a defect in the release or action of insulin, or a defect in the use of insulin by the cells.

Type I, or insulin-dependent, diabetes is caused by a deficiency of insulin. Insulin injections are required to prevent ketosis and maintain life. This form of the disease is characterized by the classic symptoms of diabetes: excessive thirst, excessive urination, extreme hunger, and weight loss.

Type II, non–insulin-dependent, diabetes is the most common form and occurs most frequently in obese people older than age 40 years. It is caused mainly by insulin resistance defects in the tissues that use insulin; insulin resistance frequently decreases when the obese person loses weight.

The terms *borderline diabetes* and *chemical diabetes* are not used today. A person has or does not have diabetes depending on the blood sugar level. People with blood glucose levels between normal and diabetic are said to have impaired glucose tolerance and are not considered to have diabetes.

Sources of blood glucose, the primary source of fuel in the body, are carbohydrates, proteins, and fat, but especially carbohydrates.

The conversion of glucose to energy occurs within body cells; getting glucose into the cell requires insulin and insulin receptors.

Type I diabetes is caused by a genetic defect in the immune system coupled with environmental factors such as viruses.

In the absence of insulin, glucose cannot be converted to energy. As a result, protein and fat are burned at an excessive rate, leading to ketoacidosis, a life-threatening condition.

Obesity and heredity are the two major factors in the development of type II diabetes. Heredity is a more important factor in type II diabetes than in type I diabetes.

The main goals of treatment are to restore the body's ability to use carbohydrates properly and to prevent vascular complications of the disease.

Hyperglycemia is toxic to the body.

The management of diabetes involves achieving a balance of three elements: food, physical activity, and insulin (either injected or endogenous).

Two or more injections of insulin are needed daily in type I diabetes. Both animal and human insulins are available; human insulin is less likely to cause problems.

The DCCT proved that tight control of blood glucose levels can dramatically decrease diabetes complications.

Tight control of blood glucose requires intensive insulin therapy—three or more insulin injections daily and frequent monitoring of blood glucose levels.

Conventional insulin therapy usually involves two injections of a mixed dose of regular and intermediate-acting insulins.

Most type II diabetes can be controlled by management of diet, exercise, and physical stress; sometimes oral hypoglycemic agents are used. Insulin may be necessary during periods of stress such as surgery.

Physical activity improves the ability of the body to use glucose and lowers insulin requirements in well-controlled diabetes; improved circulation and muscle tone are additional benefits. In type I diabetes, however, exercise is encouraged but tends to complicate glucose control.

Self-monitoring of blood glucose provides a means of evaluating the effects of the treatment plan, makes tight control safe, and motivates the client.

The goals of nutritional management are to normalize blood glucose and blood lipids, to provide an appropriate caloric intake, to prevent and treat short-term and long-term complications, and to provide a nutritionally adequate diet.

The recommended composition of the meal plan in diabetes is protein, 10% to 20%; saturated fat, less than 10%; total fat and carbohydrate, according to metabolic needs; and cholesterol, 300 mg or less.

Protein recommendations are moderate but not as restricted as previous recommendations.

Fiber recommendations are the same as those for the general public: 20 to 35 g.

Saturated fats and cholesterol are restricted as a means of delaying the progress of premature atherosclerosis, a frequent diabetes complication.

The new guidelines emphasize total carbohydrate rather than the specific type of carbohydrate.

The effect of various carbohydrate foods on the blood glucose level does not depend on whether the food contains complex or simple carbohydrates but on many other factors that affect absorption of the food.

Sucrose affects blood glucose in a manner similar to bread, rice, and potatoes.

Priorities differ: in type I diabetes, consistency in the timing, quantity, and quality of meals and snacks is most important when conventional insulin therapy is used; more flexibility is possible with intensive insulin therapy, although an initial period of consistency is useful. In type II diabetes emphasis is on achieving blood glucose, serum lipid, and blood pressure goals; weight loss is one of various strategies for achieving these goals.

The diet in diabetes must be adapted as much as possible to the client's food preferences and lifestyle; in no other condition is individualized dietary treatment more important.

Various strategies can be used to achieve goals of nutrition therapy; the exchange list system (see Chapter 22) frequently used provides variety while maintaining consistency.

Carbohydrate counting is a strategy that focuses attention on the nutrient primarily responsible for the rise in glucose levels after a meal.

Normally, blood glucose levels will not be affected by moderate use of alcohol when diabetes is well controlled. For people using insulin, one or two alcoholic beverages (1 oz alcohol) in a day can be ingested with meals. The alcoholic beverages are taken in addition to the usual meal plan and should not be substituted for other food.

The person taking insulin should always eat when drinking alcohol to avoid hypoglycemia.

Nutritive sweeteners are considered to have the same effect on blood glucose as sucrose.

Nonnutritive sweeteners approved by the FDA are safe to use.

People with type I diabetes and people taking oral hypoglycemic pills should always carry a readily available source of carbohydrate to eat in case a meal is delayed.

The person taking insulin should eat extra food before, and possibly during and after, engaging in a strenuous activity to prevent hypoglycemia.

When the person with diabetes who is taking insulin or glucose-lowering pills is too ill to consume usual foods, sugar-containing liquids and solid foods may need to be given; insulin or pills should not be omitted.

Diabetic coma results from uncontrolled diabetes and requires immediate medical treatment so that insulin and fluid therapy can be administered.

Hypoglycemia (insulin shock) results from too much insulin caused by too large a dose of insulin or an oral hypoglycemic agent, too little food or a delayed meal, or too much strenuous exercise without increases in food intake; a quick source of sugar is the required treatment.

Diabetes increases the risk of pregnancy complications. Strict blood sugar control, self-monitoring of blood glucose, and new techniques in obstetric care have greatly improved the chances of a successful pregnancy.

The diet for the insulin-dependent child must be changed as the child's growth and energy needs and lifestyle change; consistency in the timing, quantity, and quality of food is important in achieving good blood glucose control.

Clients with diabetes are responsible for managing the treatment of their own disease; a good educational program is necessary to prepare them for this task.

Education is best provided in stages according to the individual's needs.

Diabetes self-management training is now a standard of basic medical care.

KEYS TO LEARNING

STUDY–DISCUSSION QUESTIONS

1. You are attempting to help an elderly woman understand what foods are included on each exchange list. Her eyesight is failing and she has difficulty reading the printed lists. Prepare a chart or booklet to illustrate the most commonly used items in each exchange list.

2. Make two different meal selections from the hospital selective menu that follows for a client with diabetes whose meal plan allows for three lean meat exchanges, two starch exchanges, one fruit exchange, one vegetable exchange, two fat exchanges, and one milk exchange? Use exchange lists in Display 22-6. Be sure to give the quantity of each food that should be provided.
   - Beef bouillon
   - Cream of mushroom soup
   - Broiled flounder
   - Fried chicken
   - Cottage cheese (lowfat) and fresh fruit salad plate
   - Tomato juice
   - Lima beans
   - Baked potato
   - Asparagus tips
   - Tossed salad with lemon or with French dressing
   - Dinner roll
   - Bread, white or whole-wheat
   - Margarine
   - Jelly
   - Apple pie
   - Graham crackers
   - Fresh grapes
   - Milk
   - Coffee
   - Tea

3. What is the priority in the nutritional management of type I diabetes? How is this accomplished?

4. What is the priority in the nutritional management of type II diabetes? Explain.

5. What procedure is followed in your hospital for replacing food not eaten by the client taking insulin or oral hypoglycemic agents?

6. An obese client with type II diabetes tells you that he is a "mild" diabetic and does not have to watch what he eats. How would you answer him?

CASE STUDY 1

Mark, a 20-year-old college student, works part-time in the billing department of a rehabilitation center. When he was diagnosed as having type I diabetes 6 years ago, he had suddenly developed a voracious appetite and at the same time was losing weight. He then began to get thirsty and was getting up many times during the night to urinate. At that point, he realized that something was wrong and went to see his family physician, who made the diagnosis of type I diabetes.

Mark commutes to school and lives at home with his parents. He eats out about eight meals per week—six lunches and two dinners—in cafeterias and fast-food restaurants. He does not take routine snacks during the day or at bedtime but only when he feels he needs them. He eats two eggs every day for breakfast and at least 6 oz of meat, fish, or poultry for supper.

Mark lifts weights for 1 hour four times a week and rides a stationary bicycle for 20 minutes three times a week. Mark describes himself as chubby as a child. His present weight of 190 lb is his highest, but he feels good at this weight. Mark is 5 ft, 11 inches, tall and has a medium frame.

Mark takes human insulin in two doses: 24 units of NPH insulin and eight units of regular insulin before breakfast, and eight units of NPH insulin and five units of regular insulin before dinner. He is concerned about the wide fluctuation in blood glucose levels he is experiencing. His blood glucose frequently is in the high 200s before bedtime, but he often gets hypoglycemic symptoms before lunch and dinner. When that happens, Mark admits he tends to eat anything in sight. Mark is mainly concerned about the wide fluctuations in blood glucose levels.

1. When Mark was diagnosed, what symptoms of diabetes did he experience? What caused these symptoms?
2. With the information provided here, how do you think Mark's diet compares with each of the American Diabetes Association nutrition recommendations for meal planning?
3. What is the greatest priority as far as diet is concerned?
4. What might be the cause of Mark's hypoglycemia before meals? How can this be corrected?
5. The dietitian planned a 3000-kcal diet for Mark. Of the calories in the diet, 55% comprise carbohydrate. Calculate the number of grams of carbohydrate in his meal plan.
6. Mark has agreed to change his usual breakfast routine to reduce its fat and cholesterol content. His new breakfast plan is one fruit exchange, four starch/bread exchanges, two fat exchanges, and one skim milk exchange. Plan two breakfasts using these exchanges.
7. Mark has heard about the results of the DCCT and he wants to begin intensive insulin therapy. He also likes the increased flexibility in the timing of meals that this would afford him. He plans to use carbohydrate counting. Count the carbohydrate in Mark's breakfast. Assuming that Mark's insulin/carbohydrate ratio at breakfast is 1 unit of insulin to every 12 g of carbohydrate, how much regular insulin before breakfast would Mark require?

CASE STUDY 2

Dorothy is a 50-year-old white woman who works as a secretarial assistant. She lives with her husband and her 24-year-old daughter. She has had brief episodes of blurred vision lately, which she attributes to a need for new glasses. She is seeking medical attention because of frequent urination and a burning sensation when urinating. A random blood glucose test in the doctor's office revealed a blood glucose level of 225 mg/dL. She also complains of a pins-and-needles sensation in her feet. The doctor has found her ankle reflexes to be diminished. She was of normal weight as a child and weighed 103 lb when she married at age 22 years. She gained weight after each of three pregnancies. Dorothy has gained an additional 20 lb since she had a hysterectomy 4 years ago. Dorothy is 5 ft, 2 inches, tall, weighs 171 lb, and has a medium frame. She attended a diet group 2 years ago and lost 18 lb, but she has regained that and more. Dorothy's mother, who is 73 years old, has diabetes and is grossly obese.

Dorothy is too tired when she gets home from work to do anything but cook. After dinner she watches television until bedtime.

Dorothy is anxious to lose weight. She has cut down on starches. She says she eats very little. She has juice before she leaves the house in the morning, occasionally a pastry or muffin at the 10:00 AM coffee break, and a small tossed salad or a cup of soup for lunch. She is famished when she gets home at 5:15 PM and picks at food while she is cooking and also during the evening. She admits to having a substantial dinner. She and her husband eat out at least three times a week for dinner.

1. What symptoms of type II diabetes does Dorothy exhibit?
2. A C-peptide profile revealed that Dorothy was making plenty of insulin. Why, then, does Dorothy have diabetes?
3. What is the greatest priority in Dorothy's treatment? Explain your answer.
4. Dorothy would like to weigh 120 lb again. What do you think of this weight goal? What advice would you give?
5. What changes in diet may improve her blood glucose level?
6. What other lifestyle changes would help Dorothy's diabetes?
7. Because her diabetes has only recently been diagnosed, why is Dorothy experiencing signs of neuropathy so soon?
8. Dorothy's friend has told her not to worry about the diabetes. Because Dorothy is not taking in-

sulin, it must not be too serious. What do you think of this advice? Why?

9. Dorothy has been prescribed one of the second generation hypoglycemic pills. What do these pills do?

10. Dorothy's daughter is going food shopping. She says she will buy the dietetic foods her mother needs. What would you tell her?

11. What advice should be given Dorothy's daughter about her own health?

BIBLIOGRAPHY

BOOKS AND PAMPHLETS

American Diabetes Association/ American Dietetic Association. Exchange lists for meal planning. Rev. ed. Alexandria, VA: American Diabetes Association; Chicago: American Dietetic Association, 1995.

American Diabetes Association. Medical management of insulin-dependent (type I) diabetes. Alexandria, VA: American Diabetes Association, 1994.

American Diabetes Association. Medical management of non–insulin-dependent (type II) diabetes. Alexander, VA: American Diabetes Association, 1994.

PERIODICALS

American Diabetes Association. Nutrition recommendations and principles for people with diabetes mellitus. J Am Diet Assoc 1994;94:504.

American Diabetes Association. Position statement: implications of the Diabetes Control and Complications Trial. Diabetes 1993;42:1555.

American Diabetes Association. Position statement: standards of medical care for patients with diabetes mellitus. Diabetes Care 1994;17:616.

Anderson EJ, Richardson M, Castle G. Nutrition interventions for intensive therapy in the Diabetes Control and Complications Trial. J Am Diet Assoc 1993;93:768.

Babionê L. SMBG: The underused nutrition counseling tool in diabetes management. Diabetes Spectrum 1994;7;196.

Brackenridge BP. Carbohydrate gram counting: a key to accurate mealtime boluses in intensive diabetes therapy. Practical Diabetology 1992;11:2:22.

Connell JE, Thomas-Dobersen D. Nutritional management of children and adolescents with insulin-dependent diabetes mellitus: a review by the Diabetes Care and Education Dietetic Practice Group. J Am Diet Assoc 1991;91:1556.

Franz MJ, Horton ES, Bantle JP, et al. Technical review: nutrition principles for the management of diabetes and related complications. Diabetes Care 1994;17:490.

Franz MJ, Maryniuk MD. Position of the American Dietetic Association: use of nutritive and nonnutritive sweeteners. J Am Diet Assoc 1993;93:816.

Gregory RP, Davis DL. Use of carbohydrate counting for meal planning in type I diabetes. Diabetes Educator 1994;20:406.

Heiman H. Coming to America. Diabetes Forecast 1994;47:8:20.

Jornsay D, Cypress M. Tight control: the new standard of care. Diabetes Self-Management 1994;11:1:22.

Tinker LF. Diabetes mellitus—a priority health care issue for women. J Am Diet Assoc 1994;94:976.

Tinker LF, Heins JM, Holler HJ. Commentary and translation: 1994 nutrition recommendations for diabetes. J Am Diet Assoc 1994;94:507.

C H A P T E R

25

Nutrition Therapy in Cardiovascular Disease: Atherosclerosis

KEY TERMS

angina pectoris severe choking pain in the chest commonly caused by a decrease in the blood supply to the heart muscle

arteriosclerosis hardening of the arteries caused by disease

atherosclerosis disorder involving the lining of the arterial walls in which yellowed patches of fat and cholesterol are deposited, forming plaques that decrease the size of the lumen

cerebral hemorrhage/stroke destruction of brain tissue due to rupture or blockage of a blood vessel in the brain by an abnormal material, such as a clot or fat globules

hyperlipidemia elevation in the level of one or more of the fatty substances that circulate in the bloodstream, such as cholesterol and triglycerides

hyperlipoproteinemia elevation in the level of one or more of the lipoprotein groups in the blood

lipoprotein combination of fat and protein that makes possible the transport of fat in the bloodstream

myocardial infarction heart damage due to a lack of oxygen and nutrients in the heart muscle

risk factor habit, trait, or condition that is associated with an increased chance of developing a disease

sequestrant substance that separates or removes another substance

OBJECTIVES

After completing this chapter, the student will be able to:

1. Identify the risk factors, lipid and nonlipid, for coronary heart disease (CHD).
2. Discuss the strategies recommended by the National Cholesterol Education Program for identifying people at risk due to elevated blood cholesterol and low HDL-cholesterol (high-density lipoprotein cholesterol). Specifically, the student will describe
   - who should be tested and how often
   - what tests should be done
   - the classification of risk based on total cholesterol, HDL-cholesterol, and LDL-cholesterol (low-density lipoprotein cholesterol) for people without CHD and for people with established CHD.
3. State the goals of treatment for elevated blood cholesterol and the methods used to treat the condition.
4. Discuss the significance of low levels of HDL-cholesterol and methods used to treat the condition.
5. Describe the characteristics of cholesterol-lowering meal planning.
6. Give practical suggestions for reducing saturated fat and cholesterol in the diet.
7. Discuss the significance of elevated triglyceride levels and factors that contribute to high levels.
8. Give the recommendations for identifying children

and adolescents at high risk for developing premature atherosclerosis as adults and give the classification of total and LDL-cholesterol levels in children and adolescents with a positive family history.

In the United States, diseases of the heart and blood vessels are the leading cause of death in people older than age 35 years; atherosclerosis and hypertension account for 90% of these deaths. Although premature deaths from coronary heart disease (CHD) have been substantially reduced in the past 20 years, more than 500,000 Americans die from this disease each year. About 1¼ million Americans suffer heart attacks each year and millions more have angina pectoris. In addition, a significant number of people are unaware that they have CHD. The total cost including both direct (illness care) and indirect (lost earnings and productivity) of CHD is estimated to be between $50 and $100 billion annually. Nutrition therapy in the treatment of atherosclerosis is discussed in this chapter and the treatment of hypertension and congestive heart failure is discussed in Chapter 26.

CHARACTERISTICS OF ATHEROSCLEROSIS

Atherosclerosis is a form of *arteriosclerosis,* commonly called *hardening of the arteries.* Although it may begin early in life, symptoms may not appear until middle age or beyond. By this time, the disease usually has progressed to an advanced stage.

The main characteristic of atherosclerosis is a thickening of the inner wall of the artery. This thickening is due to the buildup of cholesterol, fat, and other substances on the arterial wall. The deposits first take the form of streaks within the inner lining of the artery. They then gradually enlarge to form plaques, or patches. The passageway through which the blood flows becomes increasingly narrow, hindering or completely cutting off blood flow to the tissues. Complete blockage usually occurs when a blood clot forms at a point where the artery is seriously narrowed (Fig. 25-1).

Both the nutrition of the tissues and the removal of waste products from the tissues supplied by the affected blood vessels are hampered. Eventually, the tissues and organs become damaged. When the arteries feeding the heart muscle itself are involved, the condition is called *coronary heart disease (CHD). Myocardial infarction, coronary thrombosis,* and *heart attack* are names given to the heart damage that results from a blockage of the blood supply to the heart muscle. When atherosclerosis occurs in blood vessels a distance from the heart, such as the legs, it is called *peripheral vascular disease.* A cerebral hemorrhage, or stroke, occurs when there is blockage of a blood vessel that supplies the brain. Atherosclerosis also may be involved in angina pectoris, aneurysm (dilation or ballooning) of the abdominal aorta, and gangrene of the extremities.

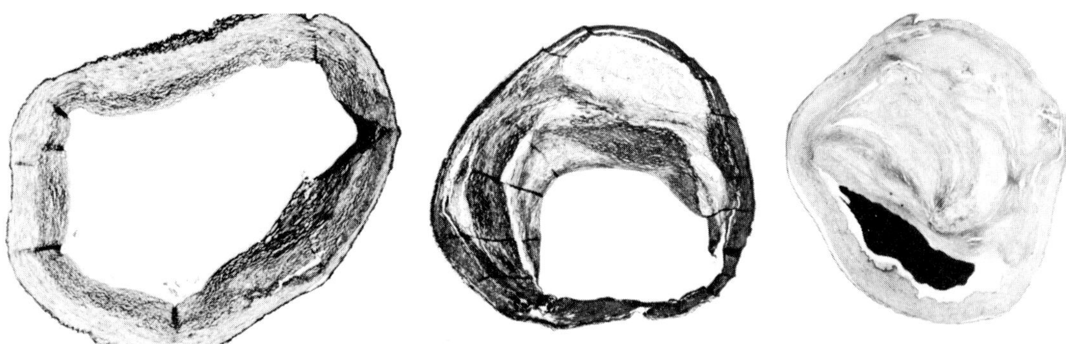

FIGURE 25-1

(*Left*) Normal artery. (*Center*) Fatty deposits in vessel wall. (*Right*) Plugged artery with fatty deposits and clot. *(Courtesy of the American Heart Association.)*

DEFINITIONS

Hyperlipidemia, or elevated blood lipids, is an abnormal rise in levels of serum cholesterol, triglycerides, or specific lipoproteins. The elevation may be due to primary causes (inherited disorders), secondary causes (conditions such as diabetes and obesity), or eating habits and other lifestyle factors. The following is a brief review of the lipids involved in atherosclerosis.

CHOLESTEROL

Cholesterol is a fatlike, soft, waxy substance. It has important functions in the body as a component of cell membranes and as a precursor of hormones, vitamin D, and bile. Cholesterol is present in all parts of the body, including the brain and nervous tissue. Blood cholesterol comes from two sources: synthesis by the body and the diet. The cholesterol level in the blood is determined partly by inheritance and partly by factors such as diet, calorie balance, and level of physical activity. Even if the diet were totally lacking in cholesterol, the liver would manufacture enough for the body's needs.

TRIGLYCERIDE

Triglyceride is the fat found in food and is the main component of adipose tissue. It also is found in blood plasma. Triglyceride that circulates in the plasma comes from fats in the diet or from fats manufactured in the body from sources of energy such as carbohydrate. If more calories are consumed in a meal than those needed immediately by the tissues, the excess is converted to triglyceride. It is then transported to fat cells for storage. Between meals, triglyceride is released from adipose tissue to meet energy needs. Hormones regulate the release of triglyceride from adipose tissue.

LIPOPROTEINS

Cholesterol and triglycerides are insoluble in water. They are carried in the blood by protein. These combinations of lipids and protein circulating in the blood are called *lipoproteins.* The term *hyperlipoproteinemia* refers to an elevation in the level of one or more lipoproteins.

Three major groups of lipoproteins are found in the blood of a *fasting* individual: *low-density lipoprotein (LDL), high-density lipoprotein (HDL),* and *very low-density lipoprotein (VLDL).* A fourth group, called *chylomicrons,* is composed mostly of fat from a recent meal.

Most cholesterol is carried by two lipoprotein groups: LDL-cholesterol and HDL-cholesterol. LDLs are rich in cholesterol and carry 60% to 70% of the serum cholesterol. HDLs have a high percentage of protein and carry 20% to 30% of total cholesterol. VLDLs are rich in triglycerides that are synthesized by the body and contain 10% to 15% of the total serum cholesterol.

If the LDLs are not reduced, cholesterol and fat build up in the arteries, contributing to atherosclerosis. LDL-cholesterol increases risk for CHD and is called *bad cholesterol.* Because HDLs carry serum cholesterol back to the liver for processing and removal from the body, they are referred to as *good cholesterol.* High levels of HDL-cholesterol reduce the risk for CHD. For this reason, a high HDL-cholesterol level of 60 mg/dL or greater is considered a negative risk factor.

RISK FACTORS FOR CORONARY HEART DISEASE

LIPID RISK FACTORS

ELEVATED BLOOD CHOLESTEROL

An elevated serum LDL-cholesterol level is a strong risk factor for CHD. A large body of epidemiologic (population) studies has supported a direct relationship between the level of serum LDL-cholesterol and the rate of CHD. In one research study, men with highest serum cholesterol levels had CHD death rates five times those of men with the lowest cholesterol levels (Fig. 25-2). When elevated blood cholesterol is combined with other risk factors, the risk for CHD increases even more.

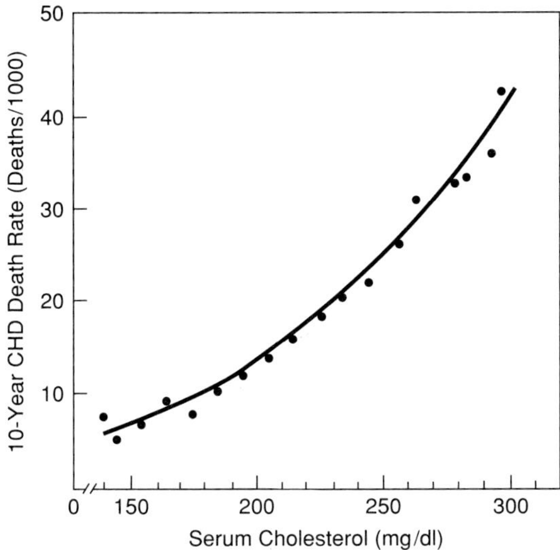

FIGURE 25-2

Relationship between serum cholesterol level and CHD death rate. *(National Cholesterol Education Program. Report of the Expert Panel on Population Strategies for Blood Cholesterol Reduction. Bethesda, MD: National Institutes of Health, National Heart, Lung, and Blood Institute, 1990:7. NIH publication 90-3046.)*

In addition, research has shown that lowering LDL-cholesterol levels decreases the risk for CHD. Recent studies have shown that cholesterol-lowering therapy slows the progression of coronary atherosclerosis and, in some individuals, even produces a regression of the disease. Relatively short-term research studies have indicated that a 2% reduction in CHD rates results from each 1% reduction in serum cholesterol level. Long-term cholesterol lowering may result in as much as a 3% reduction in CHD rates for every 1% reduction in serum cholesterol.

LOW LEVELS OF HIGH DENSITY LIPOPROTEINS

Low levels of HDL-cholesterol—below 35 mg/dL—are a significant risk factor for CHD, apart from LDL-cholesterol and other factors. It appears that for every 1 mg/dL decrease in HDL-cholesterol (good cholesterol), the risk for CHD increases 2% to 3%. A number of factors contribute to low HDL-cholesterol levels including inherited influences, cigarette smoking, lack of exercise, obesity, and certain drugs (beta-blocking agents, anabolic steroids, and progestational agents).

On the other hand, elevated levels of HDL-cholesterol protect against CHD. An HDL-cholesterol of 60 mg/dL or greater is considered a negative risk factor, and one risk factor is subtracted if the client has an HDL-cholesterol of this level.

ELEVATED TRIGLYCERIDES

Increased risk for CHD due to elevated triglycerides apart from cholesterol and HDL levels is unclear mostly because of a lack of research focused specifically on triglycerides. However, a conference of authorities in the field of CHD convened in 1992 by the National Institutes of Health indicated that triglyceride reduction should be a part of therapy for abnormal lipid levels that increase the risk for CHD. Triglycerides are discussed in the section Elevated Triglycerides.

OTHER LIPOPROTEIN FACTORS

Other components of the lipoprotein system may affect CHD risk. Knowledge of these substances is incomplete. They include apolipoproteins B and A-I, remnants of chylomicrons and VLDL, and intermediate-density lipoproteins.

RISK DUE TO ESTABLISHED CHD AND OTHER ATHEROSCLEROTIC DISEASE

People who have established heart disease or other atherosclerotic disease are five to seven times more at risk for subsequent heart attack and death than the general population. Other atherosclerotic disease includes atherosclerosis of the aorta, the arteries to the limbs, or the carotid artery.

NONLIPID RISK FACTORS

In preventing CHD, a number of nonlipid risk factors must be considered also. Some of these factors can be modified; others cannot. Although some risk factors such as sex or family history of premature CHD cannot be changed, they signal the need for more intensive efforts to lower serum cholesterol. The first goal of therapy is to reduce those risk factors such as smoking cessation, control of hypertension, weight reduction, and increased physical activity that can be modified.

SMOKING

Smoking cigarettes, including low-tar or low-nicotine varieties, is a strong risk factor for CHD and other atherosclerotic diseases. Within 1 year after stopping smoking, a major reduction in risk occurs.

HYPERTENSION

Elevated blood pressure, defined as a blood pressure of 140/90 mm Hg or above or taking a medication for hypertension, is associated with increased rates of cardiovascular disease. Treatment of hypertension significantly reduces the risk for CHD but does not completely reverse it.

OBESITY

A body mass index of more than 27 is associated with an increased risk for CHD in both sexes. The increased risk appears to be due to the metabolic effect of obesity such as glucose intolerance, hypertension, decreased HDL-cholesterol, and increased LDL-cholesterol and triglycerides. The risk produced by obesity apart from these associated conditions is unknown.

Obesity characterized by an accumulation of fat in the abdominal area (android or apple-shaped obesity) is especially associated with lipid disorders, hypertension, and other risk factors. Greater emphasis should be placed on weight reduction for people with this type of obesity.

LACK OF PHYSICAL ACTIVITY

Regular, moderate physical activity has a protective effect on the heart. *Moderate activity* is defined by the National Cholesterol Education Program as brisk walking for 30 minutes daily or running for 30 minutes three times a week. The beneficial effect of exercise may be due both to direct effects on the heart and blood vessels and also to its positive effects on HDL-cholesterol, hypertension, and weight.

AGE

The risk for CHD increases with age. However, symptoms of CHD are relatively rare until men reach their mid-forties and women reach their mid-fifties. Research has indicated that lowering LDL-cholesterol can be beneficial even in people who have advanced atherosclerotic disease.

GENDER

Men in their forties are at four times the risk of dying from CHD than women of the same age; the risk for men is two times greater by age 70 years. After menopause, the risk for CHD increases progressively until, eventually, as many women as men die from CHD. Generally, before menopause, women are at very low risk for CHD.

After menopause women tend to have higher LDL-cholesterol levels than men of the same age. However, the higher cholesterol level does not appear to have as great an influence on cardiovascular or total mortality as it does in men. Because women tend to have elevated HDL-cholesterol (good) levels, this may offset the effects of elevated LDL-cholesterol levels.

FAMILY HISTORY OF PREMATURE CHD

A positive family history of premature CHD is an important risk factor. A family history is positive if clinical CHD or sudden death has occurred in a first-degree male relative (father, brother, or son) before age 55 years and in a first-degree female relative (mother, sister, or daughter) before age 65 years. A person who has both an elevated LDL-cholesterol level and a positive family history is likely to have an inherited lipoprotein disorder. The health history of second-degree relatives (grandparents, aunts, or uncles) is also useful information.

DIABETES MELLITUS

Diabetes, both insulin-dependent (type I) and non--insulin-dependent (type II), increases the risk for CHD. This increased risk may be due, in part, to abnormal serum lipid levels that tend to occur in the disease. However, something in the diabetic state itself apparently contributes to CHD. Men with diabetes are three times at greater risk for CHD than those men without diabetes. In women with diabetes, the increased risk is even higher.

RACE

Coronary heart disease rates are 3% to 70% higher in African Americans than whites of the same age up through age 74 years. The reason for this difference is unclear. LDL-cholesterol levels are similar in both races, and African Americans actually have higher levels of protective HDL levels. The higher incidence of hypertension, diabetes mellitus, and cigarette smoking among African Americans may be some of the factors involved. Efforts to reduce serum cholesterol and other CHD risk factors are especially important for African Americans and also for Hispanics, Asian and Pacific Islanders, and American Indians.

POPULATION APPROACH TO BLOOD CHOLESTEROL REDUCTION

The National Cholesterol Education Program aims to prevent CHD by using two major strategies. One is the client-centered approach, which concentrates on identifying individuals at high risk—those who have elevated blood cholesterol. This individualized approach is the focus of this chapter. The other strategy is the population or public health approach, which aims to lower the average cholesterol level throughout the population by promoting changes in eating habits and physical activity levels.

The dietary recommendations of the National Cholesterol Education Program Population Panel have been presented throughout the normal nutrition sections of this book and are emphasized in Chapter 14. The Dietary Guidelines for Americans embody the recommendations of the Population Panel for all healthy Americans older than age 2 years: less than 10% of calories from saturated fatty acids, an average of 30% of total calories or less from all fat, dietary energy levels sufficient to reach and maintain a desirable body weight, and less than 300 mg/day of cholesterol.

INDIVIDUALIZED APPROACH: NEW CHOLESTEROL GUIDELINES

In 1993, the Second Report of the Expert Panel on Detection, Evaluation, and Treatment of High Blood Cholesterol in Adults (Adult Treatment Panel II) was issued. It presented updated National Cholesterol Education Program recommendations for individualized cholesterol management. The report reemphasized that an elevated blood cholesterol, specifically LDL-cholesterol, increases the risk for CHD; that diet therapy is the first line of treatment; and that drug therapy should be reserved only for high-risk people. The report also offered new recommendations regarding the treatment of CHD in the 1990s. These recommendations include

- more aggressive cholesterol-lowering treatment for people who already have CHD or other atherosclerotic disease
- consideration of age in addition to sex as a major risk factor: 45 years or older in men and 55 years or older in women
- more attention to HDL-cholesterol as a CHD risk factor by including HDL-cholesterol with total cholesterol as part of initial screening
- increased emphasis on weight loss and physical activity as part of the nutrition therapy of elevated serum cholesterol
- delay of drug therapy in men younger than age 35 years and premenopausal women with elevated LDL levels (160 to 220 mg/dL) who are otherwise at low risk
- increased emphasis on nondrug cholesterol-lowering therapy for otherwise healthy post-

menopausal women and elderly people who have elevated blood cholesterol levels.

INITIAL SCREENING BASED ON TOTAL CHOLESTEROL AND HDL-CHOLESTEROL

PRIMARY PREVENTION (PEOPLE WITHOUT A HISTORY OF CHD)

In its 1993 report, the Adult Treatment Panel II of the National Cholesterol Education Program recommended that total cholesterol and HDL-cholesterol be measured at least every 5 years in adults aged 20 years and older. These measurements can be taken in the nonfasting state.

For people without CHD, the results for total cholesterol are classified as follows: desirable, less than 200 mg/dL; borderline-high, 200 to 239 mg/dL; and high, 240 mg/dL and above. An HDL-cholesterol level below 35 mg/dL is defined as low and is considered a CHD risk factor (Table 25-1).

In addition to this classification, recommendations for treatment are based on whether certain additional risk factors are present. These risk factors are given in Display 25-1. Based on the results of initial screening, the following two courses of action are recommended:

1. *Repeat screening in the future* for
   - people with desirable total cholesterol and HDL-cholesterol 35 mg/dL or greater—repeat screening in 5 years
   - people with moderately high total cholesterol (200 to 239 mg/dL) and HDL-cholesterol 35 mg/dL or greater and less than two other risk factors—repeat screening in 1 to 2 years.
2. *Proceed to lipoprotein analysis* (classification then based on LDL-cholesterol level) for
   - people with an HDL-cholesterol level below 35 mg/dL regardless of total cholesterol level
   - people with moderately high blood cholesterol and two or more other risk factors, regardless of HDL level
   - people with total blood cholesterol of 240 mg/dL or higher, regardless of HDL level.

SECONDARY PREVENTION (PEOPLE WITH CHD OR OTHER ATHEROSCLEROTIC DISEASE)

For prevention of further CHD problems in adults who have CHD or other atherosclerotic disease, lipoprotein analysis is required. Classification and treatment is then based on LDL-cholesterol level.

CLASSIFICATION BASED ON LDL-CHOLESTEROL

Once the client is determined to be at substantial risk based on the initial screening, the focus of attention shifts from total to LDL-cholesterol. The amount of serum LDL-cholesterol is the most accurate predictor of CHD risk. A lipoprotein blood analysis requiring a 9- to 12-hour fast is then done. Lipoprotein analysis measures fasting levels of total cholesterol, total triglycerides, and HDL-cholesterol. From these values, the LDL-cholesterol is calculated using the formula given in Display 25-2. LDL-cholesterol levels of 160 or greater are classified as high risk; 130 to 159 mg/dL, as borderline-high risk; and below 130 mg/dL, as desirable.

The LDL-cholesterol evaluation should be part of a complete clinical evaluation so that the possible

TABLE 25-1 INITIAL CLASSIFICATION BASED ON TOTAL CHOLESTEROL AND HDL-CHOLESTEROL

Total Cholesterol	
<200 mg/dL	Desirable blood cholesterol
200–239 mg/dL	Borderline-high blood cholesterol
≥240 mg/dL	High blood cholesterol
HDL-Cholesterol	
<35 mg/dL	Low HDL-cholesterol

(National Cholesterol Education Program, Expert Panel. Second report of the Expert Panel on the Detection, Evaluation, and Treatment of High Blood Cholesterol in Adults (Adult Treatment Panel II). Bethesda, MD: National Institutes of Health, National Heart, Lung, and Blood Institute. NIH publication No. 93–3095, 1993:0–4.

DISPLAY 25-1 RISK STATUS BASED ON PRESENCE OF CHD RISK FACTORS OTHER THAN LDL-CHOLESTEROL

POSITIVE RISK FACTORS

- Age:

  Male: ≥45 years
  Female: ≥55 years or premature menopause without estrogen replacement therapy

- Family history of premature CHD (definite myocardial infarction or sudden death before age 55 years in father or other male first-degree relative, or before age 65 years in mother or other female first-degree relative)
- Current cigarette smoking
- Hypertension (≥140/90 mm Hg,* or on antihypertensive medication)
- Low HDL-cholesterol (<35 mg/dL*)
- Diabetes mellitus

NEGATIVE RISK FACTOR†

- High HDL-cholesterol (≥60 mg/dL)

High risk, defined as a net of two or more CHD risk factors, leads to more vigorous intervention. *Age* (defined differently for men and for women) is treated as a risk factor because rates of CHD are higher in elderly people than in young people, and in men than in women of the same age. Obesity is not listed as a risk factor because it operates through other risk factors that are included (hypertension, hyperlipidemia, decreased HDL-cholesterol, and diabetes mellitus), but it should be considered a target for intervention. Physical inactivity is similarly not listed as a risk factor, but it too should be considered a target for intervention, and physical activity is recommended as desirable for everyone.

* Confirmed by measurements on several occasions.

† If the HDL-cholesterol level is ≥60 mg/dL, subtract one risk factor (because high HDL-cholesterol levels decrease CHD risk).

(National Cholesterol Education Program, Expert Panel. Second report of the Expert Panel on the Detection, Evaluation, and Treatment of High Blood Cholesterol in Adults (Adult Treatment Panel II). Bethesda, MD: National Institutes of Health, National Heart, Lung, and Blood Institute, 1993:1–11. NIH publication 93-3095.)

cause of the elevated LDL-cholesterol level can be determined. Possible causes include another disease, medication, an inherited disorder, and lifestyle factors.

PRIMARY PREVENTION

People without CHD and with LDL-cholesterol levels below 130 mg/dL need no further evaluation or medical therapy and are advised to be reevaluated in 5 years. People without CHD and with LDL-cholesterol levels of 130 to 159 mg/dL who have fewer than two other risk factors are given dietary and exercise instruction and are advised to be reevaluated in 1 year. People without CHD and with LDL-cholesterol of 160 mg/dL or greater and those with borderline-high LDL-cholesterol (130 to 159 mg/dL) who have two or more risk factors should be clinically evaluated and cholesterol-lowering therapy started.

SECONDARY PREVENTION

For people who have CHD or other clinical atherosclerotic disease, the desirable LDL-cholesterol level is 100 mg/dL or lower. These clients require individualized counseling regarding diet and physical activity and at least annual reevaluation. If LDL-cholesterol levels remain at 130 mg/dL or greater, drug treatment may be considered.

DISPLAY 25-2 CALCULATING THE LDL-CHOLESTEROL LEVEL*

Lipoprotein analysis is done after a 12-hour fast. The results provide total cholesterol, HDL-cholesterol, and triglyceride levels. The LDL-cholesterol level is calculated using these results.

FORMULA FOR ESTIMATING LDL-CHOLESTEROL

Estimated LDL-cholesterol = Total cholesterol − HDL-cholesterol − (triglycerides ÷ 5)

Example: The lipoprotein analysis of Mr. Q age 42 years, was as follows:

Total cholesterol	229 mg/dL
Triglycerides	91 mg/dL
HDL-cholesterol	54 mg/dL

LDL-cholesterol is calculated as follows:

229 − 54 − (91 ÷ 5) = 175 − 18.2

LDL-cholesterol, calculated = 156.8 mg/dL

* Note: This formula cannot be used for triglycerides > 400 mg/dL.

TREATMENT OF ELEVATED BLOOD CHOLESTEROL

GOALS

The minimum goals of treatment are to reduce LDL levels to

- below 160 mg/dL for people without CHD and without two other risk factors
- below 130 mg/dL for people without CHD and with two or more risk factors
- 100 mg/dL or below for people with CHD or other atherosclerotic disease.

These are minimum goals; if possible, lower levels should be achieved. Treatment decisions based on LDL-cholesterol are given in Table 25-2.

NUTRITION THERAPY

Dietary change is the basic treatment for elevated blood cholesterol. The goals of therapy are to lower LDL-cholesterol to acceptable levels and simultaneously maintain a nutritionally adequate diet. The details of dietary treatment are discussed in the section Nutrition Therapy in the Treatment of Elevated Blood Cholesterol.

Diet plays a major role in the blood cholesterol level. Among the factors that the individual can control, diet has the greatest effect. Saturated fat raises blood cholesterol more than any other dietary factor. The cholesterol in the diet also has an important effect.

DRUG THERAPY

If nutrition therapy and increased physical activity fail to bring LDL-cholesterol below 190 mg/dL in people without CHD risk factors and below 160 mg/dL in people with two or more CHD risk factors, drug therapy is considered.

Under certain circumstances, the physician may consider it necessary to use cholesterol-lowering drugs at a lower LDL-cholesterol level. Drug therapy is not a substitute for diet. Cholesterol-lowering medications are more effective when combined with diet. Generally, intensive nutrition therapy is used for at least 6 months before drug therapy is begun. Every effort is made to lower cholesterol levels through diet, weight control, exercise, and cessation of smoking before drugs are used. For people with LDL-cholesterol levels well above 220 mg/dL, drug therapy may be started once intensive diet therapy has begun.

Drug therapy is usually prescribed for middle-aged and older people who are at high risk for CHD. Drug therapy is usually delayed until an older age for adult men younger than age 35 years and premenopausal women without other risk factors who have LDL-cholesterol levels in the 190 mg to 220 mg/dL range.

If a decision is made to use drugs, safer drugs such as bile acid sequestrants are used at the lowest effective doses. Bile acid sequestrants (cholestyramine and colestipol) are the first choice in moderately elevated cholesterol, in primary prevention,

TABLE 25-2 TREATMENT DECISIONS BASED ON LDL-CHOLESTEROL

RISK STATUS OTHER THAN LDL CHOLESTEROL	INITIATION LEVEL	LDL GOAL
DIETARY THERAPY		
Without CHD and with fewer than 2 risk factors	≥160 mg/dL	<160 mg/dL
Without CHD and with 2 or more risk factors	≥130 mg/dL	<130 mg/dL
With CHD	>100 mg/dL	≤100 mg/dL
DRUG TREATMENT	**CONSIDERATION LEVEL**	**LDL GOAL**
Without CHD and with fewer than 2 risk factors	≥190 mg/dL*	<160 mg/dL
Without CHD and with 2 or more risk factors	≥160 mg/dL	<130 mg/dL
With CHD	≥130 mg/dL†	≤100 mg/dL

* In men younger than age 35 years and premenopausal women with LDL-cholesterol levels 190–219 mg/dL, drug therapy should be delayed, except in high-risk clients such as those with diabetes.

† In CHD patients with LDL-cholesterol levels 100–129 mg/dL, the physician should exercise clinical judgment in deciding whether to initiate drug treatment.

National Cholesterol Education Program, Expert Panel. Second report of the Expert Panel on the Detection, Evaluation, and Treatment of High Blood Cholesterol in Adults (Adult Treatment Panel II). Bethesda, MD: National Institutes of Health, Heart, Lung, and Blood Institute. NIH publication No. 93–3095, 1993:0–5.

and in young adult men and premenopausal women. They are effective and have been found to be safe on a long-term basis. The bile sequestrants are not absorbed from the gastrointestinal tract and therefore are not toxic to the body's internal systems. They bind with bile (cholesterol) in the intestinal tract and remove it from the body. They may cause constipation and other gastrointestinal problems and may interfere with the absorption of other medications.

Nicotinic acid is effective in lowering cholesterol and triglycerides and in raising HDL-cholesterol levels. However, in some clients, its use may be limited due to flushing and itching of the skin, gastrointestinal disturbances, liver toxicity, elevated blood glucose, and excessive excretion of uric acid.

The statins (lovastatin, pravastatin, and simvastatin) are a class of drugs that inhibit the enzyme that promotes synthesis of LDL-cholesterol. Their long-term safety has not been established. The statins are used in severe forms of elevated cholesterol and for the greatest reduction of LDL levels in people with CHD.

Fibric acids such as gemfibrozil are effective in lowering triglycerides but do not produce substantial reductions in LDL-cholesterol. They are sometimes useful in people who have elevations of both cholesterol and triglycerides. Probucol is another drug that is not as effective as others in lowering LDL-cholesterol.

Estrogen replacement in postmenopausal women can be used as an alternative to drug therapy or used along with it. Estrogens lower LDL-cholesterol and raise HDL-cholesterol levels. Estrogens may have side effects and, when not used with progestins, may increase risk for uterine cancer.

NUTRITION THERAPY IN THE TREATMENT OF ELEVATED BLOOD CHOLESTEROL

GENERAL GUIDELINES

Nutrition therapy is the basic element of a treatment plan to lower serum cholesterol. Dietary factors most responsible for a high serum cholesterol level are a high intake of saturated fat, a high intake of cholesterol, and an excessive caloric intake that leads to obesity. The general goals of nutrition therapy are to reduce CHD risk by reducing saturated fat and cholesterol in the diet and by reducing caloric intake to an appropriate level. These modifications must be made while maintaining a nutritionally adequate diet.

Weight reduction and increased physical activity are important components of CHD risk-reduction therapy. In addition to reducing LDL-cholesterol levels, weight reduction and exercise are effective in reducing triglycerides, raising HDL-cholesterol, reducing blood pressure, and decreasing the risk for diabetes mellitus.

The National Cholesterol Education Program has advised a two-step approach to nutrition therapy. These diets reduce saturated fat and cholesterol in a stepwise fashion. The Step I Diet is composed of 30% or less of calories from total fat, 8% to 10% of total calories from saturated fat, and less than 300 mg/day of cholesterol. If the minimal goals are not met after following the Step I Diet for 3 months, the client's eating habits are reassessed, and he or she proceeds to the Step II Diet or to another trial on the Step I Diet. The Step II Diet requires the reduction of saturated fat to less than 7% of total calories and cholesterol to less than 200 mg/day (Table 25-3).

Because the Step I Diet is similar to the recommendations for the general public advocated by the Surgeon General's Report on Nutrition and Health and by the National Cholesterol Education Program, American Heart Association, and other health organizations, many clients may already be following a Step I Diet at the time of detection. If this is the case for a particular client, he or she should proceed directly to the Step II Diet.

Elderly high-risk clients with elevated LDL-cholesterol levels can benefit from dietary modifications, because elevated LDL concentrations continue to contribute to the development of atherosclerosis. The value of dietary modifications, however, must be weighed against possible adverse effects on the elderly person's appetite and food intake. The Step I Diet may be appropriate and well accepted by elderly people, but overly restrictive meal plans should be avoided.

EXPECTED RESPONSE TO NUTRITION THERAPY

Response to nutrition therapy is estimated based on research studies conducted on various groups of healthy people. Adherence to a Step I Diet reduces serum cholesterol levels 3% to 14%. Progressing to the Step II Diet will reduce cholesterol another 3%

TABLE 25-3 DIETARY THERAPY OF ELEVATED BLOOD CHOLESTEROL

	RECOMMENDED INTAKE	
NUTRIENT*	STEP I DIET	STEP II DIET
Total fat	30% or less of total calories	30% or less of total calories
Saturated fatty acids	8% to 10% of total calories	<7% of total calories
Polyunsaturated fatty acids	Up to 10% of total calories	Up to 10% of total calories
Monounsaturated fatty acids	Up to 15% of total calories	Up to 15% of total calories
Carbohydrates	55% or more of total calories	55% or more of total calories
Protein	Approximately 15% of total calories	Approximately 15% of total calories
Cholesterol	<300 mg/day	<200 mg/day
Total calories	To achieve and maintain desirable weight	To achieve and maintain desirable weight

* Calories from alcohol are not included.

National Cholesterol Education Program, Expert Panel. Second report of the Expert Panel on the Detection, Evaluation, and Treatment of High Blood Cholesterol in Adults (Adult Treatment Panel II). Bethesda, MD: National Institutes of Health, National Heart, Lung, and Blood Institute. 1993: II–2. NIH publication No. 93–3095.

to 7%. Clients with elevated blood cholesterol levels tend to consume more saturated fat and cholesterol than the average person and usually have a greater response to nutrition therapy than individuals with low serum cholesterol levels. The response to dietary change is greatly increased by weight reduction in people who are overweight.

TIMETABLE

The cholesterol-lowering effect of the Step I Diet in a particular client should be determined at 4 to 6 weeks and again at 3 months after starting the diet. If the serum cholesterol goal is not achieved after 3 months, adherence to the diet is assessed. If the client has been adhering to the Step I Diet, the client is then advanced to the more intensive Step II Diet. On the Step II Diet, the cholesterol levels are measured after 4 to 6 weeks and at 3 months of therapy. If goals are met, long-term monitoring begins. If goals are not met, the saturated fat and total fat (if weight loss is needed) can be further reduced. If the LDL-cholesterol level remains considerably higher than the goal, drug therapy is considered. A minimum of 6 months of intensive nutrition therapy and counseling should be used in primary prevention before adding drug therapy. Drug therapy may be added sooner if LDL-cholesterol is greater than 220 mg/dL.

CHARACTERISTICS OF CHOLESTEROL-LOWERING MEAL PLANNING

The purpose of nutrition therapy is to reduce saturated fat and cholesterol sufficiently to achieve the desired LDL-cholesterol level. Weight reduction, if achievable for a particular client, is another important goal of nutrition therapy because obesity contributes to a high serum cholesterol in many people. Nutrition therapy aims to achieve these permanent changes in eating habits while simultaneously maintaining a nutritious and palatable diet.

NUTRITIONALLY ADEQUATE

The diet should contain a variety of foods to meet the Recommended Dietary Allowances (RDAs) for nutrients. The diet emphasizes fruits, vegetables, legumes, whole-grain and enriched breads and cereals, and unrefined grain products, all of which provide vitamins, minerals, fiber, and complex carbohydrates. Legumes are high in protein and fiber. Poultry and fish are good sources of protein, B vitamins, and minerals. Although meat fat must be reduced, lean meats can be included in reasonable amounts (5 to 6 oz/day). Red meats are valuable for their iron and zinc content. Nonfat milk is rich in calcium and protein, and its use in encouraged.

REDUCED TOTAL FAT

The typical American diet derives 36% to 37% of total calories from fat. The fat content of the Step I and Step II Diets is less than 30% of total calories. The main purpose of limiting total fat is to promote the reduction of saturated fat. Because fats are the most concentrated source of calories, reducing fat also promotes weight reduction. Calories lost through fat reduction can be replaced by eating more carbohydrates or the saturated fat can be reduced without calorie replacement. Some authorities have recommended a reduction in total fat to 20% to 25% of calories. This total fat reduction will reduce saturated fat even more and is more likely to promote weight loss.

Effective cholesterol-lowering diets containing 30% to 35% of calories from fat can be used for people who find lower fat diets unacceptable. In these diets, monounsaturated fats replace the saturated fats.

Dietary fat contains fatty acids that are either *saturated* or *unsaturated,* terms that refer to the chemical structure of the fatty acids (see Chapter 8). Unsaturated fatty acids are further classified as either polyunsaturated or monounsaturated. Foods contain a mixture of three fatty acids, but usually one predominates. When the food contains mostly saturated fatty acids, it is referred to as a *saturated fat.* A food that contains a large proportion of polyunsaturated fatty acids is referred to as *polyunsaturated fat.* It is important to remember that all fats regardless of their fatty acids composition are the most concentrated source of energy and can cause weight gain if consumed in excessive amounts.

REDUCED SATURATED FAT

Saturated fat raises blood cholesterol more than anything else in the diet. Saturated fats contain three fatty acids that are mostly responsible for their cholesterol-raising effect: lauric, myristic, and palmitic acids. In most people, saturated fats have little effect on triglyceride and HDL-cholesterol levels.

Lowering saturated fat in the diet is the best way to lower blood cholesterol. In the Step I Diet, saturated fat composes 8% to 10% of total calories and in the Step II Diet, saturated fat composes less than 7% of total calories. The average client will have to reduce their saturated fat intake by one third to one half to meet these requirements.

Animal fats are the primary source of saturated fat in the American diet. About two thirds of the saturated fat comes from the butterfat in products such as whole milk, 2%-fat milk, ice cream, cream butter, and cheese and from the fat of beef, lamb, pork, and poultry. The remaining saturated fat comes from plant sources. Three plant sources high in saturated fats are coconut oil, palm-kernel oil, and palm oil. Although these fats continue to be used in some commercial foods, overall, Americans do not consume large quantities of these oils.

Some saturated fat is produced in the process of *hydrogenation,* in which vegetable oil is converted to a more solid fat. However, the saturated fat produced is stearic acid, which does not raise LDL-cholesterol levels.

TRANS FATTY ACIDS

Hydrogenation also converts some of the polyunsaturated fat to monounsaturated fat in the form of oleic acid and trans fatty acids, one of which is elaidic acid. Research has indicated that trans fatty acids raise LDL-cholesterol almost as much as cholesterol-raising fatty acids do. People with elevated cholesterol levels are advised to limit their intake of hydrogenated shortenings, some margarines, and other foods that contain hydrogenated fats. Soft tub or liquid margarines have a lower trans fatty acid content than hard stick margarines. However, even hard stick margarine does not raise blood cholesterol as much as butter. Soft margarine is still considered a better choice than butter.

MONOUNSATURATED FATS

For many years, monounsaturated fats were not thought to affect serum cholesterol. Recent evidence, however, has suggested that monounsaturated fats, composed mainly of oleic acid, can cause a significant decrease in LDL-cholesterol levels. Olive oil, canola oil, and high-oleic forms of sunflower seed and safflower oils are the monounsaturated fats recommended. Monounsaturated fats compose up to 15% of total calories in the Step I and Step II Diets. Much monounsaturated fat is consumed with animal fats. When animal fats are restricted, a larger portion can come from the monounsaturated vegetable oils.

POLYUNSATURATED FATS

Polyunsaturated fats are classified into two major categories: omega-6 and omega-3 fatty acids. The omega-6 fatty acids, composed mainly of linoleic acid, are the most common in the American diet. Vegetable oils rich in linoleic acid are soybean, corn, sesame, and high-linoleic forms of sunflower seed and safflower oils. Previously, high intakes of polyunsaturated fats were recommended because of their cholesterol-lowering effects. Because of questions about the safety of long-term use of large amounts of linoleic acid, however, a limit of 10% of total calories is recommended and even less is considered desirable.

Omega-3 fatty acids are composed mainly of eicosapentaenoic acid and docosahexaenoic acid. Although the omega-3 fatty acids have been found to lower blood triglyceride levels when given in high doses, they do not seem to be useful in reducing LDL-cholesterol levels. The major source of omega-3 fatty acids is the fish oils. Because of questions regarding their safety and long-term effect, fish oil supplements are not recommended. See Key Issues in Chapter 9.

Some fish, such as herring, salmon, and mackerel, are rich sources of omega-3 fatty acids. Apart from the omega-3 fatty acid content of fish, fish of any type is a good choice because it is low in saturated fat. Some studies of population groups have indicated that frequent consumption of fish is associated with a low incidence of heart disease.

REDUCED CHOLESTEROL

Dietary cholesterol raises serum cholesterol but to what degree varies from person to person. Dietary cholesterol may increase the cholesterol-raising effect of saturated fat and may also increase CHD risk apart from its cholesterol-raising effect.

Cholesterol is found *only* in animal foods. Cholesterol and saturated fat are not synonymous. They are separate factors in the diet—a fact about which the general public has been confused, partly because of past commercial advertising. The cholesterol content of food is found in both muscle and fat and, therefore, in both lowfat and high-fat animal foods (see Table 25-4). Although a food is low in fat, it may be high in cholesterol, as is the case with liver.

Cholesterol is found in eggs, dairy products, meat, poultry, fish, and shellfish. Rich sources of cholesterol are egg yolk and organ meats, such as liver, sweetbread, and brain. Some shellfish, such as shrimp, are moderately high in cholesterol but low in saturated fat. Shrimp can be consumed within the recommended cholesterol intake. The use of egg yolks should be limited. Organ meats are high in cholesterol and should be avoided entirely or used only occasionally.

MODERATE PROTEIN

Protein accounts for approximately 15% of calories in both the Step I and Step II Diets. Any type of protein food that is low in saturated fats may be used. Some nutrition authorities have advised that excessive intake of protein over the long term may be unhealthy. Thus, keeping protein at a moderate level—10% to 20% of total caloric intake—is suggested.

INCREASED CARBOHYDRATE

Carbohydrate, especially in the form of complex carbohydrates, is increased to replace the calories lost in the reduction of saturated fat. Carbohydrates account for 55% or more of the calories. Breads, pasta, rice, cereals, dried peas and beans, fruits, and vegetables are good sources of carbohydrates, fiber, vitamins, and minerals.

Carbohydrate foods are lower in calories than high-fat foods. Care must be taken, however, not to add high-fat foods such as butter, rich sauces, or whole milk to the carbohydrate foods.

If fats are reduced much below 30% of total calories, replacement of fats with carbohydrates may lead to the elevation of triglycerides and a reduction in HDL-cholesterol level. Authorities have disagreed on the value of diets that are high in carbohydrate.

CALORIES REDUCED TO ACHIEVE WEIGHT LOSS

For people who are obese, caloric restriction is important. Obesity is associated with elevated blood cholesterol and is by itself a risk factor for CHD. Weight reduction lowers LDL-cholesterol and blood triglyceride levels in many people. It also raises HDL-cholesterol. Regular exercise in conjunction with moderate caloric restriction is the best means of reducing weight. Regular exercise lowers blood triglycerides and raises HDL-cholesterol levels; it may possibly lower LDL-cholesterol levels.

FIBER

A total fiber intake of 20 to 35 g/day has been recommended by nutrition authorities primarily as a means of promoting normal gastrointestinal functioning. The gastrointestinal benefits are due mostly to insoluble fiber such as wheat bran.

Soluble fiber, on the other hand, has some cholesterol-lowering properties. Soluble fiber binds with bile salts and bile acids (which contain cholesterol) and prevents the reabsorption of cholesterol into the bloodstream. Soluble fiber is found in oats, barley, legumes, and some fruits and vegetables. Psyllium seed husks found in bulk laxatives also contain soluble fiber.

It is recommended that approximately 25% (approximately 5-9 g) of the 20 to 35 g/day of total fiber come from soluble fiber. This amount can be achieved through liberal consumption of fruits and vegetables and whole-grain products. This amount of soluble fiber will produce only a small reduction in serum cholesterol. Further reduction may be

TABLE 25-4 FAT, SATURATED FAT, CHOLESTEROL, AND IRON CONTENT OF MEAT, FISH, AND POULTRY IN 3-OZ PORTIONS COOKED WITHOUT ADDED FAT

SOURCE	TOTAL FAT (G/3 OZ)	SATURATED FAT (G/3 OZ)	CHOLESTEROL (MG/3 OZ)	IRON (MG/3 OZ)
Lean Red Meats				
Beef (rump roast, shank, bottom round, sirloin)	4.2	1.4	71	2.5
Lamb (shank roast, sirloin roast, shoulder roast, loin chops, sirloin chops, center leg chop)	7.8	2.8	78	1.9
Pork (sirloin cutlet, loin roast, sirloin roast, center roast, butterfly chops, loin chops)	11.8	4.1	77	1.0
Veal (blade roast, sirloin chops, shoulder roast, loin chops, rump roast, shank)	4.9	2.0	93	1.0
Organ Meats				
Liver				
Beef	4.2	1.6	331	5.8
Calf	5.9	2.2	477	2.2
Chicken	4.6	1.6	537	7.2
Sweetbread	21.3	7.3	250	1.3
Kidney	2.9	0.9	329	6.2
Brains	10.7	2.5	1747	1.9
Heart	4.8	1.4	164	6.4
Poultry				
Chicken (without skin)				
Light (roasted)	3.8	1.1	72	0.9
Dark (roasted)	8.3	2.3	79	1.1
Turkey (without skin)				
Light (roasted)	2.7	0.9	59	1.1
Dark (roasted)	6.1	2.0	72	2.0
Fish				
Haddock	0.8	0.1	63	1.1
Flounder	1.3	0.3	58	0.3
Salmon	7.0	1.7	54	0.3
Tuna, light, canned in water	0.7	0.2	25	1.3
Shellfish				
Crustaceans				
Lobster	0.5	0.1	61	0.3
Crabmeat				
Alaskan king crab	1.3	0.1	45	0.6
Blue crab	1.5	0.2	85	0.8
Shrimp	0.9	0.2	166	2.6

(Continued)

TABLE 25-4 *(continued)*

Source	Total Fat (g/3 oz)	Saturated Fat (g/3 oz)	Cholesterol (mg/3 oz)	Iron (mg/3 oz)
Mollusks				
Abalone	1.3	0.3	144	5.4
Clams	1.7	0.2	57	23.8
Mussels	3.8	0.7	48	5.7
Oysters	4.2	1.3	93	10.2
Scallops	1.2	0.1	27	2.6
Squid	2.4	0.6	400	1.2

(National Cholesterol Education Program, Expert Panel. Second report of the Expert Panel on the Detection, Evaluation, and Treatment of High Blood Cholesterol in Adults (Adult Treatment Panel II). Bethesda, MD: National Institutes of Health, National Heart, Lung, and Blood Institute. 1993:II–18. NIH publication 93-3095.)

achieved through the use of soluble fiber supplements (oat bran, gums, or psyllium).

VITAMINS

Recent research has indicated that oxidation of LDL in the artery increased its capacity to promote atherosclerosis. The potential of the antioxidant vitamins C, E, and beta carotene to prevent atherosclerosis and other diseases is being investigated. Data presently are insufficient to recommend the use of antioxidant vitamin supplements. The liberal use of fruits and vegetables, especially those rich in beta carotene and vitamin C, is recommended.

SODIUM

Restriction of sodium to no more than 2400 mg/day, as recommended for the general public, is supported by the National Cholesterol Education Program.

ALCOHOL

Populations that consume moderate amounts of alcohol tend to have lower CHD rates than those that abstain from alcohol. Alcohol has both beneficial and adverse effects on lipoprotein metabolism. Alcohol increases serum triglyceride levels and also raises HDL levels. Whether this rise in HDL caused by alcohol protects against CHD is unknown. Because of this uncertainty and the well-known problems associated with alcohol, alcohol is not recommended for the prevention of CHD.

IMPLEMENTING CHOLESTEROL-LOWERING NUTRITION THERAPY

The cholesterol-lowering meal planning described in this chapter is used for people with hyperlipidemia and atherosclerosis. It also is recommended as a safe and prudent way of eating for all healthy American adults as a means of preventing heart and blood vessel disease.

TEAM APPROACH

Successful nutrition intervention in the treatment of elevated serum cholesterol requires a team approach. The physicians play a significant role in helping clients become motivated and in organizing a team effort. The physician identifies for each client the risk factors and describes to the client his or her risk category of elevated serum cholesterol. The physician discusses the treatment plan and emphasizes the importance of dietary change. The physician also monitors the response to dietary change and the overall management.

Nurses and other health professionals, if appropriately trained, can assist in dietary assessment and initial dietary education and can monitor adherence. If the client fails to lower cholesterol adequately, the client should be referred to a dietitian. In some cases, the client may be referred to a dietitian from the outset of nutrition therapy.

NUTRITION COUNSELING STRATEGIES

The dietitian takes a careful detailed food history so that the client's lifestyle, food preferences, and food preparation techniques can be determined. Whenever possible, substitutes are suggested for favorite foods. Changes in diet and eating habits frequently are made in a gradual, stepwise fashion. The ultimate goal is a permanent change in eating habits.

For clients who do not need to restrict calories or carbohydrates, a diet list such as the one in Table 25-5 may be used in diet counseling. Many clients with hyperlipidemia, however, require caloric restriction to achieve or maintain ideal body weight, and some require carbohydrate control, such as when triglyceride levels are elevated or the individual has diabetes. For these clients, an exchange list system is more suitable. An exchange list designed specifically for lowering cholesterol or the Exchange Lists for Meal Planning (see Display 22-6) may be used. When the Exchange Lists for Meal Planning are used, the following modifications are made: only skim milk and skim milk products and very lean and lean meat exchanges are used; choices on the fat exchange list are limited to those that are monounsaturated and polyunsaturated; and foods that are high in cholesterol, such as egg yolks and organ meats, are limited or omitted. The total fat content of the diet is controlled by limiting the number of meat and fat exchanges permitted. See Display 24-1, Modifying the Exchange Lists for Lowfat, Low-Cholesterol Meal Planning.

Another diet method involves counting the grams of total fat and saturated fat consumed daily. Clients are given a fat allotment and can eat whatever they want as long as they do not exceed the allotment. Clients learn what changes need to be made to stay within the fat allowance. Display 25-3 gives tips for reducing fat in the diet. Counting grams of fat, especially when total fat is reduced to 20% to 25% of calories, can be an effective and less restrictive method for achieving weight loss.

RECOMMENDED DIETARY CHANGES

The amount of total fat and saturated fat will differ depending on the total caloric level of the diet. For each client, the maximum amount of total fat and saturated fat should be estimated based on the client's estimated caloric needs. The fat allotments given in Table 25-6 are maximum amounts; ideally, intakes should be below these levels.

For most people, adapting to the Step I Diet does not require drastic changes in food choices. The client can substitute foods that are lower in saturated fat and cholesterol. To decrease saturated fat, total fat, and cholesterol, emphasis is on vegetables, fruits, breads, cereals, rice, legumes, pasta, skim milk and skim milk products, and lean meat, poultry, and fish. No major food groups are omitted. Dairy products and meats should be included; however, lowfat or nonfat dairy products and lean meats should be chosen. The calcium provided by dairy products and the iron and zinc provided by red meats are important nutrients.

Using Low Fat Cooking Methods

Cooking methods that add little fat should be used. These include steaming, baking, poaching, broiling, braising, grilling, stir-frying in small amounts of fat, and microwave cooking. Foods can be cooked without fat by using nonstick pans and by using nonfat cooking spray. Limit fried foods and avoid frying in saturated fat. Foods can be kept moist by using water, broth, wine, or nonfat or lowfat sauces in cooking. Soups and stews should be chilled after cooking and the congealed fat that forms on the top should be removed.

Moderate amounts of liquid vegetable oils high in unsaturated fatty acids (canola, olive, corn, safflower, soybean, rice bran, and peanut) can be used in food preparation within the total fat allotment.

Using Food Labels

Clients should be shown how to use food labeling information to make appropriate food choices. Labeling regulations that became effective in 1994

TABLE 25-5 EXAMPLES OF FOODS TO CHOOSE OR DECREASE FOR THE STEP I AND STEP II DIETS*

FOOD GROUP	CHOOSE	DECREASE
Lean meat, poultry, and fish (≤5–6 oz/day)	Beef, pork, lamb: lean cuts well trimmed before cooking	Beef, pork, lamb: regular ground beef, fatty cuts, spare ribs, organ meats
	Poultry without skin	Poultry with skin, fried chicken
	Fish, shellfish	Fried fish, fried shellfish
	Processed meat prepared from lean meat (e.g., lean ham, lean frankfurters, lean meat with soy protein or carrageenan)	Regular luncheon meat (e.g., bologna, salami, sausage, frankfurters)
Eggs (≤4 yolks/week Step I; ≤2 yolks/week, Step II)	Egg whites (two whites can be substituted for one whole egg in recipes), cholesterol-free egg substitute	Egg yolks (if >4/week on Step I or if >2/week on Step II); includes eggs used in cooking and baking
Lowfat dairy products (2–3 servings/day)	Milk: skim, ½%, or 1% fat (fluid, powdered, evaporated) buttermilk	Whole milk (fluid, evaporated, condensed), 2% fat milk (lowfat milk), imitation milk
	Yogurt: nonfat or lowfat yogurt or yogurt beverages	Whole-milk yogurt, whole-milk yogurt beverages
	Cheese: lowfat natural or processed cheese	Regular cheeses (American, blue, Brie, cheddar, Colby, Edam, Monterey Jack, whole-milk mozzarella, Parmesan, Swiss), cream cheese, Neufchâtel cheese
	Lowfat or nonfat varieties (e.g., cottage cheese: lowfat, nonfat, or dry curd [0 to 2% fat])	Cottage cheese (4% fat)
	Frozen dairy dessert: ice milk, frozen yogurt (lowfat or nonfat)	Ice cream
	Lowfat coffee creamer Lowfat or nonfat sour cream	Cream, half-and-half, whipping cream, nondairy creamer, whipped topping, sour cream
Fats and oils (≤6–8 tsp/day)	Unsaturated oils: safflower, sunflower, corn, soybean, cottonseed, canola, olive, peanut	Coconut oil, palm kernel oil, palm oil
	Margarine made from unsaturated oils listed previously, light or diet margarine, especially soft or liquid forms	Butter, lard, shortening, bacon fat, hard margarine
	Salad dressings made with unsaturated oils listed previously, lowfat or fat-free	Dressings made with egg yolk, cheese, sour cream, whole milk
	Seeds and nuts: peanut butter, other nut butters	Coconut
Breads and cereals (6 or more servings/day)	Breads: whole-grain bread, English muffins, bagels, buns, corn or flour tortilla	Bread in which eggs, fat, or butter are a major ingredient; croissants
	Cereals: oat, wheat, corn, multigrain	Most granolas
	Pasta	
	Rice	
	Dry beans and peas	
	Crackers, lowfat: animaltype, graham, soda crackers, breadsticks, melba toast	High-fat crackers
	Homemade baked goods using unsaturated oil, skim or 1% milk, and egg substitute: quick breads, biscuits, cornbread, muffins, bran muffins, pancakes, waffles	Commercial baked pastries, muffins, biscuits
Soups	Reduced-fat or lowfat and reduced-sodium varieties (e.g., chicken or beef noodle, minestrone, tomato, vegetable, potato, reduced-fat soups made with skim milk)	Soup containing whole milk, cream, meat fat, poultry fat, or poultry skin

(Continued)

TABLE 25-5 *(continued)*

FOOD GROUP	CHOOSE	DECREASE
Vegetables (3–5 servings/day)	Fresh, frozen, or canned, without added fat or sauce	Vegetables fried or prepared with butter, cheese, or cream sauce
Fruits (2–4 servings/day)	Fruit: fresh, frozen, canned, or dried	Fried fruit or fruit served with butter or cream sauce
	Fruit juice: fresh, frozen, or canned	
Sweets and modified fat desserts	Beverages: fruit-flavored drinks, lemonade, fruit punch	
	Sweets: sugar, syrup, honey, jam, preserves, candy made without fat (e.g., candy corn, gumdrops, hard candy), fruit-flavored gelatin	Candy made with milk chocolate, coconut oil, palm kernel oil, palm oil
	Frozen desserts: lowfat and nonfat yogurt, ice milk, sherbet, sorbet, fruit ice, popsicles	Ice cream and frozen treats made with ice cream
	Cookies, cake, pie, pudding prepared with egg whites, egg substitute, skim milk or 1% milk, and unsaturated oil or margarine; gingersnaps; fig and other fruit bar cookies, fat-free cookies; angel food cake	Commercial-baked pies, cakes, doughnuts, high-fat cookies, cream pies

* Careful selection of processed foods is necessary to stay within the guideline of sodium <2400 mg/day.

(National Cholesterol Education Program, Expert Panel. Second report of the Expert Panel on the Detection, Evaluation, and Treatment of High Blood Cholesterol in Adults (Adult Treatment Panel II). Bethesda, MD: National Institutes of Health, National Heart, Lung, and Blood Institute, 1993:II-11–II-13. NIH publication 93-3095.)

DISPLAY 25-3 PRACTICAL MEAL PLANNING GUIDELINES FOR LOWERING SERUM CHOLESTEROL LEVELS

Adjust calorie intake to achieve and maintain a reasonable weight.

Limit total fat to less than 30% of total calories. To reduce total fat and saturated fat,

- limit meat, poultry, and fish to no more than a total of 5 oz to 6 oz/day
- use fish and light-meat chicken and turkey more often
- choose lean cuts of meat, trim fat, and use cooking methods that reduce fat
- use meatless or low-meat main dishes
- use skim or 1% fat milk and avoid or limit dairy products containing butterfat including butter, ice cream, regular cheese, and whole and 2% fat milk
- practice lowfat cooking techniques: bake, broil, steam, grill, roast on a rack, stir-fry, and microwave. Also, remove skin from poultry, trim visible fat from meat and poultry, skim fat from soups, stews, and gravies, and steam vegetables in water or broth, avoid sautéing in fat
- limit table and cooking fats to no more than 6 tsp to 8 tsp/day, depending on total calorie intake

Read labels carefully. Avoid saturated vegetable fats such as coconut oil, palm oil, and palm kernel oil. Also avoid hydrogenated fats including stick margarines, which contain cholesterol-raising trans fatty acids.

Limit high-cholesterol foods such as egg yolks and use organ meats (e.g., liver, sweet bread, kidney, and heart) rarely, if at all.

Be aware that some breadstuffs contain considerable quantities of fat, including biscuits, muffins, croissants, waffles, pancakes, butter rolls, and crackers.

Use liquid or soft margarine in place of butter. (These margarines contain less trans fatty acids than stick margarine and continue to be a better choice than butter.)

Increase intake of whole-grain breads and cereals, legumes, fruits, and vegetables to replace high-fat foods.

TABLE 25-6 MAXIMUM DAILY INTAKE OF FAT AND SATURATED FATTY ACIDS TO ACHIEVE THE STEP I AND STEP II DIETS*

	TOTAL CALORIE LEVEL							
FAT COMPONENT	1600	1800	2000	2200	2400	2600	2800	3000
Total fat (g)†	53	60	67	73	80	87	93	100
Saturated fat: Step I (g)‡	18	20	22	24	27	29	31	33
Saturated fat: Step II (g)‡	12	14	16	17	19	20	22	23

* The average daily energy intake for women is about 1800 kcal; for men, about 2500 kcal.

† Total fat of both diets = 30% of calories (estimated by multiplying calorie level of the diet by 0.3 and dividing the product by 9 kcal/g).

‡ The recommended intake of saturated fat on the Step I Diet should be 8% to 10% of total calories and less than 7% for the Step II Diet.

(National Cholesterol Education Program, Expert Panel. Second report of the Expert Panel on the Detection, Evaluation, and Treatment of High Blood Cholesterol in Adults (Adult Treatment Panel II). Bethesda, MD: National Institutes of Health, National Heart, Lung, and Blood Institute, 1993:II–14. NIH publication No. 93–3095.)

make it possible for clients to determine the total fat, saturated fat, and cholesterol content of one portion of almost all processed foods. The "% Daily Value" column indicates what percentage the food contributes to the maximum amount of fat (30% of total calories) recommended for a 2000-kcal diet. People consuming more or less than 2000 kcal can be shown how to use this information as a guide.

In the past, the public has been misled by terms such as *no cholesterol* and *light* because there were no legal definitions for this advertising hype. Now, label regulations spell out what terms can be used to describe the level of a nutrient in a food and how they can be used. Terms such as *lean* and *extra lean* used to describe the fat content of meat, poultry, seafood, and game meats are also clearly defined. Definitions for descriptive terms used on labels are given in Display 22-3.

MAKING SPECIFIC CHOICES

Meat, Poultry, Fish, and Shellfish

All meat, poultry, fish, and shellfish contain some saturated fat and cholesterol. The best way to control the fat and cholesterol content is to choose the leanest cuts and to limit the amount eaten to 5 oz or 6 oz/day.

Lean cuts of red meat include extra-lean ground beef, sirloin tip, round steak, rump roast, arm roast, center cut ham, loin chops, Canadian bacon, and tenderloin. People should trim all the fat on the outside of meat before cooking and should cook the meat so that the fat within it drains out during cooking. Beef is graded by the US Department of Agriculture as prime, choice, or select (formerly called good). Prime is the top grade and has the most fat because it is well marbled. Choice grade has less marbling and select grade has even less.

Ground meat should be extra lean and drained well after cooking. Very lean meat can also be ground at home or ground to order by a butcher. Ground turkey is usually very lean if it does not contain turkey skin or fat. Special reduced-fat ground meats with fillers such as carrageenan added may be used.

Fatty meats such as regular ground hamburger, bacon, bologna, hot dogs, salami, sausage, and other processed meats are high in saturated fat: 60% to 80% of their calories come from fat. They should be eaten infrequently. Lowfat varieties with no more than 3 g fat per ounce may be used. Increasingly, lowfat processed meats are on the market. Total fat and saturated fat content can be found on the "Nutrition Facts" panel of the label. If not packaged, ask the store personnel for this information.

Liver, sweetbread, and kidney are low in fat but rich in cholesterol. Their use should be avoided or severely limited. Brains should be avoided because of their high fat and extremely high cholesterol content.

Light meat chicken, Cornish hen, and turkey are low in saturated fat if the skin and globules of fat under the skin are removed. They are a good substitute for red meat, but are not as rich in iron. Goose, duck, and some processed poultry products such as turkey bologna and turkey hot dogs may be high in saturated fat and should be limited. Processed meats made from poultry are acceptable if they contain no more than 3 g of fat per ounce.

Fish is lower in saturated fat and cholesterol than meat and poultry. Some varieties of shellfish, such as shrimp and crayfish, are moderately high in cholesterol. All shellfish has less fat than meat, poultry, and most fish. Even shellfish that is moderately high in cholesterol can be eaten within the cholesterol level of the diet. Furthermore, meat, fish, and poultry should not be covered with rich sauces, and frying should be limited.

Dairy Products

Whole milk and products made with butterfat are rich sources of saturated fat. Whole-milk cheeses have more saturated fat than red meat. Even 2% fat milk has a considerable amount of fat (5 g of fat per 8-oz serving), and some cheeses labeled part-skim have as much fat as many whole-milk cheeses.

Skim or 1% fat milk and nonfat or lowfat yogurt is recommended. Fat-free and lowfat (1% to 2%) cottage cheese and imitation cheeses produced from vegetable oils can be substituted for natural and processed cheeses. Lowfat cheeses containing 3 g or less of fat per ounce can be substituted for meat in the diet. The total of meat, fish, poultry, and lowfat cheese should not exceed 5 oz to 6 oz/day. Evaporated skim milk can be substituted in recipes for heavy cream; lowfat yogurt and lowfat cottage cheese can be substituted in recipes for cream and sour cream. Avoid cream substitutes such as nondairy coffee creamers, whipped toppings, and nondairy sour cream substitutes; made with coconut, palm, or palm-kernel oil, which are highly saturated.

Fats and Oils

Animals fats such as butter, lard, and beef fat and vegetable fats such as coconut oil, palm oil, and palm-kernel oil are high in saturated fat and should be avoided. The nutrition label provides the saturated fat content of food products. Careful reading of labels is important.

Unsaturated vegetable oils and fats may be used but should be limited to about 6 to 8 tsp/day. Acceptable vegetable oils include corn, cottonseed, olive, canola, safflower, soybean, and sunflower. Peanut oil is not as desirable but may be used in small amounts.

Margarines that are soft or liquid, preferably light or diet varieties, should be selected. Margarines that have a high percentage of liquid oil (twice as much polyunsaturated as saturated) are a better choice than butter. Mayonnaise and salad dressings usually are made from unsaturated fats. Solid vegetable shortening should be avoided.

Seeds, nuts, peanut butter, olives, and avocados are high in mostly unsaturated fat. These foods as well as other fats and oils, even if they are unsaturated, must be limited because they are high in calories and consist almost entirely of fat.

Eggs

Egg yolks, high in cholesterol (approximately 215 mg), are limited to four per week in the Step I Diet and to two per week in the Step II Diet. This limitation includes egg yolks used in cooking or processed food. Egg whites contain no fat or cholesterol. Egg whites frequently can be substituted for egg yolks in recipes. Commercial egg substitutes also may be used.

Vegetables and Fruits

Fruits and vegetables have no fat, except for olives and avocados, and no cholesterol because they are not animal foods. They generally are low in calories and rich in vitamins, minerals, and fiber, and their use should be emphasized. If vegetables are prepared with butter, cream, or cheese, however, they may be high in saturated fat.

Breads, Cereals, Pasta, Rice, and Dried Peas and Beans

These products are low in fat and have no cholesterol. Dried peas and beans are good sources of protein. Pasta, rice, legumes, and vegetables can be combined with small amounts of meat, poultry, and seafood to stretch the meat allowance. They should not be eaten with butter, cream, cheese sauces, or gravies that contain fat. Care must be taken to avoid breadstuffs that are sources of hidden fats, such as some muffins and crackers, croissants, and fancy breads and biscuits.

Snacks

Lowfat snack choices include graham crackers, rye crisp, melba toast, soda crackers, pretzels, lowfat or fat-free crackers, breadsticks, English muffins, fruit, ready-to-eat cereals, vegetables, fat-free corn or potato chips, and popcorn that is air popped or popped in small amounts of vegetable oil. Check the label to determine the total fat and saturated fat content of microwave popcorn; some "light" varieties are very low in fat.

Desserts and Sweets

Cookies generally containing little fat are animal crackers, fig and other fruit bars, gingersnaps, and molasses cookies. Many fat free and reduced-fat varieties are now available. Other lowfat desserts are fruits, lowfat or nonfat fruit yogurt, fruit ices, sherbet, angel food cake, lowfat or nonfat frozen yogurt, and ice milk. Packaged commercial desserts now have their nutritive content, including the total fat and saturated fat content, given on the label. Desserts can also be homemade using acceptable ingredients such as egg whites or egg substitutes, skim milk, unsaturated oil, or margarine.

Lowfat candies are hard candy, gum drops, jelly beans, and candy corn. Avoid those containing milk chocolate and tropical oils (coconut, palm, and palm-kernel oils).

Eating Away From Home

A detailed discussion of useful ordering techniques and healthful choices when eating out is found in Chapter 14. Key Issues in Chapter 14 also provide a discussion of fast foods.

OTHER LIPID DISORDERS

ELEVATED TRIGLYCERIDES

The relationship between elevated triglycerides (*hypertriglyceridemia*) and CHD is complex. It is uncertain, also, whether the connection between these two conditions is due to the capacity of triglycerides themselves to promote atherosclerosis or to the consequences of high triglycerides such as a low HDL level (HDL levels tend to go down when triglycerides are elevated). Apparently, some forms of elevated triglycerides carry less of a risk than others.

The National Cholesterol Education Program in its 1993 Adult Treatment Panel II report classified triglyceride levels as follows:

CATEGORY	SERUM TRIGLYCERIDE LEVEL
Normal	<200 mg/dL
Borderline-high	200 mg to 400 mg/dL
High	400 mg to 1000 mg/dL
Very high	>1000 mg/dL

Many cases of borderline-high hypertriglyceridemia are due to environmental or secondary causes that raise the plasma triglyceride level. Obesity is the most common cause. Other causes include excessive alcohol intake, diabetes, chronic renal disease, liver disease, and some drugs, such as thiazide diuretics, beta-blocking agents, estrogens (including oral contraceptives), and retinoids. Borderline-high triglycerides also may be due to inherited lipid disorders.

DIETARY TREATMENT

Lifestyle changes, including weight control, consumption of a diet low in saturated fat and cholesterol, increased physical activity, and restriction of alcohol, are the main means of therapy for borderline-high triglycerides. Weight control is an important component of nutrition therapy for both borderline-high and high triglyceride levels.

Triglycerides are produced in the liver from carbohydrate and alcohol. In some people, even moderate amounts of alcohol increase serum triglyceride levels. Alcohol is eliminated or strictly limited when serum triglycerides are elevated. Even in diets in which carbohydrate constitutes half or more of total calories, triglycerides usually can be controlled as long as calories are not excessive and the carbohydrates are mostly complex. Very lowfat, high-carbohydrate diets, however, may increase the serum triglyceride level of people classified as having borderline hypertriglyceridemia. It is recommended that fat reduction not go beyond the Step I Diet. In some cases, the carbohydrate content of this diet may be too high; carbohydrate may need to be reduced and fat increased (in the form of monounsaturated fat). Lipid-lowering drugs may be considered for elevated triglycerides, depending on family history of CHD and other risk factors.

Very high triglyceride levels (more than 1000 mg/dL) are usually due to a combination of genetic and secondary (diabetes, drugs, alcohol, or obesity) factors. Clients with these levels are at high risk of developing pancreatitis (inflammation of the pancreas).

Secondary factors must be treated; for example, the client must improve control of diabetes mellitus, avoid alcohol, or discontinue use of drugs that raise triglyceride levels. A very lowfat diet in which fat constitutes 10% to 20% of calories from fat is necessary to prevent pancreatitis. The diet must be maintained on a long-term basis. In rare cases, people may have a genetic defect in which there is a deficiency of lipoprotein lipase, the enzyme that clears dietary fats from the blood. In this disorder, dietary fat must be reduced to less than 10% of total calories. If nutrition therapy and removal of aggravating drugs do not bring triglyceride levels down, triglyceride-lowering drugs are added.

REDUCED HDLS

An HDL-cholesterol level below 35 mg/dL is a risk factor for CHD independent of the other lipid levels. Causes of reduced HDLs include heavy cigarette smoking, obesity, lack of exercise, elevated triglycerides, certain drugs (anabolic steroids and beta-blocking agents), and poorly understood genetic factors.

Treatment involves making changes in those causes that are reversible, such as weight loss, increased exercise, and smoking cessation. HDL-lowering drugs may be stopped or replaced with other drugs.

If the client has hypertension or diabetes mellitus, attention is given to controlling blood pressure and blood glucose levels. If the LDL-cholesterol level is elevated also, the first priority is to reduce LDL-cholesterol levels.

INHERITED LIPOPROTEIN DISORDERS

Inherited lipoprotein disorders may be severe and complicated. Special testing may be required to make an accurate diagnosis. The client frequently is referred to a specialist for diagnosis and treatment. The type of diet needed depends on the specific lipid abnormalities present. Frequently, a diet similar to the Step II Diet is used. Clients with severely elevated triglycerides require intensive dietary treatment as described earlier. Clients with inherited lipid disorders frequently do not respond adequately to diet therapy alone. Drugs frequently are required.

ELEVATED CHOLESTEROL LEVELS IN CHILDREN AND ADOLESCENTS

Strong evidence exists that CHD, the major cause of death in the United States, has its beginnings in childhood. Various studies have indicated that the atherosclerotic process is influenced by elevated blood cholesterol level in children as it is in adults. Also, children and adolescents with elevated blood cholesterol levels are more likely than the general population to have elevated levels as adults.

In 1991, the National Cholesterol Education Program Expert Panel on Blood Cholesterol Levels in Children and Adolescents issued recommendations on two levels—a population approach intended for all healthy children older than age 2 years and an individualized approach intended for children at high risk. The population approach aims to reduce the average level of blood cholesterol among all American children older than age 2 years and adolescents by promoting changes in eating habits. See the discussion in the section Population Approach to Blood Cholesterol Reduction. The dietary recommendations made by the panel are embodied in the Dietary Guidelines for Americans, discussed in the normal nutrition sections of this book, with emphasis in Chapter 14. The recommendations for children at risk follow.

INDIVIDUALIZED APPROACH

The individualized approach aims to identify and treat children and adolescents who are at greatest risk of having elevated blood cholesterol as adults and an increased risk for CHD. The panel recommended selectively screening, as part of regular health care, children and adolescents who have a family history of early cardiovascular or other atherosclerotic disease or at least one parent with high serum cholesterol of 240 mg/dL or higher.

The purpose of this selective screening is to identify children with LDL-cholesterol levels that are likely to promote premature CHD in adulthood. The classification of total cholesterol and LDL-cholesterol in children and adolescents is given in Table 25-7. Total cholesterol is measured in children and adolescents who have at least one parent with a high serum cholesterol level. If the result is 170 mg/dL or greater (borderline or high), a lipoprotein analysis is obtained. If the young person is being tested due to a history of premature cardiovascular disease in a parent or grandparent, a lipoprotein analysis is used as the initial screening mechanism.

Based on the LDL-cholesterol results, the following recommendations are made:

- LDL-cholesterol below 110 mg/dL (acceptable): Provide educational material regarding healthy eating habits and reduction of other risk factors and repeat lipoprotein analysis in 5 years.
- LDL-cholesterol 110 to 129 mg/dL (borderline): Initiate Step I Diet and provide other risk reduction advice; repeat lipoprotein analysis in 1 year.
- LDL-cholesterol 130 mg/dL or higher: Child or adolescent evaluated for possible secondary causes and family disorders and all family members screened; initiate Step I Diet, followed, if necessary, by Step II Diet.

If, after a trial of 6 months to 1 year of nutrition therapy, the LDL-cholesterol remains 190 mg/dL or higher or 160 mg/dL or higher in children who have a positive family history of premature cardiovascular disease or who have two or more risk factors, drug therapy may be considered for children aged 10 years and older. The drugs currently used for treating children are the bile acid sequestrants, which act by binding bile acids in the intestinal tract.

TABLE 25-7 Classification of Total and LDL-Cholesterol Levels in Children and Adolescents From Families With Hypercholesterolemia or Premature Cardiovascular Disease

Category	Total Cholesterol (mg/dL)	LDL-Cholesterol (mg/dL)
Acceptable	<170	<110
Borderline	170–199	110–129
High	≥ 200	≥ 130

(National Cholesterol Education Program Expert Panel on Blood Cholesterol Levels in Children and Adolescents, Highlights of the report of the Expert Panel on Blood Cholesterol Levels in Children and Adolescents. Bethesda, MD: National Institutes of Health, National Heart, Lung, and Blood Institute, 1991:6. NIH publication No. 91–2731.)

KEYS TO PRACTICAL APPLICATION

Encourage all your adult clients to have a serum cholesterol and HDL-cholesterol screening according to the guidelines of the National Cholesterol Education Program.

Help your client believe in the importance of reducing risk factors for CHD. The risks are real.

Emphasize the importance of weight loss in cases in which it appears achievable. Excessive caloric intake is an important factor in the development of elevated cholesterol, elevated triglyceride, and low HDL-cholesterol levels. Overweight also contributes to the development of hypertension, another important risk factor.

Assure your client that, in most cases, cholesterol can be lowered by nutrition therapy.

Encourage your client to get adequate exercise and to quit smoking.

Help your client understand the difference between saturated fat and cholesterol in foods. Many people think fat and cholesterol are synonymous.

Educate clients to understand that reducing saturated fat in the diet reduces blood cholesterol more effectively than modifying any other component of the diet. Tell them what foods contain saturated fat. Give them simple guidelines for reducing total fat and saturated fat (see Display 24-4).

Encourage your clients to follow the principles of the Step I Diet. It is a prudent and safe way to prevent heart and vascular disease for all healthy Americans over 2 years of age.

Concentrate on the positive aspects of the required dietary change. Fat- and cholesterol-modified meals can be tasty and nutritious; acceptable substitutes often can be found for well-liked foods that must be omitted. Seek the help of a dietitian in assisting the client to become creative in meal planning and food preparation.

Remember that meat need not be omitted on a cholesterol-lowering diet; it is valuable for its iron and zinc content. However, special attention must be given to selecting lean cuts, preparation techniques that reduce the fat in meat, and portion size (limit meat, fish, and poultry to 5 to 6 oz/day).

Encourage cholesterol screening for children and adolescents who have a parent with an elevated cholesterol level (240 mg/dL or greater) or who have a family history of early cardiovascular disease (parent or grandparent).

KEY IDEAS

Complications of atherosclerosis are the greatest cause of death in the United States.

Three CHD risk factors that cannot be changed are age, sex, and family history of cardiovascular disease.

Nonlipid risk factors that can be modified include diet, cigarette smoking, hypertension, obesity, physical inactivity, and diabetes mellitus (blood glucose control can be improved).

Blood cholesterol comes from synthesis by the body and from the diet.

Cholesterol and triglycerides are insoluble in water. They are transported in the blood by protein. These combinations of protein and lipids are called lipoproteins. There are four types of lipoprotein.

Most of the cholesterol in the plasma is carried by two lipoprotein groups: LDL and HDL.

Because LDL-cholesterol is responsible for fat buildup in the arteries, it is called bad cholesterol. HDL-cholesterol carries blood cholesterol back to the liver for removal from the body; it is called good cholesterol.

Studies have shown conclusively that elevated blood cholesterol levels lead to the early development of atherosclerosis and CHD. The risk increases in proportion to the amount the cholesterol is elevated.

HDL-cholesterol levels less than 35 mg/dL are a significant independent risk factor; HDL-cholesterol levels of 60 mg/dL or greater are considered a negative risk factor—one risk factor is subtracted.

Total cholesterol and HDL-cholesterol should be measured at least every 5 years in adults aged 20 years and older.

Risk is classified according to total cholesterol levels as follows: desirable, less than 200 mg/dL; borderline-high, 200 to 239 mg/dL; and high, 240 mg/dL and greater.

Risk is classified as high if HDL-cholesterol is below 35 mg/dL; a subsequent lipoprotein analysis is recommended.

Clients classified as high risk because of high total serum cholesterol or a borderline-high serum cholesterol and the presence of two or more other risk factors are given a lipoprotein blood analysis.

Whether medical treatment for high serum cholesterol is necessary in primary prevention is based on LDL-cholesterol classifications: desirable, less than 130 mg/dL; borderline risk, 130 to 159 mg/dL; and high risk, over 160 mg/dL.

A desirable LDL-cholesterol level in secondary prevention is 100 mg/dL or lower; an LDL-cholesterol level of 130 mg/dL or greater may require drug treatment.

Elevated blood lipids may be inherited disorders or may be due to other factors, such as diabetes, obesity, eating habits, and medications.

Of the factors an individual can control, diet has the greatest effect on serum cholesterol.

Dietary treatment is the primary treatment for elevated blood cholesterol; drugs are added if diet fails to bring cholesterol down to target levels.

Saturated fat raises blood cholesterol more than anything else in the diet.

Cholesterol in the diet also raises blood cholesterol in some people.

Dietary treatment involves a two-step approach. If goals are not met on the Step I Diet in 3 months, the client progresses to the Step II Diet (see Table 25-5).

Cholesterol is found only in animal foods—in both high-fat and lowfat animal foods.

Characteristics of the cholesterol-lowering diet are
- reduced total fat
- reduced saturated fat
- unsaturated fat, preferably monounsaturated fat, substituted for part of the saturated fat
- reduced cholesterol
- increased carbohydrate
- increased soluble fiber
- calories reduced to achieve a reasonable weight, if it appears achievable.

Triglyceride levels between 200 to 400 mg/dL are classified as borderline-high, 400 to 1000 mg/dL as high, and greater than 1000 mg/dL as very high.

Dietary therapy for borderline-high triglyceride levels include weight control, restriction of alcohol, and improved blood glucose control in people with diabetes. Increased physical activity also is recommended. Fat reduction should not go beyond the Step I Diet because the high carbohydrate level of diets lower in fat may increase blood triglyceride levels.

For clients with severely elevated triglycerides (more than 1000 mg/dL) or high chylomicron levels, very lowfat diets (fat constitutes 10% to 20% of total calories) are necessary to prevent pancreatitis.

Treatment of low HDL-cholesterol includes weight loss, increased exercise, smoking cessation, stoppage of HDL-lowering drugs, and optimal control of hypertension and diabetes, if present.

Cholesterol screening is recommended for children and adolescents who have a family history of cardiovascular or atherosclerotic disease or at least one parent with an elevated blood cholesterol of 240 mg/dL or greater.

Treatment of elevated cholesterol in children and adolescents involves use of the Step I and Step II Diets.

For children and adolescents at risk because of family history, total cholesterol less than 170 mg/dL is acceptable, 170 to 199 mg/dL is borderline, and 200 mg/dL or greater is high. LDL-cholesterol levels less than 110 mg/dL are classified as acceptable; 110 to 129 mg/dL, as borderline; and 130 mg/dL or greater, as high.

KEYS TO LEARNING

STUDY–DISCUSSION QUESTIONS

1. The cholesterol in food is not the only source of cholesterol in the body. What is the other source? What dietary changes can lower blood cholesterol levels?
2. Write a menu for 2 days for a client on the Step I Diet (see Table 25-5). Assume that your client is a 42-year-old male college professor. Also assume that he is limited to 6 oz of meat or a substitute and six fat exchanges daily. Use the monounsaturated and polyunsaturated fat exchanges in the Exchange Lists for Meal Planning in Display 22-6. In class, discuss any problems you encountered in completing this assignment. In your opinion, what aspects of this diet would be most difficult for the client to accept?
3. Discuss food buying practices and food preparation techniques aimed at reducing saturated fat in meat and poultry.
4. Discuss ways of making food flavorful without the addition of fat.
5. What advice would you give a client who is on a lowfat, low-cholesterol, fat-controlled diet about the purchase of commercial products and convenience foods? How can the client use nutrition labeling to meet the goals of the Step I and Step II diets?
6. What changes should be made to reduce the cholesterol content of the diet?

CASE STUDY

Mr. M is a 38-year-old accounts manager for a nationwide real estate firm. He works in the corporate headquarters located in a large city.

He spends 1 week a month visiting affiliate offices scattered throughout the United States. During a cholesterol-screening program offered by his company, his cholesterol level was found to be 260 mg/dL. He made an appointment for a comprehensive physical examination with his physician, whom he had not seen in several years. The following data were noted:

Physical Data	
Weight	215 lb
Height	70 inches
Blood pressure	140/90 mm Hg
Pulse	Regular, 70 beats/minute
Laboratory Data	
Hemoglobin	15.1 g/dL
Blood urea nitrogen	18 mg/dL
Creatinine	0.9 mg/dL
Total cholesterol	260 mg/dL
HDL-cholesterol	27 mg/dL
Triglycerides	145 mg/dL

Mr. M drives to work in the city, a $1^1/_4$ hour drive from his suburban home. He smokes heavily and drinks 6 to 10 cups of coffee daily. He does not eat breakfast at home but has a bagel with cream cheese or a couple of Danish pastries when he gets to the office. His typical weekend breakfast is two or three eggs, home fries, and two slices of toast or coffee cake. Sometimes he has eggs with waffles or pancakes.

He usually orders a sandwich or hamburger platter for lunch from a nearby deli. This platter comes with coleslaw, macaroni or potato salad, or potato chips. He usually eats at his desk. If he has a business lunch, he eats a full-course meal, but usually orders fish, which he likes very much. He also is fond of vegetables.

Mr. M frequently leaves the office at 6 PM or later for his trip home. He may buy a fast-food meal on the turnpike to eat in the car on the way home. When he arrives home, he may relax for a while and at about 9 PM has a meal of leftovers or munches on cheese, crackers, chips, or fruit. When he has dinner with the family he has a generous portion of meat, fish, or poultry; a liberal portion of pasta, rice, or potatoes; a vegetable; and, always, a salad. He is fond of Italian foods, especially lasagna and Italian sausage.

His physical exercise consists mainly of yard work and playing ball with his children on weekends. During the summer, he enjoys boating.

1. Using the formula in Display 25-1, calculate Mr. M's LDL-cholesterol level. How would he be classified in regard to CHD risk?

2. List other serious risk factors presented in Mr. M's history.
3. What factors do you think contribute to the low HDL-cholesterol level? What lifestyle changes would be advisable?
4. What are some positive aspects of Mr. M's eating habits? What are the problem eating habits?
5. Using the diet guidelines in Table 25-5, write a menu for 2 days for Mr. M. Incorporate as much of his present meal pattern as possible.

BIBLIOGRAPHY

BOOKS

Feldman EB. Nutrition and diet in the management of hyperlipidemia and atherosclerosis. In: Shils ME, Olson JA, Shike M. Eds. Modern nutrition in health and disease. 8th ed. Philadelphia: Lea and Febiger, 1994:1298–1316.

National Cholesterol Education Program, Expert Panel. Second report of the Expert Panel on Detection, Evaluation, and Treatment of High Blood Cholesterol in Adults (Adult Treatment Panel II). Bethesda, MD: National Institutes of Health, National Heart, Lung, and Blood Institute, 1993. NIH publication 93-3095.

National Cholesterol Education Program. Highlights of the Expert Panel on Blood Cholesterol Levels in Children and Adolescents. Bethesda MD: National Institutes of Health, National Heart, Blood, and Lung Institute, 1991. NIH publication 91-2731.

National Cholesterol Education Program. Report of the Expert Panel on Population Strategies for Blood Cholesterol Reduction. Bethesda, MD: National Institutes of Health, National Heart, Lung, and Blood Institute, 1990. NIH publication 90-3046.

PERIODICALS

Angotti CM, Levine MS. Review of 5 years of a combined dietary and physical fitness intervention for control of serum cholesterol. J Am Diet Assoc 1994;94:634.

Asherio A, Hennekens CH, Buring JE. Trans-fatty acids intake and risk of myocardial infarction. Circulation 1994;94:1:94.

Chait A, Brunzell JD, Denke MA, et al. Rationale of the diet-heart statement of the American Heart Association: Report of the Nutrition Committee. Circulation 1994;88:3008.

Curtis AE, Musgrave KO, Klimis-Tavantzis A. A food frequency questionnaire that rapidly and accurately assesses intake of fat, saturated fat, cholesterol, and energy. J Am Diet Assoc 1992;92:1517.

Glore SR, Van Treeck D, Knehaus AW, et al. Soluble fiber and serum lipids: a literature review. J Am Diet Assoc 1994;94:425.

Gore JM, Dalen JE. Cardiovascular disease. JAMA 1994;271:1660.

Greene GW, Rossi SR, Reed GR, et al. Stages of change for reducing dietary fat to 30% of energy or less. J Am Diet Assoc 1994;94:1105.

Johnson CC, Nicklas TA, Arbert ML, et al. Behavioral counseling and contracting methods for promoting cardiovascular health in families. J Am Diet Assoc 1992;92:479.

Judd JT, Clevidence BA, Muesing RA, et al. Dietary trans-fatty acids: effects on plasma lipids and lipoproteins of healthy men and women. Am J Clin Nutr 1994;59:861.

La Rosa JC, Applegate W, Crouse JR, et al. Cholesterol lowering in the elderly: results of the Cholesterol Reduction In Seniors Program (CRISP) pilot study. Arch Intern Med 1994;154:529.

Peters JR, Quiter ES, Brekke M, et al. The Eating Pattern Assessment Tool: a simple instrument for assessing dietary fat and cholesterol intake. J Am Diet Assoc 1994;94:1008.

Schuler G, Hambrecht R, Schlierf G, et al. Exercise and low fat diet: effects on progression of coronary artery disease. Circulation 1992;86:7:1.

Steinberg D, Pearson TA, Kuller LH. Alcohol and atherosclerosis. Ann Intern Med 1991;114:967.

Wylie-Rosett J, Swencionis C, Peters MH, et al. A weight reduction intervention that optimizes use of practitioner's time, lowers glucose level, and raises HDL-cholesterol level in older adults. J Am Diet Assoc 1994;94:37.

CHAPTER

26

Nutrition Therapy in Cardiovascular Disease: Acute Illness, Congestive Heart Failure, and Hypertension

KEY TERMS

acute severe; occurring suddenly
ascites accumulation of fluid in the abdominal cavity
compensation counterbalancing of a defect
congestive heart failure failure of the heart to maintain an adequate output, causing reduced blood flow to the tissues; the result is a disproportionate amount of blood accumulating in the lungs or the systemic circulation
decompensation failure to counterbalance a defect
edema accumulation of fluid in the tissues
hypertension abnormally high blood pressure
pulmonary edema accumulation of fluid in the lungs
sodium-sensitive person person who experiences a reduction in blood pressure when sodium is restricted

OBJECTIVES

After completing this chapter, the student will be able to:

1. Give at least four dietary measures that may be taken to rest the heart during the acute stage of cardiovascular disease.
2. Explain the role of sodium restriction in congestive heart failure.
3. Give three diseases or conditions in addition to congestive heart failure in which fluid retention is a characteristic and sodium may be controlled.
4. Discuss the role of dietary factors in managing hypertension.
5. Give examples of the sodium naturally present in food and the sodium added to food.
6. Discuss the water supply and medications as sources of sodium.
7. Give two educational approaches that might be used in assisting clients to control sodium.
8. Give five food selection techniques in managing a sodium-controlled diet.
9. Explain the food labeling regulations regarding sodium. Define these descriptive terms: *sodium-free, low-sodium, very low-sodium, reduced-sodium* or *less sodium.*
10. Give three techniques for making sodium-controlled meals more flavorful.

Clients with cardiovascular disease usually require some type of modified diet. Obese clients are usually placed on a calorie-controlled diet. Achievement of ideal weight or below is an essential part of treatment. Weight loss reduces the workload of the heart and tends to reduce blood pressure and blood lipid levels. Clients with edema and hypertension may require sodium control. Those whose blood lipid levels are elevated are placed on fat-controlled diets (see Chapter 25). Any associated condition, such as diabetes or kidney disease, also must be considered. Frequently, the diet ordered is a combination of two or more modifications, such as a 1500-kcal, 2000-mg sodium diet.

ACUTE VERSUS CHRONIC HEART DISEASE

disease may surface without warning, as in a heart attack, or it may be chronic, occurring as a gradually decreasing ability of the heart to maintain normal blood circulation. Heart disease most frequently is caused by atherosclerosis (see Chapter 25). If, despite some damage, the heart is able to maintain a nearly normal blood circulation, a state of *compensation* is said to exist. If the heart is severely damaged and is no longer able to maintain adequate circulation to the tissues, the heart is said to be in *decompensation* and congestive heart failure occurs.

ACUTE CARDIOVASCULAR DISEASE

Most people admitted to coronary care units have had myocardial infarctions (heart attacks). Symptoms such as shortness of breath, fatigue, chest pain, and abdominal distention are frequent in acute stages of cardiovascular disease. The immediate treatment objective is to rest the heart so that it can heal and be restored to normal functioning. The following six dietary changes are made to rest the heart as much as possible:

1. Calories frequently are restricted, even for clients who are not obese. Smaller meals reduce the workload of the heart.
2. A liquid diet is given for the first 24 hours or so because liquids are easily digested. Only small amounts of liquid are given at one time. When their conditions improve, clients progress to a soft diet.
3. Foods that cause gaseous discomfort are avoided. Care must be taken to determine whether clients have an intolerance for milk, which may cause gastric distress or diarrhea.
4. Very hot and very cold foods are avoided. Extremes of temperature can adversely affect the cardiac muscle.
5. Foods containing stimulants such as caffeine usually are avoided because they may increase the heart rate.
6. Some clients may need to be fed to conserve their strength.

Regardless of the consistency of a client's diet—liquid, soft, or regular—foods usually are controlled in cholesterol and modified in fat. Sodium also may be controlled.

As clients recuperate and begin to readjust to their usual activities, dietary modifications frequently are continued. Clients are advised to gradually lose weight, if necessary, and to continue a cholesterol-lowering diet. Control of sodium intake frequently is advised.

CONGESTIVE HEART FAILURE

Congestive heart failure occurs when the heart loses a significant amount of its normal pumping power and is unable to pump blood efficiently. Congestive failure results from injury to the heart muscle due to atherosclerosis, infarction, hypertension, a birth defect, or rheumatic fever. The oxygen supply becomes inadequate because blood flow to the lungs is slowed. There is shortness of breath and chest pain with exertion.

The slowed circulation causes more fluid than normal to escape from the capillaries into the tissue spaces, where it is held rather than returned to the circulation. Sodium excretion is reduced because blood flow to the kidneys is diminished. Thus, sodium accumulates and causes further fluid retention, resulting in edema, especially pulmonary edema. Breathing becomes even more difficult and the heart is stressed still further.

To treat the edema, sodium is controlled. Diuretics (medications that increase urine volume) are prescribed to increase fluid and sodium excretion. Digitalis is given to strengthen the contractions of the heart, which promotes fluid and sodium excretion. In mild heart failure, sodium control alone may effectively prevent edema.

In addition to sodium restriction and medication, oxygen therapy and limited activity may be other forms of treatment. Use of caffeine and alcohol may be limited because they may cause an increased heart rate and arrhythmias. Small, frequent meals and eating slowly may reduce the workload of the heart. Weight loss in obese clients usually improves management of the disease. A high potassium diet may be indicated if the frequent use of diuretics leads to excessive potassium loss (see the section Potassium Replacement).

EDEMA

Normally, the body maintains a constant ratio of sodium to water. When this balance is upset and more sodium is retained, more fluid also is retained. Most of the excess sodium and fluid accumulates in the extracellular spaces. When fluid retention becomes visible, the condition is called *edema*. Swelling of the fingers and ankles and puffiness around the eyes are characteristic of edema. Sometimes fluid accumulates in the lungs (pulmonary edema) or in the abdominal cavity (ascites). Because of the close association between fluid and sodium, sodium restriction is effective in treating conditions in which too much fluid is retained.

HYPERTENSION

Hypertension, or high blood pressure, places heavy stress on the heart and other organs, including the brain, eyes, and kidneys. It is one of the controllable risk factors for cardiovascular disease and stroke. Undetected and uncontrolled hypertension contributes to the occurrence of heart attack, heart failure, stroke, renal failure, and aortic aneurysm. Each year, more than 1.25 million Americans, half of them younger than age 65 years, have heart attacks, and another half million have strokes. Hypertension contributes to both of these conditions. About 60 million people in the United States have hypertension, including 39 million who are younger than age 65 years. The incidence of hypertension increases with age and is more prevalent among African Americans (38%) than white Americans (29%).

In about 95% of cases, the cause of the hypertension is unknown. In such cases, the disorder is referred to as *essential* or *primary hypertension.* In the remaining cases, the hypertension is secondary to another disorder, such as disease of the kidneys or adrenal glands. Renal diseases account for 40% of the cases of secondary hypertension. Another large percentage of secondary hypertension occurs in women using oral contraceptives.

Blood pressure, as it is commonly measured, is the pressure in the artery of the upper arm. The upper number recorded is the systolic pressure, resulting from the contraction of the heart muscle. The lower number is the diastolic pressure, resulting from the relaxation phase of the heartbeat. Hypertension is diagnosed when, on several occasions, the systolic pressure is greater than 140 mm Hg and the diastolic pressure is 90 mm Hg or more. The degree of severity of high blood pressure is based on the diastolic pressure, as follows: mild hypertension, 90 to 104 mm Hg; moderate hypertension, 105 to 115 mm Hg; and severe hypertension, 115 mm Hg or higher. A sudden sustained rise in usual blood pressure, even if within normal limits, should be discussed with a physician.

Hypertension is influenced by many factors, including heredity, race, body weight, activity level, cigarette smoking, psychological stress, and diet. African Americans, people with a family history of hypertension, and all people older than age 55 years have increased risk.

Secondary hypertension is treated by correcting or controlling the underlying cause. Essential hypertension is treated by caloric reduction in people who are obese, sodium control, moderate exercise, stress reduction, and, if these measures do not produce the desired effect, antihypertensive medication.

Drugs for controlling blood pressure are being used more cautiously because of an increased awareness of their potential side effects. Among these adverse effects are elevated blood glucose, uric acid, and lipid levels and decreased potassium levels. More attention is being given to dietary and behavioral treatment instead. An average drop of about 5 mm Hg systolic pressure and 4 mm Hg diastolic pressure results when sodium intake is cut in half. Although this drop in blood pressure is small, it is significant, especially for those with mild hypertension. In many cases, this drop in blood pressure is enough to bring it down to normal.

Food intake appears to affect hypertension in two ways. Increased caloric intake increases sympathetic nervous system activity, which can elevate blood pressure by various mechanisms. For example, increased sympathetic nervous system activity can cause a constriction of blood vessels and an increase in the heart rate. The second effect of food involves the kidney. In some people with hypertension, the kidneys may be unable to excrete normal amounts of sodium at normal blood pressure levels. As a result, body sodium and blood volume increase and blood pressure rises to a point at which sodium is excreted.

OBESITY AND BLOOD PRESSURE

Weight reduction is the major form of therapy for hypertension. Even in childhood and adolescence, people who are in the highest percentile for weight usually have the highest blood pressure. In societies in which people do not gain weight as they get older, blood pressure usually remains stable throughout life. The degree to which blood pressure is reduced by weight loss depends on how high the blood pressure was initially and the amount of weight loss. Substantial reductions in blood pressure, greater than 40 mm Hg systolic and 20 mm Hg diastolic, are common. Other health benefits of weight loss, such as reduction in blood lipids and reduced blood glucose levels, also reduce risk of coronary heart disease. Weight control is discussed in detail in Chapter 23.

SODIUM AND BLOOD PRESSURE

Because the cause of essential hypertension is unknown, the methods used to prevent and treat it are controversial. There is wide agreement that achieving and maintaining ideal weight are important in treating hypertension. There is controversy, however, about the relation of sodium to the prevention and treatment of this disorder.

For some time, sodium restriction has been prescribed in the treatment of hypertension. Its possible benefit has been attributed to a reduction of fluid volume and to the effects of decreased levels of sodium in sodium-sensitive people. A moderate restriction of sodium appears to produce small decreases in blood pressure among 60% of people with hypertension. Weight reduction combined with sodium restriction significantly reduces blood pressure and should be the primary goal for this population.

PREVENTING HYPERTENSION

Substantial evidence has supported sodium control as a means of preventing hypertension. Populations with a high salt (sodium chloride) intake, 6 g or more daily, have a high incidence of hypertension and experience a rise in blood pressure with age. Populations that consume less than 4.5 g/day of salt have a low incidence of hypertension and little or no rise in blood pressure with age.

It is estimated that 10% to 20% of the general population is sodium sensitive. Because there presently is no biologic marker to identify sodium sensitivity, moderate sodium restriction by the general public is considered prudent.

OTHER DIETARY FACTORS AFFECTING BLOOD PRESSURE

Alcohol in excess of one or two standard-sized drinks (1 oz of alcohol) a day raises blood pressure. Standard-sized drinks are 12 oz of regular beer, 5 oz of wine, or $1^1/_2$ oz of distilled whiskey (each of which contains approximately $^1/_2$ oz. alcohol).

Research studies have suggested that increased intakes of potassium, calcium, magnesium, fiber, and polyunsaturated fats may reduce blood pressure. The evidence about potassium appears to be the strongest. Studies on animals and of population groups have indicated that the risk of stroke-related death is reduced as potassium intake increases. Low-sodium, high-potassium intake is associated with the lowest blood pressure levels and the lowest incidence of strokes. Some studies have shown that adding 2 to 3 g of potassium to a diet that already contains about that much lowers diastolic blood pressure 3 to 5 mm Hg.

SODIUM-CONTROLLED DIETS

The purpose of a sodium-controlled meal plan is to treat hypertension in sodium-sensitive people and to promote loss of excess fluids in edema and ascites. Moderation in sodium intake also is recommended for the general population as a means of preventing hypertension in susceptible individuals. Unfortunately, no means exists to identify susceptible individuals. Because there apparently is no advantage to consuming large amounts of sodium, moderating sodium intake is reasonable advice. In 1989, the National Academy of Sciences Committee on Diet and Health recommended that the daily intake of sodium chloride (table salt) be limited to 6 g, which represents 2.4 g (2400 mg) of sodium. The 10th edition of *Recommended Dietary Allowances* set a safe estimated *minimum* intake of sodium at 0.5 g (500 mg) per day.

A sodium-controlled diet limits the intake of sodium from food and fluids to a physician-prescribed level. The sodium level in such a plan may be as low as 250 mg/day or as high as 4500 mg/day. The physician's diet prescription states the amount of sodium in grams, milligrams, or milliequivalents (mEq; 1 mEq of sodium = 23 mg; 45 mEq of sodium = 1035 mg [i.e., 45 × 23]) that the client may have daily.

The use of terms such as *low-salt, salt-free,* or *salt-poor* to describe a sodium-controlled diet is discouraged, because these terms do not accurately convey the level of sodium desired. The terms also give the false impression that table salt is the only source of sodium that needs to be considered.

The general categories of sodium control are as follows: 250 mg/day, very severe (rarely used); less than 1000 mg/day, severe; 1000 to 2400 mg/day, moderate; 2400 to 4500 mg/day or more, mild. Levels of 2000 to 3000 mg/day of sodium are most commonly prescribed.

Diets that are severely controlled in sodium include only the sodium that occurs naturally in food. Even then, foods such as milk, meat, fish, poultry, and eggs must be limited to specific amounts. In contrast, diets containing 1000 to 4500 mg/day include some salt-containing foods or the use of salt in small quantities, depending on the level of restriction and the client's preferences.

Sodium-controlled meal plans thus differ considerably, depending on the level of control. It is important that the health worker find out what level of sodium is involved before attempting to assist clients with their diet. Otherwise, efforts to help may just confuse them.

MILD SODIUM RESTRICTION

The sodium level of a mild sodium-controlled diet may range from 2400 to 4500 mg. The foods permitted depend on the sodium level ordered by the physician. Generally speaking, light salting of food is permitted, and foods processed with moderate amounts of sodium are permitted.

CONTROLLING SODIUM INTAKE

SOURCES OF SODIUM

The sources of sodium are food, the water supply, and medicine.

FOOD

Sodium is a mineral that is found naturally in food. It also is added to many foods and beverages, primarily as sodium chloride (table salt). Most of the sodium in the American diet comes from this source. The largest percentage of salt (as much as 75%) comes from salt added to food in processing. People with diets high in processed foods have the highest salt intakes; those whose diets emphasize fresh fruits, vegetables, and legumes have the lowest salt intake.

Sodium Naturally Present in Food

Animal foods such as meat, fish, poultry, milk, and eggs have the highest natural sodium content. Milk is surprisingly high in sodium, at 120 mg/cup, compared with fruit, which has 2 mg per ½-cup serving. Fruits contain little sodium, and vegetables range from low to relatively high in natural sodium. Insignificant amounts are found in animal fats, vegetable oils, and cereal grains, provided no salt or sodium compound is added in processing or preparation. Diets that call for a high protein intake (2 g/kg of body weight daily) and are severely restricted in sodium (1000 mg/day or less) are difficult to carry out because of the high natural sodium content of animal protein foods. Table 26–1 lists the average natural sodium content of foods in the major food groups.

Sodium Added to Food

Table salt and other sodium-containing compounds used in food preservation and processing and in cooking add much sodium to the average diet (Fig. 26-1). A 3-oz portion of fresh cooked pork contains 59 mg of sodium; an equal portion of cured cooked ham contains 1114 mg of sodium.

Table salt is 39% sodium. One level teaspoon of table salt contains about 1950 mg of sodium. Because moderate sodium-controlled diets limit daily intake of sodium in all food and beverages to 1000 to 2400 mg, it is evident that salt must be omitted from the diet or used in only limited quantities. Monosodium glutamate (MSG) also must be restricted in the diet; one level teaspoon contains about 500 mg of sodium. Salt, MSG, and other sodium compounds are used extensively in the commercial processing and preservation of food. Sodium added in this way is the largest source in food.

The sodium content of some processed foods, such as ham or potato chips, is obvious. The sodium content of most processed foods is not quite so apparent. A few examples of less obvious sodium additives are sodium alginate, which produces a smooth texture in ice cream and chocolate milk drinks; the salt solution used in the sorting of frozen peas during processing; and sodium benzoate,

TABLE 26-1 NATURAL SODIUM CONTENT OF FOOD GROUPS* (AVERAGE VALUES)

FOOD	HOUSEHOLD MEASURE	SODIUM (APPROXIMATE MG)
Milk, whole, low-fat, skim	8 oz (1 cup)	120
**Milk, low-sodium	8 oz (1 cup)	7
Meat, fish, poultry	1 oz	25
Egg	1	60
Vegetable	½ cup	9
Fruit	Varies	2
Starch/bread, unsalted	Varies	5
Fat exchanges, unsalted	Varies	Negligible

* Foods produced, processed, or prepared without the addition of any sodium compound.

** Natural sodium content removed by a process that exchanges potassium for sodium.

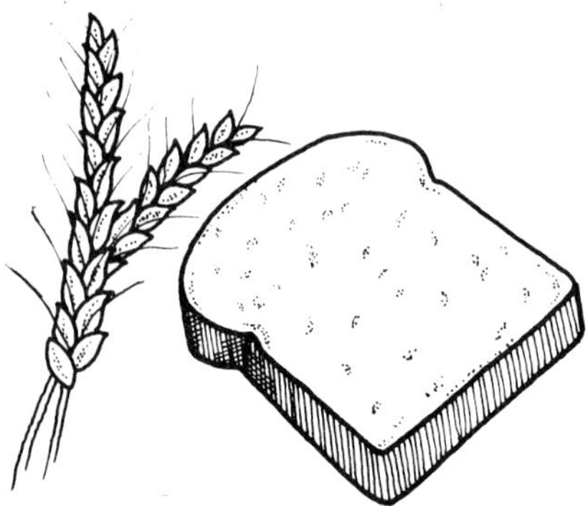

A slice of regular bread contains about 125 mg of sodium.

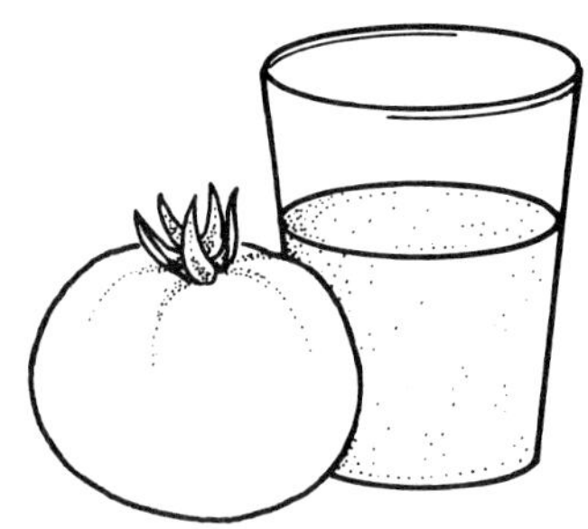

A half cup of canned tomato juice contains about 440 mg of sodium.

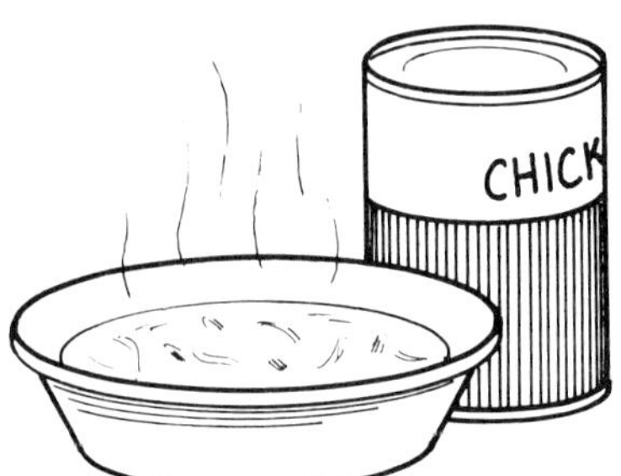

One cup of chicken noodle soup (canned, condensed, diluted with water) contains 1100 mg of sodium.

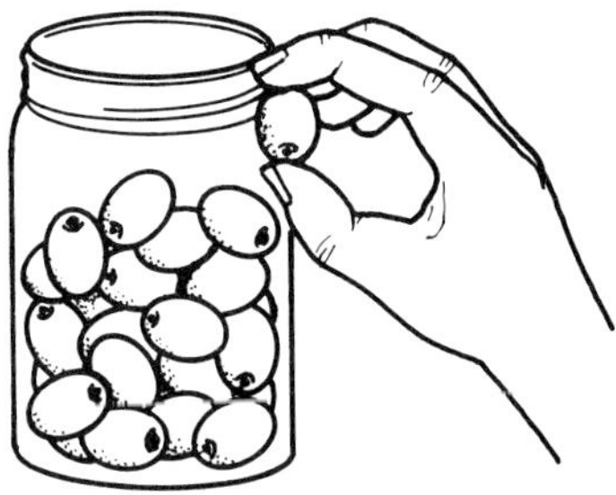

Just one large olive contains 130 mg of sodium.

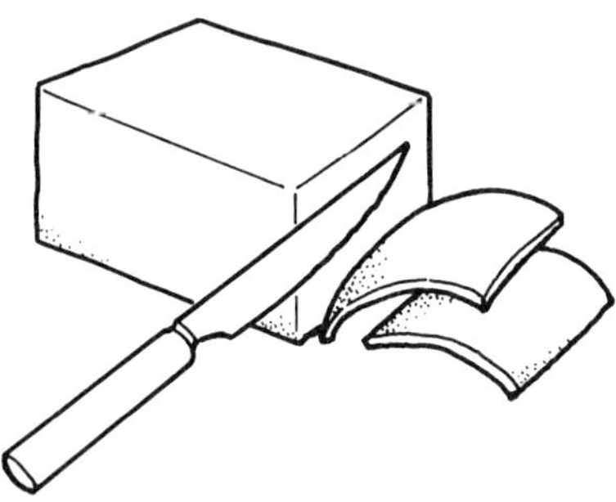

One ounce of processed American cheese contains about 400 mg sodium.

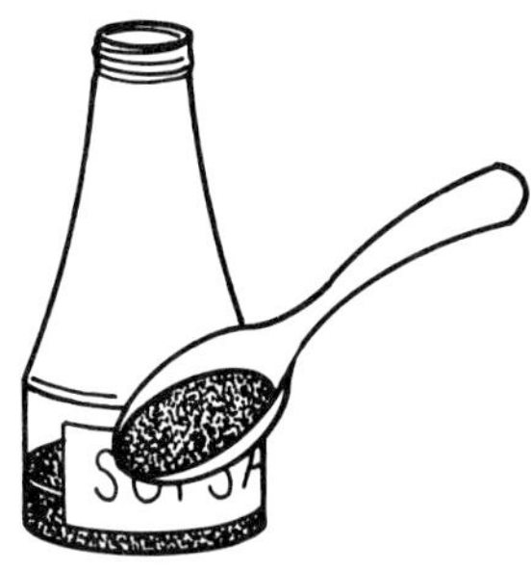

One tablespoon of soy sauce contains 1000 mg of sodium.

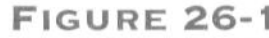

FIGURE 26-1

Processed foods add much sodium to the diet.

a preservative used in some jellies. A salty taste is not necessarily a good guide to how much sodium a food contains.

Most canned foods, packaged mixes, frozen dinners, frozen vegetables with sauces and seasonings added, frozen waffles, pizza, and other convenience foods have sodium added in one form or another. Display 26-1 shows the sodium content of representative foods in each of the food groups.

DISPLAY 26-1 QUICK GUIDE TO THE SODIUM CONTENT OF FOODS

Specific food items may be higher or lower, so always check product labels for more accurate values.

BREADS, CEREALS, RICE, PASTA

Bread, 1 slice	110–175
Baking powder biscuit, 1	300
English muffin, 1/2	130
Bagel, 1/2	145
Cracker, saltine type, 2 squares	80
Ready-to-eat cereal, 1 oz	trace*–350
Cooked cereal, pasta, rice (unsalted), 1/2 cup	<5
Flavored rice mix, cooked, 1/2 cup	250–390

VEGETABLES

Fresh or frozen vegetables (cooked without salt), 1/2 cup	<70
Vegetables, canned or frozen with sauce, 1/2 cup	140–460
Tomato juice, canned, 3/4 cup	660

FRUITS

Fruits (fresh, frozen, canned), 1/2 cup	<10

MILK, YOGURT, CHEESE

Milk, 1 cup	120
Buttermilk (salt added), 1 cup	260
Yogurt, 8 oz	165
Yogurt, fruited, 8 oz	130
Natural cheese	
Blue cheese, 1 oz	395
Cheddar cheese, 1 oz	175
Swiss cheese, 1 oz	75
Cottage cheese (regular and lowfat), 1/2 cup	440
Process cheese and cheese spreads, 1 oz	350–450

MEAT, POULTRY, FISH, DRY BEANS, EGGS, NUTS

Fresh meat, poultry, finfish, cooked, 3 oz	<90
Shellfish, 3 oz	100–300
Tuna, canned, 3 oz	300
Ham, 3 oz	1025
Sausage, 2 oz	735
Boiled ham, 2 oz	750
Bologna, 2 oz	580
Frankfurter, 1 1/2 oz	480
Dry beans, home cooked (unsalted), 1/2 cup	<10
Dry beans, canned, 1/2 cup	440
Egg, 1 large	65
Peanut butter, 1 tbsp	80

FATS, DRESSINGS

Oil, 1 tbsp	0
Vinegar, 1 tbsp	<5
Mayonnaise, 1 tbsp	80
Prepared salad dressings, 1 tbsp	105–220
Salted butter or margarine, 1 tsp	45
Unsalted butter or margarine, 1 tsp	<5

CONDIMENTS

Ketchup, chili sauce, tartar sauce, steak sauce, 1 tbsp	100–230
Mustard, prepared, 1 tsp	65
Soy sauce, 1 tsp	345
Soy sauce, lower sodium, 1 tsp	200
Salt, 1 tsp	2325

SNACKS, CONVENIENCE FOODS

Canned and dehydrated soups, 1 cup	630–1300
Lower sodium versions	Read label
Canned and frozen main dishes, 8 oz	500–1570
Lower sodium versions	Read label
Unsalted nuts and popcorn, 1 oz	<5
Salted nuts, potato chips, corn chips, 1 oz	120–240

* Shredded wheat and puffed wheat and rice cereals have only a trace of sodium per ounce.

(US Dept of Agriculture, Human Nutrition Information Service. Use salt and sodium only in moderation. Washington, DC: US Government Printing Office, 1993. Home and Garden bulletin 253-7:7.)

WATER

Most community water systems contain less than 20 mg of sodium per liter. In some communities, drinking water may have a high sodium content, as much as 200 mg or more per liter. Water softeners installed in the home add sodium. The local health department or local heart association can provide information about the sodium content of water in a particular community. In some cases, the use of distilled water may be necessary.

MEDICATION

Clients who need to restrict sodium should consult their physician before taking any unprescribed medicine or home remedy. Alkalizers for indigestion, headache remedies, cough medicine, laxatives, and others may contain sodium. A commonly used antacid contains 700 mg of sodium per dose. Home remedies such as baking soda (sodium bicarbonate) and rhubarb and baking soda are high in sodium. (Chewing tobacco also contains sodium; a 2-oz plug contains about 960 mg.)

NUTRITION COUNSELING

The aims of medical nutrition therapy are to bring sodium intake down to the prescribed level, provide adequate nutrients to meet nutritional needs, respect the client's personal food preferences, be practical and realistic, and achieve any other necessary diet modifications.

EDUCATIONAL APPROACHES

Several methods can be used to assist clients in controlling their sodium intake. Clients may be given general guidelines accompanied by lists of foods to include and to avoid. An example of such a teaching aid designed to limit sodium to 2000 mg is given in Display 26-2. Another method, the exchange list system, is useful when calories or specific nutrients as well as sodium must be controlled, as in weight reduction, diabetes, and protein-restricted diets (in renal disease).

Still another approach is the sodium point system, which involves converting the sodium prescription, given in milligrams, to sodium points (milliequivalents). Each sodium point is equal to 23 mg; for example, a sodium-controlled diet of 2000 mg/day is 87 points. Clients count the sodium points of the foods they eat, keeping within the allotted sodium points. Clients are given a sodium counter listing the sodium points in most foods. The sodium content of a processed food is given in milligrams on the label; the number of milligrams is divided by 23 to determine the sodium point value.

USING LOW-SODIUM EXCHANGE LISTS

Because low-sodium diets frequently are accompanied by control of calories or of specific energy nutrients, as in weight reduction or diabetes, the exchange list method has been adapted for use in sodium-controlled diets. In any particular diet, clients are permitted to have a specified number of exchanges (or units) from each list. The number of exchanges depends on nutritional needs, level of sodium control, food preferences, and other diet modifications, and level of caloric control. Exchange lists for low-sodium meal planning can be obtained from: The American Dietetic Association, 216 West Jackson Boulevard, Suite 700, Chicago, Illinois 60606–6995 or from local offices of the American Heart Association.

FOOD SELECTION

MILK

Because of its high natural sodium content, milk usually is limited to 2 cups/day on diets that contain 500 to 1000 mg/day of sodium. Skim milk, homemade unsalted buttermilk, and reconstituted evaporated milk contain the same amount of sodium as fresh whole milk. Cultured, salted buttermilk is higher in sodium and usually is omitted. Ice cream, sherbet, fountain drinks such as shakes and malteds, chocolate milk, and instant cocoa mixes have sodium compounds added. Ice cream or sherbet occasionally can be substituted for milk.

A special low-sodium milk is used on diets that restrict sodium to 250 mg/day. It contains more po-

DISPLAY 26-2 GUIDELINES FOR FOOD SELECTION FOR 2000-mg SODIUM DIET

FOOD CATEGORY	RECOMMENDED	EXCLUDED
Beverages	Milk (limit to 16 oz/day), buttermilk (limit to 1 cup/week); eggnog; all fruit juices; low-sodium, salt-free vegetable juices	Malted milk, milk shake, chocolate milk; regular vegetable or tomato juices; commercially softened water used for drinking or cooking
Breads and cereals	Enriched white, wheat, rye, and pumpernickel bread, hard rolls, and dinner rolls; muffins, cornbread, pancakes and waffles; most dry cereals, cooked cereal without added salt; unsalted crackers and breadsticks; low-sodium or homemade bread crumbs	Breads, rolls, and crackers with salted tops; quick breads; instant hot cereals; commercial bread stuffing; self-rising flour and biscuit mixes; regular bread crumbs or cracker crumbs
Desserts and sweets	All; desserts and sweets made with milk should be within allowance	None
Fats	Butter or margarine; vegetable oils; unsalted salad dressings; light, sour, and heavy cream	Regular salad dressings containing bacon fat, bacon bits, and salt pork; snack dips made with instant soup mixes or processed cheese
Fruits	Most fresh, frozen, and canned fruits	Fruits processed with salt or sodium-containing compounds
Meats and meat substitutes	Any fresh or frozen beef, lamb, pork, poultry, fish; some shellfish; canned tuna or salmon, rinsed; eggs and egg substitutes; low-sodium cheese including low-sodium ricotta and cream cheese; low-sodium cottage cheese; regular yogurt; low-sodium peanut butter; dried peas and beans; frozen dinners (<500 mg sodium)	Any smoked, cured, salted, koshered, or canned meat, fish, or poultry including bacon, chipped beef, cold cuts, ham, hot dogs, sausage, sardines, anchovies, marinated herring, and pickled meats; crab, lobster; frozen breaded meats; pickled eggs; regular hard and processed cheese; cheese spreads and sauces; salted nuts
Potatoes and potato substitutes	White or sweet potatoes; squash; enriched rice, barley, noodles, spaghetti, macaroni, and other pastas cooked without salt; homemade bread stuffing	Commercially prepared potato, rice, or pasta mixes; commercial bread stuffing
Soups	Low-sodium commercially canned and dehydrated soups, broths, and bouillons; homemade broth soups without added salt and made with allowed vegetables; cream soups within milk allowance	Regular canned or dehydrated soups, broths, or bouillon

(Continued)

DISPLAY 26-2 GUIDELINES FOR FOOD SELECTION FOR 2000-mg SODIUM DIET
(Continued)

FOOD CATEGORY	RECOMMENDED	EXCLUDED
Vegetables	Fresh, frozen vegetables and low-sodium canned vegetables	Regular canned vegetables, sauerkraut, pickled vegetables, and others prepared in brine; frozen vegetables in sauces; vegetables seasoned with ham, bacon, or salt pork
Miscellaneous	Salt substitute with physician's approval; pepper, herbs, spices; vinegar, lemon, or lime juice; low-sodium soy sauce; hot pepper sauce; low-sodium condiments (ketchup, chili sauce, mustard); fresh ground horseradish; unsalted tortilla chips, pretzels, potato chips, popcorn	Any seasoning made with salt including garlic salt, celery salt, onion salt, and seasoned salt; sea salt, rock salt, kosher salt; meat tenderizers; MSG, regular soy sauce, barbecue sauce, teriyaki sauce, steak sauce, Worcestershire sauce, and most flavored vinegars; canned gravy and mixes; regular condiments; salted snack foods

(Chicago Dietetic Association and South Suburban Dietetic Association. Manual of clinical dietetics. Chicago: The American Dietetic Association, 1992:503.)

tassium than regular milk and therefore cannot be used if potassium is restricted, as in some renal disorders.

MEAT, FISH, AND POULTRY

Unless there is a protein restriction, most diets permit at least 4 or 5 oz/day of meat, fish, or poultry. Brain, kidney, and shellfish have a higher sodium content than other meat and fish.

Saltwater fish (except shellfish) and freshwater fish may be used in the sodium-controlled diet. All fresh fish should be thoroughly rinsed before being cooked because fish frequently is transported to market in a salt solution. If possible, fresh fish that has not been put through a brine solution should be purchased. All salted, smoked, and canned meats, fish, and poultry are avoided, including ham, bacon, luncheon meats, and sausage.

Reduced-sodium varieties of foods such as ham and luncheon meats are readily available in supermarkets. The consumer must read labels and ask questions of store delicatessan personnel to find out how much sodium the foods contain. In some cases even reduced sodium foods may have too much sodium for a particular sodium level.

EGGS AND CHEESE

Most of the sodium in eggs is in the whites. Cheese is high in sodium. Processed cheeses such as American cheese, cheese food, and cheese spread have twice as much sodium as cheddar cheese. Some natural cheeses, such as Roquefort, blue, feta, Camembert, and Gorgonzola, are saltier than others.

On diets with only mild sodium control, limited amounts of natural cheese usually are permitted. Processed cheeses and highly salted natural cheeses usually are avoided in all sodium-restricted diets. Low-sodium cheeses are available. Each product must be evaluated separately to determine the amount that can be substituted for meat. The sodium contents of the products differ, and some may exceed the sodium content of the meat they replace. Regular salted cottage cheese, including lowfat varieties, is high in sodium. A $^1/_2$-cup portion contains 450 mg of sodium. Unsalted, dry-curd cottage cheese is low in sodium and may be used even in diets that restrict sodium to 500 mg/day, if substituted for meat.

VEGETABLES

The natural sodium content of vegetables ranges from about 9 to 70 mg per $^1/_2$ cup. Vegetables that have a high natural sodium content must be omitted on diets of 500 mg/day of sodium or less. These include beets, beet greens, carrots, spinach, celery, white turnips, chard, and frozen peas. It is possible to allow for limited quantities on diets of more than 500 mg/day of sodium. Usually there is no restriction of **unsalted** fresh, frozen or canned vegetables on diets of more than 1000 mg of sodium.

Vegetables should be fresh, frozen, or canned without the addition of salt or another sodium compound. Salt usually is not added to plain frozen vegetables. Starchy vegetables such as peas and lima beans, however, frequently are sorted in a brine solution before being frozen and thus, have a sodium content of about 70 mg per $^1/_2$ cup cooked. Frozen vegetables that have sauces, mushrooms, or nuts added are much higher in sodium than the plain varieties.

All regular canned vegetables and vegetable juices have salt added. On diets of 2000 mg/day or more of sodium, clients can reduce the sodium content of canned vegetables sufficiently by rinsing them in water, straining them, and reheating them in unsalted tap water. Many canned products with no added salt are available on the market.

FRUITS

Most fruits are low in sodium—about 2 mg per serving. Small amounts of salt sometimes are added to frozen and canned fruits to prevent darkening, and some canned and frozen fruits, as well as canned tomatoes, are dipped in sodium hydroxide so they can be peeled easily. Sodium sulfite frequently is added to dried fruit.

BREADS AND CEREALS

Cereal grains such as wheat flour, cornmeal, barley, and rice are low in natural sodium. When they are made into breads, breakfast cereals, and bakery products, however, salt and other sodium compounds usually are added (see Display 26-1).

Unsalted bread, matzo, and melba toast generally are available in food markets. Regular crackers, even those made with unsalted tops, are made with a dough that contains salt and leavening agents that contain sodium. On moderate sodium-controlled diets, regular salted bread and breadstuffs are usually permitted. Those breadstuffs with salted tops are avoided.

Cooked cereals such as farina, oatmeal, and hominy grits are low in sodium if cooked without salt; however, some quick-cooking and most instant varieties of these cereals have sodium compounds added. Check the labels. Puffed rice, puffed wheat, shredded wheat, wheat germ, and some brands of granola have no sodium added. Some ready-to-eat cereals have as much as 340 mg of sodium in a cup. Pasta, rice, tapioca, white and sweet potatoes, corn, and dried peas and beans are low in sodium when prepared without salt or other sodium compounds.

FAT

Oils, unsalted butter, unsalted margarine, and unsalted nuts are low in sodium (see Display 26-1).

MISCELLANEOUS FOODS

Sugar and honey have negligible amounts of sodium. The artificial sweeteners composed of sodium saccharin contain 3.5 mg of sodium in a 1-g packet, a negligible amount.

Sodium compounds are added to beverage mixes, fountain beverages, commercial candies, molasses, corn syrup, commercial puddings, and gelatin desserts. Soft drinks may be high in sodium because of the sodium content of the water in the area in which they are manufactured.

Most condiments and seasonings are high in sodium. Most convenience foods have salt and other sodium compounds added. TV dinners, frozen vegetables in seasoned sauces, mixes for baked goods, meat extenders, meat substitutes made from textured vegetable protein, seasoned bread stuffing, packaged dinners, and flavored rice mixes are examples of those high in sodium.

FOOD PREPARATION

Many clients find it difficult to accept a sodium-controlled diet. Low-salt foods may taste flat to them, and the thought of restricting favorite foods for the rest of their lives is unpleasant. Salt is a much overworked seasoning. Clients may not be aware of the many other ways in which food can be seasoned and flavored. Spices, herbs, and other flavoring aids are listed in Display 26-3.

DISPLAY 26-3 FLAVOR IDEAS FOR SODIUM-CONTROLLED DIETS

MAY BE USED

- Allspice
- Almond extract
- Anise seed
- Angostura bitters
- Basil
- Bay leaf
- Bouillon cubes (low-sodium)
- Caraway seeds
- Cardamon
- Chili powder
- Chives
- Cinnamon
- Cloves
- Cumin
- Curry
- Dill
- Fennel
- Garlic
- Ginger
- Horseradish (prepared without salt)
- Juniper
- Lemon juice or extract
- Mace
- Maple extract
- Marjoram
- Mint
- Mustard, dry powder
- Nutmeg
- Onion, fresh, or powder (not onion salt)
- Orange extract
- Oregano
- Paprika
- Parsley
- Pepper
- Peppermint extract
- Poppy seeds
- Poultry seasoning
- Purslane
- Rosemary
- Saccharin
- Saffron
- Sage
- Salt substitutes (only with doctor's approval)
- Savory
- Sesame seeds
- Sugar*
- Tarragon
- Thyme
- Turmeric
- Vanilla
- Vinegar
- Walnut extract
- Wine (not cooking wine)

AVOID

- Baking soda
- Barbecue sauce
- Bouillon cubes, regular
- Celery salt
- Chili sauce
- Garlic salt
- Horseradish (prepared with salt)
- Ketchup
- Meat sauces
- Meat tenderizers
- MSG
- Mustard, prepared
- Olives
- Onion salt
- Pickles
- Relishes
- Salad dressings (commercial)
- Salt
- Soy sauce
- Worcestershire sauce
- Cooking wine (has salt added)

* Unless limited for other reasons such as weight control.

Meat, fish, and poultry may be made more flavorful with the use of low-sodium marinades and sauces and with the use of fruit as a flavoring aid. Low-sodium mixtures of certain wines or vinegar, vegetable oil, and permitted herbs and spices may be used as a marinade for meat and poultry and as a basting mixture during meat preparation. Cooking wine should be avoided because it contains added salt. Meat, fish, or poultry may be cooked in a low-sodium tomato sauce.

A sweet-and-sour sauce made of diluted vinegar and sugar and seasoned with grated onion, spices, and herbs can be used to flavor vegetables. A pinch of sugar added while vegetables are cooking also can enhance flavor. Herbs may be sprinkled on vegetables after cooking.

For people on severe sodium-controlled meal plans, low-sodium breadstuffs may be necessary. If this is the case, appetizing baked goods can be made with yeast or low-sodium baking powder, unsalted fat, and other unsalted ingredients. Low-sodium dietetic baking powder is available in grocery stores. People should follow tested recipes from low-sodium cookbooks using low-sodium baking powder rather than recipes from standard cookbooks.

It is essential that the person who is responsible for food preparation in the client's household receive counseling along with the client. The dietitian is alert to cultural eating habits that may interfere with the diet, and provides suggestions for modifying favorite cultural foods so that they may be included. Health care workers also need to know the eating habits that are part of the client's cultural background so they can give support to the instruction provided (see Chapter 15).

FOOD LABELING

Clients who must restrict sodium severely or moderately need to avoid all or most foods that have sodium compounds added. The current Food and Drug Administration (FDA) labeling regulations have taken the guesswork out of selecting processed foods. The sodium content is a required component on the "Nutrition Facts" panel of the food labels of virtually all (about 90%) of processed food. In addition to listing the milligrams of sodium per serving of the product, the "% Daily Value" is also given. The reference daily value for sodium is 2400 mg regardless of caloric intake. For example, a serving of a product that has 300 mg of sodium would also be expressed as 13% of the Daily Value for sodium.

All foods that have more than one ingredient must list all ingredients on the label, including standardized foods (foods such as mayonnaise, jelly, and ketchup made according to prescribed recipes), which were exempt before May 8, 1993. Previously, the use of sodium additives in these standardized foods was not evident to the consumer because the manufacturer did not have to list the ingredients on the label.

SODIUM-MODIFIED FOODS

The link between sodium and the increased risk of hypertension is an FDA-approved health claim and can appear on the labels of foods that meet the criteria for *low-sodium*. This descriptive term as well as other terms for sodium-modified products are given in Display 26-4.

In recent years, consumer demand has led to the production of a wide variety of low-sodium processed foods. For some clients, foods such as low-sodium tuna and salmon, low-sodium canned vegetables, low-sodium cheese, and low-sodium peanut butter may add variety and convenience to the diet. These foods usually are more expensive than the regular foods they replace, however.

Clients should not assume that all sodium-modified foods can be included in their diet. Some foods labeled *reduced-sodium,* although lower in sodium than regular food, may still contain too much to be included in a specific diet. Clients should be instructed to check the serving size given on the label and compare it with the portion size they use.

DISPLAY 26-4 SODIUM LABELING

LABELING TERM	DEFINITION
Sodium-free	<5 mg per serving
Very low-sodium	≤35 mg per serving
Low-sodium	≤140 mg per serving
Reduced-sodium; less sodium	At least 25% less per serving than the reference food

SALT SUBSTITUTES

Salt substitutes should be used only with the physician's permission. The substitutes, available in drug stores and food markets, contain potassium or ammonium in place of sodium. In kidney disorders, potassium salt may be prohibited, and in severe liver disease, ammonium salt must be avoided. Morton's Light Salt and Papa Dash are examples of reduced-sodium substitutes. They cannot be used when sodium is severely restricted.

EATING OUT

People on diets controlling sodium to 1000 mg/day can eat out occasionally and keep within their sodium prescription if they choose foods carefully. When eating meals in restaurants and cafeterias on a regular basis, however, they would require a sodium level of 3000 to 5000 mg/day would be required to achieve variety and nutritional balance. Maintaining more severe sodium control would require choosing from a quite limited selection of foods. Suggestions for controlling sodium when dining out are given in Display 26-5.

EDUCATIONAL MATERIALS

Food lists and recipe pamphlets usually are given to clients if they receive diet instruction in a hospital, community agency, or nutrition counseling service. Physicians or clients with their physician's authorization may obtain instructional materials from the lo-

DISPLAY 26-5 TIPS FOR CONTROLLING SODIUM WHEN DINING OUT

Plan ahead. Choose restaurants that prepare food by request. Ask restaurant personnel if they would

- prepare a dish without added salt or MSG
- limit portion sizes of meat, fish, and poultry to 4 oz to 6 oz
- omit gravy and sauces from any entrée or side dish
- prepare a dish using unsaturated vegetable oil instead of salted butter or margarine.

Obtain dining guides from local chapters of the American Heart Association (AHA). These guides list restaurants that prepare foods that meet AHA dietary guidelines.

Ask about how food is prepared if descriptions are not given on the menu.

When ordering from a menu, do the following:

- Select simply prepared foods, which are best, such as baked, broiled, roasted, grilled, steamed, or poached without sauces, breadings or batters.
- Avoid processed meats, cheese, and mixed dishes such as stews and casseroles.
- Avoid hollandaise, tomato and cream sauces, and all gravies, and items described as au gratin or scalloped.
- Request that food be prepared without salt. Bring your own spice blend, salt-free seasoning, or salt substitute.
- Select fruit or fruit juices as an appetizer. Avoid vegetable juices and all soups.
- Use vinegar and oil or carry your own low-sodium salad dressing or request that regular salad dressings be served "on the side" and use them sparingly.
- For sandwiches, choose lean fresh meats and poultry such as lean roast beef or sliced turkey instead of processed meats and meat salads.
- Request fruit, lettuce, tomatoes, and onion as sandwich accompaniments in place of dill pickles, potato chips, and olives.
- Choose fresh vegetables instead of canned. Choose baked potato; ask for unsalted margarine.
- Request lemon slices to season food.
- For dessert, choose fresh fruit or a small dish of ice cream, sherbet, or gelatin.

In fast-food restaurants, choose plain hamburger or a roast beef sandwich. Use lettuce, tomato, and onion for garnish. Avoid pickles, mustard, cheese, ketchup, and special sauces.

In salad bars, choose fruits and fresh vegetables. Avoid bacon bits, pickles, cheese, meat salads, and canned vegetables. Use vinegar and oil, lemon juice, or carry your own low-sodium dressing.

When traveling by air, notify airline reservation office 24 hours in advance of your flight of your need for a low-sodium meal. Inform flight attendant of your request when you board the airplane.

cal chapter of the American Heart Association. Meal plans, menu suggestions, food buying and food preparation ideas, and guides for eating out are included in these booklets. Clients can purchase a low-sodium cookbook entitled *The American Heart Association's Low Salt Cookbook* from local chapters of the American Heart Association and in bookstores.

POTASSIUM REPLACEMENT

The continued use of diuretics such as thiazides and furosemide in the treatment of hypertension and water retention may cause excessive loss of potassium in the urine. Potassium is essential to life; if loss is severe, death may follow.

Potassium can be replaced by medication or liberal quantities of potassium-rich foods. It is preferable to avoid potassium deficiency by means of a high-potassium diet than to use potassium supplements. Potassium medication has an unpleasant taste and is irritating to the gastrointestinal tract.

Most fruits, fresh vegetables, whole-grain cereals, dried peas and beans, lentils, and unsalted meats are good low-sodium sources of potassium. A medium-sized banana and 1 cup of orange juice can add more than 800 mg of potassium to the diet. Display 11–3 provides a list of potassium-rich foods.

Because there is substantial evidence that a liberal potassium intake may play a role in reducing high blood pressure, a potassium-rich diet should be encouraged for everyone. Eating more natural, unprocessed foods is required. When foods are highly processed, the potassium is leached out and sodium is added. Taking potassium supplements, unless prescribed by a physician, should be avoided. Excessive amounts of potassium are toxic and can cause cardiac arrest.

KEYS TO PRACTICAL APPLICATION

Be sure you know the level of sodium restriction prescribed for your clients before advising them about foods they can or cannot have. Low-sodium diets differ depending on the level of sodium control. Advice that conflicts with their diet will confuse clients.

Be aware of the sodium content of processed foods. Many clients think of sodium restriction only in terms of the salt shaker. They frequently need help recognizing processed foods that have a high-sodium content.

Show clients how the sodium-controlled diet has reduced their edema and body weight or decreased their blood pressure. Help them understand why these changes are beneficial.

Encourage clients to try new ways of flavoring food if they find it difficult to adjust to the taste of unsalted foods. Become familiar with the many spices, herbs, and other flavoring aids that clients can use.

Advise clients to discuss the use of nonprescription drugs with their physician. These medications are an unexpected and frequently overlooked source of sodium.

Avoid use of the terms *salt-free* or *low-salt* when referring to sodium-controlled diets. These terms are inaccurate and give the false impression that table salt is the only food ingredient about which to be concerned.

Advise clients not to use a salt substitute without their physician's approval. Salt substitutes may be harmful for some clients.

Help clients identify sodium-modified foods that may be useful for them. Become familiar with the sodium labeling terms in Display 26-4.

KEY IDEAS

Diet changes frequently are prescribed in the treatment of cardiovascular disease. Diets associated with cardiovascular disease are sodiumcontrolled, fat-controlled, and weight-reducing diets.

In the acute stages of cardiovascular disease, changes in diet are made to rest the heart as much as possible. Small, low-calorie meals with easily digested consistency are given and gas-forming foods are avoided. The client may be fed by another person, if necessary.

Hypertension places heavy strain on the heart, brain, eyes, and kidneys. It contributes to the occurrence of heart attacks, strokes, aortic aneurysms, and renal failure.

Being an African American, having a family history of hypertension, and being older than age 55 years increases the risk of developing hypertension.

Weight reduction is important in the treatment of hypertension for obese people.

Sodium is controlled to prevent or treat edema and hypertension; control also may increase the effectiveness of diuretic drugs and make it possible to reduce drug dosages. The importance of sodium control in the prevention and treatment of hypertension is controversial.

Alcohol in excess of one or two standard-sized drinks a day raises blood pressure.

Research studies have suggested that potassium, calcium, magnesium, fiber, and polyunsaturated fat may affect blood pressure control.

The 10th edition of the *Recommended Dietary Allowances* has recommended 500 mg/day of sodium as a safe minimum intake. The Committee on Diet and Health has recommended a maximum intake of 2400 mg/day.

Sources of sodium include food (sodium may be naturally present or added in processing), water, and medications.

Animal foods—meat, fish, poultry, milk, and eggs—have a high natural sodium content; vegetables range from low to relatively high; fruits, animal fats, vegetable oils, and unprocessed cereal grains are low in natural sodium.

The addition of salt and other sodium-containing compounds to food considerably increases the sodium content of the average diet; salt and other sodium additives in commercial food processing are the greatest source of sodium.

The sodium content of drinking water varies considerably; in some areas, distilled water may be necessary for drinking and cooking. Water softeners add much sodium to the water supply.

Antacids and other over-the-counter medications and home remedies can add much sodium to daily intake.

Diet prescriptions should specify the level of sodium desired; terms such as *salt-free, salt-poor,* and *low-salt* are inaccurate and falsely give the impression that table salt is the only substance of concern.

Sodium-controlled diets differ, depending on the amount of sodium permitted. Diets that restrict sodium to less than 1000 mg/day include only naturally occurring sodium; diets of 1000 mg/day and more include some salt-containing foods or the use of salt in limited quantities, depending on the level of control.

The Exchange Lists for Meal Planning can be adapted for use in sodium-restricted diets; each item within a particular exchange contains about the same amount of sodium as well as protein, fat, and carbohydrate.

A diet containing a specific quantity of sodium may be planned in a number of ways, depending on the client's nutritional needs, lifestyle, and preferences.

Commercial low-sodium foods may be useful for some clients. Guidance should be given so that clients can determine whether a specific low-sodium food is suitable.

Salt substitutes should be used only with a physician's permission.

It is unrealistic to expect clients to comply with a diet that restricts sodium to less than 3000 mg/day if they eat out on a regular basis.

Some diuretics may cause excessive loss of potassium. Prevention of potassium deficiency by means of a high-potassium diet is preferred to the use of potassium supplements, which have undesirable side effects.

Most fruits, fresh vegetables, whole-grain breads and cereals, legumes, and meat are good sources of potassium.

Virtually all processed foods give the sodium content in milligrams on the label. Descriptive terms are clearly defined (see Display 26-4).

KEYS TO LEARNING

STUDY–DISCUSSION QUESTIONS

1. Using the sodium values of the food groups in Table 26-1 and the values for regular bread given in Display 26-1, calculate the sodium content of a meal plan composed of the following exchanges:
   - 2 cups skim milk
   - 6 ounces of meat, fish, or poultry
   - 3 servings of vegetables
   - 4 servings of fruit
   - 7 servings of starch/bread (four of these servings are regular salted bread).
   - 5 teaspoons unsalted fat

   Plan one day's menu using this plan. Describe the flavoring aids you might use to make the items on your menu more appealing.
2. Investigate the low-sodium foods sold in your supermarket. What kinds of foods did you find? Check the labels for sodium content in an average serving. Are there any foods you believe might not be permitted on some sodium-controlled diets even though they are labeled *low-sodium* or *reduced-sodium?* Select one or two of these items and compare their cost with equal quantities of the regular food they are meant to replace. For example, compare the price of low-sodium bread with that of a loaf of regular bread.
3. Prepare at home one of your favorite vegetables without adding salt or another sodium additive. Taste the unsalted food. Then divide the vegetable into two or three portions. Flavor each of these portions with a different salt substitute and taste. (Your instructor will help you obtain samples of salt substitutes.)
4. What would you tell a client who asked for a salt substitute?
5. Select two members of your class to visit the local chapter of the American Heart Association. What nutrition services does the association provide for clients? Discuss your visit with the class.
6. Classify the following foods as (1) high in natural sodium, (2) low in natural sodium, or (3) high in sodium content due to sodium additives: milk, canned pears, fresh spinach, fresh pork chops, bologna, orange juice, farina, puffed wheat, chocolate malted, prepared mustard, American cheese, canned beef stew, canned tuna fish, corn flakes, broccoli, fresh mackerel.
7. Discuss with the class your experiences with clients on sodium-controlled diets. What factors seem to affect their ability to adjust to sodium-controlled diets?
8. Rest is one of the most important considerations in acute heart disease. How can the diet be changed to decrease the workload of the heart?
9. Increased potassium intake frequently is necessary for people taking diuretic medication. List five foods that are rich sources of potassium.

CASE STUDY

Mr. A is a 42-year-old electrician. He has his own business and has several employees. He occasionally goes out on a job, but more frequently dispatches and supervises his employees and does paperwork in the office.

Mr. A is 5 ft, 10 inches tall, has a large frame, and weighs 220 lb. In recent doctor's visits, his blood pressure has been consistently in the 140 to 150 over 90 to 100 mm Hg range. Mr. A fears the potential problems associated with blood pressure medication. The doctor told Mr. A that his blood pressure could probably be controlled if he loses weight and reduces his sodium intake to about 2000 mg/day. Mr. A agreed to try this approach and was given a 6-month period to do so.

Mr. and Mrs. A met with the dietitian. Mr. A told the dietitian that he could not understand why his blood pressure was elevated. He had not salted his food for more than a year. Mrs. A does not use salt in cooking. Mr. A recalled the following food intake for the previous day:

Breakfast:	Orange juice	6 oz
	Scrambled eggs	Two
	Biscuit	One
	Sausage	2-oz patty
	Black coffee	1 cup
Lunch (purchased at a luncheonette):	American cheese sandwich	2 oz to 3 oz of cheese
	Lettuce and tomato for sandwich	
	Dill pickle	One quarter of a whole pickle
	Potato chips	1-oz bag
	Skim milk	8-oz carton
Midafternoon:	Apple	One
Dinner:	Fresh pork roast	4 oz to 5 oz
	Pork gravy (from dry mix)	¼ cup
	Sauerkraut	½ cup
	Stuffing for pork (commercial ready mix)	½ cup
	Stewed tomatoes (canned)	½ cup
	Rye bread	One slice
	Margarine, salted	2 tsp
	Cherry pie	One sixth of an 8-inch pie
	Tea	
Evening:	Popcorn (commercial)	3 cups
	Crackers with peanut butter	Six; 1 tbsp of peanut butter
	Skim milk	1 cup

1. Do you think Mr. A's diet is low in sodium? Generally speaking, what is the major source of sodium in this day's menu?
2. Rewrite the menu so that it meets the 2000 mg/day sodium limit.
3. How would you flavor specific items in your revised menu?
4. Mr. A likes spicy foods such as chili, sausage, barbecued chicken, and ribs. What specific suggestions can you provide for making his food more flavorful without the addition of salt?

BIBLIOGRAPHY

BOOKS AND PAMPHLETS

Chicago Dietetic Association and South Suburban Dietetic Association. Manual of clinical dietetics. 4th ed. Chicago: The American Dietetic Association, 1992:493–510.

Kotchen TA, Kotchen JM. Nutrition, diet, and hypertension. In: Shils ME, Olson JA, Shike M. Eds. Modern nutrition in health and disease. 8th ed. Philadelphia: Lea and Febiger, 1994:1287–1297.

National Academy of Sciences, National Research Council, Committee on Diet and Health, Food and Nutrition Board. Diet and health: implications for reducing chronic disease risk (executive summary). Washington, DC: National Academy Press, National Academy of Sciences, National Research Council, Food and Nutrition Board. Recommended dietary allowances. 10th ed. Washington, DC: National Academy Press, 1989.

US Dept of Agriculture, Human Nutrition Information Service. Use salt and sodium only in moderation. Washington, DC: US Government Printing Office, 1993. Home and Garden bulletin 253-7.

PERIODICALS

Davis BR, Blaufox MD, Oberman A, et al. Reduction in long term antihypertensive medication requirements: effects of weight reduction by dietary intervention in overweight persons with mild hypertension. Arch Intern Med 1993;153:1773.

Dustan HP. Obesity and hypertension. Diabetes Care 1991;14–488.

Neaton JD, Grimm RH, Prineas RJ, et al. Treatment of mild hypertension study: final results. JAMA 1993;270:713.

Tjoa HI, Kaplan NM. Nonpharmacological treatment of hypertension in diabetes. Diabetes Care 1991;14:229.

CHAPTER

27

Nutrition Therapy in Renal Disease

KEY TERMS

albumin protein found in the blood as serum albumin; it is the chief protein in the fluid portion of the blood (serum) that separates from red blood cells after clotting

anuria suppression of urine

catheter tube that can be inserted into the body; used to instill and drain dialysate in a peritoneal dialysate exchange

clinical trials research studies

dialysate solution used to draw out waste products and restore electrolyte balance across a semipermeable membrane in the dialysis treatment

dialysis treatment for the removal of waste products and restoration of electrolyte balance; used in end-stage renal disease

diuresis removal of excess fluid through increased urination; diuretic medication often used

dry weight (estimated) solid body weight after dialysis without signs of excess fluid retention

dwell time length of time one dialysate exchange remains in the abdominal cavity during peritoneal dialysis treatments

epoetin-alpha recombinant deoxyribonucleic acid (DNA)–produced erythropoietin that has the same biologic effects as erythropoietin produced by the body

erythropoietin glycoprotein produced in the kidney that stimulates red blood cell production

hematuria passage of urine containing blood

hemodialysis removal of toxins, electrolytes, and fluid from the blood by circulating it through a dialyzer (artificial kidney) outside of the body

hyperkalemia abnormally high blood potassium level

oliguria reduction in the quantity of urine

peritoneal dialysis removal of toxins, electrolytes, and fluid by instilling dialysate into the abdominal cavity and draining it out by gravity; types of peritoneal dialysis include **intermittent peritoneal dialysis,** the exchange of dialysate several times (usually three times) a week, lasting 10 to 12 hours; **continuous ambulatory peritoneal dialysis,** four exchanges of dialysate with prolonged dwell times daily; and **continuous cycling peritoneal dialysis,** several exchanges of dialysate every night with one long dwell time during the day

peritoneum membrane that lines the abdominal cavity

peritonitis inflammation of the peritoneum usually due to infection

proteinuria presence of protein, usually albumin, in the urine

renal pertaining to the kidneys

uremia set of symptoms associated with advanced renal disease; symptoms include nausea, vomiting, weakness, a bitter or metallic taste, itching, and edema

OBJECTIVES

After reading this chapter, the student will be able to:

1. Discuss the normal physiology of the kidney, describe the differences between acute and chronic renal failure, and list two major causes of renal failure.
2. Identify the techniques for conservative management of chronic renal failure.
3. Discuss the differences in protein requirements between conservative management, hemodialysis, and peritoneal dialysis.
4. Identify causes of and treatments for
   - anemia in renal disease
   - renal osteodystrophy or uremic bone disease
   - protein-calorie malnutrition
5. Explain the relationship between dietary sodium and fluid weight gain in hemodialysis.
6. List the names of vitamins and minerals that need to be supplemented in renal failure.
7. Name six nondietary causes of hyperkalemia. Address the appropriate action to correct each problem.
8. Explain the dietary differences between the dialysis diet and diet after transplantation.
9. Discuss the dietary modifications used in the treatment of kidney stones.
10. Describe the roadblocks to dietary compliance for clients with renal disease. Explain methods for assisting these clients.

In early chronic renal failure, dietary modifications along with blood pressure control and tight glycemic control in clients with diabetes can significantly delay the progressive decline in renal function. Early identification and treatment must be the focus of the health care team.

In the past, nutrition therapy for end-stage renal disease, in which kidney function is severely impaired, was aimed primarily at prolonging the client's life. Today, in addition to prolonging life, dialysis permits clients to maintain a near-normal degree of activity, which frequently includes a near-normal work schedule. The success of dialysis treatment depends largely on the client's adherence to a prescribed diet.

Because a condition that was once 100% fatal is now treatable with dialysis, the number of clients who require treatment has grown considerably. More than 165,000 people in the United States are now undergoing treatment for end-stage renal disease. Some clients receive kidney transplants; others remain on dialysis indefinitely.

PHYSIOLOGY OF THE KIDNEY

Each kidney is composed of about 1 million functioning units called *nephrons* (Fig. 27-1). Each nephron contains a cluster of tiny blood vessels or

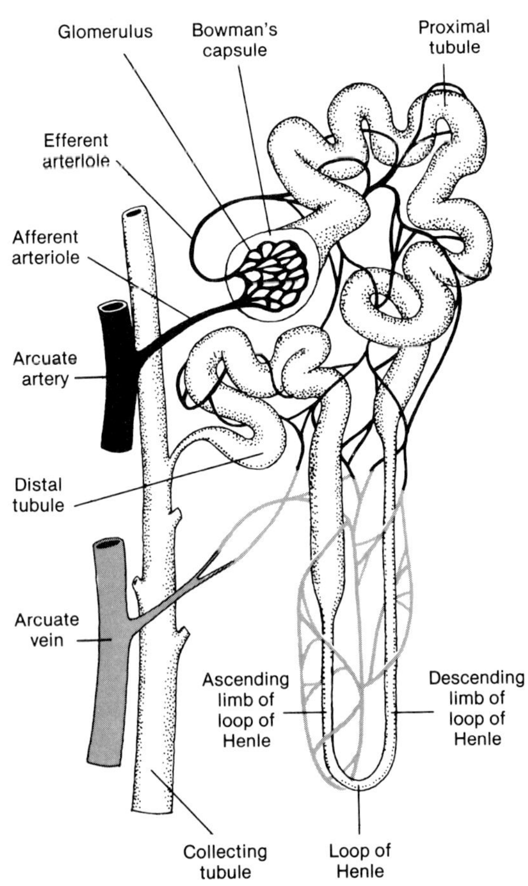

FIGURE 27-1

Simplified diagram of a nephron.

capillaries, called a *glomerulus,* and a long, winding tubule (convoluted tubule) that extends from the glomerulus to a collecting duct. The beginning of the convoluted tubule, called *Bowman's capsule,* surrounds the glomerulus. One tiny blood vessel supplies the glomerulus with blood; another drains it. As the blood passes through the glomerulus, a mixture of water and other small molecules (glucose, amino acids, sodium chloride, and waste products) passes directly from the blood, through the capillary walls, and into Bowman's capsule. In adults, the 2 million nephrons form filtrate at the rate of about 80 mL to 120 mL/min. As the filtrate passes through the convoluted tubule, about 99% of the water and most of the small molecules are returned to the blood.

Under normal conditions, substances the body needs, such as sodium, potassium, and glucose, are returned to the bloodstream, and toxic substances are expelled in the urine. Toxic substances include the waste products of protein metabolism: urea, uric acid, sulfate, creatinine, and organic acids. In this manner, the kidneys maintain the normal composition and volume of the blood and eliminate body wastes.

The kidneys also have metabolic and hormonal functions. They are involved in the breakdown of protein, the production of ammonia (which controls body acidity), glucose metabolism, and the conversion of toxic substances to harmless ones. Hormonal activities include the secretion of renin, which affects blood pressure, and of the hormone erythropoietin, which stimulates the bone marrow to produce red blood cells. The kidneys also play an essential role in converting the inactive form of vitamin D to the active form necessary for normal calcium metabolism.

RENAL DISEASES

Given the functions of the kidneys, it is not difficult to understand the serious effects of renal failure. Excretion of poisonous wastes and regulation of water and acid–base balance are disturbed; furthermore, high blood pressure, anemia, and bone disease may follow.

Diseases of the kidney may be due to genetic defects, infections, or a chronic disease such as hypertension, atherosclerosis, or diabetic nephropathy. Not all renal diseases become chronic. Some may be acute, followed by healing; others may recur and eventually lead to renal failure.

GLOMERULONEPHRITIS

Glomerulonephritis is inflammation of the glomeruli. Damage to the glomeruli causes hematuria and proteinuria. Other symptoms may include edema, nitrogen retention, oliguria, and hypertension. Glomerulonephritis frequently follows other infections, especially of the upper respiratory tract. Recovery usually is complete. In some cases, the disease progresses and becomes chronic, with progressive loss of renal function.

RENAL FAILURE

In renal failure, the kidney is no longer able to excrete waste products normally and maintain normal blood composition. Nitrogen-containing wastes accumulate; acidosis and electrolyte abnormalities occur. The secretion of urine lessens or stops completely (anuria). Renal failure may be acute, followed by healing, or may be chronic.

ACUTE RENAL FAILURE

Acute renal failure involves the complete stoppage of renal function in a person whose kidneys have been functioning adequately. X-rays usually reveal that the kidneys and urinary tract are normal in size. The condition is most often the result of a recent trauma to the kidneys that destroys the renal tubules. A sudden loss of blood supply to the kidneys due to trauma, hypotension, severe burns and burn shock, or complications of surgery is a common cause. Other causes include a recent streptococcal infection or exposure to toxic chemicals such as cleaning solvents and pesticides.

The symptoms appear suddenly. Little or no urine is produced, and the client is severely ill. Dialysis frequently is used until renal function is restored in 1 to 8 weeks.

CHRONIC RENAL FAILURE

Chronic renal failure occurs when the kidneys become permanently damaged. Healthy renal tissue is replaced by scar tissue. The damage may occur over a period of months or over a period of years or even decades. On x-rays, the kidneys appear shrunken, except in the case of polycystic renal disease, in which the cysts give the kidneys a swollen appearance.

Several stages of *renal insufficiency*, or the progressive decline of renal function, have been defined: mild (40% to 80% of normal function); moderate (15% to 40% of normal); and severe (10% to 15% or less of normal). When 90% or more of normal renal function is lost, the condition is called *end-stage renal disease*. Laboratory tests used to determine the level of renal function include creatinine clearance and serum concentrations of creatinine and urea nitrogen. Renal function usually is expressed as the *glomerular filtration rate*, which is the quantity of filtrate formed by the kidneys per minute. As the glomerular filtration rate decreases, the quantity of nitrogen-containing waste products in the blood increases. When the normal glomerular filtration rate of 80 to 120 mL/min decreases to 20 mL/min or less, symptoms appear. These symptoms may include fatigue, anemia, weight loss, hypertension, and bone and joint pain. As the condition worsens, other symptoms such as nausea, vomiting, severe itching, numbness and tingling, convulsions, easy bruising, and congestive heart failure develop. The term *uremia* is used to describe this advanced stage of renal failure. The outcome is fatal unless dialysis or a kidney transplant is available.

The following are causes of end-stage renal disease:

- diseases such as diabetes and systemic lupus erythematosis, which affect the entire body system; renal damage is one part of the disease process
- high blood pressure, which causes damage to the kidneys' blood vessels
- disease of the glomerulus, such as glomerulonephritis
- inherited diseases such as polycystic renal disease
- diseases that obstruct renal function, such as kidney stones
- abuse of pain relievers or street drugs.

The term *nephrotic syndrome* refers to renal disease characterized by large quantities of protein in the urine, severe edema, low serum protein levels, elevated cholesterol and other serum lipid levels, and anemia. The disease is caused by degenerative changes in the capillaries of the kidneys that permit the passage of protein into the filtrate. Albumin is the principal protein excreted. Sodium and water are retained. Fluid retention may be so severe that it masks the tissue wasting due to breakdown of tissue protein. The degree of malnutrition may not be apparent until diuresis has occurred.

Diabetes and hypertension are the primary diseases responsible for chronic renal failure (Table 27-1). The overall occurrence of end-stage renal disease has risen steadily since 1982; the increase due to diabetes and hypertension has exceeded the overall increase.

TABLE 27-1 END-STAGE RENAL DISEASE INCIDENCE IN 1990

PRIMARY DISEASE CAUSING END-STAGE RENAL DISEASE	NO.	% OF TOTAL
Diabetes	15,383	34.1
Hypertension	12,903	28.6
Glomerulonephritis	5595	12.4
Cystic kidney diseases	1365	3.0
Other urologic diseases	2217	4.9
Other identifiable diseases	2694	6.0
Cause unknown	2268	5.0
Cause missing	2728	6.0
Total	45,153	100.0

(National Institutes of Health, National Institute of Diabetes and Digestive and Kidney Disease, U.S. Renal Data System. *USRDS 1993 annual data report*. Produced by USRDS Coordinating Center. NIH Publication No. 93-3176; p. XVI. Bethesda, MD: March, 1993.)

TREATMENT OF CHRONIC RENAL FAILURE

The treatment of chronic renal failure involves three phases: conservative management, hemodialysis or peritoneal dialysis, and transplantation.

CONSERVATIVE MANAGEMENT

Conservative management includes the use of diet and medication. In April 1994, the National Institute of Diabetes and Digestive and Kidney Disease and the National Institutes of Health held a symposium to review current research and "to develop a broadly based set of recommendations for the management of patients with progressive renal disease, based on the recently completed clinical trials, and the world's literature." The completed trials, which were reviewed, included the Modification of Diet in Renal Disease Trial, the Diabetes Control and Complications Trial, and the Captopril Study; other pertinent ongoing studies were also reviewed. Several recommendations came out of the symposium, including restriction of dietary protein depending on the glomerular filtration rate, moderate intake of sodium, tight blood glucose control for people with diabetes, and strict control of hypertension. With careful attention to these treatment modes, dialysis often can be delayed until only 5% to 10% of normal renal function remains.

DIET

A protein-controlled diet is used for clients with decreased renal function, acute renal failure, or end-stage renal disease who are not undergoing dialysis treatment. Total protein intake is controlled so that the accumulation in the blood of protein metabolism waste products (which are excreted by the kidney) is minimized. Other goals include promoting good nutritional status as well as a positive energy balance so that dietary protein can be used for tissue maintenance and repair instead of being used for energy. Dietary phosphorus levels are often low when dietary protein is controlled. Phosphorus binders may be needed when serum phosphorus levels are elevated to reduce the risk of renal osteodystrophy. Adjustments of potassium, sodium, and fluids are made, depending on the client's needs.

PROTEIN

The amount of protein recommended is based on the glomerular filtration rate. When glomerular filtration is at or greater than 55 mL/min, the amount of dietary protein recommended is 0.8 g/kg of ideal body weight. A glomerular filtration rate of 25 to 55 mL/min indicates a dietary protein restriction of 0.6 g/kg. A protein allowance of 0.6 g/kg translates to a daily total of 35 to 40 g of protein for most individuals. In rare instances, the protein may be reduced to 20 g/day; however, in the Modification of Diet in Renal Disease Trial, this very low protein diet did not significantly slow the progression of renal disease.

Of the protein, 65% is given in the form of proteins of high biologic value, that is, those containing the highest percentage of essential amino acids. Milk and eggs contain the highest quality protein. Meat also contains high-quality protein but has a higher percentage of nonessential amino acids. The major protein sources in diets containing only 20 g of protein are milk and eggs. In diets permitting higher levels of protein, small amounts of meat are added.

Foods that contain nonessential amino acids are reduced to as low a level as possible. This reduction forces the body to use the nitrogen in the urea, which has accumulated in abnormal amounts, to produce the nonessential amino acids. In this way, the urea level of the blood decreases and the distressing symptoms of uremia lessen. Foods containing protein of low biologic value include breads, cereals, cereal products, vegetables, and fruit. Even the small amounts of protein in fruits must be counted.

ENERGY

Providing enough calories to meet the clients' energy needs is absolutely essential. If energy needs are not met, tissue protein is broken down to supply energy. The end products produced by the breakdown of protein tissue, like the breakdown of food protein, add to the nitrogen-containing waste products.

Energy is supplied by carbohydrates and fats, which do not involve the kidneys in the elimination of waste products. Maintenance of an adequate caloric intake is essential if the diet is to be effective; 35 kcal/kg is recommended for an individual at ideal body weight. The caloric requirements will vary if body weight is above or below ideal body weight.

Because regular bread, pasta, cereals, and desserts made with flour contain protein, these foods cannot be permitted in quantities sufficient to meet energy needs on diets restricted to less than 60 g/day of protein.

Low-protein carbohydrate foods that are practically protein free and low in sodium and potassium have been developed for use on low-protein diets. These products include wheat starch, low-protein baking mix, low-protein bread, low-protein pastas, and low-protein hot cereal. Recipes are available for making baked goods using wheat starch and low-protein baking mixes. The structure, flavor, and texture of these foods differ from those made with regular flour and are unacceptable to some clients. Moreover, these products are expensive and not easily obtained; clients may need help in learning how to obtain and use them advantageously. Special starch products may not be necessary for clients whose protein prescription is 60 g/day or more.

Other than the specially developed low-protein starch products, only pure fats and pure sugars are free of protein. For this reason, fats and sugars are used to make up the remainder of the client's caloric needs after the protein quota is reached. Even clients with diabetes who have chronic renal failure may need to eat foods higher in fat and sugar than normally recommended in diabetes. In such cases, insulin levels are adjusted to promote blood glucose control.

Commercial supplements that are high calorie, protein free, and low in potassium and sodium may be used to achieve adequate caloric intake. These products include Polycose (Ross Laboratories), Sumacal (Sherwood Medical) and Moducal (Mead Johnson Nutritional Group).

SODIUM

The sodium level of the diet is individualized and depends on fluid retention and blood pressure control. Control of sodium also helps control thirst when fluids are restricted. Sodium usually is restricted to 2000 to 4000 mg/day (see Chapter 25).

POTASSIUM

The potassium level of the diet also depends on client needs. If potassium excretion is impaired, potassium is restricted. This usually is unnecessary in the renal insufficiency stage of chronic renal failure.

PHOSPHORUS

Phosphorus restriction usually accompanies protein restriction. Phosphorus usually is restricted to 800 to 1000 mg/day, but can range from 600 to 1200 mg/day. Milk, meat, fish, poultry, eggs, whole-grain breads and cereals, nuts, dried peas and beans, dried fruits, chocolate, and cocoa are high in phosphorus and are carefully controlled.

FLUIDS

Fluid intake is adjusted to the body's ability to eliminate fluid. The normal intake for adults ranges from 2000 to 2500 mL/day. As long as no water is retained, normal water intake is encouraged. If the kidney becomes unable to concentrate urine and excessive fluid is lost, increased intake of fluids is ordered.

VITAMIN AND MINERAL SUPPLEMENTS

Supplementation of water-soluble vitamins is recommended. *A Clinical Guide to Nutrition in End-stage Renal Disease* advises the following: pyridoxine, or B_6 (10 mg); riboflavin (1.8 to 2.0 mg); niacin (20 mg); thiamine (1.5 to 2.0 mg); pantothenic acid (10 mg); B_{12} (3 to 6 mcg); and biotin (200 to 300 mcg). Folate is supplied at 0.8 mg to 1.0 mg, a dose which is therapeutic and requires a prescription.

A maximum of 60 mg vitamin C is recommended to avoid metabolism of excess ascorbic acid to oxalate, which increases risk of kidney stone formation. Vitamin A supplements are not given because serum retinol-binding protein and vitamin

A are often elevated in uremia. Vitamin E is recommended at 10 International Units.

Most clients on epoetin-alpha therapy eventually require iron supplements; as much as 100 mg elemental iron may be recommended. The increase in hemoglobin synthesis resulting from epoetin-alpha therapy is accompanied by an increased use of iron. To ensure sufficient iron stores to support the accelerated rate of red blood cell production, the iron status of all clients is evaluated before beginning this form of therapy and also periodically during therapy.

Zinc may be beneficial when dysgeusia (loss of taste) occurs. The recommended level is 15 mg. Calcium and vitamin D supplements may need to be provided, and are discussed in the section Phosphorus, Calcium, and Vitamin D.

MEDICATION

Clients with chronic renal disease take substantial quantities of both prescription and nonprescription drugs. Those drugs containing sodium or potassium or affecting phosphate absorption are particularly important in nutrition care. Many clients develop a mild acidosis because of a decreased ability to excrete hydrogen ions. Some require medications to correct this condition.

Results of the Diabetes Control and Complications Trial provided exciting evidence that tight blood glucose control can reduce the incidence of and can slow the progression of diabetic complications, including nephropathy for people with insulin-dependent diabetes (type I). The Captopril Study brought more good news to people with diabetes by demonstrating that captopril (an angiotensin-converting enzyme inhibitor) can protect against deterioration of renal function as well as provide excellent blood pressure control. Compliance with insulin regimen and blood pressure medication is essential in the conservative management of chronic renal failure.

PHOSPHATE BINDERS

In cases in which diet is insufficiently effective in controlling serum phosphorus levels, medication is used to bind phosphorus in the intestinal tract and prevent its absorption. Hyperphosphatemia usually starts when glomerular filtration rate falls below 25 mL/min. Calcium carbonate and calcium acetate are the most commonly used binders. In most cases they have replaced aluminum-based medications. To be effective, they must be taken with meals. Many clients find such medication difficult to take because it has an unpleasant taste, may be hard to swallow, requires excess fluid, and may cause constipation. The physician may prescribe stool softeners to alleviate constipation.

TREATMENT OF ANEMIA IN CHRONIC RENAL FAILURE

As renal function declines, the occurrence of chronic, often debilitating, anemia increases. Because of an insufficient number of red blood cells, the amount of oxygen reaching the brain, heart, and other organs and tissues is reduced, leading to symptoms such as fatigue, angina, and shortness of breath. The cause of this anemia (called *anemia of chronic renal failure*) is the reduced production of erythropoietin by the failing kidney.

In June 1989, the Food and Drug Administration approved the marketing of a recombinant deoxyribonucleic acid (DNA)–produced erythropoietin called *epoetin-alpha* (Epogen, manufactured by Amgen). This medication has the same biologic effects as the erythropoietin the body produces. Epoetin-alpha can prevent or reverse anemia of chronic renal failure by increasing red blood cell production. The most serious side effect is a rise in blood pressure during the period when the hematocrit is rising. The blood pressure of clients on epoetin-alpha must be monitored carefully.

Treatment with epoetin-alpha has greatly improved the quality of life of people with renal disease. Energy and activity levels improve and clients experience a sense of well-being.

TREATMENT OF END-STAGE RENAL DISEASE

DIALYSIS

The two basic types of dialysis are hemodialysis and peritoneal dialysis. In *hemodialysis,* the client's blood is circulated outside of the body through an artificial kidney or *dialyzer* (Fig. 27-2). The dialyzer has two compartments that are separated by a semipermeable membrane: one compartment is for blood; the other, for the dialysate solution. Through the process of diffusion, unwanted substances such as urea are removed from the blood and needed substances such as bicarbonate are restored. Ultrafiltration also occurs to remove excess water. A permanent opening into the blood vessel is surgically created to provide blood flow into the dialyzer. Hemodialysis occurs two or three times a week; each treatment lasts 2 to 4 hours.

Peritoneal dialysis involves instilling dialysate into the peritoneal (abdominal) cavity, allowing the dialysate to dwell for a period, and then draining the fluid by gravity. The peritoneal membrane acts as the semipermeable membrane, allowing for the removal of wastes and excess electrolytes and fluid. The toxins are removed by their movement from the many peritoneal capillaries into the dialysate. The dialysate enters the abdominal cavity through a catheter inserted into the client's abdomen. Each time the dialysate is drained, toxins, electrolytes, and fluid are removed. Infection is a danger with this method.

Peritoneal dialysis is a slower, gentler, and more continuous dialysis process than hemodialysis. It permits the client to be more independent and generally to maintain residual renal function longer. It also provides an alternative for people who cannot tolerate hemodialysis.

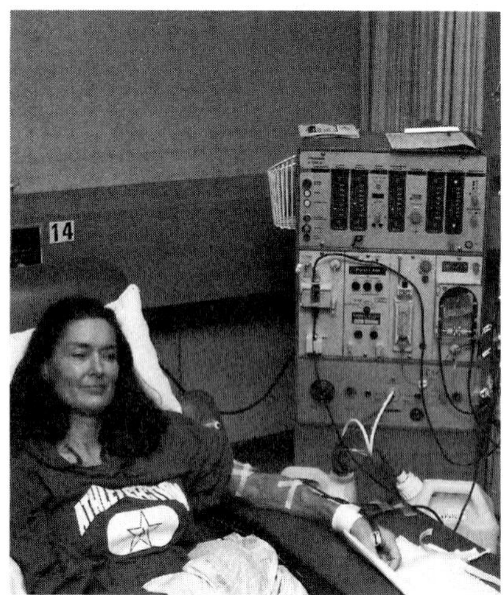

FIGURE 27-2

Dialysis has become a lifesaving procedure for many people in renal failure.

Several choices for treatment by peritoneal dialysis can be performed at a health care center or at home. *Intermittent peritoneal dialysis* involves exchange of the dialysate several times a week. The sessions last 10 to 12 hours.

Continuous ambulatory peritoneal dialysis has gradually replaced intermittent peritoneal dialysis as the preferred home treatment. In this type of peritoneal dialysis, the peritoneal dialysis solution is continuously present in the peritoneal cavity, interrupted only for drainage and instillation of fresh dialysate. The client generally has four exchanges daily. The dialysate is exchanged every 4 to 5 hours during the day; it is allowed to dwell in the peritoneal cavity for about 8 hours at night. The exchanges take about 30 to 35 minutes.

Continuous cycling peritoneal dialysis is the reverse of continuous ambulatory peritoneal dialysis. It allows for more freedom during the day. A cycler machine produces five or six exchanges per night lasting $2\frac{1}{2}$ hours each. About 2 liters of dialysate remain in the peritoneal cavity for 12 to 15 hours during the day until the nightly routine begins.

Although there are psychological and some medical advantages favoring peritoneal dialysis over hemodialysis, long-term use of peritoneal dialysis has been associated with progressive wasting and malnutrition. Poor appetite due to inadequate removal of waste products, continuous glucose load from dialysate (contains dextrose), and a feeling of fullness may contribute to wasting. Losses of protein and other nutrients through the dialysate occur and can quickly deplete muscle and organ protein stores, especially during episodes of peritonitis (Display 27-1). Aggressive nutrition intervention and counseling can help alleviate some of these problems.

DIET IN HEMODIALYSIS

Successful hemodialysis depends on more than treatments several times a week. The client will need to work with specific nutrition requirements to maintain or regain good health.

DISPLAY 27-1 MALNUTRITION IN CLIENTS RECEIVING DIALYSIS

FACTORS LEADING TO PROTEIN-CALORIE MALNUTRITION

- Anorexia, resulting in inadequate intake of nutrients
- Decreased palatability of food resulting from dietary restrictions, that is, for sodium, potassium, and phosphorus
- Increased catabolism resulting from metabolic or hormonal factors that promote net degradation of protein
- Decreased anabolism resulting from decreased biologic activity of anabolic hormones such as insulin and insulin-like growth factors as well as increased circulating levels of catabolic hormones such as glucagon and parathyroid
- Underlying illnesses or intercurrent hospitalizations
- Abnormalities in the metabolism of individual amino acids
- Intradialytic hypotensive episodes, postdialysis fatigue, and simply the time on dialysis away from nutrient intake
- Loss of 5 g to 8 g of free amino acids and 3 g to 4 g of bound amino acids into the dialysate.

(Burrowes JD, Levin NW. Morbidity and mortality in dialysis patients. Dietetic Currents 1992;19:3:10.)

PROTEIN

Clients on hemodialysis require more protein—1.1 to 1.4 g/kg of ideal body weight daily—to replace amino acids lost in dialysis and maintain nitrogen balance. At least 50% of the protein should be of high biologic value. Excessive accumulation of urea waste products between dialysis treatments also must be avoided; however, elevated blood urea nitrogen levels often indicate the need for more dialysis rather than overconsumption of protein.

ENERGY

Energy requirements vary among people who receive hemodialysis. A daily caloric intake of 30 to 35 kcal/kg of body weight is needed for people who are at a desirable weight. The recommended daily caloric intake for overweight people is 20 to 30 kcal/kg of desirable body weight and for underweight people, 35 to 50 kcal/kg. A liberal intake of carbohydrate and fat frequently is necessary to provide sufficient calories.

It is often difficult for clients receiving hemodialysis to get adequate calories and protein. The dialysis treatment itself is often scheduled at a time when meals are normally eaten. After treatment, the client may be tired, weak, nauseated, and uninterested in catching up on the lost meal. Over time, the inadequate intake of calories and protein will lead to negative nitrogen balance and poor nutritional status.

POTASSIUM

Serum potassium levels must be carefully monitored because high or low levels can result in abnormal heart rhythm or cardiac arrest. The dialysis treatment removes potassium, creating the potential for too low a level.

Potassium restriction ranges from 1500 to 3000 mg/day (the normal range is 2000 to 6000 mg/day). Potassium is distributed widely in foods (Display 11-3). Most potassium-rich foods are limited; some are omitted from the diet. Clients who use a salt substitute may benefit from counseling to find the lowest potassium salt substitutes available.

Potassium salts are highly soluble in water, so potassium can be reduced by slicing or dicing the food into small pieces, soaking it in water for a least 2 hours, and then discarding the liquid. The food is then cooked in a large quantity of fresh water, which is again discarded. This process is called *leaching*. Vegetables lend themselves well to this procedure. Canning also reduces potassium content. Canned foods should be well drained and the liquid discarded. When evaluating hyperkalemia (high blood potassium level), it is also important to consider nondietary causes (Display 27-2).

SODIUM

Sodium is limited to 2000 to 3000 mg/day for hemodialysis. Excessive intake leads to thirst, increased blood pressure, and fluid retention.

DISPLAY 27-2 NONDIETARY CAUSES OF HYPERKALEMIA

CAUSE	PROCESS
Chronic constipation	Decreased excretion of potassium by way of gastrointestinal tract
Laboratory error (false positive result)	Hemolyzed blood sample
Acidosis	As arterial pH increases, serum potassium levels increase
Lack of insulin; elevated blood glucose	Potassium shifts out of cells with hyperosmolarity
Catabolic events, such as muscle wasting, infection, malnutrition	Tissue breakdown releases potassium
Drug interactions	Penicillin, beta-blocking agents, angiotensin-converting enzyme inhibitors, steroids

FLUIDS

Fluid is restricted to 700 to 1000 mL/day plus the volume of urine output. Fluid is restricted so that weight gain due to fluid retention is no greater than $\frac{1}{2}$ to 1 kg (1 lb to 2 lb) in 24 hours. Fluids include all substances that are liquid at room temperature: water, juice, milk, tea, coffee, soup, soft drinks, ice, water ice, sherbet, ice cream, and gelatin desserts.

In the health care facility, successful control of fluids requires good communication between dietary and nursing services. Attention must be given not only to the amount of fluid a client with renal disease receives, but to the fluid itself. For example, orange juice contains significant amounts of potassium and canned tomato juice is high in sodium; even small quantities of these fluids, in addition to those normally included in the diet, would cause problems.

Nursing care includes measures to relieve the sensation of thirst, such as frequent cleansing and lubrication of the mouth. Extraordinary fluid losses, as through vomiting or diarrhea, should be accurately measured so that fluid can be increased to make up for them. Diversionary activities can help take clients' minds off their thirst.

PHOSPHORUS, CALCIUM, AND VITAMIN D

Some clients new to dialysis who have been followed by a medical team will know about phosphorus, calcium, and phosphate binders. Other will have little or no knowledge.

In end-stage renal disease, the calcium level falls and the phosphorus level rises excessively. A major cause of this imbalance is the failure of the diseased kidneys to produce the active form of vitamin D, which is needed for the absorption of calcium from the intestinal tract. The decreased ability of the kidneys to excrete phosphorus is another part of the problem. The body attempts to maintain a specific ratio of calcium to phosphorus in the blood serum. Any increase in one causes a decrease in the other. When serum phosphorus levels are elevated in kidney disease, serum calcium falls. The parathyroid gland responds to this change in levels by secreting a hormone that stimulates the release of calcium from bone tissue. Because bone is calcium phosphate, the breakdown of bone to release calcium also releases phosphorus, and a vicious cycle develops. Left untreated, *osteodystrophy,* also called *uremic bone disease,* results.

Dietary phosphorus is generally restricted to 12 to 17 mg/kg. This restriction may be difficult to achieve when the client requires high levels of protein to prevent wasting. Aggressive use of phosphate binders then becomes imperative.

Dietary calcium is often inadequate to maintain calcium balance; therefore, calcium supplementation of 1400 to 1600 mg/day is needed. Phosphate binders composed of calcium carbonate and calcium acetate are generally used to achieve this balance.

The active form of vitamin D (calcitriol) can be given as an oral supplement (Rocaltrol) or as an intravenous medication (Calcijex) during the hemodialysis treatment. Use of vitamin D in this manner suppresses the activity of the parathyroid gland and improves intestinal absorption of calcium.

VITAMINS

Vitamin requirements are similar to those discussed in the section Conservative Management under the heading Diet.

FIBER

Constipation due to medications, fluid restrictions, and lack of activity is a chronic problem for people with renal disease. It is recommended that these clients take 20 to 25 g of dietary fiber; this amount, however, is often difficult to achieve within the framework of the renal diet. A fiber supplement may be required.

DIET IN PERITONEAL DIALYSIS

The nutrition requirements for peritoneal dialysis are different than hemodialysis or conservative management. The dialysate in peritoneal dialysis contains dextrose in concentrations of 1.5%, 2.25%, and 4.25%. Exchanges are available in 1- to 3-liter bags. The caloric level of the diet must allow for calories absorbed from the dialysate; 60% to 80% of the dextrose can be absorbed. Energy requirements are similar to hemodialysis. People with diabetes may require changes in medications to maintain blood glucose control.

Dietary protein must not only meet protein needs and replace losses that occur during peritoneal dialysis but also avoid the excessive accumulation of waste products. The usual protein requirement is 1.2 to 1.3 g/kg of ideal body weight. If the client is malnourished or is losing body tissue, up to 1.5 g/kg may be required. At least half of the protein should be of high biologic value.

Protein losses through the dialysate increase with peritonitis. Fever and infection associated with peritonitis also increases the need for protein and calories. Frequent peritonitis greatly increases the risk for protein-calorie malnutrition. Supplementation with high-calorie, high-protein products may be beneficial. Commercially available products include Nepro (Ross Laboratories), Ensure Plus (Ross Laboratories), Resource Plus (Sandoz Nutrition Corp.), and Nutren 1.5 (Clintec Nutrition Co.).

In intermittent peritoneal dialysis, sodium is limited to about 2000 mg/day. Fluid is limited to prevent weight gains of more than 2 lb/day between dialysis treatments, assuming dialysis occurs three times a week. In continuous ambulatory peritoneal dialysis, sodium and fluid allowances are determined by fluid balance and blood pressure.

The potassium content of the diet depends on need. Factors that influence the potassium requirement include the extent to which potassium can be cleared from the blood, dialysate composition, the level of remaining renal function, the frequency of dialysis treatments or the number of dialysate exchanges daily, and the individual's serum potassium level. Some clients on continuous ambulatory peritoneal dialysis do not need potassium restriction, and some may need potassium supplements. Requirements for calcium, phosphorus, vitamin and mineral supplements, and fiber are similar to those for hemodialysis.

DIET FOLLOWING KIDNEY TRANSPLANTATION

Dietary modifications usually are required after kidney transplantation. The diet is less restrictive than that used during dialysis, however. The duration of these modifications varies.

Medication used to prevent the body from rejecting the new kidney may cause complications, including decreased resistance to infection, hypertension, elevated blood sugar, elevated blood lipids, obesity, and gastric ulcer. These complications are treatable by diet. Steroids, cyclosporine, and azathioprine are the medications most commonly prescribed. The amount prescribed is decreased gradually until a maintenance level is reached.

Steroids promote breakdown of muscle tissue, causing more high-quality protein to be needed in the diet immediately after transplant. The need for protein generally decreases when lower doses of steroids are achieved. Steroids also create glucose intolerance. Carbohydrates, especially concentrated sweets, may need to be limited. Increased sodium retention is a common side effect of steroid therapy. This leads to water retention and may cause a rise in blood pressure. Sodium restriction must be individualized.

The use of steroids may increase appetite. Many people have an improved appetite after a kidney transplantation. The tendency to gain excessive weight must be controlled, because obesity increases the risk of heart disease, diabetes, and high blood pressure. Foods high in fat and sugar should be limited.

Cyclosporine may cause a rise in blood pressure, requiring sodium restriction. It also may produce a rise in blood urea nitrogen, which may require protein and potassium control.

Increased calcium may be needed after transplantation to replace bone tissue lost during chronic renal failure. Sometimes phosphate is lost after transplantation and replacement is needed. The use of lowfat or skim dairy products that supply both calcium and phosphorus is encouraged. Calcium and/or phosphorus supplements may be prescribed.

People with diabetes may require a diet higher in protein and lower in carbohydrate after a kidney transplantation. The diet after transplantation changes as medication, blood values, weight, and blood pressure change.

TOOLS FOR DIETARY INSTRUCTION

Various methods can be used to control nutrients in renal disease. Some methods use counting systems with points or grams of protein, sodium, and potassium as a way to monitor and control intake. Recently, the National Renal Diet was completed by members of the Renal Dietitians Practice Group of the American Dietetic Association and the National Kidney Foundation Council on Renal Nutrition. The diet uses exchange lists and diet plans to guide clients in their food choices. This information, which provides structure and standardization, can be obtained from the American Dietetic Association, 216 West Jackson Boulevard, Suite 800, Chicago, IL 60606–6995.

When deciding what method of meal planning to present to a client, take time to assess the client and find out how he or she will learn best. Once that is established, it will be easier to find the right teaching tools.

DIET IN KIDNEY STONE DISORDERS

Kidney stones develop when calcium salts, uric acid, and other substances crystallize in the urinary tract and form masses. They usually occur in multiples, rather than singly. Kidney stones, which range in size from a pinhead to a golf ball, obstruct the urinary system and can lead to infection.

Most stones develop in the kidney. Some migrate to the ureter or bladder, where they continue to grow. Kidney stones occur most often in the industrialized nations of Western Europe and North America.

The five major types of kidney stones are calcium oxalate, calcium phosphate, uric acid, cystine, and struvite (infected), as well as stones of mixed types. Uric acid, cystine, and struvite stones can sometimes be dissolved by changing the acidity or alkalinity of the urine. Of all kidney stones, 75% to 80% contain calcium, which cannot be dissolved.

The symptoms may include blood in the urine, a persistent urinary infection, severe pain starting in the kidney or lower abdomen that later may move to the groin, burning, and the urge to pass urine often.

A number of factors increase the risk of kidney stones in susceptible people. Among these factors are male sex, middle age, immobilization, excessive sweating, a hot climate, reduced fluid intake, excess dietary sodium, genetic disorders that increase urine calcium and oxalate, and urinary tract infections.

In a recent study, men who had the highest calcium intake were found to be one third less likely to develop kidney stones. The mechanism underlying this result is thought to be that liberal amounts of calcium will bind with oxalate in the intestinal tract, making it unabsorbable. As a result, the oxalate is excreted in the feces rather than the urine. Excess oxalate and not excess calcium may be responsible for kidney stones. Not all authorities have accepted this theory. More research is needed.

Most of the stones that leave the kidney pass through the ureter in 3 to 6 weeks. Remaining stones may be removed by various techniques. In a new nonsurgical treatment called *extracorporeal shock wave lithotripsy*, the client is placed in a water bath or on a cushion filled with water. The stones are located using x-rays. High-energy shock waves are then used to break down the stones into gravel that can be passed out of the body in the urine.

The objective of medical treatment is to prevent recurrent kidney stone formation. Most clients with kidney stones have abnormal levels of certain substances in their urine, such as calcium, oxalate, citrate, or uric acid. Dietary treatment and a high fluid intake can help bring those levels into normal range. Blood and urine tests can help diagnose the specific cause for the stone formation. Depending on the cause, the client may need to make one or more of the following dietary modifications:

- Limit foods high in oxalate, such as eggplant, sweet potatoes, wheat germ, rhubarb, chocolate, and tea and avoid vitamin C supplements because they promote the excretion of oxalate in the urine and thus promote stone formation.
- Reduce sodium intake to prevent hypercalcinuria (excessive excretion of calcium in the urine).
- Avoid excessive animal protein to prevent high levels of uric acid and low levels of citrate in the urine. Citrate tends to prevent stone formation.
- Restrict calcium intake if the client has increased intestinal absorption of calcium.
- Increase fluid intake to dilute the concentration of substances that tend to form kidney stones.

CLIENT EDUCATION

Health care workers play an important role in helping clients accept nutrition therapy for renal disease. This is no easy task. Clients are asked to make drastic changes in eating habits and to eat all the food served, even when they are nauseated and have no appetite, they may feel depressed, and both they and their families are under great stress. Through a positive outlook and approach, health care workers can help clients understand the benefits of their nutrition therapy and encourage them to see that the results of feeling better and remaining active are worth the difficulties involved.

Planning the diet is the dietitian's responsibility. Clients may need help relieving the monotony of the diet, making the food palatable, and planning meals for special occasions. The dietitian's services should be available at all times.

The problems of following controlled diets are real. Foods must be weighed and measured, choices are limited, portion sizes of favorite foods such as meats may be extremely small, and time and skill are required to prepare special foods. Many clients on dialysis do not follow their diets. After an initial period of hopefulness, they may become depressed, which they may express through loss of appetite or by overeating. Clients sometimes decide to live it up by eating whatever they want with the full knowledge of the resultant serious complications. Health care workers must accept clients without judging them and simultaneously must try to find ways to motivate them.

Self-help groups for clients with renal disease help these people share their frustrations and exchange ideas on how to cope with various aspects of their disease, including diet. The National Kidney Foundation (2 Park Avenue, New York, NY 10016) provides educational services for both lay and professional groups. The American Association of Kidney Patients (Suite LL1, One Davis Boulevard, Tampa, FL 33606) also is a valuable resource for clients. This association publishes a newsletter called *Renalife*.

KEYS TO PRACTICAL APPLICATION

Encourage and persuade clients to eat all the food on their diets so that they consume adequate calories. Help them understand that adequate caloric consumption prevents the breakdown of body tissue, thus lightening the load on the kidney and preventing malnutrition.

Listen to the client for reports of social changes that may alter nutrition status.

Correct any misconceptions about diets that require protein restriction. Most of the protein permitted should be of high biologic value. Some people erroneously believe that low protein means a reduction in meat, fish, and poultry in favor of cereals, vegetables, and fruit. The opposite is true.

Carefully measure fluid output as well as intake. If no allowance is made for fluid lost in vomiting and diarrhea, a client may suffer unnecessarily from thirst.

Share your observations of the client's eating habits with the dietitian. Let the dietitian know what foods are better accepted than others.

Show acceptance and understanding for clients who do not follow their diet. Keep trying to find ways to motivate them. Use a positive approach. Do not criticize or judge.

Report changes to other health care workers and medical team members that pertain to changes in dry weight status or other biochemical changes.

KEY IDEAS

Renal disease may be acute, followed by healing, or chronic, eventually leading to renal failure.

Diabetes and hypertension are the primary diseases responsible for end-stage renal disease.

Most clients with chronic renal disease develop chronic anemia caused by the reduced production of erythropoietin by the failing kidney. The introduction of epoetin-alpha, a medication that has the same biologic effects as erythropoietin, has greatly improved the quality of life of people with chronic renal disease.

Dietary treatment in renal disease aims to replace nutrients lost in abnormal amounts, reduce nutrients retained in abnormal amounts, and maintain as good a nutritional status as possible.

Dietary treatment varies depending on the nature and cause of the disease. Dietary changes depend on the level of renal function, as follows:

- In conservative, management, protein is decreased when urea accumulates in the blood.
- Sodium is restricted when hypertension and edema are present.
- Potassium is increased when excessive amounts are excreted, and restricted when it accumulates in the blood, as in severe renal failure.
- Phosphorus is restricted when blood levels of phosphorus increase and when calcium levels decrease. The imbalance between these two minerals leads to uremic bone disease. In addition to dietary restriction of phosphorus, phosphate-binding medication and supplements of calcium and vitamin D are given.
- Fluid is adjusted according to the body's ability to eliminate it.
- Iron supplements and multivitamins are given. An increased need for iron accompanies epoetin-alpha therapy because of increased hemoglobin synthesis; iron supplements usually are needed.

Maintaining an adequate caloric intake is absolutely essential to prevent the breakdown of tissue protein, which adds to the accumulation of nitrogen-containing waste products and causes wasting of body tissue.

The Modification of Diet in Renal Disease Trial was designed to determine whether dietary protein and phosphorus restriction along with strict control of blood pressure affects the progression of chronic renal disease.

Dietary management in advanced renal failure requires the control of protein, sodium, potassium, phosphorus, and fluid. The diet for clients on dialysis usually is less restrictive than for those not on dialysis.

On protein-restricted diets, refined sugars and fats are used to make up the caloric deficit after the protein quota is reached. Clients with diabetes may have diets higher in sugar and fat than normally recommended in diabetes. When acceptable to the client, the client may use low-protein wheat starch products.

In renal failure, most of the protein in the diet is of high biologic value. Nonessential amino acids are reduced to a minimum, forcing the body to use the nitrogen in the urea to produce nonessential amino acids.

In renal failure without dialysis, protein restriction ranges from 0.6 to 0.8 g/day/kg of ideal body weight. Sixty-five percent of this amount is of high biologic value.

Protein intake during dialysis is more liberal: 1.1 to 1.4 g/kg of ideal body weight during hemodialysis and 1.2 to 1.3 g/kg or more during peritoneal dialysis. At least 50% is of high biologic value.

Potassium restriction involves limiting foods high in potassium. Soaking and cooking vegetables in large quantities of water and then discarding the cooking liquid reduces the potassium content of the food.

Milk intake is limited because of its high phosphorus content. Protein foods are high in phosphorus.

Fluid orders require the careful attention and cooperation of both the nursing and dietary departments.

Medication used to prevent the body from rejecting the new kidney after transplantation may cause complications that require dietary modification. These modifications may include sodium restriction, increased protein, and reduced carbohydrate.

To prevent recurrent kidney stone formation, dietary modifications may be useful. Depending on the cause of the stone formation, dietary modifications may include reduced oxalate, protein, calcium, and sodium intakes. Maintaining a high fluid intake is extremely important.

Compliance with the complex nutrition therapy required in renal disease is difficult; encouragement, support, and understanding are needed.

KEYS TO LEARNING

STUDY–DISCUSSION QUESTIONS

1. When is protein increased in renal disease? When is it restricted? When protein is restricted to low levels (20 to 60 g/day), it should be provided mostly in the form of high-quality protein, and foods containing nonessential amino acids should be reduced to a minimum. Why? What foods are used to provide needed calories?
2. Why is it essential that clients with renal disease consume an adequate number of calories? Discuss in class the problems of nausea and lack of appetite, which frequently accompany renal disease. Under these circumstances, what can health professionals do to promote the intake of adequate quantities of food?
3. What foods can be used to increase calories in the diet without significantly increasing protein, sodium, or potassium? Have a tasting party of low-protein starch products, a low-protein dairy drink, and high-carbohydrate, low-

electrolyte supplements. Include products you have made with the low-protein baking mix. Ask the dietitian from the renal unit in your hospital to help you obtain samples of these products.

4. Ask the physician, dietitian, or nurse from the renal unit in your hospital to discuss with the class the benefits and also the problems that have resulted from the use of the new drug epoetin-alpha.
5. Both excessive loss and excessive retention of potassium can occur in renal disease. Explain the serious effects of each condition. What foods are involved in potassium restriction? Describe the food preparation method by which the potassium content of vegetables can be reduced.
6. Fluids are restricted in renal failure. Why? How is the permitted amount determined? Not only the amount of fluid but also the kind of fluid offered the client is important. Explain.
7. Ask the dietitian from the renal unit in your hospital to discuss ways of promoting dietary compliance among clients on dialysis.
8. Ask the social worker assigned to the renal unit to discuss with the class the social problems associated with chronic renal disease, dialysis, and kidney transplantation.

BIBLIOGRAPHY

BOOKS

Council on Renal Nutrition of the National Kidney Foundation. McCann L. Ed. Pocket guide to nutritional assessment of the adult renal patient. New York: National Kidney Foundation, 1993.

Levine DZ. Care of the renal patient. 2nd ed. Philadelphia: WB Saunders, 1992.

National Institutes of Health, National Institute of Diabetes and Digestive and Kidney Diseases, US Renal Data System. USRDS 1993 annual data report. Produced by USRDS Coordinating Center, NIH Publication No. 93–3176. Bethesda, MD: March, 1993.

Mahan LK, Arlin MT. Krause's food, nutrition and diet therapy. 8th ed. Philadelphia: WB Saunders, 1992.

Stover J. Ed. A clinical guide to nutrition in end-stage renal disease. 2nd ed. Chicago: The American Dietetic Association, 1994.

PERIODICALS

Beto JA. Highlights of the consensus conference on prevention of progression in chronic renal disease: implications for disease practice. J Renal Nutr 1994;4:3:122.

Beto JA, Bansal VK. Hyperkalemia: evaluating dietary and non-dietary etiology. J Renal Nutr 1992;2:1:28.

Bradley RP. The National Renal Diet. Contemp Dialysis & Nephrology. 1993;14:7:26.

Juneja G. Idiopathic calcium oxalate lithiasis in a recurrent stone-forming patient. J Renal Nutr 1992;2:4:165.

Klair S, Levey AS, Beck GJ, Caggiula AW, Hunsicker L, Kusek JW, Striker G. The effects of dietary protein restriction and blood pressure control on the progression of chronic renal disease. N Engl J Med 1994;330:877.

CHAPTER

28

Nutrition Therapy in Gastrointestinal Disease

KEY TERMS

diarrhea frequent passing of watery stool

diverticula abnormal sacs or pouches that form in the walls of the colon

endoscope small flexible tubelike instrument with a light at the end of it—allows doctor to see esophagus, stomach, duodenum, and colon and to perform biopsies, take photographs, and perform procedures that would otherwise require surgery

endoscopic describes a procedure in which an endoscope is used.

enteropathy any intestinal disease

gluten vegetable protein found in wheat and other grains

malabsorption failure to absorb nutrients from the intestinal tract

medium-chain triglyceride manufactured oil that is digested and absorbed differently from the usual dietary fats and is helpful in treating malabsorption disorders

peritonitis inflammation of the lining of the abdominal cavity usually due to perforation

prokinetic agent drug that promotes the motor function of a region or regions of the gastrointestinal tract

residue material remaining in the intestinal tract after digestion has occurred; it includes not only undigested or unabsorbed food but also dead cells from the gastrointestinal tract, intestinal bacteria, and products produced by bacteria

steatorrhea excess fat in the stool

OBJECTIVES

After completing this chapter, the student will be able to:

1. Discuss current concepts regarding the cause of most peptic ulcers.
2. Define and distinguish between *residue* and *fiber*.
3. Give the indications for use and characteristics of a low-fiber, residue-restricted diet and a high-fiber diet.
4. Discuss the causes, symptoms, and components of medical nutrition therapy for each of the following disorders of the gastrointestinal tract:
   - gastroesophageal reflux disease
   - peptic ulcer
   - gastroparesis
   - lactose intolerance
   - gluten-sensitive enteropathy, or celiac sprue
   - inflammatory bowel disease
   - diverticulosis
   - irritable bowel syndrome
   - hepatitis and cirrhosis
   - gallbladder disease
   - pancreatitis.

The digestive system involves a complex system of organs that are responsible for converting the food we eat into the nutrients required by the body for life. More people in the United States are hospitalized for diseases of the digestive tract than for any other group of disorders. Only in recent years have researchers begun to uncover the causes of the most illusive aspects of digestive diseases.

Many of the ideas once associated with some gastrointestinal diseases have been found to be false. Diseases once thought to be caused by emotional factors have been found to be the result of bacteria, or of viruses interacting with the body's immune system, or disturbances in the motility patterns of the digestive organs.

This chapter covers medical nutrition therapy in the more common diseases of the gastrointestinal tract and the accessory organs (liver, pancreas, and gallbladder). Although the accessory organs are not part of the gastrointestinal tract, they are part of the digestive system and play vital roles in the digestion and absorption of food. Gastrointestinal disorders caused by cystic fibrosis and galactosemia, which occur primarily in infancy and childhood, are discussed in Chapters 17 and 18. Diet therapy related to surgery of the gastrointestinal tract is covered in Chapter 29. Discussions of intestinal gaseousness and constipation are found in Chapters 6 and 21.

DISEASES OF THE UPPER GASTROINTESTINAL TRACT

GASTROESOPHAGEAL REFLUX DISEASE

Gastroesophageal reflux disease is a common disorder in which there is a backflow of gastric contents into the esophagus. This backflow from the stomach consists of partially digested food, enzymes, bile, and acids. The most common symptom of gastroesophageal reflux disease is *heartburn*—a burning sensation that begins behind the breastbone and radiates upward to the neck. Often there is a sensation of food coming back into the mouth accompanied by a bitter or acid taste; this sensation usually occurs after eating or when lying down. Respiratory symptoms such as nocturnal coughing, wheezing, and hoarseness can be caused by esophageal reflux. It may also produce symptoms similar to angina. The presence of heart disease must be ruled out as a cause of the pain before a diagnosis of gastroesophageal reflux can be made.

Gastroesophageal reflux occurs when the muscle between the esophagus and stomach, called the lower esophageal sphincter, relaxes abnormally or is weak and fails to keep the esophagus closed to prevent the backup of stomach contents (Fig. 28-1). The abnormally low muscle tone of the lower esophageal sphincter can be caused by increased intra-abdominal pressure from coughing or straining; pregnancy; intake of fatty foods, chocolate, peppermint, and onions; cigarette smoking; and the use of certain drugs including isoproterenol, theophylline, calcium channel blockers, anticholinergics and benzodiazepines. In addition to lower esophageal sphincter dysfunction, the occurrence and severity of symptoms are also affected by the type and amount of fluid brought up from the

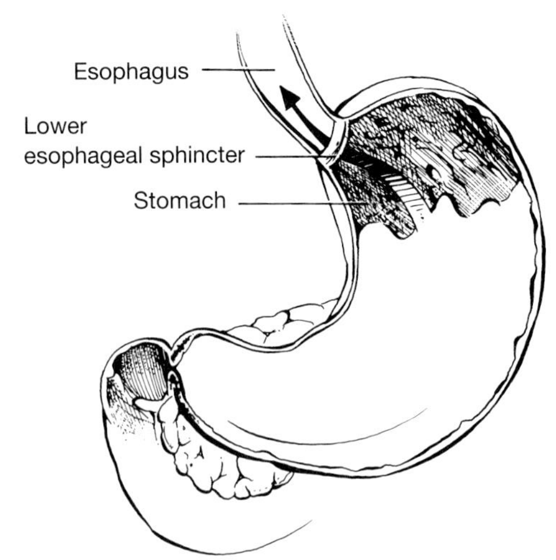

FIGURE 28-1

The cause of heartburn. Relaxation of the lower esophageal sphincter muscle can permit gastric juice to escape from the stomach into the esophagus, where it can harm the esophageal lining. *Taken from: The Johns Hopkins Medical Letter, Health After 50 1993; Nov., 1993, p. 3.*

stomach, the clearing action of the esophagus, the neutralizing affect of the saliva, and other factors.

Gastroesophageal reflux disease can occasionally result in serious complications. *Esophagitis,* an irritation or inflammation of the esophagus can occur due to repeated exposure of the esophageal tissue to stomach acid and enzymes. Foods that promote acid production or those that may directly irritate the lining of the esophagus further are avoided. These foods include citrus fruits and citrus juices, tomato-based products, coffee, and alcohol. The esophagitis can lead to esophageal bleeding, ulcers, and even a narrowing (stricture) of the esophagus, which can make swallowing difficult. Some people develop a condition known as *Barrett's esophagus,* in which the lining of the esophagus becomes severely damaged. It is thought to be a precursor of cancer. Pulmonary disease and hoarseness are also possible complications.

TREATMENT

The main objective of therapy is to reduce the backflow of gastric acid into the esophagus. Because the cause and severity of the disease varies widely from client to client, treatment must be individualized.

Treatment progresses in three phases. Phase 1 consists of antacid therapy to relieve symptoms and lifestyle changes involving diet modification, smoking cessation, elevation of the bed, and avoidance of certain medications (Display 28-1). Clients who do not improve adequately with these measures progress to phase 2 therapy, which involves using histamine$_2$ (H_2) receptor antagonists that reduce gastric acid production. Currently there are four H_2 antagonists drugs available: cimetidine, famotidine, nizatidine, and ranitidine. Another approach at this stage is to increase the strength of the lower esophageal sphincter muscle with motility drugs that cause the stomach contents to empty more rapidly. Phase 3 therapy is necessary for 5% to 10% of clients with gastroesophageal reflux disease who do not respond to treatment phases 1 or 2. Phase 3 therapy involves the use of the acid inhibitor omeprazole, which can produce almost total absence of gastric acid. Another option is *fundoplication,* a surgical procedure that increases pressure in the lower esophagus. Lifestyle changes including dietary changes possibly beneficial for all clients affected by gastroesophageal reflux disease are given in Display 28-1.

HIATAL HERNIA

A *hiatal hernia* is a condition in which the portion of the stomach adjoining the esophagus is pushed through the diaphragm (Fig. 28-2), causing an out-

DISPLAY 28-1 LIFESTYLE CHANGES BENEFICIAL IN GASTROESOPHAGEAL REFLUX DISEASE

- Avoid large meals and bedtime snacks.
- Avoid lying down for at least 3 to 4 hours after meals.
- Limit consumption of foods that lower esophageal sphincter pressure including onions, chocolate, peppermint, and fatty foods.
- Limit consumption of foods that irritate the lining of the esophagus or stimulate gastric acid production including citrus fruits and juice, tomato-based products, coffee, and alcohol.
- Elevate the head of the bed 6 inches.
- Decrease or stop smoking.
- Reduce weight, if overweight.
- Avoid prolonged activities that increase abdominal pressure such as straining, lifting, and repeated bending.
- Wear loose-fitting garments.
- Avoid medications that increase intra-abdominal pressure (e.g., anticholinergics, theophylline, and calcium channel blockers) or irritate the esophageal lining (e.g., tetracycline, quinidine, potassium chloride, nonsteroidal anti-inflammatory drugs, and iron salts). Consult a physician first, however, before making any of these changes.

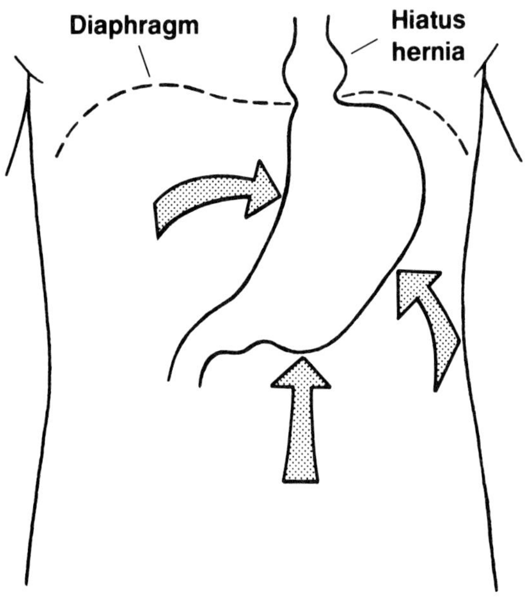

FIGURE 28-2

In hiatal hernia, pressure within the stomach (*arrows*) promotes regurgitation of gastric fluid into the esophagus.

pouching of a portion of the stomach into the chest cavity. Normally, the diaphragm acts as a muscular partition separating the chest cavity from the stomach. The majority of people older than age 60 years have small hiatal hernias, and, in most cases, the hiatal hernia does not cause problems. The most frequent known cause of hiatal hernia is an increased pressure in the abdominal cavity produced by coughing, vomiting, straining at stool, or sudden physical exertion. Pregnancy, obesity, or excess fluid in the abdomen also contributes to this condition.

In some people, hiatal hernia is accompanied by weakness of the lower esophageal sphincter. As a result, the stomach contents regurgitate into the esophagus, causing esophagitis. Treatment, which is the same as that described for gastroesophageal reflux disease, is important in relieving the discomfort and pain associated with this condition (see Display 28-1). As in gastroesophageal reflux disease, treatment of the esophagitis is necessary to prevent ulcers from forming and other serious effects. When healed, these ulcers leave scars that can seriously impair swallowing.

If esophagitis persists, surgery may be performed to restore the stomach to its proper position and strengthen the area around the opening in the diaphragm. Surgery may also be performed if the hiatal hernia is in danger of becoming strangulated, that is, constricted in such a way as to cut off the blood supply.

INDIGESTION

Symptoms of indigestion include heartburn, frequent belching, and a feeling of fullness. Because these can be symptoms of organic disease, a person who experiences them frequently should seek a physician's advice. When no organic disease is found, the condition is said to be functional. Indigestion may be due to emotional factors, poor eating habits, such as a high-fat diet, and hurried and irregular mealtimes (see the section Indigestion and the section Gaseousness in Chapter 6; see also the section Gastroesophageal Reflux Disease and the section Gastroparesis in this chapter).

PEPTIC ULCER DISEASE

Peptic ulcer affects as many as 25 million Americans at some point in their lifetime. About 75% of people with ulcers will have a recurrence of the disorder within 1 to 2 years.

A *peptic ulcer* is an open sore in the upper gastrointestinal tract usually occurring near the *pylorus,* the opening between the stomach and small intestine. An ulcer on the stomach side of the pylorus is called a *gastric ulcer;* one on the duodenal side is called a *duodenal ulcer* (see Figure 28-3). Both are known as peptic ulcers because of the role the enzyme pepsin plays in their development.

The usual symptom is a burning or gnawing pain that occurs when the stomach is empty and from 1 to 3 hours after meals. The pain is relieved by ingestion of food or nonabsorbable antacids. In some cases, hemorrhage, which may develop if the ulcer is not treated, is the first sign. If the ulcer

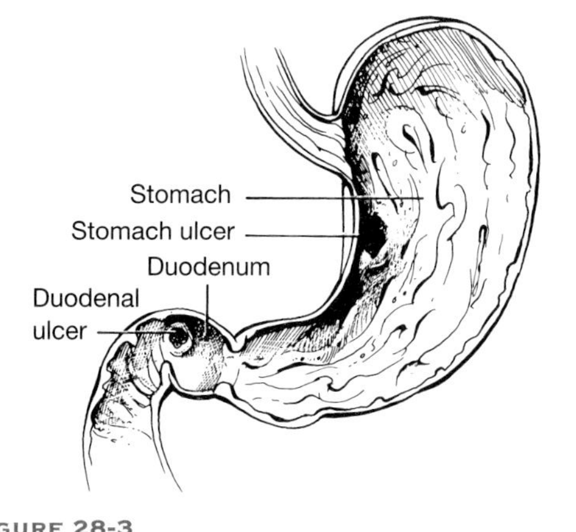

FIGURE 28-3

Places where stomach and duodenal ulcers commonly form.

erodes a small blood vessel, the blood may seep out slowly, eventually causing anemia, weakness, tiredness, and dizziness. If the damaged blood vessel is large, the bleeding is more rapid and the situation is dangerous. Tarry black stools, fainting, vomiting of blood, or sudden collapse may occur. Immediate medical attention, possibly requiring surgery, is necessary.

Other serious complications of peptic ulcers include perforation and obstruction. Sometimes the ulcer will penetrate completely through the wall of the stomach or duodenum, spilling digested food and bacteria from the digestive tract into the sterile abdominal cavity. *Peritonitis,* an inflammation of the abdominal cavity lining, results and immediate hospitalization and surgery are required. Obstruction, caused by swelling and scarring due to ulcers in the end of the stomach or first part of the duodenum, can prevent food from leaving the stomach. Endoscopic balloon dilation or surgery may be necessary to correct the problem.

DEVELOPMENT OF PEPTIC ULCERS

Under normal conditions, a healthy environment is maintained in the stomach despite the secretion of strong digestive juices by numerous glands. This is due to a balance between *aggressive factors* which are destructive to the stomach lining and *defensive factors,* which protect the stomach lining. These digestive juices contain hydrochloric acid, the primary aggressive factor, and pepsinogen (converted to the enzyme pepsin in the presence of acid), which together chemically break down food protein. Mucus, another gastric secretion, protects the stomach lining from being digested by hydrochloric acid and pepsin. Mucus contains *mucin,* a substance that neutralizes acid and holds acid away from stomach lining and reduces pepsin formation. Other defensive factors that strengthen the ability of the mucosal linings to resist acid damage are blood flow to the mucosa, bicarbonate secretion, and prostaglandin synthesis.

When the acid–pepsin reaction overpowers the protective action of the mucus lining, an ulcer develops. Exactly why this occurs is unknown, but a combination of factors apparently is involved. Cigarette smoking, the use of nonsteroidal anti-inflammatory drugs (e.g., aspirin and ibuprofen), and genetic factors appear to play a role in the formation of peptic ulcers by lowering the resistance of the mucosal lining. Recently, the bacterium *Helicobacter* pylori has been identified as a significant factor in weakening the body's mucosal defense mechanisms.

Bacterial Infection (Helicobacter pylori*)*

The bacterium *H. pylori* apparently plays a major role in the development of peptic ulcer disease. This bacterial infection is also linked to *gastritis,* an inflammation of the stomach lining.

H. pylori adheres to the stomach lining and may not be found for years. This bacterium is able to withstand the powerful stomach acidity by secreting the enzyme *urease,* which creates an alkaline environment surrounding the bacteria in the stomach. The bacteria penetrate the protective mucus layer and cause tissue damage and inflammation by stimulating the release of cytotoxins (poisons that attack cells) and enzymes that weaken the stomach lining.

In some people, the inflammation resulting from *H. pylori* may not cause any symptoms. In others, the bacteria may cause an increased release of the hormone gastrin after eating, which, in turn, causes increased gastric secretion. The hyperacidity spills into the duodenum, which causes the development of cells such as those in the stomach lining (duodenal gastric metaplasia). *H. pylori* lodges in these cells, leading to an ulcer. Both the acidity and the bacteria work together to cause duodenal ulcers. Diagnosis of *H. pylori* infection can be made by various methods, among which are several highly accurate blood tests for *H. pylori* antibodies.

Involvement of Lifestyle Factors

Smoking. Cigarette smoking is strongly associated with increased risk of gastric and duodenal ulcer. Smoking also delays the healing of an ulcer and promotes relapse after treatment.

Nonsteroidal Anti-Inflammatory Drugs. Long-term use of nonsteroidal anti-inflammatory drugs also increases the risk of developing a stomach ulcer, possibly by inhibiting the stomach's production of prostaglandins, substances that may protect the gastric mucosa. In most cases, the ulcers disappear once the medication is stopped.

Stress. Contrary to previous opinion, people under emotional stress are not more likely to develop peptic ulcers. However, people under severe physical stress such as severe burns or major surgery are at high risk of developing peptic ulcers.

Genetics. The risk of developing peptic ulcers seems to increase in people whose blood relations have the disease. Whether this is the effect of genetics, similar environment, or bacterial infection is unknown.

Diet. There is no evidence that certain foods cause peptic ulcers. Some foods seem to relieve the pain caused by ulcers, but do not cause or prevent recurrence of ulcers.

The stimulants caffeine and theobromine increase the secretion of gastric acid and may increase the pain of an existing ulcer. These stimulants are found in coffee, tea, cola beverages, and chocolate. Both decaffeinated and regular coffee also contain an unidentified substance other than caffeine that stimulates gastric secretion.

TREATMENT

For clients who have peptic ulcers and test positive for *H. pylori*, 2 weeks of therapy with combinations of bismuth and antimicrobial drugs can successfully cure the *H. pylori* infection and reduce the rate of ulcer recurrence in up to 90% of clients. In addition to these medications, antihistamine receptor antagonists such as cimetidine and ranitidine are usually added to relieve ulcer symptoms.

People who are not infected with *H. pylori* or for whom antibiotic therapy is inappropriate are treated with medications that reduce stomach acid to allow faster healing. H_2-blockers cimetidine, ranitidine, and famotidine increase the pH of the stomach more than food does and maintain a high pH at night. Another drug, sucralfate, acting at the ulcer site, shields the ulcer from acid and pepsin. In an acid environment, sucralfate becomes a highly condensed, viscous, adhesive substance that sticks to the ulcer surface.

Nutrition Therapy

Medical experts in the field of gastrointestinal disease believe that diet has no specific role to play in the treatment of ulcers. Although food also neutralizes acid and reduces pain, these beneficial effects are only temporary because foods both stimulate and neutralize gastric acidity. Proteins, as other foods, first stimulate acid secretion; the protein then buffers the acid as the acid begins to break it down. The products that result from this breakdown of protein again stimulate gastric secretion which is responsible for the pain experienced 1–3 hours after meals by people with peptic ulcers. Avoidance of smoking is recommended, as is the avoidance of foods that are strong stimulants of gastric acid: coffee (both regular and decaffeinated), tea, chocolate, and caffeinated soft drinks. Alcohol usually is omitted or restricted. Other than these restrictions, clients who are taking medication should be able to tolerate all foods without discomfort.

Sometimes the dietary approach ordered by the physician depends on the client's needs. Some clients expect dietary restrictions and feel more confident with them. Although there is no evidence that fatty, acidic, or spicy foods will harm people with ulcers, some people find those foods cause discomfort.

In the past, the bland diet and its variations were used in the treatment of peptic ulcers and other gastrointestinal disorders. The bland diet was low in fiber and connective tissue, restricted spices and condiments, and included only foods that were simply prepared. If used today, the diet is made as nonrestrictive as possible and is tailored to the individual's needs; there are few restrictions that apply to all people.

Care must be taken to meet clients' nutritional needs, especially if foods are omitted because of individual intolerances. Adequate amounts of protein and ascorbic acid are especially important because these nutrients promote healing. If citrus fruits are not tolerated, a vitamin C supplement should be prescribed. If blood loss has occurred, supplementation of iron also may be necessary.

GASTROPARESIS

Gastroparesis, delayed gastric emptying, is a motility disorder of the stomach in which the movement of the stomach contents into the duodenum is abnormally slow. Symptoms include early satiety (feeling of fullness), bloating and distention after eating, and nausea often accompanied by vomiting and abdominal pain. Abdominal discomfort is a common complaint; pain is not a significant factor. In gastroparesis, clients may vomit food that was eaten hours previously.

Various diseases, conditions, and medications can cause gastroparesis. The three most common causes are diabetes mellitus, prior peptic ulcer disease surgery, and gastroparesis of unknown origin. Gastroparesis is a complication of longstanding diabetes mellitus and is present in up to 75% of people with insulin-dependent diabetes mellitus (type I) and is probably related to nerve damage in the gastrointestinal tract caused by the diabetes. Gastroparesis often causes difficulty in controlling blood glucose levels because of the irregular manner in which food passes from the stomach to the small intestine, where most nutrient absorption occurs. In addition to symptoms, diseases and medications in the client's medical history that predispose a person to gastroparesis are considered. Radiographic and endoscopic studies are done to rule out the possibility of a mechanical obstruction of the stomach, duodenum, or small intestine. Bezoar (a solid mass of undigested material) formation and the presence of old food particles are signs of a severe gastric emptying disorder. In the absence of such obvious signs, a radioscope gastric emptying scan may be done to make a diagnosis of gastroparesis.

TREATMENT

The goals of treatment are to reduce symptoms and to maintain hydration and nutrition. The underlying medical condition, if any, must be diagnosed and treated appropriately or the offending drug eliminated; an alternative medication may be given. Hydration and electrolyte problems are corrected. Nausea and vomiting may be treated directly with medication.

A *prokinetic agent,* a drug that promotes the motility of the stomach, is given to control symptoms. This medication is usually given 30 minutes before meals and in the evening. Not all clients respond to the prokinetic agents.

Nutrition Therapy

Small frequent meals of easily digested foods are advised. High-fiber solid foods should be avoided and the fat and lactose in the diet should be decreased. Providing foods in liquid form promotes gastric emptying. Commercial liquid formulas or home-prepared blended meals may be helpful for some clients. Sometimes tube feedings that bypass the stomach and go directly to the small intestine may be necessary.

MODIFICATION OF FIBER AND RESIDUE IN DISEASES OF THE DIGESTIVE SYSTEM

The discussion that follows in this chapter covers diseases of the small and large intestines. In some cases, fiber and residue may be restricted to rest the affected organ; in others, fiber is increased to promote motility and prevent or reduce recurrence of the disorder. Sometimes both modifications will be used for the same disease—each modification for a different phase of the disease.

The terms *fiber* and *residue* are not synonymous. *Residue* refers to the total solid material in the feces, including undigested and unabsorbable components of the diet, sloughed cells from the gastrointestinal tract, intestinal bacteria, and products generated by bacteria. Residue usually pertains to the amount of fecal output regardless of whether the food remains in the colon after digestion. For example, prune juice does not produce a residue in the colon but it is considered a high-residue food because it contains a natural laxative that results in an increased stool volume. Milk also increases stool volume, even though it does not contain fiber. For these reasons, prune juice and milk may be omitted from some fiber- and residue-restricted diets. Tender or ground meats free of tough connective tissue, fats such as butter, margarine, and oil, and refined carbohydrates such as white flour, spaghetti, macaroni, noodles, rice, refined breads and cereals, and sugar add little residue to fecal material.

Fiber refers to indigestible carbohydrate and *lignin,* the part of plants that is not digested by the human digestive tract. Fiber is responsible for most of the residue in the colon. Foods that contain fiber are fruits, vegetables, nuts, and whole-grain cereals and breads. All plant foods contain fiber, but the amount varies from those that are high, such as wheat bran, to those that are low, such as potatoes without the skin and bananas. Whole-grain cereals in the form of unprocessed bran, unrefined wheat cereals, and whole-wheat and rye flours are the most important sources of fiber in food.

The fiber content of fruits and vegetables can be reduced in various ways. Young, tender vegetables have less fiber than mature ones. Cooked foods have softer fiber and create less bulk than raw ones. Peels from fruits and vegetables such as apples, pears, and potatoes can be removed. Fruits and vegetables can be strained to remove much of the fiber.

Prescribed diets vary slightly from one health facility to another. Health care workers should become familiar with the residue-restricted diets served in their facility.

FIBER AND RESIDUE RESTRICTION

Some disorders may require a fiber- and residue-restricted diet to prevent blockage of a narrowed gastrointestinal tract or to reduce the frequency and volume of fecal output. This modification is used during acute phases of ulcerative colitis, Crohn's disease, diverticulitis, or when partial blockage of the gastrointestinal tract occurs. This diet is also required during preparation for colon surgery and the immediate postsurgical period.

The minimal-residue diet contains no fruits, vegetables, or whole-grain breads and cereals. Both milk and prune juice are omitted. Strained fruit and vegetable juices may be permitted in limited amounts. This diet is followed in preparation for or following bowel surgery, or when the colon is so inflamed that any colon expansion or bowel movement causes pain. The diet is inadequate in some vitamins and minerals, for which supplements may be ordered.

The more commonly prescribed fiber- and residue-restricted diet includes cooked tender vegetables and cooked or canned fruits without skins or seeds. Ripe bananas usually are permitted, as are tender whole meats. Milk and prunes and prune juice frequently are omitted. This diet is followed as the client progresses after bowel surgery or in the treatment of inflammatory bowel disease (Table 28-1). When symptoms of the inflammatory bowel disease subside, the client is usually encouraged to gradually resume a normal diet.

HIGH-FIBER DIET

A high-fiber diet is used in the treatment of gastrointestinal diseases to decrease pressure within the gastrointestinal tract and to increase fecal bulk with absorption of water to normalize peristalsis and regularity of bowel movements. Fiber also has metabolic effects important in the treatment of cardiovascular disease and colon cancer (see Chapters 25 and 30). The value of a high-fiber diet in diabetes as a means of reducing blood glucose levels has recently been questioned (see Chapter 24). Several

TABLE 28-1 Guidelines for Food Selection for Fiber- and Residue-Restricted Diet

Food Category	Recommended	May Cause Distress
Beverages	Coffee, tea, carbonated beverages, strained fruit drinks; limit milk and foods containing milk to 2 cups/day as needed*	Any containing fruit or vegetable pulp; prune juice*
Breads	Refined breads, rolls, biscuits, muffins, crackers; pancakes or waffles; plain pastries	Any made with whole-grain flour, bran, seeds, nuts, coconut, or raw or dried fruits; cornbread, graham crackers
Cereals	Refined cooked cereals including grits and farina; refined cereals including puffed rice and puffed wheat	Oatmeal; any whole-grain, bran, or granola cereal; any containing seeds, nuts, coconut, or dried fruit
Desserts and sweets	Plain cakes and cookies; pie made with allowed fruits; plain sherbet, fruit ice, frozen pops, yogurt, gelatin, and custard; jelly, plain hard candy, and marshmallows; ice cream within 2 cups/day milk allowance*	Any made with whole-grain flour, bran, seeds, nuts, coconut, or dried fruit
Fats	Margarine, butter, salad oils and dressings, mayonnaise; bacon; plain gravies	Any containing whole-grain flour, bran, seeds, nuts, coconut, or dried fruit
Fruits	Most canned or cooked fruits; applesauce, fruit cocktail; ripe banana	Dried fruit; all berries; most raw fruit
Meats and meat substitutes	Ground or well-cooked, tender beef, lamb, ham, veal, pork, poultry, fish, organ meats; eggs and cheese	Tough fibrous meats with gristle;* any made with whole-grain ingredients, seeds, or nuts; dried beans, peas, lentils, legumes, peanut butter
Potatoes and potato substitutes	Cooked white and sweet potatoes without skin; white rice; refined pasta	All others
Soups	Bouillon, broth, or cream soups made with allowed vegetables, noodles, rice, or flour	All others
Vegetables	Most well-cooked and canned vegetables without seeds, except those excluded; lettuce, if tolerated	Sauerkraut, winter squash, and peas; most raw vegetables and vegetables with seeds
Miscellaneous	Salt, pepper, sugar, spices, herbs, vinegar, ketchup, mustard	Nuts, coconut, seeds, and popcorn

* These foods are not necessarily high in fiber, but may increase colonic residue; assess patient food tolerance and limit as needed.
If indicated, colonic residue may be further reduced by excluding all forms of fruits and vegatables with the exception of strained fruit and vegetable juices and white potatoes without skin, and by excluding all milk products.

(Chicago Dietetic Association and South Suburban Dietetic Association. Manual of clinical dietetics. Chicago: The American Dietetic Association, 1992:406.)

major diseases have been associated with a lack of fiber in the diet, including diverticular disease, colon cancer, constipation, and irritable bowel syndrome.

Although there is no Recommended Dietary Allowance (RDA) for fiber, the general opinion of authorities has been that the present average fiber intake ranging from 12 g/day for women to 18 g/day for men is too low. The American Dietetic Association has advised an intake of 20 to 35 g/day from a variety of food sources and not from fiber supplements.

The compounds that compose fiber are of two general types: water soluble and water insoluble.

The physiologic effects of these two types differ. Water-soluble fiber dissolves in water and forms a gel-like consistency in the digestive tract. It slows the movement of food along the digestive tract. Water-insoluble fiber holds water in the intestinal tract, thus increasing bulk. It tends to speed movement through the gastrointestinal tract. Foods contain both soluble and insoluble fiber; some foods are better sources of soluble fiber, whereas others contain mostly insoluble fiber. Eating a variety of plant foods ensures getting the benefits of both types of fiber. (See Chapter 8 for a more detailed discussion of fiber.)

The high-fiber diet emphasizes fiber-rich foods including fruits, legumes, vegetables, and whole-grain breads and cereals. Display 8-4 provides the average fiber content per serving of foods in these various food groups. Display 8-5 demonstrates how a high-fiber diet can be achieved in a gradual, step-wise fashion.

Fiber should be increased very gradually to reduce possible adverse effects such as bloating, flatulence, cramps, and diarrhea. Increased fiber consumption should always be accompanied by adequate fluids—at least eight 8-oz glasses daily. If adverse effects persist, the physician should be consulted. High-fiber diets are not recommended for people with gastroparesis.

DISEASES OF THE SMALL AND LARGE INTESTINES

Malabsorption is poor digestion and absorption of a nutrient or nutrients in the small intestine. It may be caused by increased peristalsis due to infection, a lack of digestive enzymes, a lack of bile, or defects in the lining of the small intestine. Symptoms such as weight loss in adults, retarded growth in infants and children, abdominal bloating, abdominal cramps, diarrhea, and steatorrhea frequently are present.

Most of the protein, digestible carbohydrate, and fat in food are absorbed in the small intestine. These substances never reach the colon except in situations of malabsorption. Nutrition therapy in diseases of the large intestine necessitates changes related to the residue of food that remains in the colon after digestion and absorption have occurred.

DIARRHEA

Diarrhea is a common symptom of gastrointestinal disease; it is not a disease in itself. It may be described as the passing of stools that are liquid or semiliquid and more frequent than normal. Because of increased peristalsis, nutrients pass too rapidly through the gastrointestinal tract to be absorbed properly. If the diarrhea continues for a prolonged period, serious losses of fluid, electrolytes, and nutrients may result. See section Clinical Applications, Dehydration, in Chapter 13.

In the acute stages of diarrhea caused by infection, a clear liquid diet (see Chapter 3) is given for a brief period, followed by a fiber-restricted diet until the client has recovered. Diarrhea resulting from lactase deficiency requires dietary changes related to the cause. If the diarrhea has been long-standing, the client usually needs a high-protein, high-calorie diet supplemented by vitamins and minerals.

LACTOSE INTOLERANCE

Lactose intolerance is the inability to digest milk sugar. People with this disorder experience bloating, flatulence (gaseousness), cramping, nausea, and sometimes diarrhea. The symptoms begin about 30 minutes to 2 hours after eating or drinking food containing lactose. The condition is caused by a deficiency of the enzyme lactase, which is needed to reduce lactose to glucose and galactose, the forms of sugar the body can absorb. When the lactose is not digested, it continues on through the digestive tract to the large intestine, where the lactose is fermented by bacteria. This fermentation causes the formation of lactic acid, short-chain fatty acids, carbon dioxide, and hydrogen gas. The presence of these fermentation products cause the symptoms of the disorder.

Although a small percentage of infants are born with lactase deficiency, most people with the condition have adequate levels of lactase at birth and acquire the disorder after early childhood or as adults. Between 30 and 50 million American adults are lactose intolerant. It occurs more frequently among certain ethnic and racial populations: 75% of all African Americans and American Indians and 90% of Asian Americans are lactose intolerant. It is least common among people of Northern European descent. Lactose intolerance also may develop in people who have undergone gastrointestinal surgery or have had gastrointestinal diseases such as celiac sprue and colitis. Three tests are commonly used to measure the absorption of lactose: the lactose tolerance test, the hydrogen breath test, and the stool acidity test (used for infants and children).

TREATMENT

Infants and young children with lactase deficiency should not consume any foods containing lactose. For lactose intolerance of infancy, lactose-free formulas are prescribed. These may be made from soybean, meat-based, or protein mixtures. Care must be taken to avoid commercially prepared baby food products that contain milk or nonfat dry milk solids. Complete information about baby foods and their lactose composition can be obtained by writing to baby food manufacturers.

The amount of lactose that can be tolerated differs greatly from one person to another. Each person must learn by trial and error how much he or she can tolerate. Most affected people do produce some lactase and can tolerate small amounts of milk (about $^{1}/_{2}$ cup) with meals and in foods such as butter, margarine, and baked goods, and even ice cream. Some people are able to tolerate yogurt with active cultures. Although yogurt is fairly high in lactose, the bacterial cultures it contains produce some of the lactase required for proper digestion. Processed and soft cheeses (American cheese, cottage cheese) often have milk solids added and may not be tolerated. Aged cheeses (cheddar, Swiss) have little lactose and usually are well tolerated.

For people with severe lactose intolerance, all sources of lactose are omitted from the diet—milk and foods containing milk, such as ice cream, milk chocolate, caramel, regular margarine, creamed soups and other creamed dishes, and bakery products. Table 28-2 shows the calcium and lactose content in common foods. Hidden sources of lactose include

- bread and other baked goods
- processed breakfast cereals
- instant potatoes, soups, and breakfast drinks
- margarine
- lunch meats (other than kosher)
- salad dressing
- candies and other snacks
- mixes for pancakes, biscuits, cookies, and so forth.

Labels of commercial products must be checked carefully, not only for milk and lactose but also for such ingredients as whey, curds, milk by-products, dry milk solids, and nonfat dry milk powder. Lactose is used as a base in 20% of prescription drugs and 6% of over-the-counter drugs. These products affect only people with a severe lactose intolerance.

Bagels, French bread, and Italian bread usually are milk free, as are bread, frankfurters, and margarine sold in Kosher markets. Many diet margarines also do not contain milk.

For people who need to severely restrict lactose or who want to have more liberal amounts of dairy products, lactose enzymes are available in liquid form to add to milk or in chewable form. Lactose-reduced and lactose-free milks and other products to which the lactase enzymes have been added are readily available.

Calcium Requirements

In lactose intolerance, care must be taken to see that recommended intakes of calcium (see Chapter 11) are being met by consuming small portions of milk or other dairy products frequently over the day (if tolerated) by use of lactose-reduced dairy products, by increasing consumption of nondairy sources of calcium (see Table 28-2), by using calcium supplements, or by combining these alternatives. Provision for adequate vitamin D must also be made

TABLE 28-2 CALCIUM AND LACTOSE CONTENT IN COMMON FOODS

	CALCIUM CONTENT*	LACTOSE CONTENT†
Vegetables		
Broccoli (pieces cooked), 1 cup	94–177 mg	0
Chinese cabbage (bok choy, cooked), 1 cup	158 mg	0
Collard greens (cooked), 1 cup	148–357 mg	0
Kale (cooked), 1 cup	94–179 mg	0
Turnip greens (cooked), 1 cup	194–249 mg	0
Dairy Products		
Ice cream/ice milk, 8 oz	176 mg	6–7 g
Milk (whole, lowfat, skim, buttermilk), 8 oz	291–316 mg	12–13 g
Processed cheese, 1 oz	159–219 mg	2–3 g
Sour cream, 4 oz	134 mg	4–5 g
Yogurt (plain), 8 oz	274–415 mg	12–13 g
Fish/Seafood		
Oysters (raw), 1 cup	226 mg	0
Salmon with bones (canned), 3 oz	167 mg	0
Sardines, 3 oz	371 mg	0
Shrimp (canned), 3 oz	98 mg	0
Other		
Molasses, 2 tbsp	274 mg	0
Tofu (processed with calcium salts), 3 oz	225 mg	0

* Nutritive value of foods. Values vary with methods of processing and preparation.

† Derived from American Dietetic Association. *Lactose intolerance: a resource including recipes* (Food Sensitivity Series). Chicago: American Dietetic Association, 1985.

(US Dept of Health and Human Services, Public Health Service, National Institutes of Health, National Digestive Diseases Information Clearinghouse. Lactose intolerance (Fact Sheet). Washington, DC: US Government Printing Office, 1991. NIH publication 91-2751.)

because fortified milk is a major food source of this vitamin.

GLUTEN-SENSITIVE ENTEROPATHY (CELIAC SPRUE)

Gluten-sensitive enteropathy is a disease of the small intestine in which there is a sensitivity to *gliadin,* a protein fraction of gluten that is found in wheat, rye, barley, and oats. The disorder is also referred to as *nontropical sprue, celiac sprue,* or *celiac disease.* The exact cause of the disease is unknown, but interactions between immunologic, genetic, environmental, and dietary factors have been suggested.

When the affected person eats food containing gliadin, the mucosa of the jejunum becomes flat and thickened, losing the normal fingerlike projections of the villi and the tremendous absorptive area they provide. Absorption of all nutrients is thus greatly reduced.

Symptoms of the disease include distention, flatulence, diarrhea, steatorrhea, and weight loss. The malabsorption of fat results in steatorrhea and the malabsorption of carbohydrates leads to the production of gas and foul-smelling stool due to fermentation of the carbohydrate by bacteria. The malabsorption and resulting diarrhea cause a severe loss of all nutrients, and the resulting malnutrition is responsible for the other symptoms such as extreme weight loss, muscle wasting, and anorexia. Lactose intolerance is also a side effect of the disease.

TREATMENT: GLUTEN-RESTRICTED, GLIADIN-FREE DIET

The removal of all sources of gliadin—wheat, rye, oats, and barley—brings about gradual improvement in the intestinal mucosa. Although rice and corn also contain gluten, they are free of the offending gliadin fraction and can be used. For this reason, *gluten-restricted, gliadin-free diet* is more accurate terminology than gluten-free diet. See Display 28-2 for a list of foods allowed on this diet.

Children may respond more quickly than adults. Improvements may be quicker if fat is restricted for 1 or 2 months after the diagnosis. During this period, the use of medium-chain triglycerides (manufactured, easily absorbed fats) may be useful in increasing caloric intake without inducing steatorrhea. Once the mucosa regains its normal structure, more liberal amounts of fat, lactose, and other sugars usually can be tolerated. The client must be advised that lifelong avoidance of gliadin-containing foods is necessary to avoid symptoms and the damage to the intestinal mucosa.

Eliminating wheat products from the diet is not an easy task; all products made with wheat must be eliminated. These products include white and whole-wheat breads and rolls; breaded foods; stuffing; macaroni; spaghetti; noodles; cookies; cakes; wheat cereals; quick breads such as pancakes, waffles, and muffins; and gravies and cream sauces thickened with wheat flour. Because wheat products are used widely in commercially prepared foods, clients must read the ingredients label carefully and with considerable knowledge of the sources of various food additives. Such products as Postum, malted milk, and Ovaltine contain cereal grains. Beer and ale may also contain cereal grain. Gluten may be present in such minor ingredients as vegetable gum, stabilizers, preparations of monosodium glutamate (MSG), hydrolyzed vegetable protein, emulsifiers, malt, and other flavorings.

Labeling regulations that became effective May 8, 1993, require that the manufacturer give the source of protein in protein hydrolysate, whether used for flavor or other purposes. Thus, the specific protein such as "hydrolyzed corn protein" or "hydrolyzed wheat protein" must be given. Only those protein hydrolysates from soy or corn should be used in celiac sprue. Rice, corn, potato, and soy flour are substituted for the omitted cereal grains. A gliadin-free flour mixture can be substituted for equivalent amounts of wheat flour in most recipes. The mixture, composed of 2 cups rice flour, $^{2}/_{3}$ cup potato flour, and $^{1}/_{3}$ cup tapioca, can be prepared at home or purchased from companies that sell specialty diet products. Cornmeal, hominy grits, rice, cream of rice, popcorn, puffed rice, and other ready-to-eat corn and rice cereals as long as they contain malt flavoring derived from corn and not barley can be used. Gravies, cream sauces, and desserts can be thickened with cornstarch or potato flour.

Clients with gluten-sensitive enteropathy need help in identifying foods that contain gliadin and using substitutes for wheat flour effectively. The also need emotional support to adhere rigidly to a gluten-restricted, gliadin-free diet for a lifetime. Several organizations have excellent resources about this disease, diet, and support groups. Clients should be encouraged to contact the organizations given in Display 28-3.

INFLAMMATORY BOWEL DISEASE

Inflammatory bowel disease is a group of chronic disorders that cause inflammation and ulceration in the small and large intestines. They have the following common characteristics: there is no known cause or cure and flare-ups occur sporadically, followed by a period without symptoms. Crohn's disease and ulcerative colitis are the two most common inflammatory bowel conditions. The major difference between the two appears to be the extent of damage to the gastrointestinal tract.

Ulcerative colitis is an inflammation of the colon. The areas of ulceration may involve only part of the rectum or colon or the entire large intestine. Only the outermost area of the intestinal wall is affected.

The inflammation in *Crohn's disease* (also called *ileitis* or *regional enteritis*) usually involves the lower part (ileum) of the small intestine. However, it may

DISPLAY 28-2 FOODS ALLOWED ON A GLUTEN-RESTRICTED, GLIADIN-FREE DIET

GRAIN GROUP

Breads: Specially prepared using cornmeal, cornstarch, potato starch, rice flour, arrowroot, tapioca, soy or other bean flours
Cereals: Cornmeal, cream of rice, grits, hominy; corn or rice ready-to-eat cereals containing malt flavoring derived from corn (not barley), puffed rice

MILK GROUP

Milk, cream, natural cheese, plain yogurt

FRUIT AND VEGETABLE GROUP

Fresh, frozen, canned, or dried without added thickeners

MEAT AND MEAT SUBSTITUTES GROUP

Legumes, nuts, seeds: Plain dried peas, beans, lentils, plain nuts and nut butters, plain seeds
Meat, fish, poultry, eggs: Plain, fresh, or frozen

OTHER FOODS

Beverages: Carbonated beverages, coffee and tea (avoid instant types), cocoa, juice drinks
Desserts: Custard; fruit ice; meringue; fruit whips; gelatin; puddings made with arrowroot, cornstarch, rice, tapioca; rennet dessert, specially prepared baked goods
Fats: Butter, margarine, mayonnaise, oils, shortening
Snacks: Corn chips, olives, pickles, potato chips, popcorn
Soups: Clear meat and vegetable soups, homemade soups using allowed ingredients
Sweets: Corn syrup, honey, jam, jelly, molasses, sugar
Seasonings: Salt, pepper, and other plain spices and herbs; vinegar; wine

Combine allowed ingredients as desired to make many interesting foods.

Additional processed foods may be gluten restricted, gliadin free. Check ingredients carefully as follows:

Hydrolyzed vegetable protein: Only those from corn or soy (specific protein source must be given on label)
Flour and cereal products: Only rice flour, corn flour, cornmeal, or potato flour
Malt or malt flavoring: Only those derived from corn
Starch: Refers to cornstarch (permitted ingredient) when found on labels of US manufacturers
Modified food starch: Only arrowroot, corn, potato, maize, tapioca
Vegetable gum: Only carob or locust bean; cellulose gum; gum arabic; gum tragacanth; xanthan gum; guar gum
Soy sauce, soy sauce solids: Only those without wheat
Monoglycerides and diglycerides: Only those using a gliadin-free carrier
Monosodium glutamate: Only US domestic-made brands, derived from sugar beets

(Suitor CJ, Crowley MF. Nutrition: principles and application in health promotion. Philadelphia: JB Lippincott, 1984; Hartsook, EI. Gluten-restricted, gliadin- and prolamin-free diet instruction. Seattle, WA: Gluten Intolerance Group of North America, 1992.)

DISPLAY 28-3 ORGANIZATIONS PROVIDING INFORMATION FOR PEOPLE WITH CELIAC SPRUE

American Celiac Society
Dietary Support Coalition
58 Musano Court
West Orange, NJ 07052–4114
(201) 325-8837

Celiac Disease Foundation
P.O. Box 1265
Studio City, CA 91614-0265
(213) 654-4085

The Gluten Intolerance Group of North America
P.O. Box 23053
Seattle, WA 98102-0353
(206) 325-6980

Celiac Sprue Association/USA, Inc.
P.O. Box 31700
Omaha, NE 68131-0700
(402) 558-0600

These organizations have excellent resources about celiac sprue, diet, and celiac sprue support groups.

also affect other parts of the digestive tract including the mouth, esophagus, stomach, and large intestine. In Crohn's disease, the inflammation appears to be more penetrating and, therefore, more damaging to the intestinal mucosa.

Inflammatory bowel disease occurs most often in people aged 15 to 40 years and appears to run in some families. Although the exact causes of these diseases are unknown, various theories have been proposed, which include genetic, infectious, environmental, immunologic, and nutritional factors. The current leading theory is that some agent, possibly a virus or an atypical bacterium, interacts with the body's immune system to trigger an inflammatory reaction in the intestinal wall. There is no evidence that emotional stress, personality disorder, or sensitivity to certain foods cause these disorders.

During the acute phases, the most common symptoms are abdominal pain and bloody diarrhea. Anemia can result if bleeding is severe. Other symptoms include fever, nausea, vomiting, fatigue, and weight loss. Sometimes problems outside the digestive tract—skin lesions, joint pain, inflamed eyes, and liver disorders—develop that are linked to the inflammatory bowel disease, possibly due to immune system triggers. In colitis, the client may have 15 to 20 stools a day. The effect of inflammatory bowel diseases on the individual's nutritional status is profound. Nutrients are poorly absorbed, fluids and electrolytes are lost in diarrhea, and protein and iron are lost in bleeding. The individual may be seriously underweight. Children with inflammatory bowel disease are sometimes more severely affected than adults, with slowed growth and delayed sexual maturation.

The most common complication is blockage of the intestine caused by swelling and fibrous scar tissue. Crohn's disease can also cause deep ulcer tracts, called *fistulas,* that penetrate through the bowel wall into surrounding tissues and nearby organs. Fistulas are associated with pockets of infection or abscesses.

About 20% to 25% of clients with ulcerative colitis require surgery to remove the diseased portion of the colon because of massive bleeding or chronic debilitation. The surgery cures the colitis condition. In Crohn's disease, however, the disease can be helped but not cured by surgery. The inflammation tends to return in areas that adjoin the portion of the intestine that has been removed.

TREATMENT

At present, there is no cure for inflammatory bowel disease. In the case of ulcerative colitis, there may be remissions for months or even years. For most clients, though, the symptoms eventually return.

The goals of therapy are to correct nutritional deficiencies, control inflammation, and relieve abdominal pain, diarrhea, and rectal bleeding. More serious cases may require adrenal steroids or other drugs that affect the immune system. Additional drugs may be given to relax the client and relieve pain, diarrhea, or infection. The client should also receive needed emotional and psychological support.

Nutrition Therapy

In addition to the loss of nutrients caused by decreased absorption and excessive gastrointestinal losses, the client's poor food intake contributes to the malnutrition associated with an inflammatory bowel disease. Because of the distressing symptoms that follow meals, people with an inflammatory bowel disease may severely restrict what they eat. They require much patience, understanding, and encouragement from the health care team. Frequent evaluation of the diet by the dietitian is important.

No particular diet has been found to prevent or treat these diseases. However, symptoms of these diseases can be relieved and nutritional status enhanced by dietary measures. Medical nutrition therapy is adapted to the individual's needs. Foods that can be tolerated differ widely from one person to another and from one time to another in the same individual. Usually, a minimum-residue or low-fiber diet is given during the acute phases of these diseases. This diet reduces peristalsis and the frequency and volume of fecal output, preventing irritation of the colon and thus permitting it to heal. It also reduces the risk of obstruction in an intestine that is narrowed due to swelling. As the client's condition improves, he or she is encouraged to resume a normal diet. Clients who do not have intestinal narrowing may benefit from a fiber-rich diet. If increased fiber is recommended, the increase should be made carefully and gradually.

Intolerance to lactose is a frequent occurrence in an inflammatory bowel disease and the prevalence is especially high in clients who have extensive involvement of the disease in the small intestine. In such clients, restriction of dietary lactose reduces cramps and diarrhea. Most clients can tolerate small amounts of milk (up to 1 cup/day). Use of dairy products to which lactase has been added or use of lactase tablets with meals may be helpful (see the section Lactose Intolerance earlier in this chapter.)

Clients with Crohn's disease that involves the small intestine, especially clients who have had resections, have poor absorption of fat. This fat malabsorption is largely responsible for the diarrhea and for the loss of calcium, magnesium, and possibly zinc, and the excessive absorption of oxalate that may lead to kidney stone formation. Clients who have steatorrhea benefit from decreasing fat to moderate levels. If more severe fat restriction is required, clients may benefit from the use of medium-chain triglycerides.

Nutrient supplements are almost always necessary due to the malabsorption, dietary restrictions, blood loss, and drug–nutrient interactions. Prolonged reductions in the intake of milk, fruits, and vegetables may require supplements of calcium, ascorbic acid, folate, and other nutrients. Clients with extensive Crohn's disease or resection of the ileum usually do not absorb vitamin B_{12} normally and require intramuscular injections of B_{12}. Long-term use of steroids results in negative calcium balance. These are just a few examples of the specific nutrient deficiencies that may require attention in inflammatory bowel disease.

Intensive Nutritional Support

The nutritional management of clients who have severe symptoms that do not respond to medical treatment is a challenge. Lactose-free, fiber-free nutritional liquid formulas can be used to supplement meals or as a complete diet. If given as a complete source of calories and nutrients, these liquid formulas provide partial rest for the intestinal tract and can be given by mouth or by tube. These high-caloric formulas, such as Resource Plus (Sandoz Nutrition Corp.), Ensure Plus (Ross Laboratories), Nutren 1.5 (Clintec Nutrition Co.), and Sustacal (Mead Johnson Nutritional Group), work best for clients with mild to moderate involvement.

If the client has moderate to severe disease, an elemental diet or total parenteral nutrition (total nutritional needs supplied intravenously) may be indicated. The use of an elemental diet administered by nasogastric tube in these cases, especially in children with growth failure, has greatly improved nutritional status and promoted catch-up growth. The elemental diet is a liquid formula composed of the essential nutrients in an easily absorbed form and leaves no residue in the intestinal tract (see Chapter 29). The elemental diet may be given by continuous nasogastric infusion during the night, which allows the child or adult to pursue normal school or work and family activities during the day. Total parenteral nutrition is usually used in those cases in which only a small portion of the intestine is functioning or when there is near-complete obstruction of the intestine.

DIVERTICULOSIS

Diverticulosis is a common disorder occurring in 10% of people older than age 40 years and in nearly 50% of people older than age 60 years. Diverticulosis is often discovered during intestinal examination for another reason.

Diverticulosis is characterized by outpouchings, called *diverticula,* in the wall of the large intestine. Outpouchings are about this size of large peas (Fig. 28-4). Some people may have no symptoms, whereas others may experience lower abdominal pain, especially in the lower left side, and distention. If the diverticula become inflamed, a condition known as *diverticulitis* develops. Bleeding of the colon mucosa also may occur.

Sometimes diverticulitis can be a serious problem. Clients with diverticulitis may be hospitalized and treated with bed rest, antibiotics, pain relievers, and intravenous fluids. The majority of clients recover from these acute episodes. In some cases, the diverticulitis results in large abscesses, blockage of the colon, or perforation of the intestinal wall, causing peritonitis or abscesses in the abdomen. Such infections can be fatal if not treated quickly. Only about 20% of people who are found to have diverticula develop diverticulitis and only a small percentage of those have serious complications.

It has been suggested that diverticulosis is caused by a lack of natural fiber, or roughage, in the diet; thus, fecal material is small, hard, and dry, causing movement to slow and pressure to increase in the colon. The pressure and the straining required when passing stools forces the lining out through weak spots in the muscle covering the colon, consequently forming pouches.

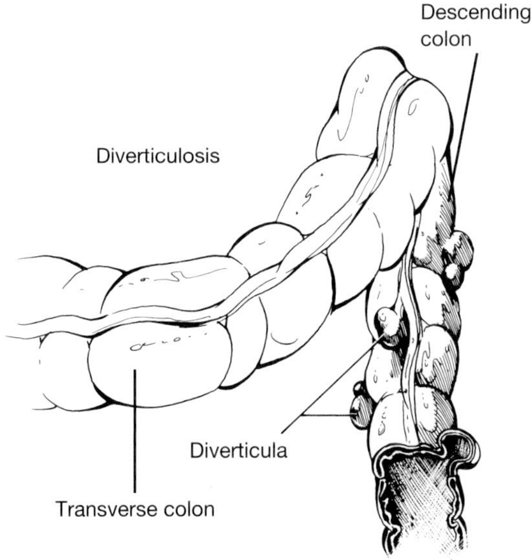

FIGURE 28-4

Diverticula in the walls of the large intestine.

TREATMENT

A high-fiber diet is followed to prevent constipation and thus prevent pressure from building up in the walls of the colon. As little as 2 tbsp of unprocessed wheat bran or $^1/_2$ to $^3/_4$ cup of breakfast cereal that is high in bran (e.g., All-Bran or Bran Buds [Kellogg] or 100% Bran [Nabisco]) can increase fecal bulk and promote faster movement along the digestive tract. Although raw fruits and vegetables and legumes are good sources of fiber, they apparently are not as effective as wheat bran in increasing fecal bulk. A small amount (about 1 to 2 tsp) of wheat bran should be taken at first; this amount is increased gradually over about 4 weeks until the desired amount is reached. The wheat bran can be added to cereal, yogurt, and other foodstuffs. The client also should drink plenty of fluids. Clients may be advised to avoid nuts, seeds, hulls (e.g., popcorn), and berries (strawberries, blueberries, raspberries, and blackberries) because particles from these foods may become trapped in the diverticula and cause pain. Improved movement in the colon as a result of a high-fiber diet may make such restriction unnecessary. Recommendations should be adapted to each client's tolerance level.

High-fiber foods should be discontinued if severe abdominal pain and fever develop, and the physician should be contacted. During an acute attack of diverticulitis, with fever, bleeding, and pain, a liquid diet or a minimal- or moderate-residue diet is given. Severe diverticulitis requires rest of the colon. Antibiotics and fluids are provided intravenously.

IRRITABLE BOWEL SYNDROME

Irritable bowel syndrome is a complex motility disorder influenced by both physical factors and emotional stress. The disturbance is characterized by abdominal pain and spasm, bloating, and abnormal bowel movements. Some people experience constipation, others experience diarrhea, and some experience diarrhea alternating with constipation. Women with irritable bowel syndrome appear to have more symptoms during menstrual periods.

The term *irritable* refers to the unusual sensitivity of the nerve endings lining the colon and the hyperactivity of the nerves that control the muscles of the intestinal tract. As a result, the colon responds in an exaggerated way to normal physical and emotional events.

Individuals react differently to the disorder—some consider it a minor annoyance, whereas others find it to be disabling, causing enough discomfort to alter daily activities and performance. Most people are able to control symptoms through diet, stress management, and, in some cases, medication.

TREATMENT

Evaluation of stress level and food habits is the first step in treating the disorder. Overwork, poor sleep habits, excessive use of caffeine, alcohol, and tobacco can be sources of stress. Large meals and high-fat meals are often identified as triggers of irritable bowel syndrome. Wheat, corn, and MSG will trigger symptoms as will almost any food or additive in a particular person. Keeping a food and symptom diary for 1 week is a useful tool in identifying triggering foods.

Adequate rest and exercise are important factors in reducing stress and have a beneficial effect on irritable bowel syndrome. Increasing fiber including bran or a psyllium preparation can help regulate bowel function. An excessive intake of fiber should be avoided, however, because it may trigger symptoms in people with diarrhea-predominant irritable bowel syndrome. Reducing fats, reducing the quantity of food at meals, and avoiding foods known to be triggers are all prudent measures. The use of laxatives should be avoided. Mental health counseling and relaxation training are also helpful elements of treatment.

When these measures fail, medications such as antispasmodics, antidepressants, and antianxiety medications can be prescribed. The potential for dependence on laxatives or tranquilizers is a major concern and must be carefully monitored.

DISEASES OF THE ACCESSORY ORGANS OF DIGESTION

DISEASES OF THE LIVER

Any liver disease is devastating to the body. This is not surprising in view of the essential functions the liver performs. Nutrients, with few exceptions, are carried by the bloodstream to the liver before they are distributed to the other body tissues. The liver changes the nutrients to a form that is most useful to the body; it stores some of them, such as iron, copper, vitamins A and D, and glucose, in the form of glycogen; it detoxifies poisonous substances; and it synthesizes protein enzymes, plasma proteins, and the waste product urea from nitrogen (resulting from amino acid metabolism).

The amount of protein permitted clients with liver disease depends on their condition; changes are necessary as clinical status changes. Nutrition therapy is complicated by the fact that, although protein is needed to rebuild damaged liver cells, protein metabolism in severe liver disease is so distorted that ammonia and other products of protein metabolism accumulate to abnormal levels in the blood. These substances are toxic to the central nervous system, which can lead to serious complications.

HEPATITIS

Hepatitis is an inflammation of the liver. It usually is caused by a virus but also may result from parasites, obstruction, alcohol, or other substances toxic to the liver. In hepatitis, liver cells are damaged, and replacement of the cells occurs too slowly for the organ to function normally. In milder cases, injury to liver tissue is reversible; in more severe cases, injury to liver cells is so extensive that liver failure and death result.

The most common types of acute viral hepatitis are hepatitis A and hepatitis B. Hepatitis A, formerly called infectious hepatitis, is contracted through drinking water, food, or sewerage. Hepatitis B, formerly called serum hepatitis, is a more severe form and is transmitted by transfusion from a carrier, unsterile needles, saliva, blood, and semen. In 3% to 10% of cases, the disease becomes chronic. Carriers of hepatitis B are at increased risk of developing liver cancer. People at high risk of contracting the disease such as intravenous drug users and health care workers should be immunized by hepatitis B vaccine.

Regardless of the type of hepatitis, the symptoms include nausea, anorexia, right upper quadrant pain, dark urine, and jaundice. Carbohydrate metabolism is frequently abnormal and both hypoglycemia and hyperglycemia may occur. Fasting hypoglycemia may result from decreased glycogen stores and elevated serum insulin. Hyperglycemia may result from insulin resistance. Nutrition therapy and bed rest are the main forms of treatment. Antiviral drugs may be given to reduce liver cell injury.

CIRRHOSIS

Cirrhosis is a term applied to all forms of liver disease in which there is extensive loss of liver cells. The cells are lost faster than they are replaced, seriously impairing liver function. The active liver cells are replaced by scar tissue (connective tissue), which impairs blood circulation through the liver. The loss of normal liver tissue impairs the processing of nutrients, hormones, drugs, and toxins by the liver. Also impaired is the production of protein and other vital body substances made by the liver.

In 1991, chronic liver disease and cirrhosis was the ninth leading cause of death and the seventh leading cause by disease. In the United States, chronic alcoholism is the most common cause. Other causes include chronic viral hepatitis; a number of metabolic disorders including cystic fibrosis, hemochromatosis (excess iron storage), Wilson's disease (excess copper storage), and galactosemia; obstruction of bile ducts; and chemical or drug poisoning.

Few symptoms may occur at first. As the number of functioning liver cells declines and distortion of the liver due to scarring occurs, the person experiences fatigue, weakness, exhaustion, nausea, appetite loss, and weight loss. With diminished production of the serum protein albumin, water accumulates in the legs (edema) or abdomen (ascites). In later stages, jaundice and intense itching (due to the deposit of bile products in the skin) may occur.

In advanced cirrhosis, there is extensive loss of liver cells with disruption in blood flow through the liver. The liver is unable to metabolize protein normally or to detoxify the ammonia that enters the blood from the intestinal tract. As a result, ammonia and other toxins accumulate in the blood. These substances are toxic to the central nervous system and cause hepatic encephalopathy, which is characterized by symptoms of drowsiness, apathy, personality changes, a fecal odor to the breath, flapping tremors of the hands and tongue when extended, and disorientation. If it is untreated, coma and then death follow.

Another serious problem is portal hypertension caused by obstruction of the portal vein that flows through the liver. The obstruction of blood flow causes pressure to build up in the portal vein. The body attempts to find a way around the liver through the development of new blood vessels that may form in the stomach and esophagus. These new blood vessels may become enlarged *(varices)* and may rupture, causing serious bleeding in the stomach and esophagus.

Nutrition Therapy

The purpose of nutrition therapy is to maintain or improve nutritional status by providing adequate calories and protein to maintain positive nitrogen balance and to promote regeneration of new tissue. Nutrition therapy simultaneously aims to prevent further aggravation of liver disease, including hepatic encephalopathy. Nutrition intervention is also directed to other complications of liver disease such as hypoglycemia, hyperglycemia, fluid imbalance, and esophageal varices.

Therapy must be individualized according to client needs. Protein is restricted depending on the type of disorder and the degree of liver failure. Sodium, potassium, and fluids may also need to be controlled.

In Hepatitis and Early Cirrhosis. Dietary treatment in hepatitis and early cirrhosis requires a normal diet with adequate calories and a moderate level of protein—70 to 80 g/day or less. Authorities have cautioned that the need to restore protein and the potential risk of precipitating hepatic encephalopathy must be carefully considered. Positive nitrogen balance can be achieved with less dietary protein than was previously thought. The amount of dietary protein that can be tolerated by an individual will vary from one time to another. Sparing protein by providing adequate calories in the form of carbohydrate and fat is important.

Achieving these dietary goals may appear to be a simple task; however, nausea, diarrhea, fever, and fatigue interfere with food intake. In the early stages of hepatitis, the nausea and vomiting may necessitate the use of tube feedings and parenteral fluids. Much encouragement and persuasion are needed to get clients to eat enough food. The nurse and dietitian must work together closely to provide the kinds and amounts of food most acceptable to the client and to ensure environmental conditions that promote appetite. Food intake usually is increased when six small meals are given rather than three large meals. The amount of food eaten should be carefully observed and recorded.

Meeting caloric needs is a basic requirement. If calories supplied by carbohydrates and fats are inadequate, proteins from food and from body cells are broken down to supply energy, consequently decreasing the protein available for cell replacement. A caloric intake of 2500 kcal/day or more (about 35 to 40 kcal/kg of body weight) is offered. The level may be more than 3000 kcal/day if fever is high and weight loss is extensive.

Most of the energy is supplied by carbohydrate and fat. Fat is usually not restricted unless the client experiences steatorrhea. In such a case, fats are restricted to 30 to 40 g/day. The diet may be supplemented with medium-chain triglycerides (MCT Oil: Mead Johnson) if additional calories are needed.

In Advanced Cirrhosis. Protein intake should be sufficient to achieve positive nitrogen balance. Korsten and Leiber have advised that positive nitrogen balance in clients with cirrhosis can be attained with dietary protein of .74 g/kg of body weight, similar to the RDA of .8 g/kg. To relieve symptoms of encephalopathy, protein may be reduced to .5 g/kg of ideal body weight or 50 g/day. If improvement does not occur, dietary protein may be reduced to 10 to 20 g/day. As protein is decreased, increased amounts of carbohydrate and possibly fats are necessary to ensure an adequate energy intake. If caloric intake is inadequate, body protein must be broken down to supply energy, and blood ammonia levels will increase. As the client's condition improves, protein is added gradually and in small quantities. Some clients may need to restrict protein intake to 40 to 60 g/day permanently. Medication may be given also to reduce absorption of ammonia from the intestinal tract.

Sodium restriction may be necessary to alleviate edema or ascites. Sodium restriction may range from 500 to 2000 mg/day, depending on severity of the problem. Potassium may be restricted if blood levels are elevated due to poor renal function or increased if diuretics that deplete potassium are used.

If esophageal varices are present, coarse fibrous foods are excluded from the diet and foods with a smooth texture are included. Meats are ground and fruits and vegetables are pureed to make them easier to swallow. If bleeding occurs, a liquid diet is substituted. Vitamins and minerals are prescribed as needed.

In Liver Transplantation. More than 1600 people with severe symptoms or life-threatening complications are receiving liver transplants each year. Nutrition therapy aims to improve nutritional status to the extent possible before surgery and to promote wound healing, prevent and treat complications, and manage nutrition-related side effects of immunosuppressive drugs after surgery. Adequate calories (30 to 40 kcal/kg) and protein (1.5 to 2.0 g/kg) are needed to promote positive nitrogen balance. Long-term nutrition goals, once the client has recovered from the initial stress of surgery, are to prevent diabetes (as a result of drug therapy), hyperlipidemia, and excessive weight gain.

GALLBLADDER DISEASE

Gallbladder disease most frequently takes the form of *cholelithiasis* (gallstones), accompanied by *cholecystitis* (inflammation of the gallbladder). An estimated 20 million Americans have gallstones, most of whom have no symptoms. Before age 60 years, woman are twice as likely as men to develop gallstones. American Indians and Mexican Americans have a high incidence of gallstones. Obesity is a major risk factor and people who go on very low-calorie diets and lose weight rapidly are also at higher risk.

The gallbladder is a small, pear-shaped organ located in a depression on the right underside of the liver. Its primary function is to store and concentrate bile that is produced by the liver and to secrete the bile into the small intestine at the proper time for normal digestion to occur. Bile emulsifies dietary fats so that they can more easily be broken down by digestive enzymes. Bile is delivered from the liver to the gallbladder and from the gallbladder to the intestine by a series of ducts (see Figure 6-2).

Gallstones form when substances in the bile, primarily cholesterol or bile pigments, form hard, crystal-like particles that can range in size from a small particle to the size of a golf ball. Most gallstones are cholesterol stones; pigments stones are usually associated with other disorders such as cirrhosis, infections, and hereditary blood disorders such as sickle cell anemia. Pain results from cholecystitis or gallstones lodged in the cystic duct leading from the gallbladder or in the common bile duct shared by the gallbladder and liver when the gallbladder contracts. If the gallstones block digestive fluids from the pancreas, pancreatitis results. Prolonged blockage of any of these ducts can cause severe complications that can lead to death. Warning signs are fever, jaundice, and persistent pain.

Symptoms of a gallstone attack include severe pain in the upper abdomen. The pain persists for only 20 to 30 minutes or as long as several hours. The pain may radiate to the right shoulder or to the back between the shoulder blades. Abdominal distention, nausea, and vomiting may also be present. The exact cause of cholelithiasis is unknown; however, the following factors have been implicated: genetics, body weight, gallbladder motility, and diet (high fat, low fiber).

TREATMENT

Cholecystectomy, removal of the gallbladder, is the most common method of treatment. Previously, gallbladder removal involved major abdominal surgery and a considerable amount of time (3 to 6 weeks) for recuperation. Now the laparoscopic laser cholecystectomy is the most common procedure. It is much less invasive, usually requiring only an overnight stay in the hospital and several days recovery at home.

Before surgery, fat may be limited to 25 to 50 g/day to reduce contractions of the gallbladder. Only nonfat dairy products are permitted. Lean meats and meat substitutes are limited to 5 or 6 oz/day. Table and cooking fat may be excluded entirely or limited to small amounts, the equivalent of 3 to 5 tsp, depending on the fat level of the diet. Fatty meats or meat substitutes, hard cheeses, fried foods, salad dressings, gravies, nuts, and rich pastries and desserts are omitted.

After surgery, bile flows directly from the liver to the small intestine. At first, clients may feel more comfortable limiting fat, but after a month or two, they may resume a normal diet. In time, a portion of the bile duct may enlarge, providing for temporary storage of bile.

Alternative treatments are used for people who cannot tolerate surgery. They include the use of oral bile acids to dissolve small stones or extracorporeal (ultrasonic) shock wave lithotripsy, a nonevasive procedure that shatters stones and is used together with the oral bile acid medication.

PANCREATITIS

Pancreatitis, or inflammation of the pancreas, may be associated with alcoholism, infection, or other disease, or may be of unknown origin. Abdominal pain is the most common symptom; nausea, vomiting, and steatorrhea also may be present.

When the pancreas is inflamed, stimulating pancreatic secretion may cause excruciating pain. Intravenous feedings usually provide nourishment during the acute stages of the disease and rest the pancreas. High-carbohydrate liquids are the first oral feedings given. Later, small meals that consist of easily digested carbohydrate and protein, with limited fat, are given. Fats are restricted because the pancreatic enzymes necessary for their digestion are missing. The diet is bland to reduce the presence of dilute hydrochloric acid in the duodenum, which stimulates the flow of pancreatic juice. Pancreatic enzymes may be taken with meals and snacks. Medium-chain triglycerides may be included in the diet to provide additional calories. Pancreatic enzymes do not appear to be required for the digestion of this fat.

KEYS TO PRACTICAL APPLICATION

Be aware that recent research has uncovered physical causes for diseases once thought to have strong emotional and personality components.

Encourage people with repeated episodes of heartburn, indigestion, constipation, and gaseousness—seemingly harmless discomforts—to seek medical attention to rule out the possibility of a serious underlying cause.

When advising clients who have peptic ulcers or other gastric disorders, bear in mind that much of the information about the irritating characteristics of various foods has not been supported by research.

Respect clients' aversion to foods that cause them distress. Tolerance for foods differs greatly from person to person.

Encourage clients with a lactose intolerance to seek a solution to this problem. Small amounts of milk at a time, fermented milk products, or enzyme-treated milk may be tolerated. Emphasize the importance of adequate calcium intake at all ages.

Be accepting of the food aversions and food-related complaints of clients with inflammatory bowel disease. Encourage clients to eat adequate amounts of food, and see that they receive foods they like, to the extent possible.

When the use of bran in the diet has been ordered, caution clients to start with a small amount, increasing it gradually until the desired amount is reached. This gradual increase helps reduce the unpleasant side effects of high-fiber diets. Advise clients to drink plenty of fluids.

Encourage clients who are experiencing nausea and vomiting in liver disease to eat as much as they can. Help them understand why this is important. Carefully record the amount of food consumed.

KEY IDEAS

Gastrointestinal diseases previously thought to be caused by emotional factors have been found to result from bacteria or viruses interacting with the body's immune system or disturbances in motility patterns of the digestive organs.

Lifestyle modifications that may relieve symptoms in gastroesophageal reflux disease are given in Display 28-1.

Peptic ulcers develop when aggressive factors (hydrochloric acid and pepsin) overpower the defensive factors (gastric mucosa strengthened by good blood flow, bicarbonate secretion, and prostaglandin synthesis).

Factors that lower the body's mucosal defense include cigarette smoking, use of nonsteroidal anti-inflammatory drugs, genetic factors, and bacteria.

Helicobacter pylori plays a major role in the development of most peptic ulcer disease.

There is no evidence that certain foods cause peptic ulcers or prevent occurrence.

Physical stress, but not emotional stress, is strongly associated with the development of peptic ulcers.

Clients with peptic ulcers for whom antibiotic treatment is inappropriate are treated with H_2 blockers. These drugs increase the pH of the stomach more than food and for longer periods. Another drug, sucralfate,adheres to the ulcer surface and shields it from the acid environment.

Diet has no specific role to play in the treatment of ulcers. It is recommended that clients avoid alcohol and foods that are strong stimulants of gastric acid: both regular and decaffeinated coffee, tea, chocolate, and caffeinated soft drinks.

Gastroparesis is a motility disorder of the stomach in which the movement of the stomach contents into the duodenum is abnormally slow.

Treatment of gastroparesis consists of the use of prokinetic drugs and dietary modifications that promote gastric emptying such as small meals, low-fiber foods, foods in liquid form, and decreased fat and lactose.

Fiber- and residue-modified diets are used in some diseases of the lower gastrointestinal tract.

Fiber refers to indigestible carbohydrates and lignin found in plant foods; residue refers to the total solid material in the feces, including fiber and also other unabsorbed components of the diet, sloughed cells, intestinal bacteria, and by-products of bacteria.

Fiber is responsible for most of the residue in the colon.

Fiber- and residue-restricted diets reduce the frequency and volume of fecal output.

High-fiber diets increase fecal bulk, reduce pressure, and normalize peristalsis.

Most clients with lactose intolerance can tolerate small quantities of milk at a time, fermented milk products such as yogurt, or milk and milk products treated with a commercial enzyme preparation. When lactose intolerance is severe, the client must be alerted to hidden sources of lactose in foods.

The gluten-restricted, gliadin-free diet used to treat celiac sprue requires that the client avoid all wheat, rye, oats, and barley and, instead, substitute rice, corn, soy, and potato flours for wheat flour.

During acute stages of an inflammatory bowel disease, a low-residue diet may be used to prevent irritation and permit rest and healing; milk frequently is poorly tolerated. The diet must be highly individualized, because tolerance for foods differs widely from person to person.

People with a severe inflammatory bowel disease may be given an elemental diet by continuous nasogastric infusion. Sometimes total parenteral (intravenous) nutrition is necessary.

Diverticulosis is now treated by high-fiber diets rather than by the low-residue diets used in the past. Wheat bran has been found to be the most effective form of fiber. During an acute attack of diverticulitis, a minimal- or moderate-residue diet is given.

In irritable bowel syndrome, the colon responds in an exaggerated way to normal physical and emotional events. *Irritable* refers to unusually sensitive nerves that line the intestinal tract.

Reducing fat, having smaller meals, avoiding "trigger" foods, and increasing fiber may be beneficial in irritable bowel syndrome. Other recommendations include adequate rest and exercise, mental health counseling, and relaxation training.

In hepatitis and early cirrhosis, the diet is moderate in protein; in advanced cirrhosis, protein is restricted to 20 to 60 g/day as a means of preventing hepatic coma. Supplying sufficient calories is extremely important at all stages of liver disease; however, symptoms of nausea, vomiting, and abdominal distress make the ingestion of adequate amounts of food difficult.

Ascites, a frequent complication of cirrhosis, requires severe sodium restriction. With esophageal varices, food must be smooth in texture—finely ground or pureed.

Surgery is the most common treatment for cholelithiasis; a fat-restricted diet is frequently advised before surgery. Most people can gradually resume a normal diet after surgery.

Total parenteral nutrition usually provides nourishment during the acute stages of pancreatitis. When oral feedings are tolerated, the diet is low in fat and bland to avoid stimulating the flow of pancreatic enzymes. Medium-chain triglyceride oil may be used to provide additional calories. Pancreatic enzyme medication may be taken with meals and snacks.

KEYS TO LEARNING

STUDY–DISCUSSION QUESTIONS

1. A client is diagnosed as having gastrointestinal reflux disease. What diet and lifestyle changes might relieve symptoms of this disease?
2. Ask your hospital's dietitian to discuss with the class the changes that have occurred in the treatment of peptic ulcer in recent years. What dietary modifications, if any, are being ordered by physicians for people with this disease?
3. Assume that you are counseling a client who has severe lactose intolerance. What foods would you advise this person to avoid? What alternatives can you recommend for achieving adequate calcium intake?
4. What effect does the gliadin fraction of gluten have on the jejunal mucosa of the client with celiac sprue? What are the characteristic symptoms of this disease? Plan a gluten-free menu for 1 day for a 30-year-old engineer who eats her lunch in the cafeteria at work using Display 28-2 as a guide.
5. Plan a 1-day menu consisting of three meals and two between-meal snacks for a hospitalized client on a fiber- and residue-restricted diet, following the dietary guidelines of your hospital.
6. What foods contribute fiber, or roughage, to the diet? Why is fiber thought to be beneficial in the treatment of diverticulosis? Plan a 1-day menu that contains approximately 30 g fiber using Table 8-4 as a guide in calculating the fiber content of food.
7. Discuss the dietary changes necessary in each of the following complications of cirrhosis: ascites, esophageal bleeding, and hepatic coma.
8. In your hospital, how many grams of fat are included in the lowfat diet usually served to clients with gallbladder disease? What foods supply this fat?

BIBLIOGRAPHY

BOOKS

Chicago Dietetic Association and South Suburban Dietetic Association. Manual of clinical dietetics. 4th ed. Chicago: The American Dietetic Association, 1992.

Korsten MA, Lieber CS. Nutrition in pancreatic and liver disorders. In: Shils ME, Olson JA, Shike M. Eds. Modern nutrition in health and disease. 8th ed. Philadelphia: Lea and Febiger, 1994:1066–1080.

Meyer JH. The stomach and nutrition. In: Shils ME, Olson JA, Shike M. Eds. Modern nutrition in health and disease. 8th ed. Philadelphia: Lea and Febiger, 1994:1029–1035.

Turtel PS, Shike M. Diseases of the small bowel. In: Shils ME, Olson JA, Shike M. Eds. Modern nutrition in health and disease. 8th ed. Philadelphia: Lea and Febiger, 1994:1050–1059.

PERIODICALS

Bouthillier L, Seidman EG. Growth failure in children with impaired gut function. RD 1991;11:3:1.

Camilleri M. A guide to the treatment of GI motility disorders. Drug Therapy 1991; 21:12:15.

Deckman RC, Cheskin LJ. Diverticular disease in the elderly. J Am Geriatr Soc 1993;41:986.

DeCross AJ, Peura DA. Role of *H. pylori* in peptic ulcer disease. Contemp Gastroenterol 1992;5:4:18.

Elfrink RJ, Miedema BW. Colonic diverticula. Postgrad Med 1992;92:6:97.

Hendricks KM, Williams E, Stoker TW, et al. Dietary intake of adolescents with Crohn's disease. J Am Diet Assoc 1994; 94:441.

Lieber CS. Herman Award Lecture 1993: a personal perspective on alcohol, nutrition, and the liver. Am J Clin Nutr 1993; 58:430.

Montes RG, Perman JA. Lactose intolerance: pinpointing the source of nonspecific gastrointestinal symptoms. Postgrad Med 1991;89:8:175.

Parkman HP, Fisher RS. Gastroparesis: diagnostic and therapeutic management. Practical Gastroenterol 1993;17:2:18.

Roth B, Ippoliti A, DeMuster T. Choosing the right option for acute GERD. Contemp Gastroenterol 1991;4:5:36.

Steinhart MJ. Irritable bowel syndrome: how to relieve symptoms enough to improve daily function. Postgrad Med 1992;91:6:315.

Sullivan, M, Sitrin MD. Nutrition in Crohn's disease: support or primary therapy? RD 1991;11:1:1.

Sutherland JE. Gastroesophageal reflux disease. Postgrad Med 1991;89:7:45.

Tripodi J, Burakoff R. Diabetic gastroparesis. Practical Diabetology 1994;13:1:4.

CHAPTER

29

Nutrition Therapy Related to Surgery and Following Burns; Alternative Feeding Methods

KEY TERMS

elemental diet liquid formula that provides the essential nutrients in a form that is easily absorbed and leaves no residue in the intestinal tract

enteral nutrition delivery of nutrients directly into the stomach or the small intestine

enterostomy procedure in which the small intestine is opened and a tube is brought through the abdominal wall

ileus loss of intestinal peristalsis

isotonic solution characterized by osmotic pressure equal to that of another solution (usually normal plasma)

nasoenteral running from the nose to the gastrointestinal tract

needle catheter jejunostomy fine feeding tube is introduced through a large-bore needle into the jejunum

parenteral nutrition delivery of nutrients intravenously into circulation, hence bypassing the intestinal tract

percutaneous endoscopic gastrostomy procedure in which a feeding tube is placed into the stomach and brought through the abdominal wall with the use of an endoscope

peripheral veins small-diameter veins that supply the extremities (arms and legs)

polymeric the form of nutrients before digestion; prepared with whole protein and starch

repletion the act of restoring or replacing what is lacking

stoma opening created by surgery between a body passageway and the body surface

viscosity a property of fluid; usually referred to as viscous or thick

OBJECTIVES

After completing this chapter, the student will be able to:

1. Describe the effects catabolism has on the body.
2. Identify the client's nutrient needs following surgery.
3. Describe the symptoms associated with dumping syndrome and also describe the nutritional management.
4. Calculate the client's total energy needs using the Harris-Benedict equation adjusted for activity and injury.
5. Calculate the protein needs using the calorie/nitrogen ratio.
6. Identify clients who are at greatest risk for nutritional complications following small bowel resection.
7. List three possible nutrition problems associated with poor bile salt absorption.
8. Calculate an adult client's approximate fluid needs.

9. Describe the fluid needs of the client with an ostomy.
10. Discuss the burn client's general nutrient needs.
11. Define enteral and parenteral nutrition and give the conditions for which each is indicated.
12. Distinguish between the different types of enteral feeding formulas available.
13. Describe how osmolality influences product selection.
14. List the three methods by which enteral feedings can be administered.
15. Describe the difference between peripheral parenteral nutrition and central parenteral nutrition.

NUTRITION IN SURGERY

Among the most critically ill clients are those who have undergone surgery or have experienced acute injury such as severe burns. Meeting the clients' nutritional needs is a challenge to the health care team that requires a high degree of skill and cooperation. Without proper nutrition care, recovery may be delayed or may not proceed normally.

NUTRITION IN PREPARATION FOR SURGERY

Preoperative improvement in the nutritional status of a poorly nourished client who is scheduled to undergo surgery lessens the possibility of later complications. Well-nourished surgical clients have many advantages: they heal more quickly, are better able to fight infection, lose less muscle tissue, and enjoy a greater sense of well-being than clients who are poorly nourished.

In some instances, a client's poor nutritional state may be a consequence of the disease itself, as in cancer of the stomach or esophagus, which interferes with the intake and use of food. If the client is poorly nourished and if the surgery is not an emergency, a high-protein, high-calorie diet may be ordered to improve nutritional status. Methods of feeding that can improve the nutritional status of a severely malnourished client are available (see the section Alternative Feeding Methods).

In addition to malnourished people, extremely obese people are surgical risks. They may not recover from anesthesia in the normal way and may have breathing difficulties, which increase the risk of lung complications. The obese person's extra blood vessels, which nourish the extra adipose tissue, increase the work of the heart. Furthermore, adipose tissue heals more slowly and is more prone to infection than muscle tissue. Sometimes the physician delays surgery until the obese client loses a specified amount of weight. A minimal-residue diet may be ordered for several days before gastrointestinal surgery to reduce the residue (material that remains after digestion) in the intestine (see Chapter 28).

Usually, nothing is permitted by mouth for a minimum of 8 hours before surgery so that the stomach is free of food. Food in the stomach during surgery or recovery from anesthesia could be vomited or aspirated and could cause postoperative dilation of the stomach. In the case of emergency surgery, the contents of the stomach are removed by gastric suction.

NUTRITION FOLLOWING SURGERY

The stress response by the body following surgery or injury can be divided into three phases. These phases are characterized by hormonal changes that occur in response to the physiologic stress. Immediately following surgery, the body is in a catabolic state. During this period, metabolism is greatly increased and breakdown of body tissue results in urinary nitrogen and potassium losses. Hormonal control influences the kidneys to retain fluid and sodium to support circulating blood volume. Body fat is the primary source of energy. Peristalsis and absorption in the gastrointestinal tract are reduced. If the loss of body protein is great, wound healing is delayed, the ability of immune system to fight infection is impaired, and the recovery period is prolonged. The extent of the catabolic effect on the body depends on the type and level of stress.

In the anabolic phase that follows, positive nitrogen balance is reestablished as the lean body tissue that was lost is gradually restored. Weight is slowly regained. Excess sodium and water are excreted, and potassium is retained. Peristalsis returns to normal. This phase usually begins within 3 to 6 days of surgery or injury. In cases of complex surgery or severe burns, the anabolic phase may be delayed.

In the final phase, fat lost during the catabolic phase is restored. This period of convalescence may last 2 to 3 months.

POSTOPERATIVE CARE

Postoperative nutrition care includes maintenance of fluid and electrolyte balance and provision of adequate energy, protein, vitamins, and minerals.

Fluid and Electrolyte Balance

The first priority is maintaining fluid and electrolyte balance. Immediately after surgery, fluids and electrolytes are administered intravenously. Intravenous solutions of 5% or 10% dextrose are commonly given and may include vitamins and medications. No food or fluids are given by mouth until peristalsis has returned and the gastrointestinal tract is functioning. Oral fluids, generally as a clear liquid diet, provide the client with calories in the form of carbohydrate, electrolytes, mainly sodium and potassium, and fluids. In general, the fluid requirement for an adult is approximately 30 to 35 mL/kg of body weight per day. However, a clear liquid diet is inadequate in almost all nutrients.

Calories

Postoperative nutrition care must be individualized. The type of nutrition intervention used depends on the type of surgery, function of the gastrointestinal tract, and client's nutritional status. In the immediate postoperative period, intravenous solutions of 5% or 10% dextrose supply the client with only minimal energy. However, if the individual is well nourished before surgery, has no complications, and is expected to eat by postoperative day 4 or 5, this amount of nutrients may be adequate. The cost associated with more aggressive nutrition support for this short period must be considered.

After surgery, the adult male weighing 70 kg (154 lb) requires 30 to 35 kcal/kg of body weight per day (2100 to 2450 calories/day). The Harris-Benedict equation, which represents basal energy expenditure (BEE), is also frequently used. Total energy requirements can be calculated using the BEE with activity or injury factors added (Display 29-1).

If calories are inadequate for an extended period, wound healing and all other aspects of recovery are hindered. Without sufficient calories, body proteins cannot be synthesized. Instead, dietary proteins and body proteins are used to produce glucose and body fat is used as the main energy source.

Protein

Adequate amounts of protein are essential for wound healing, as well as to protect the liver from damage and promote resistance to infection. Following severe injury, such as extensive burns, large amounts of muscle tissue can be lost in 1 day. Following surgery, blood loss and tissue damage both result in considerable protein loss. Significant protein loss also can result from the wasting of bone and muscle when the body is immobilized. Getting the client up and out of bed is extremely important in promoting a positive nitrogen balance for the rebuilding of lean body tissue. Sufficient protein and calories must be provided for anabolism to occur.

In most circumstances, 1.0 to 1.5 g of protein per kilogram of body weight per day, or about 80 to 100 g/day, is sufficient for clients who have been well nourished. Many adult Americans ordinarily consume these amounts, so this intake is not difficult to achieve. In clients with poor absorption or extensive injury, protein needs are greater; 1.5 to 2.0 g/kg of body weight per day may be required.

When planning a high-calorie, high-protein diet, determining the calorie to nitrogen (kcal/*N*) ratio can be used to assure there is adequate protein for repletion. Generally, this ratio is determined using energy from carbohydrate and fat (nonprotein calories) to support protein synthesis. A kcal/*N* ratio of 100 to 200 kcal (nonprotein) per gram of nitrogen meets the needs of moderately to severely

DISPLAY 29-1 DETERMINATION OF ENERGY AND PROTEIN REQUIREMENTS IN STRESS

STEP 1. DETERMINE TOTAL ENERGY REQUIREMENT IN STRESS.

Total energy requirements = BEE × activity factor × injury factor

BEE (male) = 66.47 + (13.75 × W) + (5.0 × H) − (6.76 × age)

BEE (female) = 655.1 + (9.56 × W) + (1.85 × H) − (4.68 × age)

W = weight in kg and *H* = height in cm

ACTIVITY FACTORS*	INJURY FACTORS*
1.2 Confined to bed	1.2 Minor operation
1.3 Out of bed	1.35 Skeletal trauma
	1.6 Major sepsis
	2.1 Severe burn

STEP 2. USING CALORIC REQUIREMENT CALCULATED ABOVE, DETERMINE THE PROTEIN REQUIREMENT.

The relationship between calories and protein is expressed as the calorie/nitrogen ratio. Approximately 6.25 g of protein yields 1 g nitrogen. The goal is to provide enough non-protein calories (from carbohydrate and fat) to ensure that protein is used for tissue building and not as a source of energy. A ratio of 150 kcal to 1 g of nitrogen meets the needs of most clients during physical stress. Based on this ratio, protein requirement is figured as follows:

Estimated caloric need ÷ 150 = Estimated nitrogen need

Estimated nitrogen need (g) × 6.25 = Estimated protein need[†]

Example: To determine protein need of client requiring 2750 kcal:

2750 ÷ 150 = 18.3 g Nitrogen

18.3 g N × 6.25 = 114.4 g Protein

*Activity and injury factors are from Long CL et al: Metabolic response to injury and illness: Estimation of energy and protein needs from indirect calorimetry and nitrogen balance. J Parenter Enteral Nutr 3:452, 1979.

[†]Protein/Nitrogen Conversion:
Nitrogen to protein: nitrogen (g) × 6.25 = protein (g)
Protein to nitrogen: protein (g) ÷ 6.25 = nitrogen (g)

(Adapted from Mahan LK, Arlin MT. *Krause's food, nutrition, and diet therapy.* 8th ed. Philadelphia: WB Saunders, 1992.)

stressed individuals. Generally, 6.25 g of protein contain 1 g of nitrogen. This calculation is given in Display 29-1.

Vitamins and Minerals

Vitamin K is necessary for blood clotting and plays an essential role in the first stage of wound healing. Adequate amounts of vitamin C are needed to produce collagen. Vitamin A, zinc, copper, and iron are also essential for proper wound healing. The B-complex vitamins, as well as various minerals, are required for protein metabolism and energy demands associated with tissue repair.

Phosphorus and potassium are lost as a result of body tissue breakdown. Abnormal sodium and chloride metabolism may occur due to vomiting, diarrhea, drainage of fluid from the incision, renal failure, or other conditions that sometimes occur after surgery. Clinical signs and laboratory studies are used to monitor electrolyte status. Electrolyte imbalances are corrected with intravenous fluid and electrolyte therapy.

Excessive blood loss or malabsorption of iron may result in iron-deficiency anemia. A diet high in protein and ascorbic acid together with iron medication is prescribed. Transfusions are necessary if hemoglobin levels are severely reduced.

FEEDING METHODS

In most cases, the client will be able to resume oral feedings within 24 to 48 hours after the postoperative period when the gastrointestinal tract returns to normal. Bowel sounds and flatus usually indicate the passage of postoperative ileus. A clear liquid diet such as broth and gelatin is introduced and, if tolerated, the client may progress to full liquids or solid foods. Clear liquids are given initially because fluids pose fewer risks than solids, should aspiration occur as a result of vomiting. If adequate nutritional intake cannot be achieved by mouth, enteral tube feedings or parenteral intravenous feedings need to be initiated (see the section Alternative Feeding Methods). For clients with a condition that requires a modified diet, such as diabetes or cardiovascular disease, a diet appropriate to that condition is given.

Whatever feeding method is used, refeeding the client who has been severely malnourished for many days should be done slowly and the individual monitored for *"refeeding syndrome."* Rapid refeeding may cause an overload on the heart and blood vessels, gastrointestinal problems may occur, and low insulin levels may result in carbohydrate intolerance. In a severely malnourished person, the blood pressure and the amount of blood pumped by the heart per minute are lower than normal. Also, digestive enzymes may be restored more slowly after surgery.

Nutrition care of the client suffering from acute stress following surgery, critical illness, or severe injury should be carefully monitored to ensure adequate nutrition is provided. The client who was malnourished before the acute stress provides the greatest challenge. The increased metabolic needs and depressed immunity in this group increases the risk of other medical complications such as multiple organ system dysfunction or failure (MOSF). In this complication, decreased lung function or acute respiratory distress syndrome, acute renal failure, liver failure, or gastrointestinal ileus or stress ulcer may occur. Early identification of the high-risk client and early nutrition intervention should be a priority in critical care. Once the nutrition care plan has been established, ongoing evaluation of the adequacy of the nutrition care is essential.

DIET AFTER GASTROINTESTINAL SURGERY

GASTRECTOMY

A *gastrectomy* is an operation for the removal of all or part of the stomach. Diet therapy following a gastrectomy aims to avoid or minimize possible postoperative problems. After surgery and when peristalsis has returned, the client is given ice or small sips of water. Warm water may be better tolerated than ice or cold water by some individuals. As the ice or water is tolerated, the amount of fluid given is gradually increased. The client is then progressed to solid foods. The diet should be bland, easy to digest, and provided in six to eight small feedings per day. Each client's nutritional needs will differ depending on the extent of the surgery, the client's nutritional status, and individual tolerances to food.

DUMPING SYNDROME

Following a gastrectomy, the contents of the stomach tend to pass more rapidly than normal from the stomach into the small intestine. As undigested food enters the jejunum, the food mass draws water from the circulating blood volume to become diluted. As a result, blood volume drops. In addition, sugars are absorbed more quickly and overstimulate the release of insulin by the pancreas, causing blood sugar levels to drop. Consequently, the client experiences nausea, cramps, diarrhea, lightheadedness, and extreme weakness 10 to 15 minutes after eating. This is known as the *dumping syndrome.*

Nutritional management of the postgastrectomy client must be individualized. In general, the diet should be high in protein and moderate in fat. Simple carbohydrates should be limited and complex carbohydrates increased. Dry meals tend to be better tolerated. Fluids should be offered 30 to 60 minutes after the meal. Small frequent meals (six to eight per day) are recommended. Sources of the dietary fiber pectin, such as unsweetened applesauce, may help control diarrhea associated with dumping syndrome. If milk is not tolerated, lactose-free products are used. For some clients, fats may not be tolerated and steatorrhea results. For these clients, medium-chain triglycerides may be needed. Medium-chain triglycerides do not require digestion and are absorbed directly into portal circulation. The diet should be modified to meet the client's specific nutritional needs and tolerances. Many clients will be able to resume a normal diet; however, some clients may need to continue a modified diet.

INTESTINAL SURGERY

SMALL BOWEL RESECTION

Intestinal surgery or small bowel resection may be required as treatment for disease, disorder, or injury. It involves removal of a portion of the small or large intestine and causes loss of the surface through which nutrients are absorbed. The malnutrition and dehydration that results from the malabsorption and diarrhea is known as the *short-bowel syndrome.* Nutrition care and management of the client depends on the extent of the resection and if the absorptive surface of the remaining small bowel portion has adapted. Clients with 70% to 80% of their small bowel resectioned or who have only the duodenum will require intensive nutrition intervention. These clients will generally require long-term parenteral nutrition support.

After surgery, intravenous fluids and electrolytes are given to replace losses. The method of feeding should be determined by the extent of the surgery and the client's overall nutritional status. Clients with massive resectioning of the small bowel require parenteral nutrition support. Other clients may require enteral tube feedings, which are gradually progressed to oral feedings. Small oral feedings that are lactose and sucrose free may be better tolerated. New foods should be introduced slowly and small, frequent feedings are recommended. Clients who are able to receive oral intake are gradually tapered off from nutrition support. It is important to monitor the client closely to assure that adequate nutrition is being received during the transition period.

Clients who have had their ileum removed will require vitamin B_{12} injections. In addition, because bile salts are poorly absorbed, steatorrhea may be a problem and fat-soluble vitamins may need to be given. The nutrition care of the client who has undergone small bowel resection needs to be individually assessed for protein, energy, vitamin, mineral, and fluid needs.

OSTOMIES

Serious cases of ulcerative colitis, Crohn's disease, and diverticulitis may require surgical removal of the entire colon, rectum, and anus. As a result, a small opening, or *stoma,* is formed through the abdominal wall to the intestine. Digestive wastes are eliminated through this opening into an attached pouch. An *ileostomy* is performed when the entire colon, rectum, and anus must be removed. When the rectum and anus are removed, a *colostomy* is done.

Waste material from the ileum is fluid and drains almost continuously. There is considerable loss of fluid, sodium, potassium, and other nutrients. The client may also need a lowfat diet and fat-soluble vitamins. Attention to the fluid and electrolyte needs for the client with an ileostomy is important, especially in the beginning when the risk for dehydration is great. The client should be encouraged to consume liberal amounts of fluid, at least 2 qt/day. In addition, adequate sodium and potassium should be provided in the diet.

Once liquids are tolerated, the client can begin solid foods. A bland, low-residue diet is recommended, and new foods should be introduced slowly. As the surgical site heals, the fiber content of the diet may be advanced. However, certain foods may increase gas production and cause odors.

Foods that tend to cause these problems include cabbage, broccoli, dried beans, and onions. In addition, certain fiber-types may need to be avoided so that the stoma does not become blocked. Foods that tend to block the stoma include dried fruit, corn, popcorn, coconut, skins and seeds of fruits and vegetables, and nuts. Thorough chewing of food reduces the risk of blockage. The nutritional management of clients with ostomies should be individualized. If a food is not tolerated at first, it may be reintroduced later. For the client with a permanent ostomy, extra support and understanding from the health care team will help to relieve some of the fears and anger that may be associated with this problem.

RECTAL SURGERY

Clear liquids followed by a low-residue diet may be ordered for a short period following rectal surgery. Sometimes a low-residue, semisynthetic diet is used. Keeping residue to a minimum delays bowel movements until healing has begun. Later, the client can be instructed on a high-fiber diet with adequate fluid.

NUTRITION IN BURN TREATMENT

The rate of tissue breakdown and loss of body fat and other nutrient stores is faster in serious burns than in any other disease process. Most causes of burns are thermal, resulting from flames, explosions, hot liquids, or hot metals. Other causes of burns include electricity, chemicals, or radioactive energy. In the immediate hours following the injury, fluid replacement is essential to restore volume.

In the phase that follows, the body's metabolic rate is markedly elevated and the body is in a catabolic state. This period may last several days to weeks until the wound is covered with skin grafting or healing has begun. Providing adequate nutrition care for the burn client is of primary importance. Unless positive nitrogen balance is achieved, wound healing cannot occur, the risk for infection becomes greater, and protein-calorie malnutrition ensues.

Careful nutrition assessment is important. Body weight is the most often used parameter to assess nutritional status. Body weight is a good way to evaluate the effectiveness of nutrition care in the burn client. However, it must be interpreted initially with caution because of the fluid changes that occur. In addition, nutritional assessment may be difficult because serum albumin, prealbumin, and transferrin are all affected by burn injury.

The burn client's calorie needs are directly related to extent and depth of the injury and the individual's size. Energy needs may range from 3000 to 5000 kcal/day for adults. Several formulas are available to determine caloric needs and are based on the total body surface area burned. Generally, the "rule of nines" is used to determine the total percentage of body burn (Display 29-2). The Curreri formula provides a simple estimate of the adult burn client's energy needs:

$$(25 \text{ kcal} \times \text{kg of body weight}) + (40 \text{ kcal} \times \text{percent of total body surface area burned})$$

For example, the estimated energy need of a client weighing 160 lb who has a burn covering 23% of his body would be:

$$(25 \text{ kcal} \times 73) + (40 \text{ kcal} \times 23) = 1825 \text{ kcal} + 920 \text{ kcal} = 2745 \text{ kcal}$$

For burns over 50% of the total body surface area, use a constant of 50% for the percentage of the total body surface area to prevent overestimation of calories.

Protein needs are increased in the burn client. Protein is needed to replace nitrogen losses from the wound and urine and to promote wound healing. Daily protein needs may range from 1.5 to 3.0 g/kg of body weight. Fat should provide between 30% and 40% of the total calories. Additional vitamins and minerals are needed to promote wound healing and replace losses. Supplementation of vitamin C is required because of its role in wound healing. In addition, vitamin A and zinc may be

DISPLAY 29-2 "RULE OF NINES": DETERMINING TOTAL BURN SURFACE AREA

QUANTIFYING BURNS

To get a quick estimate of the total area of a burn, use the "rule of nines." It divides the body into multiples of nine, as shown here. To determine the total percentage of body burn, add the percentages listed for each area of the body.

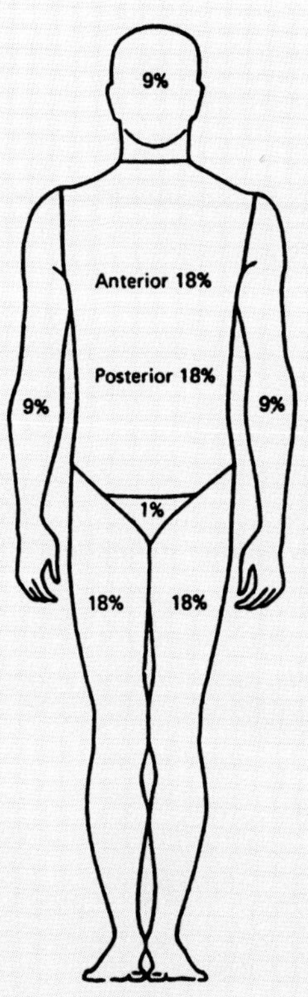

CHILD

BODY PART	% TOTAL BODY SURFACE
Arm	9
Head and neck	18
Anterior trunk	18
Posterior trunk	18
Leg	14

ADULT

BODY PART	% TOTAL BODY SURFACE
Arm	9
Head	9
Leg	18
Anterior trunk	18
Posterior trunk	18
Perineum	1

(Calistro, A. Burn care basics and beyond. RN 1993;56:3:29.)

necessary but should be monitored for toxicity. Folate is needed for protein synthesis. B-complex vitamins are needed to meet the demands of the high metabolic rate. During acute injury and infection, iron supplementation is not recommended. Potassium, phosphorus, and magnesium should be carefully monitored.

Initiation of nutrition support should begin as soon as possible. The method of feeding depends on several criteria, such as the ability of the client to take foods by mouth, gastrointestinal tract function, the extent and location of the burn, the client's age, the preburn nutritional status, and the client's overall medical condition. Clients who are able to eat should be provided with a high-calorie, high-protein diet. Milk shakes and supplemental beverages can help to provide the extra calories. For clients with extensive burns, nutritional requirements can seldom be met by oral feedings. In this case, a combination of oral diet with enteral tube feedings may be necessary. If there is injury to the mouth, face, or respiratory or gastrointestinal tract, total parenteral nutrition may be required.

ALTERNATIVE FEEDING METHODS

Under certain circumstances in which the client is unable or unwilling to eat adequate amounts of food, alternative feeding methods must be used to satisfy nutritional needs. Nutrition is necessary for the body's physiologic functions. When protein-calorie malnutrition exists, optimum healing and recovery from illness cannot proceed.

LIQUID SUPPLEMENTS

When a client's voluntary food intake meets at least two thirds of his or her needs, the balance usually can be satisfied using liquid supplements. These supplements may include common, milk-based drinks such as milk shakes and instant breakfast drinks, which are fortified with vitamins and minerals. Eggs, if added to drinks or formulas, should be pasteurized; raw eggs should be avoided because of the danger of salmonella food poisoning. Commercially produced liquid formulas are available that are nutritionally complete. Some of these formulas are milk-based and others are lactose free for people who are lactose intolerant. The commercial formulas provide 240 to 480 kcal per 8-oz portion. In quantities sufficient to cover energy needs, these formulas can satisfy the client's total nutritional needs. Formulas more often are used as supplements to add calories and nutrients to the food the client already is eating. Table 29-1 lists some liquid formulas.

When digestion and absorption of food are a problem, chemically defined or elemental formulas may be used. These formulas are described in the section Types of Formulas. Elemental diets are difficult to take orally because of their objectionable taste. Acceptance of even the good-tasting formulas sometimes becomes a problem, especially with long-term use. Alternating brands or flavors may help to relieve boredom. Flavor packets are also available.

Single-nutrient supplemental products called modules supply one nutrient that can be used to add extra protein, carbohydrate, or fat to the diet. These products can often be added to beverages, cooked foods such as mashed potatoes or pudding, or a commercial supplement.

ENTERAL TUBE FEEDINGS

Enteral tube feedings are liquified foods fed through a tube inserted into the stomach or small intestine. They are used when the gastrointestinal tract is functioning but the client is unwilling or unable to eat normally. For example, the client may be unable to chew or swallow following surgery of the mouth, neck, or esophagus; the gastrointestinal tract may be impaired so that nutrients are required in predigested forms; nutrient needs may be so great that the client cannot consume at least two thirds of his or her nutritional needs orally; or the client may refuse to eat, as in anorexia nervosa.

If the gastrointestinal tract is adequately functioning, enteral tube feedings rather than intrave-

TABLE 29-1 FORMULAS* USED TO ENHANCE CALORIE AND PROTEIN INTAKE

SUPPLEMENT	PROTEIN (G/1000 ML)	CONCENTRATION (KCAL/ML)	OSMOLALITY (MOSM/KG)	VOLUME TO MEET RDA†	MANUFACTURER
POLYMERIC					
Whole-protein, milk-based; form: powder mixed with lowfat milk					
Carnation Instant Breakfast	48	0.93	590	N/A	Clintec
Carnation Diet Instant Breakfast	63	0.70	500	N/A	Clintec
Forta Shake	58	1.2	N/A	N/A	Ross
Delmark Instant Breakfast	52	1.22	796	N/A	Sandoz
Whole-protein, lactose-free (<1.5 kcal/mL); form: liquid					
Nutren 1.0	40	1.0	340	1500	Clintec
Osmolite	35.2	1.06	300	1887	Ross
Attain	40	1.0	300	1250	Sherwood Medical
Isocal	32	1.06	300	1890	Mead Johnson
Ensure	35.2	1.06	470	1887	Ross
Whole-protein, lactose-free, with fiber; form: liquid					
Nutren 1.0 With Fiber	40	1.0	360	1500	Clintec
Sustacal With Fiber	43	1.06	480	1420	Mead Johnson
Ensure With Fiber	36	1.1	480	1530	Ross
Fiberlan	42	1.2	310	1250	Elan Pharmaceutical
Profiber	40	1.0	300	1500	Sherwood Medical
Blenderized (lactose-free‡); form: liquid					
Compleat Regulat	42.8	1.07	450	1500	Sandoz
Compleat Modified‡	42.8	1.07	300	1500	Sandoz
Vitaneed	40	1.0	300	1500	Sherwood Medical
Whole-protein, high-calorie, lactose-free (>1.5 kcal/mL); form: liquid					
Nutren 1.5	40	1.5	410–590	1000	Clintec
Nutren 2.0	40	2.0	710	750	Clintec
Ensure Plus	36.6	1.5	690	1420	Ross Laboratories
Magnacal	35	2.0	590	1000	Sherwood Medical
Comply	40	1.5	410	1000	Sherwood Medical
Sustacal HC	41	1.5	650	1200	Mead Johnson
Whole-protein, high-nitrogen, lactose-free; form: liquid (powder‡)					
Isocal HN	42	1.06	300	1179	Mead Johnson
Ensure HN	42	1.06	470	1321	Ross
Osmolite HN	42	1.06	300	1321	Ross
Promote	62.4	1.0	350	1250	Ross
Isotein HN‡	57	1.19	300	1770	Sandoz
Whole-protein, high-calorie, high-nitrogen, lactose-free; form: liquid					
Isocal HCN	38	2.0	690	1000	Mead Johnson
Ensure Plus HN	41.7	1.5	650	947	Ross
Two Cal HN	41.7	2.0	690	950	Ross
Trauma Cal	55	1.5	490	2000	Mead Johnson

(Continued)

TABLE 29-1 *(continued)*

Supplement	Protein (g/1000 ml)	Concentration (kcal/ml)	Osmolality (mOsm/kg)	Volume to Meet RDA†	Manufacturer
OLIGOMERIC/MONOMERIC					
Partially and Fully Hydrolyzed Formulas; form: liquid (powder‡)					
Peptamen Diet	40	1.0	270	1500	Clintec
Reabilan	31.5	1.0	350	3000	Elan Pharmaceutical
Vital HN	41.7	1.0	500	1500	Ross
Criticare HN	36	1.06	650	1890	Mead Johnson
Tolerex‡	21	1.0	550	3160	Sandoz
Vivonex TEN‡	38	1.0	630	2000	Sandoz
SPECIALLY DESIGNED, DISEASE-SPECIFIC					
Form: liquid (powder‡)					
Portagen‡ (fat malabsorption)	41	1.0	N/A	N/A	Mead Johnson
Stresstein‡ (critical care)	58	1.2	910	2000	Sandoz
Travasorb Renal‡ (renal failure)	17	1.35	590	N/A	Clintec
Amin Aid‡ (renal failure)	10	2.0	700	N/A	Kendall McGaw
Nepro (renal)	34.9	2.0	635	947	Ross
Hepatic Aid II (liver disease)	38	1.2	560	N/A	Kendall McGaw
Travasorb Hepatic Diet (liver disease)	26.7	1.1	600	2060	Clintec
Nutrivent (pulmonary)	45	1.5	450	1000	Clintec
Pulmocare (pulmonary)	41.7	1.5	465	947	Ross
Glucerna (abnormal glucose tolerance)	41.8	1.0	375	1422	Ross

MODULAR PRODUCTS AVAILABLE

Protein	Carbohydrate	Fat
Promod (Ross Laboratories)	Moducal (Mead Johnson)	MCT Oil (Mead Johnson)
Nutrisource Protein (Sandoz)	Polycose (Ross Laboratories)	Microlipid (Sherwood Medical)
Casec (Mead Johnson)	Sumacal (Sherwood Medical)	Nutrisource MCT (Corpak)
Nutrisource Amino Acids (Sandoz)		

NA, not applicable.

* Products may vary. Consult manufacturer for changes in formulary and new product lines.

† Volume (ml) to meet 100% of the recommended dietary allowance (RDA) for vitamin and minerals.

‡ Powder products mixed with water following package directions.

(Adapted from: Clintec. Enteral product reference guide. Deerfield, IL: Clintec Nutrition Company, 1992; Mahan LK, Arlin MT. Krause's food, nutrition and diet therapy. 8th ed. Philadelphia: WB Saunders, 1992.)

nous therapy is the method of choice. Enteral tube feedings help to maintain the integrity of the gastrointestinal tract. Using the GI tract assures that absorption and the use of nutrients continues in the normal way. In addition, enteral tube feedings also provides the GI tract stimulation needed to protect against *bacterial translocation.* In this process, microbes cross the protective surface of the intestine and enter the lymphatic system, where they are taken up into the general body circulation. When nutrients are introduced directly into the bloodstream, as in parenteral nutrition, disorders of protein, carbohydrate, and fat metabolism or infection are more likely to occur. Enteral tube feedings have lower associated risks, are more economical, and are easier to administer than parenteral nutrition. In addition, enteral tube feedings do not require a trained maintenance team. Enteral tube feedings should not be used when there is a mechanical obstruction or malfunction of the gastrointestinal tract, prolonged ileus, or when severe diarrhea or vomiting occurs.

Careful planning is needed to assure that the client receives his or her required nutrient needs daily. A common problem for the hospitalized client is the frequent interruption of the feeding for diagnostic tests or other procedures. Clients at high risk for malnutrition should be monitored closely to avoid this problem.

TYPES OF FORMULAS

The formula chosen depends on the client's needs. These needs include the client's ability to digest and absorb nutrients, placement of the tube (stomach versus intestine) and the feeding equipment needed, nutrient requirements, any fluid or electrolyte restrictions, and individual intolerances (e.g., allergies or lactose intolerance).

A number of commercial formulas are available. Products that contain nutrients in their natural, undigested form are referred to as *polymeric (or intact) formulas.* Standard, fiber-containing, blenderized, concentrated, and high-nitrogen commercial formulas fall into this category. Standard polymeric formulas are either milk based or lactose free. Fiber-containing formulas contain natural food sources of fiber, are generally lactose free, and help to prevent diarrhea or constipation that may occur with tube feedings. Commercial blenderized formulas contain food normally included in the diet, such as meats, vegetables, fruits, nonfat dry milk, and pasteurized eggs. Concentrated formulas are calorically dense providing 1.5–2.0 kcal/mL instead of the 1.0–1.2 kcal/mL in standard formulas. When the client's caloric needs are high, or fluid must be restricted, concentrated formulas are used. High-nitrogen formulas are higher in protein, providing at least 15% of the total calories of the formula as protein. Whatever type of polymeric formula selected, the client must be able to digest and absorb nutrients adequately.

Polymeric formulas have a moderate-to-low osmolality, except for the concentrated and high-protein formulas. Osmolality is important in selecting a product. *Osmolality,* expressed in terms of milliosmoles per kilogram (mOsm/kg), refers to the number of particles per kilogram of solution. The greater the number of particles in solution and the greater their size, the greater the pressure exerted by the fluid. Normal plasma osmolality is approximately 300 mOsm/kg. In general, polymeric formulas tend to have osmolalities approximately the same as plasma. These products may also be referred to as *isotonic formulas.*

A second type of formula used is the *monomeric formula,* which is partially or fully hydrolyzed or predigested. Oligomeric/monomeric formulas contain protein, fat, and carbohydrate that have been reduced to a simpler chemical form to make them more easily digested. *Elemental formulas* contain protein, fat, and carbohydrate in their basic units (amino acids, fatty acid, and simple sugars) and do not require digestion. Because elemental formulas are fully hydrolyzed, they are absorbed directly without pancreatic enzymes. Many of these products use medium-chain triglycerides as the fat source. Predigested formulas are useful for people who have gastrointestinal conditions that limit their ability to digest food or who have a reduced area for nutrient absorption. These formulas also leave little residue and may be used to rest the large intestine. Oligomeric/monomeric formulas have higher osmolalities and are more expensive than most polymeric formulas.

Another group of formulas includes specialty or disease-specific products. These products are formulated for nutritional management of diabetes, pulmonary, renal, or immune-compromised diseases. The modular formulas mentioned earlier provide a single nutrient. Modular formulas can be added to other formulas to modify the protein, fat, or carbohydrate ratio of the final product.

Standard commercial tube feeding formulas supply about 1 kcal/mL; thus, 1500 mL of formula provides 1500 kcal. Concentrated formulas provide 1.5 to 2.0 kcal/mL. Most of the formulas provide the daily RDAs for vitamins and minerals when a specific amount of formula is given. When using less than the specified amount, or when specialty or modular formulas are used, the client's vitamin/mineral needs must be considered.

Health care facilities use commercial formulas because they are more convenient than having to prepare the feedings and they provide savings in labor, improved quality control, and the reduced risk for contamination. Although commercial products are prepared under sterile conditions, once the product is open, proper storage and handling is essential to prevent contamination. Policies regarding the length of time a formula is to be held or left to hang should be enforced.

FEEDING SITES

Usually, a nasoenteric tube is used to administer tube feedings. Nasoenteric tube feedings are used for short-term feeding generally 3 to 4 weeks. The tube is passed into the nose, down the throat, and into the stomach or small intestine. Nasogastric tube placement should be considered for the client who is medically stable and not at risk for aspiration, esophageal reflux, or gastric ileus. In critically ill clients, the incidence of gastroparesis (lack of movement in the stomach) and aspiration is higher. For these clients, the tube should be placed past the pylorus into the duodenum or jejunum. Figure 29-1 illustrates common nasoen-

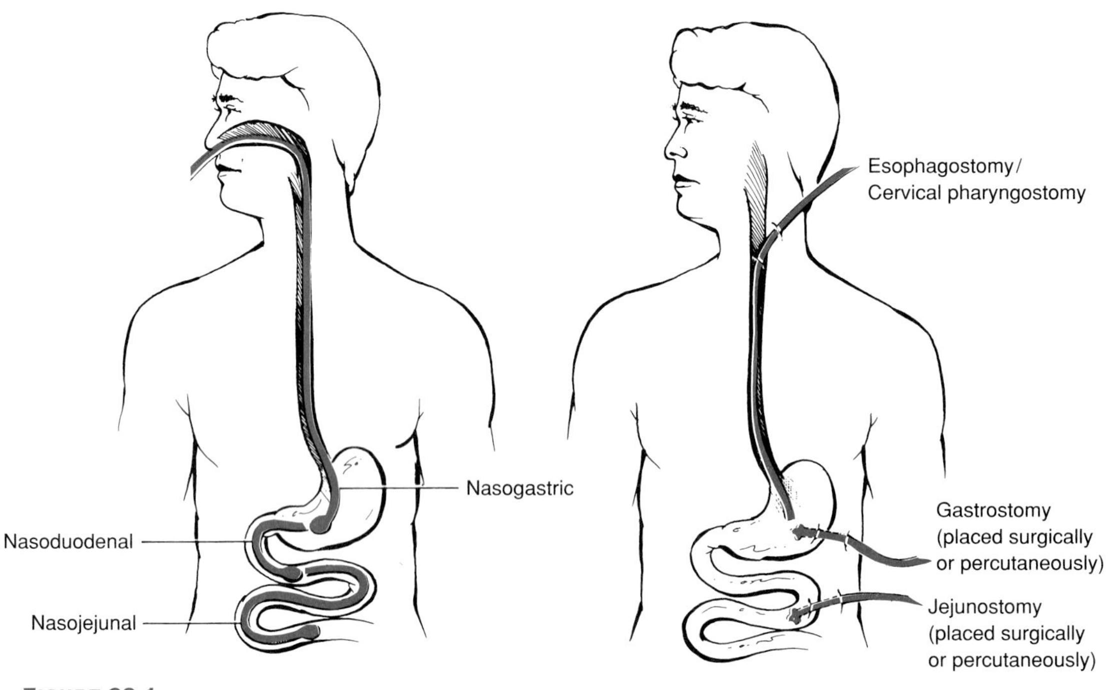

FIGURE 29-1

Common access sites for enteral tube feedings.

tric feeding sites: nasogastric, nasoduodenal, and nasojejunal.

Nasoenteric tubes are made of soft nonreactive material such as silicone rubber or polyurethane, and are reasonably well tolerated for short-term feeding. The diameter of the feeding tube is described in French units (Fr). Each unit is 0.33 mm. Most nasoenteric tubes are 8 to 12 Fr. The tips of the feeding tubes may be weighted to aid in tube placement and help prevent dislodgment. The placement of the feeding tube is checked by abdominal x-rays before feedings are begun. Figure 29-2 illustrates nasoenteral tube insertion.

In clients who require tube feedings for more than 4 weeks, stomas are created surgically to allow the tube to enter. Tube enterosotomies in which the tube is brought through the intestinal wall are preferred for long-term use. Tube enterostomies are used to avoid irritation of the mucous membranes of the nose and throat or when disease or surgery of the mouth, throat, or neck makes it impossible for a tube to be passed through this area. Conventional tube enterostomies are surgically placed under general anesthesia. The different types of enterostomies include a cervical pharyngostomy, esophagostomy, gastrostomy, and a jejunostomy. Figure 29-1 illustrates these tube placements.

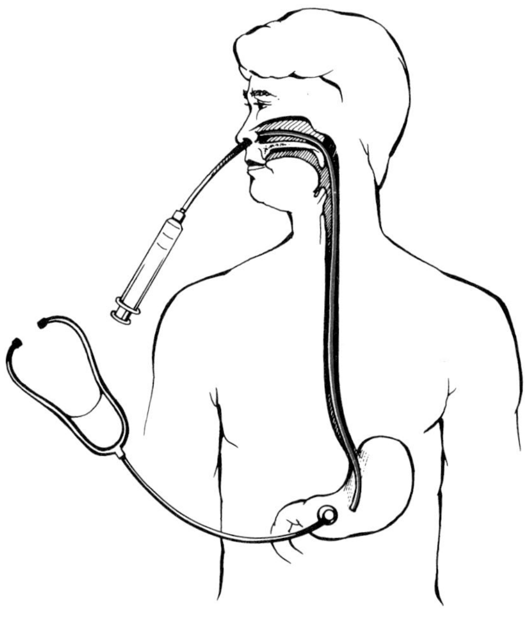

FIGURE 29-2

Technique of nasoenteral catheter insertion.

An alternative to the traditional gastrostomy or jejunostomy is the percutaneous endoscopic gastrostomy (PEG) or percutaneous endoscopic jejunostomy (PEJ). These are generally considered to be nonsurgical procedures performed under local anesthesia. A PEG is a feeding tube that is placed percutaneously (through the skin) into the stomach using an endoscope for guidance. The tube is placed through the mouth into the stomach and pulled out through the abdominal wall. The tube is then secured in place by a rubber bumper or a balloon catheter. Figure 29-3 illustrates PEG insertion. Clients with abdominal obesity may not be suitable for a PEG because of the difficulty in making the percutaneous puncture. A PEJ is a modification of the PEG in which a small feeding tube is passed into the small bowel.

A jejunostomy should be used as the feeding site in clients who have had gastroesophageal or abdominal surgery and for those at risk for aspiration. Jejunostomies are generally placed during intestinal surgery. The advantage of feeding into the jejunum is to begin early enteral feedings. Jejunal recovery from paralytic ileus associated with abdominal surgery occurs more quickly than in the upper gastrointestinal tract. Another technique used is the needle catheter jejunostomy (NCJ) in which a fine catheter or tube is placed into the jejunum through a large-bore needle. Because the diameter of these tubes is small (6 Fr or less) for feeding, a low-viscosity formula should be used to prevent clogging.

Advanced feeding placement techniques such as the NCJ and feeding formulas now make it possible to give enteral nutrition support early postoperatively or within 36 hours to the severely stressed client suffering from trauma, shock, or sepsis, or the client with malnutrition. Early enteral nutritional support appears to have many advantages in helping to preserve lean body mass, prevent gastric atrophy, maintain immune function, and promote wound healing. It also reduces the need for more costly parenteral nutrition support.

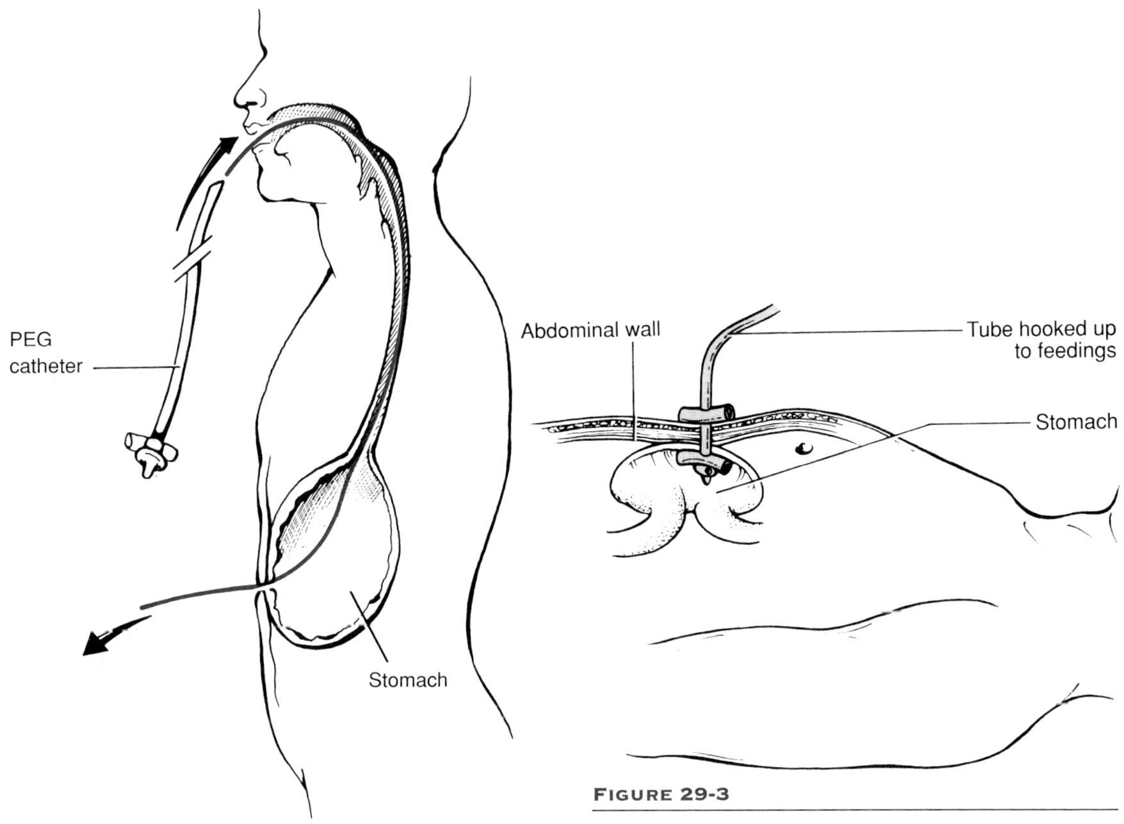

FIGURE 29-3

Percutaneous endoscopic gastrostomy (PEG).

DELIVERY METHODS

Continuous drip and intermittent feedings are two commonly used feeding delivery methods. Continuous feeding provides the formula continuously over a 16- to 24-hour period. Intermittent feeding involves giving a prescribed amount of formula for short periods (15 to 30 minutes) at regular intervals throughout the day (e.g., every 1 or 2 hours). Both methods can be administered by gravity drip or by an enteral infusion pump to control flow rate. Another method, although not as commonly used, is bolus feedings. Bolus feedings involve giving 250 to 350 mL of formula six times per day with about 3 hours between feedings. Bolus feedings should only be given by the nasogastric route. Checking gastric residuals (amount of formula left in the stomach) is especially important when bolus feedings are given.

For critically ill clients, continuous feeding is preferred. It is better tolerated, results in smaller residuals, reduces the possibility for aspiration, decreases stool frequency, and helps one achieve nutritional goals more quickly. Continuous drip feedings are preferred when feedings are introduced past the pylorus into the duodenum or jejunum.

The concentration of the formula and the rate of infusion depend on the location of the feeding tube, osmolality of the formula, and client's nutritional status. In general, formulas with osmolalities 300 to 500 mOsm/kg can be at initiated full strength with the volume increased slowly. Hyperosmolar formulas greater than 500 mOsm/kg tend to draw water from the circulatory system to dilute the solution in the intestinal tract. As a result, the client may become weak, feel distended, and have diarrhea. Hyperosmolar formulas should be initiated at half strength and the volume gradually increased. Volume and concentration should not be increased simultaneously. Malnourished clients should be monitored closely when a hyperosmolar formula is being given.

MONITORING

Many products today come in ready-to-use prefilled bags. For formulas that need to be poured into a feeding bag or a container, ensure that all equipment is clean. Do not add fresh formula to formula already hanging. Feeding formulas provide an excellent environment for bacterial growth, which may lead to gastrointestinal infection. Furthermore, change administration tubing and the feeding bag daily.

The client must receive adequate fluid for the waste products of protein metabolism to be excreted in the urine. Fluid intake must be observed especially carefully in elderly people. Close supervision and careful recording of protein intake and fluid intake and output are always necessary. Adults generally require 1 ml of water per calorie fed. Fluid needs should be individualized.

The nutrition support team should monitor the client carefully to see that nutritional goals are being met and to treat complications, if they develop. The client usually is weighed daily. Fluid and electrolytes are checked, as are other indicators of nutritional status such as serum albumin and transferrin levels, and total lymphocyte count. Although not routinely performed, skinfold thickness and midarm muscular circumference can be useful assessment parameters (see Chapter 2). The dietitian conducts calorie counts to determine what percentage of the total calories ordered are actually consumed.

COMPLICATIONS

Gastrointestinal problems are the most common problems associated with tube feedings. Delayed emptying of the stomach is common in critically ill clients; medication that speeds movement in the stomach may be prescribed. Diarrhea, another common complication, may be caused by a hyperosmolar formula, antibiotics or other medications, or bacterial infection. The treatment depends on the cause. Aspiration is a serious complication. Pneumonia can develop if stomach contents enter the lungs. Placing the feeding tube in the intestine instead of the stomach, elevating the head of the bed to 30 degrees, and periodically measuring gastric residual (so that excessive amounts do not accumulate) are ways of preventing aspiration. Metabolic complications such as fluid and electrolyte imbalance are easily corrected if the client is carefully monitored. Mechanical problems can result from irritation of the gastrointestinal tract by the tube itself or from a clogged tube.

Other problems involve client acceptance. Many people object to the insertion of a feeding tube. Once the tube is inserted, a hostile or disoriented client may pull it out. Sometimes the tube is dislodged only partially, so the displacement may be hard to detect. As a result, aspiration and tissue damage may occur, and nutrients may be lost. Placement of the tube must be checked before each feeding. The reasons for the tube feeding should be explained thoroughly to the client and his or her family before the tube is inserted.

PARENTERAL NUTRITION

Parenteral nutrition (PN) is the term used when nutrients are given intravenously. The term *total parenteral nutrition (TPN)* is used when the client's total nutrient needs are being given intravenously. These solutions are usually hyperosmolar and must be centrally infused into the superior vena cava. TPN may also be referred to as *central parenteral nutrition (CPN)*; the terms *TPN* and *CPN* are often used interchangeably. PN administered peripherally into a vein is known as *peripheral parenteral nutrition (PPN)*.

PN involves the delivery of water, dextrose (glucose), amino acids, fats, vitamins, minerals, and electrolytes directly into systemic circulation or the vein. PN is indicated if the gastrointestinal tract cannot be used or if its use is contraindicated, if enteral feedings are inadequate, in cases of severe malnutrition with a malfunctioning gut, or if the client is in an extreme state of catabolism and use of the gastrointestinal tract will be delayed more than 5 to 7 days. PN may be used as the only method of feeding or in combination with enteral feedings.

Successful PN requires a highly skilled nutrition support team, which may include a physician, nurse specialist, registered dietitian, pharmacist, social worker, and physical therapist. A clinical nutrition specialist and the physician determine and monitor the composition of the nutrient solutions. A trained pharmacist prepares and specially trained nurses administer the solutions.

If the client on PN is not receiving anything by mouth, the mucous lining of the oral cavity may become dry and irritated. Good oral care is a comfort to the client. The mouth should be moistened and cleansed, and the teeth brushed regularly.

PERIPHERAL PARENTERAL NUTRITION

For clients whose nutritional needs are moderate and who are unable to consume adequate calories by the enteral route (oral or tube feeding), or if a central vein catheter is not recommended, PPN may be implemented. PPN is considered as a short-term (less than 2 weeks) method of PN. In PPN, partial or TPN support may be delivered by means of a needle inserted into a peripheral vein on the arm or the hand. PPN solutions may provide approximately 1800 to 2000 kcal/day when fat is used. The concentration of dextrose in PPN solutions is limited because the risk of phlebitis to the peripheral vein. In general, the final solution of dextrose should be no more than 10%. A dextrose–amino acid solution may be co-infused with a fat emulsion, or a total nutrient mixture (three-in-one) system can be used. PPN should not be used on clients who have poor veins resulting from severe malnutrition or disease.

CENTRAL PARENTERAL NUTRITION

For clients who are severely malnourished or who have high nutritional needs, and for those who require intravenous feedings for extended periods, TPN must be administered into a larger central vein. Insertion of the central vein line is a surgical procedure. It can be performed at the bedside under strict sterile conditions. The catheter is inserted into the subclavian or jugular vein and passed into the superior vena cava. This vein is selected because the TPN solution is hypertonic (high osmolarity) and must enter the body in a region of high blood flow so that the solution is rapidly diluted.

Long-term access is possible when the catheter is tunneled subcutaneously away from the insertion, making home parenteral nutrition (HPN) a more common practice today. Total nutrient mixtures are frequently used in home parenteral nutrition.

COMPLICATIONS

PN sometimes is associated with serious complications related to insertion of the catheter, infection, and metabolic problems. Infections, either bacterial or fungal, may occur at the catheter insertion site. The infection may enter the bloodstream, causing sepsis, a serious blood infection. The PN solution is an excellent medium for the growth of bacteria and fungi. It should be refrigerated until used and should not be hung for more than 24 hours. Metabolic complications include abnormal electrolyte levels and elevated liver enzymes. Sometimes the problems are technical, as when the catheter tips puncture the blood vessel wall. Blood clots may form, or air, fluid, or blood may accumulate in the chest cavity. Improvements in PN solutions and administration have helped to reduce the risk of complications.

TRANSITIONAL FEEDING

Once the need for enteral tube feedings or intravenous nutrition diminishes, the client is gradually transferred to an oral diet. As oral intake increases, the alternative feeding method is reduced. The client should be taking adequate amounts of food by mouth before the tube feeding or intravenous nutrition is totally discontinued. Sometimes a client on PN makes the transition to tube feeding and then to oral feeding. Tube feedings and PN can be continued at home, if necessary.

PROVIDING PSYCHOLOGICAL SUPPORT

Clients who are tube fed or who receive PN usually are critically ill and often are depressed and frightened. It is not difficult to imagine the stress created by the feeding method itself; in addition, the client is denied the pleasures and the social and emotional satisfactions associated with eating.

Correct techniques, procedures, and formulas must be followed. Good care, however, goes beyond these mechanical details and considers the client's psychological needs as well. Showing kindness, understanding, concern, and encouragement also is part of the health team's responsibility.

KEYS TO PRACTICAL APPLICATION

See that diet orders are carried out accurately before surgery. Feeding clients when they should not be fed or providing the wrong diet may require a delay in surgery.

Check trays carefully. Serious complications can result if the client receives the wrong diet after surgery.

Follow instructions accurately when feeding someone who has been undernourished for many days. The severely undernourished body cannot adjust immediately to a normal amount of food. Small amounts are given at first and increased gradually.

Use sanitary techniques when preparing or handling tube feedings. Be sure that the equipment used is the proper equipment needed and is clean. Do add fresh formula to formula that has been hanging.

Provide good oral care for the client who is not being fed by mouth.

Record food and fluid intake accurately. This information is necessary to evaluate the adequacy of nutrition care.

Show understanding and encourage the client who is receiving enteral tube feedings or PN. These extreme feeding methods are stressful for clients.

KEY IDEAS

The client who is well nourished before surgery has a great advantage; when possible, the nutritional status of a poorly nourished person is improved before surgery. Weight loss may be required of the obese client.

In preparation for surgery, no food is given after the evening meal and no fluids are given after midnight of the day before surgery. This timing may be adjusted when surgery is scheduled late in the day.

The body response to surgery or injury is characterized by three phases: breakdown, recovery, and fat gain.

Maintaining fluid and electrolyte balance is the first priority after surgery.

Following surgery and acute injury, the need for calories, protein, vitamins, and minerals is much higher than normal.

Body fat reserves are the primary source of energy in the early postoperative period. If calories remain inadequate for long periods, protein is used for energy rather than for repair and rebuilding of tissue. All aspects of recovery are hindered as a result.

In most cases, food may be taken by mouth 1 to 4 days after surgery; however, some situations require enteral tube feedings or PN.

Refeeding of the client who has been severely undernourished for many days should be carried out gradually and cautiously to avoid cardiovascular overload and gastrointestinal problems.

Feeding methods after surgery should be individualized. Intravenous solutions of 5% and 10% dextrose are used primarily to restore fluid balance.

Liquid supplements are given to boost the nutrient intake of clients who are able to consume at least two thirds of their nutrient needs voluntarily.

When an alternative feeding method is required, enteral tube feeding is preferred over PN.

The feeding formula chosen depends on the client's needs. There are two general types of formulas: polymeric (intact) formulas, which contain nutrients in their natural, undigested form, and oligomeric/monomeric (hydrolyzed) formulas, which contain protein, fat, and carbohydrate that have been reduced to a simpler chemical form to make them more easily digested. Elemental formulas, a type of hydrolyzed formula, contain protein, fat, and carbohydrate in their basic forms and require no digestion.

Hydrolyzed formulas require little digestion and leave practically no residue; they are used when there is poor absorption or to rest the large intestine. They may be given by tube or by mouth.

Hydrolyzed formulas have higher osmolalities. Hyperosmolar formulas greater than 500 mOsm/kg should be started at half strength.

Standard commercial formulas supply about 1 kcal/mL; more concentrated formulas provided 1.5 or 2 kcal/mL.

The feeding sites for tube feedings are nasogastric for short-term use and gastrostomy or jejunostomy (openings at points along the intestinal tract) for long-term use. Other methods include percutaneous endoscopic gastrostomy (PEG), percutaneous endoscopic jejunostomy (PEJ), and needle catheter jejunostomy (NCJ).

The three methods for tube feeding frequency are continuous feeding, intermittent feeding, and bolus administration.

Aspiration, pneumonia, and gastrointestinal problems are the most serious complications of enteral tube feedings.

Measures that can help prevent aspiration include placing the feeding tube in the small intestine instead of the stomach, elevating the head of the bed to 30 degrees, measuring gastric residuals periodically, and using the continuous-drip method of delivery.

TPN refers to intravenous feedings that meet the client's total nutritional needs. It can be provided by peripheral vein if the use is short term and nutritional needs are moderate; for long-term use and when nutritional needs are great, central vein TPN is used.

Serious infection at the catheter insertion site, which may enter the bloodstream, is the most serious complication of PN.

Careful monitoring of enteral tube feeding and PN is necessary to see that nutritional needs are being met and to uncover complications as soon as possible.

Clients receiving large quantities of protein need adequate fluid intake so that waste products of protein metabolism can be excreted properly.

Good oral care for the client fed by tube or intravenously is important. Without such care, the mouth becomes dry and irritated.

Clients being fed by extreme measures such as enteral tube feedings or PN are in great need of psychological support—kindness, understanding, and encouragement.

The amounts of food and fluid consumed either by mouth or by tube or PN following surgery or severe injury should be carefully monitored and recorded.

The postgastrectomy diet is designed to counteract development of the dumping syndrome. A bland, easy-to-digest diet, offered in six to eight small feedings is better tolerated. Fluids should be consumed between meals.

Removal of a large portion of the small intestine entails great loss of the intestinal surface, through which nutrients are absorbed, making good nutritional status difficult to maintain. The client is fed by PN or by tube for an extended period following surgery.

Nutritional needs of clients with severe burns are far above normal and are rarely met by oral feeding alone. Enteral tube feedings or PN is necessary.

KEYS TO LEARNING

STUDY–DISCUSSION QUESTIONS

1. Review the foods served on the clear liquid diet and on the full liquid diet (see Chapter 3). Why is the first postoperative feeding a clear liquid diet? Why is it important for the clear liquid diet to be advanced? Why is it so important that the client receive the correct diet after surgery?
2. Meeting the clients' nutritional needs is extremely important to their recovery. Why, then, should refeeding of the severely malnourished client be started slowly and cautiously?
3. What factors are involved in choosing a formula for a client who will receive enteral tube feedings? What adverse reactions may a client experience from tube feedings? How can these be prevented? Discuss the importance of adequate water intake.
4. Why are raw eggs not used in tube feedings or supplemental beverages such as eggnogs? What is used in their place?
5. What commercial supplemental liquids are used most frequently in your hospital? Why have these particular products been chosen? What types of supplemental beverages are prepared in the hospital?
6. What is the nutrition assessment protocol at your hospital for clients who are at high risk for malnutrition.
7. How many clients are presently on enteral tube feedings in your hospital? What commercial formulas are being used in each of these cases? Why have these particular products been chosen?
8. What are the sanitary procedures for the handling and administration of enteral tube feedings in your hospital?
9. Present to the class a case study of the nutrition care of a tube-fed client or a client on PN. Include in your report the following information: the reason the client is receiving this alternative feeding method (i.e., diagnosis and current medical condition) the kind of feeding given, the nutritional content (protein, fat, carbohydrate, and calories) of the client's average daily intake, the average daily fluid intake, any adverse reactions, and the client's psychological outlook. Evaluate your case based on information in this chapter. Identify problems and give recommendations, if appropriate.
10. Describe the symptoms of the dumping syndrome. Why do they occur? What changes in diet help alleviate the problem?
11. What is short-bowel syndrome? What type of enteral feeding formula would you select for a client with this syndrome? Why?
12. Discuss the extraordinary nutritional needs of severely burned clients. What are the methods of providing nutrients for these clients? Estimate the caloric needs of an adult female client weighing 135 lb who has burns covering one leg and the posterior trunk using the Curreri formula and rule of nines in the section Nutrition In Burn Treatment.

BIBLIOGRAPHY

BOOKS AND PAMPHLETS

American Dietetic Association. Handbook of clinical dietetics. 2nd ed. New Haven, CT: Yale University Press, 1992.

Chicago Dietetic Association and South Suburban Dietetic Association. Manual of clinical dietetics. 4th ed. Chicago: The American Dietetic Association, 1992.

Clintec. Enteral product reference guide. Deerfield, IL: Clintec Nutrition Co., 1992.

Fischer J. Total parenteral nutrition. 2nd ed. Boston: Little, Brown, 1991.

Ideno K. Enteral nutrition. In: Gottschlich M, Materese L, Shronts E. Eds. Nutrition support dietetic core curriculum. 2nd ed. Silver Spring, MD: ASPEN Publishers, 1993:71–104.

Jeejeebhoy KN. Intestinal disorders. In: Shils ME, Olson JA, Shike M. Eds. Modern nutrition in health and disease. Vol. 2. 8th ed. Philadelphia: Lea and Febiger, 1994:1036–1042.

Mahan LK, Arlin MT. Krause's food, nutrition and diet therapy. 8th ed. Philadelphia: WB Saunders, 1992.

Page C, Hardin T, Melnik G. Nutritional assessment and support: a primer. 2nd ed. Baltimore: Williams & Wilkins, 1994.

Rosenberg I, Mason JB. Inflammatory bowel disease. In: Shils ME, Olson JA, Shike M. Eds. Modern nutrition in health and disease. Vol. 2. 8th ed. Philadelphia: Lea and Febiger, 1994:1043–1059.

Shike M. Enteral feeding. In: Shils ME, Olson JA, Shike M. Eds. Modern nutrition in health and disease. Vol. 2. 8th ed. Philadelphia: Lea and Febiger, 1994:1417–1429.

Shils M. Parenteral nutrition. In: Shils ME, Olson JA, Shike M. Eds. Modern nutrition in health and disease. Vol. 2. 8th ed. Philadelphia: Lea and Febiger, 1994:1430–1458.

Skipper A, Marian M. Parenteral nutrition. In: Gottschlich M, Materese L, Shronts E. Eds. Nutrition support dietetic core curriculum. 2nd ed. Silver Spring, MD: ASPEN Publishers, 1993:105–123.

PERIODICALS

Alexander JW. Early enteral nutrition. RD: Essential News for Dietitians from Sandoz Nutrition 1994;14:2:4.

Bloch A. Creative enteral access in the cancer patient. Support Line (Dietitians in Nutrition Support Newsletter) 1994;16:4:1.

Calistro A. Burn care basics and beyond. RN 1993;56:3:26.

Charney P, Martindale R. Early enteral nutrition support in metabolic stress. RD: Essential News for Dietitians from Sandoz Nutrition 1994;14:2:1.

Charney P, Martindale R. Early postoperative enteral nutrition: feasibility and recommendations. RD: Essential News for Dietitians from Sandoz Nutrition 1993;13:1:1, 4.

Carroll P. Care of the burn patient. Part I: metabolic and nutritional considerations. Top Clin Nutr 1992;7:2:51.

Carroll P. Care of the burn patient. Part II: guidelines for nutritional intervention. Top Clin Nutr 1992;7:2:60.

Curreri P. Assessing the nutritional needs for the burned patient. J Trauma 1990;30:12(suppl): 20.

Eisenberg P. Gastrostomy and jejunostomy tubes. RN 1994;57:11:54.

Juskelis D. Starvation in patients: guidelines for refeeding. RD: Essential News for Dietitians from Sandoz Nutrition 1991;11:2:1.

Konstantinides N, Lehmann S. The impact of nutrition on wound healing. Crit Care Nurs 1993;13:5:33.

McCrae J, O'Shea R, Udine L. Parenteral nutrition: hospital to home. J Am Diet Assoc 1993;93:664.

Posa P. Nutrition support of the critically ill patient: bedside strategies for successful patient outcomes. Crit Care Nurs Quarterly 1994;16:4:61.

CHAPTER

30

Nutrition Therapy in Cancer, AIDS, and Other Special Problems

KEY TERMS

allergen any substance that causes an allergic reaction

allergy adverse reaction of body tissue to specific substances that are harmless to most people

anaphylactic relating to severe hypersensitivity (or allergic reaction)

antibodies protein substances produced by the body in response to the presence of an allergen

cachexia complex syndrome of anorexia, biochemical abnormalities, malnutrition, and wasting occurring in advanced stages of disease

corticosteroids steroids produced by the adrenal gland

encephalopathy disease of the brain

endometrial relating to mucous membrane lining the uterus

immunologic pertaining to immunity; resistant to harmful agents or organisms

malignant tending to grow worse, resist treatment, and result in death

metastasis transfer of disease from one part of the body to another not directly connected to it; spread is by the lymph or bloodstream

mucositis inflammation of the mucous membranes of the oral mucosa

palliative alleviating suffering; relieving symptoms of a disease without curing it

prognosis prediction of the disease outcome

remission temporary lessening or absence of disease symptoms

temporomandibular joint joint between the temporal (temple) and mandibular (jaw) bones

OBJECTIVES

After completing this chapter, the student will be able to:

1. Describe cancer cachexia and discuss the factors that affect the cancer client's ability to eat.
2. List ways to increase the protein and calorie content of the diet to help meet the nutritional needs of clients with wasting diseases.
3. Discuss the dietary recommendations for reducing risk factors associated with cancer.
4. Identify the nutritional complications associated with acquired immunodeficiency syndrome and describe how to modify the diet or meals for clients with oral inflammation, diarrhea, or fat malabsorption.
5. Describe how nutrition plays a role in the care of the client with chronic obstructive pulmonary disease and tuberculosis.
6. Define *food allergy* and list the foods most often associated with severe anaphylactic reactions.
7. Using food package labels, identify hidden forms of milk, egg, corn, and legumes commonly used in the manufacturing of food products.
8. Describe the "on–off" phenomenon of Parkinson's

disease and how diet plays a role in the medical management of this disease.

9. Describe the nutritional concerns and considerations for clients with severe arthritis.
10. Define *functional hypoglycemia* and plan a 1-day sample meal plan.
11. List the population groups at highest risk for drug–nutrient interaction and briefly state why they are at risk.
12. Describe the drug–nutrient interaction that occurs when foods containing tyramine- and dopamine- are consumed together with monoamine oxidase inhibitors.
13. List the seven monoamine oxidase inhibitors that require a tyramine- and dopamine-controlled diet.

CANCER

Cancer is a general term for a malignant *tumor,* an abnormal growth of cells that spreads to neighboring tissue. Tumors have no useful purpose and grow at the expense of healthy tissue. Some cancer cells may break away from the original tumor and spread by the lymph or bloodstream to distant body parts, a process called *metastasis.*

Cancer is the second leading cause of death in the United States. Heredity, viruses, environmental factors, and immunologic factors appear to be involved in the development of cancer, but the exact cause is unknown. Surgery, radiation, and chemotherapy are the primary means of treatment. Other treatment forms include biologic response modifiers (i.e., interleukin and interferon) and bone marrow transplantation. Any one or a combination of these methods may be used.

Like all cells, malignant cells require energy and nutrients to maintain themselves and to grow. This requirement probably is responsible for the weight loss and reduction of body fat that may occur early in cancer even though the client does not change caloric intake or physical activity level. If the disease does not respond to treatment, the continued metabolic demands of cancer cells, anorexia (loss of appetite), nausea, vomiting, and other nutrition-related problems lead to extreme weight loss, anemia, malnutrition, and a complete collapse of body processes. This extreme state of malnutrition and body wasting is called *cancer cachexia.*

NUTRITION CARE

The short-term goal is to provide the best nutritional support possible by treating symptoms, maintaining a reasonable body weight, correcting nutritional deficiencies brought on by the cancer and its treatments, and correcting fluid and electrolyte imbalances. Frequent problems are the retention of body water, increased extracellular water, increased total body sodium, decreased amounts of intracellular water and body potassium, and glucose intolerance.

Long-term nutrition goals depend on the long-term medical goals. Clients who have a poor prognosis and are not receiving anticancer treatment are given supportive or palliative care. This involves making the client comfortable and providing emotional support for the client and his or her family.

Aggressive nutritional support is provided for clients who are responding to cancer therapy or surgery. The primary goal is to prevent weight loss. Clients who can maintain their weight or minimize weight loss improve their response to cancer treatment and their survival rate.

Clients who are on high-calorie, high-protein diets are better able to withstand the side effects of the types of cancer therapy and may be able to tolerate higher doses of drugs than clients who are not on such diets. A balanced diet can help the client maintain strength and fight infection. Displays 30-1 and 30-2 give suggestions for increasing protein and caloric intake. These suggestions must be adapted to the individual client's needs and tolerances. The nutritional goals can be accomplished by one or a combination of the following: an adequate intake of food by means of regular meals or regular meals plus supplemental feedings, tube feedings, or parenteral (intravenous) nutrition.

The nutritional support selected depends on the stage of the disease, the client's nutritional status, the degree to which the gastrointestinal tract is functioning, and how well the client can chew, swallow, and self-feed. Feeding by mouth is the

DISPLAY 30-1 HINTS FOR ADDING PROTEIN TO THE DIET

Protein can be added to the diet without increasing the volume of food eaten.

- Add 2 tbsp of nonfat dry milk to the regular amount of milk called for in recipes, for added protein.
- Use milk fortified with nonfat dry milk for cooking and drinking.
- Add nonfat dry milk to hot or cold cereals, scrambled eggs, soups, gravies, ground meat (for meat patties, meat balls, and meatloaf), casserole dishes, desserts, and baked goods.
- Use milk or half-and-half instead of water when making soup, cereals, instant cocoa, puddings, and canned soups. Soy formulas may also be used.
- Add instant breakfast to hot or cold milk or milk shakes.
- Add diced or ground meat to soups and casseroles.
- Add cheese, cottage cheese, or tofu to scrambled eggs or an omelet.
- Add grated cheese or chunks of cheese to sauces, vegetables, soups, and casseroles.
- Add cream cheese or peanut butter to butter on hot bread.
- Add cooked cubed shrimp, canned tuna, crab meat, diced ham, or sliced boiled eggs to sauces and serve over rice, cooked noodles, buttered toast, or hot biscuits.
- Choose dessert recipes that contain eggs, such as sponge and angel food cake, egg custard, bread pudding, and rice pudding.
- Add peanut butter to sauces or use it on crackers, waffles, or celery sticks.

method of choice. Commercial food supplements frequently are added to the diet to increase caloric and protein intake. A wide variety of supplements are available: lactose-free, lowfat, high-protein, and low-sodium supplements (see Table 29-1 for a list of commercial supplements). Bland-tasting formulas may be more acceptable than sweet or flavored products. If possible, offer the client a small taste of the different products available. If sufficient calories cannot be taken by mouth, enteral tube feedings or total parenteral nutrition may be indicated (see Chapter 29).

Whatever the method of feeding, nutrition care must be individualized and adapted to each client's special needs. The dietitian considers eating problems that are likely to result from therapy or disease progression and often makes changes to prevent these problems.

DISPLAY 30-2 HINTS FOR ADDING CALORIES TO THE DIET

- Use 1 tsp of butter or margarine to add 45 kcal. Mix it into hot foods such as soups, vegetables, mashed potatoes, cooked cereal, and rice.
- Use mayonnaise, which has 100 kcal/tbsp—almost twice as much as salad dressing—in salads, with eggs, and with lettuce on sandwiches.
- Use peanut butter, which has protein as well as calores—1 tbsp is 90 kcal. Spread it on fruit such as apple, banana, or pear, or stuff celery with it.
- Use honey, jam, or preserves on toast, pancakes, waffles, or French toast or add to desserts such as pudding or pound cake.
- Use sour cream and yogurt on vegetables such as potatoes, beans, carrots, and squash. Try them in gravies or as a salad dressing for fruit.
- Use sour cream as a dip for fresh vegetables. Add sour cream to mashed potatoes, main dishes, and sauces for vegetables. For a good dessert, scoop it on fresh fruit, add brown sugar, and let it sit in the refrigerator for a while. One level tablespoon of sour cream is 25 kcal.
- Add heavy cream, which is about 50 kcal/fluid tbsp, to pies, fruit, puddings, hot chocolate, gelatin dessert, and other desserts.
- Add marshmallows to fruit or hot chocolate.
- Have snacks ready to eat. Nuts, dried fruits, candy, popcorn, crackers and cheese, granola, ice cream, and popsicles all make good snacks. Milk shakes add calories and are especially easy to make with a blender.
- Use powdered coffee creamers, which add calories without volume. Add them to gravy, soup, milk shakes, and hot cereals.
- Include meat, chicken, and fish, which are higher in calories when breaded than when broiled or roasted plain.
- Add raisins, dates, or chopped nuts and brown sugar to hot or cold cereals for a snack.

FACTORS THAT AFFECT NUTRITIONAL STATUS

The major nutritional problem in cancer is the client's unwillingness or inability to eat enough food. Anorexia, nausea and vomiting, early satiety (fullness), extreme tiredness, and pain and discomfort associated with eating all play a part. These symptoms may be caused by the disease itself or by the treatment, especially radiation and chemotherapy. Most cancer drugs cause nausea and vomiting, and many cause diarrhea. Today, antiemetic drugs are frequently given at the time of treatment to help control these side effects.

ANOREXIA

Anorexia may be due in part to changes in taste sensation. The client may complain that food is tasteless or unpalatable. Some clients have a decreased ability to taste salt, sugar, or acid. Some find that food tastes bitter. Even the smell of food may cause nausea. *Dysgeusia,* an alteration in taste perception, is not uncommon in clients undergoing cancer treatment.

An uncomfortable sense of fullness after the first meal of the day also interferes with eating. This feeling has been attributed to a delay in the emptying time of the stomach, possibly due to a decrease in digestive enzymes, loss of stomach muscle, and other physiologic changes.

Extreme tiredness is another hindrance to eating. Loss of muscle tissue accounts for much of the weight loss that occurs in cancer, giving rise to fatigue, weakness, and inactivity. Chemotherapy and radiation are tiring because they damage normal tissue as well as cancer cells.

In a study conducted by Feuz and Rapin involving 116 older people with terminal cancer, consumption of food by mouth was possible by making certain changes in treatment. The most important of these changes was to control pain and distressing symptoms (e.g., constipation) and adapt the food to the client's condition and tastes. As a result of these changes, 92% of the clients could eat until the day they died.

The following suggestions may help increase the food consumption of clients with cancer:

- Create a pleasant mealtime atmosphere; arrange food attractively on the plate; encourage clients to eat with family and friends.
- Encourage clients to suggest foods they think would appeal to them.
- Have nutritious food readily available so that clients may eat when their appetite is good rather than according to a set meal schedule.
- Alter seasonings by adding more sugar, salt, or tart flavors to food (unless these seasonings must be avoided). Encourage clients to try using herbs and other seasonings and wine and beer in cooking.
- Encourage clients to try cold foods rather than hot ones. (Heat intensifies the odor of food.) Meats may be more acceptable cold than hot.
- Use dairy products, legumes, and peanut butter if clients will not or do not eat meat.
- Encourage clients to eat well on days they feel well
- Encourage clients to eat small meals frequently if they feel uncomfortably full after eating larger amounts of food.
- Encourage clients to rest before eating when they are extremely tired. Light exercise, such as a short walk, may be helpful between meals.
- Avoid pressuring clients to eat. Pressure may intensify the anorexia.
- Easily digested high-carbohydrate foods such as toast and crackers may be better tolerated during periods of nausea.

PAIN AND DISCOMFORT ASSOCIATED WITH EATING

The tumor location can intensify nutritional problems. Surgery of the tongue and larynx impairs swallowing, gastric surgery may cause the dumping syndrome, and tumors of the intestine and accessory organs lead to problems in digestion, absorption, and metabolism (see Chapter 29).

Pain experienced during eating due to ulceration or inflammation of the mouth and esophagus is particularly distressing. Clients with mucositis should avoid foods that are acidic, salty, spicy, dry, or very hot to reduce irritation and discomfort. Pureed and liquid foods may be better tolerated. Pain medication given at the appropriate time to bring relief at mealtime, or a local anesthetic applied to the mouth or pharynx, can improve food intake.

Radiation treatments of the head and neck may damage salivary glands so that saliva cannot be produced. An artificial saliva, similar in composition to natural saliva, may be ordered. This saliva is kept in a plastic squeeze bottle and used as necessary. Artificial saliva also helps reduce the severe dental decay that usually occurs after radiation of the head and neck.

When mouth dryness (*xerostomia*) is a problem, moist food or dry foods mixed with sauces, gravies, and fats should be served. Offer liquids with meals to make the food easier to chew.

RESPONSIBILITIES OF THE HEALTH TEAM

The health care worker who is aware of the eating problems that may arise in cancer will respect the client's likes and dislikes and understand that tolerances for food may change from meal to meal. Nursing and dietary personnel must do all they can to help the client consume a reasonable amount of food. No one diet or nutrition plan can suit all clients' needs; nutrition care must be individualized.

Problems that interfere with eating, such as pain, difficulty chewing and swallowing, and nausea, should be reported to the physician immediately so that changes can be made. The client's food intake, including foods and beverages eaten at meals, food supplements, and food provided by family and friends, should be carefully checked and recorded. Observations should be made as inconspicuously as possible so that clients are not constantly reminded of their eating problems. They usually are well aware of and extremely worried about them.

LINK BETWEEN DIET AND CANCER

Research has indicated that nutritional factors most likely are involved in the development of some cancers. Nutritional deficiencies as well as excesses have been implicated.

The dietary factors that have been evaluated for their possible link to cancer risk include intake of fat, total calories, lack of fiber, foods low in vitamin A and carotenoids, and alcohol. Possible roles for vitamin C, vitamin E, selenium, protein, and salt-cured, salt-pickled, and smoked foods also have been proposed.

In 1989, the National Research Council Committee on Diet and Health in the publication *Diet and Health: Implications for Reducing Chronic Disease Risk* made the following six recommendations regarding diet and cancer risk:

1. Reduce total fat to 30% or less of total calories. Evidence from epidemiologic and animal studies has indicated that high-fat diets are associated with higher risk of several cancers, especially colon, prostate, and breast cancer.
2. Eat five or more servings of vegetables and fruits, especially green and yellow vegetables and citrus fruits, every day. Just what factors are responsible for the protective action of these foods against cancer of the lungs, stomach, and large intestine has not been fully determined. Their fiber content is one possibility. There is strong evidence, however, that a low intake of carotenoids, present in green and yellow vegetables, contributes to an increased risk of lung cancer. (Vitamin C, folate, and selenium in fruits and vegetables also appear to play an important role.)
3. Maintain protein intake at moderate levels. Diets high in meat have been associated with increased risk of breast and colon cancer. Whether adverse effects in epidemiologic studies are due to the protein per se or to other factors, such as the high fat content or the low level of plant foods in these diets, is unknown.
4. Balance food intake and physical activity to maintain appropriate body weight. Excess weight is associated with the increased risk of endometrial cancer.
5. Avoid alcohol. If consumed, limit consumption to less than 1 oz of pure alcohol in 1 day. This amount is contained in two cans of beer, two small glasses of wine, or two average cocktails. Alcohol consumption is associated with an in-

creased risk of cancers of the oral cavity, pharynx, esophagus, and larynx, especially when combined with cigarette smoking. Some evidence has linked alcohol with liver cancer and moderate beer drinking with rectal cancer.

6. Consume salty, highly processed salty, salt-preserved, and salt-pickled foods sparingly. Frequent consumption may increase the risk of stomach cancer.

In 1991, the American Cancer Society published similar guidelines on diet, nutrition, and cancer. However, the recommendation for total fat intake was less specific. The past suggestion of 30% or less total calories from fat was not included because of the potential benefits a further reduction of fats might have.

AIDS

Acquired immunodeficiency syndrome (AIDS) was first recognized and classified in 1981. The syndrome is caused by a human T-cell lymphotropic retrovirus referred to as *human immunodeficiency virus* (HIV). HIV infects *T cells,* white blood cells that protect the body from infection and other diseases. When the body loses its T-cell function, the person becomes susceptible to many life-threatening infections and certain cancers.

Today, an estimated 1 million people in the United States are infected with HIV. Poor nutrition may be a factor in the progression of AIDS. However, nutrition counseling and intervention may help delay that progression. Good nutrition helps to maintain the functioning of our body's immune system.

Chronic body wasting is a characteristic feature of AIDS. Weight loss, lean body tissue loss, hypoalbuminemia, decreased iron-binding capacity, and selenium deficiency are all complications associated with the malnutrition AIDS causes. Clients with AIDS have increased nutritional requirements due to infections and decreased intake and poor absorption of nutrients. Infection increases the body's basal metabolic rate and the loss of body protein. Clients with AIDS are always at risk of infection. As the disease progresses, periods of severe illness followed by periods of general good health are not uncommon. Good nutrition care is essential to help preserve lean body mass, maintain weight and strength, improve the body's response to medications, and maintain the client's self-image.

NUTRITIONAL PROBLEMS AND TREATMENT

Factors that hinder the client with AIDS from maintaining a good nutritional status are decreased appetite, oral complications and pain while eating, neurologic problems, and gastrointestinal complications. Of these factors, decreased appetite is a major problem. Respiratory infections and gastrointestinal problems often cause anorexia. The most common respiratory infection, *Pneumocystis carinii pneumonia,* is usually the first onset of AIDS. The client may be severely ill but tends to recover. *P. carinii* pneumonia is treated with sulfamethoxazole–trimethoprim (Bactrim) and pentamidine, which may cause nausea, vomiting, and taste changes. The worry and anxiety brought on by the diagnosis of AIDS and its social and financial implications also can seriously depress appetite.

Techniques for increasing food intake include: encouraging small, frequent meals instead of larger meals, keeping snacks and nutritious beverages at the bedside, using high-calorie, high-protein liquid supplements, administering drugs after meals rather than before or during meals, and making the most of days when the client is feeling well. Providing foods on regular dishes instead of disposables may promote food intake.

Oral and esophageal pain results from sores and inflammation in the mouth and esophagus caused by fungal, viral, and bacterial infections. Oral cavity disease is common in AIDS. These factors may make eating painful. The healthcare worker must determine what foods the client can tolerate. Generally, highly seasoned and acidic foods and very hot or very cold foods are avoided. Soft or blended foods may be better tolerated. Nutritionally complete liquid formulas are more easily consumed and increase the nutrient intake. Although nasogastric tube feedings may be useful, the presence of the tube may be too irritating to the esophageal lesions.

Some degree of neurologic impairment occurs in most clients with AIDS over the course of the disease. This impairment may be due to infections of the central nervous system or to AIDS encephalopathy, which is thought to be caused by direct HIV infections of the brain. Confusion and dementia, impaired motor ability, and difficulty swallowing may result from the neurologic complications. These symptoms further reduce the client's ability to consume a nutritionally adequate diet.

Meal trays may need to be simplified for the confused client. Depending on the circumstances, special eating utensils (see Chapter 3) and changes in food consistency for the client with dysphagia (see Chapter 21) may be necessary. Close monitoring and encouragement are necessary for neurologically impaired clients. In advanced cases, the client may need to be fed or may require tube feeding.

Gastrointestinal complications in the form of diarrhea and malabsorption are among the major nutritional problems occurring in clients with AIDS. These symptoms sometimes are due to infections that can be effectively treated. In other cases, the infections may be resistant to treatment, the cause of the diarrhea may be unknown, or the diarrhea may be the result of medication.

If the cause of the diarrhea can be readily treated, total parenteral nutrition may be provided while the colon is given a chance to rest and heal. If the cause is unknown, treatment aims to relieve symptoms. Dietary changes might include a low-lactose diet or a lowfat, low-fiber, caffeine-free diet for controlling diarrhea. Fermented diary products may help prevent bacterial overgrowth. In cases of fat malabsorption, medium-chain triglycerides can be used. Clients with ulcerative lesions may need a low-fiber diet. Fluid intake is important because of the large volume of fluid lost in the stool. If the diarrhea does not respond to treatment, the client's comfort is the primary goal of nutrition therapy.

Polymeric or whole-protein formulas can be used by clients without diarrhea or malabsorption. When malabsorption exists, hydrolyzed or elemental formulas that are easily digested and absorbed may be given by mouth or by tube feeding, or parenteral nutrition may be provided. If elemental diets are given orally, their acceptance can be improved by adding flavorings and sugar and serving with ice or frozen as a slush.

Complications of AIDS differ from one individual to another. Early intervention, counseling, and individualized nutrition care plans can help to delay the severity of the malnutrition caused by AIDS.

NUTRITION GOALS

Clients with AIDS are highly sensitive to other people's feelings toward them. Establishing a supportive, nonjudgmental, trusting relationship is an important aspect of care. Many clients with AIDS are well informed about their disease and take an active role in making decisions about their care. Clients should be involved in nutrition care planning. Nutrition counseling should include principles for healthy eating, tips for managing poor appetite and early satiety, and proper food safety and sanitation principles for home food preparation. There is no known cure for AIDS; clients frequently want to try unconventional diets and food treatments they have heard about. Nutrition counseling should also provide the client with guidelines for evaluating nutrition information. As long as these diets meet nutrition goals, clients should be allowed to follow the diet of their choice. Frequently, these diets or therapies can be manipulated to provide a nutritionally adequate diet. If the unproven nutritional practices are harmful, the matter should be thoroughly discussed and the shortcomings in relation to nutrition goals should be demonstrated.

FOOD SERVICE ISSUES

Education of dietary staff is needed to allay fears about caring for clients with AIDS and to stress the importance of a caring, nonjudgmental attitude on the part of all personnel. Whenever possible, meals should be provided on regular dishes to help clients feel less socially isolated. HIV does not live long outside the body. It is inactivated by disinfectants or heat used in usual institutional dishwashing procedures. Saliva has not been documented as a means of transmitting the disease. Any dishes that have been exposed to blood; bodily excretions, or vomitus, however, should not be handled by dietary personnel until the dishes have been cleared of these materials.

Precautionary procedures of the institution's infectious disease control policy should be followed. These procedures are dictated by the extent of the infections that accompany AIDS.

CHRONIC OBSTRUCTIVE PULMONARY DISEASE

Chronic obstructive pulmonary disease (COPD) describes a group of conditions in which chronic obstruction of airflow within the lungs occurs. This obstruction reduces the airflow of oxygen into the lungs and limits the exchange of carbon dioxide removal. Chronic bronchitis, emphysema, bronchiectasis, and cystic fibrosis are all forms of COPD. These progressive diseases lead to destruction of lung tissue with permanent impairment of lung function. Clients with COPD need nutrition education and counseling early in the medical management of the disease. Good nutrition will help maintain muscle function of the lungs and help maintain the body's resistance to infection.

Weight loss is common in COPD. It may be related to the client's inability to consume adequate calories and protein because of shortness of breath or anorexia caused by the medications used, or the medications themselves may cause gastric upset. Encouraging the client to eat small meals will help to maintain body weight and assure that adequate nutrients are consumed. Early satiety is a common problem with these clients. Offering fluids between meals rather than with meals may help prevent clients from filling up too soon. A fluid restriction may need to be considered in clients with congestive heart failure, edema, or ascites. Many clients find that breakfast and lunch are better tolerated than dinner. If so, the client may need tips for simple, light, quick, and nourishing meals at dinner time.

In severe cases of COPD, especially if the client is ventilator dependent, nutrition therapy must be carefully planned. In this case, the *respiratory quotient (RQ)*, which is the ratio of carbon dioxide produced and oxygen consumed, can be evaluated. A high RQ increases carbon dioxide production, therefore placing more demands on the respiratory system, making breathing or weaning from the ventilator more difficult. Carbohydrate, protein, and fat are metabolized in the body to carbon dioxide and water. The *oxidation,* or burning of the energy nutrients, results in specific RQs: carbohydrate, 1.0; protein, 0.8; and fat, 0.7. The RQ of a mixed diet of carbohydrate, protein, and fat is 0.85. The highest RQ, 1.01–1.20, occurs when excessive caloric intake leads to the deposit of fat in the body. In determining the ventilator-dependent client's nonprotein calorie needs, the fat has a lower RQ value than carbohydrate and has been shown to be of value as an energy source. In addition, total calories must be considered. Excess calories will also contribute to the respiratory system workload. On the other hand, inadequate calories may lead to further loss of lean body mass, wasting of the respiratory muscles, and hypoalbuminemia. The risk for pulmonary edema and infections such as pneumonia are increased.

In feeding the COPD client with poor intake, oral supplemental feedings help to provide the malnourished client with extra calories and protein. If enteral tube feedings are indicated, a calorically dense formula can be used. Formulas that are higher in fat than carbohydrate should be considered. Fat modulars can also be added to formulas to improve the ratio of protein, fat, and carbohydrate. Clients with respiratory conditions on enteral tube feedings should always be fed past the pylorus because of the high risk of aspiration. If parenteral nutrition is indicated, the glucose concentration, total volume of the solution, and total calories given need to be carefully considered.

TUBERCULOSIS

Tuberculosis (TB) is caused by *Myobacterium,* a rod-shaped bacteria that commonly infect the respiratory tract, although other organs can be affected. This chronic illness is one of the oldest diseases known, and occurs worldwide. In the United States, the population at highest risk for TB includes poorly nourished and immune-compromised individuals, such as alcoholic clients, homeless people, substance abusers, immigrants from endemic areas, people with HIV or AIDS, and individuals with chronic illnesses. There has recently been a resurgence of a drug-resistant form of TB.

For the hospitalized client with TB, a nutrition assessment will help identify the presence of malnutrition. Nutrition care should be individualized, especially for the client with TB who has another chronic illness such as diabetes. Providing a balanced diet with snacks between meals will help provide the extra calories and protein these clients often need. Oral liquid supplements can also be incorporated into the client's meal plan. Weight loss commonly occurs with the onset of TB; thus, weight maintenance or weight gain should be a goal of the client's nutrition care. Because TB is a chronic illness, promoting good nutritional practices and avoiding alcohol will help the client in the long term. Clients with TB are generally on medications for 4 months to 1 year. The most commonly used drugs in the treatment of TB are isoniazid, rifampin, and pyrimethamine. Isoniazid and pyrimethamine may cause nausea and anorexia. Clients on isoniazid should receive a vitamin B_6 (pyridoxine) supplement. Supplementation of vitamin D may be needed when rifampin is used, and clients treated with pyrimethamine may require additional folate. Clients who have a drug-resistant form of TB require longer, more intensive medication treatment.

FOOD ALLERGY

Abdominal pain, asthmatic attack, headache, and rash are typical symptoms of people with food allergy. About one third of the estimated 35 million Americans suffering from allergy have a sensitivity to food. In some cases, treatment involves avoiding foods that have no effect on nutritional status. If the offending food is a nutritionally important one or one that is widely used in food processing, however, treatment can be difficult, especially in the case of infants and children who are allergic to foods such as milk, wheat, or eggs.

An allergy is an adverse reaction to substances called *allergens.* This reaction causes the production of *antibodies,* which are proteins. In the case of an infectious disease, antibodies are protective. In allergic conditions, however, the type of antibody produced after exposure to the allergen (e.g., pollen, penicillin, or pork) is not protective. When the antibodies interact with the allergen, certain chemicals are released that cause the allergic symptoms. Allergic symptoms usually do not appear on first contact. It takes considerable exposure to an allergen before enough antibodies are formed to cause symptoms. A true food allergy (or hypersensitivity) involves the immune system, usually immunoglobulin E mediated.

In the case of food allergy, antibodies trigger allergic symptoms every time a person eats a particular food. Sometimes the food does not even have to be eaten to cause symptoms—inhaling its aroma or having an injection of a related product may be enough.

Foods that commonly cause allergic reactions are fish and seafood, berries, nuts, eggs, cereals, milk, beef, pork, chocolate, legumes such as beans and peanuts, and fresh fruits in the peach family. A person may be allergic to foods that belong to a single family of plants. For example, a person who is allergic to cantaloupe also may be allergic to pumpkin and cucumber.

The symptoms associated with food allergy are urticaria (hives), eczema, vomiting, diarrhea, asthma, rhinitis (hay fever), and migraine headache. In severe reactions, angioedema (gigantic swellings of body tissue), cardiovascular collapse, and shock can occur. These anaphylactic reactions are life threatening. The allergic symptoms may appear immediately or may be delayed until several hours after the food has been eaten. Peanuts, tree nuts, fish, shellfish, and cow's milk are the foods most often associated with severe anaphylactic reactions.

Food allergies may develop in people of any age, although infants and young children are especially susceptible. The tendency to develop an allergy appears to be inherited. Physical and emotional stress may aggravate the condition.

The food or foods causing the allergic reaction are identified by a diet history, physical examination, immunologic tests, elimination diets, and food challenges. No single test can diagnose a food allergy. Diagnosis is based on accumulated evidence.

FOOD HISTORY AND DIAGNOSTIC PROCEDURES

A thorough history of foods eaten and of the occurrence of symptoms often reveals possible allergens. The client may be asked to keep a diary of all items consumed as well as a record of symptoms. All items taken by mouth should be entered in the food diary, including beverages, gums, candies, vitamins, and nonprescription medications.

Skin tests may be helpful in efforts to isolate suspected foods. Food extracts are rubbed into scratches on the skin or injected under the skin. If redness or swelling occurs, the food is considered to be a possible allergen. A food giving a positive skin test should not be considered the definite cause of allergic symptoms, however. The results of skin tests must be evaluated in the light of information in the medical history. Skin tests may help in determining the type of elimination diet that should be tried.

Once a list of suspected foods has been established, the physician may order an *elimination diet.* This diet omits the suspected food or foods for 7 to 14 days. Relief from symptoms should occur within this time. The suspected foods are then slowly added to the diet one at a time for identification of those that cause symptoms. If a food containing an allergen is consumed, symptoms appear, usually within 7 days, and subside again when the food is eliminated.

If the elimination diet fails to identify the allergen or if the allergic symptoms are severe, an elemental diet preparation (see Chapter 29) may be given as the only source of nourishment. This diet eliminates all food allergens. Suspected foods are then added one at a time. Elimination diets should only be used short-term because of the possible nutritional inadequacies.

Another way to confirm the diagnosis of food allergy is a food challenge. A double-blind placebo-controlled food challenge provides the most unbiased test. Both the doctor and client are unaware of the substance being tested. The client takes dehydrated foods and placebos that look alike placed in opaque capsules. Symptoms are carefully observed and recorded by a neutral observer. In a single-blind study, the client does not know what food is being tested and the doctor does.

TREATMENT AND COUNSELING

Once the food or foods causing the allergy have been identified, they are avoided either partially or completely. The extent to which a food is eliminated from the diet depends on its nutritional importance and the severity of the client's symptoms. Allergy to milk, wheat, or eggs, for example, is difficult to deal with because these foods are basic to the American diet and are used widely in food processing.

Sometimes the changes that occur when the offending food is cooked make it more tolerable. For example, some people who are allergic to milk or eggs may be able to tolerate small quantities of these foods in baked goods. Clients who cannot tolerate the food in any form may use a food substitute. When a substitute for a nutritionally important food is unavailable or is not accepted, use of vitamin or mineral supplements may be necessary. Careful meal planning is important to assure that all nutritional requirements are being met when several food allergies are present. This is especially important when the client is a young child or adolescent.

The client and family must be made aware of all sources of the food to be avoided, including hidden sources (e.g., dry milk powder in frankfurters).

The client must be instructed to read food package labels carefully to identify the allergen (Display 30-3). If a substitute food can be used, such as rice flour in place of wheat flour, the client needs to know where to obtain the substitute and how to use it in food preparation. Display 30-4 lists several books for clients with food sensitivities.

Labeling regulations that became effective in 1994 are more user friendly for people with food allergy. All ingredients must be listed on all processed, packaged foods including standardized foods that were previously exempt. Also, manufacturers must list by name all color additives certified by the Food and Drug Administration. *Casein* must be identified on labels as a milk derivative and protein hydrolysates must be listed by their common names and their source must be identified, such as *hydrolyzed corn protein* or *hydrolyzed casein.* See

DISPLAY 30-3 TERMS ON LABELS THAT INDICATE THE PRESENCE OF COMMON ALLERGENS

COMMON ALLERGEN	TERMS	COMMON ALLERGEN	TERMS
Milk	Buttermilk	Corn	Corn flour
	Casein		Corn meal
	Caseinate		Corn oil
	Casein hydrolysate		Corn solids
	Cottage cheese		Cornstarch
	DMS [dried milk solids]		Corn sweeteners
	Lactate solids		Corn syrup
	Lactalbumin		Grits
	Milk by-products		High-fructose corn syrup
	Milk chocolate		Maize
	Milk solid pastes		Sorbitol
	Nonfat dry milk		Vegetable gum
	Sour cream		Vegetable oil
	Sweetened condensed milk		Vegetable starch
	Whey or whey solids	Legume	Food gums from the legume family
Egg	Albumin		Acacia gum
	Dried egg solids		Arabic gum
	Dried egg white		Carob
	Egg powder		Karaya gum
	Egg solids		Locust bean gum
	Egg yolks		Tragacanth
	Globulin		Hydrolyzed vegetable protein
	Ovomucin		Soy
	Ovomucoid		Lecithin
	Vitellin		Soya flour
			Soy concentrate
			Soy milk
			Soy oil
			Soybean oil
			Soy protein
			Soy protein isolate
			TVP [textured vegetable protein]
			Vegetable protein concentrate

(Kendall P, Gloeckner J. Managing food allergies and sensitivities. Top Clin Nutr 1994;9:4:1–10.)

DISPLAY 30-4 RECOMMENDED BOOKS FOR CLIENTS WITH FOOD SENSITIVITES

Allergy Information Association. *The Allergy Cookbook: Diets Unlimited for Limited Diet.* Toronto, Canada: Methuen Publications, 1985.

Allergy Information Association. *The Allergy Cookbook: Foods for Festive Occasions.* Toronto, Canada: Methuen Publications, 1985.

Dobler ML. *Food Allergies.* Chicago, IL: American Dietetic Association, 1991.

Dong FM. *All About Food Allergy.* Philadelphia: George F Stickley Co, 1984.

Food Allergy Network. *The Food Allergy News Cookbook.* Fairfax, VA: The Food Allergy Network, 1992.

Johns SB. *The Allergy Guide to Brand-Name Foods and Food Additives.* New York: New American Library, 1988.

Jones MH. *The Allergy Self-Help Cookbook.* Emmaus, PA: Rodale Press, 1984.

Moyer J. *Cooking for the Allergic Child.* Bellefonte, PA: Grove Printing, 1987.

Nonken PP, Hirsch SR. *The Allergy Cookbook and Food-Buying Guide.* New York: Warner Books, 1982.

Rudoff C. *The Allergy Baker.* Menlo Park, CA: Prologue Publications, 1981.

Rudoff C. *The Allergy Cookie Jar.* Menlo Park, CA: Prologue Publications, 1985.

Rudoff C. *The Allergy Gourmet.* Menlo Park, CA: Prologue Publications, 1983.

Weiss L. *The Kitchen Magician.,* Milford, MI: Prosperity Publishing, 1986.

Williams ML. *Cooking Without—Recipes for the Allergic Child (and Family).* Ambler, PA: Gimball Corporation, 1989.

Yoder ER. *Allergy-Free Cooking.* Reading, MA: Addison-Wesley, 1987.

(Carroll P. Guidelines for counseling patients with food sensitivities. Top Clin Nutr 1994;9:3:35.)

Chapter 4 for labeling regulations to protect sulfite-sensitive people.

The physician may try to desensitize the client to an allergy-causing food, especially if the food is nutritionally important. Desensitization is the development of tolerance for an allergy-causing food by the ingestion of controlled doses of the allergen that are minute at first and are increased by tiny amounts over an extended period. If symptoms occur, dosage remains at the last level that did not produce symptoms.

SPECIFIC ALLERGIES

MILK ALLERGY

Allergy to milk occurs most often in children younger than age 2 years. Many children outgrow this allergy. Infants who have a severe allergic reaction are given milk-free commercial infant formulas made with either a soybean or meat base. These milk-free formulas are similar in calories and nutrients to other infant formulas and provide the essentials for adequate growth.

When solid foods are added, parents must be counseled to read labels carefully to avoid foods containing nonfat dry milk. For children or adults with severe milk allergy, all foods containing milk or nonfat dry milk may have to be avoided. Clients should be alerted to hidden sources of milk, such as frankfurters, luncheon meats, and chocolate. If, on the food label, the product is marked *pareve,* the product does not contain milk.

Supplements of calcium, vitamin D, and riboflavin are necessary for children who do not accept milk substitutes. Adults may also require calcium supplements.

WHEAT ALLERGY

Allergy to wheat requires that many foods commonly used in the American diet be avoided. The client must be made aware of hidden sources of wheat, such as malted milk; luncheon meats, frankfurters, and sausage, in which wheat has been used as a filler; canned and frozen dinners; beer; and commercial soups. Some wheat flour is commonly added to rye, cornmeal, and oat breads. Rice flour, potato flour, and cornstarch may be used as a substitute for wheat flour.

EGG ALLERGY

Eggs are used widely in commercial products. Baking powder and foaming beverages may contain egg whites. Eggs are used in the preparation of mayonnaise, cooked salad dressing, and hollandaise sauce; in many baked goods; in desserts such as ice cream, puddings, meringues, and candies; and in malted beverages and other preparations.

ARTHRITIS

About 32 million people in the United States suffer from various forms of arthritis. The symptoms of arthritis (inflammation of the joint) occur in more than 100 different diseases. Among the most frequent and serious forms of arthritis are osteoarthritis and rheumatoid arthritis.

Osteoarthritis is caused by degenerative changes in the cartilage in the joints, especially in the spine and knees. The client's diet should be adequate in all essential nutrients and moderately reduced in calories to prevent obesity, if activity is restricted. If the client already is obese, a diet that is more restricted in calories is necessary.

Rheumatoid arthritis is a chronic inflammatory disorder characterized by progressive deformity and destruction of the joints. The disease is systemic, involving the body as a whole; its cause is unknown. Deformities of the hands, elbows, shoulders, and temporomandibular joint limit clients' ability to shop, prepare food, and feed themselves. The deformities may even limit the client's ability to open and close the mouth and to chew food. Symptoms other than those involving the joints include increased metabolic rate caused by the inflammatory process; alterations in digestion and absorption; anemia; Sjögren's syndrome (see Chapter 21), occurring in 10% to 15% of clients; and osteoporosis and osteomalacia. Drug therapy is the main aspect of treatment. Remission may occur and may last for 1 day, 1 month, 1 year, or longer.

The client with rheumatoid arthritis is considered to be at high risk for malnutrition. There is no special diet to treat this disease. Nutrition therapy is directed at treating symptoms, complications (e.g., weight loss and anemia), and drug-related side effects, and at dealing with physical limitations that hinder the consumption of an adequate diet. Special considerations in meal planning include adequate protein and calories especially during periods of inflammation and a salt restriction, which may be necessary with use of nonsteroidal anti-inflammatory drugs. These drugs may cause water retention or leg edema. Good nutritional status cannot always be maintained by normal meals and snacks. In such cases, nutrition supplements, tube feedings, or parenteral nutrition may become necessary (see Chapter 29). A complete assessment of the client's ability to perform tasks associated with activities of daily living such as self-feeding and meal preparation should be done. The use of special equipment for self-feeding may be recommended (see Chapter 3).

There is no known dietary means of preventing or curing these forms of arthritis. Some arthritic diseases, such as rheumatoid arthritis, involve the immune system. Scientists are beginning to understand how nutrition influences immune mechanisms. Research is now being conducted in this area and in other aspects of nutrition and arthritic diseases. Sometimes joint pain is caused by food allergy, which may explain why some people get relief when they eliminate certain foods. Unfortunately, people with arthritis seeking relief from this painful disease spend millions of dollars annually for worthless products, such as filtered sea water and alfalfa tablets.

PARKINSON'S DISEASE

Parkinson's disease (PD) is a progressive neurodegenerative disease that affects approximately 1 million Americans. The medical treatment for PD involves managing the symptoms and slowing its progression. Clients with PD suffer from tremors, impaired ability or slowness in moving muscles (bradykinesia), rigidity, and postural instability. In the later stages of the disease, falling and moments of "freezing" or total inability to control muscle coordination may occur. PD is related to an inadequate amount of the neurotransmitter dopamine. The primary drug used in PD is levodopa, a precursor to dopamine in the body that acts like a natural neurotransmitter. However, as the disease progresses, the ability of levodopa to keep the client stable is reduced. When this occurs, the client with severe PD may experience the *"on–off" phenomenon*. This effect is characterized by periods when the client benefits from the drug "on" and periods where the levodopa has worn "off."

Nutrition therapy for the client with severe PD involves a low-protein diet to help control the "on–off" periods. Levodopa is an amino acid, and during absorption of proteins from a meal, the ability of the drug to be absorbed is reduced. Thus, a lower protein diet may help to promote better drug absorption and improve drug effectiveness. Clients may also find that the type of protein in the diet, animal versus plant, may affect the drug. Plant protein may enhance the length of the "on" period. For any client on a low-protein diet, careful meal planning must be considered to assure that adequate calories and nutrients are received. If the PD client takes a vitamin/mineral supplement, it would be important for the client to know to avoid supplementation of vitamin B_6 (pyridoxine), which reduces the effectiveness of levodopa.

Special consideration should be given to the client's ability to self-feed. Observing the client at mealtimes may help to identify if special feeding equipment is required. Understanding the stage of the client's illness in the progression of PD is important. Supportive care and assistance should be provided during periods of muscular incoordination.

GOUT

Gout involves abnormal metabolism of a group of compounds called *purines*. The end result of this abnormality is that uric acid becomes deposited as salts in soft tissue and joints, where it causes great pain. These deposits can destroy joint tissue, leading to chronic arthritis.

Drugs, for the most part, have replaced diet therapy in the treatment of gout. However, diet therapy should be designed to promote weight loss if the client is obese, limit protein to moderate intake, reduce alcohol, and provide adequate fluid. Fat may also need to be restricted to help control elevated triglycerides. Clients may be advised to avoid substances high in purines such as liver, kidney, brain, sweetbreads, fish roe, sardines, and anchovies, and to limit intake of foods moderately high in purines such as meats, seafood, dried beans, lentils, spinach, and peas.

Weight loss is an important goal but should be accomplished gradually. Rapid weight loss increases blood levels of uric acid and can provoke an acute attack of gout.

HYPERTHYROIDISM

Hyperthyroidism is caused by excessive secretion of the hormone thyroxine, which regulates metabolism. In hyperthyroidism, the metabolic rate may be as much as 50% higher than normal. Symptoms include weight loss, increased appetite, nervousness, and bulging eyeballs.

Until a normal metabolic rate is established by means of medication or surgery, the diet must meet the client's increased energy needs. The client may require as many as 3000 to 4000 kcal/day to prevent excessive weight loss. Stimulants such as coffee, tea, alcohol, and tobacco are omitted or limited. Substantial between-meal snacks in addition to regular meals are necessary.

HYPOGLYCEMIA (HYPERINSULINISM)

Hypoglycemia, a low blood glucose level, is a symptom rather than a disease state. It is characterized by weakness, palpitations, anxiety, sweating, and extreme hunger. In severe cases, brain function may be impaired, causing confusion, amnesia, blurred vision, and, ultimately, convulsions and coma. Hypoglycemia is caused by an excessive amount of insulin circulating in the bloodstream.

The two general types of hypoglycemia are *food-stimulated hypoglycemia,* which occurs 2 to 4 hours after the person has eaten, and *fasting hypoglycemia,* which develops in the fasting state and is not associated with eating. (Fasting hypoglycemia, which can be caused by drugs or various disease states, is not discussed in this chapter). Food-stimulated hypoglycemia may develop in early diabetes or after gastrectomy. Hypoglycemia in early diabetes is treated by a meal plan used in diabetes management. Dietary treatment following a gastrectomy is discussed in Chapter 29.

Food-stimulated hypoglycemia also may occur without evidence of organic disease. Referred to as *functional* (or *reactive*) *hypoglycemia,* it is caused by an overproduction of insulin by the pancreas in response to the absorption of glucose. Symptoms appear about 2 hours after a meal. The symptoms disappear on eating.

The diagnosis of functional hypoglycemia is made on the basis of documented low blood sugar levels that coincide with symptoms. The purpose of the diet is to provide adequate energy without overstimulating the pancreas to produce insulin. In the past, a high-protein, high-fat diet was prescribed because proteins and fats are more slowly digested and more slowly converted to glucose than carbohydrates. This is no longer advocated, because a high-fat diet has been shown to interfere with insulin use and is now contrary to what is considered a healthy diet.

Current dietary recommendations involve eating smaller meals (five to six) and eating high-fiber complex carbohydrate snacks between meals and at bedtime. Although unrefined complex carbohydrate foods are encouraged, they are limited to specific amounts at each feeding and are distributed among meals and snacks throughout the day. Foods containing refined simple carbohydrates are avoided. These foods include jams, jellies, table sugar, honey, syrup, molasses, pies, cakes, cookies, candies, pastries, and regular soda. Complex carbohydrates are increased, especially those that are high in fiber, such as fruits, vegetables, legumes, and whole grains. Foods high in soluble fiber—oats, barley, some fruits and vegatables, and legumes—are encouraged because they slow the absorption of carbohydrate foods. The fat content of the diet is decreased. Caffeinated foods and beverages should be avoided because they frequently produce the same symptoms as hypoglycemia. Alcohol also is avoided because it lowers blood glucose, especially on an empty stomach. Display 30-5 gives a sample menu for the person with functional hypoglycemia.

DISPLAY 30-5 DIET FOR FUNCTIONAL HYPOGLYCEMIA

CHARACTERISTICS

- Lowfat
- Increased complex carbohydrates high in fiber, especially soluble fiber
- Carbohydrate distributed in small frequent meals throughout the day
- No simple, refined carbohydrate
- No alcohol or caffeine

SAMPLE MENU

BREAKFAST
1/2 cup of oatmeal
1 slice of whole-wheat toast
1 tsp of margarine
1/2 banana
1/2 cup of skim milk

MIDMORNING SNACK
3 graham cracker squares
1/2 cup of skim milk

LUNCH
1/2 cup of water-packed tuna
1 tbsp to 2 tbsp of light mayonnaise
2 slices of whole-wheat bread
Carrot sticks
1/2 cup of skim milk

MIDAFTERNOON SNACK
3 cups of popcorn
1 tsp of margarine
1 small apple

SUPPER
3 oz baked chicken
2/3 cup of brown rice
1/2 cup of broccoli
1 tsp of margarine
Tossed salad with 1 tbsp of French dressing
1/2 cup of skim milk

EVENING SNACK
1/2 cup of bran flakes
1/2 cup of skim milk

FOOD AND DRUG INTERACTIONS

Some drugs interfere with nutritional status, and foods, in turn, may interfere with response to a drug. For example, the effectiveness of some antibiotics is reduced when they are taken with meals; in contrast, other medications, such as iron preparations, are best taken with meals to lessen gastrointestinal upset. Display 30-6 shows several drug–nutrient interactions (see also Table 21-1). Health care workers should be aware of the possibility of harmful interactions between food and drugs.

The people at greatest risk of undesirable drug-nutrient interaction are those taking medication for long periods, those taking two or more medications, and those who are not eating well. Poorly nourished people are less likely to have nutrient stores that can overcome a challenge imposed by a drug. Elderly people fall into the high-risk category. They are the highest drug users, taking at least half of the total drugs consumed in the United States, including both prescription drugs and over-the-counter drugs, which they tend to use excessively. Physiologic changes that occur with increased age also make elderly clients more prone to adverse reaction. Aging slows the metabolism of certain drugs in the liver and slows the elimination of drugs from the body. Elderly people may discontinue taking required drugs because the drugs are ineffective. This ineffectiveness may be due to preventable drug–nutrient interactions.

Drugs can affect an individual's intake of food by depressing appetite or inducing nausea and vomiting. A drug may hinder absorption of a nutrient in the gastrointestinal tract or it may interfere with the action of the nutrient after it is absorbed.

DISPLAY 30-6 EXAMPLES OF DRUG–NUTRIENT INTERACTIONS

DRUGS	INDICATION	POSSIBLE EFFECTS
Mineral oil	Constipation	Reduced absorption of fat-soluble vitamins
Aspirin	Rheumatoid disorders	Gastrointestinal bleeding leading to iron deficiency anemia
Thiazide diuretics	Cardiovascular disease	Increased potassium and magnesium excretion
Corticosteroids	Inflammation	Increased vitamin D metabolism leading to accelerated bone loss; decreased glucose tolerance; gastric ulceration; increased excretion of vitamin C, potassium, and zinc; increased vitamin B_6 requirement
Oral contraceptive steroids	Birth control	Reduced blood serum levels of folate, vitamin B_6, riboflavin, and ascorbic acid; increased blood serum levels of vitamin A, iron, and copper; increased absorption of calcium
Antacids that contain aluminum hydroxide	Indigestion, heartburn	Depletion of phosphorus, calcium, vitamin D
Antibiotics	Infection	Decreased synthesis of vitamin K, folate
Cholestyramine	Elevated blood cholesterol	Reduced absorption of vitamins A, D, E, and K

For example, the nutritional status of clients undergoing chemotherapy for cancer may be so severely upset that the therapy may have to be interrupted. On the other hand, certain foods or dietary patterns may affect drug action by altering drug absorption, metabolism, or excretion.

TYRAMINE- AND DOPAMINE-CONTROLLED DIET

The interaction between monoamine oxidase inhibitor (MAO or MAOI) drugs and foods high in tyramine and dopamine is an example of the potentially serious consequences of drug–nutrient interactions. Tyramine and dopamine are *monoamines,* protein substances that cause blood vessels to constrict, resulting in an abnormal elevation of blood pressure. Normally these substances are harmless because they are rapidly detoxified by an enzyme in the body called *monoamine oxidase.* However, when certain drugs such as MAOIs are taken, this reaction is blocked. If foods high in tyramine are consumed while on this medication, a hypertensive crisis may result. Symptoms include a headache or pounding head, nausea, vomiting, choking sensations, and palpitations. In some cases, strokes have occurred. The severity of the reaction depends on the drug dosage and the amount of tyramine in the food.

People taking monoamine oxidase inhibitors (Display 30-7) should follow a tyramine- and dopamine-controlled diet. A food may have a high natural tyramine content or may obtain it through aging or spoiling, processes that increase the tyramine content by protein breakdown. Food and drink that is fermented or aged contains tyramine in large amounts and should be avoided. Foods high in tyramine include red wines, especially Chianti and vermouth wines, beer and ale, aged cheese, dry sausages, pickled herring and other pickled or smoked fish, sauerkraut, overripe or spoiled fruit, liver, and Brewer's yeast. Pods of broad beans such as fava beans and Italian green beans are the only foods known to be high in dopamine. Caffeine-containing foods are limited because in large amounts they may cause hypertension and cardiac arrhythmias in people taking monoamine oxidase inhibitors. A good practice to recommend to the client is that only fresh foods be consumed. Clients should not eat foods that are old, aged, or fermented, or for which the shelf life has expired.

DISPLAY 30-7 MONOAMINE OXIDASE INHIBITORS THAT REQUIRE A TYRAMINE- AND DOPAMINE-CONTROLLED DIET

GENERIC NAME	TRADEMARK
Furazolidone	Furoxone (Norwich Eaton)
Isocarboxazid	Marplan (Roche)
Pargyline hydrochloride and methyclothiazine	Eutron (Abbott)
Pargyline hydrochloride	Eutonyl (Abbott)
Phenelzine sulfate	Nardil (Parke-Davis)
Procarbazine	Matulane (Roche)
Tranylcypromine sulfate	Parnate (Smith, Kline & French)

Twin Cites District Dietetic Association, Manual of clinical nutrition. ed. Minneapolis: Chronimed/DCI Publishing, 1988.)

KEYS TO PRACTICAL APPLICATION

Create a pleasant mealtime atmosphere for clients with cancer, shield them from food odors they find nauseating, be alert to foods they accept as well as those they reject, and provide good oral care. Do all you can to increase clients' food intake.

Establish a helping relationship with cancer clients; avoid nagging or pressuring them to eat.

Establish a helping relationship with AIDS clients; remember that a judgmental attitude on the part of the healthcare worker will destroy such a relationship.

Offer food choices to clients with poor appetites due to illness or medications.

Ensure that the client with a food allergy is aware of hidden sources of the offending food.

Encourage a well-balanced diet and the maintenance of normal weight in clients with arthritis; discourage fad products promoted as cures.

Offer feeding assistance to clients with severe arthritis or Parkinson's disease who are unable to feed themselves.

Check with your supervisor about the timing of medication in relation to food intake and about mixing medication with fruit juice, milk, or other foods to avoid drug–food interactions.

KEY IDEAS

Cancer cells require energy and nutrients; they grow at the expense of healthy tissue.

The purpose of nutrition care in clients with cancer is to counteract the nutritional deficiencies caused by the cancer and the cancer treatment.

Maintaining or improving the cancer client's nutritional status improves the response to treatment, may make possible higher doses of medication, helps maintain strength and body weight, and helps fight infection.

The kind of nutrition support chosen—oral, tube feeding, or total parenteral nutrition—depends on the client's nutritional status, the degree to which the gastrointestinal tract is functioning, the ability to chew, swallow, and self-feed, and the stage of the disease.

The major nutrition problem in cancer is the inability of the client to eat a sufficient quantity of food.

Symptoms such as anorexia, taste changes, nausea, vomiting, early satiety, extreme tiredness, and pain and discomfort associated with eating are responsible for the decline in food intake among people with cancer.

The primary nutrition goal in cancer is to prevent weight loss.

Pureed and liquid foods are the foods most likely to be tolerated in clients with ulceration and inflammation of the mouth and esophagus; acidic, salty, spicy, and dry foods should be avoided.

When mouth dryness is a problem, moist foods or dry food mixed with sauces, gravies, and fats are tolerated best.

Nutrition care in cancer must be highly individualized; no one diet or feeding program can be applied to every client.

Although dietary factors most likely are involved in the development of cancer, the exact causes have not been determined. Substantial evidence has supported the following recommendations: decrease fat intake; increase consumption of fruits and vegetables, especially green and yellow vegetables and citrus fruits; have a moderate protein intake; control weight; avoid alcohol; and reduce the intake of salty, highly processed salty, salt-preserved, and salt-pickled foods.

The causes of malnutrition in AIDS are increased nutritional requirements due to infections and decreased intake and poor absorption of nutrients.

Factors that contribute to poor nutritional status in AIDS are decreased appetite, pain while eating, neurologic problems, and gastrointestinal complications.

A supportive, nonjudgmental trusting relationship is the most important factor in the care of people with AIDS; clients should take an active role in making decisions about their care.

AIDS is not transmitted during the preparation and serving of food. Usual dishwashing procedures in the hospital, which include correct water temperatures and sanitizing solutions, provide adequate decontamination.

Clients with COPD need adequate protein and calories to prevent weight loss and lung muscle weakness.

TB is a bacterial infection that commonly infects the lungs. The populations at greatest risk are poorly nourished and immune-compromised people.

Drugs commonly used in the treatment of TB often require supplementation of vitamin B_6, vitamin D, and folate.

Fat is an important energy source in COPD because its metabolism produces less carbon dioxide than either protein or carbohydrate.

Diagnosis of food allergy is based on accumulated evidence from a diary of items consumed and the occurrence of symptoms, as well as skin tests, food challenges, and elimination diets.

Treatment of food allergy involves partial or complete avoidance of the offending food or, possibly, the development of a tolerance for the food through desensitization.

Counseling involves informing the client with an allergy of the sources of the offending food, with special emphasis on hidden sources and the use of substitute foods.

Diet can neither prevent nor cure arthritis; the diet for people with arthritis should be adequate in all essential nutrients and reduced in calories for obese people.

A high-protein diet may reduce the effectiveness of levodopa in clients who are being treated with the drug for Parkinson's disease. Supplements of vitamin B_6 should not be given to clients on levodopa.

Drugs have replaced diet in the treatment of gout; foods high in purines sometimes are avoided.

Weight control, alcohol reduction, and control of elevated triglycerides are important aspects of gout treatment.

Rapid weight loss increases blood levels of uric acid and can bring on an acute attack of gout in people prone to the disease.

In hyperthyroidism, a high-calorie diet (3000 to 4000 kcal/day or more) may be necessary until a normal metabolic rate is established; foods containing stimulants are avoided or eliminated from the diet.

Functional hypoglycemia, caused by excessive production of insulin following meals, is treated with a diet low in fat and high in complex carbohydrates. Carbohydrates are distributed in small, frequent meals throughout the day. Refined simple carbohydrates and alcohol and caffeine are avoided.

Drugs may adversely affect an individual's nutritional status, and food may interfere with the effectiveness of a drug.

People taking monoamine oxidase inhibitor drugs must avoid foods high in tyramine and dopamine to prevent the occurrence of a hypertensive crisis.

KEYS TO LEARNING

STUDY–DISCUSSION QUESTIONS

1. What factors interfere with eating in clients with cancer? Discuss your own observations regarding nutrition care in cancer. What measures have you found to be helpful in improving a client's appetite?
2. How do the complications of AIDS affect nutritional status? Discuss how common nutrition problems are treated.
3. What explanation would you give employees who are concerned about providing nondisposable tray service for AIDS clients?
4. Describe how to increase protein and calories in the diet of a client with cancer, AIDS, COPD, TB, or arthritis.
5. Discuss how medications influence the client's ability to eat. Suggest ways in which you could help the client to eat more.
6. What is an elimination diet? How is it used? What test for food allergy is used most frequently in your hospital? What foods does it include? What is a double-blind food challenge?
7. Plan a 1-day menu for a 6-year-old who is allergic to wheat.
8. Investigate and evaluate food fads associated with arthritis.
9. Why is rapid weight loss dangerous in people with gout?
10. As a class, develop a set of guidelines to help a client prevent harmful food–drug interactions.

BIBLIOGRAPHY

BOOKS AND PAMPHLETS

American Dietetic Association. Handbook of clinical dietetics. 2nd ed. New Haven, CT: Yale University Press, 1992.

Bollet A. Nutrition and diet in rheumatic diseases. In: Shils ME, Olson JA, Shike M. Eds. Modern nutrition in health and disease. Vol. 2. 8th ed. Philadelphia: Lea and Febiger, 1994:1362–1372.

Chicago Dietetic Association and South Suburban Dietetic Association. Manual of clinical dietetics. 4th ed. Chicago: The American Dietetic Association, 1992.

Mahan LK, Arlin MT. Krause's food, nutrition and diet therapy. 8th ed. Philadelphia: WB Saunders, 1992.

National Academy of Sciences, National Research Council, Food and Nutrition Board, Committee on Diet and Health. Diet and health: implications for reducing chronic disease risk (executive summary). Washington, DC: National Academy Press, 1989.

National Center for Health Statistics. Healthy people 2000: review, 1993. Hyattsville, MD: US Public Health Service.

Sande M, Volberding P. The medical management of AIDS. Philadelphia: WB Saunders, 1992.

Schwartz D. Pulmonary failure. In: Gottschlich M, Materese L, Shronts, E. Eds. Nutrition support dietetic core curriculum. 2nd ed. Silver Spring, MD: ASPEN Publishers, 1993:251–260.

PERIODICALS

American Dietetic Association. Position of the American Dietetic Association and the Canadian Dietetic Association: nutrition intervention in the case of persons with human immunodeficiency virus infection. J Am Diet Assoc 1994;94:9:1042.

Anderson J. Tips when considering the diagnosis of food allergy. Top Clin Nutr 1994;9:3:11.

Bal G, Foerster S. Changing the American diet. Cancer 1991;67:2671.

Carroll P. Guidelines for counseling patients with food sensitivities. Top Clin Nutr 1994;9:3:33.

Charuhas P. Dietary management during antitumor therapy of cancer patients. Top Clin Nutr 1993;9:1:42.

Feuz A, Rapin C. An observational study of the role of pain control and food adaptation of elderly patients with terminal cancer. J Am Diet Assoc 1994;94:767.

Heimburger D, Hensrud D. Nutritional factors in cancer prevention. Support Line: Dietitians in Nutrition Support Newsletter 1994;16:4:6.

Hubbard R, Will A, & Peterson G. Evaluating dietary effects of plant and animal protein on the "on–off" effect in Parkinson's patients. Parkinson Report 1992;13:4:6.

Kendall P, Gloeckner J. Managing food allergies and sensitivities. Top Clin Nutr 1994;9:3:1.

Pahwa R, Koller W. A rational polypharmacy approach to Parkinson's. Internal Medicine 1994;15:7:52.

Pincus J. The role of dietary protein in managing fluctuations. Drugs & Nutrients in Neurology (special report) 1994;Feb:16–23.

Pinto J. The pharmacokinetic and pharmacodynamic interactions of food and drugs. Top Clin Nutr 1991;6:3:14.

Reichman L. Multidrug-resistant tuberculosis: meeting the challenges. Hosp Pract 1994; 29:5:85.

Tangney C. A review of low-protein and high-carbohydrate diets in Parkinson's disease. Drugs & Nutrients in Neurology (Special Report) 1994;Feb:24.

Timbo B, Tollefon L. Nutrition: a cofactor in HIV disease. J Am Diet Assoc 1994;94:9:1018.

Tougher-Decker R. Nutritional considerations in rheumatoid arthritis. J Am Diet Assoc 1988;88:327.

APPENDIX A

Metropolitan Life Height and Weight Tables

TABLE A-1 Height and Weight Tables

MEN					WOMEN				
HEIGHT		SMALL	MEDIUM	LARGE	HEIGHT		SMALL	MEDIUM	LARGE
Feet	**Inches**	FRAME	FRAME	FRAME	**Feet**	**Inches**	FRAME	FRAME	FRAME
5	2	128–134	131–141	138–150	4	10	102–111	109–121	118–131
5	3	130–136	133–143	140–153	4	11	103–113	111–123	120–134
5	4	132–138	135–145	142–156	5	0	104–115	113–126	122–137
5	5	134–140	137–148	144–160	5	1	106–118	115–129	125–140
5	6	136–142	139–151	146–164	5	2	108–121	118–132	128–143
5	7	138–145	142–154	149–168	5	3	111–124	121–135	131–147
5	8	140–148	145–157	152–172	5	4	114–127	124–138	134–151
5	9	142–151	148–160	155–176	5	5	117–130	127–141	137–155
5	10	144–154	151–163	158–180	5	6	120–133	130–144	140–159
5	11	146–157	154–166	161–184	5	7	123–136	133–147	143–163
6	0	149–160	157–170	164–188	5	8	126–139	136–150	146–167
6	1	152–164	160–174	168–192	5	9	129–142	139–153	149–170
6	2	155–168	164–178	172–197	5	10	132–145	142–156	152–173
6	3	158–172	167–182	176–202	5	11	135–148	145–159	155–176
6	4	162–176	171–187	181–207	6	0	138–151	148–162	158–179

(Source of basic data: 1979 Build Study, Society of Actuaries and Association of Life Insurance Medical Directors of America, 1980. Reprinted from Metropolitan Life Insurance Company, Medical Department, Health and Safety Education Division. Copyright 1993)

To approximate your frame size, see Displays 2-1 and 2-2.

APPENDIX B

Recommended Dietary Allowances

TABLE B-1 Food and Nutrition Board, National Academy of Sciences—National Research Council Recommended Dietary Allowances, Revised 1989 (Designed for the maintenance of good nutrition of practically all healthy people in the U.S.)

							FAT-SOLUBLE VITAMINS				
CATEGORY	AGE (YR) OR CONDITION	WEIGHT* (KG)	WEIGHT* (LB)	HEIGHT* (CM)	HEIGHT* (IN)	PROTEIN (G)	VITAMIN A (μg RE)‡	VITAMIN D (μg)§	VITAMIN E (mg α-TE)¶	VITAMIN K (μg)	VITAMIN C (mg)
Infants	0.0–0.5	6	13	60	24	13	375	7.5	3	5	30
	0.5–1.0	9	20	71	28	14	375	10	4	10	35
Children	1–3	13	29	90	35	16	400	10	6	15	40
	4–6	20	44	112	44	24	500	10	7	20	45
	7–10	28	62	132	52	28	700	10	7	30	45
Males	11–14	45	99	157	62	45	1000	10	10	45	50
	15–18	66	145	176	69	59	1000	10	10	65	60
	19–24	72	160	177	70	58	1000	10	10	70	60
	25–50	79	174	176	70	63	1000	5	10	80	60
	51+	77	170	173	68	63	1000	5	10	80	60
Females	11–14	46	101	157	62	46	800	10	8	45	50
	15–18	55	120	163	64	44	800	10	8	55	60
	19–24	58	128	164	65	46	800	10	8	60	60
	25–50	63	138	163	64	50	800	5	8	65	60
	51+	65	143	160	63	50	800	5	8	65	60
Pregnant						60	800	10	10	65	70
Lactating											
1st 6 mo						65	1300	10	12	65	95
2nd 6 mo						62	1200	10	11	65	90

TABLE B-1 *(continued)*

WATER-SOLUBLE VITAMINS						MINERALS						
THIAMIN (mg)	RIBOFLAVIN (mg)	NIACIN (mg NE)‖	VITAMIN B_6 (mg)	FOLATE (μg)	VITAMIN B_{12} (μg)	CALCIUM (mg)	PHOSPHORUS (mg)	MAGNESIUM (mg)	IRON (mg)	ZINC (mg)	IODINE (μg)	SELENIUM (μg)
0.3	0.4	5	0.3	25	0.3	400	300	40	6	5	40	10
0.4	0.5	6	0.6	35	0.5	600	500	60	10	5	50	15
0.7	0.8	9	1.0	50	0.7	800	800	80	10	10	70	20
0.9	1.1	12	1.1	75	1.0	800	800	120	10	10	90	20
1.0	1.2	13	1.4	100	1.4	800	800	170	10	10	120	30
1.3	1.5	17	1.7	150	2.0	1200	1200	270	12	15	150	40
1.5	1.8	20	2.0	200	2.0	1200	1200	400	12	15	150	50
1.5	1.7	19	2.0	200	2.0	1200	1200	350	10	15	150	70
1.5	1.7	19	2.0	200	2.0	800	800	350	10	15	150	70
1.2	1.4	15	2.0	200	2.0	800	800	350	10	15	150	70
1.1	1.3	15	1.4	150	2.0	1200	1200	280	15	12	150	45
1.1	1.3	15	1.5	180	2.0	1200	1200	300	15	12	150	50
1.1	1.3	15	1.6	180	2.0	1200	1200	280	15	12	150	55
1.1	1.3	15	1.6	180	2.0	800	800	280	15	12	150	55
1.0	1.2	13	1.6	180	2.0	800	800	280	10	12	150	55
1.5	1.6	17	2.2	400	2.2	1200	1200	320	30	15	175	65
1.6	1.8	20	2.1	280	2.6	1200	1200	355	15	19	200	75
1.6	1.7	20	2.1	260	2.6	1200	1200	340	15	16	200	75

The allowances, expressed as average daily intakes over time, are intended to provide for individual variations among most normal persons as they live in the United States under usual environmental stresses. Diets should be based on a variety of common foods in order to provide other nutrients for which human requirements have been less well defined. See text for detailed discussion of allowances and of nutrients not tabulated.

* Weights and heights of Reference Adults are actual medians for the U.S. population of the designated age, as reported by NHANES II. The median weights and heights of those under 19 years of age were taken from Hamill et al. (1979) (see pages 16–17). The use of these figures does not imply that the height-to-weight ratios are ideal.

‡ Retinol equivalents. 1 RE = 1 μg retinal or 6 μg B-carotene.

§ As cholecalciferol. 10 μg cholecalciferol = 400 IU of vitamin D.

¶ α-Tocopherol equivalents. 1 mg d-α-tocopherol = 1 α-TE.

‖ 1 NE (niacin equivalent) is equal to 1 mg of niacin or 60 mg of dietary tryptophan.

(National Research Council, Subcommittee on the Tenth Edition of the RDAs. Recommended dietary allowances. 10th ed. Washington, DC: National Academy Press, 1989).

APPENDIX C

Recommended Nutrient Intakes for Canadians

TABLE C-1 Health Canada–Nutrition Recommendations

Age	Sex	Weight (kg)	Protein (g)	Vitamin A (RE)	Vitamin D (μg)	Vitamin E (mg)	Vitamin C (mg)
0–4 mo	M,F	6	12*	400	10	3	20
5–12 mo	M,F	9	12	400	10	3	20
1 yr	M,F	11	13	400	10	3	20
2–3 yr	M,F	14	16	400	5	4	20
4–6 yr	M,F	18	19	500	5	5	25
7–9 yr	M	25	26	700	2.5	7	25
	F	25	26	700	2.5	6	25
10–12 yr	M	34	34	800	2.5	8	25
	F	36	36	800	2.5	7	25
13–15 yr	M	50	49	900	2.5	9	30§
	F	48	46	800	2.5	7	30§
16–18 yr	M	62	58	1000	2.5	10	40§
	F	53	47	800	2.5	7	30§
19–24 yr	M	71	61	1000	2.5	10	40§
	F	58	50	800	2.5	7	30§
25–49 yr	M	74	64	1000	2.5	9	40§
	F	59	51	800	2.5	6	30§
50–74 yr	M	73	63	1000	5	7	40§
	F	63	54	800	5	6	30§
75+ yr	M	69	59	1000	5	6	40§
	F	64	55	800	5	5	30§
Pregnancy							
1st trimester			+5	0	+2.5	+2	0
2nd trimester			+15	0	+2.5	+2	+10
3nd trimester			+24	0	+2.5	+2	+10
Lactation			+22	+400	+2.5	+3	+25

TABLE C-1 *(continued)*

FOLATE (μG)	VITAMIN B_{12} (μG)	CALCIUM (MG)	PHOSPHORUS (MG)	MAGNESIUM (MG)	IRON (MG)	IODINE (μG)	ZINC (MG)
25	0.3	250†	150	20	0.3‡	30	2‡
40	0.4	400	200	32	7	40	3
40	0.5	500	300	40	6	55	4
50	0.6	550	350	50	6	65	4
70	0.8	600	400	65	8	85	5
90	1.0	700	500	100	8	110	7
90	1.0	700	500	100	8	95	7
120	1.0	900	700	130	8	125	9
130	1.0	1100	800	135	8	110	9
175	1.0	1100	900	185	10	160	12
170	1.0	1000	850	180	13	160	9
220	1.0	900	1000	230	10	160	12
190	1.0	700	850	200	12	160	9
220	1.0	800	1000	240	9	160	12
180	1.0	700	850	200	13	160	9
230	1.0	800	1000	250	9	160	12
185	1.0	700	850	200	13	160	9
230	1.0	800	1000	250	9	160	12
195	1.0	800	850	210	8	160	9
215	1.0	800	1000	230	9	160	12
200	1.0	800	850	210	8	160	9
+200	+0.2	+500	+200	+15	0	+25	+6
+200	+0.2	+500	+200	+45	+5	+25	+6
+200	+0.2	+500	+200	+45	+10	+25	+6
+100	+0.2	+500	+200	+65	0	+50	+6

* Protein is assumed to be from breast milk and must be adjusted for infant formula.

† Infant formula with high phosphorus should contain 375 mg of calcium.

‡ Breast milk is assumed to be the source of the mineral.

§ Smokers should increase vitamin C by 50%.

(Health Canada, Nutrition recommendations: A report of the Scientific Review Committee, Reproduced with permission of the Minister of Supply and Services Canada, 1994.)

APPENDIX

D

The Scientific Review Committee: Defining the Canadian Diet

The Scientific Review Committee conducted an in-depth study of nutrition recommendations for Canadians and the recommended nutrient intakes for Canadians, to incorporate new research findings that might contribute to a healthier diet. The ultimate purpose of the review was to provide guidance to Canadians over 2 years of age in making food choices that will supply recommended levels of essential nutrients while reducing the risk of chronic disease.

The Committee adopted the following key statements as the Nutrition Recommendations for Canadians.

NUTRITION RECOMMENDATIONS FOR CANADIANS*

- *The Canadian diet should provide energy consistent with the maintenance of body weight within the recommended range.*
- *The Canadian diet should include essential nutrients in amounts recommended.*
- *The Canadian diet should include no more than 30% of energy as fat (33 g/1000 kcal or 39 g/5000 kJ) and no more than 10% as saturated fat (11 g/1000 kcal or 13 g/5000 kJ).*
- *The Canadian diet should provide 55% of energy as carbohydrate (138 g/1000 kcal or 165 g/5000 kJ) from a variety of sources.*
- *The sodium content of the Canadian diet should be reduced.*
- *The Canadian diet should include no more than 5% of total energy as alcohol, or two drinks daily, whichever is less.*
- *The Canadian diet should contain no more caffeine than the equivalent of four regular cups of coffee per day.*
- *Community water supplies containing less than 1 mg/L should be fluoridated to that level.*

More fully, the key findings were:

- *The Canadian diet should provide energy consistent with the maintenance of body weight within the recommended range.* Physical activity should be appropriate to circumstances and capabilities. Both longevity and the incidence of a number of chronic diseases are associated adversely with body weights above or below the recommended range. There is, thus, a health benefit to controlling weight, but a possible downside to control by energy intake alone. Physical activity should also play a role. While the importance of maintaining some activity throughout life can be stressed, it is not possible to specify a level of physical activity appropriate for the whole population. As a general guideline it is desirable that adults, for as long as possible, maintain an activity level that permits an energy intake of at least 1800 kcal or 7.6 MJ/day while keeping weight within the recommended range.
- *The Canadian diet should include essential nutrients in amounts recommended.* One of the reasons for including physical activity as a desirable element in weight control is the increasing difficulty in meeting the recommended nutrient intake (RNI) as energy intake falls below 1800 kcal or 7.6 MJ/day. While it is important that the diet provide the recommended amounts of nutrients, it should be understood that no evidence was found that intakes in excess of the

(Nutrition recommendations: A call to action: Health Canada 1990. Reproduced with permission of Minister of Supply and Services Canada, 1995.)

*Over 2 years of age.

RNIs confer any health benefit. There is no general need for supplements except for vitamin D for infants and folic acid during pregnancy. Vitamin D supplementation might be required for elderly persons not exposed to the sun, and iron for pregnant women with low iron stores. It should be noted that while the habitual intake of certain nutrients, for example, protein and vitamin C, greatly exceeds the RNI, there is no reason to suggest that present intakes can be reduced.

- *The Canadian diet should include no more than 30% of energy as fat (33 g/1000 kcal or 39 g/5000 kJ) and no more than 10% as saturated fat (11 g/1000 kcal or 13 g/5000 kJ).* Diets high in fat have been associated with a high incidence of heart disease and certain types of cancer and a reduction in total fat intake is an important way to reduce the intake of saturated fat. The evidence linking saturated fat intake with elevated blood cholesterol and the risk of heart disease is among the most persuasive of all diet/disease relationships and was an important factor in establishing the recommended dietary pattern. Dietary cholesterol, though not as influential in affecting levels of blood cholesterol, is not without importance. A reduction in cholesterol intake normally will accompany a reduction in total fat and saturated fat. The recommendation to reduce total fat intake does not apply to children under the age of 2 years.
- *The Canadian diet should provide 55% of energy as carbohydrate (138 g/1000 kcal or 165 g/5000 kJ) from a variety of sources.* Sources selected should provide complex carbohydrates, a variety of dietary fibre and β-carotene. Carbohydrate is the preferred replacement for fat as a source of energy since protein intake already exceeds requirements. There are a number of reasons why the increased carbohydrate calories should be in the form of complex carbohydrates. Diets high in complex carbohydrates have been associated with a lower incidence of heart disease and cancer, and are sources of dietary fibre and of β-carotene.
- *The sodium content of the Canadian diet should be reduced.* The present food supply provides sodium in an amount greatly exceeding requirements. While there is insufficient evidence to support a quantitative recommendation, potential benefit would be expected from a reduction in current sodium intake. Consumers are encouraged to reduce the use of salt (sodium chloride) in cooking and at the table, but individual efforts will be relatively ineffective unless the food industry makes a determined effort to reduce the sodium content of processed and prepared food. A diet rich in fruits and vegetables will ensure an adequate intake of potassium.
- *The Canadian diet should include no more than 5% of total energy as alcohol, or two drinks daily, whichever is less.* There are many reasons to limit the use of alcohol. From the nutritional point of view, alcohol dilutes the nutrient density of the diet and can undermine the consumption of RNIs. The deleterious influence of alcohol on blood pressure provides more urgent reason for moderation. During pregnancy it is prudent to abstain from alcoholic beverages because a safe intake is not known with certainty.
- *The Canadian diet should contain no more caffeine than the equivalent of four regular cups of coffee per day.* This is a prudent measure in view of the increased risk of cardiovascular disease associated with high intakes of caffeine.
- *Community water supplies containing less than 1 mg/L should be fluoridated to that level.* Fluoridation of community water supplies has proven to be a safe, effective, and economical method of improving dental health.

The report of the Scientific Review Committee is valuable to researchers, educators, students, practitioners, and policy-makers. From the range of scientific and technical sources consulted, the Committee provided the scientific basis for healthy eating in Canada.

CANADA'S GUIDELINES FOR HEALTHY EATING*

- *Enjoy a VARIETY of foods.*
- *Emphasize cereals, breads, other grain products, vegetables and fruits.*
- *Choose lower fat dairy products, leaner meats and foods prepared with little or no fat.*
- *Achieve and maintain a healthy body weight by enjoying regular physical activity and healthy eating.*
- *Limit salt, alcohol, and caffeine.*

*For healthy Canadians over 2 years of age.

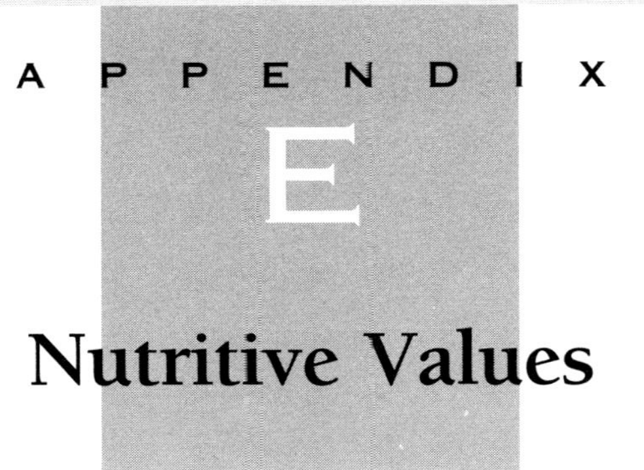

APPENDIX E

Nutritive Values

TABLE E-1 Nutritive Value of the Edible Part of Food*
(footnotes on p. 682)
(nutrients in indicated quantity)

ITEM	FOODS, APPROXIMATE MEASURES, UNITS, AND WEIGHT (WEIGHT OF EDIBLE PORTION ONLY)	WEIGHT (G)	WATER (%)	FOOD ENERGY (KCAL)	PROTEIN (G)	FAT (G)	FATTY ACIDS SATURATED (G)	MONOUNSATURATED (G)	POLYUNSATURATED (G)	CHOLESTEROL (MG)	CARBOHYDRATE (G)	CALCIUM (MG)	PHOSPHORUS (MG)	IRON (MG)	POTASSIUM (MG)	SODIUM (MG)	VITAMIN A VALUE (IU)	VITAMIN A VALUE (RE)	THIAMIN (MG)	RIBOFLAVIN (MG)	NIACIN (MG)	ASCORBIC ACID (MG)
BEVERAGES																						
Alcoholic																						
		0,000	000	0.000	00	000	000.0	0C0.0	000.0	0,000	000	000.0	000.0	00.0^{00}	000.0	$0,000^{00}$	$00,000^{00}$	$0,000^{00}$	00.0^{00}	00.0^{00}	$00\ 0^{00}$	000^{00}
Beer																						
Regular	12 fl oz	360	92	150	1	0	0.0	0.0	0.0	0	13	14	50	0.1	115	18	0	0	0.02	0.09	1.8	0
Light	12 fl oz	355	95	95	1	0	0.0	0.0	0.0	0	5	14	43	0.1	64	11	0	0	0.03	0.11	1.4	0
Gin, rum, vodka, whiskey																						
80-proof	1-$^1/_2$ fl oz	42	67	95	0	0	0.0	0.0	0.0	0	Tr	Tr	Tr	Tr	1	Tr	0	0	Tr	Tr	Tr	0
86-proof	1-$^1/_2$ fl oz	42	64	105	0	0	0.0	0.0	0.0	0	Tr	Tr	Tr	Tr	1	Tr	0	0	Tr	Tr	Tr	0

90-proof	1-1/2 fl oz	42	62	110	0	0	0.0	0.0	0.0	0	Tr	Tr	Tr	Tr	1	Tr	0	0	Tr	Tr	Tr	0
Wines																						
Dessert	3-1/2 fl oz	103	77	140	Tr	0	0.0	0.0	0.0	0	8	8	9	0.2	95	9	([1])	([1])	0.01	0.02	0.2	0
Table																						
Red	3-1/2 fl oz	102	88	75	Tr	0	0.0	0.0	0.0	0	3	8	18	0.4	113	5	([1])	([1])	0.00	0.03	0.1	0
White	3-1/2 fl oz	102	87	80	Tr	0	0.0	0.0	0.0	0	3	9	14	0.3	83	5	([1])	([1])	0.00	0.01	0.1	0
Carbonated[2]																						
Club soda	12 fl oz	355	100	0	0	0	0.0	0.0	0.0	0	0	18	0	Tr	0	78	0	0	0.00	0.00	0.0	0
Cola type																						
Regular	12 fl oz	369	89	160	0	0	0.0	0.0	0.0	0	41	11	52	0.2	7	18	0	0	0.00	0.00	0.0	0
Diet, artifically sweetened	12 fl oz	355	100	Tr	0	0	0.0	0.0	0.0	0	Tr	14	39	0.2	7	[3]32	0	0	0.00	0.00	0.0	0
Ginger ale	12 fl oz	366	91	125	0	0	0.0	0.0	0.0	0	32	11	0	0.1	4	29	0	0	0.00	0.00	0.0	0
Grape	12 fl oz	372	88	180	0	0	0.0	0.0	0.0	0	46	15	0	0.4	4	48	0	0	0.00	0.00	0.0	0
Lemon-lime	12 fl oz	372	89	155	0	0	0.0	0.0	0.0	0	39	7	0	0.4	4	33	0	0	0.00	0.00	0.0	0
Orange	12 fl oz	372	88	180	0	0	0.0	0.0	0.0	0	46	15	4	0.3	7	52	0	0	0.00	0.00	0.0	0
Pepper type	12 fl oz	369	89	160	0	0	0.0	0.0	0.0	0	41	11	41	0.1	4	37	0	0	0.00	0.00	0.0	0
Root beer	12 fl oz	370	89	165	0	0	0.0	0.0	0.0	0	42	15	0	0.2	4	48	0	0	0.00	0.00	0.0	0
Cocoa and chocolate-flavored beverages																						
See Dairy Products.																						
Coffee																						
Brewed	6 fl oz	180	100	Tr	Tr	Tr	Tr	Tr	Tr	0	Tr	4	2	Tr	124	2	0	0	0.00	0.02	0.4	0
Instant, prepared (2 tsp powder plus 6 fl oz water)	6 fl oz	182	99	Tr	Tr	Tr	Tr	Tr	Tr	0	1	2	6	0.1	71	Tr	0	0	0.00	0.03	0.6	0
Fruit drinks, noncarbonated																						
Canned																						
Fruit punch drink	6 fl oz	190	88	85	Tr	0	0.0	0.0	0.0	0	22	15	2	0.4	48	15	20	2	0.03	0.04	Tr	[4]61
Grape drink	6 fl oz	187	86	100	Tr	0	0.0	0.0	0.0	0	26	2	2	0.3	9	11	Tr	Tr	0.01	0.01	Tr	[4]64
Pineapple-grapefruit juice drink	6 fl oz	187	87	90	Tr	Tr	Tr	Tr	Tr	0	23	13	7	0.9	97	24	60	6	0.06	0.04	0.5	[4]110
Frozen																						
Lemonade concentrate																						
Undiluted	6 fl oz	219	49	425	Tr	Tr	Tr	Tr	Tr	0	112	9	13	0.4	153	4	40	4	0.04	0.07	0.7	66
Diluted with 4-1/3 parts water by volume	6 fl oz	185	89	80	Tr	Tr	Tr	Tr	Tr	0	21	2	2	0.1	30	1	10	1	0.01	0.02	0.2	13
Limeade concentrate																						
Undiluted	6 fl oz	218	50	410	Tr	Tr	Tr	Tr	Tr	0	108	11	13	0.2	129	Tr	Tr	Tr	0.02	0.02	0.2	26
Diluted with 4-1/3 parts water by volume	6 fl oz	185	89	75	Tr	Tr	Tr	Tr	Tr	0	20	2	2	Tr	24	Tr	Tr	Tr	Tr	Tr	Tr	4
Fruit juices																						
See type under Fruits and Fruit Juices.																						
Milk beverages																						
See Dairy Products.																						
Tea																						
Brewed	8 fl oz	240	100	Tr	Tr	Tr	Tr	Tr	Tr	0	Tr	0	2	Tr	36	1	0	0	0.00	0.03	Tr	0
Instant, powder, prepared																						
Unsweetened (1 tsp powder plus 8 fl oz water)	8 fl oz	241	100	Tr	Tr	Tr	Tr	Tr	Tr	0	1	1	4	Tr	61	1	0	0	0.00	0.02	0.1	0

(Continued)

TABLE E-1 *(continued)*

ITEM	FOODS, APPROXIMATE MEASURES, UNITS, AND WEIGHT (WEIGHT OF EDIBLE PORTION ONLY)	WEIGHT (G)	WATER (%)	FOOD ENERGY (KCAL)	PROTEIN (G)	FAT (G)	FATTY ACIDS SATURATED (G)	FATTY ACIDS MONOUNSATURATED (G)	FATTY ACIDS POLYUNSATURATED (G)	CHOLESTEROL (MG)	CARBOHYDRATE (G)	CALCIUM (MG)	PHOSPHORUS (MG)	IRON (MG)	POTASSIUM (MG)	SODIUM (MG)	VITAMIN A VALUE (IU)	VITAMIN A VALUE (RE)	THIAMIN (MG)	RIBOFLAVIN (MG)	NIACIN (MG)	ASCORBIC ACID (MG)
Sweetened (3 tsp powder plus 8 fl oz water)	8 fl oz	262	91	85	Tr	Tr	Tr	Tr	Tr	0	22	1	3	Tr	49	Tr	0	0	0.00	0.04	0.1	0
DAIRY PRODUCTS																						
Butter																						
See Fats and Oils.																						
Cheese																						
Natural																						
Blue	1 oz	28	42	100	6	8	5.3	2.2	0.2	21	1	150	110	0.1	73	396	200	65	0.01	0.11	0.3	0
Camembert (3 wedges per 4-oz container)	1 wedge	38	52	115	8	9	5.8	2.7	0.3	27	Tr	147	132	0.1	71	320	350	96	0.01	0.19	0.2	0
Cheddar																						
Cut pieces	1 oz	28	37	115	7	9	6.0	2.7	0.3	30	Tr	204	145	0.2	28	176	300	86	0.01	0.11	Tr	0
	1 in³	17	37	70	4	6	3.6	1.6	0.2	18	Tr	123	87	0.1	17	105	180	52	Tr	0.06	Tr	0
Shredded	1 cup	113	37	455	28	37	23.8	10.6	1.1	119	1	815	579	0.8	111	701	1,200	342	0.03	0.42	0.1	0
Cottage (curd not pressed down)																						
Creamed (cottage cheese, 4% fat)																						
Large curd	1 cup	225	79	235	28	10	6.4	2.9	0.3	34	6	135	297	0.3	190	911	370	108	0.05	0.37	0.3	Tr
Small curd	1 cup	210	79	215	26	9	6.0	2.7	0.3	31	6	126	277	0.3	177	850	340	101	0.04	0.34	0.3	Tr
With fruit	1 cup	226	72	280	22	8	4.9	2.2	0.2	25	30	108	236	0.2	151	915	280	81	0.04	0.29	0.2	Tr
Lowfat (2%)	1 cup	226	79	205	31	4	2.8	1.2	0.1	19	8	155	340	0.4	217	918	160	45	0.05	0.42	0.3	Tr
Uncreamed (cottage cheese dry curd, less than 1/2% fat)	1 cup	145	80	125	25	1	0.4	0.2	Tr	10	3	46	151	0.3	47	19	40	12	0.04	0.21	0.2	0
Cream	1 oz	28	54	100	2	10	6.2	2.8	0.4	31	1	23	30	0.3	34	84	400	124	Tr	0.06	Tr	0
Feta	1 oz	28	55	75	4	6	4.2	1.3	0.2	25	1	140	96	0.2	18	316	130	36	0.04	0.24	0.3	0
Mozzarella, made with																						
Whole milk	1 oz	28	54	80	6	6	3.7	1.9	0.2	22	1	147	105	0.1	19	106	220	68	Tr	0.07	Tr	0
Part skim milk (low moisture)	1 oz	28	49	80	8	5	3.1	1.4	0.1	15	1	207	149	0.1	27	150	180	54	0.01	0.10	Tr	0
Muenster	1 oz	28	42	105	7	9	5.4	2.5	0.2	27	Tr	203	133	0.1	38	178	320	90	Tr	0.09	Tr	0
Parmesan, grated																						
Cup, not pressed down	1 cup	100	18	455	42	30	19.1	3.7	0.7	79	4	1,376	807	1.0	107	1,861	700	173	0.05	0.39	0.3	0
Tablespoon	1 tbsp	5	18	25	2	2	1.0	0.4	Tr	4	Tr	69	40	Tr	5	93	40	9	Tr	0.02	Tr	0
Ounce	1 oz	28	18	130	12	9	5.4	2.5	0.2	22	1	390	229	0.3	30	528	200	49	0.01	0.11	0.1	0
Provolone	1 oz	28	41	100	7	8	4.8	2.1	0.2	20	1	214	141	0.1	39	248	230	75	0.01	0.09	Tr	0
Ricotta, made with																						
Whole milk	1 cup	246	72	430	28	32	20.4	8.9	0.9	124	7	509	389	0.9	257	207	1,210	330	0.03	0.48	0.3	0

Part skim milk	1 cup	246	74	340	28	19	12.1	5.7	0.6	76	13	669	449	1.1	307	307	1,060	278	0.05	0.46	0.2	0
Swiss	1 oz	28	37	105	8	8	5.0	2.1	0.3	26	1	272	171	Tr	31	74	240	72	0.01	0.10	Tr	0
Pasteurized process cheese																						
American	1 oz	28	39	105	6	9	5.6	2.5	0.3	27	Tr	174	211	0.1	46	406	340	82	0.01	0.10	Tr	0
Swiss	1 oz	28	42	95	7	7	4.5	2.0	0.2	24	1	219	216	0.2	61	388	230	65	Tr	0.08	Tr	0
Pasteurized process cheese food, American	1 oz	28	43	95	6	7	4.4	2.0	0.2	18	2	163	130	0.2	79	337	260	62	0.01	0.13	Tr	0
Pasteurized process cheese spread, American	1 oz	28	48	80	5	6	3.8	1.8	0.2	16	2	159	202	0.1	69	381	220	54	0.01	0.12	Tr	0
Cream, sweet																						
Half-and-half (cream and milk)	1 cup	242	81	315	7	28	17.3	8.0	1.0	89	10	254	230	0.2	314	98	1,050	259	0.08	0.36	0.2	2
	1 tbsp	15	81	20	Tr	2	1.1	0.5	0.1	6	1	16	14	Tr	19	6	70	16	0.01	0.02	Tr	Tr
Light, coffee, or table	1 cup	240	74	470	6	46	28.8	13.4	1.7	159	9	231	192	0.1	292	95	1,730	437	0.08	0.36	0.1	2
	1 tbsp	15	74	30	Tr	3	1.8	0.8	0.1	10	1	14	12	Tr	18	6	110	27	Tr	0.02	Tr	Tr
Whipping, unwhipped (volume about double when whipped)																						
Light	1 cup	239	64	700	5	74	46.2	21.7	2.1	265	7	166	146	0.1	231	82	2,690	705	0.06	0.30	0.1	1
	1 tbsp	15	64	45	Tr	5	2.9	1.4	0.1	17	Tr	10	9	Tr	15	5	170	44	Tr	0.02	Tr	Tr
Heavy	1 cup	238	58	820	5	88	54.8	25.4	3.3	326	7	154	149	0.1	179	89	3,500	1,002	0.05	0.26	0.1	1
	1 tbsp	15	58	50	Tr	6	3.5	1.6	0.2	21	Tr	10	9	Tr	11	6	220	63	Tr	0.02	Tr	Tr
Whipped topping, (pressurized)	1 cup	60	61	155	2	13	8.3	3.9	0.5	46	7	61	54	Tr	88	78	550	124	0.02	0.04	Tr	0
	1 tbsp	3	61	10	Tr	1	0.4	0.2	Tr	2	Tr	3	3	Tr	4	4	30	6	Tr	Tr	Tr	0
Cream, sour																						
	1 cup	230	71	495	7	48	30.0	13.9	1.8	102	10	268	195	0.1	331	123	1,820	448	0.08	0.34	0.2	2
	1 tbsp	12	71	25	Tr	3	1.6	0.7	0.1	5	1	14	10	Tr	17	6	90	23	Tr	0.02	Tr	Tr
Cream products, imitation (made with vegetable fat)																						
Sweet																						
Creamers																						
Liquid (frozen)	1 tbsp	15	77	20	Tr	1	1.4	Tr	Tr	0	2	1	10	Tr	29	12	[5]10	[5]1	0.00	0.00	0.0	0
Powdered	1 tsp	2	2	10	Tr	1	0.7	Tr	Tr	0	1	Tr	8	Tr	16	4	Tr	Tr	0.00	Tr	0.0	0
Whipped topping																						
Frozen	1 cup	75	50	240	1	19	16.3	1.2	0.4	0	17	5	6	0.1	14	19	[5]650	[5]65	0.00	0.00	0.0	0
	1 tbsp	4	50	15	Tr	1	0.9	0.1	Tr	0	1	Tr	Tr	Tr	1	1	[5]30	[5]3	0.00	0.00	0.0	0
Powdered, made with whole milk	1 cup	80	67	150	3	10	8.5	0.7	0.2	8	13	72	69	Tr	121	53	[5]290	[5]39	0.02	0.09	Tr	1
	1 tbsp	4	67	10	Tr	Tr	0.4	Tr	Tr	Tr	1	4	3	Tr	6	3	[5]10	[5]2	Tr	Tr	Tr	Tr
Pressurized	1 cup	70	60	185	1	16	13.2	1.3	0.2	0	11	4	13	Tr	13	43	[5]330	[5]33	0.00	0.00	0.0	0
	1 tbsp	4	60	10	Tr	1	0.8	0.1	Tr	0	1	Tr	1	Tr	1	2	[5]20	[5]2	0.00	0.00	0.0	0
Sour dressing (filled cream type product, nonbutterfat)	1 cup	235	75	415	8	39	31.2	4.6	1.1	13	11	266	205	0.1	380	113	20	5	0.09	0.38	0.2	2
	1 tbsp	12	75	20	Tr	2	1.6	0.2	0.1	1	1	14	10	Tr	19	6	Tr	Tr	Tr	0.02	Tr	Tr
Ice cream.																						
See Milk desserts, frozen.																						
Ice milk.																						
See Milk desserts, frozen.																						

(Continued)

TABLE E-1 *(continued)*

ITEM	FOODS, APPROXIMATE MEASURES, UNITS, AND WEIGHT (WEIGHT OF EDIBLE PORTION ONLY)	WEIGHT (G)	WATER (%)	FOOD ENERGY (KCAL)	PROTEIN (G)	FAT (G)	FATTY ACIDS: SATURATED (G)	MONOUNSATURATED (G)	POLYUNSATURATED (G)	CHOLESTEROL (MG)	CARBOHYDRATE (G)	CALCIUM (MG)	PHOSPHORUS (MG)	IRON (MG)	POTASSIUM (MG)	SODIUM (MG)	VITAMIN A VALUE (IU)	VITAMIN A VALUE (RE)	THIAMIN (MG)	RIBOFLAVIN (MG)	NIACIN (MG)	ASCORBIC ACID (MG)
Milk																						
Fluid																						
Whole (3.3% fat)	1 cup	244	88	150	8	8	5.1	2.4	0.3	33	11	291	228	0.1	370	120	310	76	0.09	0.40	0.2	2
Lowfat (2%)																						
No milk solids added	1 cup	244	89	120	8	5	2.9	1.4	0.2	18	12	297	232	0.1	377	122	500	139	0.10	0.40	0.2	2
Milk solids added, label claim less than 10 g of protein per cup	1 cup	245	89	125	9	5	2.9	1.4	0.2	18	12	313	245	0.1	397	128	500	140	0.10	0.42	0.2	2
Lowfat (1%)																						
No milk solids added	1 cup	244	90	100	8	3	1.6	0.7	0.1	10	12	300	235	0.1	381	123	500	144	0.10	0.41	0.2	2
Milk solids added, label claim less than 10 g of protein per cup	1 cup	245	90	105	9	2	1.5	0.7	0.1	10	12	313	245	0.1	397	128	500	145	0.10	0.42	0.2	2
Nonfat (skim)																						
No milk solids added	1 cup	245	91	85	8	Tr	0.3	0.1	Tr	4	12	302	247	0.1	406	126	500	149	0.09	0.34	0.2	2
Milk solids added, label claim less than 10 g of protein per cup	1 cup	245	90	90	9	1	0.4	0.2	Tr	5	12	316	255	0.1	418	130	500	149	0.10	0.43	0.2	2
Buttermilk	1 cup	245	90	100	8	2	1.3	0.6	0.1	9	12	285	219	0.1	371	257	80	20	0.08	0.38	0.1	2
Canned																						
Condensed, sweetened	1 cup	306	27	980	24	27	16.8	7.4	1.0	104	166	868	775	0.6	1,136	389	1,000	248	0.28	1.27	0.6	8
Evaporated																						
Whole milk	1 cup	252	74	340	17	19	11.6	5.9	0.6	74	25	657	510	0.5	764	267	610	136	0.12	0.80	0.5	5
Skim milk	1 cup	255	79	200	19	1	0.3	0.2	Tr	9	29	738	497	0.7	845	293	1,000	298	0.11	0.79	0.4	3
Dried																						
Buttermilk	1 cup	120	3	465	41	7	4.3	2.0	0.3	83	59	1,421	1,119	0.4	1,910	621	260	65	0.47	1.89	1.1	7
Nonfat, instantized																						
Envelope, 3.2 oz, net wt.[6]	1 envelope	91	4	325	32	1	0.4	0.2	Tr	17	47	1,120	896	0.3	1,552	499	[7]2,160	[7]646	0.38	1.59	0.8	5
Cup	1 cup	68	4	245	24	Tr	0.3	0.1	Tr	12	35	837	670	0.2	1,160	373	[7]1,610	[7]483	0.28	1.19	0.6	4
Milk beverages																						
Chocolate milk (commercial)																						
Regular	1 cup	250	82	210	8	8	5.3	2.5	0.3	31	26	280	251	0.6	417	149	300	73	0.09	0.41	0.3	2
Lowfat (2%)	1 cup	250	84	180	8	5	3.1	1.5	0.2	17	26	284	254	0.6	422	151	500	143	0.09	0.41	0.3	2
Lowfat (1%)	1 cup	250	85	160	8	3	1.5	0.8	0.1	7	26	287	256	0.6	425	152	500	148	0.10	0.42	0.3	2
Cocoa and chocolate-flavored beverages																						
Powder containing nonfat dry milk	1 oz	28	1	100	3	1	0.6	0.3	Tr	1	22	90	88	0.3	223	139	Tr	Tr	0.03	0.17	0.2	Tr
Prepared (6 oz water plus 1 oz powder)	1 serving	206	86	100	3	1	0.6	0.3	Tr	1	22	90	88	0.3	223	139	Tr	Tr	0.03	0.17	0.2	Tr
Powder without nonfat dry milk	$^3/_4$ oz	21	1	75	1	1	0.3	0.2	Tr	0	19	7	26	0.7	136	56	Tr	Tr	Tr	0.03	0.1	Tr

Prepared (8 oz whole milk plus 3/4 oz powder)	1 serving	265	81	225	9	9	5.4	2.5	0.3	33	30	298	254	0.9	508	176	310	76	0.10	0.43	0.3	3
Eggnog (commercial)	1 cup	254	74	340	10	19	11.3	5.7	0.9	149	34	330	278	0.5	420	138	890	203	0.09	0.48	0.3	4
Malted milk																						
Chocolate																						
Powder	3/4 oz	21	2	85	1	1	0.5	0.3	0.1	1	18	13	37	0.4	130	49	20	5	0.04	0.04	0.4	0
Prepared (8 oz whole milk plus 3/4 oz powder)	1 serving	265	81	235	9	9	5.5	2.7	0.4	34	29	304	265	0.5	500	168	330	80	0.14	0.43	0.7	2
Natural																						
Powder	3/4 oz	21	3	85	3	2	0.9	0.5	0.3	4	15	56	79	0.2	159	96	70	17	0.11	0.14	1.1	0
Prepared (8 oz whole milk plus 3/4 oz powder)	1 serving	265	81	235	11	10	6.0	2.9	0.6	37	27	347	307	0.3	529	215	380	93	0.20	0.54	1.3	2
Shakes, thick																						
Chocolate	10 oz	283	72	335	9	8	4.8	2.2	0.3	30	60	374	357	0.9	634	314	240	59	0.13	0.63	0.4	0
Vanilla	10 oz	283	74	315	11	9	5.3	2.5	0.3	33	50	413	326	0.3	517	270	320	79	0.08	0.55	0.4	0
Milk desserts, frozen																						
Ice cream, vanilla																						
Regular (about 11% fat)																						
Hardened	1/2 gal	1,064	61	2,155	38	115	71.3	33.1	4.3	476	254	1,406	1,075	1.0	2,052	929	4,340	1,064	0.42	2.63	1.1	6
	1 cup	133	61	270	5	14	8.9	4.1	0.5	59	32	176	134	0.1	257	116	540	133	0.05	0.33	0.1	1
	3 fl oz	50	61	100	2	5	3.4	1.6	0.2	22	12	66	51	Tr	96	44	200	50	0.02	0.12	0.1	Tr
Soft serve (frozen custard)	1 cup	173	60	375	7	23	13.5	6.7	1.0	153	38	236	199	0.4	338	153	790	199	0.08	0.45	0.2	1
Rich (about 16% fat), hardened	1/2 gal	1,188	59	2,805	33	190	118.3	54.9	7.1	703	256	1,213	927	0.8	1,771	868	7,200	1,758	0.36	2.27	0.9	5
	1 cup	148	59	350	4	24	14.7	6.8	0.9	88	32	151	115	0.1	221	108	900	219	0.04	0.28	0.1	1
Ice milk, vanilla																						
Hardened (about 4% fat)	1/2 gal	1,048	69	1,470	41	45	28.1	13.0	1.7	146	232	1,409	1,035	1.5	2,117	836	1,710	419	0.61	2.78	0.9	6
	1 cup	131	69	185	5	6	3.5	1.6	0.2	18	29	176	129	0.2	265	105	210	52	0.08	0.35	0.1	1
Soft serve (about 3% fat)	1 cup	175	70	225	8	5	2.9	1.3	0.2	13	38	274	202	0.3	412	163	175	44	0.12	0.54	0.2	1
Sherbet (about 2% fat)	1/2 gal	1,542	66	2,160	17	31	19.0	8.8	1.1	113	469	827	594	2.5	1,585	706	1,480	308	0.26	0.71	1.0	31
	1 cup	193	66	270	2	4	2.4	1.1	0.1	14	59	103	74	0.3	198	88	190	39	0.03	0.09	0.1	4
Yogurt																						
With added milk solids																						
Made with lowfat milk																						
Fruit-flavored[8]	8 oz	227	74	230	10	2	1.6	0.7	0.1	10	43	345	271	0.2	442	133	100	25	0.08	0.40	0.2	1
Plain	8 oz	227	85	145	12	4	2.3	1.0	0.1	14	16	415	326	0.2	531	159	150	36	0.10	0.49	0.3	2
Made with nonfat milk	8 oz	227	85	125	13	Tr	0.3	0.1	Tr	4	17	452	355	0.2	579	174	20	5	0.11	0.53	0.3	2
Made with whole milk	8 oz	227	88	140	8	7	4.8	2.0	0.2	29	11	274	215	0.1	351	105	280	68	0.07	0.32	0.2	1
Without added milk solids																						
EGGS																						
Eggs, large (24 oz per dozen)																						
Raw																						
Whole, without shell	1	50	75	75	6	5	1.6	1.9	0.7	213	1	25	89	0.7	60	63	320	95	0.03	0.25	Tr	0
White	1	33	88	15	4	0	0.0	0.0	0.0	0	Tr	2	4	Tr	48	55	0	0	Tr	0.15	Tr	0
Yolk	1	17	49	60	3	5	1.6	1.9	0.7	213	Tr	23	81	0.6	16	7	320	97	0.03	0.11	Tr	0
Cooked																						
Fried in margarine	1	46	69	90	6	7	1.9	2.7	1.3	211	1	25	89	0.7	61	162	390	114	0.03	0.24	Tr	0
Hard-cooked, shell removed	1	50	75	75	6	5	1.6	2.0	0.7	213	1	25	86	0.6	63	62	280	84	0.03	0.26	Tr	0
Poached	1	50	75	75	6	5	1.5	1.9	0.7	212	1	25	89	0.7	60	140	320	95	0.02	0.22	Tr	0

(Continued)

TABLE E-1 *(continued)*

ITEM	FOODS, APPROXIMATE MEASURES, UNITS, AND WEIGHT (WEIGHT OF EDIBLE PORTION ONLY)	WEIGHT (G)	WATER (%)	FOOD ENERGY (KCAL)	PROTEIN (G)	FAT (G)	FATTY ACIDS SATURATED (G)	FATTY ACIDS MONOUNSATURATED (G)	FATTY ACIDS POLYUNSATURATED (G)	CHOLESTEROL (MG)	CARBOHYDRATE (G)	CALCIUM (MG)	PHOSPHORUS (MG)	IRON (MG)	POTASSIUM (MG)	SODIUM (MG)	VITAMIN A VALUE (IU)	VITAMIN A VALUE (RE)	THIAMIN (MG)	RIBOFLAVIN (MG)	NIACIN (MG)	ASCORBIC ACID (MG)
Scrambled (milk added) in margarine	1	61	73	100	7	7	2.2	2.9	1.3	215	1	44	104	0.7	84	171	420	119	0.03	0.27	Tr	Tr
FATS AND OILS																						
Butter (4 sticks per lb)																						
Stick	1/2 cup	113	16	810	1	92	57.1	26.4	3.4	247	Tr	27	26	0.2	29	[9]933	[10]3,460	[10]852	0.01	0.04	Tr	0
Tablespoon (1/8 stick)	1 tbsp	14	16	100	Tr	11	7.1	3.3	0.4	31	Tr	3	3	Tr	4	[9]116	[10]430	[10]106	Tr	Tr	Tr	0
Pat (1 in square, 1/3 in high; 90 per lb)	1	5	16	35	Tr	4	2.5	1.2	0.2	11	Tr	1	1	Tr	1	[9]41	[10]150	[10]38	Tr	Tr	Tr	0
Fats, cooking (vegetable shortenings)	1 cup	205	0	1,810	0	205	51.3	91.2	53.5	0	0	0	0	0.0	0	0	0	0	0.00	0.00	0.0	0
	1 tbsp	13	0	115	0	13	3.3	5.8	3.4	0	0	0	0	0.0	0	0	0	0	0.00	0.00	0.0	0
Lard	1 cup	205	0	1,850	0	205	80.4	92.5	23.0	195	0	0	0	0.0	0	0	0	0	0.00	0.00	0.0	0
	1 tbsp	13	0	115	0	13	5.1	5.9	1.5	12	0	0	0	0.0	0	0	0	0	0.00	0.00	0.0	0
Margarine																						
Imitation (about 40% fat), soft	8 oz	227	58	785	1	88	17.5	35.6	31.3	0	1	40	31	0.0	57	[11]2,178	[12]7,510	[12]2,254	0.01	0.05	Tr	Tr
	1 tbsp	14	58	50	Tr	5	1.1	2.2	1.9	0	Tr	2	2	0.0	4	[11]134	[12]460	[12]139	Tr	Tr	Tr	Tr
Regular (about 80% fat)																						
Hard (4 sticks per lb)																						
Stick	1/2 cup	113	16	810	1	91	17.9	40.5	28.7	0	1	34	26	0.1	48	[11]1,066	[12]3,740	[12]1,122	0.01	0.04	Tr	Tr
Tablespoon (1/8 stick)	1 tbsp	14	16	100	Tr	11	2.2	5.0	3.6	0	Tr	4	3	Tr	6	[11]132	[12]460	[12]139	Tr	0.01	Tr	Tr
Pat (1 in square, 1/3 in high; 90 per lb)	1	5	16	35	Tr	4	0.8	1.8	1.3	0	Tr	1	1	Tr	2	[11]47	[12]170	[12]50	Tr	Tr	Tr	Tr
Soft	8 oz	227	16	1,625	2	183	31.3	64.7	78.5	0	1	60	46	0.0	86	[11]2,449	[12]7,510	[12]2,254	0.02	0.07	Tr	Tr
	1 tbsp	14	16	100	Tr	11	1.9	4.0	4.8	0	Tr	4	3	0.0	5	[11]151	[12]460	[12]139	Tr	Tr	Tr	Tr
Spread (about 60% fat)																						
Hard (4 sticks per lb)																						
Stick	1/2 cup	113	37	610	1	69	15.9	29.4	20.5	0	0	24	18	0.0	34	[11]1,123	[12]3,740	[12]1,122	0.01	0.03	Tr	Tr
Tablespoon (1/8 stick)	1 tbsp	14	37	75	Tr	9	2.0	3.6	2.5	0	0	3	2	0.0	4	[11]139	[12]460	[12]139	Tr	Tr	Tr	Tr
Pat (1 in square, 1/3 in high; 90 per lb)	1	5	37	25	Tr	3	0.7	1.3	0.9	0	0	1	1	0.0	1	[11]50	[12]170	[12]50	Tr	Tr	Tr	Tr
Soft	8 oz	227	37	1,225	1	138	29.1	71.5	31.3	0	0	47	37	0.0	68	[11]2,256	[12]7,510	[12]2,254	0.02	0.06	Tr	Tr
	1 tbsp	14	37	75	Tr	9	1.8	4.4	1.9	0	0	3	2	0.0	4	[11]139	[12]460	[12]139	Tr	Tr	Tr	Tr

Food	Measure																					
Oils, salad or cooking																						
Corn	1 cup	218	0	1,925	0	218	27.7	52.8	128.0	0	0	0	0	0.0	0	0	0	0	0.00	0.00	0.0	0
	1 tbsp	14	0	125	0	14	1.8	3.4	8.2	0	0	0	0	0.0	0	0	0	0	0.00	0.00	0.0	0
Olive	1 cup	216	0	1,910	0	216	29.2	159.2	18.1	0	0	0	0	0.0	0	0	0	0	0.00	0.00	0.0	0
	1 tbsp	14	0	125	0	14	1.9	10.3	1.2	0	0	0	0	0.0	0	0	0	0	0.00	0.00	0.0	0
Peanut	1 cup	216	0	1,910	0	216	36.5	99.8	69.1	0	0	0	0	0.0	0	0	0	0	0.00	0.00	0.0	0
	1 tbsp	14	0	125	0	14	2.4	6.5	4.5	0	0	0	0	0.0	0	0	0	0	0.00	0.00	0.0	0
Safflower	1 cup	218	0	1,925	0	218	19.8	26.4	162.4	0	0	0	0	0.0	0	0	0	0	0.00	0.00	0.0	0
	1 tbsp	14	0	125	0	14	1.3	1.7	10.4	0	0	0	0	0.0	0	0	0	0	0.00	0.00	0.0	0.0
Soybean oil, hydrogenated (partially	1 cup	218	0	1,925	0	218	32.5	93.7	82.0	0	0	0	0	0.0	0	0	0	0	0.00	0.00	0.0	0
hardened)	1 tbsp	14	0	125	0	14	2.1	6.0	5.3	0	0	0	0	0.0	0	0	0	0	0.00	0.00	0.0	0
Soybean-cottonseed oil blend,	1 cup	218	0	1,925	0	218	39.2	64.3	104.9	0	0	0	0	0.0	0	0	0	0	0.00	0.00	0.0	0
hydrogenated	1 tbsp	14	0	125	0	14	2.5	4.1	6.7	0	0	0	0	0.0	0	0	0	0	0.00	0.00	0.0	0
Sunflower	1 cup	218	0	1,925	0	218	22.5	42.5	143.2	0	0	0	0	0.0	0	0	0	0	0.00	0.00	0.0	0
	1 tbsp	14	0	125	0	14	1.4	2.7	9.2	0	0	0	0	0.0	0	0	0	0	0.00	0.00	0.0	0
Salad dressings																						
Commercial																						
Blue cheese	1 tbsp	15	32	75	1	8	1.5	1.8	4.2	3	1	12	11	Tr	6	164	30	10	Tr	0.02	Tr	Tr
French																						
Regular	1 tbsp	16	35	85	Tr	9	1.4	4.0	3.5	0	1	2	1	Tr	2	188	Tr	Tr	Tr	Tr	Tr	Tr
Low carlorie	1 tbsp	16	75	25	Tr	2	0.2	0.3	1.0	0	2	6	5	Tr	3	306	Tr	Tr	Tr	Tr	Tr	Tr
Italian																						
Regular	1 tbsp	15	34	80	Tr	9	1.3	3.7	3.2	0	1	1	1	Tr	5	162	30	3	Tr	Tr	Tr	Tr
Low carlorie	1 tbsp	15	86	5	Tr	Tr	Tr	Tr	Tr	0	2	1	1	Tr	4	136	Tr	Tr	Tr	Tr	Tr	Tr
Mayonnaise																						
Regular	1 tbsp	14	15	100	Yr	11	1.7	3.2	5.8	8	Tr	3	4	0.1	5	80	40	12	0.00	0.00	Tr	0
Imitation	1 tbsp	15	63	35	Tr	3	0.5	0.7	1.6	4	2	Tr	Tr	0.0	2	75	0	0	0.00	0.00	0.0	0
Mayonnaise type	1 tbsp	15	40	60	Tr	5	0.7	1.4	2.7	4	4	2	4	Tr	1	107	30	13	Tr	Tr	Tr	0
Tartar sauce	1 tbsp	14	34	75	Tr	8	1.2	2.6	3.9	4	1	3	4	0.1	11	182	30	9	Tr	Tr	0.0	Tr
Thousand island																						
Regular	1 tbsp	16	46	60	Tr	6	1.0	1.3	3.2	4	2	2	3	0.1	18	112	50	15	Tr	Tr	Tr	0
Low calorie	1 tbsp	15	69	25	Tr	2	0.2	0.4	0.9	2	2	2	3	0.1	17	150	50	14	Tr	Tr	Tr	0
Salad dressings																						
Prepared from home recipe																						
Cooked type[13]	1 tbsp	16	69	25	1	2	0.5	0.6	0.3	9	2	13	14	0.1	19	117	70	20	0.01	0.02	Tr	Tr
Vinegar and oil	1 tbsp	16	47	70	0	8	1.5	2.4	3.9	0	Tr	0	0	0.0	1	Tr	0	0	0.00	0.00	0.0	0
FISH AND SHELLFISH																						
Clams																						
Raw, meat only	3 oz	85	82	65	11	1	0.3	0.3	0.3	43	2	59	138	2.6	154	102	90	26	0.09	0.15	1.1	9
Canned, drained solids	3 oz	85	77	85	13	2	0.5	0.5	0.4	54	2	47	116	3.5	119	102	90	26	0.01	0.09	0.9	3
Crabmeat																						
Canned	1 cup	135	77	135	23	3	0.5	0.8	1.4	135	1	61	246	1.1	149	1,350	50	14	0.11	0.11	2.6	0
Fish sticks																						
Frozen, reheated, (stick, 4 by 1 by $^{1}/_{2}$ in)	1	28	52	70	6	3	0.8	1.4	0.8	26	4	11	58	0.3	94	53	20	5	0.03	0.05	0.6	0

(Continued)

TABLE E-1 *(continued)*

ITEM	FOODS, APPROXIMATE MEASURES, UNITS, AND WEIGHT (WEIGHT OF EDIBLE PORTION ONLY)	WEIGHT (G)	WATER (%)	FOOD ENERGY (KCAL)	PROTEIN (G)	FAT (G)	FATTY ACIDS SATURATED (G)	MONOUNSATURATED (G)	POLYUNSATURATED (G)	CHOLESTEROL (MG)	CARBOHYDRATE (G)	CALCIUM (MG)	PHOSPHORUS (MG)	IRON (MG)	POTASSIUM (MG)	SODIUM (MG)	VITAMIN A VALUE (IU)	(RE)	THIAMIN (MG)	RIBOFLAVIN (MG)	NIACIN (MG)	ASCORBIC ACID (MG)
Flounder or sole																						
Baked, with lemon juice																						
With butter	3 oz	85	73	120	16	6	3.2	1.5	0.5	68	Tr	13	187	0.3	272	145	210	54	0.05	0.08	1.6	1
With margarine	3 oz	85	73	120	16	6	1.2	2.3	1.9	55	Tr	14	187	0.3	273	151	230	69	0.05	0.08	1.6	1
Without added fat	3 oz	85	78	80	17	1	0.3	0.2	0.4	59	Tr	13	197	0.3	286	101	30	10	0.05	0.08	1.7	1
Haddock																						
Breaded, fried[14]	3 oz	85	61	175	17	9	2.4	3.9	2.4	75	7	34	183	1.0	270	123	70	20	0.06	0.10	2.9	0
Halibut																						
Broiled, with butter and lemon juice	3 oz	85	67	140	20	6	3.3	1.6	0.7	62	Tr	14	206	0.7	441	103	610	174	0.06	0.07	7.7	1
Herring																						
Pickled	3 oz	85	59	190	17	13	4.3	4.6	3.1	85	0	29	128	0.9	85	850	110	33	0.04	0.18	2.8	0
Ocean perch																						
Breaded, fried[14]	1 fillet	85	59	185	16	11	2.6	4.6	2.8	66	7	31	191	1.2	241	138	70	20	0.10	0.11	2.0	0
Oysters																						
Raw, meat only (13–19 medium Selects)	1 cup	240	85	160	20	4	1.4	0.5	1.4	120	8	226	343	15.6	290	175	740	223	0.34	0.43	6.0	24
Breaded, fried[14]	1	45	65	90	5	5	1.4	2.1	1.4	35	5	49	73	3.0	64	70	150	44	0.07	0.10	1.3	4
Salmon																						
Canned (pink), solids and liquid	3 oz	85	71	120	17	5	0.9	1.5	2.1	34	0	[15]167	243	0.7	307	443	60	18	0.03	0.15	6.8	0
Baked (red)	3 oz	85	67	140	21	5	1.2	2.4	1.4	60	0	26	269	0.5	305	55	290	87	0.18	0.14	5.5	0
Smoked	3 oz	85	59	150	18	8	2.6	3.9	0.7	51	0	12	208	0.8	327	1,700	260	77	0.17	0.17	6.8	0
Sardines																						
Atlantic, canned in oil, drained solids	3 oz	85	62	175	20	9	2.1	3.7	2.9	85	0	[15]371	424	2.6	349	425	190	56	0.03	0.17	4.6	0
Scallops																						
Breaded, frozen, reheated	6	90	59	195	15	10	2.5	4.1	2.5	70	10	39	203	2.0	369	298	70	21	0.11	0.11	1.6	0
Shrimp																						
Canned, drained solids	3 oz	85	70	100	21	1	0.2	0.2	0.4	128	1	98	224	1.4	104	1,955	50	15	0.01	0.03	1.5	0
French fried (7 medium)[16]	3 oz	85	55	200	16	10	2.5	4.1	2.6	168	11	61	154	2.0	189	384	90	26	0.06	0.09	2.8	0
Trout																						
Broiled, with butter and lemon juice	3 oz	85	63	175	21	9	4.1	2.9	1.6	71	Tr	26	259	1.0	297	122	230	60	0.07	0.07	2.3	1

Tuna																						
Canned, drained solids																						
Oil pack, chunk light	3 oz	85	61	165	24	7	1.4	1.9	3.1	55	0	7	199	1.6	298	303	70	20	0.04	0.09	10.1	0
Water pack, solid white	3 oz	85	63	135	30	1	0.3	0.2	0.3	48	0	17	202	0.6	255	468	110	32	0.03	0.10	13.4	0
Tuna salad[17]	1 cup	205	63	375	33	19	3.3	4.9	9.2	80	19	31	281	2.5	531	877	230	53	0.06	0.14	13.3	6
FRUITS AND FRUIT JUICES																						
Apples																						
Raw																						
Unpeeled, without cores																						
2-3/4-in diam. (about 3 per lb with cores)	1	138	84	80	Tr	Tr	0.1	Tr	0.1	0	21	10	10	0.2	159	Tr	70	7	0.02	0.02	0.1	8
3-1/4-in diam. (about 2 per lb with cores)	1	212	84	125	Tr	1	0.1	Tr	0.2	0	32	15	15	0.4	244	Tr	110	11	0.04	0.03	0.2	12
Peeled, sliced	1 cup	110	84	65	Tr	Tr	0.1	Tr	0.1	0	16	4	8	0.1	124	Tr	50	5	0.02	0.01	0.1	4
Dried, sulfured	10 rings	64	32	155	1	Tr	Tr	Tr	0.1	0	42	9	24	0.9	288	[18]56	0	0	0.00	0.10	0.6	2
Apple juice																						
Bottled or canned[19]	1 cup	248	88	115	Tr	Tr	Tr	Tr	0.1	0	29	17	17	0.9	295	7	Tr	Tr	0.05	0.04	0.2	[20]2
Applesauce																						
Canned																						
Sweetened	1 cup	255	80	195	Tr	Tr	0.1	Tr	0.1	0	51	10	18	0.9	156	8	30	3	0.03	0.07	0.5	[20]4
Unsweetened	1 cup	244	88	105	Tr	Tr	Tr	Tr	Tr	0	28	7	17	0.3	183	5	70	7	0.03	0.06	0.5	[20]3
Apricots																						
Raw, without pits (about 12 per lb with pits)	3	106	86	50	1	Tr	Tr	0.2	0.1	0	12	15	20	0.6	314	1	2,770	277	0.03	0.04	0.6	11
Canned (fruit and liquid)																						
Heavy syrup pack	1 cup	258	78	215	1	Tr	Tr	0.1	Tr	0	55	23	31	0.8	361	10	3,170	317	0.05	0.06	1.0	8
	3 halves	85	78	70	Tr	Tr	Tr	Tr	Tr	0	18	8	10	0.3	119	3	1,050	105	0.02	0.02	0.3	3
Juice pack	1 cup	248	87	120	2	Tr	Tr	Tr	Tr	0	31	30	50	0.7	409	10	4,190	419	0.04	0.05	0.9	12
	3 halves	84	87	40	1	Tr	Tr	Tr	Tr	0	10	10	17	0.3	139	3	1,420	142	0.02	0.02	0.3	4
Dried																						
Uncooked (28 large or 37 medium halves per cup)	1 cup	130	31	310	5	1	Tr	0.3	0.1	0	80	59	152	6.1	1,791	13	9,410	941	0.01	0.20	3.9	3
Cooked, unsweetened, fruit and liquid	1 cup	250	76	210	3	Tr	Tr	0.2	0.1	0	55	40	103	4.2	1,222	8	5,910	591	0.02	0.08	2.4	4
Apricot nectar																						
Canned	1 cup	251	85	140	1	Tr	Tr	0.1	Tr	0	36	18	23	1.0	286	8	3,300	330	0.02	0.04	0.7	[20]2
Avocados																						
Raw, whole, without skin and seed																						
California (about 2 per lb with skin and seed)	1	173	73	305	4	30	4.5	19.4	3.5	0	12	19	73	2.0	1,097	21	1,060	106	0.19	0.21	3.3	14
Florida (about 1 per lb with skin and seed)	1	304	80	340	5	27	5.3	14.8	4.5	0	27	33	119	1.6	1,484	15	1,860	186	0.33	0.37	5.8	24
Bananas																						
Raw, without peel																						
Whole (about 2-1/2 per lb with peel)	1	114	74	105	1	1	0.2	Tr	0.1	0	27	7	23	0.4	451	1	90	9	0.05	0.11	0.6	10

(Continued)

TABLE E-1 *(continued)*

ITEM	FOODS, APPROXIMATE MEASURES, UNITS, AND WEIGHT (WEIGHT OF EDIBLE PORTION ONLY)	WEIGHT (G)	WATER (%)	FOOD ENERGY (KCAL)	PROTEIN (G)	FAT (G)	FATTY ACIDS SATURATED (G)	MONOUNSATURATED (G)	POLYUNSATURATED (G)	CHOLESTEROL (MG)	CARBOHYDRATE (G)	CALCIUM (MG)	PHOSPHORUS (MG)	IRON (MG)	POTASSIUM (MG)	SODIUM (MG)	VITAMIN A VALUE (IU)	(RE)	THIAMIN (MG)	RIBOFLAVIN (MG)	NIACIN (MG)	ASCORBIC ACID (MG)
Sliced	1 cup	150	74	140	2	1	0.3	0.1	0.[illegible]	0	35	9	30	0.5	594	2	120	12	0.07	0.15	0.8	14
Blackberries																						
Raw	1 cup	144	86	75	1	1	0.2	0.1	0.1	0	18	46	30	0.8	282	Tr	240	24	0.04	0.06	0.6	30
Blueberries																						
Raw	1 cup	145	85	80	1	1	Tr	0.1	0.3	0	20	9	15	0.2	129	9	150	15	0.07	0.07	0.5	19
Frozen, sweetened	10 oz	284	77	230	1	Tr	Tr	0.1	0.2	0	62	17	20	1.1	170	3	120	12	0.06	0.15	0.7	3
	1 cup	230	77	185	1	Tr	Tr	Tr	0.1	0	50	14	16	0.9	138	2	100	10	0.05	0.12	0.6	2
Cantaloup																						
See Melons.																						
Cherries																						
Sour, red, pitted, canned, water pack	1 cup	244	90	90	2	Tr	0.1	0.1	0.1	0	22	27	24	3.3	239	17	1,840	184	0.04	0.10	0.4	5
Sweet, raw, without pits and stems	10	68	81	50	1	1	0.1	0.2	0.2	0	11	10	13	0.3	152	Tr	150	15	0.03	0.04	0.3	5
Cranberry juice cocktail																						
Bottled, sweetened	1 cup	253	85	145	Tr	Tr	Tr	Tr	0.1	0	38	8	3	0.4	61	10	10	1	0.01	0.04	0.1	[21]108
Cranberry sauce																						
Sweetened, canned, strained	1 cup	277	61	420	1	Tr	Tr	0.1	0.2	0	108	11	17	0.6	72	80	60	6	0.04	0.06	0.3	6
Dates																						
Whole, without pits	10	83	23	230	2	Tr	0.1	0.1	Tr	0	61	27	33	1.0	541	2	40	4	0.07	0.08	1.8	0
Chopped	1 cup	178	23	490	4	1	0.3	0.2	Tr	0	131	57	71	2.0	1,161	5	90	9	0.16	0.18	3.9	0
Figs																						
Dried	10	187	28	475	6	2	0.4	0.5	1.0	0	122	269	127	4.2	1,331	21	250	25	0.13	0.16	1.3	1
Fruit cocktail																						
Canned, fruit and liquid																						
Heavy syrup pack	1 cup	255	80	185	1	Tr	Tr	Tr	0.1	0	48	15	28	0.7	224	15	520	52	0.05	0.05	1.0	5
Juice pack	1 cup	248	87	115	1	Tr	Tr	Tr	Tr	0	29	20	35	0.5	236	10	760	76	0.03	0.04	1.0	7
Grapefruit																						
Raw, without peel, membrane and seeds (3-3/4-in diam., 1 lb 1 oz, whole, with refuse)	1/2	120	91	40	1	Tr	Tr	Tr	Tr	0	10	14	10	0.1	167	Tr	[22]10	[22]1	0.04	0.02	0.3	41
Canned, sections with syrup	1 cup	254	84	150	1	Tr	Tr	Tr	0.1	0	39	36	25	1.0	328	5	Tr	Tr	0.10	0.05	0.6	54

Grapefruit juice																						
Raw	1 cup	247	90	95	1	Tr	Tr	Tr	0.1	0	23	22	37	0.5	400	2	20	2	0.10	0.05	0.5	94
Canned																						
Unsweetened	1 cup	247	90	95	1	Tr	Tr	Tr	0.1	0	22	17	27	0.5	378	2	20	2	0.10	0.05	0.6	72
Sweetened	1 cup	250	87	115	1	Tr	Tr	Tr	0.1	0	28	20	28	0.9	405	5	20	2	0.10	0.06	0.8	67
Frozen concentrate, unsweetened																						
Undiluted	6 fl oz	207	62	300	4	1	0.1	0.1	0.2	0	72	56	101	1.0	1,002	6	60	6	0.30	0.16	1.6	248
Diluted with 3 parts water by volume	1 cup	247	89	100	1	Tr	Tr	Tr	0.1	0	24	20	35	0.3	336	2	20	2	0.10	0.05	0.5	83
Grapes																						
European type (adherent skin), raw																						
Thompson seedless	10	50	81	35	Tr	Tr	0.1	Tr	0.1	0	9	6	7	0.1	93	1	40	4	0.05	0.03	0.2	5
Tokay and Emperor, seeded types	10	57	81	40	Tr	Tr	0.1	Tr	0.1	0	10	6	7	0.1	105	1	40	4	0.05	0.03	0.2	6
Grape juice																						
Canned or bottled	1 cup	253	84	155	1	Tr	0.1	Tr	0.1	0	38	23	28	0.6	334	8	20	2	0.07	0.09	0.7	[20]Tr
Frozen concentrate, sweetened:																						
Undiluted	6 fl oz	216	54	385	1	1	0.2	Tr	0.2	0	96	28	32	0.8	160	15	60	6	0.11	0.20	0.9	[21]179
Diluted with 3 parts water by volume	1 cup	250	87	125	Tr	Tr	0.1	Tr	0.1	0	32	10	10	0.3	53	5	20	2	0.04	0.07	0.3	[21]60
Kiwifruit																						
Raw, without skin (about 5 per lb with skin)	1	76	83	45	1	Tr	Tr	0.1	0.1	0	11	20	30	0.3	252	4	130	13	0.02	0.04	0.4	74
Lemons																						
Raw, without peel and seeds (about 4 per lb with peel and seeds)	1	58	89	15	1	Tr	Tr	Tr	0.1	0	5	15	9	0.3	80	1	20	2	0.02	0.01	0.1	31
Lemon juice																						
Raw	1 cup	244	91	60	1	Tr	Tr	Tr	Tr	0	21	17	15	0.1	303	2	50	5	0.07	0.02	0.2	112
Canned or bottled, unsweetened	1 cup	244	92	50	1	1	0.1	Tr	0.2	0	16	27	22	0.3	249	[23]51	40	4	0.10	0.02	0.5	61
	1 tbsp	15	92	5	Tr	Tr	Tr	Tr	Tr	0	1	2	1	Tr	15	[23]3	Tr	Tr	0.01	Tr	Tr	4
Frozen, single-strength, unsweetened	6 fl oz	244	92	55	1	1	0.1	Tr	0.2	0	16	20	20	0.3	217	2	30	3	0.14	0.03	0.3	77
Lime juice																						
Raw	1 cup	246	90	65	1	Tr	Tr	Tr	0.1	0	22	22	17	0.1	268	2	20	2	0.05	0.02	0.2	72
Canned, unsweetened	1 cup	246	93	50	1	1	0.1	0.1	0.2	0	16	30	25	0.6	185	[23]39	40	4	0.08	0.01	0.4	16
Mangos																						
Raw, without skin and seed (about 1-$^1/_2$ per lb with skin and seed)	1	207	82	135	1	1	0.1	0.2	0.1	0	35	21	23	0.3	323	4	8,060	806	0.12	0.12	1.2	57
Melons																						
Raw, without rind and cavity contents																						
Cantaloupe, orange-fleshed (5-in diam., 2-$^1/_3$ lb, whole, with rind and cavity contents)	$^1/_2$	267	90	95	2	1	0.1	0.1	0.3	0	22	29	45	0.6	825	24	8,610	861	0.10	0.06	1.5	113
Honeydew (6-$^1/_2$-in diam., 5-$^1/_4$ lb, whole, with rind and cavity contents)	$^1/_{10}$	129	90	45	1	Tr	Tr	Tr	0.1	0	12	8	13	0.1	350	13	50	5	0.10	0.02	0.8	32
Nectarines																						
Raw, without pits (about 3 per lb with pits)	1	136	86	65	1	1	0.1	0.2	0.3	0	16	7	22	0.2	288	Tr	1,000	100	0.02	0.06	1.3	7

(Continued)

TABLE E-1 *(continued)*

ITEM	FOODS, APPROXIMATE MEASURES, UNITS, AND WEIGHT (WEIGHT OF EDIBLE PORTION ONLY)	WEIGHT (G)	WATER (%)	FOOD ENERGY (KCAL)	PROTEIN (G)	FAT (G)	FATTY ACIDS: SATURATED (G)	FATTY ACIDS: MONOUNSATURATED (G)	FATTY ACIDS: POLYUNSATURATED (G)	CHOLESTEROL (MG)	CARBOHYDRATE (G)	CALCIUM (MG)	PHOSPHORUS (MG)	IRON (MG)	POTASSIUM (MG)	SODIUM (MG)	VITAMIN A VALUE (IU)	VITAMIN A VALUE (RE)	THIAMIN (MG)	RIBOFLAVIN (MG)	NIACIN (MG)	ASCORBIC ACID (MG)
Oranges																						
Raw																						
Whole, without peel and seeds (2-5/8-in diam., about 2-1/2 per lb, with peel and seeds)	1	131	87	60	1	Tr	Tr	Tr	Tr	0	15	52	18	0.1	237	Tr	270	27	0.11	0.05	0.4	70
Sections without membranes	1 cup	180	87	85	2	Tr	Tr	Tr	Tr	0	21	72	25	0.2	326	Tr	370	37	0.16	0.07	0.5	96
Orange juice																						
Raw, all varieties	1 cup	248	88	110	2	Tr	0.1	0.1	0.1	0	26	27	42	0.5	496	2	500	50	0.22	0.07	1.0	124
Canned, unsweetened	1 cup	249	89	105	1	Tr	Tr	0.1	0.1	0	25	20	35	1.1	436	5	440	44	0.15	0.07	0.8	86
Chilled	1 cup	249	88	110	2	1	0.1	0.1	0.2	0	25	25	27	0.4	473	2	190	19	0.28	0.05	0.7	82
Frozen concentrate																						
Undiluted	6 fl oz	213	58	340	5	Tr	0.1	0.1	0.1	0	81	68	121	0.7	1,436	6	590	59	0.60	0.14	1.5	294
Diluted with 3 parts water by volume	1 cup	249	88	110	2	Tr	Tr	Tr	Tr	0	27	22	40	0.2	473	2	190	19	0.20	0.04	0.5	97
Orange and grapefruit juice																						
Canned	1 cup	247	89	105	1	Tr	Tr	Tr	Tr	0	25	20	35	1.1	390	7	290	29	0.14	0.07	0.8	72
Papayas																						
Raw, 1/2-in cubes	1 cup	140	86	65	1	Tr	0.1	0.1	Tr	0	17	35	12	0.3	247	9	400	40	0.04	0.04	0.5	92
Peaches																						
Raw																						
Whole, 2-1/2-in diam., peeled, pitted (about 4 per lb with peels and pits)	1	87	88	35	1	Tr	Tr	Tr	Tr	0	10	4	10	0.1	171	Tr	470	47	0.01	0.04	0.9	6
Sliced	1 cup	170	88	75	1	Tr	Tr	0.1	0.1	0	19	9	20	0.2	335	Tr	910	91	0.03	0.07	1.7	11
Canned, fruit and liquid																						
Heavy syrup pack	1 cup	256	79	190	1	Tr	Tr	0.1	0.1	0	51	8	28	0.7	236	15	850	85	0.03	0.06	1.6	7
	1 half	81	79	60	Tr	Tr	Tr	Tr	Tr	0	16	2	9	0.2	75	5	270	27	0.01	0.02	0.5	2
Juice pack	1 cup	248	87	110	2	Tr	Tr	Tr	Tr	0	29	15	42	0.7	317	10	940	94	0.02	0.04	1.4	9
	1 half	77	87	35	Tr	Tr	Tr	Tr	Tr	0	9	5	13	0.2	99	3	290	29	0.01	0.01	0.4	3
Peaches																						
Dried																						
Uncooked	1 cup	160	32	380	6	1	0.1	0.4	0.6	0	98	45	190	6.5	1,594	11	3,460	346	Tr	0.34	7.0	8
Cooked, unsweetened, fruit and liquid	1 cup	258	78	200	3	1	0.1	0.2	0.3	0	51	23	98	3.4	826	5	510	51	0.01	0.05	3.9	10
Frozen, sliced, sweetened	10 oz	284	75	265	2	Tr	Tr	0.1	0.2	0	68	9	31	1.1	369	17	810	81	0.04	0.10	1.9	[21]268
	1 cup	250	75	235	2	Tr	Tr	0.1	0.2	0	60	8	28	0.9	325	15	710	71	0.03	0.09	1.6	[21]236

Food	Measure																					
Pears																						
Raw, with skin, cored																						
Bartlett, 2-$^1/_2$-in diam. (about 2-$^1/_2$ per lb with cores and stems)	1	166	84	100	1	1	Tr	0.1	0.2	0	25	18	18	0.4	208	Tr	30	3	0.03	0.07	0.2	7
Bosc, 2-$^1/_2$-in diam. (about 3 per lb with cores and stems)	1	141	84	85	1	1	Tr	0.1	0.1	0	21	16	16	0.4	176	Tr	30	3	0.03	0.06	0.1	6
D'Anjou, 3-in diam. (about 2 per lb with cores and stems)	1	200	84	120	1	1	Tr	0.2	0.2	0	30	22	22	0.5	250	Tr	40	4	0.04	0.08	0.2	8
Canned, fruit and liquid																						
Heavy syrup pack	1 cup	255	80	190	1	Tr	Tr	0.1	0.1	0	49	13	18	0.6	166	13	10	1	0.03	0.06	0.6	3
	1 half	79	80	60	Tr	Tr	Tr	Tr	Tr	0	15	4	6	0.2	51	4	Tr	Tr	0.01	0.02	0.2	1
Juice pack	1 cup	248	86	125	1	Tr	Tr	Tr	Tr	0	32	22	30	0.7	238	10	10	1	0.03	0.03	0.5	4
	1 half	77	86	40	Tr	Tr	Tr	Tr	Tr	0	10	7	9	0.2	74	3	Tr	Tr	0.01	0.01	0.2	1
Pineapple																						
Raw, diced	1 cup	155	87	75	1	1	Tr	0.1	0.2	0	19	11	11	0.6	175	2	40	4	0.14	0.06	0.7	24
Canned, fruit and liquid																						
Heavy syrup pack:																						
Crushed, chunks, tidbits	1 cup	255	79	200	1	Tr	Tr	Tr	0.1	0	52	36	18	1.0	265	3	40	4	0.23	0.06	0.7	19
Slices	1	58	79	45	Tr	Tr	Tr	Tr	Tr	0	12	8	4	0.2	60	1	10	1	0.05	0.01	0.2	4
Juice pack																						
Chunks or tidbits	1 cup	250	84	150	1	Tr	Tr	Tr	0.1	0	39	35	15	0.7	305	3	100	10	0.24	0.05	0.7	24
Slices	1	58	84	35	Tr	Tr	Tr	Tr	Tr	0	9	8	3	0.2	71	1	20	2	0.06	0.01	0.2	6
Pineapple juice																						
Unsweetened, canned	1 cup	250	86	140	1	Tr	Tr	Tr	0.1	0	34	43	20	0.7	335	3	10	1	0.14	0.06	0.6	27
Plantains																						
Without peel																						
Raw	1	179	65	220	2	1	0.3	0.1	0.1	0	57	5	61	1.1	893	7	2,020	202	0.09	0.10	1.2	33
Cooked, boiled, sliced	1 cup	154	67	180	1	Tr	0.1	Tr	0.1	0	48	3	43	0.9	716	8	1,400	140	0.07	0.08	1.2	17
Plums																						
Without pits																						
Raw																						
2-$^1/_8$-in diam. (about 6-$^1/_2$ per lb with pits)	1	66	85	35	1	Tr	Tr	0.3	0.1	0	9	3	7	0.1	114	Tr	210	21	0.03	0.06	0.3	6
1-$^1/_2$-in diam. (about 15 per lb with pits)	1	28	85	15	Tr	Tr	Tr	0.1	Tr	0	4	1	3	Tr	48	Tr	90	9	0.01	0.03	0.1	3
Canned, purple, fruit and liquid																						
Heavy syrup pack	1 cup	258	76	230	1	Tr	Tr	0.2	0.1	0	60	23	34	2.2	235	49	670	67	0.04	0.10	0.8	1
	3	133	76	120	Tr	Tr	Tr	0.1	Tr	0	31	12	17	1.1	121	25	340	34	0.02	0.05	0.4	1
Juice pack	1 cup	252	84	145	1	Tr	Tr	Tr	Tr	0	38	25	38	0.9	388	3	2,540	254	0.06	0.15	1.2	7
	3	95	84	55	Tr	Tr	Tr	Tr	Tr	0	14	10	14	0.3	146	1	960	96	0.02	0.06	0.4	3
Prunes																						
Dried																						
Uncooked	4 extra large or 5 large	49	32	115	1	Tr	Tr	0.2	0.1	0	31	25	39	1.2	365	2	970	97	0.04	0.08	1.0	2
Cooked, unsweetened, fruit and liquid	1 cup	212	70	225	2	Tr	Tr	0.3	0.1	0	60	49	74	2.4	708	4	650	65	0.05	0.21	1.5	6
Prune juice																						
Canned or bottled	1 cup	256	81	180	2	Tr	Tr	0.1	Tr	0	45	31	64	3.0	707	10	10	1	0.04	0.18	2.0	10

(Continued)

TABLE E-1 *(continued)*

ITEM	FOODS, APPROXIMATE MEASURES, UNITS, AND WEIGHT (WEIGHT OF EDIBLE PORTION ONLY)	WEIGHT (G)	WATER (%)	FOOD ENERGY (KCAL)	PROTEIN (G)	FAT (G)	FATTY ACIDS SATURATED (G)	FATTY ACIDS MONOUNSATURATED (G)	FATTY ACIDS POLYUNSATURATED (G)	CHOLESTEROL (MG)	CARBOHYDRATE (G)	CALCIUM (MG)	PHOSPHORUS (MG)	IRON (MG)	POTASSIUM (MG)	SODIUM (MG)	VITAMIN A VALUE (IU)	VITAMIN A VALUE (RE)	THIAMIN (MG)	RIBOFLAVIN (MG)	NIACIN (MG)	ASCORBIC ACID (MG)
Raisins																						
Seedless																						
Cup, not pressed down	1 cup	145	15	435	5	1	0.2	Tr	0.2	0	115	71	141	3.0	1,089	17	10	1	0.23	0.13	1.2	5
Packet, 1/2 oz (1-1/2 tbsp)	1	14	15	40	Tr	Tr	Tr	Tr	Tr	0	11	7	14	0.3	105	2	Tr	Tr	0.02	0.01	0.1	Tr
Raspberries																						
Raw	1 cup	123	87	60	1	1	Tr	0.1	0.4	0	14	27	15	0.7	187	Tr	160	16	0.04	0.11	1.1	31
Frozen, sweetened	10 oz	284	73	295	2	Tr	Tr	Tr	0.3	0	74	43	48	1.8	324	3	170	17	0.05	0.13	0.7	47
	1 cup	250	73	255	2	Tr	Tr	Tr	0.2	0	65	38	43	1.6	285	3	150	15	0.05	0.11	0.6	41
Rhubarb																						
Cooked, added sugar	1 cup	240	68	280	1	Tr	Tr	Tr	0.1	0	75	348	19	0.5	230	2	170	17	0.04	0.06	0.5	8
Strawberries																						
Raw, capped, whole	1 cup	149	92	45	1	1	Tr	0.1	0.3	0	10	21	28	0.6	247	1	40	4	0.03	0.10	0.3	84
Frozen, sweetened, sliced	10 oz	284	73	275	2	Tr	Tr	0.1	0.2	0	74	31	37	1.7	278	9	70	7	0.05	0.14	1.1	118
	1 cup	255	73	245	1	Tr	Tr	Tr	0.2	0	66	28	33	1.5	250	8	60	6	0.04	0.13	1.0	106
Tangerines																						
Raw, without peel and seeds (2-3/8-in diam., about 4 per lb, with peel and seeds)	1	84	88	35	1	Tr	Tr	Tr	Tr	0	9	12	8	0.1	132	1	770	77	0.09	0.02	0.1	26
Canned, light syrup, fruit and liquid	1 cup	252	83	155	1	Tr	Tr	Tr	0.1	0	41	18	25	0.9	197	15	2,120	212	0.13	0.11	1.1	50
Tangerine juice																						
Canned, sweetened	1 cup	249	87	125	1	Tr	Tr	Tr	0.1	0	30	45	35	0.5	443	2	1,050	105	0.15	0.05	0.2	55
Watermelon																						
Raw, without rind and seeds																						
Piece (4 by 8 in wedge with rind and seeds; 1/16 or 32-2/3-lb melon, 10 by 16 in)	1	482	92	155	3	2	0.3	0.2	1.0	0	35	39	43	0.8	559	10	1,760	176	0.39	0.10	1.0	46
Diced	1 cup	160	92	50	1	1	0.1	0.1	0.3	0	11	13	14	0.3	186	3	590	59	0.13	0.03	0.3	15
GRAIN PRODUCTS																						
Bagels																						
Plain or water, enriched, 3-1/2-in diam.[24]	1	68	29	200	7	2	0.3	0.5	0.7	0	38	29	46	1.8	50	245	0	0	0.26	0.20	2.4	0

Barley																						
Pearled, light, uncooked	1 cup	200	11	700	16	2	0.3	0.2	0.9	0	158	32	378	4.2	320	6	0	0	0.24	0.10	6.2	0
Biscuits																						
Baking powder, 2-in diam. (enriched flour, vegetable shortening)																						
From home recipe	1	28	28	100	2	5	1.2	2.0	1.3	Tr	13	47	36	0.7	32	195	10	3	0.08	0.08	0.8	Tr
From mix	1	28	29	95	2	3	0.8	1.4	0.9	Tr	14	58	128	0.7	56	262	20	4	0.12	0.11	0.8	Tr
From refrigerated dough	1	20	30	65	1	2	0.6	0.9	0.6	1	10	4	79	0.5	18	249	0	0	0.08	0.05	0.7	0
Breadcrumbs																						
Enriched																						
Dry, grated	1 cup	100	7	390	13	5	1.5	1.6	1.0	5	73	122	141	4.1	152	736	0	0	0.35	0.35	4.8	0
Soft. See White bread.																						
Breads																						
Boston brown bread, canned, slice, 3-1/4 in by 1/2 in[25]	1	45	45	95	2	1	0.3	0.1	0.1	3	21	41	72	0.9	131	113	[26]0	[26]0	0.06	0.04	0.7	0
Cracked-wheat bread (3/4 enriched wheat flour, 1/4 cracked wheat flour)[25]																						
Loaf, 1 lb	1	454	35	1,190	42	16	3.1	4.3	5.7	0	227	295	581	12.1	608	1,966	Tr	Tr	1.73	1.73	15.3	Tr
Slice (18 per loaf)	1	25	35	65	2	1	0.2	0.2	0.3	0	12	16	32	0.7	34	106	Tr	Tr	0.10	0.09	0.8	Tr
Toasted	1	21	26	65	2	1	0.2	0.2	0.3	0	12	16	32	0.7	34	106	Tr	Tr	0.07	0.09	0.8	Tr
French or Vienna bread, enriched[25]																						
Loaf, 1 lb	1	454	34	1,270	43	18	3.8	5.7	5.9	0	230	499	386	14.0	409	2,633	Tr	Tr	2.09	1.59	18.2	Tr
Slice																						
French, 5 by 2-1/2 by 1 in	1	35	34	100	3	1	0.3	0.4	0.5	0	18	39	30	1.1	32	203	Tr	Tr	0.16	0.12	1.4	Tr
Vienna, 4-3/4 by 4 by 1/2 in	1	25	34	70	2	1	0.2	0.3	0.3	0	13	28	21	0.8	23	145	Tr	Tr	0.12	0.09	1.0	Tr
Italian bread, enriched																						
Loaf, 1 lb	1	454	32	1,255	41	4	0.6	0.3	1.6	0	256	77	350	12.7	336	2,656	0	0	1.80	1.10	15.0	0
Slice, 4-1/2 by 3-1/4 by 3/4 in	1	30	32	85	3	Tr	Tr	Tr	0.1	0	17	5	23	0.8	22	176	0	0	0.12	0.07	1.0	0
Mixed grain bread, enriched[25]																						
Loaf, 1 lb	1	454	37	1,165	45	17	3.2	4.1	6.5	0	212	472	962	14.8	990	1,870	Tr	Tr	1.77	1.73	18.9	Tr
Slice (18 per loaf)	1	25	37	65	2	1	0.2	0.2	0.4	0	12	27	55	0.8	56	106	Tr	Tr	0.10	0.10	1.1	Tr
Toasted	1	23	27	65	2	1	0.2	0.2	0.4	0	12	27	55	0.8	56	106	Tr	Tr	0.08	0.10	1.1	Tr
Breads																						
Oatmeal bread, enriched[25]																						
Loaf, 1 lb	1	454	37	1,145	38	20	3.7	7.1	8.2	0	212	267	563	12.0	707	2,231	0	0	2.09	1.20	15.4	0
Slice (18 per loaf)	1	25	37	65	2	1	0.2	0.4	0.5	0	12	15	31	0.7	39	124	0	0	0.12	0.07	0.9	0
Toasted	1	23	30	65	2	1	0.2	0.4	0.5	0	12	15	31	0.7	39	124	0	0	0.09	0.07	0.9	0
Pita bread, enriched, white, 6-1/2-in diam.	1	60	31	165	6	1	0.1	0.1	0.4	0	33	49	60	1.4	71	339	0	0	0.27	0.12	2.2	0
Pumpernickel (2/3 rye flour, 1/3 enriched wheat flour)[25]																						
Loaf, 1 lb	1	454	37	1,160	42	16	2.6	3.6	6.4	0	218	322	990	12.4	1,966	2,461	0	0	1.54	2.36	15.0	0
Slice, 5 by 4 by 3/8 in	1	32	37	80	3	1	0.2	0.3	0.5	0	16	23	71	0.9	141	177	0	0	0.11	0.17	1.1	0
Toasted	1	29	28	80	3	1	0.2	0.3	0.5	0	16	23	71	0.9	141	177	0	0	0.09	0.17	1.1	0
Raisin bread, enriched[25]																						
Loaf, 1 lb	1	454	33	1,260	37	18	4.1	6.5	6.7	0	239	463	395	14.1	1,058	1,657	Tr	Tr	1.50	2.81	18.6	Tr
Slice (18 per loaf)	1	25	33	65	2	1	0.2	0.3	0.4	0	13	25	22	0.8	59	92	Tr	Tr	0.08	0.15	1.0	Tr
Toasted	1	21	24	65	2	1	0.2	0.3	0.4	0	13	25	22	0.8	59	92	Tr	Tr	0.06	0.15	1.0	Tr

(Continued)

TABLE E-1 *(continued)*

ITEM	FOODS, APPROXIMATE MEASURES, UNITS, AND WEIGHT (WEIGHT OF EDIBLE PORTION ONLY)	WEIGHT (G)	WATER (%)	FOOD ENERGY (KCAL)	PROTEIN (G)	FAT (G)	FATTY ACIDS SATURATED (G)	MONOUNSATURATED (G)	POLYUNSATURATED (G)	CHOLESTEROL (MG)	CARBOHYDRATE (G)	CALCIUM (MG)	PHOSPHORUS (MG)	IRON (MG)	POTASSIUM (MG)	SODIUM (MG)	VITAMIN A VALUE (IU)	(RE)	THIAMIN (MG)	RIBOFLAVIN (MG)	NIACIN (MG)	ASCORBIC ACID (MG)
Rye bread, light (²/₃ enriched wheat flour, ¹/₃ rye flour)[25]																						
Loaf, 1 lb	1	454	37	1,190	38	17	3.3	5.2	5.5	0	218	363	658	12.3	926	3,164	0	0	1.86	1.45	15.0	0
Slice, 4-³/₄ by 3-³/₄ by ⁷/₁₆ in	1	25	37	65	2	1	0.2	0.3	0.3	0	12	20	36	0.7	51	175	0	0	0.10	0.08	0.8	0
Toasted	1	22	28	65	2	1	0.2	0.3	0.3	0	12	20	36	0.7	51	175	0	0	0.08	0.08	0.8	0
Wheat bread, enriched[25]																						
Loaf, 1 lb	1	454	37	1,160	43	19	3.9	7.3	4.5	0	213	572	835	15.8	627	2,447	Tr	Tr	2.09	1.45	20.5	Tr
Slice (18 per loaf)	1	25	37	65	2	1	0.2	0.4	0.3	0	12	32	47	0.9	35	138	Tr	Tr	0.12	0.08	1.2	Tr
Toasted	1	23	28	65	3	1	0.2	0.4	0.3	0	12	32	47	0.9	35	138	Tr	Tr	0.10	0.08	1.2	Tr
White bread, enriched[25]																						
Loaf, 1 lb	1	454	37	1,210	38	18	5.6	6.5	4.2	0	222	572	490	12.9	508	2,334	Tr	Tr	2.13	1.41	17.0	Tr
Slice (18 per loaf)	1	25	37	65	2	1	0.3	0.4	0.2	0	12	32	27	0.7	28	129	Tr	Tr	0.12	0.08	0.9	Tr
Toasted	1	22	28	65	2	1	0.3	0.4	0.2	0	12	32	27	0.7	28	129	Tr	Tr	0.09	0.08	0.9	Tr
Slice (22 per loaf)	1	20	37	55	2	1	0.2	0.3	0.2	0	10	25	21	0.6	22	101	Tr	Tr	0.09	0.06	0.7	Tr
Toasted	1	17	28	55	2	1	0.2	0.3	0.2	0	10	25	21	0.6	22	101	Tr	Tr	0.07	0.06	0.7	Tr
Cubes	1 cup	30	37	80	2	1	0.4	0.4	0.3	0	15	38	32	0.9	34	154	Tr	Tr	0.14	0.09	1.1	Tr
Crumbs, soft	1 cup	45	37	120	4	2	0.6	0.6	0.4	0	22	57	49	1.3	50	231	Tr	Tr	0.21	0.14	1.7	Tr
Whole-wheat bread[25]																						
Loaf, 1 lb	1	454	38	1,110	44	20	5.8	6.8	5.2	0	206	327	1,180	15.5	799	2,887	Tr	Tr	1.59	0.95	17.4	Tr
Slice (16 per loaf)	1	28	38	70	3	1	0.4	0.4	0.3	0	13	20	74	1.0	50	180	Tr	Tr	0.10	0.06	1.1	Tr
Toasted	1	25	29	70	3	1	0.4	0.4	0.3	0	13	20	74	1.0	50	180	Tr	Tr	0.08	0.06	1.1	Tr
Bread stuffing (from enriched bread), prepared from mix																						
Dry type	1 cup	140	33	500	9	31	6.1	13.3	9.6	0	50	92	136	2.2	126	1,254	910	273	0.17	0.20	2.5	0
Moist type	1 cup	203	61	420	9	26	5.3	11.3	8.0	67	40	81	134	2.0	118	1,023	850	256	0.10	0.18	1.6	0
Breakfast cereals																						
Hot type, cooked																						
Corn (hominy) grits																						
Regular and quick, enriched	1 cup	242	85	145	3	Tr	Tr	0.1	0.2	0	31	0	29	[27]1.5	53	[28]0	[29]0	[29]0	[27]0.24	[27]0.15	[27]2.0	0
Instant, plain	1 pkt	137	85	80	2	Tr	Tr	Tr	0.1	0	18	7	16	[27]1.0	29	343	0	0	[27]0.18	[27]0.08	[27]1.3	0
Cream of Wheat																						
Regular, quick, instant	1 cup	244	86	140	4	Tr	0.1	Tr	0.2	0	29	[30]54	[31]43	[30]10.9	46	[31,32]5	0	0	[30]0.24	[30]0.07	[30]1.5	0
Mix'n Eat, plain	1 pkt	142	82	100	3	Tr	Tr	Tr	0.1	0	21	[30]20	[30]20	[30]8.1	38	241	[30]1,250	[30]376	[30]0.43	[30]0.28	[30]5.0	0
Malt-O-Meal	1 cup	240	88	120	4	Tr	Tr	Tr	0.1	0	26	5	[30]24	[30]9.6	31	[33]2	0	0	[30]0.48	[30]0.24	[30]5.8	0
Oatmeal or rolled oats																						
Regular, quick, instant, nonfortified	1 cup	234	85	145	6	2	0.4	0.8	1.0	0	25	19	178	1.6	131	[34]2	40	4	0.26	0.05	0.3	0
Instant, fortified																						

Plain	1 pkt	177	86	105	4	2	0.3	0.6	0.7	0	18	[27]163	133	[27]6.3	99	[27]285	[27]1,510	[27]453	[27]0.53	[27]0.28	[27]5.5	0
Flavored	1 pkt	164	76	160	5	2	0.3	0.7	0.8	0	31	[27]168	148	[27]6.7	137	[27]254	[27]1,530	[27]460	[27]0.53	[27]0.38	[27]5.9	Tr
Breakfast cereals																						
Ready to eat																						
All-Bran (about $^1/_3$ cup)	1 oz	28	3	70	4	1	0.1	0.1	0.3	0	21	23	264	[30]4.5	350	320	[30]1,250	[30]375	[30]0.37	[30]0.43	[30]5.0	[30]15
Cap'n Crunch (about $^3/_4$ cup)	1 oz	28	3	120	1	3	1.7	0.3	0.4	0	23	5	36	[27]7.5	37	213	40	4	[27]0.50	[27]0.55	[27]6.6	0
Cheerios (about 1-$^1/_4$ cup)	1 oz	28	5	110	4	2	0.3	0.6	0.7	0	20	48	134	[30]4.5	101	307	[30]1,250	[30]375	[30]0.37	[30]0.43	[30]5.0	[30]15
Corn Flakes (about 1-$^1/_4$ cup)																						
Kellogg's	1 oz	28	3	110	2	Tr	Tr	Tr	Tr	0	24	1	18	[30]1.8	26	351	[30]1,250	[30]375	[30]0.37	[30]0.43	[30]5.0	[30]15
Toasties	1 oz	28	3	110	2	Tr	Tr	Tr	Tr	0	24	1	12	[27]0.7	33	297	[30]1,250	[30]375	[30]0.37	[30]0.43	[30]5.0	0
40% Bran Flakes																						
Kellogg's (about $^3/_4$ cup)	1 oz	28	3	90	4	1	0.1	0.1	0.3	0	22	14	139	[30]8.1	180	264	[30]1,250	[30]375	[30]0.37	[30]0.43	[30]5.0	0
Post (about $^2/_3$ cup)	1 oz	28	3	90	3	Tr	0.1	0.1	0.2	0	22	12	179	[30]4.5	151	260	[30]1,250	[30]375	[30]0.37	[30]0.43	[30]5.0	0
Froot Loops (about 1 cup)	1 oz	28	3	110	2	1	0.2	0.1	0.1	0	25	3	24	[30]4.5	26	145	[30]1,250	[30]375	[30]0.37	[30]0.43	[30]5.0	[30]15
Golden Grahams (about $^3/_4$ cup)	1 oz	28	2	110	2	1	0.7	0.1	0.2	Tr	24	17	41	[30]4.5	63	346	[30]1,250	[30]375	[30]0.37	[30]0.43	[30]5.0	[30]15
Grape-Nuts (about $^1/_4$ cup)	1 oz	28	3	100	3	Tr	Tr	Tr	0.1	0	23	11	71	1.2	95	197	[30]1,250	[30]375	[30]0.37	[30]0.43	[30]5.0	0
Honey Nut Cheerios (about $^3/_4$ cup)	1 oz	28	3	105	3	1	0.1	0.3	0.3	0	23	20	105	[30]4.5	99	257	[30]1,250	[30]375	[30]0.37	[30]0.43	[30]5.0	[30]15
Lucky Charms (about 1 cup)	1 oz	28	3	110	3	1	0.2	0.4	0.4	0	23	32	79	[30]4.5	59	201	[30]1,250	[30]375	[30]0.37	[30]0.43	[30]5.0	[30]15
Nature Valley Granola (about $^1/_3$ cup)	1 oz	28	4	125	3	5	3.3	0.7	0.7	0	19	18	89	0.9	98	58	20	2	0.10	0.05	0.2	0
100% Natural Cereal (about $^1/_4$ cup)	1 oz	28	2	135	3	6	4.1	1.2	0.5	Tr	18	49	104	0.8	140	12	20	2	0.09	0.15	0.6	0
Product 19 (about $^3/_4$ cup)	1 oz	28	3	110	3	Tr	Tr	Tr	0.1	0	24	3	40	[30]18.0	44	325	[30]5,000	[30]1,501	[30]1.50	[30]1.70	[30]20.0	[30]60
Raisin Bran																						
Kellogg's (about $^3/_4$ cup)	1 oz	28	8	90	3	1	0.1	0.1	0.3	0	21	10	105	[30]3.5	147	207	[30]960	[30]288	[30]0.28	[30]0.34	[30]3.9	0
Post (about $^1/_2$ cup)	1 oz	28	9	85	3	1	0.1	0.1	0.3	0	21	13	119	[30]4.5	175	185	[30]1,250	[30]375	[30]0.37	[30]0.43	[30]5.0	0
Rice Krispies (about 1 cup)	1 oz	28	2	110	2	Tr	Tr	Tr	0.1	0	25	4	34	[30]1.8	29	340	[30]1,250	[30]375	[30]0.37	[30]0.43	[30]5.0	[30]15
Shredded Wheat (about $^2/_3$ cup)	1 oz	28	5	100	3	1	0.1	0.1	0.3	0	23	11	100	1.2	102	3	0	0	0.07	0.08	1.5	0
Special K (about 1-$^1/_3$ cup)	1 oz	28	2	110	6	Tr	Tr	Tr	Tr	Tr	21	8	55	[30]4.5	49	265	[30]1,250	[30]375	[30]0.37	[30]0.43	[30]5.0	[30]15
Super Sugar Crisp (about $^7/_8$ cup)	1 oz	28	2	105	2	Tr	Tr	Tr	0.1	0	26	6	52	[30]1.8	105	25	[30]1,250	[30]375	[30]0.37	[30]0.43	[30]5.0	0
Sugar Frosted Flakes, Kellogg's																						
(about $^3/_4$ cup)	1 oz	28	3	110	1	Tr	Tr	Tr	Tr	0	26	1	21	[30]1.8	18	230	[30]1,250	[30]375	[30]0.37	[30]0.43	[30]5.0	[30]15
Sugar Smacks (about $^3/_4$ cup)	1 oz	28	3	105	2	1	0.1	0.1	0.2	0	25	3	31	[30]1.8	42	75	[30]1,250	[30]375	[30]0.37	[30]0.43	[30]5.0	[30]15
Total (about 1 cup)	1 oz	28	4	100	3	1	0.1	0.1	0.3	0	22	48	118	[30]18.0	106	352	[30]5,000	[30]1,501	[30]1.50	[30]1.70	[30]20.0	[30]60
Trix (about 1 cup)	1 oz	28	3	110	2	Tr	0.2	0.1	0.1	0	25	6	19	[30]4.5	27	181	[30]1,250	[30]375	[30]0.37	[30]0.43	[30]5.0	[30]15
Wheaties (about 1 cup)	1 oz	28	5	100	3	Tr	0.1	Tr	0.2	0	23	43	98	[30]4.5	106	354	[30]1,250	[30]375	[30]0.37	[30]0.43	[30]5.0	[30]15
Buckwheat flour																						
Light, sifted	1 cup	98	12	340	6	1	0.2	0.4	0.4	0	78	11	86	1.0	314	2	0	0	0.08	0.04	0.4	0
Bulgur																						
Uncooked	1 cup	170	10	600	19	3	1.2	0.3	1.2	0	129	49	575	9.5	389	7	0	0	0.48	0.24	7.7	0
Cakes prepared from cake mixes with enriched flour[35]																						
Angel food																						
Whole cake, 9-$^3/_4$-in diam. tube cake	1	635	38	1,510	38	2	0.4	0.2	1.0	0	342	527	1,086	2.7	845	3,226	0	0	0.32	1.27	1.6	0
Piece, $^1/_{12}$ of cake	1	53	38	125	3	Tr	Tr	Tr	0.1	0	29	44	91	0.2	71	269	0	0	0.03	0.11	0.1	0
Coffeecake, crumb																						
Whole cake, 7-$^3/_4$ by 5-$^5/_8$ by 1-$^1/_4$ in	1	430	30	1,385	27	41	11.8	16.7	9.6	279	225	262	748	7.3	469	1,853	690	194	0.82	0.90	7.7	1
Piece, $^1/_6$ of cake	1	72	30	230	5	7	2.0	2.8	1.6	47	38	44	125	1.2	78	310	120	32	0.14	0.15	1.3	Tr
Devil's food with chocolate frosting																						
Whole, 2-layer cake, 8- or 9-in diam.	1	1,107	24	3,755	49	136	55.6	51.4	19.7	598	645	653	1,162	22.1	1,439	2,900	1,660	498	1.11	1.66	10.0	1
Piece, $^1/_{16}$ of cake	1	69	24	235	3	8	3.5	3.2	1.2	37	40	41	72	1.4	90	181	100	31	0.07	0.10	0.6	Tr
Cupcake, 2-$^1/_2$-in diam.	1	35	24	120	2	4	1.8	1.6	0.6	19	20	21	37	0.7	46	92	50	16	0.04	0.05	0.3	Tr

(Continued)

TABLE E-1 *(continued)*

ITEM	FOODS, APPROXIMATE MEASURES, UNITS, AND WEIGHT (WEIGHT OF EDIBLE PORTION ONLY)	WEIGHT (G)	WATER (%)	FOOD ENERGY (KCAL)	PROTEIN (G)	FAT (G)	FATTY ACIDS SATURATED (G)	MONOUNSATURATED (G)	POLYUNSATURATED (G)	CHOLESTEROL (MG)	CARBOHYDRATE (G)	CALCIUM (MG)	PHOSPHORUS (MG)	IRON (MG)	POTASSIUM (MG)	SODIUM (MG)	VITAMIN A VALUE (IU)	VITAMIN A VALUE (RE)	THIAMIN (MG)	RIBOFLAVIN (MG)	NIACIN (MG)	ASCORBIC ACID (MG)
Gingerbread																						
Whole cake, 8 in square	1	570	37	1,575	18	39	9.6	16.4	10.5	6	291	513	570	10.8	1,562	1,733	0	0	0.86	1.03	7.4	1
Piece, $^1/_9$ of cake	1	63	37	175	2	4	1.1	1.8	1.2	1	32	57	63	1.2	173	192	0	0	0.09	0.11	0.8	Tr
Cakes prepared from cake mixes with enriched flour[35]																						
Yellow with chocolate frosting																						
Whole, 2-layer cake, 8- or 9-in diam.	1	1,108	26	3,735	45	125	47.8	48.8	21.8	576	638	1,008	2,017	15.5	1,208	2,515	1,550	465	1.22	1.66	11.1	1
Piece, $^1/_{16}$ of cake	1	69	26	235	3	8	3.0	3.0	1.4	36	40	63	126	1.0	75	157	100	29	0.08	0.10	0.7	Tr
Cakes prepared from home recipes using enriched flour																						
Carrot, with cream cheese frosting[36]																						
Whole cake, 10-in diam. tube cake	1	1,536	23	6,175	63	328	66.0	135.2	107.5	1183	775	707	998	21.0	1,720	4,470	2,240	246	1.83	1.97	14.7	23
Piece, $^1/_{16}$ of cake	1	96	23	385	4	21	4.1	8.4	6.7	74	48	44	62	1.3	108	279	140	15	0.11	0.12	0.9	1
Fruitcake, dark[36]																						
Whole cake, 7-$^1/_2$-in diam., 2-$^1/_4$-in high tube cake	1	1,361	18	5,185	74	228	47.6	113.0	51.7	640	783	1,293	1,592	37.6	6,138	2,123	1,720	422	2.41	2.55	17.0	504
Piece, $^1/_{32}$ of cake, $^2/_3$-in arc	1	43	18	165	2	7	1.5	3.6	1.6	20	25	41	50	1.2	194	67	50	13	0.08	0.08	0.5	16
Plain sheet cake[37]																						
Without frosting																						
Whole cake, 9-in square	1	777	25	2,830	35	108	29.5	45.1	25.6	552	434	497	793	11.7	614	2,331	1,320	373	1.24	1.40	10.1	2
Piece, $^1/_9$ of cake	1	86	25	315	4	12	3.3	5.0	2.8	61	48	55	88	1.3	68	258	150	41	0.14	0.15	1.1	Tr
With uncooked white frosting																						
Whole cake, 9-in square	1	1,096	21	4,020	37	129	41.6	50.4	26.3	636	694	548	822	11.0	669	2,488	2,190	647	1.21	1.42	9.9	2
Piece, $^1/_9$ of cake	1	121	21	445	4	14	4.6	5.6	2.9	70	77	61	91	1.2	74	275	240	71	0.13	0.16	1.1	Tr
Pound[38]																						
Loaf, 8-$^1/_2$ by 3-$^1/_2$ by 3-$^1/_4$ in	1	514	22	2,025	33	94	21.1	40.9	26.7	555	265	339	473	9.3	483	1,645	3,470	1,033	0.93	1.08	7.8	1
Slice, $^1/_{17}$ of loaf	1	30	22	120	2	5	1.2	2.4	1.6	32	15	20	28	0.5	28	96	200	60	0.05	0.06	0.5	Tr
Cakes, commercial, made with enriched flour																						
Pound																						
Loaf, 8-$^1/_2$ by 3-$^1/_2$ by 3 in	1	500	24	1,935	26	94	52.0	30.0	4.0	1100	257	146	517	8.0	443	1,857	2,820	715	0.96	1.12	8.1	0
Slice, $^1/_{17}$ of loaf	1	29	24	110	2	5	3.0	1.7	0.2	64	15	8	30	0.5	26	108	160	41	0.06	0.06	0.5	0
Snack cakes																						
Devil's food with creme filling (2 small cakes per pkg)	1	28	20	105	1	4	1.7	1.5	0.6	15	17	21	26	1.0	34	105	20	4	0.06	0.09	0.7	0
Sponge with creme filling (2 small cakes per pkg)	1	42	19	155	1	5	2.3	2.1	0.5	7	27	14	44	0.6	37	155	30	9	0.07	0.06	0.6	0
White with white frosting																						
Whole, 2-layer cake, 8- or 9-in diam.	1	1,140	24	4,170	43	148	33.1	61.6	42.2	46	670	536	1,585	15.5	832	2,827	640	194	3.19	2.05	27.6	0

Piece, 1/16 of cake	1	71	24	260	3	9	2.1	3.8	2.6	3	42	33	99	1.0	52	176	40	12	0.20	0.13	1.7	0
Yellow with chocolate frosting																						
Whole, 2-layer cake, 8- or 9-in diam.	1	1,108	23	3,895	40	175	92.0	58.7	10.0	609	620	366	1,884	19.9	1,972	3,080	1,850	488	0.78	2.22	10.0	0
Piece, 1/16 of cake	1	69	23	245	2	11	5.7	3.7	0.6	38	39	23	117	1.2	123	192	120	30	0.05	0.14	0.6	0
Cheesecake																						
Whole cake, 9-in diam.	1	1,110	46	3,350	60	213	119.9	65.5	14.4	2053	317	622	977	5.3	1,088	2,464	2,820	833	0.33	1.44	5.1	56
Piece, 1/12 of cake	1	92	46	280	5	18	9.9	5.4	1.2	170	26	52	81	0.4	90	204	230	69	0.03	0.12	0.4	5
Cookies made with enriched flour																						
Brownies with nuts																						
Commercial, with frosting, 1-1/2 by 1-3/4 by 7/8 in	1	25	13	100	1	4	1.6	2.0	0.6	14	16	13	26	0.6	50	59	70	18	0.08	0.07	0.3	Tr
From home recipe, 1-3/4 by 1-3/4 by 7/8 in[36]	1	20	10	95	1	6	1.4	2.8	1.2	18	11	9	26	0.4	35	51	20	6	0.05	0.05	0.3	Tr
Chocolate chip																						
Commercial, 2-1/4-in diam., 3/8 in thick	4	42	4	180	2	9	2.9	3.1	2.6	5	28	13	41	0.8	68	140	50	15	0.10	0.23	1.0	Tr
Cookies made with enriched flour																						
Chocolate chip																						
From home recipe, 2-1/3-in diam.[25]	4	40	3	185	2	11	3.9	4.3	2.0	18	26	13	34	1.0	82	82	20	5	0.06	0.06	0.6	0
From refrigerated dough, 2-1/4-in diam., 3/8 in thick	4	48	5	225	2	11	4.0	4.4	2.0	22	32	13	34	1.0	62	173	30	8	0.06	0.10	0.9	0
Fig bars, square, 1-5/8 by 1-5/8 by 3/8 in or rectangular, 1-1/2 by 1-3/4 by 1/2 in	4	56	12	210	2	4	1.0	1.5	1.0	27	42	40	34	1.4	162	180	60	6	0.08	0.07	0.7	Tr
Oatmeal with raisins, 2-5/8-in diam., 1/4 in thick	4	52	4	245	3	10	2.5	4.5	2.8	2	36	18	58	1.1	90	148	40	12	0.09	0.08	1.0	0
Peanut butter cookie, from home recipe, 2-5/8-in diam.[25]	4	48	3	245	4	14	4.0	5.8	2.8	22	28	21	60	1.1	110	142	20	5	0.07	0.07	1.9	0
Sandwich type (chocolate or vanilla), 1-3/4-in diam., 3/8 in thick	4	40	2	195	2	8	2.0	3.6	2.2	0	29	12	40	1.4	66	189	0	0	0.09	0.07	0.8	0
Shortbread																						
Commercial	4	32	6	155	2	8	2.9	3.0	1.1	27	20	13	39	0.8	38	123	30	8	0.10	0.09	0.9	0
From home recipe[38]	2	28	3	145	2	8	1.3	2.7	3.4	0	17	6	31	0.6	18	125	300	89	0.08	0.06	0.7	Tr
Sugar cookie, from refrigerated dough, 2-1/2-in diam., 1/4 in thick	4	48	4	235	2	12	2.3	5.0	3.6	29	31	50	91	0.9	33	261	40	11	0.09	0.06	1.1	0
Vanilla wafers, 1-3/4-in diam., 1/4 in thick	10	40	4	185	2	7	1.8	3.0	1.8	25	29	16	36	0.8	50	150	50	14	0.07	0.10	1.0	0
Corn chips	1 oz	28	1	155	2	9	1.4	2.4	3.7	0	16	35	52	0.5	52	233	110	11	0.04	0.05	0.4	1
Cornmeal																						
Whole-ground, unbolted, dry form	1 cup	122	12	435	11	5	0.5	1.1	2.5	0	90	24	312	2.2	346	1	620	62	0.46	0.13	2.4	0
Bolted (nearly whole-grain), dry form	1 cup	122	12	440	11	4	0.5	0.9	2.2	0	91	21	272	2.2	303	1	590	59	0.37	0.10	2.3	0
Degermed, enriched																						
Dry form	1 cup	138	12	500	11	2	0.2	0.4	0.9	0	108	8	137	5.9	166	1	610	61	0.61	0.36	4.8	0
Cooked	1 cup	240	88	120	3	Tr	Tr	0.1	0.2	0	26	2	34	1.4	38	0	140	14	0.14	0.10	1.2	0
Crackers[39]																						
Cheese																						
Plain, 1 in square	10	10	4	50	1	3	0.9	1.2	0.3	6	6	11	17	0.3	17	112	20	5	0.05	0.04	0.4	0

(Continued)

TABLE E-1 *(continued)*

ITEM	FOODS, APPROXIMATE MEASURES, UNITS, AND WEIGHT (WEIGHT OF EDIBLE PORTION ONLY)	WEIGHT (G)	WATER (%)	FOOD ENERGY (KCAL)	PROTEIN (G)	FAT (G)	FATTY ACIDS SATURATED (G)	FATTY ACIDS MONOUNSATURATED (G)	FATTY ACIDS POLYUNSATURATED (G)	CHOLESTEROL (MG)	CARBOHYDRATE (G)	CALCIUM (MG)	PHOSPHORUS (MG)	IRON (MG)	POTASSIUM (MG)	SODIUM (MG)	VITAMIN A VALUE (IU)	VITAMIN A VALUE (RE)	THIAMIN (MG)	RIBOFLAVIN (MG)	NIACIN (MG)	ASCORBIC ACID (MG)
Sandwich type (peanut butter)	1	8	3	40	1	2	0.4	0.8	0.3	1	5	7	25	0.3	17	90	Tr	Tr	0.04	0.03	0.6	0
Graham, plain, 2-1/2 in square	2	14	5	60	1	1	0.4	0.6	0.4	0	11	6	20	0.4	36	86	0	0	0.02	0.03	0.6	0
Melba toast, plain	1	5	4	20	1	Tr	0.1	0.1	0.1	0	4	6	10	0.1	11	44	0	0	0.01	0.01	0.1	0
Rye wafers, whole-grain, 1-7/8 by 3-1/2 in	2	14	5	55	1	1	0.3	0.4	0.3	0	10	7	44	0.5	65	115	0	0	0.06	0.03	0.5	0
Saltines[40]	4	12	4	50	1	1	0.5	0.4	0.2	4	9	3	12	0.5	17	165	0	0	0.06	0.05	0.6	0
Snack-type, standard	1	3	3	15	Tr	1	0.2	0.4	0.1	0	2	3	6	0.1	4	30	Tr	Tr	0.01	0.01	0.1	0
Wheat, thin	4	8	3	35	1	1	0.5	0.5	0.4	0	5	3	15	0.3	17	69	Tr	Tr	0.04	0.03	0.4	0
Whole-wheat wafers	2	8	4	35	1	2	0.5	0.6	0.4	0	5	3	22	0.2	31	59	0	0	0.02	0.03	0.4	0
Croissants																						
Made with enriched flour, 4-1/2 by 4 by 1-3/4 in	1	57	22	235	5	12	3.5	6.7	1.4	13	27	20	64	2.1	68	452	50	13	0.17	0.13	1.3	0
Danish pastry																						
Made with enriched flour																						
Plain without fruit or nuts																						
Packaged ring, 12 oz	1	340	27	1,305	21	71	21.8	28.6	15.6	292	152	360	347	6.5	316	1,302	360	99	0.95	1.02	8.5	Tr
Round piece, about 4-1/4-in diam., 1 in high	1	57	27	220	4	12	3.6	4.8	2.6	49	26	60	58	1.1	53	218	60	17	0.16	0.17	1.4	Tr
Ounce	1 oz	28	27	110	2	6	1.8	2.4	1.3	24	13	30	29	0.5	26	109	30	8	0.08	0.09	0.7	Tr
Fruit, round piece	1	65	30	235	4	13	3.9	5.2	2.9	56	28	17	80	1.3	57	233	40	11	0.16	0.14	1.4	Tr
Doughnuts																						
Made with enriched flour																						
Cake type, plain, 3-1/4-in diam., 1 in high	1	50	21	210	3	12	2.8	5.0	3.0	20	24	22	111	1.0	58	192	20	5	0.12	0.12	1.1	Tr
Yeast-leavened, glazed, 3-3/4-in diam., 1-1/4 in high	1	60	27	235	4	13	5.2	5.5	0.9	21	26	17	55	1.4	64	222	Tr	Tr	0.28	0.12	1.8	0
English muffins																						
Plain, enriched	1	57	42	140	5	1	0.3	0.2	0.3	0	27	96	67	1.7	331	378	0	0	0.26	0.19	2.2	0
Toasted	1	50	29	140	5	1	0.3	0.2	0.3	0	27	96	67	1.7	331	378	0	0	0.23	0.19	2.2	0
French toast																						
From home recipe	1	65	53	155	6	7	1.6	2.0	1.6	112	17	72	85	1.3	86	257	110	32	0.12	0.16	1.0	Tr
Macaroni																						
Enriched, cooked (cut lengths, elbows, shells)																						

Firm stage (hot)	1 cup	130	64	190	7	1	0.1	0.1	0.3	0	39	14	85	2.1	103	1	0	0	0.23	0.13	1.8	0
Tender stage																						
Cold	1 cup	105	72	115	4	Tr	0.1	0.1	0.2	0	24	8	53	1.3	64	1	0	0	0.15	0.08	1.2	0
Hot	1 cup	140	72	155	5	1	0.1	0.1	0.2	0	32	11	70	1.7	85	1	0	0	0.20	0.11	1.5	0
Muffins made with enriched flour																						
2-1/2-in diam., 1-1/2 in high																						
From home recipe																						
Blueberry[25]	1	45	37	135	3	5	1.5	2.1	1.2	19	20	54	46	0.9	47	198	40	9	0.10	0.11	0.9	1
Bran[36]	1	45	35	125	3	6	1.4	1.6	2.3	24	19	60	125	1.4	99	189	230	30	0.11	0.13	1.3	3
Corn (enriched, degermed cornmeal and flour)[25]	1	45	33	145	3	5	1.5	2.2	1.4	23	21	66	59	0.9	57	169	80	15	0.11	0.11	0.9	Tr
From commercial mix (egg and water added)																						
Blueberry	1	45	33	140	3	5	1.4	2.0	1.2	45	22	15	90	0.9	54	225	50	11	0.10	0.17	1.1	Tr
Bran	1	45	28	140	3	4	1.3	1.6	1.0	28	24	27	182	1.7	50	385	100	14	0.08	0.12	1.9	0
Corn	1	45	30	145	3	6	1.7	2.3	1.4	42	22	30	128	1.3	31	291	90	16	0.09	0.09	0.8	Tr
Noodles																						
(Egg noodles), enriched, cooked	1 cup	160	70	200	7	2	0.5	0.6	0.6	50	37	16	94	2.6	70	3	110	34	0.22	0.13	1.9	0
Noodles																						
Chow mein, canned	1 cup	45	11	220	6	11	2.1	7.3	0.4	5	26	14	41	0.4	33	450	0	0	0.05	0.03	0.6	0
Pancakes, 4-in diam.																						
Buckwheat, from mix (with buckwheat and enriched flours), egg and milk added	1	27	58	55	2	2	0.9	0.9	0.5	20	6	59	91	0.4	66	125	60	17	0.04	0.05	0.2	Tr
Plain																						
From home recipe using enriched flour	1	27	50	60	2	2	0.5	0.8	0.5	16	9	27	38	0.5	33	115	30	10	0.06	0.07	0.5	Tr
From mix (with enriched flour), egg, milk, and oil added	1	27	54	60	2	2	0.5	0.9	0.5	16	8	36	71	0.7	43	160	30	7	0.09	0.12	0.8	Tr
Piecrust																						
Made with enriched flour and vegetable shortening, baked																						
From home recipe, 9-in diam.	1 piecrust for 2-crust pie	180	15	900	11	60	14.8	25.9	15.7	0	79	25	90	4.5	90	1,100	0	0	0.54	0.40	5.0	0
From mix, 9-in diam.	1 piecrust for 2-crust pie	320	19	1,485	20	93	22.7	41.0	25.0	0	141	131	272	9.3	179	2,602	0	0	1.06	0.80	9.9	0
Pies, piecrust made with enriched flour, vegetable shortening, 9-in diam.																						
Apple																						
Whole	1	945	48	2,420	21	105	27.4	44.4	26.5	0	360	76	208	9.5	756	2,844	280	28	1.04	0.76	9.5	9
Piece, 1/6 of pie	1	158	48	405	3	18	4.6	7.4	4.4	0	60	13	35	1.6	126	476	50	5	0.17	0.13	1.6	2
Blueberry																						
Whole	1	945	51	2,285	23	102	25.5	44.4	27.4	0	330	104	217	12.3	945	2,533	850	85	1.04	0.85	10.4	38
Piece, 1/6 of pie	1	158	51	380	4	17	4.3	7.4	4.6	0	55	17	36	2.1	158	423	140	14	0.17	0.14	1.7	6
Cherry																						
Whole	1	945	47	2,465	25	107	28.4	46.3	27.4	0	363	132	236	9.5	992	2,873	4,160	416	1.13	0.85	9.5	0
Piece, 1/6 of pie	1	158	47	410	4	18	4.7	7.7	4.6	0	61	22	40	1.6	166	480	700	70	0.19	0.14	1.6	0
Creme																						

(Continued)

TABLE E-1 *(continued)*

ITEM	FOODS, APPROXIMATE MEASURES, UNITS, AND WEIGHT (WEIGHT OF EDIBLE PORTION ONLY)	WEIGHT (G)	WATER (%)	FOOD ENERGY (KCAL)	PROTEIN (G)	FAT (G)	FATTY ACIDS SATURATED (G)	FATTY ACIDS MONOUNSATURATED (G)	FATTY ACIDS POLYUNSATURATED (G)	CHOLESTEROL (MG)	CARBOHYDRATE (G)	CALCIUM (MG)	PHOSPHORUS (MG)	IRON (MG)	POTASSIUM (MG)	SODIUM (MG)	VITAMIN A VALUE (IU)	VITAMIN A VALUE (RE)	THIAMIN (MG)	RIBOFLAVIN (MG)	NIACIN (MG)	ASCORBIC ACID (MG)
Whole	1	910	43	2,710	20	139	90.1	23.7	6.4	46	351	273	919	6.8	796	2,207	1,250	391	0.36	0.89	6.4	0
Piece, 1/6 of pie	1	152	43	455	3	23	15.0	4.0	1.1	8	59	46	154	1.1	133	369	210	65	0.06	0.15	1.1	0
Custard																						
Whole	1	910	58	1,985	56	101	33.7	40.0	19.1	1010	213	874	1,028	9.1	1,247	2,612	2,090	573	0.82	1.91	5.5	0
Piece, 1/6 of pie	1	152	58	330	9	17	5.6	6.7	3.2	169	36	146	172	1.5	208	436	350	96	0.14	0.32	0.9	0
Lemon meringue																						
Whole	1	840	47	2,140	31	86	26.0	34.4	17.6	857	317	118	412	8.4	420	2,369	1,430	395	0.59	0.84	5.0	25
Piece, 1/6 of pie	1	140	47	355	5	14	4.3	5.7	2.9	143	53	20	69	1.4	70	395	240	66	0.10	0.14	0.8	4
Peach																						
Whole	1	945	48	2,410	24	101	24.6	43.5	26.5	0	361	95	274	11.3	1,408	2,533	6,900	690	1.04	0.95	14.2	28
Piece, 1/6 of pie	1	158	48	405	4	17	4.1	7.3	4.4	0	60	16	46	1.9	235	423	1,150	115	0.17	0.16	2.4	5
Pies																						
Piecrust made with enriched flour, vegetable shortening, 9-in diam.																						
Pecan																						
Whole	1	825	20	3,450	42	189	28.1	101.5	47.0	569	423	388	850	27.2	1,015	1,823	1,320	322	1.82	0.99	6.6	0
Piece, 1/6 of pie	1	138	20	575	7	32	4.7	17.0	7.9	95	71	65	142	4.6	170	305	220	54	0.30	0.17	1.1	0
Pumpkin																						
Whole	1	910	59	1,920	36	102	38.2	40.0	18.2	655	223	464	628	8.2	1,456	1,947	22,480	2,493	0.82	1.27	7.3	0
Piece, 1/6 of pie	1	152	59	320	6	17	6.4	6.7	3.0	109	37	78	105	1.4	243	325	3,750	416	0.14	0.21	1.2	0
Pies																						
Fried																						
Apple	1	85	43	255	2	14	5.8	6.6	0.6	14	31	12	34	0.9	42	326	30	3	0.09	0.06	1.0	1
Cherry	1	85	42	250	2	14	5.8	6.7	0.6	13	32	11	41	0.7	61	371	190	19	0.06	0.06	0.6	1
Popcorn																						
Popped																						
Air-popped, unsalted	1 cup	8	4	30	1	Tr	Tr	0.1	0.2	0	6	1	22	0.2	20	Tr	10	1	0.03	0.01	0.2	0
Popped in vegetable oil, salted	1 cup	11	3	55	1	3	0.5	1.4	1.2	0	6	3	31	0.3	19	86	20	2	0.01	0.02	0.1	0
Sugar syrup coated	1 cup	35	4	135	2	1	0.1	0.3	0.6	0	30	2	47	0.5	90	Tr	30	3	0.13	0.02	0.4	0
Pretzels																						
Made with enriched flour																						
Stick, 2-1/4 in long	10	3	3	10	Tr	Tr	Tr	Tr	Tr	0	2	1	3	0.1	3	48	0	0	0.01	0.01	0.1	0
Twisted, dutch, 2-3/4 by 2-5/8 in	1	16	3	65	2	1	0.1	0.2	0.2	0	13	4	15	0.3	16	258	0	0	0.05	0.04	0.7	0
Twisted, thin, 3-1/4 by 2-1/4 by 1/4 in	10	60	3	240	6	2	0.4	0.8	0.6	0	48	16	55	1.2	61	966	0	0	0.19	0.15	2.6	0
Rice																						

Brown, cooked, served hot	1 cup	195	70	230	5	1	0.3	0.3	0.4	0	50	23	142	1.0	137	0	0	0	0.18	0.04	2.7	0
White, enriched																						
Commercial varieties, all types																						
Raw	1 cup	185	12	670	12	1	0.2	0.2	0.3	0	149	44	174	5.4	170	9	0	0	0.81	0.06	6.5	0
Cooked, served hot	1 cup	205	73	225	4	Tr	0.1	0.1	0.1	0	50	21	57	1.8	57	0	0	0	0.23	0.02	2.1	0
Instant, ready-to-serve, hot	1 cup	165	73	180	4	0	0.1	0.1	0.1	0	40	5	31	1.3	0	0	0	0	0.21	0.02	1.7	0
Parboiled																						
Raw	1 cup	185	10	685	14	1	0.1	0.1	0.2	0	150	111	370	5.4	278	17	0	0	0.81	0.07	6.5	0
Cooked, served hot	1 cup	175	73	185	4	Tr	Tr	Tr	0.1	0	41	33	100	1.4	75	0	0	0	0.19	0.02	2.1	0
Rolls, enriched																						
Commercial																						
Dinner, 2-1/2-in diam., 2 in high	1	28	32	85	2	2	0.5	0.8	0.6	Tr	14	33	44	0.8	36	155	Tr	Tr	0.14	0.09	1.1	Tr
Frankfurter and hamburger (8 per 11-1/2-oz pkg.)	1	40	34	115	3	2	0.5	0.8	0.6	Tr	20	54	44	1.2	56	241	Tr	Tr	0.20	0.13	1.6	Tr
Hard, 3-3/4-in diam., 2 in high	1	50	25	155	5	2	0.4	0.5	0.6	Tr	30	24	46	1.4	49	313	0	0	0.20	0.12	1.7	0
Hoagie or submarine, 11-1/2 by 3 by 2-1/2 in	1	135	31	400	11	8	1.8	3.0	2.2	Tr	72	100	115	3.8	128	683	0	0	0.54	0.33	4.5	0
From home recipe																						
Dinner, 2-1/2-in diam., 2 in high	1	35	26	120	3	3	0.8	1.2	0.9	12	20	16	36	1.1	41	98	30	8	0.12	0.12	1.2	0
Spaghetti																						
Enriched, cooked																						
Firm stage, "al dente," served hot	1 cup	130	64	190	7	1	0.1	0.1	0.3	0	39	14	85	2.0	103	1	0	0	0.23	0.13	1.8	0
Tender stage, served hot	1 cup	140	73	155	5	1	0.1	0.1	0.2	0	32	11	70	1.7	85	1	0	0	0.20	0.11	1.5	0
Toaster pastries	1	54	13	210	2	6	1.7	3.6	0.4	0	38	104	104	2.2	91	248	520	52	0.17	0.18	2.3	4
Tortillas																						
Corn	1	30	45	65	2	1	0.1	0.3	0.6	0	13	42	55	0.6	43	1	80	8	0.05	0.03	0.4	0
Waffles																						
Made with enriched flour, 7-in diam.																						
From home recipe	1	75	37	245	7	13	4.0	4.9	2.6	102	26	154	135	1.5	129	445	140	39	0.18	0.24	1.5	Tr
From mix, egg and milk added	1	75	42	205	7	8	2.7	2.9	1.5	59	27	179	257	1.2	146	515	170	49	0.14	0.23	0.9	Tr
Wheat flours																						
All-purpose or family flour, enriched																						
Sifted, spooned	1 cup	115	12	420	12	1	0.2	0.1	0.5	0	88	18	100	5.1	109	2	0	0	0.73	0.46	6.1	0
Unsifted, spooned	1 cup	125	12	455	13	1	0.2	0.1	0.5	0	95	20	109	5.5	119	3	0	0	0.80	0.50	6.6	0
Cake or pastry flour, enriched, sifted, spooned	1 cup	96	12	350	7	1	0.1	0.1	0.3	0	76	16	70	4.2	91	2	0	0	0.58	0.38	5.1	0
Self-rising, enriched, unsifted, spooned	1 cup	125	12	440	12	1	0.2	0.1	0.5	0	93	331	583	5.5	113	1,349	0	0	0.80	0.50	6.6	0
Whole-wheat, from hard wheats, stirred	1 cup	120	12	400	16	2	0.3	0.3	1.1	0	85	49	446	5.2	444	4	0	0	0.66	0.14	5.2	0
LEGUMES, NUTS, AND SEEDS																						
Almonds, shelled																						
Slivered, packed	1 cup	135	4	795	27	70	6.7	45.8	14.8	0	28	359	702	4.9	988	15	0	0	0.28	1.05	4.5	1
Whole	1 oz	28	4	165	6	15	1.4	9.6	3.1	0	6	75	147	1.0	208	3	0	0	0.06	0.22	1.0	Tr

(Continued)

TABLE E-1 *(continued)*

ITEM	FOODS, APPROXIMATE MEASURES, UNITS, AND WEIGHT (WEIGHT OF EDIBLE PORTION ONLY)	WEIGHT (G)	WATER (%)	FOOD ENERGY (KCAL)	PROTEIN (G)	FAT (G)	FATTY ACIDS SATURATED (G)	FATTY ACIDS MONOUNSATURATED (G)	FATTY ACIDS POLYUNSATURATED (G)	CHOLESTEROL (MG)	CARBOHYDRATE (G)	CALCIUM (MG)	PHOSPHORUS (MG)	IRON (MG)	POTASSIUM (MG)	SODIUM (MG)	VITAMIN A VALUE (IU)	VITAMIN A VALUE (RE)	THIAMIN (MG)	RIBOFLAVIN (MG)	NIACIN (MG)	ASCORBIC ACID (MG)
Beans																						
Dry																						
Cooked, drained																						
Black	1 cup	171	66	225	15	1	0.1	0.1	0.5	0	41	47	239	2.9	608	1	Tr	Tr	0.43	0.05	0.9	0
Great Northern	1 cup	180	69	210	14	1	0.1	0.1	0.6	0	38	90	266	4.9	749	13	0	0	0.25	0.13	1.3	0
Lima	1 cup	190	64	260	16	1	0.2	0.1	0.5	0	49	55	293	5.9	1,163	4	0	0	0.25	0.11	1.3	0
Pea (navy)	1 cup	190	69	225	15	1	0.1	0.1	0.7	0	40	95	281	5.1	790	13	0	0	0.27	0.13	1.3	0
Pinto	1 cup	180	65	265	15	1	0.1	0.1	0.5	0	49	86	296	5.4	882	3	Tr	Tr	0.33	0.16	0.7	0
Canned, solids and liquid																						
White with																						
Frankfurters (sliced)	1 cup	255	71	365	19	18	7.4	8.8	0.7	30	32	94	303	4.8	668	1,374	330	33	0.18	0.15	3.3	Tr
Pork and tomato sauce	1 cup	255	71	310	16	7	2.4	2.7	0.7	10	48	138	235	4.6	536	1,181	330	33	0.20	0.08	1.5	5
Pork and sweet sauce	1 cup	255	66	385	16	12	4.3	4.9	1.2	10	54	161	291	5.9	536	969	330	33	0.15	0.10	1.3	5
Red kidney	1 cup	255	76	230	15	1	0.1	0.1	0.6	0	42	74	278	4.6	673	968	10	1	0.13	0.10	1.5	0
Black-eye peas																						
Dry, cooked (with residual cooking liquid)	1 cup	250	80	190	13	1	0.2	Tr	0.3	0	35	43	238	3.3	573	20	30	3	0.40	0.10	1.0	0
Brazil nuts																						
Shelled	1 oz	28	3	185	4	19	4.6	6.5	6.8	0	4	50	170	1.0	170	1	Tr	Tr	0.28	0.03	0.5	Tr
Carob flour	1 cup	140	3	255	6	Tr	Tr	0.1	0.1	0	126	390	102	5.7	1,275	24	Tr	Tr	0.07	0.07	2.2	Tr
Cashew nuts																						
Salted																						
Dry roasted	1 cup	137	2	785	21	63	12.5	37.4	10.7	0	45	62	671	8.2	774	[41]877	0	0	0.27	0.27	1.9	0
	1 oz	28	2	165	4	13	2.6	7.7	2.2	0	9	13	139	1.7	160	[41]181	0	0	0.06	0.06	0.4	0
Roasted in oil	1 cup	130	4	750	21	63	12.4	36.9	10.6	0	37	53	554	5.3	689	[42]814	0	0	0.55	0.23	2.3	0
	1 oz	28	4	165	5	14	2.7	3.1	2.3	0	8	12	121	1.2	150	[42]177	0	0	0.12	0.05	0.5	0
Chestnuts																						
European (Italian), roasted, shelled	1 cup	143	40	350	5	3	0.6	1.1	1.2	0	76	41	153	1.3	847	3	30	3	0.35	0.25	1.9	37
Chickpeas																						
Cooked, drained	1 cup	163	60	270	15	4	0.4	0.9	1.9	0	45	80	273	4.9	475	11	Tr	Tr	0.18	0.09	0.9	0
Coconut																						
Raw																						

Piece, about 2 by 2 by $^1/_2$ in	1	45	47	160	1	15	13.4	0.6	0.2	0	7	6	51	1.1	160	9	0	0	0.03	0.01	0.2	1
Shredded or grated	1 cup	80	47	285	3	27	23.8	1.1	0.3	0	12	11	90	1.9	285	16	0	0	0.05	0.02	0.4	3
Dried, sweetened, shredded	1 cup	93	13	470	3	33	29.3	1.4	0.4	0	44	14	99	1.8	313	244	0	0	0.03	0.02	0.4	1
Filberts																						
(Hazelnuts), chopped	1 cup	115	5	725	15	72	5.3	56.5	6.9	0	18	216	359	3.8	512	3	80	8	0.58	0.13	1.3	1
	1 oz	28	5	180	4	18	1.3	13.9	1.7	0	4	53	88	0.9	126	1	20	2	0.14	0.03	0.3	Tr
Lentils																						
Dry, cooked	1 cup	200	72	215	16	1	0.1	0.2	0.5	0	38	50	238	4.2	498	26	40	4	0.14	0.12	1.2	0
Macadamia nuts																						
Roasted in oil, salted	1 cup	134	2	960	10	103	15.4	80.9	1.8	0	17	60	268	2.4	441	[43]348	10	1	0.29	0.15	2.7	0
	1 oz	28	2	205	2	22	3.2	17.1	0.4	0	4	13	57	0.5	93	[43]74	Tr	Tr	0.06	0.03	0.6	0
Mixed nuts																						
With peanuts, salted																						
Dry roasted	1 oz	28	2	170	5	15	2.0	8.9	3.1	0	7	20	123	1.0	169	[44]190	Tr	Tr	0.06	0.06	1.3	0
Roasted in oil	1 oz	28	2	175	5	16	2.5	9.0	3.8	0	6	31	131	0.9	165	[44]185	10	1	0.14	0.06	1.4	Tr
Peanuts																						
Roasted in oil, salted	1 cup	145	2	840	39	71	9.9	35.5	22.6	0	27	125	734	2.8	1,019	[45]626	0	0	0.42	0.15	21.5	0
	1 oz	28	2	165	8	14	1.9	6.9	4.4	0	5	24	143	0.5	199	[45]122	0	0	0.08	0.03	4.2	0
Peanut butter	1 tbsp	16	1	95	5	8	1.4	4.0	2.5	0	3	5	60	0.3	110	75	0	0	0.02	0.02	2.2	0
Peas																						
Split, dry, cooked	1 cup	200	70	230	16	1	0.1	0.1	0.3	0	42	22	178	3.4	592	26	80	8	0.30	0.18	1.8	0
Pecans																						
Halves	1 cup	108	5	720	8	73	5.9	45.5	18.1	0	20	39	314	2.3	423	1	140	14	0.92	0.14	1.0	2
	1 oz	28	5	190	2	19	1.5	12.0	4.7	0	5	10	83	0.6	111	Tr	40	4	0.24	0.04	0.3	1
Pine nuts																						
(Pinyons), shelled	1 oz	28	6	160	3	17	2.7	6.5	7.3	0	5	2	10	0.9	178	20	10	1	0.35	0.06	1.2	1
Pistachio nuts																						
Dried, shelled	1 oz	28	4	165	6	14	1.7	9.3	2.1	0	7	38	143	1.9	310	2	70	7	0.23	0.05	0.3	Tr
Pumpkin and squash kernels																						
Dry, hulled	1 oz	28	7	155	7	13	2.5	4.0	5.9	0	5	12	333	4.2	229	5	110	11	0.06	0.09	0.5	Tr
Refried beans																						
Canned	1 cup	290	72	295	18	3	0.4	0.6	1.4	0	51	141	245	5.1	1,141	1,228	0	0	0.14	0.16	1.4	17
Sesame seeds																						
Dry, hulled	1 tbsp	8	5	45	2	4	0.6	1.7	1.9	0	1	11	62	0.6	33	3	10	1	0.06	0.01	0.4	0
Soybeans																						
Dry, cooked, drained	1 cup	180	71	235	20	10	1.3	1.9	5.3	0	19	131	322	4.9	972	4	50	5	0.38	0.16	1.1	0
Soy products																						
Miso	1 cup	276	53	470	29	13	1.8	2.6	7.3	0	65	188	853	4.7	922	8,142	110	11	0.17	0.28	0.8	0
Tofu, piece 2-$^1/_2$ by 2-$^3/_4$ by 1 in	1	120	85	85	9	5	0.7	1.0	2.9	0	3	108	151	2.3	50	8	0	0	0.07	0.04	0.1	0

(Continued)

TABLE E-1 *(continued)*

ITEM	FOODS, APPROXIMATE MEASURES, UNITS, AND WEIGHT (WEIGHT OF EDIBLE PORTION ONLY)	WEIGHT (G)	WATER (%)	FOOD ENERGY (KCAL)	PROTEIN (G)	FAT (G)	FATTY ACIDS SATURATED (G)	FATTY ACIDS MONOUNSATURATED (G)	FATTY ACIDS POLYUNSATURATED (G)	CHOLESTEROL (MG)	CARBOHYDRATE (G)	CALCIUM (MG)	PHOSPHORUS (MG)	IRON (MG)	POTASSIUM (MG)	SODIUM (MG)	VITAMIN A VALUE (IU)	VITAMIN A VALUE (RE)	THIAMIN (MG)	RIBOFLAVIN (MG)	NIACIN (MG)	ASCORBIC ACID (MG)
Sunflower seeds																						
Dry, hulled	1 oz	28	5	160	6	14	1.5	2.7	9.3	0	5	33	200	1.9	195	1	10	1	0.65	0.07	1.3	Tr
Tahini	1 tbsp	15	3	90	3	8	1.1	3.0	3.5	0	3	21	119	0.7	69	5	10	1	0.24	0.02	0.8	1
Walnuts																						
Black, chopped	1 cup	125	4	760	30	71	4.5	15.9	46.9	0	15	73	580	3.8	655	1	370	37	0.27	0.14	0.9	Tr
	1 oz	28	4	170	7	16	1.0	3.6	10.6	0	3	16	132	0.9	149	Tr	80	8	0.06	0.03	0.2	Tr
English or Persian, pieces or chips	1 cup	120	4	770	17	74	6.7	17.0	47.0	0	22	113	380	2.9	602	12	150	15	0.46	0.18	1.3	4
	1 oz	28	4	180	4	18	1.6	4.0	11.1	0	5	27	90	0.7	142	3	40	4	0.11	0.04	0.3	1
MEAT AND MEAT PRODUCTS																						
Beef, cooked																						
Cuts braised, simmered, or pot roasted																						
Relatively fat such as chuck blade																						
Lean and fat, piece, 2-$^{1}/_{2}$ by 2-$^{1}/_{2}$ by $^{3}/_{4}$ in	3 oz	85	43	325	22	26	10.8	11.7	0.9	87	0	11	163	2.5	163	53	Tr	Tr	0.06	0.19	2.0	0
Lean only	2.2 oz	62	53	170	19	9	3.9	4.2	0.3	66	0	8	146	2.3	163	44	Tr	Tr	0.05	0.17	1.7	0
Relatively lean, such as bottom round																						
Lean and fat, piece, 4-$^{1}/_{8}$ by 2-$^{1}/_{4}$ by $^{1}/_{2}$ in	3 oz	85	54	220	25	13	4.8	5.7	0.5	81	0	5	217	2.8	248	43	Tr	Tr	0.06	0.21	3.3	0
Lean only	2.8 oz	78	57	175	25	8	2.7	3.4	0.3	75	0	4	212	2.7	240	40	Tr	Tr	0.06	0.20	3.0	0
Ground beef, broiled, patty, 3 by $^{5}/_{8}$ in																						
Lean	3 oz	85	56	230	21	16	6.2	6.9	0.6	74	0	9	134	1.8	256	65	Tr	Tr	0.04	0.18	4.4	0
Regular	3 oz	85	54	245	20	18	6.9	7.7	0.7	76	0	9	144	2.1	248	70	Tr	Tr	0.03	0.16	4.9	0
Heart, lean, braised	3 oz	85	65	150	24	5	1.2	0.8	1.6	164	0	5	213	6.4	198	54	Tr	Tr	0.12	1.31	3.4	5
Liver, fried, slice, 6-$^{1}/_{2}$ by 2-$^{3}/_{8}$ by $^{3}/_{8}$ in[47]	3 oz	85	56	185	23	7	2.5	3.6	1.3	410	7	9	392	5.3	309	90	[48]30,690	[48]9,120	0.18	3.52	12.3	23
Roast, oven cooked, no liquid added																						
Relatively fat, such as rib																						
Lean and fat, 2 pieces, 4-$^{1}/_{8}$ by 2-$^{1}/_{4}$ by $^{1}/_{4}$ in	3 oz	85	46	315	19	26	10.8	11.4	0.9	72	0	8	145	2.0	246	54	Tr	Tr	0.06	0.16	3.1	0
Lean only	2.2 oz	61	57	150	17	9	3.6	3.7	0.3	49	0	5	127	1.7	218	45	Tr	Tr	0.05	0.13	2.7	0
Relatively lean, such as eye of round																						
Lean and fat, 2 pieces, 2-$^{1}/_{2}$ by 2-$^{1}/_{2}$ by $^{3}/_{8}$ in	3 oz	85	57	205	23	12	4.9	5.4	0.5	62	0	5	177	1.6	308	50	Tr	Tr	0.07	0.14	3.0	0
Lean only	2.6 oz	75	63	135	22	5	1.9	2.1	0.2	52	0	3	170	1.5	297	46	Tr	Tr	0.07	0.13	2.8	0

Steak																						
Sirloin, broiled																						
Lean and fat, piece, 2-1/2 by 2-1/2 by 3/4 in	3 oz	85	53	240	23	15	6.4	6.9	0.6	77	0	9	186	2.6	306	53	Tr	Tr	0.10	0.23	3.3	0
Lean only	2.5 oz	72	59	150	22	6	2.6	2.8	0.3	64	0	8	176	2.4	290	48	Tr	Tr	0.09	0.22	3.1	0
Beef, canned corned	3 oz	85	59	185	22	10	4.2	4.9	0.4	80	0	17	90	3.7	51	802	Tr	Tr	0.02	0.20	2.9	0
Beef, dried chipped	2.5 oz	72	48	145	24	4	1.8	2.0	0.2	46	0	14	287	2.3	142	3,053	Tr	Tr	0.05	0.23	2.7	0
Lamb, Cooked																						
Chops, (3 per lb with bone):																						
Arm, braised																						
Lean and fat	2.2 oz	63	44	220	20	15	6.9	6.0	0.9	77	0	16	132	1.5	195	46	Tr	Tr	0.04	0.16	4.4	0
Lean only	1.7 oz	48	49	135	17	7	2.9	2.6	0.4	59	0	12	111	1.3	162	36	Tr	Tr	0.03	0.13	3.0	0
Loin, broiled																						
Lean and fat	2.8 oz	80	54	235	22	16	7.3	6.4	1.0	78	0	16	162	1.4	272	62	Tr	Tr	0.09	0.21	5.5	0
Lean only	2.3 oz	64	61	140	19	6	2.6	2.4	0.4	60	0	12	145	1.3	241	54	Tr	Tr	0.08	0.18	4.4	0
Leg, roasted																						
Lean and fat, 2 pieces, 4-1/8 by 2-1/4 by 1/4 in	3 oz	85	59	205	22	13	5.6	4.9	0.8	78	0	8	162	1.7	273	57	Tr	Tr	0.09	0.24	5.5	0
Lean only	2.6 oz	73	64	140	20	6	2.4	2.2	0.4	65	0	6	150	1.5	247	50	Tr	Tr	0.08	0.20	4.6	0
Rib, roasted																						
Lean and fat, 3 pieces, 2-1/2 by 2-1/2 by 1/4 in	3 oz	85	47	315	18	26	12.1	10.6	1.5	77	0	19	139	1.4	224	60	Tr	Tr	0.08	0.18	5.5	0
Lean only	2 oz	57	60	130	15	7	3.2	3.0	0.5	50	0	12	111	1.0	179	46	Tr	Tr	0.05	0.13	3.5	0
Pork, cured, cooked																						
Bacon																						
Regular slice	3	19	13	110	6	9	3.3	4.5	1.1	16	Tr	2	64	0.3	92	303	0	0	0.13	0.05	1.4	6
Canadian-style slice	2	46	62	85	11	4	1.3	1.9	0.4	27	1	5	136	0.4	179	711	0	0	0.38	0.09	3.2	10
Ham, light cure, roasted																						
Lean and fat, 2 pieces, 4-1/8 by 2-1/4 by 1/4 in	3 oz	85	58	205	18	14	5.1	6.7	1.5	53	0	6	182	0.7	243	1,009	0	0	0.51	0.19	3.8	0
Lean only	2.4 oz	68	66	105	17	4	1.3	1.7	0.4	37	0	5	154	0.6	215	902	0	0	0.46	0.17	3.4	0
Ham, canned, roasted, 2 pieces, 4-1/8 by 2-1/4 by 1/4 in	3 oz	85	67	140	18	7	2.4	3.5	0.8	35	Tr	6	188	0.9	298	908	0	0	0.82	0.21	4.3	[49]19
Luncheon meat																						
Canned, spiced or unspiced, slice, 3 by 2 by 1/2 in	2	42	52	140	5	13	4.5	6.0	1.5	26	1	3	34	0.3	90	541	0	0	0.15	0.08	1.3	Tr
Chopped ham (8 slices per 6 oz pkg)	2	42	64	95	7	7	2.4	3.4	0.9	21	0	3	65	0.3	134	576	0	0	0.27	0.09	1.6	[49]8
Cooked ham (8 slices per 8-oz pkg)																						
Regular	2	57	65	105	10	6	1.9	2.8	0.7	32	2	4	141	0.6	189	751	0	0	0.49	0.14	3.0	[49]16
Extra lean	2	57	71	75	11	3	0.9	1.3	0.3	27	1	4	124	0.4	200	815	0	0	0.53	0.13	2.8	[49]15
Pork, fresh, cooked																						
Chop, loin (cut 3 per lb with bone)																						
Broiled																						
Lean and fat	3.1 oz	87	50	275	24	19	7.0	8.8	2.2	84	0	3	184	0.7	312	61	10	3	0.87	0.24	4.3	Tr
Lean only	2.5 oz	72	57	165	23	8	2.6	3.4	0.9	71	0	4	176	0.7	302	56	10	1	0.83	0.22	4.0	Tr
Pan fried																						
Lean and fat	3.1 oz	89	45	335	21	27	9.8	12.5	3.1	92	0	4	190	0.7	323	64	10	3	0.91	0.24	4.6	Tr
Lean only	2.4 oz	67	54	180	19	11	3.7	4.8	1.3	72	0	3	178	0.7	305	57	10	1	0.84	0.22	4.0	Tr

(Continued)

TABLE E-1 *(continued)*

ITEM	FOODS, APPROXIMATE MEASURES, UNITS, AND WEIGHT (WEIGHT OF EDIBLE PORTION ONLY)	WEIGHT (G)	WATER (%)	FOOD ENERGY (KCAL)	PROTEIN (G)	FAT (G)	FATTY ACIDS SATURATED (G)	FATTY ACIDS MONOUNSATURATED (G)	FATTY ACIDS POLYUNSATURATED (G)	CHOLESTEROL (MG)	CARBOHYDRATE (G)	CALCIUM (MG)	PHOSPHORUS (MG)	IRON (MG)	POTASSIUM (MG)	SODIUM (MG)	VITAMIN A VALUE (IU)	VITAMIN A VALUE (RE)	THIAMIN (MG)	RIBOFLAVIN (MG)	NIACIN (MG)	ASCORBIC ACID (MG)
Ham (leg), roasted																						
Lean and fat, piece, 2-1/2 by 2-1/2 by 3/4 in	3 oz	85	53	250	21	18	6.4	8.1	2.0	79	0	5	210	0.9	280	50	10	2	0.54	0.27	3.9	Tr
Lean only	2.5 oz	72	60	160	20	8	2.7	3.6	1.0	68	0	5	202	0.8	269	46	10	1	0.50	0.25	3.6	Tr
Rib, roasted																						
Lean and fat, piece, 2-1/2 by 3/4 in	3 oz	85	51	270	21	20	7.2	9.2	2.3	69	0	9	190	0.8	313	37	10	3	0.50	0.24	4.2	Tr
Lean only	2.5 oz	71	57	175	20	10	3.4	4.4	1.2	56	0	8	182	0.7	300	33	10	2	0.45	0.22	3.8	Tr
Shoulder cut, braised																						
Lean and fat, 3 pieces, 2-1/2 by 2-1/2 by 1/4 in	3 oz	85	47	295	23	22	7.9	10.0	2.4	93	0	6	162	1.4	286	75	10	3	0.46	0.26	4.4	Tr
Lean only	2.4 oz	67	54	165	22	8	2.8	3.7	1.0	76	0	5	151	1.3	271	68	10	1	0.40	0.24	4.0	Tr
Sausages																						
(See also Luncheon meats.)																						
Bologna, slice (8 per 8-oz pkg)	2	57	54	180	7	16	6.1	7.6	1.4	31	2	7	52	0.9	103	581	0	0	0.10	0.08	1.5	[49]12
Braunschweiger, slice (6 per 6-oz pkg)	2	57	48	205	8	18	6.2	8.5	2.1	89	2	5	96	5.3	113	652	8,010	2,405	0.14	0.87	4.8	[49]6
Brown and serve (10–11 per 8-oz pkg), browned	1	13	45	50	2	5	1.7	2.2	0.5	9	Tr	1	14	0.1	25	105	0	0	0.05	0.02	0.4	0
Frankfurter (10 per 1-lb pkg), cooked (reheated)	1	45	54	145	5	13	4.8	6.2	1.2	23	1	5	39	0.5	75	504	0	0	0.09	0.05	1.2	[49]12
Pork link (16 per 1-lb pkg), cooked[50]	1	13	45	50	3	4	1.4	1.8	0.5	11	Tr	4	24	0.2	47	168	0	0	0.10	0.03	0.6	Tr
Salami																						
Cooked type, slice (8 per 8-oz pkg)	2	57	60	145	8	11	4.6	5.2	1.2	37	1	7	66	1.5	113	607	0	0	0.14	0.21	2.0	[49]7
Dry type, slice (12 per 4-oz pkg)	2	20	35	85	5	7	2.4	3.4	0.6	16	1	2	28	0.3	76	372	0	0	0.12	0.06	1.0	[49]5
Sandwich spread (pork, beef)	1 tbsp	15	60	35	1	3	0.9	1.1	0.4	6	2	2	9	0.1	17	152	10	1	0.03	0.02	0.3	0
Vienna sausage (7 per 4-oz can)	1	16	60	45	2	4	1.5	2.0	0.3	8	Tr	2	8	0.1	16	152	0	0	0.01	0.02	0.3	0
Veal																						
Medium fat, cooked, bone removed																						
Cutlet, 4-1/8 by 2-1/4 by 1/2 in, braised or broiled	3 oz	85	60	185	23	9	4.1	4.1	0.6	109	0	9	196	0.8	258	56	Tr	Tr	0.06	0.21	4.6	0
Rib, 2 pieces, 4-1/8 by 2-1/4 by 1/4 in, roasted	3 oz	85	55	230	23	14	6.0	6.0	1.0	109	0	10	211	0.7	259	57	Tr	Tr	0.11	0.26	6.6	0

MIXED DISHES AND FAST FOODS

Mixed dishes

Beef and vegetable stew, from home recipe	1 cup	245	82	220	16	11	4.4	4.5	0.5	71	15	29	184	2.9	613	292	5,690	568	0.15	0.17	4.7	17
Beef potpie, from home recipe, baked, piece, 1/3 of 9-in diam. pie[51]	1	210	55	515	21	30	7.9	12.9	7.4	42	39	29	149	3.8	334	596	4,220	517	0.29	0.29	4.8	6
Chicken a la king, cooked, from home recipe	1 cup	245	68	470	27	34	12.9	13.4	6.2	221	12	127	358	2.5	404	760	1,130	272	0.10	0.42	5.4	12
Chicken and noodles, cooked, from home recipe	1 cup	240	71	365	22	18	5.1	7.1	3.9	103	26	26	247	2.2	149	600	430	130	0.05	0.17	4.3	Tr
Chicken chow mein																						
Canned	1 cup	250	89	95	7	Tr	0.1	0.1	0.8	8	18	45	85	1.3	418	725	150	28	0.05	0.10	1.0	13
From home recipe	1 cup	250	78	255	31	10	4.1	4.9	3.5	75	10	58	293	2.5	473	718	280	50	0.08	0.23	4.3	10
Chicken potpie, from home recipe, baked, piece, 1/3 of 9-in diam. pie[51]	1	232	57	545	23	31	10.3	15.5	6.6	56	42	70	232	3.0	343	594	7,220	735	0.32	0.32	4.9	5
Chili con carne with beans, canned	1 cup	255	72	340	19	16	5.8	7.2	1.0	28	31	82	321	4.3	594	1,354	150	15	0.08	0.18	3.3	8
Chop suey with beef and pork, from home recipe	1 cup	250	75	300	26	17	4.3	7.4	4.2	68	13	60	248	4.8	425	1,053	600	60	0.28	0.38	5.0	33
Macaroni (enriched) and cheese																						
Canned[52]	1 cup	240	80	230	9	10	4.7	2.9	1.3	24	26	199	182	1.0	139	730	260	72	0.12	0.24	1.0	Tr
From home recipe[38]	1 cup	200	58	430	17	22	9.8	7.4	3.6	44	40	362	322	1.8	240	1,086	860	232	0.20	0.40	1.8	1
Quiche Lorraine, 1/8 of 8-in diam. quiche[51]	1	176	47	600	13	48	23.2	17.8	4.1	285	29	211	276	1.0	283	653	1,640	454	0.11	0.32	Tr	Tr
Spaghetti (enriched) in tomato sauce with cheese																						
Canned	1 cup	250	80	190	6	2	0.4	0.4	0.5	3	39	40	88	2.8	303	955	930	120	0.35	0.28	4.5	10
From home recipe	1 cup	250	77	260	9	9	3.0	3.6	1.2	8	37	80	135	2.3	408	955	1,080	140	0.25	0.18	2.3	13
Spaghetti (enriched) with meatballs and tomato sauce																						
Canned	1 cup	250	78	260	12	10	2.4	3.9	3.1	23	29	53	113	3.3	245	1,220	1,000	100	0.15	0.18	2.3	5
From home recipe	1 cup	248	70	330	19	12	3.9	4.4	2.2	89	39	124	236	3.7	665	1,009	1,590	159	0.25	0.30	4.0	22
Fast food entrees																						
Cheeseburger																						
Regular	1	112	46	300	15	15	7.3	5.6	1.0	44	28	135	174	2.3	219	672	340	65	0.26	0.24	3.7	1
4 oz patty	1	194	46	525	30	31	15.1	12.2	1.4	104	40	236	320	4.5	407	1,224	670	128	0.33	0.48	7.4	3
Chicken, fried. See Poultry and Poultry Products.																						
Enchilada	1	230	72	235	20	16	7.7	6.7	0.6	19	24	97	198	3.3	653	1,332	2,720	352	0.18	0.26	Tr	Tr
English muffin, egg, cheese, and bacon	1	138	49	360	18	18	8.0	8.0	0.7	213	31	197	290	3.1	201	832	650	160	0.46	0.50	3.7	1
Fish sandwich																						
Regular, with cheese	1	140	43	420	16	23	6.3	6.9	7.7	56	39	132	223	1.8	274	667	160	25	0.32	0.26	3.3	2
Large, without cheese	1	170	48	470	18	27	6.3	8.7	9.5	91	41	61	246	2.2	375	621	110	15	0.35	0.23	3.5	1
Hamburger																						
Regular	1	98	46	245	12	11	4.4	5.3	0.5	32	28	56	107	2.2	202	463	80	14	0.23	0.24	3.8	1
4 oz patty	1	174	50	445	25	21	7.1	11.7	0.6	71	38	75	225	4.8	404	763	160	28	0.38	0.38	7.8	1
Pizza, cheese, 1/8 of 15-in diam. pizza[51]	1	120	46	290	15	9	4.1	2.6	1.3	56	39	220	216	1.6	230	699	750	106	0.34	0.29	4.2	2
Roast beef sandwich	1	150	52	345	22	13	3.5	6.9	1.8	55	34	60	222	4.0	338	757	240	32	0.40	0.33	6.0	2
Taco	1	81	55	195	9	11	4.1	5.5	0.8	21	15	109	134	1.2	263	456	420	57	0.09	0.07	1.4	1
POULTRY AND POULTRY PRODUCTS																						
Chicken																						
Fried, flesh, with skin[53]																						
Batter dipped																						

(Continued)

TABLE E-1 *(continued)*

ITEM	FOODS, APPROXIMATE MEASURES, UNITS, AND WEIGHT (WEIGHT OF EDIBLE PORTION ONLY)	WEIGHT (G)	WATER (%)	FOOD ENERGY (KCAL)	PROTEIN (G)	FAT (G)	FATTY ACIDS: SATURATED (G)	FATTY ACIDS: MONOUNSATURATED (G)	FATTY ACIDS: POLYUNSATURATED (G)	CHOLESTEROL (MG)	CARBOHYDRATE (G)	CALCIUM (MG)	PHOSPHORUS (MG)	IRON (MG)	POTASSIUM (MG)	SODIUM (MG)	VITAMIN A VALUE (IU)	VITAMIN A VALUE (RE)	THIAMIN (MG)	RIBOFLAVIN (MG)	NIACIN (MG)	ASCORBIC ACID (MG)
Breast, $^1/_2$ breast (5.6 oz with bones)	4.9 oz	140	52	365	35	18	4.9	7.6	4.3	119	13	28	259	1.8	281	385	90	28	0.16	0.20	14.7	0
Drumstick (3.4 oz with bones)	2.5 oz	72	53	195	16	11	3.0	4.6	2.7	62	6	12	106	1.0	134	194	60	19	0.08	0.15	3.7	0
Flour coated																						
Breast, $^1/_2$ breast (4.2 oz with bones)	3.5 oz	98	57	220	31	9	2.4	3.4	1.9	87	2	16	228	1.2	254	74	50	15	0.08	0.13	13.5	0
Drumstick (2.6 oz with bones)	1.7 oz	49	57	120	13	7	1.8	2.7	1.6	44	1	6	86	0.7	112	44	40	12	0.04	0.11	3.0	0
Roasted, flesh only																						
Breast, $^1/_2$ breast (4.2 oz with bones and skin)	3.0 oz	86	65	140	27	3	0.9	1.1	0.7	73	0	13	196	0.9	220	64	20	5	0.06	0.10	11.8	0
Drumstick, (2.9 oz with bones and skin)	1.6 oz	44	67	75	12	2	0.7	0.8	0.6	41	0	5	81	0.6	108	42	30	8	0.03	0.10	2.7	0
Stewed, flesh only, light and dark meat, chopped or diced	1 cup	140	67	250	38	9	2.6	3.3	2.2	116	0	20	210	1.6	252	98	70	21	0.07	0.23	8.6	0
Chicken liver																						
Cooked	1	20	68	30	5	1	0.4	0.3	0.2	126	Tr	3	62	1.7	28	10	3,270	983	0.03	0.35	0.9	3
Duck																						
Roasted, flesh only	$^1/_2$	221	64	445	52	25	9.2	8.2	3.2	197	0	27	449	6.0	557	144	170	51	0.57	1.04	11.3	0
Turkey																						
Roasted, flesh only																						
Dark meat, piece, 2-$^1/_2$ by 1-$^5/_8$ by $^1/_4$ in	4	85	63	160	24	6	2.1	1.4	1.8	72	0	27	173	2.0	246	67	0	0	0.05	0.21	3.1	0
Light meat, piece, 4 by 2 by $^1/_4$ in	2	85	66	135	25	3	0.9	0.5	0.7	59	0	16	186	1.1	259	54	0	0	0.05	0.11	5.8	0
Light and dark meat																						
Chopped or diced	1 cup	140	65	240	41	7	2.3	1.4	2.0	106	0	35	298	2.5	417	98	0	0	0.09	0.25	7.6	0
Pieces (1 slice white meat, 4 by 2 by $^1/_4$ in and 2 slices dark meat, 2-$^1/_2$ by 1-$^5/_8$ by $^1/_4$ in)	3	85	65	145	25	4	1.4	0.9	1.2	65	0	21	181	1.5	253	60	0	0	0.05	0.15	4.6	0
Poultry food products																						
Chicken																						
Canned, boneless	5 oz	142	69	235	31	11	3.1	4.5	2.5	88	0	20	158	2.2	196	714	170	48	0.02	0.18	9.0	3
Frankfurter (10 per 1-lb pkg)	1	45	58	115	6	9	2.5	3.8	1.8	45	3	43	48	0.9	38	616	60	17	0.03	0.05	1.4	0
Roll, light (6 slices per 6 oz pkg)	2	57	69	90	11	4	1.1	1.7	0.9	28	1	24	89	0.6	129	331	50	14	0.04	0.07	3.0	0
Turkey																						
Gravy and turkey, frozen	5 oz	142	85	95	8	4	1.2	1.4	0.7	26	7	20	115	1.3	87	787	60	18	0.03	0.18	2.6	0

Ham, cured turkey thigh meat (8 slices per 8-oz pkg)	2	57	71	75	11	3	1.0	0.7	0.9	32	Tr	6	108	1.6	184	565	0	0	0.03	0.14	2.0	0
Loaf, breast meat (8 slices per 6-oz pkg)	2	42	72	45	10	1	0.2	0.2	0.1	17	0	3	97	0.2	118	608	0	0	0.02	0.05	3.5	[54]0
Patties, breaded, battered, fried (2.25 oz)	1	64	50	180	9	12	3.0	4.8	3.0	40	10	9	173	1.4	176	512	20	7	0.06	0.12	1.5	0
Roast, boneless, frozen, seasoned, light and dark meat, cooked	3 oz	85	68	130	18	5	1.6	1.0	1.4	45	3	4	207	1.4	253	578	0	0	0.04	0.14	5.3	0
SOUPS, SUACES, AND GRAVIES																						
Soups																						
Canned, condensed																						
Prepared with equal volume of milk																						
Clam chowder, New England	1 cup	248	85	165	9	7	3.0	2.3	1.1	22	17	186	156	1.5	300	992	160	40	0.07	0.24	1.0	3
Cream of chicken	1 cup	248	85	190	7	11	4.6	4.5	1.6	27	15	181	151	0.7	273	1,047	710	94	0.07	0.26	0.9	1
Cream of mushroom	1 cup	248	85	205	6	14	5.1	3.0	4.6	20	15	179	156	0.6	270	1,076	150	37	0.08	0.28	0.9	2
Tomato	1 cup	248	85	160	6	6	2.9	1.6	1.1	17	22	159	149	1.8	449	932	850	109	0.13	0.25	1.5	68
Soups																						
Canned, condensed																						
Prepared with equal volume of water																						
Bean with bacon	1 cup	253	84	170	8	6	1.5	2.2	1.8	3	23	81	132	2.0	402	951	890	89	0.09	0.03	0.6	2
Beef borth, bouillon, consomme	1 cup	240	98	15	3	1	0.3	0.2	Tr	Tr	Tr	14	31	0.4	130	782	0	0	Tr	0.05	1.9	0
Beef noodle	1 cup	244	92	85	5	3	1.1	1.2	0.5	5	9	15	46	1.1	100	952	630	63	0.07	0.06	1.1	Tr
Chicken noodle	1 cup	241	92	75	4	2	0.7	1.1	0.6	7	9	17	36	0.8	55	1,106	710	71	0.05	0.06	1.4	Tr
Chicken rice	1 cup	241	94	60	4	2	0.5	0.9	0.4	7	7	17	22	0.7	101	815	660	66	0.02	0.02	1.1	Tr
Clam chowder, Manhattan	1 cup	244	90	80	4	2	0.4	0.4	1.3	2	12	34	59	1.9	261	1,808	920	92	0.06	0.05	1.3	3
Cream of chicken	1 cup	244	91	115	3	7	2.1	3.3	1.5	10	9	34	37	0.6	88	986	560	56	0.03	0.06	0.8	Tr
Cream of mushroom	1 cup	244	90	130	2	9	2.4	1.7	4.2	2	9	46	49	0.5	100	1,032	0	0	0.05	0.09	0.7	1
Minestrone	1 cup	241	91	80	4	3	0.6	0.7	1.1	2	11	34	55	0.9	313	911	2,340	234	0.05	0.04	0.9	1
Pea, green	1 cup	250	83	165	9	3	1.4	1.0	0.4	0	27	28	125	2.0	190	988	200	20	0.11	0.07	1.2	2
Tomato	1 cup	244	90	85	2	2	0.4	0.4	1.0	0	17	12	34	1.8	264	871	690	69	0.09	0.05	1.4	66
Vegetable beef	1 cup	244	92	80	6	2	0.9	0.8	0.1	5	10	17	41	1.1	173	956	1,890	189	0.04	0.05	1.0	2
Vegetarian	1 cup	241	92	70	2	2	0.3	0.8	0.7	0	12	22	34	1.1	210	822	3,010	301	0.05	0.05	0.9	1
Dehydrated																						
Unprepared																						
Bouillon	1 pkt	6	3	15	1	1	0.3	0.2	Tr	1	1	4	19	0.1	27	1,019	Tr	Tr	Tr	0.01	0.3	0
Onion	1 pkt	7	4	20	1	Tr	0.1	0.2	Tr	Tr	4	10	23	0.1	47	627	Tr	Tr	0.02	0.04	0.4	Tr
Prepared with water																						
Chicken noodle	1 pkt (6 fl oz)	188	94	40	2	1	0.2	0.4	0.3	2	6	24	24	0.4	23	957	50	5	0.05	0.04	0.7	Tr
Onion	1 pkt (6 fl oz)	184	96	20	1	Tr	0.1	0.2	0.1	0	4	9	22	0.1	48	635	Tr	Tr	0.02	0.04	0.4	Tr
Tomato vegetable	1 pkt (6 fl oz)	189	94	40	1	1	0.3	0.2	0.1	0	8	6	23	0.5	78	856	140	14	0.04	0.03	0.6	5
Sauces																						
From dry mix																						
Cheese, prepared with milk	1 cup	279	77	305	16	17	9.3	5.3	1.6	53	23	569	438	0.3	552	1,565	390	117	0.15	0.56	0.3	2
Hollandaise, prepared with water	1 cup	259	84	240	5	20	11.6	5.9	0.9	52	14	124	127	0.9	124	1,564	730	220	0.05	0.18	0.1	Tr
White sauce, prepared with milk	1 cup	264	81	240	10	13	6.4	4.7	1.7	34	21	425	256	0.3	444	797	310	92	0.08	0.45	0.5	3
From home recipe																						
White sauce, medium[55]	1 cup	250	73	395	10	30	9.1	11.9	7.2	32	24	292	238	0.9	381	888	1,190	340	0.15	0.43	0.8	2

(Continued)

TABLE E-1 *(continued)*

ITEM	FOODS, APPROXIMATE MEASURES, UNITS, AND WEIGHT (WEIGHT OF EDIBLE PORTION ONLY)	WEIGHT (G)	WATER (%)	FOOD ENERGY (KCAL)	PROTEIN (G)	FAT (G)	FATTY ACIDS SATURATED (G)	FATTY ACIDS MONOUNSATURATED (G)	FATTY ACIDS POLYUNSATURATED (G)	CHOLESTEROL (MG)	CARBOHYDRATE (G)	CALCIUM (MG)	PHOSPHORUS (MG)	IRON (MG)	POTASSIUM (MG)	SODIUM (MG)	VITAMIN A VALUE (IU)	VITAMIN A VALUE (RE)	THIAMIN (MG)	RIBOFLAVIN (MG)	NIACIN (MG)	ASCORBIC ACID (MG)
Ready to serve																						
Barbecue	1 tbsp	16	81	10	Tr	Tr	Tr	0.1	0.1	0	2	3	3	0.1	28	130	140	14	Tr	Tr	0.1	1
Soy	1 tbsp	18	68	10	2	0	0.0	0.0	0.0	0	2	3	38	0.5	64	1,029	0	0	0.01	0.02	0.6	0
Gravies																						
Canned																						
Beef	1 cup	233	87	125	9	5	2.7	2.3	0.2	7	11	14	70	1.6	189	1,305	0	0	0.07	0.08	1.5	0
Chicken	1 cup	238	85	190	5	14	3.4	6.1	3.6	5	13	48	69	1.1	259	1,373	880	264	0.04	0.10	1.1	0
Mushroom	1 cup	238	89	120	3	6	1.0	2.8	2.4	0	13	17	36	1.6	252	1,357	0	0	0.08	0.15	1.6	0
From dry mix																						
Brown	1 cup	261	91	80	3	2	0.9	0.8	0.1	2	14	66	47	0.2	61	1,147	0	0	0.04	0.09	0.9	0
Chicken	1 cup	260	91	85	3	2	0.5	0.9	0.4	3	14	39	47	0.3	62	1,134	0	0	0.05	0.15	0.8	3
SUGARS AND SWEETS																						
Candy																						
Caramels, plain or chocolate	1 oz	28	8	115	1	3	2.2	0.3	0.1	1	22	42	35	0.4	54	64	Tr	Tr	0.01	0.05	0.1	Tr
Chocolate																						
Milk, plain	1 oz	28	1	145	2	9	5.4	3.0	0.3	6	16	50	61	0.4	96	23	30	10	0.02	0.10	0.1	Tr
Milk, with almonds	1 oz	28	2	150	3	10	4.8	4.1	0.7	5	15	65	77	0.5	125	23	30	8	0.02	0.12	0.2	Tr
Milk, with peanuts	1 oz	28	1	155	4	11	4.2	3.5	1.5	5	13	49	83	0.4	138	19	30	8	0.07	0.07	1.4	Tr
Milk, with rice cereal	1 oz	28	2	140	2	7	4.4	2.5	0.2	6	18	48	57	0.2	100	46	30	8	0.01	0.08	0.1	Tr
Semisweet, small pieces (60 per oz)	1 cup or 6 oz	170	1	860	7	61	36.2	19.9	1.9	0	97	51	178	5.8	593	24	30	3	0.10	0.14	0.9	Tr
Sweet (dark)	1 oz	28	1	150	1	10	5.9	3.3	0.3	0	16	7	41	0.6	86	5	10	1	0.01	0.04	0.1	Tr
Fondant, uncoated (mints, candy corn, other)	1 oz	28	3	105	Tr	0	0.0	0.0	0.0	0	27	2	Tr	0.1	1	57	0	0	Tr	Tr	Tr	0
Fudge, chocolate, plain	1 oz	28	8	115	1	3	2.1	1.0	0.1	1	21	22	24	0.3	42	54	Tr	Tr	0.01	0.03	0.1	Tr
Gum drops	1 oz	28	12	100	Tr	Tr	Tr	Tr	0.1	0	25	2	Tr	0.1	1	10	0	0	0.00	Tr	Tr	0
Candy																						
Hard	1 oz	28	1	110	0	0	0.0	0.0	0.0	0	28	Tr	2	0.1	1	7	0	0	0.10	0.00	0.0	0
Jelly beans	1 oz	28	6	105	Tr	Tr	Tr	Tr	0.1	0	26	1	1	0.3	11	7	0	0	0.00	Tr	Tr	0
Marshmallows	1 oz	28	17	90	1	0	0.0	0.0	0.0	0	23	1	2	0.5	2	25	0	0	0.00	Tr	Tr	0
Custard																						
Baked	1 cup	265	77	305	14	15	6.8	5.4	0.7	278	29	297	310	1.1	387	209	530	146	0.11	0.50	0.3	1
Gelatin dessert																						
Prepared with gelatin dessert powder and water	$^1/_2$ cup	120	84	70	2	0	0.0	0.0	0.0	0	17	2	23	Tr	Tr	55	0	0	0.00	0.00	0.0	0

Honey																						
Strained or extracted	1 cup	339	17	1,030	1	0	0.0	0.0	0.0	0	279	17	20	1.7	173	17	0	0	0.02	0.14	1.0	3
	1 tbsp	21	17	65	Tr	0	0.0	0.0	0.0	0	17	1	1	0.1	11	1	0	0	Tr	0.01	0.1	Tr
Jams and preserves	1 tbsp	20	29	55	Tr	Tr	0.0	Tr	Tr	0	14	4	2	0.2	18	2	Tr	Tr	Tr	0.01	Tr	Tr
	1 packet	14	29	40	Tr	Tr	0.0	Tr	Tr	0	10	3	1	0.1	12	2	Tr	Tr	Tr	Tr	Tr	Tr
Jellies	1 tbsp	18	28	50	Tr	Tr	Tr	Tr	Tr	0	13	2	Tr	0.1	16	5	Tr	Tr	Tr	0.01	Tr	1
	1 packet	14	28	40	Tr	Tr	Tr	Tr	Tr	0	10	1	Tr	Tr	13	4	Tr	Tr	Tr	Tr	Tr	1
Popsicle																						
3-fl-oz size	1	95	80	70	0	0	0.0	0.0	0.0	0	18	0	0	Tr	4	11	0	0	0.00	0.00	0.0	0
Puddings																						
Canned																						
Chocolate	5 oz	142	68	205	3	11	9.5	0.5	0.1	1	30	74	117	1.2	254	285	100	31	0.04	0.17	0.6	Tr
Tapioca	5 oz	142	74	160	3	5	4.8	Tr	Tr	Tr	28	119	113	0.3	212	252	Tr	Tr	0.03	0.14	0.4	Tr
Vanilla	5 oz	142	69	220	2	10	9.5	0.2	0.1	1	33	79	94	0.2	155	305	Tr	Tr	0.03	0.12	0.6	Tr
Dry mix, prepared with whole milk																						
Chocolate																						
Instant	1/2 cup	130	71	155	4	4	2.3	1.1	0.2	14	27	130	329	0.3	176	440	130	33	0.04	0.18	0.1	1
Regular (cooked)	1/2 cup	130	73	150	4	4	2.4	1.1	0.1	15	25	146	120	0.2	190	167	140	34	0.05	0.20	0.1	1
Rice	1/2 cup	132	73	155	4	4	2.3	1.1	0.1	15	27	133	110	0.5	165	140	140	33	0.10	0.18	0.6	1
Tapioca	1/2 cup	130	75	145	4	4	2.3	1.1	0.1	15	25	131	103	0.1	167	152	140	34	0.04	0.18	0.1	1
Vanilla																						
Instant	1/2 cup	130	73	150	4	4	2.2	1.1	0.2	15	27	129	273	0.1	164	375	140	33	0.04	0.17	0.1	1
Regular (cooked)	1/2 cup	130	74	145	4	4	2.3	1.0	0.1	15	25	132	102	0.1	166	178	140	34	0.04	0.18	0.1	1
Sugars																						
Brown, pressed down	1 cup	220	2	820	0	0	0.0	0.0	0.0	0	212	187	56	4.8	757	97	0	0	0.02	0.07	0.2	0
White																						
Granulated	1 cup	200	1	770	0	0	0.0	0.0	0.0	0	199	3	Tr	0.1	7	5	0	0	0.00	0.00	0.0	0
	1 tbsp	12	1	45	0	0	0.0	0.0	0.0	0	12	Tr	Tr	Tr	Tr	Tr	0	0	0.00	0.00	0.0	0
	1 packet	6	1	25	0	0	0.0	0.0	0.0	0	6	Tr	Tr	Tr	Tr	Tr	0	0	0.00	0.00	0.0	0
Powdered, sifted, spooned into cup	1 cup	100	1	385	0	0	0.0	0.0	0.0	0	100	1	Tr	Tr	4	2	0	0	0.00	0.00	0.0	0
Syrups																						
Chocolate-flavored syrup or topping																						
Thin type	2 tbsp	38	37	85	1	Tr	0.2	0.1	0.1	0	22	6	49	0.8	85	36	Tr	Tr	Tr	0.02	0.1	0
Fudge type	2 tbsp	38	25	125	2	5	3.1	1.7	0.2	0	21	38	60	0.5	82	42	40	13	0.02	0.08	0.1	0
Molasses, cane, blackstrap	2 tbsp	40	24	85	0	0	0.0	0.0	0.0	0	22	274	34	10.1	1,171	38	0	0	0.04	0.08	0.8	0
Table syrup (corn and maple)	2 tbsp	42	25	122	0	0	0.0	0.0	0.0	0	32	1	4	Tr	7	19	0	0	0.00	0.00	0.0	0
VEGETABLES AND VEGETABLE PRODUCTS																						
Alfalfa seeds																						
Sprouted, raw	1 cup	33	91	10	1	Tr	Tr	Tr	0.1	0	1	11	23	0.3	26	2	50	5	0.03	0.04	0.2	3
Artichokes																						
globe or French, cooked, drained	1	120	87	55	3	Tr	Tr	Tr	0.1	0	12	47	72	1.6	316	79	170	17	0.07	0.06	0.7	9
Asparagus																						
Green																						

(Continued)

TABLE E-1 *(continued)*

ITEM	FOODS, APPROXIMATE MEASURES, UNITS, AND WEIGHT (WEIGHT OF EDIBLE PORTION ONLY)	WEIGHT (G)	WATER (%)	FOOD ENERGY (KCAL)	PROTEIN (G)	FAT (G)	FATTY ACIDS SATURATED (G)	MONOUNSATURATED (G)	POLYUNSATURATED (G)	CHOLESTEROL (MG)	CARBOHYDRATE (G)	CALCIUM (MG)	PHOSPHORUS (MG)	IRON (MG)	POTASSIUM (MG)	SODIUM (MG)	VITAMIN A VALUE (IU)	VITAMIN A VALUE (RE)	THIAMIN (MG)	RIBOFLAVIN (MG)	NIACIN (MG)	ASCORBIC ACID (MG)
Cooked, drained																						
From raw																						
Cuts and tips	1 cup	180	92	45	5	1	0.1	Tr	0.2	0	8	43	110	1.2	558	7	1,490	149	0.18	0.22	1.9	49
Spears, 1/2-in diam. at base	4	60	92	15	2	Tr	Tr	Tr	0.1	0	3	14	37	0.4	186	2	500	50	0.06	0.07	0.6	16
From frozen																						
Cuts and tips	1 cup	180	91	50	5	1	0.2	Tr	0.3	0	9	41	99	1.2	392	7	1,470	147	0.12	0.19	1.9	44
Spears, 1/2-in diam. at base	4	60	91	15	2	Tr	0.1	Tr	0.1	0	3	14	33	0.4	131	2	490	49	0.04	0.06	0.6	15
Canned, spears, 1/2-in diam. at base	4	80	95	10	1	Tr	Tr	Tr	0.1	0	2	11	30	0.5	122	[56]278	380	38	0.04	0.07	0.7	13
Bamboo shoots																						
Canned, drained	1 cup	131	94	25	2	1	0.1	Tr	0.2	0	4	10	33	0.4	105	9	10	1	0.03	0.03	0.2	1
Beans																						
Lima, immature seeds, frozen, cooked, drained																						
Thick-seeded types (Ford-hooks)	1 cup	170	74	170	10	1	0.1	Tr	0.3	0	32	37	107	2.3	694	90	320	32	0.13	0.10	1.8	22
Thin-seeded types (baby limas)	1 cup	180	72	190	12	1	0.1	Tr	0.3	0	35	50	202	3.5	740	52	300	30	0.13	0.10	1.4	10
Snap																						
Cooked, drained																						
From raw (cut and French style)	1 cup	125	89	45	2	Tr	0.1	Tr	0.2	0	10	58	49	1.6	374	4	[57]830	[57]83	0.09	0.12	0.8	12
From frozen (cut)	1 cup	135	92	35	2	Tr	Tr	Tr	0.1	0	8	61	32	1.1	151	18	[58]710	[58]71	0.06	0.10	0.6	11
Canned, drained solids (cut)	1 cup	135	93	25	2	Tr	Tr	Tr	0.1	0	6	35	26	1.2	147	[59]339	[60]470	[60]47	0.02	0.08	0.3	6
Beans, mature. See Beans, dry and Black-eyed peas, dry.																						
Bean sprouts (mung)																						
Raw	1 cup	104	90	30	3	Tr	Tr	Tr	0.1	0	6	14	56	0.9	155	6	20	2	0.09	0.13	0.8	14
Cooked, drained	1 cup	124	93	25	3	Tr	Tr	Tr	Tr	0	5	15	35	0.8	125	12	20	2	0.06	0.13	1.0	14
Beets																						
Cooked, drained																						
Diced or sliced	1 cup	170	91	55	2	Tr	Tr	Tr	Tr	0	11	19	53	1.1	530	83	20	2	0.05	0.02	0.5	9
Whole beets, 2-in diam.	2	100	91	30	1	Tr	Tr	Tr	Tr	0	7	11	31	0.6	312	49	10	1	0.03	0.01	0.3	6
Canned, drained solids, diced or sliced	1 cup	170	91	55	2	Tr	Tr	Tr	0.1	0	12	26	29	3.1	252	[61]466	20	2	0.02	0.07	0.3	7
Beet greens																						
Leaves and stems, cooked, drained	1 cup	144	89	40	4	Tr	Tr	0.1	0.1	0	8	164	59	2.7	1,309	347	7,340	734	0.17	0.42	0.7	36
Black-eyed peas																						
Immature seeds, cooked and drained																						
From raw	1 cup	165	72	180	13	1	0.3	0.1	0.6	0	30	46	196	2.4	693	7	1,050	105	0.11	0.18	1.8	3

From frozen	1 cup	170	66	225	14	1	0.3	0.1	0.5	0	40	39	207	3.6	638	9	130	13	0.44	0.11	1.2	4
Broccoli																						
Raw	1	151	91	40	4	1	0.1	Tr	0.3	0	8	72	100	1.3	491	41	2,330	233	0.10	0.18	1.0	141
Cooked, drained																						
From raw																						
Spear, medium	1	180	90	50	5	1	0.1	Tr	0.2	0	10	82	86	2.1	293	20	2,540	254	0.15	0.37	1.4	113
Spears, cut into $^1/_2$-in pieces	1 cup	155	90	45	5	Tr	0.1	Tr	0.2	0	9	71	74	1.8	253	17	2,180	218	0.13	0.32	1.2	97
From frozen																						
Piece, 4-$^1/_2$ to 5 in long	1	30	91	10	1	Tr	Tr	Tr	Tr	0	2	15	17	0.2	54	7	570	57	0.02	0.02	0.1	12
Chopped	1 cup	185	91	50	6	Tr	Tr	Tr	0.1	0	10	94	102	1.1	333	44	3,500	350	0.10	0.15	0.8	74
Brussels sprouts, cooked, drained																						
From raw, 7-8 sprouts, 1-$^1/_4$ to 1-$^1/_2$-in diam.	1 cup	155	87	60	4	1	0.2	0.1	0.4	0	13	56	87	1.9	491	33	1,110	111	0.17	0.12	0.9	96
From frozen	1 cup	155	87	65	6	1	0.1	Tr	0.3	0	13	37	84	1.1	504	36	910	91	0.16	0.18	0.8	71
Cabbage																						
Common varieties																						
Raw, coarsely shredded or sliced	1 cup	70	93	15	1	Tr	Tr	Tr	0.1	0	4	33	16	0.4	172	13	90	9	0.04	0.02	0.2	33
Cooked, drained	1 cup	150	94	30	1	Tr	Tr	Tr	0.2	0	7	50	38	0.6	308	29	130	13	0.09	0.08	0.3	36
Cabbage, Chinese																						
Pak-choi, cooked, drained	1 cup	170	96	20	3	Tr	Tr	Tr	0.1	0	3	158	49	1.8	631	58	4,370	437	0.05	0.1	0.7	44
Pe-tsai, raw, 1-in pieces	1 cup	76	94	10	1	Tr	Tr	Tr	0.1	0	2	59	22	0.2	181	7	910	91	0.03	0.04	0.3	21
Cabbage, red																						
Raw, coarsely shredded or sliced	1 cup	70	92	20	1	Tr	Tr	Tr	0.1	0	4	36	29	0.3	144	8	30	3	0.04	0.02	0.2	40
Cabbage, savoy																						
Raw, coarsely shredded or sliced	1 cup	70	91	20	1	Tr	Tr	Tr	Tr	0	4	25	29	0.3	161	20	700	70	0.05	0.02	0.2	22
Carrots																						
Raw, without crowns and tips, scraped																						
Whole, 7-$^1/_2$ by 1-$^1/_8$ in, or strips, 2-$^1/_2$ to 3 in long	1 carrot or 18 strips	72	88	30	1	Tr	Tr	Tr	0.1	0	7	19	32	0.4	233	25	20,250	2,025	0.07	0.04	0.7	7
Grated	1 cup	110	88	45	1	Tr	Tr	Tr	0.1	0	11	30	48	0.6	355	39	30,940	3,094	0.11	0.06	1.0	10
Cooked, sliced, drained																						
From raw	1 cup	156	87	70	2	Tr	0.1	Tr	0.1	0	16	48	47	1.0	354	103	38,300	3,830	0.05	0.09	0.8	4
From frozen	1 cup	146	90	55	2	Tr	Tr	Tr	0.1	0	12	41	38	0.7	231	86	25,850	2,585	0.04	0.05	0.6	4
Canned, sliced, drained solids	1 cup	146	93	35	1	Tr	0.1	Tr	0.1	0	8	37	35	0.9	261	[62]352	20,110	2,011	0.03	0.04	0.8	4
Cauliflower																						
Raw, (flowerets)	1 cup	100	92	25	2	Tr	Tr	Tr	0.1	0	5	29	46	0.6	355	15	20	2	0.08	0.06	0.6	72
Cooked, drained																						
From raw (flowerets)	1 cup	125	93	30	2	Tr	Tr	Tr	0.1	0	6	34	44	0.5	404	8	20	2	0.08	0.07	0.7	69
From frozen (flowerets)	1 cup	180	94	35	3	Tr	0.1	Tr	0.2	0	7	31	43	0.7	250	32	40	4	0.07	0.10	0.6	56
Celery, pascal type																						
Raw																						
Stalk, large outer, 8 by 1-$^1/_2$ in (at root end)	1	40	95	5	Tr	Tr	Tr	Tr	Tr	0	1	14	10	0.2	114	35	50	5	0.01	0.01	0.1	3
Pieces, diced	1 cup	120	95	20	1	Tr	Tr	Tr	0.1	0	4	43	31	0.6	341	106	150	15	0.04	0.04	0.4	8

(Continued)

TABLE E-1 ·*(continued)*

ITEM	FOODS, APPROXIMATE MEASURES, UNITS, AND WEIGHT (WEIGHT OF EDIBLE PORTION ONLY)	WEIGHT (G)	WATER (%)	FOOD ENERGY (KCAL)	PROTEIN (G)	FAT (G)	FATTY ACIDS SATURATED (G)	FATTY ACIDS MONOUNSATURATED (G)	FATTY ACIDS POLYUNSATURATED (G)	CHOLESTEROL (MG)	CARBOHYDRATE (G)	CALCIUM (MG)	PHOSPHORUS (MG)	IRON (MG)	POTASSIUM (MG)	SODIUM (MG)	VITAMIN A VALUE (IU)	VITAMIN A VALUE (RE)	THIAMIN (MG)	RIBOFLAVIN (MG)	NIACIN (MG)	ASCORBIC ACID (MG)
Collards																						
Cooked, drained																						
From raw (leaves without stems)	1 cup	190	96	25	2	Tr	0.1	Tr	0.2	0	5	148	19	0.8	177	36	4,220	422	0.03	0.08	0.4	19
From frozen (chopped)	1 cup	170	88	60	5	1	0.1	0.1	0.4	0	12	357	46	1.9	427	85	10,170	1,017	0.08	0.20	1.1	45
Corn																						
Sweet																						
Cooked, drained																						
From raw, ear 5 by 1-3/4 in	1	77	70	85	3	1	0.2	0.3	0.5	0	19	2	79	0.5	192	13	[63]170	[63]17	0.17	0.06	1.2	5
From frozen																						
Ear, trimmed to about 3-1/2 in long	1	63	73	60	2	Tr	0.1	0.1	0.2	0	14	2	47	0.4	158	3	[63]130	[63]13	0.11	0.04	1.0	3
Kernels	1 cup	165	76	135	5	Tr	Tr	Tr	0.1	0	34	3	78	0.5	229	8	[63]410	[63]41	0.11	0.12	2.1	4
Canned																						
Cream style	1 cup	256	79	185	4	1	0.2	0.3	0.5	0	46	8	131	1.0	343	[64]730	[63]250	[63]25	0.06	0.14	2.5	12
Whole kernel, vacuum pack	1 cup	210	77	165	5	1	0.2	0.3	0.5	0	41	11	134	0.9	391	[65]571	[63]510	[63]51	0.09	0.15	2.5	17
Cowpeas																						
See Black-eyed peas, immature, mature.																						
Cucumber																						
With peel, slices, 1/8 in thick (large, 2-1/8-in diam.; small, 1-3/4-in diam.)	6 large or 8 small slices	28	96	5	Tr	Tr	Tr	Tr	Tr	0	1	4	5	0.1	42	1	10	1	0.01	0.01	0.1	1
Dandelion greens																						
Cooked, drained	1 cup	105	90	35	2	1	0.1	Tr	0.3	0	7	147	44	1.9	244	46	12,290	1,229	0.14	0.18	0.5	19
Eggplant																						
Cooked, steamed	1 cup	96	92	25	1	Tr	Tr	Tr	0.1	0	6	6	21	0.3	238	3	60	6	0.07	0.02	0.6	1
Endive																						
Curly (including escarole), raw, small pieces	1 cup	50	94	10	1	Tr	Tr	Tr	Tr	0	2	26	14	0.4	157	11	1,030	103	0.04	0.04	0.2	3
Jerusalem-artichoke																						
Raw, sliced	1 cup	150	78	115	3	Tr	0.0	Tr	Tr	0	26	21	117	5.1	644	6	30	3	0.30	0.09	2.0	6

Kale																						
Cooked, drained																						
From raw, chopped	1 cup	130	91	40	2	1	0.1	Tr	0.3	0	7	94	36	1.2	296	30	9,620	962	0.07	0.09	0.7	53
From frozen, chopped	1 cup	130	91	40	4	1	0.1	Tr	0.3	0	7	179	36	1.2	417	20	8,260	826	0.06	0.15	0.9	33
Kohlrabi																						
Thickened bulb-like stems, cooked, drained, diced	1 cup	165	90	50	3	Tr	Tr	Tr	0.1	0	11	41	74	0.7	561	35	60	6	0.07	0.03	0.6	89
Lettuce																						
Raw																						
Butterhead, as Boston types																						
Head, 5-in diam	1	163	96	20	2	Tr	Tr	Tr	0.2	0	4	52	38	0.5	419	8	1,580	158	0.10	0.10	0.5	13
Leaves	1 outer or 2 inner leaves	15	96	Tr	Tr	Tr	Tr	Tr	Tr	0	Tr	5	3	Tr	39	1	150	15	0.01	0.01	Tr	1
Crisphead, as iceberg																						
Head, 6-in diam	1	539	96	70	5	1	0.1	Tr	0.5	0	11	102	108	2.7	852	49	1,780	178	0.25	0.16	1.0	21
Wedge, ¹/₄ of head	1	135	96	20	1	Tr	Tr	Tr	0.1	0	3	26	27	0.7	213	12	450	45	0.06	0.04	0.3	5
Pieces, chopped or shredded	1 cup	55	96	5	1	Tr	Tr	Tr	0.1	0	1	10	11	0.3	87	5	180	18	0.03	0.02	0.1	2
Looseleaf (bunching varieties including romaine or cos), chopped or shredded pieces	1 cup	56	94	10	1	Tr	Tr	Tr	0.1	0	2	38	14	0.8	148	5	1,060	106	0.03	0.04	0.2	10
Mushrooms																						
Raw, sliced or chopped	1 cup	70	92	20	1	Tr	Tr	Tr	0.1	0	3	4	73	0.9	259	3	0	0	0.07	0.31	2.9	2
Cooked, drained	1 cup	156	91	40	3	1	0.1	Tr	0.3	0	8	9	136	2.7	555	3	0	0	0.11	0.47	7.0	6
Canned, drained solids	1 cup	156	91	35	3	Tr	0.1	Tr	0.2	0	8	17	103	1.2	201	663	0	0	0.13	0.03	2.5	0
Mustard greens																						
Without stems and midribs, cooked, drained	1 cup	140	94	20	3	Tr	Tr	0.2	0.1	0	3	104	57	1.0	283	22	4,240	424	0.06	0.09	0.6	35
Okra pods																						
3 by ⁵/₈ in, cooked	8	85	90	25	2	Tr	Tr	Tr	Tr	0	6	54	48	0.4	274	4	490	49	0.11	0.05	0.7	14
Onions																						
Raw																						
Chopped	1 cup	160	91	55	2	Tr	0.1	0.1	0.2	0	12	40	46	0.6	248	3	0	0	0.10	0.02	0.2	13
Sliced	1 cup	115	91	40	1	Tr	0.1	Tr	0.1	0	8	29	33	0.4	178	2	0	0	0.07	0.01	0.1	10
Cooked (whole or sliced), drained	1 cup	210	92	60	2	Tr	0.1	Tr	0.1	0	13	57	48	0.4	319	17	0	0	0.09	0.02	0.2	12
Onions, spring																						
Raw, bulb (³/₈-in diam.) and white portion of top	6	30	92	10	1	Tr	Tr	Tr	Tr	0	2	18	10	0.6	77	1	1,500	150	0.02	0.04	0.1	14
Onion rings																						
Breaded, par-fried, frozen, prepared	2	20	29	80	1	5	1.7	2.2	1.0	0	8	6	16	0.3	26	75	50	5	0.06	0.03	0.7	Tr
Parsley																						
Raw	10 sprigs	10	88	5	Tr	Tr	Tr	Tr	Tr	0	1	13	4	0.6	54	4	520	52	0.01	0.01	0.1	9
Freeze-dried	1 tbsp	0.4	2	Tr	Tr	Tr	Tr	Tr	Tr	0	Tr	1	2	0.2	25	2	250	25	Tr	0.01	Tr	1

(Continued)

TABLE E-1 *(continued)*

ITEM	FOODS, APPROXIMATE MEASURES, UNITS, AND WEIGHT (WEIGHT OF EDIBLE PORTION ONLY)	WEIGHT (G)	WATER (%)	FOOD ENERGY (KCAL)	PROTEIN (G)	FAT (G)	FATTY ACIDS SATURATED (G)	MONOUNSATURATED (G)	POLYUNSATURATED (G)	CHOLESTEROL (MG)	CARBOHYDRATE (G)	CALCIUM (MG)	PHOSPHORUS (MG)	IRON (MG)	POTASSIUM (MG)	SODIUM (MG)	VITAMIN A VALUE (IU)	VITAMIN A VALUE (RE)	THIAMIN (MG)	RIBOFLAVIN (MG)	NIACIN (MG)	ASCORBIC ACID (MG)
Parsnips																						
Cooked (diced or 2 in lengths), drained	1 cup	156	78	125	2	Tr	0.1	0.2	0.1	0	30	58	108	0.9	573	16	0	0	0.13	0.08	1.1	20
Peas, edible pod																						
Cooked, drained	1 cup	160	89	65	5	Tr	0.1	Tr	0.2	0	11	67	88	3.2	384	6	210	21	0.20	0.12	0.9	77
Peas, green																						
Canned, drained solids	1 cup	170	82	115	8	1	0.1	0.1	0.3	0	21	34	114	1.6	294	[66]372	1,310	131	0.21	0.13	1.2	16
Frozen, cooked, drained	1 cup	160	80	125	8	Tr	0.1	Tr	0.2	0	23	38	144	2.5	269	139	1,070	107	0.45	0.16	2.4	16
Peppers																						
Hot chili, raw	1	45	88	20	1	Tr	Tr	Tr	Tr	0	4	8	21	0.5	153	3	[67]4,840	[67]484	0.04	0.04	0.4	109
Sweet (about 5 per lb, whole), stem and seeds removed																						
Raw	1	74	93	20	1	Tr	Tr	Tr	0.2	0	4	4	16	0.9	144	2	[68]390	[68]39	0.06	0.04	0.4	[69]95
Cooked, drained	1	73	95	15	Tr	Tr	Tr	Tr	0.1	0	3	3	11	0.6	94	1	[70]280	[70]28	0.04	0.03	0.3	[71]81
Potatoes																						
Cooked																						
Baked (about 2 per lb, raw)																						
With skin	1	202	71	220	5	Tr	0.1	Tr	0.1	0	51	20	115	2.7	844	16	0	0	0.22	0.07	3.3	26
Flesh only	1	156	75	145	3	Tr	Tr	Tr	0.1	0	34	8	78	0.5	610	8	0	0	0.16	0.03	2.2	20
Boiled (about 3 per lb, raw)																						
Peeled after boiling	1	136	77	120	3	Tr	Tr	Tr	0.1	0	27	7	60	0.4	515	5	0	0	0.14	0.03	2.0	18
Peeled before boiling	1	135	77	115	2	Tr	Tr	Tr	0.1	0	27	11	54	0.4	443	7	0	0	0.13	0.03	1.8	10
French fried, strip, 2 to 3-1/2 in long, frozen																						
Oven heated	10	50	53	110	2	4	2.1	1.8	0.3	0	17	5	43	0.7	229	16	0	0	0.06	0.02	1.2	5
Fried in vegetable oil	10	50	38	160	2	8	2.5	1.6	3.8	0	20	10	47	0.4	366	108	0	0	0.09	0.01	1.6	5
Potato products																						
Prepared																						
Au gratin																						
From dry mix	1 cup	245	79	230	6	10	6.3	2.9	0.3	12	31	203	233	0.8	537	1,076	520	76	0.05	0.20	2.3	8
From home recipe	1 cup	245	74	325	12	19	11.6	5.3	0.7	56	28	292	277	1.6	970	1,061	650	93	0.16	0.28	2.4	24
Hashed brown, from frozen	1 cup	156	56	340	5	18	7.0	8.0	2.1	0	44	23	112	2.4	680	53	0	0	0.17	0.03	3.8	10
Mashed																						
From home recipe																						
Milk added	1 cup	210	78	160	4	1	0.7	0.3	0.1	4	37	55	101	0.6	628	636	40	12	0.18	0.08	2.3	14

Milk and margarine added	1 cup	210	76	225	4	9	2.2	3.7	2.5	4	35	55	97	0.5	607	620	360	42	0.18	0.08	2.3	13
From dehydrated flakes (without milk), water, milk, butter, and salt added	1 cup	210	76	235	4	12	7.2	3.3	0.5	29	32	103	118	0.5	489	697	380	44	0.23	0.11	1.4	20
Potato salad																						
Made with mayonnaise	1 cup	250	76	360	7	21	3.6	6.2	9.3	170	28	48	130	1.6	635	1,323	520	83	0.19	0.15	2.2	25
Scalloped																						
From dry mix	1 cup	245	79	230	5	11	6.5	3.0	0.5	27	31	88	137	0.9	497	835	360	51	0.05	0.14	2.5	8
From home recipe	1 cup	245	81	210	7	9	5.5	2.5	0.4	29	26	140	154	1.4	926	821	330	47	0.17	0.23	2.6	26
Potato chips	10	20	3	105	1	7	1.8	1.2	3.6	0	10	5	31	0.2	260	94	0	0	0.03	Tr	0.8	8
Pumpkin																						
Cooked from raw, mashed	1 cup	245	94	50	2	Tr	0.1	Tr	Tr	0	12	37	74	1.4	564	2	2,650	265	0.08	0.19	1.0	12
Canned	1 cup	245	90	85	3	1	0.4	0.1	Tr	0	20	64	86	3.4	505	12	54,040	5,404	0.06	0.13	0.9	10
Radishes																						
Raw, stem ends, rootlets cut off	4	18	95	5	Tr	Tr	Tr	Tr	Tr	0	1	4	3	0.1	42	4	Tr	Tr	Tr	0.01	0.1	4
Sauerkraut																						
Canned, solids and liquid	1 cup	236	93	45	2	Tr	0.1	Tr	0.1	0	10	71	47	3.5	401	1,560	40	4	0.05	0.05	0.3	35
Seaweed																						
Kelp, raw	1 oz	28	82	10	Tr	Tr	0.1	Tr	Tr	0	3	48	12	0.8	25	66	30	3	0.01	0.04	0.1	([1])
Spirulina, dried	1 oz	28	5	80	16	2	0.8	0.2	0.6	0	7	34	33	8.1	386	297	160	16	0.67	1.04	3.6	3
Southern peas																						
See Black-eyed peas, immature.																						
Spinach																						
Raw, chopped	1 cup	55	92	10	2	Tr	Tr	Tr	0.1	0	2	54	27	1.5	307	43	3,690	369	0.04	0.10	0.4	15
Cooked, drained																						
From raw	1 cup	180	91	40	5	Tr	0.1	Tr	0.2	0	7	245	101	6.4	839	126	14,740	1,474	0.17	0.42	0.9	18
From frozen (leaf)	1 cup	190	90	55	6	Tr	0.1	Tr	0.2	0	10	277	91	2.9	566	163	14,790	1,479	0.11	0.32	0.8	23
Canned, drained solids	1 cup	214	92	50	6	1	0.2	Tr	0.4	0	7	272	94	4.9	740	[72]683	18,780	1,878	0.03	0.30	0.8	31
Spinach souffle	1 cup	136	74	220	11	18	7.1	6.8	3.1	184	3	230	231	1.3	201	763	3,460	675	0.09	0.30	0.5	3
Squash																						
Cooked																						
Summer (all varieties), sliced, drained	1 cup	180	94	35	2	1	0.1	Tr	0.2	0	8	49	70	0.6	346	2	520	52	0.08	0.07	0.9	10
Winter (all varieties), baked, cubes	1 cup	205	89	80	2	1	0.3	0.1	0.5	0	18	29	41	0.7	896	2	7,290	729	0.17	0.05	1.4	20
Sunchoke																						
See Jerusalem artichoke.																						
Sweet potatoes																						
Cooked (raw, 5 by 2 in; about 2-1/2 per lb)																						
Baked in skin, peeled	1	114	73	115	2	Tr	Tr	Tr	0.1	0	28	32	63	0.5	397	11	24,880	2,488	0.08	0.14	0.7	28
Boiled, without skin	1	151	73	160	2	Tr	0.1	Tr	0.2	0	37	32	41	0.8	278	20	25,750	2,575	0.08	0.21	1.0	26

(Continued)

TABLE E-1 *(continued)*

ITEM	FOODS, APPROXIMATE MEASURES, UNITS, AND WEIGHT (WEIGHT OF EDIBLE PORTION ONLY)	WEIGHT (G)	WATER (%)	FOOD ENERGY (KCAL)	PROTEIN (G)	FAT (G)	FATTY ACIDS SATURATED (G)	FATTY ACIDS MONOUNSATURATED (G)	FATTY ACIDS POLYUNSATURATED (G)	CHOLESTEROL (MG)	CARBOHYDRATE (G)	CALCIUM (MG)	PHOSPHORUS (MG)	IRON (MG)	POTASSIUM (MG)	SODIUM (MG)	VITAMIN A VALUE (IU)	VITAMIN A VALUE (RE)	THIAMIN (MG)	RIBOFLAVIN (MG)	NIACIN (MG)	ASCORBIC ACID (MG)
Candied, 2-1/2 by 2-in piece	1	105	67	145	1	3	1.4	0.7	0.2	8	29	27	27	1.2	198	74	4,400	440	0.02	0.04	0.4	7
Canned																						
Solid pack (mashed)	1 cup	255	74	260	5	1	0.1	Tr	0.2	0	59	77	133	3.4	536	191	38,570	3,857	0.07	0.23	2.4	13
Vacuum pack, piece 2-3/4 by 1 in	1	40	76	35	1	Tr	Tr	Tr	Tr	0	8	9	20	0.4	125	21	3,190	319	0.01	0.02	0.3	11
Tomatoes																						
Raw, 2-3/5-in diam. (3 per 12 oz pkg.)	1	123	94	25	1	Tr	Tr	Tr	0.1	0	5	9	28	0.6	255	10	1,390	139	0.07	0.06	0.7	22
Canned, solids and liquid	1 cup	240	94	50	2	1	0.1	0.1	0.2	0	10	62	46	1.5	530	[73]391	1,450	145	0.11	0.07	1.8	36
Tomato juice																						
Canned	1 cup	244	94	40	2	Tr	Tr	Tr	0.1	0	10	22	46	1.4	537	[74]881	1,360	136	0.11	0.08	1.6	45
Tomato products																						
Canned																						
Paste	1 cup	262	74	220	10	2	0.3	0.4	0.9	0	49	92	207	7.8	2,442	[75]170	6,470	647	0.41	0.50	8.4	111
Puree	1 cup	250	87	105	4	Tr	Tr	Tr	0.1	0	25	38	100	2.3	1,050	[76]50	3,400	340	0.18	0.14	4.3	88
Sauce	1 cup	245	89	75	3	Tr	0.1	0.1	0.2	0	18	34	78	1.9	909	[77]1,482	2,400	240	0.16	0.14	2.8	32
Turnips																						
Cooked, diced	1 cup	156	94	30	1	Tr	Tr	Tr	0.1	0	8	34	30	0.3	211	78	0	0	0.04	0.04	0.5	18
Turnip greens																						
Cooked, drained																						
From raw (leaves and stems)	1 cup	144	93	30	2	Tr	0.1	Tr	0.1	0	6	197	42	1.2	292	42	7,920	792	0.06	0.10	0.6	39
From frozen (chopped)	1 cup	164	90	50	5	1	0.2	Tr	0.3	0	8	249	56	3.2	367	25	13,080	1,308	0.09	0.12	0.8	36
Vegetable juice cocktail																						
Canned	1 cup	242	94	45	2	Tr	Tr	Tr	0.1	0	11	27	41	1.0	467	883	2,830	283	0.10	0.07	1.8	67
Vegetables, mixed																						
Canned, drained solids	1 cup	163	87	75	4	Tr	0.1	Tr	0.2	0	15	44	68	1.7	474	243	18,990	1,899	0.08	0.08	0.9	8
Frozen, cooked, drained	1 cup	182	83	105	5	Tr	0.1	Tr	0.1	0	24	46	93	1.5	308	64	7,780	778	0.13	0.22	1.5	6
Water chestnuts																						
Canned	1 cup	140	86	70	1	Tr	Tr	Tr	Tr	0	17	6	27	1.2	165	11	10	1	0.02	0.03	0.5	2
Baking powders for home use																						
Sodium aluminum sulfate																						
With monocalcium phosphate monohydrate	1 tsp	3	2	5	Tr	0	0.0	0.0	0.0	0	1	58	87	0.0	5	329	0	0	0.00	0.00	0.0	0

With monocalcium phosphate monohydrate, calcium sulfate	1 tsp	2.9	1	5	Tr	0	0.0	0.0	0.0	0	1	183	45	0.0	4	290	0	0	0.00	0.00	0.0	0
Straight phosphate	1 tsp	3.8	2	5	Tr	0	0.0	0.0	0.0	0	1	239	359	0.0	6	312	0	0	0.00	0.00	0.0	0
Low sodium	1 tsp	4.3	1	5	Tr	0	0.0	0.0	0.0	0	1	207	314	0.0	891	Tr	0	0	0.00	0.00	0.0	0
Catsup	1 cup	273	69	290	5	1	0.2	0.2	0.4	0	69	60	137	2.2	991	2,845	3,820	382	0.25	0.19	4.4	41
	1 tbsp	15	69	15	Tr	Tr	Tr	Tr	Tr	0	4	3	8	0.1	54	156	210	21	0.01	0.01	0.2	2
Celery seed	1 tsp	2	6	10	Tr	1	Tr	0.3	0.1	0	1	35	11	0.9	28	3	Tr	Tr	0.01	0.01	0.1	Tr
Chili powder	1 tsp	2.6	8	10	Tr	Tr	0.1	0.1	0.2	0	1	7	8	0.4	50	26	910	91	0.01	0.02	0.2	2
Chocolate																						
Bitter or baking	1 oz	28	2	145	3	15	9.0	4.9	0.5	0	8	22	109	1.9	235	1	10	1	0.01	0.07	0.4	0
Semisweet, see Candy.																						
Cinnamon	1 tsp	2.3	10	5	Tr	Tr	Tr	Tr	Tr	0	2	28	1	0.9	12	1	10	1	Tr	Tr	Tr	1
Curry powder	1 tsp	2	10	5	Tr	Tr	(1)	(1)	(1)	0	1	10	7	0.6	31	1	20	2	0.01	0.01	0.1	Tr
Garlic powder	1 tsp	2.8	6	10	Tr	Tr	Tr	Tr	Tr	0	2	2	12	0.1	31	1	0	0	0.01	Tr	Tr	Tr
Gelatin																						
Dry	1 envelope	7	13	25	6	Tr	Tr	Tr	Tr	0	0	1	0	0.0	2	6	0	0	0.00	0.00	0.0	0
Mustard																						
Prepared, yellow	1 tsp or individual packet	5	80	5	Tr	Tr	Tr	0.2	Tr	0	Tr	4	4	0.1	7	63	0	0	Tr	0.01	Tr	Tr
Olives																						
Canned																						
Green	4 medium or 3 extra large	13	78	15	Tr	2	0.2	1.2	0.1	0	Tr	8	2	0.2	7	312	40	4	Tr	Tr	Tr	0
Ripe, Mission, pitted	3 small or 2 large	9	73	15	Tr	2	0.3	1.3	0.2	0	Tr	10	2	0.2	2	68	10	1	Tr	Tr	Tr	0
Onion powder	1 tsp	2.1	5	5	Tr	Tr	Tr	Tr	Tr	0	2	8	7	0.1	20	1	Tr	Tr	0.01	Tr	Tr	Tr
Oregano	1 tsp	1.5	7	5	Tr	Tr	Tr	Tr	0.1	0	1	24	3	0.7	25	Tr	100	10	0.01	Tr	0.1	1
Paprika	1 tsp	2.1	10	5	Tr	Tr	Tr	Tr	0.2	0	1	4	7	0.5	49	1	1,270	127	0.01	0.04	0.3	1
Pepper, black	1 tsp	2.1	11	5	Tr	Tr	Tr	Tr	Tr	0	1	9	4	0.6	26	1	Tr	Tr	Tr	0.01	Tr	0
Pickles																						
Cucumber																						
Dill, medium, whole, 3-$^3/_4$ in long, 1-$^1/_4$-in diam.	1 pickle	65	93	5	Tr	Tr	Tr	Tr	0.1	0	1	17	14	0.7	130	928	70	7	Tr	0.01	Tr	4
Fresh-pack, slices 1-$^1/_2$-in diam., $^1/_4$ in thick	2 slices	15	79	10	Tr	Tr	Tr	Tr	Tr	0	3	5	4	0.3	30	101	20	2	Tr	Tr	Tr	1
Sweet, gherkin, small, whole, about 2-$^1/_2$ in long, $^3/_4$-in diam.	1 pickle	15	61	20	Tr	Tr	Tr	Tr	Tr	0	5	2	2	0.2	30	107	10	1	Tr	Tr	Tr	1
Popcorn																						
See Grain Products.																						

(Continued)

TABLE E-1 *(continued)*

ITEM	FOODS, APPROXIMATE MEASURES, UNITS, AND WEIGHT (WEIGHT OF EDIBLE PORTION ONLY)	WEIGHT (G)	WATER (%)	FOOD ENERGY (KCAL)	PROTEIN (G)	FAT (G)	FATTY ACIDS SATURATED (G)	FATTY ACIDS MONOUNSATURATED (G)	FATTY ACIDS POLYUNSATURATED (G)	CHOLESTEROL (MG)	CARBOHYDRATE (G)	CALCIUM (MG)	PHOSPHORUS (MG)	IRON (MG)	POTASSIUM (MG)	SODIUM (MG)	VITAMIN A VALUE (IU)	VITAMIN A VALUE (RE)	THIAMIN (MG)	RIBOFLAVIN (MG)	NIACIN (MG)	ASCORBIC ACID (MG)
Relish																						
Finely chopped, sweet	1 tbsp	15	63	20	Tr	Tr	Tr	Tr	Tr	0	5	3	2	0.1	30	107	20	2	Tr	Tr	0.0	1
Salt	1 tsp	5.5	0	0	0	0	0.0	0.0	0.0	0	0	14	3	Tr	Tr	2,132	0	0	0.00	0.00	0.0	0
Vinegar																						
Cider	1 tbsp	15	94	Tr	Tr	0	0.0	0.0	0.0	0	1	1	1	0.1	15	Tr	0	0	0.00	0.00	0.0	0
Yeast																						
Baker's, dry, active	1 pkg	7	5	20	3	Tr	Tr	0.1	Tr	0	3	3	90	1.1	140	4	Tr	Tr	0.16	0.38	2.0	Tr
Brewer's, dry	1 tbsp	8	5	25	3	Tr	Tr	Tr	0.0	0	3	[7,8]17	140	1.4	152	10	Tr	Tr	1.25	0.34	3.0	Tr

* Tr indicates nutrient present in trace amount. [1] Value not determined. [2] Mineral content varies depending on water source.

[3] Blend of aspartame and saccharin; if only sodium saccharin is used, sodium is 75 mg; if only aspartame is used, sodium is 23 mg.

[4] With added ascorbic acid. [5] Vitamin A value is largely from beta-carotene used for coloring.

[6] Yields 1 qt of fluid milk when reconstituted according to package directions. [7] With added vitamin A.

[8] Carbohydrate content varies widely because of amount of sugar added and amount and solids content of added flavoring. Consult the label if more precise values for carbohydrate and calories are needed.

[9] For salted butter; unsalted butter contains 12 mg sodium per stick, 2 mg per tbsp, or 1 mg per pat.

[10] Values for vitamin A are year-round average. [11] For salted margarine.

[12] Based on average vitamin A content of fortified margarine. Federal specifications for fortified margarine require a minimum of 15,000 IU per pound.

[13] Fatty acid values apply to product made with regular margarine. [14] Dipped in egg, milk, and breadcrumbs; fried in vegetable shortening.

[15] If bones are discarded, value for calcium will be greatly reduced. [16] Dipped in egg, breadcrumbs, and flour; fried in vegetable shortening.

[17] Made with drained chunk light tuna, celery, onion, pickle relish, and mayonnaise-type salad dressing.

[18] Sodium bisulfite used to preserve color; unsulfited product would contain less sodium. [19] Also applies to pasteurized apple cider.

[20] Without added ascorbic acid. For value with added ascorbic acid, refer to label. [21] With added ascorbic acid

[22] For white grapefruit; pink grapefruit have about 310 IU or 31 RE. [23] Sodium benzoate and sodium bisulfite added as preservatives.

[24] Egg bagels have 44 mg cholesterol and 22 IU or 7 RE vitamin A per bagel. [25] Made with vegetable shortening.

[26] Made with white cornmeal. If made with yellow cornmeal, value is 32 IU or 3 RE. [27] Nutrient added.

[28] Cooked without salt. If salt is added according to label recommendations, sodium content is 540 mg.

[29] For white corn grits. Cooked yellow grits contain 145 IU or 14 RE. [30] Value based on label declaration for added nutrients.

[31] For regular and instant cereal. For quick cereal, phosphorus is 102 mg and sodium is 142 mg.

[32] Cooked without salt. If salt is added according to label recommendations, sodium content is 390 mg.

[33] Cooked without salt. If salt is added according to label recommendations, sodium content is 324 mg.

[34] Cooked without salt. If salt is added according to label recommendations, sodium content is 374 mg.

[35] Excepting angel food cake, cakes were made from mixes containing vegetable shortening and frostings were made with margarine.

[36] Made with vegetable oil. [37] Cake made with vegetable shortening; frosting with margarine. [38] Made with margarine.

[39] Crackers made with enriched flour except for rye wafers and whole-wheat wafers. [40] Made with lard.

[41] Cashews without salt contain 21 mg sodium per cup or 4 mg per oz. [42] Cashews without salt contain 22 mg sodium per cup or 5 mg per oz.

[43] Macadamia nuts without salt contain 9 mg sodium per cup or 2 mg per oz. [44] Mixed nuts without salt contain 3 mg sodium per oz.

[45] Peanuts without salt contain 22 mg sodium per cup or 4 mg per oz.

[46] Outer layer of fat was removed to within approximately $^1/_2$ inch of the lean. Deposits of fat within the cut were not removed.

[47] Fried in vegetable shortening. [48] Value varies widely.

[49] Contains added sodium ascorbate. If sodium ascorbate is not added, ascorbic acid content is negligible.

[50] One patty (8 per pound) of bulk sausage is equivalent to 2 links. [51] Crust made with vegetable shortening and enriched flour.

[52] Made with corn oil. [53] Fried in vegetable shortening. [54] If sodium ascorbate is added, product contains 11 mg ascorbic acid.

[55] Made with enriched flour, margarine, and whole milk. [56] For regular pack; special dietary pack contains 3 mg sodium.

[57] For green varieties; yellow varieties contain 101 IU or 10 RE. [58] For green varieties; yellow varieties contain 151 IU or 15 RE.

[59] For regular pack; special dietary pack contains 3 mg sodium. [60] For green varieties; yellow varieties contain 142 IU or 14 RE.

[61] For regular pack; special dietary pack contains 78 mg sodium. [62] For regular pack; special dietary pack contains 61 mg sodium.

[63] For yellow varieties; white varieties contain only a trace of vitamin A. [64] For regular pack; special dietary pack contains 8 mg sodium.

[65] For regular pack; special dietary pack contains 6 mg sodium. [66] For regular pack; special dietary pack contains 3 mg sodium.

[67] For red peppers; green peppers contain 350 IU or 35 RE. [68] For green peppers; red peppers contain 4,220 IU or 422 RE.

[69] For green peppers; red peppers contain 141 mg ascorbic acid. [70] For green peppers; red peppers contain 2,740 IU or 274 RE.

[71] For green peppers; red peppers contain 121 mg ascorbic acid. [72] With added salt; if none is added, sodium content is 58 mg.

[73] For regular pack; special dietary pack contains 31 mg sodium. [74] With added salt; if none is added, sodium content is 24 mg.

[75] With no added salt; if salt is added, sodium content is 2,070 mg. [76] With no added salt; if salt is added, sodium content is 998 mg.

[77] With salt added. [78] Value may vary from 6 to 60 mg.

(United States Dept. of Agriculture, Human Nutrition Information Service. Nutritive value of foods. Washington, DC: US Government Printing Office, 1991. Home and Garden bulletin 72.)

INDEX

Numbers followed by f indicate a figure;
t indicates tabular material; d indicates a display.